W9-CEF-169

ESSENTIALS OF
FAMILY MEDICINE

FIFTH EDITION

ESSENTIALS OF
FAMILY MEDICINE

FIFTH EDITION

PHILIP D. SLOANE, MD, MPH

Elizabeth and Oscar Goodwin Distinguished Professor of Family Medicine
University of North Carolina at Chapel Hill
Chapel Hill, North Carolina

LISA M. SLATT, MEd

Associate Professor
Associate Director, Medical Student Programs
Department of Family Medicine
University of North Carolina at Chapel Hill
Chapel Hill, North Carolina

MARK H. EBELL, MD, MS

Associate Professor
Deputy Editor, *American Family Physician*
Augusta, Georgia
Medical College of Georgia

LOUIS B. JACQUES, MD

Associate Professor
Georgetown University
Washington, D.C.

MINDY A. SMITH, MD, MS

Professor, Department of Family Medicine
Michigan State University College of Human Medicine
East Lansing, Michigan
Associate Editor, *Family Medicine*

Wolters Kluwer | Lippincott Williams & Wilkins
Health

Philadelphia • Baltimore • New York • London
Buenos Aires • Hong Kong • Sydney • Tokyo

Acquisitions Editor: Donna Balado
Managing Editor: Cheryl W. Stringfellow
Marketing Manager: Jennifer Kuklinski
Production Editor: Sally Anne Glover
Designer: Stephen Druding
Compositor: Maryland Composition, Inc.
Printer: Data Reproductions Corporation

Fifth Edition

Copyright © 2008, 2002, 1998, 1993, 1988 Lippincott Williams & Wilkins, a Wolters Kluwer business.

351 West Camden Street   530 Walnut Street
Baltimore, MD 21201   Philadelphia, PA 19106

All rights reserved. This book is protected by copyright. No part of this book may be reproduced or transmitted in any form or by any means, including as photocopies or scanned-in or other electronic copies, or utilized by any information storage and retrieval system without written permission from the copyright owner, except for brief quotations embodied in critical articles and reviews. Materials appearing in this book prepared by individuals as part of their official duties as U.S. government employees are not covered by the above-mentioned copyright. To request permission, please contact Lippincott Williams & Wilkins at 530 Walnut Street, Philadelphia, PA 19106, via email at permissions@lww.com, or via website at lww.com (products and services).

9 8 7 6 5 4 3 2

Library of Congress Cataloging-in-Publication Data

Essentials of family medicine / [edited by] Philip D. Sloane ... [et al.]. — 5th ed.
       p. ; cm.
   Includes bibliographical references and index.
   ISBN 978-0-7817-8188-6
   1. Family medicine. I. Sloane, Philip D. II. Title: Family medicine.
   [DNLM: 1. Family Practice. WB 110 E78 2008]
   RC46.E88 2008
   616—dc22

                          2007006972

DISCLAIMER

Care has been taken to confirm the accuracy of the information present and to describe generally accepted practices. However, the authors, editors, and publisher are not responsible for errors or omissions or for any consequences from application of the information in this book and make no warranty, expressed or implied, with respect to the currency, completeness, or accuracy of the contents of the publication. Application of this information in a particular situation remains the professional responsibility of the practitioner; the clinical treatments described and recommended may not be considered absolute and universal recommendations.

The authors, editors, and publisher have exerted every effort to ensure that drug selection and dosage set forth in this text are in accordance with the current recommendations and practice at the time of publication. However, in view of ongoing research, changes in government regulations, and the constant flow of information relating to drug therapy and drug reactions, the reader is urged to check the package insert for each drug for any change in indications and dosage and for added warnings and precautions. This is particularly important when the recommended agent is a new or infrequently employed drug.

Some drugs and medical devices presented in this publication have Food and Drug Administration (FDA) clearance for limited use in restricted research settings. It is the responsibility of the health care provider to ascertain the FDA status of each drug or device planned for use in their clinical practice.

To purchase additional copies of this book, call our customer service department at **(800) 638-3030** or fax orders to **(301) 223-2320**. International customers should call **(301) 223-2300**.

Visit Lippincott Williams & Wilkins on the Internet: http://www.lww.com. Lippincott Williams & Wilkins customer service representatives are available from 8:30 am to 6:00 pm, EST.

To the many family physicians, past and present, who have provided state-of-the art, compassionate care to their patients and communities. Also to the families, such as the children of Dr. Oscar Goodwin of Apex, NC, who have honored one of these exemplary family physicians through generous support of academic family medicine.
P. S.

To my parents, Allan and Louise Slatt, and my husband, Alan Spanos
L. M. S.

To my wife, Laura Bierema and my late son, Lukas Willem
M. H. E.

To Tek Young Lin and Zoe Johnstone, teachers
L. B. J.

To the many students, residents, and fellows who I have been privileged to learn from and teach.
M. S.

To the many practicing family physicians who generously give of their time and expertise to teach our medical students about the pleasures and challenges of caring for people and their families.

CONTRIBUTORS

Cathleen Abbott, MD
Department of Family Medicine
Michigan State University College of Human Medicine
East Lansing, Michigan

Thomas Agresta, MD
Associate Professor
St. Francis Family Practice Residency Program
University of Connecticut Health Center
Hartford, Connecticut

Saloni Anand, MD
St. Francis Family Practice Residency Program
University of Connecticut Health Center
Hartford, Connecticut

Henry C. Barry, MD, MS
Associate Professor, Department of Family Practice
Michigan State University College of Human Medicine
East Lansing, Michigan

George R. Bergus, MD
Professor, Department of Family Medicine
University of Iowa Hospital & Clinics
Iowa City, Iowa

Derrick Blackwell, DO
Resident in Family Practice
Sparrow Hospital
Michigan State University
Lansing, Michigan

Soo Borson, MD
Professor, Department of Psychiatry and Behavioral Sciences
University of Washington School of Medicine
Seattle, Washington

Howard Brody, MD, PhD
Professor, Department of Family Medicine
Director Institute for Medical Humanities
University of Texas Medical Branch
Galveston, Texas

Larissa S. Buccolo, MD
Naval Hospital Family Practice Clinic
Jacksonville, Florida

Elizabeth A. Burns, MD, MA
Professor, Department of Family & Community Medicine
University of North Dakota School of Medicine & Health Sciences
Grand Forks, North Dakota

Kevin E. Burroughs, MD
Director of Sports Medicine
Cabarrus Family Medicine Residency Program
Concord, North Carolina

Beth A. Choby, MD
Curriculum Coordinator, Surgery and ENT
San Jacinto Methodist Hospital
Houston, Texas

Sandra C. Clark, MD
Piedmont Health Services
Carrboro, North Carolina

Remy R. Coeytaux, MD, PhD
Assistant Professor, Department of Family Medicine
University of North Carolina at Chapel Hill
Chapel Hill, North Carolina

Timothy P. Daaleman, DO, MPH
Associate Professor, Department of Family Medicine
University of North Carolina at Chapel Hill
Chapel Hill, North Carolina

Philip M. Diller, MD, PhD
Associate Professor, Residency Director, Department of Family Medicine
UC Physicians, University of Cincinnati College of Medicine
Cincinnati, Ohio

Katrina Donahue, MD, MPH
Assistant Professor, Department of Family Medicine
University of North Carolina at Chapel Hill
Chapel Hill, North Carolina

Marguerite Duane, MD, MHA
Clerkship Director, Department of Family Medicine
Georgetown University School of Medicine
Washington, DC

Mark H. Ebell, MD, MS
Associate Professor, Medical College of Georgia
Augusta, Georgia
Deputy Editor, American Family Physician

John W. Epling, Jr., MD
Associate Professor, Department of Family Medicine
Upstate Medical University
State University of New York
Syracuse, New York

Jonathan D. Ference, PharmD
Clinical Assistant Professor
Department of Pharmacy
University of Oklahoma College of Pharmacy
Oklahoma City, Oklahoma

Linda French, MD
Associate Professor, Department of Family Medicine
Michigan State University College of Human Medicine
East Lansing, Michigan

David L. Gaspar, MD
Director, Predoctoral Education
Department of Family Medicine
University of Colorado at Denver and Health Sciences Center
Aurora, Colorado

John R. Gimpel, DO, MEd
Vice President
Clinical Skills Testing
National Board of Osteopathic Medical Examiners
Philadelphia, PA

Adam O. Goldstein, MD
Professor, Department of Family Medicine
University of North Carolina at Chapel Hill
Chapel Hill, North Carolina

Gary R. Gray, DO
Family Medicine Residency Program
Natividad Medical Center
Salinas, California

Larry A. Green, MD
Director, Prescription for Health
Department of Family Medicine
University of Colorado Health Sciences Center
Aurora, Colorado

Lee A. Green, MD, MPH
Professor and Associate Chair for Information Management University of
Michigan Department of Family Medicine University of Michigan Center
for the Advancement of Clinical Research
Ann Arbor, Michigan

Robert E. Gwyther, MD, MBA
Professor, Department of Family Medicine
University of North Carolina at Chapel Hill
Chapel Hill, North Carolina

Wayne A. Hale, MD MS
Associate Professor
Department of Family Medicine
Moses H. Cone Memorial Hospital
Greensboro, North Carolina

Peter Ham, MD
Assistan Professor, Department of Family Medicine
University of Virginia
Charlottesville, Virginia

Caryl J. Heaton, DO
Associate Professor, Department of Family Medicine
UMDNJ-New Jersey Medical School
Newark, New Jersey

David Henderson, MD
Assistant Professor, St. Francis Family Practice Residency Program
University of Connecticut Health Center
Hartford, Connecticut

Melissa M. Hicks, MD
Clinical Assistant Professor
MAHEL Family Medicine Residency Program
Asheville, North Carolina

William Y. Huang, MD
Department of Family and Community Medicine
Baylor College of Medicine
Houston, Texas

William J. Hueston, MD
Department of Family Medicine
Medical University of South Carolina
Charleston, South Carolina

Mollie Kane, MD, MPH
Clinical Assistant Professor
School of Medicine and Public Health
University of Wisconsin-Madison
Madison, Wisconsin

Fareed M. Khan, MD
Assistant Professor
Family and Community Medicine
Baylor College of Medicine
Houston, Texas

Scott Kinkade, MD, MSPH
Assistant Professor, Department of Family Medicine and Community
Medicine
Southwestern Medical School
Dallas, Texas

Kathleen Klink, MD
Director, Center for Family Medicine
Columbia University College of Physicians & Surgeons
New York, New York

Charles M. Kodner MD
Associate Professor, Department of Family and Geriatric Medicine
University of Louisville School of Medicine
Louisville, Kentucky

John P. Langlois, MD
Clinical Professor
MAHEC Family Medicine Residency
Asheville, North Carolina

Allen R. Last, MD, MPH
Assistant Professor, Family and Community Medicine
Medical College of Wisconsin
Milwaukee, Wisconsin

Kenneth W. Lin, MD
Assistant Professor, Pre-Doctoral Division
Department of Family Medicine
Georgetown University School of Medicine
Washington, DC

David Little, MD
Professor, Department of Family Medicine
University of Vermont College of Medicine
Burlington, Vermont

Arch G. Mainous III, PhD
Professor, Department of Family Medicine
Medical University of South Carolina
Charleston, South Carolina

Karl E. Miller, MD
Professor and Vice Chair
Department of Family Medicine
Chattanooga Unit, UTCOM
Chattanooga, Tennessee

Donald E. Nease, Jr., MD
Associate Professor, Department of Family Medicine
University of Michigan Medical School
Ann Arbor, Michigan

Warren P. Newton, MD
Chairman and Aycock Distinguished Professor of Family Medicine
University of North Carolina at Chapel Hill
Chapel Hill, North Carolina

Mary Barth Noel, PhD, MPH, RD
Professor, Department of Family Medicine
Michigan State University College of Human Medicine
East Lansing, Michigan

Karen S. Ogle, MD
Professor, Department of Family Medicine
Michigan State University College of Human Medicine
East Lansing, Michigan

Louise Parent-Stevens, PharmD, BCPS
Clinical Assistant Professor, College of Pharmacy
University of Illinois at Chicago
Chicago, Illinois

Barbara D. Reed, MD, MSPH
Professor, Department of Family Medicine
University of Michigan Medical School
Ann Arbor, Michigan

Jeri R. Reid, MD
Assistant Professor, Department of Family and Geriatric Medicine
University of Louisville
Louisville, Kentucky

Carol E. Ripley-Moffitt
Social Research Associate, Department of Family Medicine
University of North Carolina at Chapel Hill
Chapel Hill, North Carolina

Phillip E. Rodgers, MD
Assistant Professor, Department of Family Medicine
University of Michigan Medical School
Ann Arbor, Michigan

Mary Roederer, PharmD
Assistant Professor
School of Pharmacy
University of North Carolina at Chapel Hill
Chapel Hill, North Carolina

Samuel E. Romano, PhD, MA
Department of Family Medicine
University of Michigan Health System
Chelsea Health Center
Chelsea, Michigan

Rebecca L. Rosen, MD
Family Medicine Residency Program
Natividad Medical Center
Salinas, California

Kendra L. Schwartz, MD, MSPH
Associate Professor, Department of Family Medicine
Wayne State University School of Medicine
Detroit, Michigan

Steven M. Schwartz, MD
Associate Professor, Department of Family Medicine
Georgetown University School of Medicine
Washington, DC

Thomas L. Schwenk, MD
Professor and Chair, Department of Family Medicine
University of Michigan Health System
Ann Arbor, Michigan

Allen F. Shaugnessy, PharmD
Research Assistant Professor
Department of Public Health and Family Medicine
Tufts University
Boston Massachusetts

Leslie A. Shimp, PharmD, MS
Assistant Professor, Department of Family Medicine
University of Michigan Health System
Ann Arbor, Michigan

David C. Slawson, MD
B. Lewis Barnett, Jr. Professor of Family Medicine
Director of the Center for Information Mastery
Professor, Department of Family Medicine
University of Virginia School of Medicine
Charlottesville, Virginia

Philip D. Sloane, MD
Elizabeth and Oscar Goodwin Distinguished Professor of Family Medicine
University of North Carolina at Chapel Hill
Chapel Hill, North Carolina

Mindy A. Smith, MD, MS
Professor, Department of Family Medicine
Michigan State University
East Lansing, Michigan
Associate Editor, Family Medicine

Douglas R. Smucker, MD
Associate Professor, Department of Family Medicine
University of Cincinnati
Cincinnati, Ohio

John Smucny, MD
Associate Professor, Department of Family Medicine
Upstate Medical University
State University of New York
Syracuse, New York

Kurt Stange, MD, PhD
Director, Family Medicine Research Division
Department of Family Medicine
Case Western Reserve University
Cleveland, Ohio

Beat Steiner, MD, MPH
Associate Professor, Department of Family Medicine
University of North Carolina at Chapel Hill
Chapel Hill, North Carolina

Joseph Thompson, MD
Mercy Health Partners, Mercy Family Practice
Toledo, Ohio

Margaret E. Thompson, MD
Associate Professor, Department of Family Medicine
Michigan State University College of Human Medicine
East Lansing, Michigan

Richard P. Usatine, MD
Professor, Department of Family & Community Medicine
University of Texas Health Science Center at San Antonio
San Antonio, Texas

Gregg K. Vandekieft, MD, MA
Providence St. Peter Hospital Family Medicine Residency Program
Olympia, Washington

James VanHuysen, DO
Clinical Instructor, Department of Family Medicine
Michigan State University College of Human Medicine
East Lansing, Michigan

Anthony J. Viera, MD, MPH
Assistant Professor, Department of Family Medicine
University of North Carolina at Chapel Hill
Chapel Hill, North Carolina

Dorothy E. Vura-Weis, MD, MPH
Assistant Health Officer, San Mateo County Health Department
San Mateo, California

William C. Wadland, MD, MS
Professor and Chair, Department of Family Medicine
Michigan State University College of Human Medicine
East Lansing, Michigan

Sam Weir, MD, MPH
Associate Professor, Department of Family Medicine
University of North Carolina at Chapel Hill
Chapel Hill, North Carolina

David Weismantel, MD, MS
Assistant Professor, Department of Family Practice
Michigan State University College of Human Medicine
East Lansing, Michigan

Thayer White
University of North Carolina at Chapel Hill
Chapel Hill, North Carolina

Vincent WinklerPrins, MD
Michigan State University College of Human Medicine
East Lansing, Michigan

Adam J. Zolotor, MD, MPH
Assistant Professor, Department of Family Medicine
University of North Carolina at Chapel Hill
Chapel Hill, North Carolina

The following individuals wrote the faculty and student review questions for the online database.

Judy C. Washington, MD
Assistant Director, Mountainside Family Practice Associates
Family Medicine Residency Clinical Associate Professor
UMDNJ-New Jersey Medical School
Newark, New Jersey
Examkit Question Editor

Chantal Brazeau, MD
Director of Predoctoral Education, Department of Family Medicine
Associate Professor of Psychiatry and Family Medicine
UMDNJ-New Jersey Medical School
Newark, New Jersey
Examkit Question Editor

Sital Bhargava, DO
Academic Fellow and Instructor, Department of Community and Family Medicine
Medical College of Wisconsin
Milwaukee, Wisconsin
CHAPTER 5

Douglas J. Bower, MD
Associate Professor, Department of Family and Community Medicne
Medical College of Wisconsin
Milwaukee, Wisconsin
CHAPTER 24

John R. Brill, MD, MPH
Associate Professor, Department of Family Medicine
University of Wisconsin
Milwaukee, Wisconsin
CHAPTER 25

Michael Cannon, MD, MS
Assistant Professor, Department Community and Family Medicine
Saint Louis University School of Medicine
St. Louis, Missouri
CHAPTERS 35, 39

Jan Carline, PhD
Professor, Department of Medical Education and Biomedical Informatics
University of Washington
Seattle, Washington
CHAPTERS 4, 19

Alexander W. Chessman, MD
Professor, Department of Family Medicine
Medical University of South Carolina
Charleston, South Carolina
CHAPTER 14

Heidi Chumley, MD
Assistant Professor, Department of Family Medicine
Kansas University School of Medicine
Kansas City, Kansas
CHAPTER 10

Deborah S. Clements, MD
Associate Professor, Department of Family Medicine
University of Kansas Medical Center
Kansas City, Kansas
CHAPTER 21

Mark Cucuzzella, MD
Associate Professor, Department of Family Medicine
West Virginia University
Harpers Ferry, West Virginia
CHAPTER 22

D. Todd Detar, DO
Associate Clinical Professor, Department of Family Medicine
Medical University of South Carolina
Charleston, South Carolina
CHAPTERS 7, 48, 46

Sabina Diehr, MD
Associate Professor, Department of Family and Community Medicine
Medical College of Wisconsin
Milwaukee, Wisconsin
CHAPTER 41

Stu Farber, MD
Associate Professor, Department of Family Medicine
University of Washington
Seattle, Washington
CHAPTERS 4, 19

Cha-Chi Fung, PhD
Assistant Professor, Department of Family Medicine
David Geffen School of Medicine at UCLA
Los Angeles, California
CHAPTERS 33, 34

Patrick H. Ginn, MD, MBA
Assistant Professor, Department of Family and Community Medicine
Waukesha Family Medicine Residency Program
Medical College of Wisconsin
Milwaukee, Wisconsin
CHAPTER 9

Tom Greer, MD, MPH
Associate Professor, Department of Family Medicine
University of Washington
Seattle, Washington
CHAPTERS 4, 19

Nancy E. Havas, MD
Academic Fellow in Primary Care Research
Department of Family Medicine
Medical College of Wisconsin
Milwaukee, Wisconsin
CHAPTER 36

David Henderson, MD
Assistant Professor, Department of Family Medicine
University of Connecticut
Farmington, Connecticut
CHAPTERS 15, 44

Karen Hulbert, MD
Assistant Professor, Department of Family & Community Medicine
Racine Family Practice Center
Medical College of Wisconsin
Racine, Wisconsin
CHAPTER 13

Amanda Keerbs, MD
Assistant Professor, Department of Family Medicine
University of Washington
Seattle, Washington
CHAPTERS 4, 19

Susanne M. Krasovich, MD
Assistant Professor, Department of Family and Community Medicine
Waukesha Family Medicine Residency Program
Medical College of Wisconsin
Milwaukee, Wisconsin
CHAPTER 47

David Little, MD
Professor, Department of Family Medicine
University of Vermont College of Medicine
Burlington, Vermont
CHAPTERS 31, 43

Robert Mallin, MD
Associate Professor, Department of Family Medicine
Medical University of South Carolina
Charleston, South Carolina
CHAPTER 46

Katherine Margo, MD
Assistant Professor, Department of Family Medicine and Community Health
University of Pennsylvania School of Medicine
Philadelphia, Pennsylvania
CHAPTER 50

Mary Barth Noel, PhD, MPH, RD
Professor, Department of Family Medicine
Michigan State University College of Human Medicine
East Lansing, Michigan
CHAPTER 18

Barbara J. Orr, MD
Associate Professor, Department of Family Medicine
Loma Linda University School of Medicine
Loma Linda, California
CHAPTERS 23, 37

Kayleen P. Papin, MD
Assistant Professor, Department of Family and Community Medicine
Medical College of Wisconsin
Milwaukee, Wisconsin
CHAPTER 12

Fiona Prabhu, MD
Associate Professor, Department of Family and Community Medicine
Texas Tech University Health Sciences Center--School of Medicine
Lubbock, Texas
CHAPTERS 38, 42

Jeri R. Reid, MD
Assistant Professor, Department of Family and Geriatric Medicine
University of Louisville
Louisville, Kentucky
CHAPTERS 17, 28

Donna Roberts, MD
Associate Professor, Department of Family and Geriatric Medicine
University of Louisville
Louisville, Kentucky
CHAPTER 30

Dana Romalis, MD
Instructor, Department of Family Medicine
Montefiore Medical Center
Bronx, New York
CHAPTER 20

Fredric J. Romm, MD, MPH
Associate Professor, Department of Family and Community Medicine
Medical College of Wisconsin
Milwaukee, Wisconsin
CHAPTER 16

Roger W. Schauer, MD
Associate Professor, Department of Family and Community Medicine
University of North Dakota School of Medicine & Health Sciences
Grand Forks, North Dakota
CHAPTER 29

Susan Stangl, MD, MSEd
Associate Professor, Department of Family Medicine
David Geffen School of Medicine at UCLA
Los Angeles, California
CHAPTERS 33, 34

Margaret E. Thompson, MD
Associate Professor, Department of Family Medicine
Michigan State University College of Human Medicine
East Lansing, Michigan
CHAPTER 26

Scott Tripler, MD
Associate Professor, Department of Family Medicine
Office of Medical Education
University of Rochester School of Medicine and Dentistry
Rochester, New York
CHAPTERS 45, 49

Cynthia M. Waickus, MD, PhD
Assistant Professor, Department of Family Medicine
Rush Medical College
Chicago, Illinois
CHAPTER 6

Gordon S. Walbroehl, MD
Professor, Department of Famiy Medicine
Wright State University School of Medicine
Dayton, Ohio
CHAPTER 11

Judy C. Washington, MD
Assistant Director, Mountainside Family Practice
Associate Family Medicine Program
Clinical Associate Professor, Department of Family Medicine
UMDNJ New Jersey Medical School
Verona, New Jersey
Examkit Question Editor

Jenny Walker, MD, MPH, MSW
Assistant Professor, Department of Community and Preventive Medicine
Division of Family Medicine
Mount Sinai School of Medicine
New York, New York
CHAPTER 40

Michelle Whitehurst-Cook, MD
Associate Professor, Department of Famiy Medicine
Associate Dean for Admissions
Virgina Commonwealth University School of Medicine
Richmond, Virginia
CHAPTER 51

Pamela Wiseman, MD
Assistant Professor, Department of Family and Community Medicine
Tulane University School of Medicine
New Orleans, Louisiana
CHAPTER 27

CONTENTS

Dedication   v
Contributors   vii
Preface   xvii

I Principles of Family Medicine

1. Family Medicine in Today's Changing Health Care System 3
PHILIP D. SLOANE, THAYER WHITE, LARRY GREEN, WARREN P. NEWTON, AND KURT STANGE

2. The Challenging Patient Encounter 31
SAMUEL E. ROMANO AND THOMAS L. SCHWENK

3. Information Mastery: Basing Care on the Best Available Evidence 39
ALLEN F. SHAUGHNESSY, MARK H. EBELL, AND DAVID C. SLAWSON

II Preventive Care

4. Prenatal Care 51
BETH A. CHOBY

5. Well Child and Adolescent Care 73
BEAT STEINER

6. Well Adult Care 87
STEVEN M. SCHWARTZ AND MARGUERITE DUANE

7. Palliative and End-of-Life Care 105
GREGG K. VANDEKIEFT, HOWARD BRODY, AND KAREN S. OGLE

III Common Problems

8. Approach to Common Problems in Family Medicine 119
PHILIP D. SLOANE AND MARK H. EBELL

Cardiovascular Problems

9. Chest Pain 131
LEE A. GREEN AND PHILLIP E. RODGERS

10. Chronic Cardiac Disease 149
DOUGLAS R. SMUCKER AND PHILIP M. DILLER

11. Hypertension 165
ANTHONY J. VIERA AND WARREN P. NEWTON

12. Venous Thromboembolism 179
DAVID WEISMANTEL

Problems of Children

13. Disorders of Behavior and Development 197
ADAM J. ZOLOTOR AND MOLLIE KANE

14. Fever in Infants and Preschool Children 215
VINCE WINKLERPRINS AND WILLIAM C. WADLAND

Endocrine Problems

15. Diabetes 227
SAM WEIR, KATRINA DONAHUE, AND MARY ROEDERER

16. Hyperlipidemia 247
ALLEN R. LAST AND JONATHAN D. FERENCE

17. Thyroid Disease 263
JERI R. REID

18. Nutrition and Weight Management 279
MARGARET E. THOMPSON AND MARY BARTH NOEL

Eye, Ear, Nose, and Throat Problems

19. Ear Pain 293
WILLIAM J. HUESTON AND ARCH G. MAINOUS III

20. Eye Problems 301
GARY R. GRAY AND REBECCA ROSEN

21. Sore Throat 313
MARK H. EBELL

Gastrointestinal Problems

22. Abdominal Pain 325
JOHN SMUCNY, JOHN EPLING, AND JOSEPH THOMPSON

23. Chronic Liver Disease 341
KENNETH W. LIN

24. Dyspepsia 351
WILLIAM Y. HUANG AND FAREED M. KHAN

25. Lower Intestinal Problems 365
CHARLES M. KODNER

Men's and Women's Health

26. Breast Problems 381
KENDRA L. SCHWARTZ

27. Contraception 395
LESLIE A. SHIMP AND MINDY A. SMITH

28. Dysuria 425
GEORGE R. BERGUS

29. Menstrual Syndromes 437
ELIZABETH A. BURNS AND LOUISE PARENT-STEVENS

30. Promoting Health for Women at Menopause 455
LINDA FRENCH AND CATHLEEN ABBOTT

31. Men's Health Concerns 469
ANTHONY J. VIERA AND LARISSA S. BUCCOLO

32. Relationship Issues 497
SANDRA C. CLARK AND TIMOTHY P. DAALEMAN

33. Sexually Transmitted Infections 511
KARL E. MILLER

34. Vaginitis 527
BARBARA D. REED

Musculoskeletal and Skin Problems

35. Ankle and Knee Pain 543
JAMES VANHUYSEN, DERRICK BLACKWELL, AND HENRY C. BARRY

36. Arthritis and Rheumatism 557
JOHN R. GIMPEL

37. Low Back Pain 579
SCOTT KINKADE

38. Neck Pain 589
CARYL J. HEATON

39. Shoulder Pain 601
KEVIN E. BURROUGHS

40. Dermatology 617
RICHARD P. USATINE

41. Skin Wounds: Contusions, Abrasions, Lacerations, and Ulcers 633
RICHARD USATINE AND WAYNE A. HALE

Neurologic Problems

42. Cognitive Impairment 643
JOHN P. LANGLOIS AND SOO BORSON

43. Dizziness 663
KATHLEEN KLINK

44. Fatigue, Tiredness, and Sleep Problems 681
PHILIP D. SLOANE, THOMAS AGRESTA, DAVID LITTLE, DAVID HENDERSON, AND SALONI ANAND

45. Headache 695
MELISSA M. HICKS AND REMY R. COEYTAUX

Psychiatric Problems and Substance Abuse

46. Addictions 705
ADAM O. GOLDSTEIN, ROBERT E. GWYTHER, AND CAROL E. RIPLEY-MOFFITT

47. Anxiety 721
PETER HAM

48. Depression 733
DONALD E. NEASE, JR.

Respiratory Problems

49. Allergies and Asthma 745
DOROTHY E. VURA-WEIS

50. Acute Respiratory Infections 769
ARCH G. MAINOUS III AND WILLIAM J. HUESTON

51. Chronic Obstructive Pulmonary Disease 785
DAVID L. GASPAR AND DOROTHY E. VURA-WEIS

Index   *797*

PREFACE

The fifth edition of *Essentials of Family Medicine* continues our tradition of providing learners with a state-of-the-art guide to the field. New features for this edition include

- Continued focus on an evidence-based approach to care, with chapters on Information Mastery: Basing Care on the Best Available Evidence, extensive rating of the strength of evidence supporting recommendations, and, where appropriate, algorithms outlining general approaches to common problems.
- New chapters on venous thromboembolism, liver disease, cognitive impairment, and relationship issues.
- A comprehensive introduction to the principles and science base of family medicine, and the role of the specialty in the U.S. healthcare system.
- A bank of web-based multiple choice questions, called Examkit, linked to the chapters. Faculty can use these questions to generate customized examinations.
- A web-based self-assessment for students to test their understanding of material presented in the text.

Essentials of Family Medicine is meant to be read from cover to cover and used as a basic reference by students doing third- and fourth-year clerkships in family medicine. Other professionals, including specialists in other fields, residents in family medicine, physicians' assistants, and nurse practitioners, have used it as a comprehensive introduction to the field. We hope our readers find it useful and easy to read.

As always, we welcome comments, corrections, and suggestions for the next edition. Please address them to Philip Sloane or Lisa Slatt in care of Department of Family Medicine, Aycock Building, CBₒ 7595, University of North Carolina, Chapel Hill, NC 27599.

Finally, we'd like to thank the people who have helped put this edition together. The list must include, first and foremost, our author-colleagues, who drafted chapters while pursuing busy clinical and academic lives. Special recognition goes to the outstanding efforts of Dr. Judy Washington and Dr. Chantal Brazeau, who served as editors for Examkit questions. In addition, key assistance has been provided by Linda Allred, Mary Roederer, and our editorial team at Lippincott Williams & Wilkins, including Donna Balado, Cheryl Stringfellow, Emilie Moyer, Jennifer Kuklinski, and Tenille Sands.

Philip D. Sloane
Lisa M. Slatt
Mark H. Ebell
Louis B. Jacques
Mindy A. Smith

I

Principles of Family Medicine

Family Medicine in Today's Changing Health Care System

Philip D. Sloane, Thayer White, Larry Green, Warren P. Newton, and Kurt Stange

CASE

Carleton Tenney, a 48-year-old self-employed painter, lives in a trailer with his third wife, Carla, and their 6-year-old son, Jason. Carleton has recurrent abdominal pain and a chronic cough. However, because he does not have health insurance and is skeptical of doctors, he self-medicates with over-the-counter antacids and cough syrup. Carla, a private duty nurse, is also without health insurance. Her most persistent complaint is chronic pain in her shoulders, neck, and upper back. Several months ago, when in the emergency room for a bladder infection, she was told that her blood sugar was elevated and should be rechecked. Their son, Jason, receives his immunizations and routine care at the county health department; he has asthma and occasionally is brought to an urgent care clinic when his symptoms get bad.

CLINICAL QUESTIONS

1. Recognizing that you only have limited information, please list one or more medical diagnoses and underlying behavioral issues that you suspect may underlie: a) Carleton's abdominal pain; b) Carleton's chronic cough; c) Carla's chronic pain; d) Carla's elevated blood sugar; and e) Jason's asthma.
2. Within the current United States health care system, what options exist to provide this family with care that is both affordable and in line with the principles of good primary care practice? What are those principles?
3. Would this family be better served by a primary care-based health system or a specialty-based system? Why? What is the scientific evidence supporting your answer?

HEALTH PRIORITIES: A NATIONAL PERSPECTIVE

A paradox in modern American medicine is that remarkable advancements in biomedical care exist alongside failure to address the basic health care needs of a significant portion of our population. As a result, in spite of spending almost twice as much money per capita on health care as many other countries, the United States is:

- 42nd in the world in infant mortality—behind, for example, Singapore (#1), the Czech Republic (#9), France (#12), Spain (#15), Canada (#23), Greece (#32), Italy (#37), and Cuba (#40); and

- 47th in the world in life expectancy—behind, for example, Andorra (#1), Japan (#6), Canada (#12), Spain (#19), the US Virgin Islands (#28), Guam (#37), the United Kingdom (#38), and Bosnia/Herzegovina (#44) (1).

Thus, it is clear that our high cost of care, and our preeminent position as developers of medical technology, have not translated into leadership in health outcomes.

The reason for this disparity between costs and outcomes is complex and not completely understood. What is clear is that in the future, the nation will continue to examine its system of health care provision and make adjustments, with the primary goals being more cost-effective care, improved quality of care, and more attention paid to customer satisfaction.

What *are* the nation's most pressing health care needs? The most comprehensive statement of US health priorities is *Healthy People 2010*, a 2-volume report representing a consortium of more than 350 national organizations and 250 state agencies, convened by the US Department of Health and Human Services, with the goal of guiding health policy from 2000 to 2010. That report identified the following two overriding goals for the decade: To increase the life expectancy and quality of life for all Americans, and to eliminate health disparities (2). Furthermore, the report recommended that, to advance these goals, improvements should be targeted toward the health indicators noted in Table 1.1, most of which involve behavior change at the individual level, policy and organizational changes at the health system level, and provision of improved access to health care.

Addressing National Health Priorities

To understand how health care problems are currently managed, and the role of various segments of the health care system in addressing them, it is helpful to use a population perspective. This was elucidated in the early 1960s by Kerr White, and updated in 2001 by Larry Green, et al, and is graphically portrayed in Figure 1.1. When a population perspective is used, we see that medical symptoms are very common, and that traditional medical care, and tertiary care in particular, is only a small part of the management picture (3, 4). Because most health-related decisions occur outside the hospital, it is at the community level that the rubber really hits the road in terms of addressing the health care priorities outlined in *Healthy People 2010*. Therefore, only by involving primary care and community settings can medical education and practice affect key health indicators (see Table 1.1).

TABLE 1.1   Key National Targets for Increasing Life Expectancy and Quality of Life in the United States

Health Indicator	Significance	National Goals
Regular physical activity	Reduces risk of heart disease, diabetes, and high blood pressure; increases well-being and mood	Increase participation rates
Overweight and obesity	Raises risk of high blood pressure, elevated cholesterol, diabetes, heart disease, stroke, gallbladder disease, arthritis, sleep disorders, and certain cancers	Reduce proportion of people who are overweight or obese
Cigarette smoking	Increases risk of heart disease, stroke, lung cancer, and chronic lung disease; is associated with miscarriage, premature delivery, sudden infant death syndrome, and household fires.	Reduce proportion of people who smoke
Alcohol abuse andillicit drug use	Associated with child and spouse abuse, sexually transmitted diseases, teen pregnancy, school failure, motor vehicle crashes, job failure, homelessness, and family disruption.	Increase the proportion of adolescents and adults who do not use illicit drugs or abuse alcohol
Sexual behavior	Irresponsible sexual behavior is associated with unintended pregnancy and sexually transmitted diseases (including HIV/AIDS)	Increase responsible behavior, including fewer lifetime partners and regular condom use
Depression	Impairs social function and is associated with a poorer prognosis for most medical illnesses, as well as eating disorders and alcohol and drug use.	Increase the proportion of adults with depression who receive treatment.
Injury and homicide	Leads to over $200 billion per year in health care costs, and reduces work force productivity.	Reduce incidence through preventive behaviors (e.g., seat belts, not driving while impaired, firearm safety)
Preventable infectious diseases	Vaccines are available and recommended for influenza, pneumonia, tetanus, diphtheria, pertussis, hepatitis B, polio, varicella, hemophilus influenzae type b, measles, mumps, rubella, meningococcus, and hepatitis A, however, many children and adults are not up-to-date (37)	Increase the proportion of children and adults who are up-to-date on all recommended vaccines
Access to health care	Access to care is associated with use of clinical preventive services and with early diagnosis. Predictors of access to care include having health insurance, higher incomes, and a regular primary care provider.	Increase the proportion of persons who have health insurance, a regular source of ongoing medical care, and prenatal care beginning in the first trimester

(Adapted from Healthy People 2010 (2).)

Role of Primary Care in Addressing Health Care Priorities

Primary care is defined as care "which provides integrated, accessible health care services by clinicians who are accountable for addressing a large majority of personal health care needs, developing a sustained partnership with patients, in the context of family and community" (5). Primary care providers include family physicians, general internists, general pediatricians, family nurse practitioners (and some adult care and pediatric nurse practitioners), some physician assistants, and some gynecologists. Because they provide care that is aimed at preventing adverse, costly events such as hospitalizations and further morbidity, primary care physicians are well positioned to address the major national health priorities. As will be discussed later in this chapter, there are many challenges to addressing these issues optimally at the primary care level, many involving system problems both within the primary care office and within the US health care system.

To find out what primary care physicians actually do, a comprehensive study of the activities of family physicians directly observed 4,454 patient visits to 138 family physicians in 84 practices. Among the findings of that study are (6):

- An extensive variety of common, rare, and undifferentiated problems are managed in primary care. Often, management included a diagnostic process where the patient presents with new symptoms and leaves with a new or provisional diagnosis.
- Prevention is practiced broadly in primary care visits, and not just during "physicals." During 32% of illness visits, the family physician delivers at least one preventive service

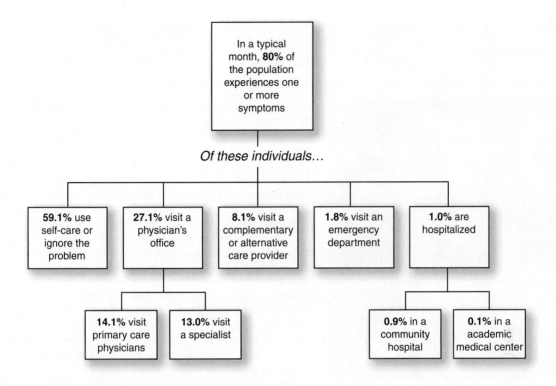

Figure 1.1 • **The ecology of medical care in the United States.**   Note that, during the course of a month, 80% of persons have one or more symptoms, but that of these only a minority seek medical attention, and fewer than 1% are hospitalized in academic medical centers. The implications of these statistics include: a) in order to have a significant impact on population health, the health care system must devote significant attention to the community level, and b) problems seen in academic medical centers represent an atypical subset of what actually presents in the community. Adapted from Green, et al, 2001 (4).

recommended by the US Preventive Services Task Force (see Box 1.1). Health habit messages are tailored toward high-risk patients and teachable moments; for example, smoking counseling is more often given in the context of smoking-related illness visits.

- Mental health problems present frequently, and are often managed in the primary care setting. For example, in 18% of visits, family physicians diagnose depression or anxiety and/or provide counseling related to these diagnoses.
- Patient education is a major part of primary care practice. Fully 90% of office visits, and 19% of visit time overall, involves patient education or health habit advice.
- Care is often provided in the context of family. Seventy percent of patients seen in these family physician visits have another family member seeing the same physician. In 18% of visits, care is provided to another family member in addition to the identified patient.
- Coordination of care is common in primary care visits. During 10% of office visits, a referral is made to a medical specialist, mental health provider, physical therapist, social worker, or other health professional.

The study also showed that family physicians have to prioritize among a broad agenda of competing opportunities, taking a patient-centered approach. By developing relationships over time, problems are addressed gradually, over many visits.

In summary, primary care practice involves a broad series

of activities that include early diagnosis, chronic disease management, acute care, mental health care, prevention, family care, and attention to community. These activities occur because of ongoing relationships between the patient and a personal physician who knows and is trusted by the patient. As we will see, when primary care is the cornerstone of the health care system, costs are lower and health outcomes are better.

Primary Care Versus Subspecialty-Based Care

In an analysis of 15 years of data from all 50 states, Barbara Starfield and her colleagues at the Johns Hopkins University School of Public Health concluded that the higher the ratio of primary care physicians to subspecialists, the better the outcomes. "Regardless of the year," they wrote, "after variable lag periods between the assessment of primary care and health outcomes, levels of analysis (state, county, or local area), or type of outcome as measured by all-cause mortality, infant mortality, low birth weight, life expectancy, and self-rated health. . . . The magnitude of improvement associated with an increase of one primary care physician per 10,000 population (a 12.6 percent increase over the current average supply) averaged 5.3 percent." Furthermore, "the supply of primary care physicians was significantly associated with lower all-cause mortality, whereas a greater supply of subspecialty physicians was associated with higher mortality."(7, 8) In contrast, subspecialist-focused care tends to lead to higher costs and poorer health outcomes. This is portrayed graphically in Figure 1.2.

BOX 1-1

Family Physician Leader Profile

Alfred Berg, MD, MPH: Leading the Effort to Develop National Prevention Guidelines

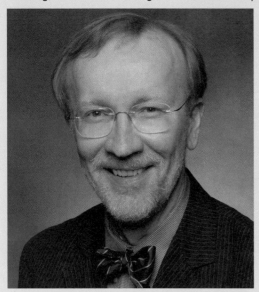

As chair of the United States Preventive Services Task Force, family physician Al Berg was responsible for making national recommendations regarding more than 40 screening and counseling interventions. "Large provider groups and insurance companies tend to follow Task Force recommendations because our decisions are made by independent panels that focus on the scientific evidence," Berg says. "In developing the recommendations, an interdisciplinary panel works together to assess the quality of the evidence and its applicability to primary care practice throughout the United States."

"Providing preventive services is an increasingly important and complex part of the primary care physician's role," Dr. Berg states. "If medical science is to improve overall population health," he notes, "then preventive services that make a difference need to be offered to all persons who will benefit from them. The Task Force's job is to evaluate specific clinical problems, such as screening for abdominal aortic aneurysms or screening for family violence, and to make recommendations regarding whether, how, and for whom these services should be offered." Task Force reports are available on line at *http:// www.ahrq.gov/clinic/prevenix.htm.*

"I worked on the Task Force for 12 years, chairing it for the last 5. It was an incredible privilege working with such a highly focused and talented group of colleagues on issues that really make a difference in the health of average people," Berg says. He served as the spokesman for more than 30 news releases, and was quoted many times in print media and on radio and television when new or controversial recommendations were released. He was featured on the Lehrer News Hour when the Task Force released a report finding the evidence insufficient to recommend for or against screening for prostate cancer.

"Assessing the quality of evidence can be difficult and tedious, but it is not all that complicated. The real challenge is in figuring out ways to incorporate effective prevention into typical practices, given the limitation of time and resources," Berg concludes. "It is important to generate new knowledge about processes and systems that actually work, leading to the potential benefits that the evidence points toward. I see this as one of the critical agendas for our future research as a discipline."

Why is this? There are several reasons. When patients have a primary care physician as the regular source of care:

• Preventive services are more consistently delivered
• Chronic diseases, such as asthma, cardiovascular disease, and diabetes, are better managed
• Acute problems are diagnosed and treated earlier
• People with low incomes tend to have greater access to care and, concomitantly, fewer disparities in health outcomes
• Primary care physicians tend to be active at a community level to improve health care resources and attitudes for both healthy patients and those with chronic diseases

As a result, hospitalization rates are lower, and overall health is better.

When patients go to a variety of subspecialists for their care, without having a primary care provider, their care tends to be fragmented and discontinuous. Furthermore, treatments focused on one body system can have unintended adverse impacts in other areas; more and more care is not necessarily best for patients. On the other hand, when access to subspecialists is severely restricted, patients often suffer symptoms for months or years without getting available treatments. Therefore, a well-functioning health care system needs both primary care providers and subspecialists.

PRINCIPLES OF GOOD PRIMARY CARE

The principles of good primary care are embodied in the principles of family medicine (see Table 1.2). They include: continuity of care, comprehensiveness, coordination of care, community orientation, prevention focus, evidence-based practice, a biopsychosocial, life-cycle perspective, and family orientation. Each is described briefly below.

Continuity of Care

The average family medicine patient has seen the same physician 20 times over the previous 5 years (6). This provision of care by the same provider over time is called *continuity of care.* However, since no physician can be available all the time, continuity of care generally needs to be shared across several providers. Mechanisms for providing this inter-provider continuity include having a medical record system that communicates personal medical information and preferences to others

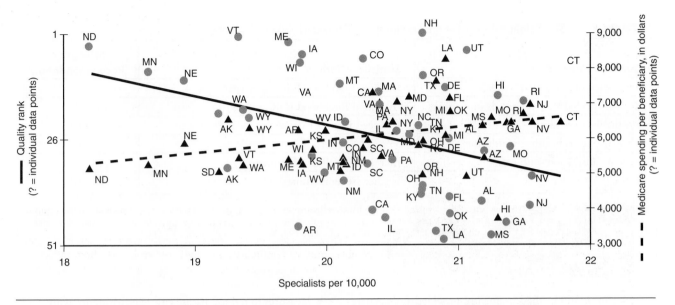

Figure 1.2 • The relationship between provider mix and quality, by state, United States, 2000. These data document that as the number of medical specialists in a state increases, the cost of care increases, and the quality of care decreases. Key: ● = state rank in Medicare indicators of quality of care (smaller values indicate better quality); ▲ = state rank in dollars spent per Medicare beneficiary. Smaller values indicate lower cost per patient. Source: Medicare claims data and Area Resource File (2003) data, as reported in: Baicker K, Chandra A. Medicare Spending, the physician workforce, and beneficiaries' quality of care. In: Iglehart JK, ed. Health affairs—Web Exclusives. Bethesda, MD: Project HOPE; 2004:184–197 (42).

(continuity of information) and, in large organizations, forming small subunits (i.e., teams) in which several providers get to know each other's patients.

Two evidence-based reviews have identified numerous favorable outcomes from continuity of care (see Table 1.3). In addition, continuity of care is associated with fuller, more satisfying relationships for the medical practice with its patients. For family physicians who practice for years in the same location, these relationships are often among the greatest sources of professional satisfaction.

Comprehensiveness

A family physician manages without referral between 85% and 90% of the patients who present for primary care. In doing so, a wide range of services are provided, including acute care, chronic disease care, preventive care, and care for biomedical and psychosocial problems (6). This provision of a wide variety of services, covering the majority of patient needs, is termed *comprehensiveness of care.*

The role of comprehensiveness in quality primary care

is clear. Comprehensiveness is a prerequisite for continuity of care and the development of trust in the provider as a reliable source of care. Furthermore, comprehensive care is convenient for the patient, as there is no need to go to multiple providers to get service. However, as health care has become more complex, the ability of a single physician or medical practice to provide comprehensive care has been challenged. For example, studies have suggested that primary care providers frequently miss opportunities to pick up on psychosocial or emotional issues, and that barriers exist to access from primary care offices to a variety of specialized services (9). In response, some primary care settings offer access to health care resources far beyond those offered by primary care physicians alone; examples include low-cost drugs, dental services, on-site physical therapy, a variety of complementary/alternative health providers, and social workers.

Coordination of Care

Primary care providers help their patients negotiate the complex health care system by serving as coordinators of care for complex patients. This process of coordination includes being aware of the variety of services available, making appropriate requests for consultation or referral, collecting and interpreting results of studies and specialist visits, and advising when additional care provision is and is not warranted. It also involves helping patients comprehend what is happening to them, by helping them integrate what are often disparate messages into a coherent whole (10).

During the 1990s, some health plans tried to exploit the care coordination role of primary care physicians by setting them up as "gatekeepers." These gatekeeping systems required patients to have a primary care referral in order to see a specialist or access a specialized service, such as physical

TABLE 1.2	Principles of Family Medicine
Continuity of care	
Comprehensiveness	
Coordination of care	
Community orientation	
Prevention focus	
Evidence-based practice	
Biopsychosocial, life-cycle perspective	
Family-centeredness	

TABLE 1.3 Relationship between Continuity of Care and Patient Outcomes

Outcome Affected	Statistical Finding	Strength of Recommendation*
Frequency of preventive visits	Increased likelihood during a year (OR = 3.41)	B
Referral of diabetics for eye examinations	Increased likelihood (OR = 2.89)	B
Hospitalization rate	Reduced from 9.1 days/year to 5.7 days/year	B
Annual rate of health expenditures	33%-36% lower	B
Patient satisfaction with care	Increased in 19 of 22 studies	B
Trust in provider	Higher (several studies)	B*

* A = consistent, good-quality patient-oriented evidence; B = inconsistent or limited-quality patient-oriented evidence; C = consensus, disease-oriented evidence, usual practice, expert opinion, or case series. For information about the SORT evidence rating system, see *http://www.aafp.org/afpsort.xml*. (Burstin and Clancy, 2004 (9); Cabana and Jee, 2004 (38); Franks and Fiscella, 1998 (39); Saultz and Aldebaiwi, 2004 (40).)

therapy; in addition, they frequently provided financial rewards to primary care physicians who had low referral rates. This system proved highly unpopular with patients and providers alike, and it led to a temporary decline in popularity of primary care careers. A variety of studies showed that gatekeeping models were ineffective in reducing referral rates and highly effective in reducing patients' trust of and satisfaction with their primary care providers and insurers. As a result, gatekeeping models have largely been abandoned, and primary care physicians are increasingly recognized for the importance of their role as active coordinators of patient care.

Community Orientation

While most of the physician's work is at the patient level, good primary care physicians also seek to improve the broader health of the community. Good medical practice requires this orientation, because what happens in homes, schools, worksites, health departments, and elsewhere in the community can have profound effects on individual health and quality of life. Often, this broader perspective is necessary for improvements in a patient's health.

Many primary care physicians throughout the United States take community involvement seriously. On a volunteer basis, they serve on school boards, act as advisors to health departments and police departments, lobby for improved pollution controls in local factories, provide medical oversight for free clinics or homeless shelters, organize pre-participation screening for athletes, and stand at the sidelines during high school football games. They consider these and other types of community activism to be part of their job. Box 1.2 provides a profile of one such physician.

Prevention Focus

Preventive care is the most common reason patient's visit a family physician's office—for prenatal care, routine adult physicals, well baby checkups, well child examinations, pre-employment physicals, visits as preparation for international travel, and examinations to certify persons for participation in sports activities or summer camp. Providing good preventive care is complex and challenging, but also very satisfying. Among the facets of preventive care are:

- Measures to reduce disease risk (e.g., assistance with smoking cessation or physical activity)
- Immunizations
- Measures to prevent morbidity in persons who have established disease (e.g., prescription of aspirin for persons with coronary artery disease or angiotensin converting enzyme (ACE) inhibitors to diabetics with microalbuinuria)
- Prevention of secondary disability in people with disease-related morbidity (e.g. post-stroke rehabilitation)

Providing and maintaining community-based preventive care is an ongoing challenge. In setting priorities, use of available scientific evidence is important and can be guided by reviews by the US Preventive Services Task Force (see Box 1.1) and other organizations. The actual delivery of preventive services at a practice and community level is, however, impaired by the large numbers of uninsured patients in the United States, and by the fact that many third-party payers do not reimburse for preventive visits. The task remains a vital one, however, and a high priority for primary care providers, and for the country. Figure 1.3 illustrates how the current breakdown in primary cares services has led to a resurgence of pertussis, a completely preventable disease.

Evidence-Based Practice

Exemplary primary care is evidence based. By this, we mean that the primary care physician has access to and uses effectively what is available in the literature to guide practice. Unfortunately, 80% of the clinical questions that arise in family medicine practice do not have adequate empirical data to be answered in a wholly "evidence-based" manner. As a result, primary care physicians must integrate different kinds of evidence, depending on logic, clinical intuition, and knowledge of the patient, family, and community to arrive at the best decisions (10).

Considerable research is ongoing to improve the evidence base of primary care. The methods are varied, transdisciplinary, and require active participation of community physicians, patients, and university-based researchers (11). As part of this research effort, more than 111 practice-based research networks have been developed (12). These networks use real-world medical practices as the setting to answer complex, yet

BOX 1-2

Family Physician Leader Profile

Adele O'Sullivan, MD: Physician as Servant Leader

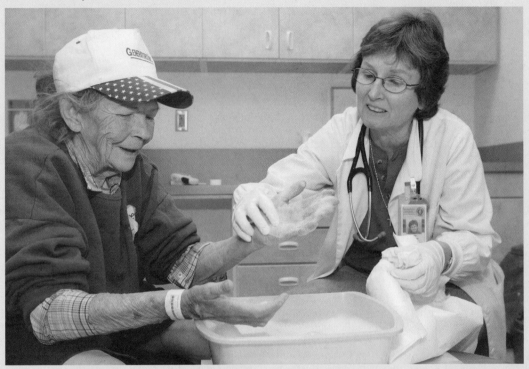

Many highly effective leaders are motivated by a desire to serve rather than to lead (41). These servant leaders do not necessarily rise to positions with high salaries and fancy titles. However, through their creativity, energy, passion, communication skills, and exemplary works, they inspire others. Often their work becomes a model from which more organizationally inclined leaders develop policies and implement broader change.

One such servant leader is Adele O'Sullivan, who was honored in 2006 as America's Family Physician of the Year. On most days Dr. O'Sullivan can be found administering medical care to the large and growing homeless population of downtown Phoenix. "My patients are people who have bottomed out in society," she states. "At one level they have nothing, but they are rich in insight into themselves, in stories, and in the resiliency to face the harsh realities of life that the rest of us are often able to ignore. For example, one of the most painful things about homelessness is the isolation, the sorrow of separation, the absence of a support network. Yet my patients maintain a dignity and honesty that I find refreshing every day."

Dr. O'Sullivan, a devout Christian, considers her medical work to be a type of ministry. "I believe that God does his work through people," she states, "and I feel lucky to be able to be one of God's agents." When caring for one of her homeless patients—for example, cleaning and dressing the feet of a diabetic, with severe peripheral neuropathy—Dr. O'Sullivan endeavors to act as though she were ministering directly to Jesus, recalling the words from the Bible, "*I was hungry and you gave me something to eat, I was thirsty and you gave me something to drink, I was a stranger and you invited me in, I needed clothes and you clothed me, I was sick and you looked after me, I was in prison and you came to visit me . . . As often as you did these things, you did them for me.*" [Matthew 25:35–36, 45] "Many of my colleagues and patients view the things I do as merely good science," Dr. O'Sullivan states, "and that perspective is fine. But for me, medicine has an added dimension, that of service to my faith."

Dr. O'Sullivan's base of operations is a clinic for the homeless, but she goes wherever she can be most effective. Every Monday evening she conducts an impromptu clinic for persons who are waiting for food at a local soup kitchen. "By meeting people where they are, I can help them view medicine as a person who cares rather than a system to be feared," she states. In addition, because of her growing recognition as one who has effectively reached a challenging population, Dr. O'Sullivan is increasingly called upon to provide guidance to organizations that seek to provide services to America's homeless.

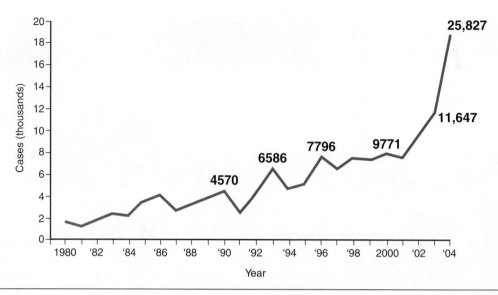

Figure 1.3 • The growth of reported cases of pertussis in the United States between 2000 and 2004. This illustrates how, when access to primary care services is impaired, critical preventive health care provision can break down, threatening public health. Note that, because pertussis is difficult to distinguish clinically from other respiratory illnesses (e.g., bronchitis) and is often treated empirically without microbiological confirmation, the actual number of cases is likely to be more than 10 times the number of reported cases. Data adapted from: Centers for Disease Control: Morbidity and Mortality Weekly Reports, 1997, 2001, 2003, and 2004.

common, clinical questions. Several journals disseminate the evidence base for family medicine, including the Journal of the American Board of Family Medicine (*www.abfm.org*) and Annals of Family Medicine (*www.annfammed.org*). Furthermore, intense efforts are ongoing to summarize the existing research data and to make them available to physicians in the office setting; Box 1.3 describes one such effort.

Biopsychosocial, Life-Cycle Perspective

Effective primary care physicians view patients from a broad perspective, taking into account physiology, physical illness, emotional health, and the social, occupational, and environmental context within which the person lives. Such a biopsychosocial approach is important because health and illness behavior are strongly colored by the personality and environment of the patient. For example, whether or not a patient will actually take a prescribed medicine will depend on many factors, such as the medication's cost, the experience of the person and others he or she knows with similar medical treatment, and the interaction between side effects and the person's needs (e.g., alertness or sexual potency).

One useful perspective for approaching patients from such a biopsychosocial perspective is to view patient's needs from the perspective outlined by psychologist Abraham Maslow. According to Maslow (see Figure 1.4), human needs must be satisfied in a specific hierarchy, with lower-level needs generally having to be addressed before an individual can successfully deal with higher challenges (13). Take, as an example, a person with a chronic illness such as HIV disease. Society's first priority would be to assure that his or her physiological needs are met—that food, shelter, warmth, and the ability to rest were available. The next priority would be to provide the person with safety and security from harm. In the case of the person with HIV disease, this would include having access to

health care services and medications, such as protease inhibitors. While not specifically discussed by Maslow, relief of pain and suffering would undoubtedly fall into either the first or second level. With these assured, the person with HIV disease would then have the energy and ability to develop and nurture satisfying interpersonal relationships, to contribute to society, and to achieve his or her greatest potential.

Family Orientation

Quality primary care must take into account the family context. By family we mean the entire range of relationships—whether or not by blood or marriage—that can comprise a patient's close social network (14, 15). Being oriented to the family context is important in medical care because most health behaviors and illness episodes involve some connection with the patient's social support network. The pregnant woman who, by the act of conception, has entwined her life with both the father and the child, and who will, because of this, see her relationship with (and view of) her mother change. The man who develops a chronic illness that will require him to perhaps eat differently or alter his recreational patterns or have less money for family incidentals. Even the healthy young athlete who twists her ankle and needs to use crutches (and, therefore, cannot drive) for a few days. These are examples of situations that present in primary care settings, in which the care of patients usually requires a family orientation. Furthermore, with more sophisticated electronic information systems and further maturation of applied genetics, it is likely that the importance of a family orientation will increase.

There are many tools available to assess and treat families, though most family physicians do the majority of their history-taking and therapeutic work with families informally. A genogram (formal family tree) can at times be helpful in under-

BOX 1-3

Bringing Evidence-Based Medicine into the Primary Care Office

Medical decision making should integrate clinical observations and in-depth knowledge of the patient with the best available research evidence. Recently, existing research has been made more available to practicing physicians through approaches that create concise practice recommendations, and grade them according to the strength of the evidence. Furthermore, the information technology needed to provide point-of-care access to such summaries has also been developed. Turning such possibilities into a reality is the ambitious goal of the Family Physicians Inquiries Network (FPIN), a unique, not-for-profit consortium of clinicians and medical librarians. "Our vision is to provide the best evidence-based answer to 80% of questions that arise in primary care practice, using electronic methods that require less than 60 seconds of a clinician's time," says Dr. Bernard Ewigman, founder of FPIN and chair of the Department of Family Medicine at the University of Chicago.

Here is how FPIN works. Suppose you see a patient with low back pain and a persistent, aggravating radiculopathy and wonder whether an epidural steroid injection (ESI) might help. In the examining room, you use your wireless computer or personal digital assistant to search FPIN-developed resources for ESIs. Every month, FPIN fields hundreds of questions from clinicians in primary care practice, and farms them out to volunteers (usually academic faculty), who develop structured, evidence-based reviews. You find that such a review of ESIs was carried out and published in a peer-reviewed publication, and that it concluded that there is no proven advantage of ESI compared with usual care, with a strength of recommendation (SOR) = "A" (i.e., based on well-done randomized trials).

By 2006, only 4 years after its founding, FPIN involved 22 universities, 78 family medicine residency programs, 80 medical librarians, 15 practice-based research networks, and nearly 3,000 individuals. In addition to providing evidence-based answers to practical clinical questions, FPIN provides scholarly training on conducting structured literature searches, performing critical appraisal, writing for publication, and editing. More information on FPIN is available at *www.fpin.org.*

Another evidence-based product, designed to provide succinct, practice-relevant data at the source of care, is InfoRetriever®. Developed by three family physicians, InfoRetriever® focuses on providing Patient-Oriented Evidence that Matters in readily-accessible, electronic format. More information on InfoRetriever® is available at *http://www.infopoems.com.*

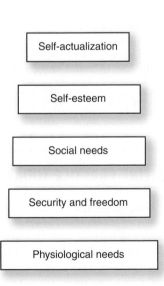

Figure 1.4 • Maslow's hierarchy of needs. According to Maslow, the lower-level (i.e., more basic) needs generally must be attended to before an individual can effectively address higher level issues. From a biopsychosocial perspective, optimal health can be viewed as similar to Maslow's concept of self-actualization (13).

standing family relationships in complex systems, but they are time-consuming, and most electronic medical record systems do not yet incorporate genograms. Charting systems that keep families together have also been used occasionally; however, though the majority of patients in family physicians' offices have another family member who sees the same physician (6), it is rare for all family members to do so. Another simple tool—the family circle—will be described in the case example below.

Case Example

To illustrate how many of the principles of family medicine described above can be applied to care of patients, we will describe the real case of a woman who did not have a personal physician, and how lack of application of these principles compromised her care. Cases such as this remain disturbingly frequent in the United States and around the world (16).

The patient was a 36-year-old named Maria, who was hospitalized for asthma. This was her sixth admission in 3 years, all for severe asthma. On the most recent three admissions, the asthma had required intensive care, and she was near death on one occasion. One of the major frustrations of the resident who admitted Maria was her lack of adherence with medication regimens. As she had a few months beforehand, she presented to the hospital severely ill and admitted to not having followed her prescribed regimen.

Maria lived 30 miles from the hospital and did not have health insurance. Primary care was sporadic and occurred in the hospital emergency department and outpatient clinics. Nowhere in her hospital chart could the name of a primary care physician be found. Each time she was transferred from the intensive care unit (ICU) back to the regular floor, her physician changed. Various specialists cared for her from time to time. A review of both outpatient and inpatient records revealed little communication between her respective physicians. The outpatient physicians did not appear aware of the number of times Maria had been hospitalized or the details of the hospitalizations, and many details of her outpatient care were not reflected in the hospital admission notes. Many of the tests ordered in one setting had been repeated in another, thus increasing the cost of care. This lack of continuity, communication, and coordination places a tremendous burden on the health care system, as well as on the patient and family.

Maria had excellent hospital care for her biological problems. There were pulmonary function tests, blood chemistries, and so on. However, nothing was listed in the chart about depressive or anxiety symptoms. Furthermore, the hospital chart did not discuss her occupation or the condition of her home. Physicians assumed that dust was present in the environment. Home health nurse and social services referrals had been ordered, but no report was available in the hospital record.

Other than discussions regarding prevention of asthma, no other preventive services were documented. The hospital and outpatient clinic records consisted entirely of acute and post-hospitalization visits, and did not provide information on whether and when PAP smears had been done, influenza vaccination had been given, or the role of diet and exercise had been discussed as prevention of osteoporosis, heart disease, and cancer. In summary, her record provided a good example of care of the disease rather than care of the patient.

At this point Maria's genogram was elicited. It showed that Maria and her husband, José, had three children. Both of Maria's parents were deceased, and her father had been an alcoholic. José's parents were both living; his mother had dementia and his father was an alcoholic. Of the children, the two girls were healthy and the boy had mild asthma. José's parents had moved into the family's two-bedroom home 3 years before.

The genogram provided a biological description of the family. To learn more about their relationships, Maria was asked to draw a family circle—a brief assessment technique in which a patient is asked to graphically represent the relationships between individuals in his or her family. The physician drew a large circle on a blank piece of paper and instructed Marie to draw her family members within or outside the circle, representing the relationships between them by how large she made the individuals and how close to each other she placed them.

Maria quickly drew her own family circle (see Figure 1.5). On one side was José (J). Behind him were his mother and father. At the other side was Maria (M), with the three children behind her.

The physician asked Maria for an interpretation, and she began to tell her story.

José and his father would begin drinking and start to pick on the son, and on occasion would beat him. Maria would become upset, and she would begin to wheeze. As her story unfolded, it became evident why her asthma had worsened 3 years before, when José's family moved in, and that every one of Maria's attacks had been triggered by drinking in the family. Once Maria became severely ill, her illness protected her

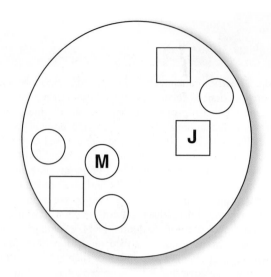

Figure 1.5 • Maria's family circle. On one side is Maria, with her three children behind her; on the other is José, with his parents behind him. See text for interpretation.

children, as it shifted attention away from her son and onto herself. It only protected them for awhile, however, and she expressed deep worry about what was happening to the children when she was not there to protect them.

Case Discussion

The majority of the problems that present to a physician's office have both medical and psychological components. While addressing the medical issues can at times lead to resolution, more often than not—and especially in severe or chronic disease—psychosocial issues also need to be addressed. To most effectively apply a biopsychosocial approach requires continuity of care, a family and community orientation, comprehensiveness, and application of the other principles of family medicine. In the case of Maria, the unfolding of her story led to a family conference, a comprehensive management plan, more attention to developing a relationship with a single provider, and, ultimately, much better management of her asthma.

FAMILY MEDICINE PRACTICE TODAY

Until the late 1960s, generalist physicians typically entered practice after a year of internship. However, as medicine became more complex, it became clear that a specialty needed to be created to consistently train physicians to perform quality primary care. The specialty was named Family Medicine, and a rigorous 3-year training requirement was established. As of 2004, there were 469 family medicine residencies in the United States, training a total of 9,373 residents (17).

The practice of family medicine today is highly varied, with men and women who complete residency training taking a variety of career paths. Careers can include outpatient and inpatient care, rural or urban settings, and community or academic medicine, in addition to fellowships in obstetrics, sports

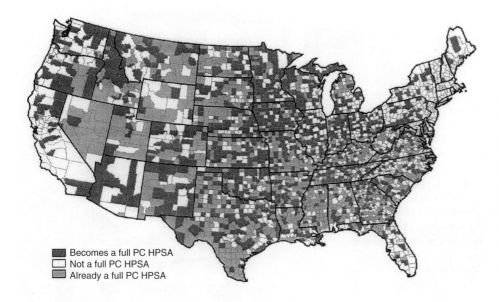

Figure 1.6 • Map of the United States showing the impact of family physicians on reducing the number of primary care health professions shortage areas (PCHPSAs). The dark shading indicates counties that would be PCHPSAs if family physicians were removed. Legend: PC = primary care; FP = family physicians; HPSA = health professional shortage area. Source: Green, L.A., et al, 2004 (18).

Legend:
- Becomes a full PC HPSA
- Not a full PC HPSA
- Already a full PC HPSA

medicine, geriatrics, and research. What all these careers share is a commitment to deliver excellent, patient-oriented primary care.

In this section we seek to demonstrate some of the many careers and lifestyles available to today's family physician. We will illustrate this diversity with examples of graduates from a single residency training program. Each of these physicians has followed a unique path that represents his or her interests and talents while upholding the basic core values of family medicine.

Rural Practice

The archetypical rural physician was and continues to be a family physician. This is because, in communities that can support only a few physicians, breadth of training and skills are valued. So indispensable is the role of family medicine in rural care that, as is shown in Figure 1.6, if all family physicians were removed, much of the rural United States would meet the federal definition of a health professions shortage area (18).

CASE EXAMPLE: DR. VICKIE INGLEDUE, JEFFERSON NORTH CAROLINA

To get a flavor of what rural practice is like, for one day we followed Dr. Vickie Ingledue, of Jefferson, North Carolina. Her day began at 6 o'clock, with Dr. Ingledue, her husband, and their children getting up and preparing for the day. After convincing 6-year-old Griffin to stop jumping on the couch long enough to eat breakfast, she pried Olivia, her 2-year-old, away from the computer, a new favorite toy, to sit down for a few bites. When both were fed and dressed, matching socks and all, and Griffin had grabbed his Spongebob backpack, Dr. Ingledue drove Griffin to school while Olivia stayed behind with her father to wait for the nanny.

Next, Dr. Ingledue headed to the second floor of Ashe Memorial Hospital, as she did nearly every day, arriving around eight. She had only two patients to see that day, and the report from the doctor on call that night told her that

both were doing well. The first, her patient for the past 7 years, was to be discharged, and Dr. Ingledue went over the diagnosis and follow-up plans with the patient and her daughter. The second, a thin 78-year-old admitted 2 nights before with a gastrointestinal bleed, was alert and stable. However, the physical therapist's note indicated that he was weak and unsteady, and, since he lived alone, recommended against his going directly home. Dr. Ingledue cautiously broached the subject with the patient, recommending a short-term rehabilitative nursing home stay, and the patient—whom she had known for several years—agreed.

After completing her documentation, Dr. Ingledue headed over to the operating room suite to assist a colleague during the Caesarian section of a patient with twins. All of the obstetric care in Jefferson is provided by fellowship-trained family physicians, and they often have to rely on each other when an extra set of hands is needed. Prior to returning to Jefferson, where she had grown up, she completed a residency in family medicine followed by a year-long fellowship in obstetrics. "I didn't want to send my patients to another doctor if they needed a C-section," Dr. Ingledue remarked.

The woman was not her patient but remembered that Dr. Ingledue had also assisted on her first C-section, 2 years before. Dr. Ingledue reviewed the records, scrubbed, and gowned for surgery. She hoped that things would go smoothly, so that she could arrive at the office in time for her first patient at 11:00. The procedure began as planned. In addition to the patient and her mother in the room, there were three doctors (one for each baby, and one for the mother), two teams of pediatric nurses, and the operating room (OR) nurses. Dr. Ingledue was there to assist at the surgery and care for the second baby after its delivery.

As they began to cut through the peritoneum, the lights went dim, and all equipment turned off. Everyone waited in silence. A nurse hurried out to find the OR supervisor. Fortunately, the surgeon had not yet started to make the low transverse uterine incision, and the babies were safe. A functioning outlet was discovered down the hall, extension cords

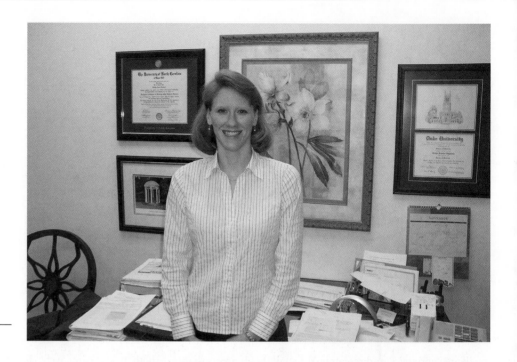

Dr. Vickie Ingledue

strung, portable lamps brought in, suction and electrocautery machines connected, and the delivery completed. Later, they discovered that an emergency circuit breaker supplying that operating suite had blown.

After passing off the first baby, Dr. Ingledue took the second. The babies—both boys— were placed in twin warmers, which had been squeezed into a storage closet that had power and had been stocked with warm blankets from down the hall. The two teams pressed together to examine the babies. The first was vigorous from the start, but the second required oxygen to keep his O_2 saturation in the 90s. His blood sugar read out in the 30s. He was unable to take oral glucose because of the oxygen hood, so an IV line was placed and a glucose drip started. The baby perked up, letting out a strong cry, and there was a collective exhale.

Dr. Ingledue finished her paperwork, checked the baby one more time, and left the hospital. At her request, in the midst of the C-section, one of the OR nurses had called ahead to request that her morning patients be rescheduled, so she found herself with time to drive into town for a sandwich and a glass of sweet tea before beginning her afternoon schedule.

On a normal day, Dr. Ingledue is in her office from about 9 to 5 and sees about 20 patients. "When I am in the room, I want each patient to feel like my only patient," she explains. As a result, she sees fewer patients per day than many rural providers, but has no plans to change her style. "I want to know my patients' lives at home," she says. "It gives me the ability to provide the best care for every family member."

Relationships that extend beyond medical diagnoses are part of what drew Dr. Ingledue to family medicine. She also draws professional satisfaction from the broad scope of medicine she delivers. "I wear a lot of hats," she quips.

When she was growing up, her town doctor shaped her ideal of what a physician should be. Today she practices alongside him. When in medical school, her appreciation of the importance of good primary care grew as she watched her

father's battle with multiple chronic diseases. "His medical care was fragmented, and he couldn't understand all the things his doctors were telling him," she explains. "I saw the family physician as someone who had the ability to tie everything together." Then, during her clinic clerkships in medical school, she enjoyed all of her rotations and didn't want to let go of any. Thus, it was the combination of a belief in the importance of primary care and a desire to practice full-scope medicine that ultimately led Dr. Ingledue into the type of practice that she has now.

"I find family medicine to be interesting, exciting, and challenging," she remarks. "You face a variety of different challenges throughout the day. You can make it whatever you want it to be."

Urban and Suburban Private Practice

Approximately two-thirds of America's family physicians practice in urban or suburban settings. Within these practices there is wide variation in physician practice patterns. Some practice "full-spectrum family medicine"—including maternity care, newborn care, hospital practice, and nursing home care. Others have outpatient-only practices. Some focus on providing complementary and alternative medicine; others on occupational health. The common denominator is having completed residency training under a rigorous, comprehensive curriculum specified by the American Board of Family Medicine, which certifies family physicians. The following case example profiles a husband and wife whose philosophy of practice blends love of medicine with devotion to family.

CASE EXAMPLE: DRS. ELIZABETH AND GREG GIBBONS, CARY, NORTH CAROLINA

It was an interest in relationships and personal interactions that drew Dr. Elizabeth Gibbons to medicine. She majored in psychology as an undergraduate, and while growing up she listened to her grandfather, a general practitioner, talk about

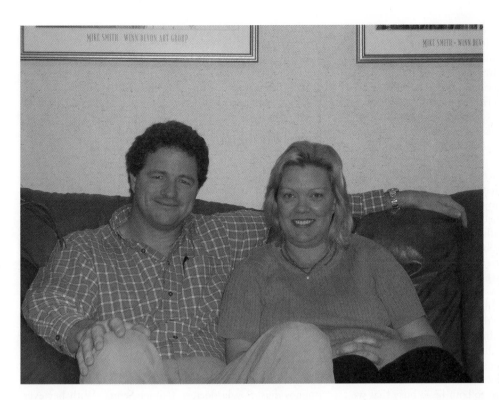

Drs. Elizabeth and Greg Gibbons

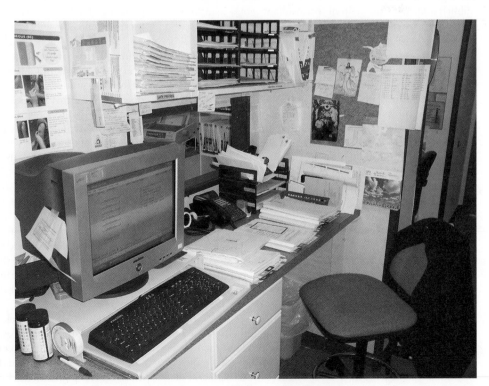

The Gibbons' office is designed to be compact and efficient.

how medicine allowed him "to see life unfolding." While in medical school she met Greg, a doctoral student pursuing a PhD in biochemistry. They began dating, later married, and their first child was born while Elizabeth was a 4th-year medical student. Meanwhile, Greg continued his biochemical studies, obtaining a doctorate and entering a post-doctoral research program. However, he was impressed by the personal satisfaction he watched Elizabeth experience, despite the long hours and hard work—so impressed, in fact, that he decided to apply to medical school.

For Greg his greatest satisfaction in training came from diagnosing and treating the patient who had multiple issues or unusual presentations. "I enjoy the challenge that comes with treating real patients. They seem to invariably have many problems that all interact and influence one another," he remarks. He chose family medicine because it offered the ability to diagnose and treat a wide variety of conditions. "When patients come to see me, they haven't been referred, and they don't have a diagnosis yet. I enjoy that challenge," he admits. By the time Greg was ready to enter residency, their second child was on the way, and Elizabeth was a full-time practicing physician. Not wanting to miss time with his children, Greg arranged to do what Elizabeth had done several years before—take a shared internship position, in which he worked half-time and finished in 2 years. "Our family is important to both of us, and we didn't want to both be so busy that we didn't have time for our children," Elizabeth comments.

Initially, Greg joined the group practice in which Elizabeth had been practicing, but this was not the ideal situation for them. Elizabeth remarks, "We enjoyed working with that group, but we did not have the flexibility we wanted to balance work and family." So, they decided to open their own practice. This would give them the flexibility they were looking for, but it meant they had to shoulder the full financial risk of managing a business. They picked a location in a growing suburb and, with the help of a consultant, got a loan, found a building, hired a staff, and began to plan the business.

Their staff now includes nurses, front desk personnel, a practice manager, and two family nurse practitioners (FNPs). The two FNPs give Greg and Elizabeth the ability to see more patients in the practice as well as maintain extended office hours. Elizabeth works one full day and 2 half-days per week. This allows her to be home when her children arrive from school and to take care of their third child, an 18-month-old infant. Greg works four 10-hour days, Monday through Thursday, giving him a 3-day weekend.

The Gibbons made the decision to have an outpatient-only practice. Every hospital in their area is staffed with hospitalists; so this was a feasible option. Although providing hospital care can be a valuable source of revenue, the Gibbons gladly gave it up to avoid long on-call nights in the emergency department. To provide after-hours service to their patients, they have partnered with another local practice. An after-hours nurse fields all calls, and those that require more consultation are forwarded to the doctor on call. Six doctors share this arrangement; so Greg and Elizabeth are on call every 6th week.

Five years into the adventure of owning their own practice, Greg and Elizabeth are still enthusiastic about their decision. They are doing well financially, and both have plenty of time to spend with their three children. Elizabeth still de-

rives joy from the relationships forged with her patients. "They give me back so much," she says. "Plus, taking care of patients is easier now than it was during residency, because I have personal relationships with them." Greg, ever the scientist, still finds a unique challenge in every patient. "You can know all the science, but patients never present like a textbook."

Community Health Centers

Across the United States, more than 1,000 Federally-qualified community health centers (CHCs) provide care in approximately 5,000 sites to more than 15 million persons, primarily of low income, often without insurance (19, 20). CHCs receive federal funding to provide a primary care "safety net" for persons with limited financial resources. Their patient population tends to include disproportionate numbers of racial and ethnic minorities, and immigrants. Studies have shown that persons residing in communities with CHCs have considerably better access to care (21), and CHCs have been credited with helping narrow the black/white and Latino/white health gap in key areas, such as infant mortality, prenatal care, and tuberculosis death rates.

CASE EXAMPLE: DR. MELISSA GILMER-SCOTT, MONCURE, NORTH CAROLINA

"Buenos dias. Soy la doctora Gilmer-Scott." With her ever-present smile, Dr. Melissa Gilmer-Scott greets her patient, a Latino woman at 30 weeks' gestation, accompanied by her husband and 2-year-old son. This is one of a dozen Spanish-speaking patients she will see in a typical day. Most are without health insurance and have little money to pay for medical care. Without the services provided by the Moncure Community Health Center many of these patients, both English- and Spanish-speaking, would have no other source of care. "The most rewarding part of my job is the 'Thank you' from my patients," Dr. Gilmer-Scott relates. "I love being able to help those no one else will help."

Since finishing her family medicine residency in 2003, Dr. Gilmer-Scott has been working for Piedmont Health Services (PHS), a network of CHCs located in central North Carolina. PHS was founded in 1970 with federal funding, and its mission is "to improve the health of the community by providing the highest quality preventive and primary health care services to individuals and families who need access to these services." The patients seen at PHS clinics are predominantly poor, with a large Spanish-speaking immigrant population. In 2004, 77% of the patients were below the federal poverty line, 48% were Latino, 48% had no insurance, and 45% had either Medicare or Medicaid. Patients without insurance are treated on a sliding fee scale according to their family income. Dr. Gilmer-Scott works at the Moncure clinic located in rural Chatham County, which has a particularly high proportion of Spanish-speaking patients due to the presence of two local poultry plants. The Moncure clinic also has a laboratory and pharmacy on-site as well as dental offices to provide these services to patients at a reduced cost.

Dr. Gilmer-Scott developed her interest in rural medicine as a medical student in West Virginia. Although she decided to leave West Virginia after graduating from medical school, Dr. Gilmer-Scott did not leave behind her desire to work with underserved populations. For her, family medicine gave her

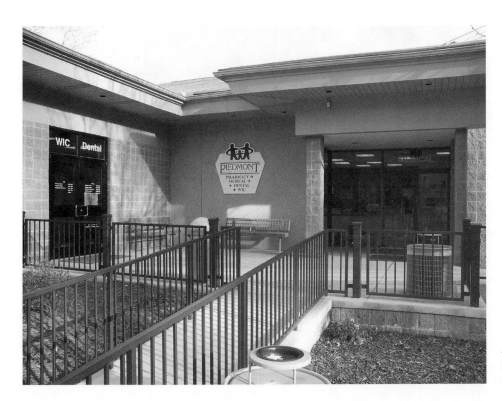

Moncure Community Health Center.

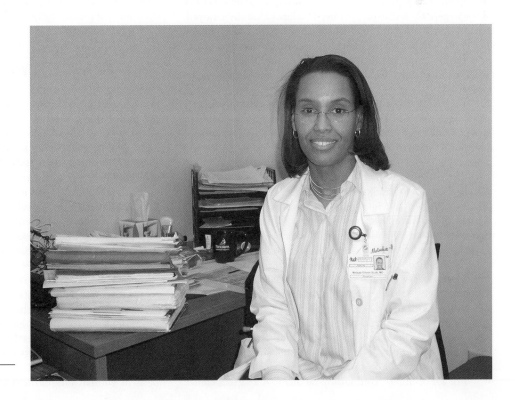

Dr. Melissa Gilmer-Scott

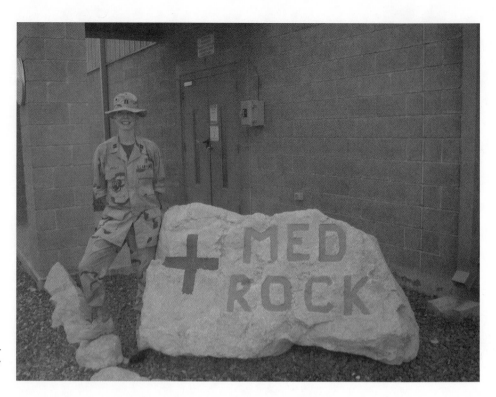

Dr. Jessica Wright, when on duty in Kuwait.

the ability to provide a broad spectrum of care to a patient population that may have nowhere else to go. By treating the whole family, she does not have to rely on the presence of other providers to fill in the gaps.

Despite her passion for working with underserved populations, when it came time to leave residency she faced some tough choices. To preserve her private life, she did not want to both live and practice in a small town. She also did not want to give up two aspects of her residency that she enjoyed, teaching and inpatient medicine. Working for PHS allowed her to do both because of its affiliation with the medical school and residency program. Once every 2 months she spends a week as attending physician on the inpatient service at the university.

Practicing medicine in a resource-poor setting presents challenges that Dr. Gilmer-Scott finds rewarding. "Most of my patients can't afford to get an MRI (magnetic resonance imaging). I have to rely on my ability to do a good history and physical." Even common laboratory tests have to be carefully considered. Because she is a salaried employee, her income is not directly tied to patient receipts; however, like all providers, she is aware of the economics of the practice and her role as a provider and income-generator. In a typical day Dr. Gilmer-Scott sees about 20 patients by 3:00, when she usually heads home to spend time with her husband and their two dogs, Nina and Simeon. One day each week she works a long shift, until 8:00. Every provider has a similar schedule, allowing the clinic to stay open late each evening, and there are also Saturday hours. As an added benefit of not being in private practice, she doesn't have to spend part of her time managing a business, which is a huge benefit for her. "I just want to practice medicine," she admits. The trade-off is that she does not have the earning potential of a private practice doctor.

For Dr. Gilmer-Scott, family medicine is a "great choice if you like to do everything." She confesses, "I get bored easily." But in the clinic "every door is a surprise."

Military Medicine

Because of their broad training and adaptability, family physicians have a major role in providing health services to US military personnel. Fifteen of the nation's 472 family medicine residency training programs are in the armed services, and thousands of practicing family physicians trained in or worked in military settings.

CASE EXAMPLE: JESSICA WRIGHT, CAPTAIN, UNITED STATES AIR FORCE, KUWAIT

Dr. Jessica Wright joined the United States Air Force after her 4th year of medical school. Like many medical students, she had amassed a small fortune in debt, and the Air Force provided immediate relief. But, really, she says, it was the intangibles that drew her to make her commitment. She was single and had not seen nearly as much of the world as she had wanted. Plus, she had always enjoyed meeting new people. "So far the experience has exceeded my expectations," she says.

At the time we interviewed her, she was in Kuwait as part of a 4-month deployment, helping to provide medical care to 3,500 soldiers, private contractors, and international troops on the Air Force base where she was stationed. "My professional responsibilities are in many ways similar to any other acute care doctor," she says. "I examine patients with cold symptoms, put on casts and splints for patients with broken bones, and evaluate chest pain. I can order labs, x-rays, and other basic tests, just like I would back home." Her work week on the base involves 10- to 12-hour shifts, 6 days per week. "One unique aspect of medical care next to a combat zone," she says, "is that I am constantly on the lookout for signs of combat fatigue in soldiers who have come in from

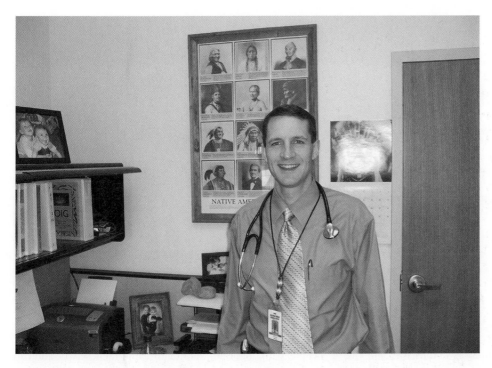

Dr. John Mohs

Iraq. Diagnosing the early signs has become a priority for military doctors."

It was off duty that the contrasts became most apparent. She lived in cinderblock dormitory-style housing. To occupy her spare time, she had access to the base's gym, theater, and library, plus scheduled events such as salsa dancing, boxing matches, or Tae-Kwon-Do lessons (taught by Korean soldiers on the base). She also participated in a unique continuing education activity—a desert survival class.

Before being sent overseas, Dr. Wright had spent the previous 2 years at Langley Air Force Base in Virginia. Other than a more structured system of authority, she did not see much difference between the Langley job and that of her husband, a family physician in private practice. She had a regular panel of patients, often seeing whole families. "It took some time for me to get used to being called ma'am and my patients standing when I entered the exam room," she says.

She likes the fact that, in the military, she does not have to worry about the economic side of medicine. All of her patients have health insurance and get free medications. On the down side, she does not have the autonomy that she would in private practice. Ultimately, however, it is the itinerant military lifestyle that will probably force her out. She will be transferred every 2 to 3 years if she stays in the Air Force, which is difficult to do with a spouse who is not military. Still, Dr. Wright has no regrets about being an Air Force physician. "There's nothing like it. I will remember this experience for the rest of my life," she says.

Public Health Service

The United States Public Health Service is a federal agency that employs many physicians. It has three main branches—the Centers for Disease Control and Prevention, the Indian Health Service (IHS), and the National Institutes of Health. The IHS, whose mission is to provide health care

to 1.8 million American Indians and Alaska Natives, employs the most primary care physicians of the Public Health Service branches and has sites in 35 states. These range from small outpatient clinics to large hospitals providing comprehensive medical services. The legislation that created the IHS was passed in 1921, but the roots of the relationship date back to the 18th century, when Native Americans were promised health care, among other things, by the federal government, in return for land.

CASE EXAMPLE: DR. JOHN MOHS, INDIAN HEALTH SERVICE, SHIPROCK NEW MEXICO

After graduating from the U. S. Naval Academy, Dr. John Mohs entered medical school at the Uniformed Services University of the Health Sciences (USUHS). There he met Kim, who would become his wife. But there was a catch. Kim was in the US Public Health Service's Commissioned Corps, but he was in the Navy, and accepting a position at USUHS obligates you to a term of service in your chosen field. The only way for them to stay together would be for one of them to switch services. So, after an extended application process, John secured a transfer into the Public Health Service.

John and Kim applied for residencies through the couples match—John in family medicine, Kim in internal medicine. After completing their respective training programs, both had a minimum 7-year commitment to the Public Health service. They chose the IHS, because they wanted to work with a traditionally underserved population, and were assigned to the Northern Navajo Medical Center.

The Navajo Nation is the largest Indian tribe in the United States, occupying a reservation the size of West Virginia. To provide medical care to the Navajo people, the IHS staffs 6 hospitals, 7 health centers, and 15 health stations. The Northern Navajo Medical Center is a 55-bed hospital and outpatient clinic. Shiprock, where the Mohs' live and work,

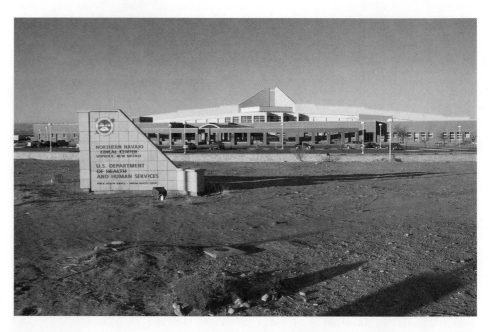

Northern Navajo Medical Center.

is an ideal launching pad for outdoors enthusiasts, and the couple take advantage of as many opportunities as time allows. "Some of the best skiing in the country is within a few hours drive," John says. "Plus, the area is full of bike trails, hiking paths, and great camping, and the desert landscape is strikingly beautiful."

It was the prospect of being able to deliver the full spectrum of family medicine that really attracted Dr. Mohs to Shiprock, however. A typical day often begins in the ICU, where clinical teaching rounds keep all staff current on critical care medicine. Next, Dr. Mohs visits his own hospital patients, usually between one and three persons, and then heads to the office, where he spends the remainder of the day treating chronic and acute conditions. Because his office is adjacent to the hospital, Dr. Mohs can take advantage of breaks in his schedule to review a non-stress test in labor and delivery or check on an unstable new admission.

After 7 years in Shiprock, Dr. Mohs was named chief of staff. He still spends the majority of his time doing clinical work, but he now gets to (or is it has to?) face the economic and administrative aspects of running a hospital. Three of the last four chiefs of staff have been family physicians, and Dr. Mohs does not think this is a coincidence. "Family physicians are used to working with different people and different personalities. We know how to compromise and negotiate," he says. In addition to juggling his responsibilities as a clinician and administrator, Dr. Mohs and his wife have their hands full at home with 4-year-old Emma and 2-year-old Oliver. Raising children in a different culture presents unique challenges in childcare and education.

It is the patients who make working for the IHS a truly unique experience. "Working with a different culture has been the most interesting part of this," Dr. Mohs relates. On the reservation, "You're in the middle of their culture. You have to buy into what they are thinking."

Traditional healing is important to many of the Navajo people, and most of Dr. Mohs' patients use some form of traditional healing. The Navajo are "very appreciative, warm people, who hold onto their culture and their beliefs, and can be pretty skeptical of western medicine," he says. "But after you build up trust, which may be after seven or eight visits, they will buy into what you are doing."

Treating diabetes, which is rampant in the Native American population, is a good example of the give and take between western and traditional medicine. Much of traditional healing for diabetes focuses on returning to the traditional Navajo lifestyle. Dr. Mohs notes, "This often results in increased physical activity and a healthier diet, with fewer high-calorie processed western foods. As a result, patients often lose weight and may not need medicine." Those patients who do need medical treatment, Dr. Mohs can send over to his wife, Kim, who is the chair of internal medicine and the director of the diabetes program. The program provides a comprehensive approach to managing patients at NNMC, nearly half of whom have diabetes.

Although they have fulfilled their 7-year obligation to the IHS, John and Kim Mohs have no plans to leave Shiprock. This is not unusual; many of their colleagues have been there longer than ten years. "I can't imagine any situation that would satisfy me more," Dr. Mohs says, "unless I was a full time woodworker."

Resort Settings

Many resorts are small towns whose populations temporarily swell during tourist season. Physicians in these settings must provide general medical care to the local population and also meet the needs of visitors. Thus, resort practice tends to include a higher proportion of urgent care than most other settings. A family physician who works in a ski resort town, for example, may treat hundreds of fractures in a season, and therefore needs to have particularly well-developed orthopedic skills. Cruise ship doctors, on the other hand, often need significant background in geriatric care. The case example below describes the life of a family physician practicing in a beach community.

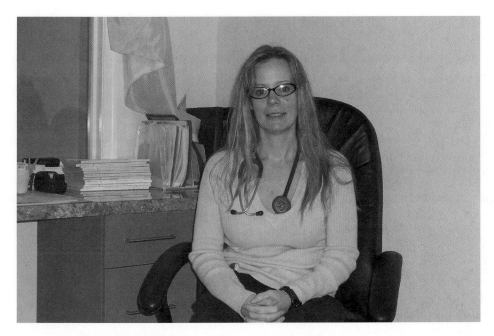

Dr. Shannon Sawin

CASE EXAMPLE: DR. SHANNON SAWIN, NAGS HEAD, NORTH CAROLINA

Dr. Shannon Sawin practices in Nags Head, on North Carolina's Outer Banks, a series of low, narrow islands bordered by the Atlantic Ocean on the east and Albemarle Sound on the west, and connected to the mainland by a long causeway with an arching bridge. The area's population swells more than tenfold in the summer, but during the rest of the year Kill Devil Hills feels surprisingly rural. The closest referral hospital is more than 2 hours away. In winter, the area's restaurants, hotels, and strip malls are largely deserted.

This massive population shift brings a unique seasonal variation to medical practices here. While the winter season is the busiest time in most practices, at Outer Banks Urgent Care (which provides more than just urgent care), these colder days provide an opportunity to catch up with the regulars and take care of any lingering preventive measures.

It was an overcast Monday in February when we visited Dr. Sawin. The previous night had seen a rare dusting of snow, and the dunes were a ghostly, glistening white. But the big news was that school would be delayed 2 hours. Fortunately, her husband, who had a flight to catch, didn't need to leave until noon and could watch the children, who range in age from age 5 to 15. Also, since this was Dr. Sawin's long workday, her in-laws, who live next door, would be available when the children returned from school.

As on most Mondays, Dr. Sawin was scheduled to work from 7:30 AM until 7:30 PM. Her contract specifies that she work 32 hours per week, and on most other days she is out by mid-afternoon. Except when the practice is down a provider, as happened not long before, when Dr. Sawin put in

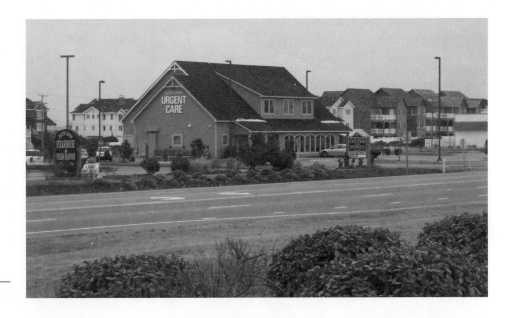

Outer Banks Urgent Care

50-hour weeks. But such is the nature of any small medical practice: you plan for what you want to do, and then do what you need to do.

The patient care area of Outer Banks Urgent Care is divided into two sections. To the right of the central nurse's station is the family medicine side. This is where the scheduled continuity patients are seen. On this particular Monday, Dr. Sawin's schedule is about half-filled with regular patients. When she has a free moment, she moves to the left of the nurse's station— the acute care side, where patients are seen on a first-come, first-served basis—and grabs the next patient's chart.

It is a middle-aged man with atypical chest pain. She completes a brief history and physical, notes that the patient is stable, estimates that his cardiac risk is low to moderate, and orders an electrocardiogram (EKG), chest x-ray, cardiac enzymes, and a complete blood count (CBC). She then returns to the family medicine side to see another continuity patient, emerging later to review the EKG. It is normal. Had there been signs of ischemic damage, however, she would have arranged transfer to the small community hospital nearby. She then rechecks her patient, who is doing well, and digs a little deeper into the past medical, family and social histories.

Medical schools often teach that the history and physical exam should be completed at one time, in a set fashion, but Dr. Sawin's clinic and urgent care setting demands that, at times, multiple patients must be evaluated simultaneously, and priorities be continuously adjusted. Her further history suggests that the illness has a strong respiratory component, and now the chest x-ray comes back showing an early pneumonia. The patient is started on a course of outpatient antibiotics, and a follow-up appointment is arranged.

The summer will bring a sharp increase in patients, and a more frenetic pace. Some of these tourists will be regulars, who have spent many summers at their Outer Banks beach houses. They will come for routine follow up, to have their protimes monitored, their blood pressures checked, and their medications adjusted. More commonly, however, summer visitors will come with acute problems ranging from sunburns to jet ski accidents to fishing boat mishaps. The clinic keeps a collection of fishhooks that have been removed from patients' shoulders, legs, feet, and practically every other body part.

"We see anyone for anything," Dr. Sawin says, describing both her clinic and her specialty. She knew heading into residency that she wanted to return to North Carolina's Outer Banks, where she had grown up, and that a broad knowledge base would be essential. "Often our community has been without a pediatrician," she says. "Rural areas like ours don't have a large enough patient population to support multiple specialists, making family physicians essential."

Multispecialty Health Systems

Multispecialty clinics arose decades ago as a means of integrating the services of many medical specialties under one roof or one administration. Initially, they tended not to involve family physicians, but over time this has changed, as the critical role of primary care in diagnosing and referring patients to specialists has been documented. Increasingly, the large multispecialty clinics have expanded to form health systems in which primary care physicians, and often family physicians,

have had a prominent role, as the following case example illustrates.

CASE EXAMPLE: DR. VANCE BROWN, CLEVELAND CLINIC HEALTH SYSTEM, STRONGSVILLE, OHIO

As medical director of Cleveland Clinic Strongsville, Dr. Vance Brown is responsible for managing 61 physicians, ranging from family medicine to plastic surgery. "Running a clinic of this size is a lot like running a company," he states. "In addition to making sure that the personnel are happy, I have to keep an eye on the bottom line." This means analyzing monthly reports on the clinic's charges and collections, and keeping tabs on the productivity of individual physicians by reviewing their relative value unit production, a standardized measure of productivity used for billing purposes. "Most of the physicians at our clinic are over the 80th percentile nationally for productivity," he states proudly.

He is also proud of the facilities; a new electronic medical record system has just been installed. An advantage to being part of a larger system is that all consults, operative reports, labs, and radiology reports are available instantly to the primary care physician, making coordination much easier. The electronic record also facilitates chronic disease management by tracking critical lab values and medication use. One feature that Dr. Brown is particularly happy with is the capability for patients to access portions of their own record and even update demographic and personal history information.

Dr. Brown first came to the Cleveland Clinic as part of a plan to increase the provision of primary care services. In addition to his role as medical director, he serves as the chair of the Cleveland Clinic's family medicine department. Under his leadership, the family medicine department has grown from 12 physicians to 57, and is still growing.

Despite a heavy administrative load, Dr. Brown continues to spend nearly half his time seeing patients. "After all," he states, "taking care of patients is the reason I got into medicine and what I still enjoy most. Not only that, but staying active is essential to maintaining my clinical skills and remaining connected to the day-to-day workings of the clinic." Serving as both a physician and a manager makes him better at both.

Dr. Brown's path to this position was not a straight one. He began medical school determined to be a basic scientist, but became captivated by clinical medicine. Upon graduation from medical school, he enrolled in and completed a residency in internal medicine at Yale, and subsequently spent 2 years training in emergency medicine at the University of California-Los Angeles (UCLA). He loved the generalism inherent in emergency medicine, the philosophy of treating everything that came through the door. "The problem," Dr. Brown remembers, "was that just when the case was getting interesting, the patient would be admitted or discharged." In addition, he missed the continuity that is central to primary care. Therefore, to round out his training as a generalist, he moved to North Carolina and completed a family medicine residency.

As Dr. Brown is quick to point out, family physicians are at the heart of many multispecialty medical settings, often taking leadership roles. Dr. Brown credits his rapid administrative rise to the skills he learned in family medicine. "At the heart of family medicine training are the skills needed to recognize and handle multiple problems simultaneously,

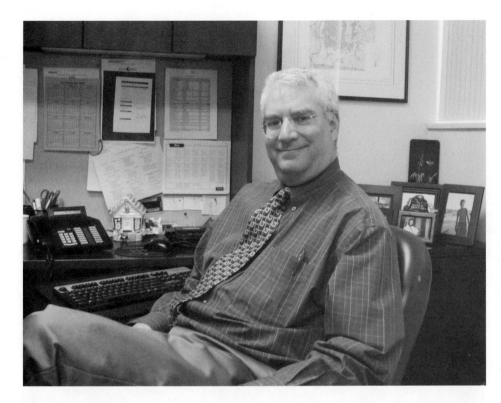

Dr. Vance Brown

while always giving heed to the personal relationship." he states. "That is essential to the leadership of any organization."

Academic Medicine

In 1969, family medicine was officially recognized as the nation's 20th medical specialty. Since then, the number of family medicine departments in medical schools has gradually increased; currently only a few medical schools do not have family medicine programs. Furthermore, because of their generalist nature, family physicians have found themselves called on frequently to teach clinical skills to medical students, and to develop innovations in medical education. The following case example profiles one such academic family physician.

CASE EXAMPLE: DR. SUSAN SKOCHELAK, UNIVERSITY OF WISCONSIN, MADISON WISCONSIN

Dr. Susan Skochelak was training to become a medical technician when, at the urging of one of her supervisory pathologists, she applied to medical school. Soon, she became not just the first generation of her family to graduate from college, but the first to attend medical school.

Pursuing family medicine was not an obvious choice for her. She trained at a large academic center, where much of the teaching was done by specialists, and many of the students chose to specialize. But she was attracted by the breadth of family medicine. She found support in a group of like-minded students who were also committed to primary care, and she still keeps in touch with many of them.

As a resident, she discovered that she had a knack for teaching. Also, as she reflected on her own training, it became increasingly clear to her that she had ideas about how medical education could be improved. This kindled an interest not just in teaching but in becoming involved in medical educa-

tion. She applied to and was accepted to receive fellowship training in the Robert Wood Johnson Clinical Scholars program, a multidisciplinary initiative designed to train future health care leaders. She loved the interdisciplinary give-and-take of the program, and was gratified to see that she could stand toe-to-toe with any other specialist. During her 2 years as a fellow, she also earned a Master's degree in public health and completed a fellowship in preventive medicine.

After completing her fellowship training, Dr. Skochelak jumped at the chance to join the faculty at the University of Wisconsin. Her passion and enthusiasm for teaching enabled her to quickly advance to the director of medical student education for the Department of Family Medicine. Under her leadership, the medical school developed several courses that were innovative at the time, and that are now standard aspects of medical education nationwide. These included a required primary care rotation for the third year and a series of integrated clinical experiences in the first 2 years. Her passion and reputation for innovation has earned Dr. Skochelak both national and international recognition, including several teaching awards and a consultant position in medical education, traveling as far away as Russia.

As her career has advanced, Dr. Skochelak has taken on new roles. "Early on I was very hands-on, designing courses, recruiting faculty, teaching students . . . now I mostly provide administrative support for curriculum development." She currently serves as the senior associate dean of academic affairs, providing support and advice to faculty and staff who are doing many of the same things she did early in her own career. She is also the principal investigator on several grants relating to medical education and health disparities in addition to her numerous administrative duties.

In her current role as an associate dean at the University

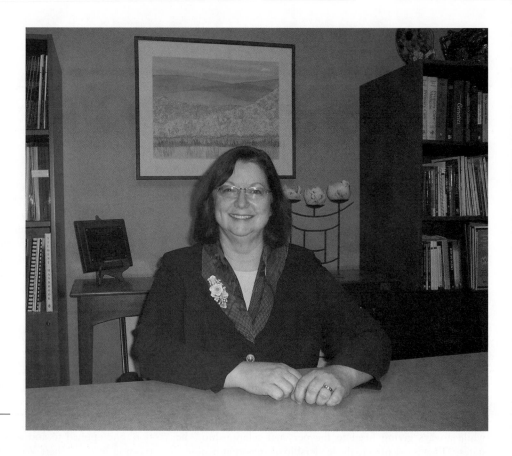

Dr. Susan Skochelak

of Wisconsin School of Medicine, Dr. Skochelak has developed programs that move medical education into community settings, establish interdisciplinary partnerships, and enhance the generalist education. "My background in family medicine helped prepare me to partner with all medical disciplines," Dr. Skochelak says. She also advises medical students, adding emphatically that she avoids trying to push anyone toward any specific career. She does believe, however, that all physicians benefit from getting a solid generalist medical training before specializing.

Although Dr. Skochelak no longer spends as much of her time directly working with medical students, she is proud of the changes she has been able to effect in their education. "I feel lucky," she says, "to have been able to make a career of something I am passionate about."

THE CHANGING HEALTH CARE SYSTEM

It is a time of crisis, change, and challenge for the US health care system. As noted previously, medical costs in the United States are the highest in the world, but outcomes are behind many other countries. Furthermore, rising medical costs are stressing the budgets of individuals, employers, and governments; the proportion of individuals without health insurance is large and growing; and prominent racial and socioeconomic disparities in health outcomes exist. At the same time, other trends are affecting the field. Health care is a business, and the need for good business acumen is critical. Technological advances continue to occur at a rapid pace, as does a generation of new knowledge through research.

Thus, a number of trends characterize today's changing health care system, and these trends will shape the practice of primary care in the future. They are listed in Table 1.4 and are described briefly below:

- **Health care as a business.** Increasingly, health care in the United States, and the physicians' role in providing care, are viewed within a business model. Health care has, of course, always been a business; however, what is different today is that the margin between expenses and receipts is less, and large businesses (e.g., the insurance industry) have more influence (22). This means that health care is being increasingly governed by the "bottom line," and financial issues tend to dominate health care policy. How time is spent needs to be accounted for, and expenses must be weighed against benefits. For example, a family

TABLE 1.4	Key Trends Affecting the Future of the US Health Care System
Health care as a business	
The need to control health care costs	
Tension between high-tech and high-touch	
Patient-directed care	
Evidence-based medicine	
Outcome-oriented reimbursement	
Globalization and outsourcing	
The aging of America	
The need to reduce health disparities	

physician who sets up a private practice must make a myriad of sophisticated business decisions, ranging from what type of medical records to use, to what kind of staff to hire (and how many), and which services to offer.

Unfortunately, the business orientation has eroded what many physicians in the past have seen as an implicit contract between medicine and society—to take care of every person's needs, regardless of ability to pay. A high priority for the future, though at present an apparently long-range one, is for medicine to achieve a better balance between business realities and service to society.

- **Concern about health care expenditures.** The US health care system is the most expensive in the world, and increases in health care expenditures far outpace the rising cost of living. As a result, health insurance is an increasing burden for US employers and for the state and federal governments, who fund Medicare and Medicaid. The challenge is that the primary cause of these rising costs is what consumers value—rapid and widespread use of disease and illness care-related technology, such as thrombolytic therapy, laparoscopic surgery, and MRIs. Another major driver of health care expenditures has been an increase in overhead expenses; administrative costs now account for about one-quarter of US health care expenditures (23). Attempts to control health care expenditures have squeezed many primary care budgets, and cost control issues are likely to continue to dominate the health care world in the future, as other sectors (e.g., education, transportation, defense) will be threatened by continued increases in health care spending.
- **Efforts to improve quality of care, and to make care more evidence-based.** Two reports by the Institute of Medicine crystallized concerns about problems with quality of care, including medical errors (24, 25). The response to these and other concerns about quality has been major efforts to monitor and improve quality, and to make care more consistent with the research evidence. "Guidelines" for care are ubiquitous, and physicians are increasingly expected to adhere to them. Research results are being made accessible to the practitioner (see Box 1.3), and consequently, providers are increasingly expected to be up-to-date.

The combined concerns about cost and quality have led to a drive toward outcome-based reimbursement, in which third-party payers monitor selected health care outcomes and reward providers based on their performance. In primary care office practice, this movement began by addressing "hard," easily measurable outcomes for which considerable evidence existed regarding their impact on health. The prototypical outcome indicator in these "pay-for-performance" systems is the hemoglobin A1c (HbA1c) test; others are rates of delivery of preventive health services (e.g., mammography in women aged 50–75). Many barriers exist to outcome-based reimbursement becoming a major factor in primary care, however, insurers remain quite interested.

- **High-tech versus high-touch.** In today's world, good medical care requires both technology and personal service. Both are high-priced, and they tend to vie for health care dollars. In hospital and nursing home care, for example, pressure ulcers can be prevented by using sophisticated alternating-pressure beds or by having staff turn, reposition, and toilet patients frequently. Similarly, in labor and delivery suites, the fetal heart rate can be monitored by attaching electronic devices to infants' heads or by having staff frequently ascultate the mother's abdomen. The US health care system favors high-tech approaches, whereas many other countries (e.g., Sweden or the Netherlands) are more inclined to use high-touch techniques.

Until now, primary care has been relatively low-tech and high-touch. However, a variety of forces are moving the primary care office into a more high-tech mode. One such technology is the electronic health record (EHR), which can incorporate such quality-improvement measures as built-in prompts for health maintenance, flowsheets for chronic disease management, and automatic evaluation of new prescriptions for drug interactions. While the appeal of EHRs is widespread, their cost-effectiveness in primary care is yet to be demonstrated.

- **Patient-directed care.** During the past several decades, medicine has moved from a paternalistic approach to one that involves shared decision making. Patients are now viewed as partners, and they increasingly want to direct their own care. In part this represents a generational shift, as the baby boomers become major consumers of health care. It also represents the result of increased access to health information, particularly through the Internet. This move toward patient-directed care will probably increase in the future, and health care providers will need to respond accordingly.
- **Globalization and outsourcing.** One of the biggest changes in the US economy in the last 15–20 years has been globalization. Increasingly, businesses and consumers have gone wherever needed to obtain a high-quality product at a low price. As a result, Americans find themselves wearing shoes manufactured in Indonesia; talking to "customer service" representatives in India; driving cars assembled in US plants, with parts manufactured in five or six different countries; and purchasing toys, games, and even American flags that have been manufactured in China.

The health care industry has also begun to feel the impact of globalization, but bigger changes are likely to occur in the coming decades. Already, dictation services, insurance inquiries, and some radiology readings have been outsourced to countries like India. In addition, consumers who must pay out-of-pocket are increasingly going out of the country for expensive elective procedures, such as atrial septal defect repairs and elective plastic surgery, which can cost 80% to 90% less when performed in Thailand, India, or Panama by graduates of US training programs. Given the need to control health care costs, the trend for greater consumer involvement in payment, and the large disparities between physician salaries in the United States compared with much of the rest of the world, it is very likely that costly medical and surgical procedures will be increasingly outsourced to other countries in the coming decades, and, as a result, that opportunities and salaries of many specialists may fall dramatically.

BOX 1-4

Family Physician Leader Profile

David Satcher, MD, PhD: From Rural Poverty to National Leadership

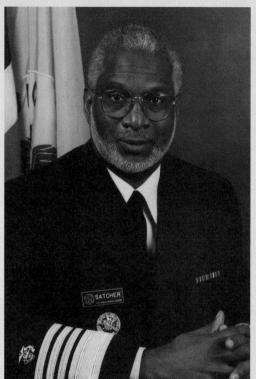

Education, hard work, and a vision of the needs of poor, underserved Americans are the keys to Dr. David Satcher's rise from humble origins to national leadership. He was born and grew up in rural Alabama. Neither of his parents had completed high school, but they taught him the value of hard work and encouraged him to pursue an education. At age 2, he fell dangerously ill with pertussis, and — because treatment at the local hospital was not an option in pre-civil-rights Alabama — his father begged the nearest black physician, Dr. Fred Jackson, to walk several miles on his day off to treat their child. The family credited Dr. Jackson with saving their son's life, and by age 6, David had decided to follow in this rural doctor's footsteps.

Teachers in the local black high school encouraged David, giving him extra assignments and supporting his application to Morehouse College in Atlanta, from which he graduated Phi Beta Kappa. He went on to receive an M.D. and a Ph.D. (in cytogenetics) from Case Western Reserve University in Cleveland, Ohio, to complete family medicine residency training at the UCLA-affiliated Santa Monica program, and to be trained in the prestigious Robert Wood Johnson Clinical Scholars program, which has prepared many physician-leaders over the past decades. After completing his training, Dr. Satcher went on to serve on the faculty of the UCLA School of Medicine, the King-Drew Medical Center, as chairman of the Department of Community Medicine and Family Practice at Morehouse School of Medicine, as president of Meharry Medical College, and as director of the Centers for Disease Control and Prevention.

Dr. Satcher served as Surgeon General of the United States from February 1998 to February 2002. In that position he actively worked to advance public understanding of the needs of poor, minority Americans, including persons with a variety of chronic medical and mental health conditions, and championed the elimination of health disparities in the nation's health care system. Under Dr. Satcher's leadership, the Surgeon General's office issued reports on tobacco use, mental health, suicide prevention, oral health, youth violence, sexual health, overweight/obesity prevention, and several aspects of minority health. In 2001 he received the Jimmy and Rosalynn Carter Award for Humanitarian Contributions to the Health of Humankind from the National Foundation for Infectious Disease.

As of June 2006, Dr. Satcher was serving as interim president of Morehouse University.

- **The aging of America.** In the year 2000, there were 35.1 million persons aged 65 and older in the United States, representing 12.4% of the population. By 2050, 92.7 million seniors are expected to live in the United States, and they will represent 20.7% of the population (26). The aging of the US population will have a far-reaching impact on the practice of medicine, as well as on other aspects of society. As a result, health care providers will increasingly orient their work toward serving the needs of the geriatric population, many of whom are afflicted with multiple health problems, and most of whom are highly interested in prevention, maintenance of function, and involvement in medical care decisions.

- **Increasing racial and ethnic diversity, and the need to reduce health disparities.** Another demographic change that will occur in the United States during the coming decades is an increasing ethnic and racial diversity. The Hispanic population is projected to increase the most—from 12.6% to 24.4% of the US population, but there will also be gains in the African American (from 12.7% to 14.6%) and Asian (from 3.8% to 8.0%) populations, with concomitant reductions in non-Hispanic whites (from 69.4% to 50.1%) (26). Currently, Hispanics and African Americans score lower on many health status indicators than whites, and an important goal (as outlined in *Healthy People 2010*) is for the health care system to work to reduce these disparities (2).

Response of Family Physicians to Changes in the Health Care System

The majority of family physicians view the current health care system as flawed. Within this system, they nonetheless make real, tangible, professionally satisfying contributions to patient and community health. In addition, family physicians play an increasingly prominent role as shapers of health policy and health system change. Box 1.4 provides a profile of one such family physician.

Like all of health care, family medicine and the other

primary care disciplines need to respond to the current and future trends in US health care. Family physicians need to take a careful look at the way they provide services and determine if more effective ways are feasible. Family medicine has been particularly proactive in conceptualizing new, improved ways of health care delivery. Some of these are outlined in the next sections.

THE FUTURE OF FAMILY MEDICINE

At the present time, the primary care system is increasingly perceived as "broken"(27). The issues were highlighted in a report by the Institute of Medicine, which argued persuasively that the quality of American health care falls short of what is needed and possible (24).

In response to these challenges, the leading professional organizations in family medicine conducted a joint study aimed at identifying new directions for the field, with the goal of better addressing the health care needs of the public. Six task forces were organized to address core values, training, delivery system innovation, role communication, health system leadership, and practice finance. They issued a series of reports, which together outline a bold, new direction for family medicine (18, 28–33). As a result, the coming decade promises to be one of excitement and innovation, as these new models are tested and refined.

Innovations in Primary Care Delivery

In addition to adhering to the basic principles of family medicine (see Table 1.2), the new model of family medicine will provide improved access for patients, make increased use of information technology, be increasingly evidence-based, assure a predictable quality of care, and be better oriented toward chronic disease care. The *Future of Family Medicine Report* highlighted a number of innovations that will help implement these changes. All of these innovations have already been implemented in selected sites around the nation; the discipline now is working to determine how best to integrate these innovations into an effective, efficient, financially viable practice model. A unifying concept behind all of these advances is the concept of the health care team; in the new model of practice, practice staff members who share responsibility for patient care are involved in continuously evaluating and improving the practice setting and integrate care across multiple settings, often with community partners. Some of the new trends in care delivery include open access scheduling, outcome-based management of chronic diseases, increased use of non-physician health care providers, EHRs, and nontraditional forms of primary care delivery.

Below we list and briefly describe a few of the innovations in primary care delivery that exist now. Few will be found in the majority of primary care practices today, but all have been implemented and are functioning in multiple sites across the United States (27):

- **Open Access Scheduling**. Open access (also known as advanced access) refers to a way of organizing a practice whereby a patient who calls for an appointment is routinely offered an appointment within a day or two. To first implement open access, a practice often must work extra hours to eliminate the patient backlog, revise sched-

uling templates to keep slots open for same-day appointments, revise telephone protocols, and schedule provider availability to correspond with consumer demand. Open access tends to be associated with reduced wait times for physician services, and with increased patient satisfaction (34).

- **Outcome-based Management of Chronic Diseases.** For many diseases (e.g., asthma, diabetes, and congestive heart failure [CHF]), randomized trials have clearly demonstrated which treatments are most effective and which outcomes are most important to monitor. Many practices have responded by developing ongoing quality improvement programs aimed at improving performance on such outcome indicators as hospitalization rates for CHF or HbA1c levels of diabetics. The most sophisticated programs have included case identification and tracking using disease registries, ongoing monitoring using integrated electronic record systems, prompts and reminders to providers, interdisciplinary care teams, and group visits.

- **Group Visits.** Group visits have emerged as a powerful, enjoyable, cost-effective method of managing certain chronic diseases, such as diabetes, and also for providing prenatal care. The visits are based on the premise that, if much of a visit is educational, it is best done in a group setting of 6–8 patients, because groups give the provider more contact time and provide opportunities for patients to learn from and support each other. The typical group visit program consists of 4–8 visits over several months, with a prearranged curriculum. Each visit includes an hour or more of group time, plus a brief individual consultation with the physician or nurse practitioner.

- **Increased Use of Nurse Practitioners, Physician Assistants, and Office Medical Assistants.** Increasingly, family physicians in community practices are becoming coordinators of health care teams that include other providers, such as nurse practitioners, physician assistants, and/or clinical pharmacists. In addition, to help keep costs down, nurses are being used less frequently in many practices, and instead, cross-trained medical office assistants do much of the everyday patient care support services. This combined team approach keeps costs low while maintaining a high level of quality.

- Electronic Health Records (**EHRs**). Perhaps the most revolutionary development in primary care delivery is the adoption of EHR systems by practices. In 2000, fewer than 10% of practices used EHR systems; by 2005, that figure was between 25% and 30%; and by 2010, 80% or more are likely to use these systems. EHRs will continue to develop and consolidate well into the next decade. However, the direction of movement is clear—toward a national record system (or series of systems), communicating seamlessly across settings (e.g., nursing home, office, hospital), and providing instant access to clinically-useful information, such as practice guidelines, standardized order sets, evidence summaries, disease tracking, prevention reminders, and drug interaction data.

- **Electronic Communication with Patients.** With more and more people having email access, physicians are increasingly communicating with patients via secure email sites. Using email can save time and patient visits; it can also help facilitate closer monitoring, for example, of day-to-day adjustments in an insulin regimen. Patients are also beginning to have access to on-line scheduling so they can pick the time that is most convenient for them rather than that which is most conveniently offered by a receptionist.

- **Low-overhead Practices, Cash-only.** Today's commercial insurance plans tend to require patients to pay much of their health care costs as deductibles; furthermore, the cost to practices of doing insurance paperwork is high. As a result, low-overhead, cash-only practices have been developed that cost the typical patient little or no more than if they billed the insurance company. Patients pay at the time of service, are given a receipt, and—if they have coverage—bill their own insurer.
- **Home Care Practices.** Another nontraditional, low-overhead form of practice is the home care practice. In these practices, one or more physicians work out of a car or van, supported by a lean infrastructure of staff, who schedule visits, phone patients for follow-up, and manage administrative paperwork. Often, home care practices are partly subsidized by one or more hospitals, because they reduce visits to the emergency department. As one home care physician wrote, "Two years ago I traded my salaried position in a traditional practice—with an office, exam rooms, not to mention a regular paycheck—for a cash-only, house-call practice that relies mostly on a car, a doctor's bag, charts, a simple fee structure and cash, which I collect at the time of service. I'm earning less per year than I did in salaried practice (because I work fewer hours now) but my hourly income is much higher— about $150 to $200 before expenses. My overhead was as high as 30% during my start-up year, but it continues to decline . . . I can deliver high-quality medical care to patients in comfort and privacy at a reasonable cost to them and with a reasonable income for me"(35).

What Will Family Medicine Look Like in 20 Years?

Any prognostication about the future of medical practice is speculation. Still, one cannot help wondering what the family medicine will look like in, say, 20 years. As was illustrated in the profiles presented earlier in this chapter, the specialty already offers a tremendous variety of practice situations and lifestyles to graduates of residency training programs. In the future, it is possible that opportunities will broaden further; for example, through the development of more part-time and job-sharing arrangements for dual-career physicians. Also, the trend toward nontraditional forms of primary care delivery—such as cash-only, home care, school-based, or workplace-based practice settings—may continue to grow. In response to America's increasing ethnic diversity, alternative practice models are likely to burgeon, integrating traditional ethnic values with modern health care principles. Many other changes are possible, such as consolidation of primary care practices into large organizations with greater bargaining power vis-à-vis insurers and hospitals (27, 36).

A key role for new family physicians in the next few years will be to further develop the new approaches to primary care that are already being pioneered. By integrating the core values of the patient-centered healer with the enabling infor-mation technologies of today, such models of care could form the basis for development of the sustainable, equitable, and effective health care system that the country is demanding.

The big, unanswered question is whether a transformational change in health care will occur, such as development of a national health care system. While such a development seems remote at this time, it is hard to imagine any change that will not continue the current focus on controlling health care expenditures, give increased attention to disease prevention, or include a prominent role for a personal physician. Given the data supporting the effectiveness and cost-effectiveness of primary care systems that include generalists with broad training, the future of family medicine appears bright indeed.

CASE DISCUSSION

The case of the Tenney family (presented at the beginning of this chapter) illustrates how psychosocial, environmental, and biomedical factors interact, and how understanding all of them is essential to making an accurate diagnosis and implementing effective treatment. Epidemiologically, because of his occupation, Mr. Tenney is at risk for alcoholism; the recurrent abdominal pain and the history of self-medication with cough syrup increase the likelihood that alcohol is a significant problem for him. Given that history, and his chronic cough, inquiry about his smoking history would also be important. Mrs. Tenney's symptoms are highly suggestive of fibromyalgia, a common musculoskeletal disease that invariably requires psychosocial, biomedical, and environmental approaches to effectively treat. Furthermore, her history is highly suggestive of type 2 diabetes, the diagnosis and treatment of which are likely to have been delayed by her lack of health insurance. Both fibromyalgia and type 2 diabetes are linked to obesity, so while we have not been given Mrs. Tenney's weight, we would be suspicious of obesity on an epidemiological basis. Jason receives adequate preventive care but does not receive ongoing primary care for his asthma, and since access to continuity of care is associated with better asthma control, lack of access to comprehensive primary care services is likely to be contributing to his asthma morbidity. Thus, improved access to quality primary health care, for example, by becoming regular patients at a community health center, would reduce long-term morbidity for this family.

REFERENCES

1. US Census Bureau Population Division, International Data Base. 2006.
2. US Department of Health and Human Services, Healthy People 2010. Conference Edition ed. 2000, Washington, DC: US Department of Health and Human Services.
3. White KL, Williams TF, Greenberg BG. The ecology of medical care. N Engl J Med. 1961; 265:885–892.
4. Green LA, et al. The ecology of medical care revisited. N Engl J Med. 2001;344(26): 2021–2025.
5. Donaldson MS, et al., Primary care: American's health in a new era. Washington, DC: National Academy Press: 1996.
6. Stange KC, et al. The value of a family physician. J Fam Pract. 1998;46(5):363–368.
7. Starfield B, Shi L, Macinko J. Contribution of primary care to health systems and health. Milbank Q. 2005;83(3):457–502.

8. Shi L, et al. The relationship between primary care, income inequality, and mortality in US States., 1980–1995. J Am Board Fam Pract. 2003;16(5):412–422.

9. Burstin H, Clancy C. Nontraditional approaches to primary care delivery. In: J. Showstack J, Rothman AA, Hassmiller SB, eds. The Future of Primary Care. San Francisco, CA: Jossey-Bass; 2004:89–108.

10. Stange KC, Miller WL, McWhinney I. Developing the knowledge base of family practice. Fam Med. 2001;33(4): 286–297.

11. Stange KC. The paradox of the parts and the whole in understanding and improving general practice. Int J Quality Health Care. 2002;14(4):267–268.

12. Green LA, Hickner J. A short history of primary care practice-based research networks: from concept to essential research laboratories. J Am Board Fam Med. 2006;19(1):1–10.

13. Maslow AH. Toward a Psychology of Being, 3rd ed. New York: John Wiley and Sons; 1999.

14. Medalie JH, Zyzanski SJ, Langa DM, Stange KC. The family in family practice: is it a reality? Results of a multi-faceted study. J Fam Pract. 1998;46(5):390–396.

15. Medalie JH, Zyzanski SJ, Goodwin MA, Stange KC. Two physician styles of focusing on the family: their relationship to patient outcomes and process of care. J Fam Pract. 2000; 49:209–215.

16. Shahady, E. Principles of family medicine: an overview. In: Sloane P, Slatt L, Curtis P, eds. Essentials of Family Medicine, 2nd ed. Baltimore, MD: Williams & Wilkins; 1993:3–8.

17. Graduate medical education. JAMA, 2005. 294(9):1129–1143.

18. Green LA, et al. Task force 1. Report of the task force on patient expectations, core values, reintegration, and the new model of family medicine. Ann Fam Med. 2004;2(Suppl 1): S33–50.

19. National Association of Community Health Centers. Available at *http://www.nachc.com*. Accessed April 25, 2006.

20. Bureau of Primary Health Care. Available at http://bphc.hrsa.gov/chc/pi.htm. Accessed April 25, 2006.

21. Hadley J, Cunningham P. Availability of safety net providers and access to care of uninsured persons. Health Serv Res. 2004;39(5):1527–1546.

22. Bodenheimer T. High and rising health care costs. Part 3: the role of health care providers. Ann Intern Med. 2005; 142(12 Pt 1):996–1002.

23. Bodenheimer T. High and rising health care costs. Part 2: technologic innovation. Ann Intern Med. 2005;142(11): 932–937.

24. Institute of Medicine. Crossing the quality chasm: a new health system for the twenty-first century. Washington, DC: National Academy Press; 2001.

25. Kohn LT, Corrigan JM, Donaldson MS, eds. To err is human: building a safer health system. Washington, DC: National Academy Press; 2000.

26. US Census Bureau. US interim projections by age, sex, race, and Hispanic origin. 2004. Available at: *http://www.census.gov/ipc/www/usinterimproj*. Accessed on May 6, 2006.

27. Newton WP, DuBard CA, Wroth TH. New developments in primary care practice. N C Med J. 2005;66(3):194–204.

28. Bucholtz JR, et al. Task force report 2. Report of the task force on medical education. Ann Fam Med. 2004;2(Suppl 1): S51–64.

29. Jones WA, et al. Task force report 3. Report of the task force on continuous personal, professional, and practice development in family medicine. Ann Fam Med. 2004;2(Suppl 1): S65–74.

30. Dickinson JC, et al. Task force report 4. Report of the task force on marketing and communications. Ann Fam Med. 2004;2(Suppl 1):S75–87.

31. Roberts RG, Snape PS, Burke K. Task force report 5. Report of the task force on family medicine's role in shaping the future health care delivery system. Ann Fam Med. 2004; 2(Suppl 1):S88–99.

32. Spann SJ. Task force report 6. Report on financing the new model of family medicine. Ann Fam Med. 2004;2(Suppl 1): S1–21.

33. Martin JC, et al. The future of family medicine: a collaborative project of the family medicine community. Ann Fam Med. 2004;2(Suppl 1):S3–32.

34. Parente DH, Pinto MB, Barber JC. A pre-post comparison of service operational efficiency and patient satisfaction under open access scheduling. Health Care Management Review. 2005;30(3):220–228.

35. Brand AL. Cashing in on house calls. Family Practice Management 2006; February: 67–68.

36. Peckham S. Primary care purchasing. Are integrated primary care provider/purchasers the way forward? Pharmacoeconomics. 1999;15(3):209–216.

37. Centers for Disease Control and Prevention. Immunization schedules. Available at: *http://www.cdc.gov/nip/recs*. Accessed April 27, 2006.

38. Cabana MD, Jee SH. Does continuity of care improve patient outcomes? J Fam Pract. 2004;53(12):974–980.

39. Franks P, Fiscella K. Primary care physicians and specialists as personal physicians. Health care expenditures and mortality experience. J Fam Pract. 1998;47(2):105–109.

40. Saultz JW, Albedaiwi W. Interpersonal continuity of care and patient satisfaction: a critical review. Ann Fam Med. 2004;2(5):445–451.

41. Greenleaf RK. Servant Leadership: A Journey into the Nature of Legitimate Power and Greatness. New York: Paulist Press; 1977.

42. Baicker K, Chandra A. The physician workforce and beneficiaries' quality of care. In: Iglehart JK, ed. Health Affairs—Web Exclusives. Bethesda, MD: Project HOPE; 2004: 184–197.

CHAPTER 2

The Challenging Patient Encounter

Samuel E. Romano and Thomas L. Schwenk

CASE

A 3rd-year medical student is asked to gather initial information and a general history from a 47-year-old woman. The student notices that her chief complaint is listed as "lump in left breast." As he enters the examination room, the woman sharply states, "I have been waiting 45 minutes.... This is unacceptable.... I took time from my work and I have to get back." The student is taken aback, but attempts to engage her and appropriately acknowledges being delayed. He begins to question her about her concerns, and her answers are curt and unhelpful. The patient alternately looks at her watch and the door, and rarely looks at the student. He becomes increasingly annoyed with her, and his remarks reflect this. The woman interrupts him and says, "Look, I don't have time for this.... If the doctor cannot see me now, I need to leave. Go get her, please." Angry now, the student leaves, finds his preceptor, and explains that the patient is upset, rude, and resistant.

CLINICAL QUESTIONS

1. What are your objectives for this encounter?
2. What were the patient's (hypothesized) objectives?
3. What strategies can help you manage this patient and other patients with whom you may have a difficult relationship?

The challenging patient encounter is neither a medical nor a psychiatric diagnosis; rather it is a disruption or potential breakdown of the usual positive and satisfying interaction between patient and physician. The challenging patient encounter can best be thought of as a syndrome of the physician-patient relationship with certain clinical or descriptive features. Although a few patients may present a challenge to all or most physicians, most patients labeled by one physician as challenging can be cared for quite effectively and often more easily by another physician. This is because both the patient and the physician bring behaviors and attitudes to the encounter that can lead to either successful and satisfying or frustrating and unproductive relationships and encounters. This chapter provides a brief review of the nature of this relationship, and the medical, psychosocial, attitudinal, behavioral, and physician correlates and predictors of this relationship.

KEY CONCEPTS FROM THE RESEARCH LITERATURE

Although there is little data-based research on this relationship, and most writing is anecdotal in nature, a few clinical studies provide some guidance regarding effective approaches to improving the outcomes of the challenging encounter. We will use this background to structure a case-based discussion of the common types of challenging relationships encountered by physicians, providing specific guidance to help you recognize and manage these situations as they arise. Existing studies can be organized using a few key principles that guide clinical practice in this important area (see Table 2.1).

Difficult Relationships Are Common

Difficult physician-patient relationships account for a substantial minority of all physician-patient contacts. They are sufficiently common and troubling to both physician and patient, however, as to deserve significant attention by physicians (1, 2). One primary care study of 627 consecutive patients found that 96 patients (15%) were rated by their physicians as difficult. These patients were significantly more likely than nondifficult patients to have a psychiatric disorder, in particular somatoform disorder, panic disorder, dysthymia, generalized anxiety, major depressive disorder, or alcohol abuse. Difficult patients had more functional impairment and greater health care use, without any difference in demographic characteristics or physical illnesses compared with nondifficult patients, and experienced lower satisfaction with care (3).

Difficult Relationships, Not Difficult Patients

There is no such entity as a difficult patient, only difficult relationships; therefore, physicians need to examine their own attitudes, beliefs, expectations, and behavior to determine how they might be contributing to such a relationship. This is supported by a study of "difficult" patients, which found that physicians with poorer attitudes and beliefs about the importance of psychosocial issues in medical care rated a far higher proportion of patient encounters as difficult than did physicians with more positive attitudes (4). Because the difficult physician-patient relationship may cause feelings of frustration, dysphoria, and anger on the part of the physician, physicians often blame patients for the problem or label them in pejorative ways (5). Early writings on the difficult patient used terms such as "hateful" (6) and discussed the use of names such as "crock" and "gomer."

interview, recognizing as she did so that this may not please the patient, and that the patient may continually try to revert to her agenda. The interview should not be looked at as a win-or-lose situation. Both the student and the patient need to accomplish their goals; it is the student's role to do so directly and in the process to consider the following truths: attentive listening is providing care; the patient's style would be a challenge for anyone working with her, including the preceptor; it is good to choose one presenting problem, gather what you can about it, then move on to the next; and frustration and anger, although understandable, can interfere with a satisfactory experience and waste your energy. Lastly, the student needs to accept that she may not be able to prepare and present to her preceptor in an ideal way. She should explain her difficulties with the interaction and ask the preceptor to suggest ways she could learn to improve her management style.

The Patient Seeking Pain Relief
CLINICAL VIGNETTE

A 42-year-old woman presents to an outpatient medical clinic with chronic right flank pain. The woman's assigned physician asks the fourth-year medical student he is working with to evaluate her. The student introduces herself and is struck by the woman's seeming agony and by her husband's agitated concern. The patient has a history of pyelonephritis and states that this pain is very similar. Her husband, a "big, burly, biker kind of guy," tells the student that she has to have Vicodin because it is the only medication that has helped her in the past. The patient tells the student that she saw her gynecologist earlier in the week, and he had given her only enough pain medication to last until today's appointment. The student expressed her concerns and offered empathy, with a reassurance that the physician would likely provide the Vicodin. On presenting the case, her preceptor suggested they check the computer for the report on the visit to the gynecologist. The report indicated that the patient had been seen 2 days previously and had been given a prescription for 30 Vicodin tablets. The student was surprised and then angry at what she felt was manipulative behavior on the part of the patient and her husband. The student expressed anxiety about having to tell the patient and her husband what they had learned. The preceptor confronted the patient while the student observed. The patient and her husband expressed denial and anger and left abruptly, with the patient stating that "no one cares."

MANAGING CHALLENGING PATIENT REQUESTS

The student involved in this case was initially influenced in her responses by the patient and her husband's apparent distress. She believed the woman's story and wanted to offer relief and reassurance. The student acknowledged that she was somewhat intimidated by the patient's husband, and that this response was both surprising and discomforting. The student had not entertained the possibility that the patient could be deceiving her, so when she read the gynecologist's note, she was shocked, then embarrassed. She then felt herself becoming angry. These reactions, coupled with her feelings about the patient's husband, contributed to her anxiety and wish to avoid confronting the patient. She was quite relieved that her preceptor was willing to deal with the situation, but the poignancy

of the patient's final comment caused the student to wonder whether she and the preceptor were prematurely judging her.

There are several possible scenarios that can be hypothesized for the patient's objectives in seeking medical care. In the first case, the patient was powerfully motivated by her pain to seek understanding, compassion, and, primarily, relief. She may have been fearful that she would not be believed and would be denied the medication that has helped her. This could have affected her decision to report information that was not accurate. Her husband's presence would have been to provide personal support, as well as to confirm the veracity of her report. When confronted by the preceptor, her feelings of shame and embarrassment could have led to her denial and decision to abruptly leave. In the second possible situation, the patient chose to present her story with both exaggeration and deception in order to obtain the opioid analgesic. It is important to recognize that in this scenario, the patient was again powerfully motivated by pain but also by addiction, and may not have understood the differences in the treatment of acute versus chronic pain. The presence of her husband could have, again, been to provide confirmation and personal support. Another possibility is that the patient and/or her husband were attempting to obtain the medication in order to sell it for a profit, or possibly for the use of the husband, who was addicted. In each of these scenarios, it is likely that the patient tried to engage the student as an ally in an effort to influence the preceptor's response. This could have accounted for, in part, the strength of the student's response when she learned that she had been deceived.

The major strategies that the student and health care provider could use to more effectively intervene in this and similar situations are listed in Table 2.3. Appropriate responses would be to offer empathy and understanding (e.g., "You certainly seem to be in a lot of pain; I understand how you would want the medication that has previously helped you."), and assurance that the treatment warranted by examination and review of the patient would be provided (e.g., "Our goal is to carefully evaluate you and decide with you what treatment would be most appropriate and helpful.").

Although it is always important to approach patients with open and honest acceptance of their problems and concerns, it is wise to learn that patients can distort things for their own gain. This does not make them bad patients, merely patients struggling with problems over which they have lost control. Another significant factor to acknowledge is the power of

---

TABLE 2.3 Key Strategies for Managing the Patient Seeking Pain Relief

- Acknowledge that patients can be deceptive.
- Understand the power of certain motivating factors, such as pain, addiction, greed, or coercion.
- Learn how and when to confront.
- Pay attention to uncomfortable feelings you may have.
- Be willing to risk losing a patient if the relationship cannot be salvaged.
- Adhere to professional standards without being unnecessarily rigid.

certain motivations. Chronic pain and addiction to medications are powerful factors that can affect the choices patients make, and how they present to you. You need to acquire and maintain empathy while you avoid getting caught in their dramas. Experience and consultation with experienced colleagues can help achieve this balance.

The art of appropriate and well-timed confrontation is an essential skill in patient encounters. It is almost always an unpleasant experience; therefore, many clinicians will try to avoid this type of exchange. Effective confrontation requires the physician to 1) deal directly and specifically with the conflict or ambiguity issue; 2) avoid accusations to reduce patient defensiveness; 3) use empathy; 4) set clear limits for what will and will not be tolerated in the medical relationship; and 5) on occasion, be willing to be wrong. It is also important to assess the potential or perceived risk that confrontation might evoke; some patients could react strongly and threateningly to confrontation. Physicians need to take this into account before proceeding, and possibly institute safety measures (e.g., be between the patient and the door; have a staff member in or outside the room).

One of the best predictors of a challenging encounter can be your own emotional reaction. It is important to identify your feelings whether they are suspicion, distrust, sympathy, or guilt. Our emotional responses may lead us to think and judge patients and patients' families in certain biased and premature ways. It can be therapeutically effective to voice our feelings to patients, for example, "I am feeling uncomfortable about what you are requesting," provided that we are willing to listen to and deal with our patients' responses.

A final strategy to consider in this case is the willingness to risk losing a patient. Patients will make many requests of physicians that may or may not be legitimate. Physicians need to assess all sources of information available to them, then respond within the structure of their personal and professional ethics. If you are denying a patient's request, you need to be prepared for an angry and/or hurt response, which may include the patient choosing to leave your practice. You need to believe that you have acted in your and the patient's best interests, but the patient may not be happy with the denial of the request and with the alternative options you offer. It is never easy when a patient chooses to leave.

The Reticent Patient
CLINICAL VIGNETTE

A 26-year-old man presents to his primary care physician's office with a 5-day history of nausea, vomiting, diarrhea, and chills. The attending physician asks his student to evaluate the patient with particular concern about dehydration and the possibility of admission for fluids. As the student prepares to go into the patient's room, his preceptor tells him, "I think he's gay, so you'd better talk with him about hepatitis and HIV testing."

The student greets the patient, who looks tired, sick, and distressed, and attempts to engage with him, and gather a history. The patient offers only "yes," "no," or "I don't know" in response to the student's questions. The student begins to feel frustrated with the patient's lack of detail in his responses and asks the patient what he thinks is going on with him. The patient's response to this is, "You're the doctor, you tell

me," which frustrates and annoys the student even more. The student is aware of avoiding questions about hepatitis and HIV risk. When he tells the patient that they need to consider hospitalization because of the dehydration, the patient states that he would like his fiancée, who is sitting in the waiting room, to join the discussion. The student is startled by this request, but agrees to let the preceptor know of the patient's wish. After presenting his findings to the preceptor, the student and preceptor invite the patient's fiancée into the room with the patient, and the decision is made to admit the patient.

MANAGING RETICENCE AND MISCOMMUNICATION

The student involved in this case had one very clear objective on entering the room; this was to complete a thorough history and examination and determine whether the patient should be hospitalized. He did not initially feel as if his questioning was affected by the preceptor's comment about the patient's sexuality. It was only during the interview, as the student found the patient reticent or withholding, that he began to think in a biased manner of the patient. The student felt frustrated, then angry with the patient, and these feelings led him to think critically about the patient and to avoid "bringing things up" related to the patient's potential risks. Therefore, the two issues that caused the student to view this case as challenging were the patient's verbal style, which the student perceived as both resistant and defiant, and the student's biased ways of thinking and responding to the patient.

It seems evident that the patient's primary objective was to obtain medical care and relief for his illness. His verbal style may reflect a general manner of relating to health care providers, or more likely, how badly he was feeling. He would have been unaware of the preceptor's comment to the student and how that may have altered the dynamics of the interview. His desire to include his fiancée in the decision making about his treatment seems understandable and warranted.

This case provides a good example of the conflict and dissatisfaction that can ensue when the objectives of both the physician and the patient are not met in a timely or comfortable manner. It also illustrates the importance of recognizing and monitoring potential biases. The strategies listed in Table 2.4 can help students and health care providers avoid these limiting and stigmatizing responses.

It is difficult, if not impossible, to determine in an initial meeting whether a patient's reticent style of responding is a

---

TABLE 2.4 Key Strategies for Management of the Reticent Patient

- Try to understand why a patient is being unresponsive.
- Be patient.
- Understand the power of empathy, and use it frequently.
- Know yourself well, and acknowledge the biases you hold.
- Be prepared to handle your responses to unexpected outcomes.

characteristic or is situational. It is, therefore, important to form a set of hypotheses to help you understand and effectively manage such a style. Illness can strongly affect a patient's ability and willingness to respond. Similarly, the anxiety of being in a medical setting or the fear of having a serious illness can alter a patient's responses. Additional issues that can affect responses include a depressive disorder, hearing impairment, and cultural or language barriers. An important strategy that could benefit any patient encounter, not just challenging ones, is the use of patience. Many newer medical interviewers will want to obtain the information they need quickly, and will view a patient who fails to respond in full detail as uncooperative. When this occurs, a physician may experience the resulting relationship as a failure, and subconsciously blame the patient.

An essential skill to learn is the ability to coach the patient to be your ally in his/her care. A phrase such as "Help me to understand what is going on with you" can be useful. Also remember that certain behaviors will change best when a secure and trusting relationship is established, and when a patient's basic needs and comfort are addressed. In all manner of human interaction, the quality of the relationship can be enhanced by the sincere and selective use of empathy. Phrases that communicate to patients that you do understand how they might be feeling, and that validate their responses, can help in many challenging encounters. Patients will be more cooperative and responsive, even while sick and in pain, when they experience the student/physician as offering caring and empathic comments (e.g., "This must be a difficult time for you." "You seem very quiet.") and attending to their comfort ("Do you need a blanket?", "Would you feel better with your head up?").

Everyone holds certain biasing responses based on our values, beliefs, culture, religion, and ethnicity, and these biases can creep into an encounter and undermine it. It is imperative in medical settings that these biases do not negatively affect our relationships with patients. Becoming frustrated, annoyed, and/or angry with patients can be a clue that one of our values or beliefs has been challenged. You must be able to recognize these triggers and to separate their influence from your responses to the patient. If your beliefs are so strong that you feel incapable of altering a biasing response, you need to transfer care of the patient to a different provider.

A final strategy from this case relates to our responses to unexpected information or outcomes. Even with the most comprehensive information we can have on a patient, there will be occasions in which new information arises and catches us off guard. In such situations, we need to be able to adjust our responses so that our surprise does not register too strongly. When it becomes apparent that the patient is aware of our response, we need to offer an apology and reasonable explanation (e.g., "I didn't mean to react so strongly, I was not aware of _____. Tell me more about this.").

GENERAL MANAGEMENT STRATEGIES

The first step in managing challenging relationships with patients is to learn to trust your negative feelings as indications that a relationship with a patient is becoming difficult. When

TABLE 2.5	A General Approach to Managing Challenging Encounters

- Define what your objectives were for the encounter (i.e., what did you hope would be achieved).
- Hypothesize what your patient's objectives were for the encounter (i.e., what was he or she seeking to accomplish).
- Identify the assumptions or expectations you brought to the interaction (i.e., what did you assume would occur).
- Attempt to define the expectations the patient may have brought to the encounter (i.e., what did he or she expect to, as opposed to hope would, happen).
- Look for the incongruities between the patient's objectives and assumptions and your own.
- Evaluate your use of communication and relationship-building skills within the encounter (i.e., engagement strategies, active listening, summarization, empathy, reflection).

this occurs, we encourage you to apply the model, presented in Table 2.5, which we used in discussing the case examples. The number of incongruities identified, and the breadth of disparity between the physician's and patient's expectations and assumptions, can help the health care provider determine the existence and severity of a challenging encounter. This awareness can guide you as you institute a treatment plan.

It is critical to note that any treatment plan or management strategy will be affected by the quality of the physician-patient relationship. You are likely to feel most comfortable incorporating these strategies when you have an established relationship with the patient. Similarly, a patient will likely be most open to hearing and responding to your attempts to alter or redirect their interaction when a caring and committed relationship exists.

Although a difficult relationship may continue to have frustrating features, it can be managed to the satisfaction of both the physician and the patient. Appropriate management goals are described in Table 2.6. These goals suggest five general management strategies.

Strategy 1: Clarify Your Professional Feelings About the Patient

In all medical care encounters, it is essential for the physician to be aware of the extent to which personal values and beliefs may be affecting responses to the patient. Being honest about one's feelings toward the patient is critical. When you feel angry, depressed, frustrated, or anxious, you should ask yourself several important questions: What does the patient do to elicit these feelings? What need does the patient have to behave this way? What is there about your motivations, values, personal history, stresses, or behaviors that may be contributing to this unproductive interaction? Consultation with colleagues and/or behavioral scientists can be very helpful in this process.

TABLE 2.6 Management Goals for the Challenging Encounter
• Minimize inappropriate "medicalization" through judicious use of diagnostic tests, therapeutic procedures, hospitalization, and referral, with greater effort to uncover depression and other psychiatric illnesses.   • Maintain physician-patient continuity to the greatest extent possible.   • Maintain professional self-esteem through the maximal use of productive and constructive physician behaviors and support.   • Focus on the more satisfying and productive aspects of the patient's personality and behavior.   • Recognize that the relationship will probably always be less satisfying than desired, but can still be productive for both physician and patient.

TABLE 2.7 Reassurance Therapy: One Model for Interacting with Challenging Patients (19)
1. Obtain a detailed description of the patient's symptoms. Ask the patient to bring in a list of concerns, and focus on the three most important symptoms at each visit.   2. Elicit the emotional meaning or content of the symptoms, such as realistic fears, irrational phobias, connections to illnesses in friends or relatives, anxiety from incomplete understanding, and anniversary reactions.   3. Perform an appropriately thorough physical examination, selectively repeating only limited portions of the examination in future visits.   4. Make a specific diagnosis, which will often include biomedical and/or psychosocial explanations.   5. Connect the symptoms to the diagnosis, and explain the particular meaning the symptoms may have to the patient.   6. Conclude with expressions of reassurance and support.

Strategy 2: Use Precise and Effective Communication

Studies have demonstrated that better physician training in the psychosocial dimensions of patient care can lead to clinical improvement in the functional outcomes of patients (5, 18). Effective strategies include:

- Requesting feedback from patients and colleagues about ways to improve communication skills
- Removing barriers to communication by understanding and adapting to the patient's communication style
- Involving family members
- Using an interpreter
- Providing for a longer initial visit to allow patients with a less direct conversational style to tell their stories
- Scheduling more frequent visits

Reassurance therapy is one model of physician-patient communication that can be used to improve interactions with challenging patients. Effective reassurance therapy involves the six steps listed in Table 2.7 (19).

Strategy 3: Have a High Index of Suspicion for Undiagnosed Psychiatric Illness

A large number of patients have undiagnosed psychiatric illness, and the lack of an accurate diagnosis frequently contributes to the development of a difficult physician-patient relationship (3, 11). The most common psychiatric diagnostic categories that can affect the physician-patient encounter are depression, substance abuse, anxiety, and personality disorders.

Strategy 4: Set Appropriate Limits and Mobilize Useful Support Systems

It is sometimes difficult for physicians to acknowledge their personal and professional limits. Within the challenging encounter, setting limits is critical. The physician must know how much he or she can give, how much time and energy can be devoted to a particular patient, and how much control the physician is comfortable relinquishing. Consultation with colleagues can be very useful, especially presenting and discussing patients the physician experiences as challenging.

Strategy 5: Hang in There

If you are "put off" by the patient, chances are that others are too, and that the patient feels isolated and alone. In such situations, the physician who continues to be engaged with the patient, providing continuity of care and continued compassion and interest, will often, over time, develop a strong trusting relationship, and the grateful patient will often become less of a "problem" as time passes. Again, it is important to keep your goals limited, but small successes over time will often lead to larger ones. Indeed, developing an effective alliance with a challenging patient is family medicine practice at its best.

CASE DISCUSSION

The student hoped that he would be able to easily engage with the patient so that he could address her concerns and gather the information he needed. He was aware that his preceptor was running behind, but because this was often the case, he did not anticipate the strength of the patient's response. Because he had appropriately apologized, he thought they could simply proceed with the interview. As he experienced her growing impatience and distraction, he became annoyed, and then angry. The anger caused him to see her as rude and resistant, which is how he presented her to the preceptor.

The patient appeared to have two major needs to be addressed in this encounter. The first was to be seen in a timely manner, because she was taking time away from work and needed to return. The second and more significant need was to have her anxiety assuaged. It is extremely important to recognize that she had discovered a problem (i.e., a lump in her breast) that worried and potentially scared her. This realistic anxiety may have affected her response to the delay, and to the student's role in trying to interview her.

REFERENCES

1. Haas LJ, Leiser JP, Magill MK, Sanyer ON. Management of the difficult patient. Am Fam Physician. 2005;72:2063–2068.
2. Kron FW, Fetters MD, Goldman EB. The challenging patient. Clin Fam Practice. 2003;5:893–903.
3. Hahn SR, Kroenke K, Spitzer RL, et al. The difficult patient: prevalence, psychopathology, and functional impairment. J Gen Intern Med. 1996;11:1–8.
4. Jackson JL, Kroenke K. Difficult patient encounters in the ambulatory clinic: clinical predictors and outcomes. Arch Intern Med. 1999;159:1069–1075.
5. Barsky AJ, Wyshak G, Latham KS, Klerman GL. Hypochondriacal patients, their physicians, and their medical care. J Gen Intern Med. 1991;6:413–419.
6. Groves JE. Taking care of the hateful patient. N Engl J Med. 1978;298:883–887.
7. John C, Schwenk TL, Roi LD, Cohen M. Medical care and demographic characteristics of "difficult" patients. J Fam Pract. 1987;24:607–610.
8. Bartlett EE. What's up doc? The patient and the malpractice suit. Risk Manage. 1987;24:607–610.
9. Levinson W, Stiles WB, Inui TS, Engle R. Physician frustration in communicating with patients. Med Care. 1993;31:285–295.
10. Schwenk TL, Marquez JT, Lefever RD, Cohen M. Physician and patient determinants of difficult physician-patient relationships. J Fam Pract. 1989;28:59–63.
11. Lin EH, Katon W, Von Korff M, et al. Frustrating patients: physician and patient perspectives among distressed high users of medical services. J Gen Intern Med. 1991;6:241–246.
12. Levinson W, Roter DL, Mullooly JP, Dull VT, Frankel RM. Physician-patient communication: the relationship with malpractice claims among primary care physicians and surgeons. JAMA. 1997;277:553–559.
13. Bartlett EE. Great expectations: a tale of malpractice. Risk Manage. 1988;35:20–21, 24, 26–27.
14. McCord RS, Floyd MR, Lang F, Young VK. Responding effectively to patient anger directed at the physician. Fam Med. 2002;34:331–336.
15. Schwenk TL, Romano SE. Managing the difficult physician-patient relationship. Am Fam Physician. 1992;46:1503–1509.
16. Gillette RD. "Problem patients": a fresh look at an old vexation. Fam Pract Management. 2000;July–August:57–61.
17. Beckman HB. "Difficult patients." In: Feldman MD, Christensen JF, eds. Behavioral Medicine in Primary Care: A Practical Guide. Stamford, CT: Appleton & Lange; 1997.
18. Smith RC. The Patient's Story. Integrated Patient-Doctor Interviewing. Boston, MA: Little, Brown and Company; 1996.
19. Sapira JD. Reassurance therapy. What to say to symptomatic patients with benign diseases. Ann Intern Med. 1972;77:603–604.

CHAPTER 3

Information Mastery: Basing Care on the Best Available Evidence

Allen F. Shaughnessy, Mark H. Ebell, and David C. Slawson

CASE

Ms. B. is a 34-year old woman who presents with a complaint of fatigue. She has no major comorbidities, and denies cold intolerance, hair loss, skin changes, heavy menses, or other symptoms. She takes a multivitamin with iron. You perform a careful history and physical examination, the results of which are completely normal. An office hemoglobin is 12.8 g/dl, well within the normal range.

CLINICAL QUESTIONS

1. You suspect depression; what is a good way to confirm this?
2. If she is depressed, what are your treatment options?
3. This case makes you think—how can you possibly stay current with the rapidly changing medical literature, in order to provide your patients with the best possible care?

INTRODUCTION

Evidence-Based Medicine

The prevailing focus in many areas of medicine is practicing what is called "evidence-based medicine." Evidence-based medicine (EBM) is ". . . an acknowledgment that there is a hierarchy of evidence and that conclusions related to evidence from controlled experiments are accorded greater credibility than conclusion grounded in other sorts of evidence."(1)

Many clinicians believe that they have always practiced in this way. However, too often decisions are actually based on local custom, habit, the teaching of experts, or what was learned (a long time ago for some!) in medical school. An evidence-based approach means that the clinician has made the effort to identify the strongest, most valid studies, is able to change his or her mind about a test or treatment when the evidence supports a change in practice, and acknowledges when the evidence available for making a decision is less than ideal. Sometimes we will have good, clear evidence to support medical practices, whereas at other times we will have relatively little information to help guide care. The trick is to know the strength of evidence available to support one's current practice and to acknowledge that level of evidence when making decisions.

Sometimes you will hear clinicians complain about the seemingly restrictive nature of EBM, thinking that it provides a "cookbook" that must be followed at all times. It doesn't.

Information alone is not all that's necessary for the compassionate, effective care of individual patients. EBM is just one aspect of clinical practice. Along with good information skills, competent clinicians must have the following:

- Good history-taking and physical examination skills
- A deep understanding of their patient's family and their community, which form the context for their care
- The ability to develop a relationship with the patient to understand his or her beliefs and values
- A practical knowledge of the availability of resources in the community

Therefore, the practice of medicine begins with a thorough understanding of the patient. EBM adds the best available evidence from the research literature. From these two complementary pieces the clinician formulates a management plan based on the patient's medical problems, his or her goals and desires, and a knowledge, derived from the best evidence, of the best way to meet these expectations and goals. Often it is a matter of helping a patient choose the best approach among valid competing alternatives. It's exciting to practice an evidence-based approach to health care. EBM provides a framework for knowing when to begin using new technologies and therapies, when to discard old ones, and how to answer questions that occur daily in the care of patients.

The evidence-based approach to patient care acknowledges that medicine is a probabilistic enterprise. Our goal should be to choose tests and treatments that have the greatest probability of helping our patients. However, even when we choose the approach with the greatest probability of success, we must remember that, although every patient has the potential to benefit, not all patients will benefit from a treatment, and some may be harmed by it. For example, we know that lowering blood pressure in hypertensive patients will make them, *on average*, have fewer cardiovascular complications than if their blood pressure elevation was left unchecked. We do not know, though, for a particular patient, that treatment of his or her blood pressure will actually make a difference. For patients with mild hypertension, 700 have to be treated each year to prevent one bad thing from happening to any one of them. For severe hypertension, this number decreases to 15. Armed with these approximations, clinicians can make better patient management choices.

For too long, physicians have relied on dogma, anecdote, and tradition to guide patient care. EBM encourages a healthy skepticism of every practice in medicine and promotes a culture of inquiry. The history of medicine is full of examples in which dogma and tradition were later proved false. For example, the use of β-blockers was absolutely prohibited in patients with heart failure based on an understanding of the pharmacology and their effect on cardiac output in otherwise normal patients. Twenty years ago all medical students learned this concept as dogma. Research into the treatment of patients with heart failure has countered this idea, showing that the use of β-blockers in these patients can decrease symptoms and mortality.

Of course, there are limitations and biases inherent in the research literature. Studies generally address narrow questions in highly selected patients. Although this is good science, it means that studies are lacking on some of the most challenging aspects of family medicine: the patient with multiple problems, and patients with vague symptoms such as fatigue and dizziness. Another limitation is that the majority of research has been conducted in referral settings and may not be applicable to a primary care population. Finally, it is worth noting that because much research funding is provided by the pharmaceutical industry, far more clinical trials have been conducted of pharmaceutical products than of alternative therapies. Thus, the absence of evidence is not evidence of absence of an effect.

The bottom line with EBM is that the patient—not pathophysiologic reasoning, schools of thought, or specialty-specific approaches—should be the center of all care decisions. Patient-outcomes that matter—decreased symptoms, better quality of life, lower mortality, and even cost—supersede tradition, anecdote, turf, authority, mental gymnastics, and other approaches that have plagued the practice of medicine.

How to Practice EBM

The practice of EBM has traditionally involved asking the right question, searching for information, evaluating its validity, and applying the information to the care of your patient. Information mastery, the practical approach to EBM that you will learn in this chapter, adds the critical step of evaluating the relevance of information before assessing validity. After all, there is no sense in doing the hard work of evaluating validity if the information is not relevant. Learning how to perform the following five steps–asking the question, searching for information, assessing its relevance, evaluating its validity, and applying the result to your patient–is crucial to applying the best information available to the care of patients.

Consider a patient with upper respiratory tract symptoms suggestive of bronchitis. Several questions could be asked about the care of this patient: should I order an x-ray to rule out pneumonia? How effective are antitussives? Should I use an antibiotic, and if so, which one? To be useful, these questions must be framed more broadly. The questions then become: Does routine use of chest radiography in patients with suspected acute bronchitis improve any clinical outcomes? Do antitussives actually reduce the frequency of cough? Do antibiotics reduce the duration of symptoms more than no treatment? Each question has the general form of population, intervention, comparison, outcomes (PICO). Keep this in mind as you ask your own clinical questions.

During a typical day of seeing patients, a family physician generates about 15 clinical questions (2). Unfortunately, most of the clinical questions that come up in practice go unanswered, and about half of those questions have answers that would have affected patient care. What we need is a way to instantly access information at the point of care that is both valid and relevant to the care of patients. It is inevitable that computers will be part of the solution.

Developing the skills necessary to use computers in medical practice will soon become as valuable (and perhaps even more so) as learning how to auscultate with a stethoscope. Computers now play a major role in medicine and have the ability to put the information necessary to answer clinical questions at our fingertips. Computers also put medical information at the fingertips of patients who may not have the skill and knowledge to know what to do with this information. Your role will be to help them obtain good information and to help them understand how to use the information they find.

Desktop and handheld computers can be used, with the proper sources, to quickly obtain validated information. The Internet offers a number of free and subscription evidence-based sites for information (see Table 3.1). You should become familiar with a few high quality sources of information, including the PubMed interface of the National Library of Medicine's Medline database.

The most useful sources of information have done steps 3 and 4 for you: they have already focused on information that is relevant to the primary care setting, and have evaluated its validity. Many will also assist with step 2 of searching for information by filtering it to include only the most useful information. In the next section, we will discuss the issues of relevance and validity in greater detail. In the fifth and final step, you must decide how to apply this information to your patient. In doing so, you should not only consider the external evidence, but also your patient's values, tolerance for risk and uncertainty, cost, and the outcomes that matter most to the patient.

INFORMATION MASTERY: EVALUATING RELEVANCE AND VALIDITY

Information mastery focuses on starting with information that has the potential to be relevant and then determining its validity, rather than the other way around (3). It also considers the myriad information sources that are available and focuses on reducing the work of searching. The first key concept of information mastery is to recognize that not all sources of information are equal, but that they differ with regard to their usefulness.

Determining the Usefulness of Medical Information

Whether reading a journal, attending a conference, or discussing a patient with a colleague, our goal is to spend the least amount of time and energy finding a useful and valid answer to our question. This useful information has three attributes: it must be relevant to our practice; it must be correct (valid); and it must take little work to obtain. These three factors can be conceptually related in the following manner:

$$\text{Usefulness of information} = \frac{\text{Relevance} \times \text{Validity}}{\text{Work}}$$

"Relevance" begins with the concept of "applicability to practice" but goes much further. It is easy to lose sight of the

TABLE 3.1   Web-based Sources of Evidence-Based Clinical Information

Site	Web address	Comment
Free		
Information Mastery Online Course	*http://www.poems.msu.edu/InfoMastery*	Free online course in Information Mastery
Centre for Evidence-Based Medicine	*http://cebm.jr2.ox.ac.uk/*	This site has useful tools and resources, including the "official" table of levels of evidence
Netting the Evidence	*http://www.shef.ac.uk/~scharr/ir/netting*	An extensive list of sites
Bandolier	*http://www.jr2.ox.ac.uk/Bandolier/index.html*	Popular British site, includes essays and features a good sense of humor
National Guidelines Clearinghouse	*www.guidelines.gov*	Repository for practice guidelines. Note that not all are evidence-based
Subscription		
InfoPOEMs and InfoRetriever	*www.infopoems.com*	Source of POEMs and decision support software for PDA and desktop computer
Gwent / Turning Research Into Practice (TRIP)	*http://www.tripdatabase.com*	Lets you search over a dozen evidence-based sites at once
The Cochrane Library	*http://www.updateusa.com/clibhome/clib.htm*	The Cochrane Library contains the Cochrane Database of Systematic Reviews, the Database of Abstracts of Reviews of Effectiveness, and The Cochrane Controlled Trials Register
ACP Journal Club	*http://www.acpjc.org/*	Abstracts of adult medicine studies with commentary
Dynamed	*http://www.dynamicmedical.com/*	A medical information database with clinical topic summaries

primary goal of medicine—helping patients live long, functional, satisfying, pain and symptom-free lives—in the deluge of medical information available to us. What we are looking for are patient-oriented evidence that matters (POEMs). POEMs come from research that evaluates the effectiveness of interventions on the outcomes that matter the most to our patients. Only 1% to 2% of original research, even in clinical journals, represents POEMs (4).

The rare POEM is scattered in among the huge number of articles that can be labeled as disease-oriented evidence (DOEs). DOEs consist of information aimed at increasing our understanding of disease—etiology, prevalence, pathophysiology, pharmacology, prognosis, etc. This information is absolutely crucial to medicine, for we would not have POEMs without it. We must have a basis of understanding how a disease "works" before we can diagnose and treat or prevent it with any certainty.

However, disease-oriented information assumes a chain of causality, linking disease-oriented outcomes such as lower blood pressure to patient-oriented outcomes such as fewer myocardial infarctions. While this chain may look convincing, links are often found to be missing or broken when the POEM is finally published. Sometimes DOEs support POEMs (e.g., treatment of hyperlipidemia with statins reduces the risk of myocardial infarction); in other cases, the POEM disproves a therapy that had been promising based on DOEs. See Table 3.2 for examples of initially promising DOEs that have not turned out to be POEMs. Finally, some cases are undecided,

as in screening for prostate cancer where we have plenty of DOEs but few POEMs.

Another way to distinguish DOEs from POEMs is to determine whether the information leads to *thinking* or *knowing*. Sometimes a test or treatment makes so much sense that we *think* it will benefit patients. However, until a clinical trial is performed, we actually don't *know* that this outcome will occur. This is an important distinction. It has been estimated, for example, that more deaths can be attributed to antiarrhythmic therapies than to the Vietnam War, because for years they were prescribed for asymptomatic arrhythmias before clinical trials showed that they did more harm than good.

Once you have identified a POEM you must weigh how common the clinical problem is in clinical practice. It is impossible to keep up with every new discovery and advance in medicine; we must instead focus on findings that are relevant to our scope of practice. In other words, POEMs dealing with issues common or important to your scope of practice have the greatest relevance.

Next we have to determine the validity of the information. Well-designed clinical studies that minimize bias are more likely to provide valid conclusions. This is the foundation of the scientific method. Unfortunately, assessing the validity of research is time-consuming and difficult without formal training and a great deal of practice. In addition, once these skills are learned, busy clinicians must not only stay current with important clinical content, but also with changes in critical appraisal techniques. For example, the value of con-

TABLE 3.2 Comparison of Disease-Oriented Evidence (DOE) with Patient-OrientedEvidence that Matters (POEM) for Common Conditions

Disease or condition	DOE	POEM
Doxazosin for blood pressure (a)	Reduces blood pressure	Increases mortality in African-Americans
Arrhythmia following acute myocardial infarction (b)	Suppresses arrhythmias	Increases mortality
Sleeping infants on their stomach or side (c)	Anatomy and physiology suggest this will decrease aspiration	Increased risk of sudden infant death syndrome.
Vitamin E for heartdisease (d)	Reduces levels of free radicals	No change in mortality
Histamine antagonists and proton-pump-inhibitors for non-ulcer dyspepsia (e)	Significantly reduce gastric pH levels	Little or no improvement in symptoms in patients with non-GERD, non-ulcer dyspepsia
Hormone replacement therapy (f)	Reduced LDL cholesterol, increased HDL cholesterol	No decrease in cardiovascular or all-cause mortality and an increase in cardiovascular events
Beta-blockers for heart failure (g)	Reduces cardiac output	Reduces mortality in moderate to severe disease

a. Major cardiovascular events in hypertensive patients randomized to doxazosin vs chlorthalidone: the antihypertensive and lipid-lowering treatment to prevent heart attack trial (ALLHAT). JAMA 2000;283:1967–1975.
b. Echt DS, Liebson PR, Mitchell LB, Peters RW, Obias-Manno D, Barker AH, et al. Mortality and morbidity in patients receiving encainide, flecainide, or placebo. N Engl J Med 1991;324:781–788.
c. Dwyer T, Ponsonby A. Sudden infant death syndrome: after the "back to sleep" campaign. Br Med J. 1996;313:180–181
d. The HOPE Investigators. Vitamin E supplementation and cardiovascular events in high risk patients. N Engl J Med 2000; 342:154–60.
e. Moaayedi P, Soo S, Deeks J, et al. Pharmacological interventions for non-ulcer dyspepsia (Cochrane Review). In: The Cochrane Library, Issue 1, 2003. Oxford: Update Software.
f. Writing Group for the Women's Health Initiative Investigators. Risks and benefits of estrogen plus progestin in healthy postmenopausal women. Principal results from the Women's Health Initiative randomized controlled trial. JAMA 2002;288:321–333.
g. Heidenreich PA, Lee TT, Massie, BM. Effect of beta-blockade on mortality in patients with heart failure: a meta-analysis of randomized controlled trials. J Am Coll Cardiol 1997;30:27–34.

cealed allocation assignment has only recently entered the EBM literature. Many family practice residencies emphasize the teaching of these skills to their residents. A free online course is available at Michigan State University (*http://www.poems.msu.edu/InfoMastery*). Excellent published guides for reviewing the medical literature are also available (5, 6).

To remain an effective clinician you need a source (or sources) of information to keep current, and a source (or sources) of information for answering clinical questions as they arise during your care of patients. You should have the skills to evaluate relevance and understand the validity assessments of others. However, with more than 20,000 original research articles and 200 to 300 POEMs published annually in the top 100 clinical journals, it is impractical to do it all yourself. Instead, you should identify one or more independent sources that survey the literature, evaluate relevance (ideally using the POEMs criteria described above), assess the article for validity and bias, and summarize it in a concise, structured format for you. Sources are even available that automatically download the latest summaries to your handheld computer. Such sources are summarized in Table 3.1.

Deciphering Research Reports

Reading an original research study can be a challenge: the language is often stilted, the articles are filled with acronyms, and the statistics can be intimidating. In the next section, we will help you understand how to interpret research results.

THERAPY

There are many biases that can invalidate the results of a study of therapy. The best studies randomize patients, increasing the likelihood that the only difference between groups is the treatment intervention. Blinding both patients and investigators and having a placebo group (or better yet an active comparator group) also improve the validity of the study. Concealing allocation to groups (i.e., making sure that neither the patient nor investigator can influence which patient receives the active treatment and which receives the comparison intervention) has recently been recognized as a critical factor in study design. This differs from blinding, which is what occurs after the study begins. Of course, the most useful studies measure patient-oriented outcomes, as noted above.

Consider the hypothetical study of green versus brown beer bottles described in Box 3-1. The first thing we have to do is determine the extent to which the observed difference could have been due to chance. The *P value* expresses this as a probability. A *P value* of 0.05, which is the typical (although somewhat arbitrary) cutoff, tells us that these findings would only occur 5 times if a study is repeated 100 times. Put another way, there is only a 5% chance that the findings represent chance rather than a real effect of the intervention on the outcome. Let's assume that the statistics found a *P value* of 0.03, which is statistically significant using the cutoff of 0.05 (i.e., there is only a 3% probability that the difference didn't

BOX 3-1

Green or Brown Beer Bottles?

Dr. Frank N. Stein, a German researcher, wants to determine whether beer in brown bottles causes a greater likelihood of auto accidents than beer in green bottles. The investigator chooses representatives of beer in green bottles and in brown bottles with similar alcohol content and decants them into identical appearing containers. He randomly divides a large group of subjects into two groups: those who are to drink beer originally in brown bottles, and those who drink green-bottled beer. After imbibing the same amount, the subjects are placed in a driving simulator and the number of accidents measured. The simulator shows that 9 of the 100 (9%) brown-bottled imbibers have an accident compared with only 3 of the 100 (3%) green-bottled gulpers.

occur by chance). Our next task is to determine the magnitude of the effect. It is not enough to know whether something works; we also need to know how well or how much it works. One way to convey the degree to which the test prevented mortality is the relative risk reduction (RRR). This number represents the percent reduction in the risk of the studied outcome achieved by use of the intervention, and in this case is 67% ([9% − 3%] / 9% = 67%). Relative risk reductions are often used because they tend to be impressively large. However, the clinical relevance of such a number sometimes can be overestimated. A better, more clinically "honest" way to look at this difference is the absolute risk reduction (ARR). This number is the risk difference between the two groups, in this case 6% (9% − 3%)

However, many people have a hard time grasping the meaning of this number because we have trouble understanding decimals, and the clinical relevance of the ARR is sometimes underestimated. A statistic that is conceptually easier to understand and apply is the number needed to treat (NNT). This number tells us how many patients need to be treated to prevent one of them from experiencing the outcome (a car accident, for example). It is easily calculated as 100%/ARR, and in this example is 100% / 6% = 16.7, rounded to 17. In

other words, for every 17 people who drank brown-bottled beer instead of green-bottled beer, one additional person would have a car accident.

The advantage of the NNT is that it is an easy number to understand, especially when comparing the effect of different interventions, and facilitates communication with patients about risk and benefit. When the likelihood of an outcome is low, NNTs will be high. NNTs will decrease as either the likelihood of the outcome increases or as the benefit of the treatment increases. Table 3.3 presents some NNTs for various medical interventions.

DIAGNOSIS

Often, a study will describe the accuracy of a diagnostic test. Tests can include history and physical examination maneuvers, clinical decision rules like the Ottawa Ankle Rules, blood tests, and imaging studies. Important factors in designing a good diagnostic test study include assembling a group of patients with an appropriate spectrum of disease (rather than identifying one group of very sick subjects and one group of perfectly healthy subjects) design, a reliable method of confirming whether or not the test was correct (the reference standard), consistent application of the reference standard to all patients in the study, blinding, and a clear description of the test and population. It is also important to evaluate the overall benefit of using the new diagnostic test. Does it change diagnosis? Does it change treatment? Does it change patient-oriented outcomes? Is it cost effective? These questions can only be answered in clinical trials where the new diagnostic test is used in one population of patients (the intervention group) and not in another (the control group).

A number of statistics are used to describe the accuracy of a diagnostic test:

- *Sensitivity (Sn)* and *specificity (Sp)* are the most widely used measures. Sensitivity is the proportion of patients with disease who have a positive test, while specificity is the proportion of patients without disease who have a negative test. Unfortunately, sensitivity and specificity aren't very useful clinically, because the definitions assume that we already know whether or not the patient has the disease in question!

  Sensitivity = # true positive test / # persons with disease
  Specificity = # true negative tests / # persons without disease

TABLE 3.3 Examples of Numbers Needed to Treat (NNT)*

Therapy	Event Prevented	Length of Follow-Up	NNT
H. pylori eradication in duodenal ulcer	Ulcer at 1 year	1 year	1.1
Finasteride for benign prostatic hypertropy	Need for one operation	2 years	39
Streptokinase and aspirin for acute MI	One death	5 weeks	20
Enalapril for class I or II CHF	One death	1 year	100
Lipid lowering in patients with CHD	One MI or stroke-related death	5 years	16
Treatment of mild hypertension	One MI, stroke, or death	1 year	700
Treatment of severe hypertension	One MI, stroke, or death	1 year	15

* The number of patients that would need to be treated to prevent one adverse clinical event during the follow-up period.

- *Positive (PPV)* and *negative predictive values (NPV)* are more useful to clinicians in the real world. The positive predictive value is the proportion of patients with a positive test who actually have disease, while the negative predictive value is the proportion of patients with a negative test who are actually free of disease:
- Positive predictive value = # with disease / # with positive test
- Negative predictive value = # without disease / # with negative test

Predictive values answer the question of how to interpret a test result. Posttest probabilities are cousins to the predictive values and tell us the probability of disease in a person with a positive or negative test (ultimately, what we want to know.) The posttest probability of a positive test is actually the positive predictive value, while the posttest probability for a negative test is the probability of disease if the test is negative (and is the converse of the negative predictive value).

Posttest probability of a positive test = # with disease / # with positive test

Posttest probability of a negative test = # with disease / # with a negative test

Both predictive values and post-test probabilities have a significant limitation, though; they change as the likelihood of disease changes.

- *Likelihood ratios* have the advantage of not changing when the likelihood of disease changes. Additionally, they allow you to describe the results of a test in more detail. The likelihood ratio for a positive test (LR +) is the probability that a finding is present in diseased patients divided by the probability that it is present in nondiseased persons (7). If a test is simply positive or negative, one can calculate a likelihood ratio for a positive test result (LR +) and a likelihood ratio for a negative test result (LR −) using the sensitivity and specificity:

LR + = Sensitivity / (100 − Specificity)
LR − = (100 − Sensitivity) / Specificity

Likelihood ratios can also be calculated for multiple levels of test results. What does that mean? As in the example of ferritin, a test can have more than two possible results (see Box 3.2). For example, a CAGE score of 4 for the diagnosis of alcoholism is associated with a much greater likelihood of disease than a score of 2, yet both are positive if you use a single cutoff of greater than one for a positive test. Table 3.4 gives some general guidelines on how to interpret likelihood ratios. Using the nomogram on the inside cover of this book, you can use likelihood ratios to convert a pretest probability to a posttest probability.

Information Sources

Numerous sources of medical information are available, each with its advantages and disadvantages. Depending on the reason, different information sources will be more useful than others, based on a balance of relevance, validity, and work. Each may have a role in specific instances.

ORIGINAL RESEARCH JOURNALS

Research journals can help us to find answers to specific questions as well as to stay abreast of new medical developments.

BOX 3-2

Interpreting the Serum Ferritin

Consider the serum ferritin test, a test for iron deficiency anemia (IDA). While laboratories generally report a single cutoff for abnormal, we know that as the serum ferritin increases, the likelihood of IDA decreases. Clearly, a serum ferritin of 2 mg/dl is more strongly associated with IDA than a ferritin of 20; yet a simple-minded single cutoff would assign the same diagnostic meaning to both values. The likelihood ratio gives us a richer way to interpret the serum ferritin. The likelihood ratio for serum ferritin ≤15 mg/dl is 51.8; for 15–24 mg/dl is 8.8; for 25–34 mg/dl is 2.5; for 35–44 mg/dl is 1.8; for 45–100 mg/dl is 0.5; and for ≥100 mg/dl is 0.08. Clearly, a value <15 rules in the diagnosis, while a value ≥100 essentially rules it out. Values in between must be interpreted in light of the patient's history, and may require additional confirmatory testing.

Original research is the information source best suited to evaluation for validity, although this process is time-consuming. It can also be difficult to find the most relevant article, and original research articles are usually not quick reading. Examples of original research journals include *JAMA, Annals of Family Medicine, BMJ*, and at least 4,000 others.

Research studies published in knowledge-creation journals can be quickly skimmed for relevance by reading the title of the article and the abstract. This initial screen should focus on three questions:

- Is the problem studied one that is common to my practice and is the intervention feasible?
- Did the authors study an outcome that patients would care about?
- Will this information, if true, require me to change my current practice?

This simple screening method will help you quickly eliminate most of the articles in research journals (3, 4).

TRANSLATION JOURNALS

Translation journals, sometimes called freebies by their detractors, consist mainly of expert reviews or opinion. *Patient*

TABLE 3.4 Interpreting a Likelihood Ratio

Likelihood Ratio	Interpretation
>10	Strong evidence to rule in disease
5–10	Moderate evidence to rule in disease
2–5	Weak evidence to rule in disease
0.5–2	No significant change in the likelihood of disease
0.2–0.5	Weak evidence to rule out disease
0.1–0.2	Moderate evidence to rule out disease
<0.1	Strong evidence to rule out disease

Care, Emergency Medicine, Hospital and Staff Physician, and many others are in this category. Articles in these publications are generally fun to read and are useful for review or for rapidly refamiliarizing yourself with a topic. The downside of these articles is that too often there is no real quality control to ensure the information is correct. Unlike systematic reviews (see below), these articles generally are written backwards, meaning the author writes his or her conclusions and then finds data to support this viewpoint, rather than looking at all of the data and arriving at a conclusion. Some journals, such as *American Family Physician*, are making a concerted effort to improve the "evidence-basedness" of their articles by providing evidence summaries to authors and requiring strength of evidence labeling.

NEWSLETTERS

Newsletters are another way to quickly process new information. *The ACP Journal Club, Bandolier, Journal Watch, FP-IM Database*, and others, provide abstracts and sometimes commentary on articles of interest to family physicians. Review services, such as *The Medical Letter* and *Primary Care Reports*, AAFP Home Study course, as well as audiotape subscription services such as the *Audio-Digest* series focus on one or a few issues each month. True *news*letters such as *Drug Therapy Update* and *Medical Sciences Bulletin* are hybrids, providing cursory reviews of the current literature along with topical news from other sources. As with any source of information, consider the relevance (how the articles are selected for the newsletter) and validity (how they are evaluated).

EMAIL SERVICES

Rather than receive a paper newsletter, many physicians prefer to receive updates via email because of their timeliness. Examples include *Daily POEMs (www.infopoems.com)* and *BMJ Updates (http://bmjupdates.mcmaster.ca/index.asp)*.

REVIEW ARTICLES

Summary reviews, such as those published in translation journals, cover a lot of ground, making in-depth discussion of individual points impossible. As a result, it is difficult to assess the validity of the information behind the conclusion, and bias, often unrecognized by the author, can creep into these reviews. In 1993, Oxman and his colleagues identified 36 review articles and applied ten criteria for evaluating the methodological rigor of the review (8). They compared the ratings of the rigor of the review among experts in the field of study with non-experts trained to critique review articles. Scores from the non-expert group were very consistent, whereas scores in the expert group were widely disparate. Additionally, reviews written by experts in a particular field consistently received lower scores than those written by non-experts. A more recent analysis of review articles on type II diabetes examined the methodological rigor of both relevance and validity assessments. It found that the average score was 1 out of a possible high score of 15, with the best score being only 5. (9)

Experts in a field should be doing original research. However, the refinement and synthesis of information should be done by individuals who are not biased (i.e., not necessarily experts in the clinical content) and who have been taught to critically evaluate original research and summarize it into

reviews. These individuals are also less likely to be dependent on research grants or speaking fees from parties with a vested interest in the conclusion.

Summary reviews also may not be current, especially in rapidly changing areas of medicine. For example, 6 years elapsed between the publication of a meta-analysis showing a pronounced decrease in mortality by thrombolytic therapy for myocardial infarction, and when the majority of reviews recommended its general use (10).

SYSTEMATIC REVIEWS AND META-ANALYSES

Systematic reviews focus on only one or two clinical questions. Writing these articles is a painstaking process, and represents the creation of new knowledge. A good systematic review has four steps: 1) identification of one or two highly focused clinical questions; 2) an exhaustive search of the world's medical literature; 3) evaluation of the quality of each article, with inclusion of only those that meet criteria for quality; and 4) synthesis of the data. The synthesis can be qualitative (a textual description of the bottom line) or quantitative (using specific statistical methods to combine the data from different studies into a single summary measure of effect, a technique called meta-analysis). Quantitative reviews should only be attempted if the outcome measures from different studies are generally the same and their study designs are similar.

Systematic reviews and meta-analyses can be a powerful tool. For example, 19 of 23 trials of the use of β-blockers after myocardial infarction did not show a statistically significant benefit to this therapy. However, when all of the trial results were analyzed together, β-blocker therapy was associated with a 23% relative reduction of the risk of death (11).

One of the best sources of this type of high quality review is the Cochrane Library *(http://www.updateusa.com/clibhome/clib.htm)*. It includes the Cochrane Database of Systematic Reviews. Each review is aimed at answering a particular question (e.g., "Are antibiotics effective in the treatment of acute bronchitis in adults?"). The methods used to identify all relevant research on this question are outlined in the review. Only results of randomized, controlled trials—the strongest form of clinical research—are used in the reviews. The Cochrane Library also includes the Database of Abstracts of Reviews of Effectiveness (DARE), a compilation of systematic reviews from other sources that meet the Cochrane's rigorous standards for systematic reviews. The Cochrane Controlled Trials Register is a database of more than 260,000 individual controlled clinical trials and their abstracts, many of which are not found in Medline.

TEXTBOOKS

Textbooks such as this one can be thought of as collections of summary reviews. They usually present the bottom-line and are sometimes hard to evaluate for validity. One thing that distinguishes this textbook is the focus on an evidence-based approach to care, which means providing detailed information to support each recommendation. Because textbooks gradually become outdated, we anticipate that textbooks of the future will increasingly use electronic methods to update themselves.

LECTURES

Clinicians often leave a continuing medical education (CME) lecture feeling they have learned something. However, a large body of research has shown that practice habits are rarely influenced by CME presentations. This has been called "Chinese-dinner memory dysfunction," which is a temporary feeling of satiety derived from "learning something" that is quickly followed by an inability to remember or apply information (12).

There are some things you can consider when evaluating the usefulness of a CME presentation. Is the topic common or important in your practice? Is the speaker focusing on patient-oriented outcomes or disease-oriented outcomes? Does the speaker cite the strength of supporting evidence for key recommendations, or does the talk appear to be based on anecdote, habit, and custom? Does the speaker refer to key evidence-based sources, such as the Cochrane Database, systematic reviews, and evidence-based guidelines, or is the survey of the literature more selective? Do not assume that the speaker is an expert who is beyond reproach. The next section should give you some insight into why experts can and must be questioned.

EXPERTS

We often turn to someone with greater experience and knowledge in a particular area when we have a question. These people are content experts. Information from a content expert tends to be quite subjective; even narrowly focused specialties, experts have a tough time agreeing. For example, in a study of radiologists who reviewed the same set of mammograms, the radiologists disagreed with one another 21% of the time (13). The same lack of agreement has been shown for histopathologic diagnosis of melanoma (62%), liver necrosis (53%), and breast cancer classification (27%) (13–15). The experts cannot be faulted for these discrepancies, for all tests have some built in imprecision, and the toughest areas are often the ones involving human interpretation.

There is another type of expert, the clinical scientist. These experts in methodology may be physicians, pharmacists, epidemiologists, or librarians who are expert at evaluating information for validity but are not necessarily content experts. They are able to give an objective assessment of the quality of information, unencumbered by the bias of experience and training.

PHARMACEUTICAL REPRESENTATIVES

These well-dressed, polite individuals present their information in an easy-to-understand fashion. The relevance and validity of their information, like any other source, should be carefully evaluated. A helpful mnemonic for gathering information about a new drug therapy is STEPS, which stands for five characteristics of a drug that determine its usefulness: Safety, Tolerability, Effectiveness, Price, and Simplicity. As you listen to a pharmaceutical representative, try to pigeonhole the information you are given into one of these five categories (Table 3.5). Many times the information you hear really doesn't fit and it can be ignored. Also, remember to focus on patient-oriented rather than disease-oriented outcomes. If you don't hear any, don't be afraid to ask for it.

PRACTICE GUIDELINES

The goal of practice guidelines (also called policies, consensus reports, or practice parameters) is to help clinicians improve the quality of care that they deliver and reduce inappropriate variation in practice. Although some guidelines come from a careful synthesis of all of the available evidence, others are developed by simply polling experts for their consensus opinion. The latter may reduce inappropriate variation in practice but do not necessarily improve the quality of care. When evaluating a guideline, look for a description of how the evidence was assembled, and make sure that the authors rate the strength of key recommendations. The best use of clinical guidelines is as suggestions governing most practice most of the time, and not as inviolable protocols. Like a master chef, you will learn to use these cookbooks as the guides that they are designed to be, taking each recipe and varying it to meet the needs of the moment.

CLINICAL EXPERIENCE

Clinical experience is often given short shrift in discussions of evidence-based medicine and information mastery. This is

TABLE 3.5 Sales Techniques Often Used to Promote Pharmaceuticals

Technique	Example
Appeal to authority: Using the opinion of an authority, not the evidence, to support a particular medication	"Dr. Knowitall, the famous cardiologist from Atlanta, prescribes our drug a lot!"
The Bandwagon appeal: Using the popularity of a medication to support its superiority	"Cephakillitall is the most widely prescribed antibiotic in the United States!"
The red herring appeal: Using factual but irrelevant information (disease-oriented evidence) to support a medication.	"Our antibiotic achieves the highest minimum inhibitory concentration in the respiratory epithelium!"
The appeal to pity: Basing a decision on emotions (pity, wishful thinking) instead of the evidence	"You've got to help me out here—our sales are really suffering this year!"
Appeal to curiosity: Similar to the red herring appeal, it is the use of a demonstration or highlighting of a non-clinical uniqueness to captivate your mind	"Our drug has a unique shape that's easy to remember!"
Error of omission: Not mentioning useful information. The STEPS acronym (see text) can help identify omissions.	"Really? A recent study showed it's no more effective than hydrochlorothiazide? I'll look into that, doctor!"

unfortunate, because clinical experience and clinical skills are central to the effective, compassionate practice of medicine. Information mastery does not tell us how to listen to a patient, take a comprehensive history, perform a physical examination, communicate effectively with patients, help them make decisions that are best for them, or deal with ethical issues. However, information mastery does help us make the best use of the information that we gather from patients, helps us streamline our clinical examination to focus on the most important elements, and helps us present the best possible array of options to our patients. The synthesis of information mastery and clinical experience is "clinical jazz," because it melds the structure and rhythm of the scientific method with the improvisation and skill of clinical practice.

USING INFORMATION TO CHANGE YOUR PRACTICE WITH CONFIDENCE

Adopting a new method of practice requires a number of steps. Even the smallest change requires an active effort. Specialists in education, sociology, and psychology have outlined several steps necessary for us to manage our own change process (Table 3.6).

Thinking while you are doing is the first step in the change process. This requires enough confidence to honestly examine your own actions but not so much self-assurance that you are unwilling to admit to imperfection.

The next step is to open your mind to the idea of change. You must embrace the attitude that change is healthy and nonthreatening. Once your mind is open, you must pay attention to feedback from patients, colleagues, and other health care professionals. Also, you must continuously reflect on your performance, learn to value the clinical questions that arise in daily practice, and make an effort to answer them with the best available evidence. The best physician asks more questions, not fewer.

One useful practice is to figure out the "state-of-the-evidence" for common problems encountered in your practice. For some problems we can feel confident in the state of knowl-

edge; for many others, our knowledge is very preliminary. For example, we have good information supporting the treatment of moderate to severe hypertension in adults. We also have good information that tells us *not* to treat asymptomatic ventricular arrhythmias. However, the treatment of peripheral neuropathy symptoms is much less clear; several agents have been shown to be effective, but none of them work consistently. Knowing the state of the evidence supporting medical practice allows you to be flexible in your approach to the care of patients. When there is good evidence of benefit, such as the treatment of high blood pressure, most patients should be treated most of the time. Conversely, when we have good evidence of harm (e.g., antiarrhythmics), most patients should *not* receive this treatment most of the time.

Good evidence is available to support only about half of what we do as physicians. This leaves much room to include personal experience, reasoning, and the preferences of patients in the decision-making process. This "evidence-based liberation" allows you to tailor care since there is no clear cut approach for some aspects of medical care.

Here's a disheartening thought: the information you have recently learned may already be outdated. The next step in the change process is to keep up with new developments in medicine.

THE RESPONSIBLE INFORMATION MASTER

In 2004, there were 45 million Americans without health care benefits. The majority of these people are the "working poor," who work in service industries and who we see daily in our trips to the mall, restaurant, or shoe store. For these people, even the basics of health care are all but out of reach. Although they can go to an emergency department when they have a stroke or heart attack, many delay these visits due to concerns over cost. More importantly, preventing these catastrophic events is usually not an option. Our health care system is set up to serve those who have appropriate insurance coverage rather than those people who don't. In other words, we ration health care—not in terms of what services we provide, but rather in terms of who is able to get those services at all. Put another way, we ration at the people level rather than at the service level.

Because resources are not unlimited, we must decrease the amount of money spent by each person on health care to allow more people access to that care. Note that controlling costs does not have to mean denying needed services. Instead, treating patients correctly the first time, based on the best information, can control costs. In other words, improving the quality of care can result in cost savings.

This is a difficult concept to accept. Many patients and many clinicians believe that doing more for a patient must always be better. However, recent evidence has clearly shown a point of diminishing return, and even increasing harm, as a result of ever increasing services. An unnecessary CT scan that finds a questionable lesion, that requires a biopsy, that results in a complication, has harmed that patient. The widely prescribed cyclo-oxygenase-2 (COX-2) inhibitors were ten times as expensive as acetaminophen or naproxen sodium, were no better at reducing pain, and actually caused tens of

---

TABLE 3.6	Steps to Affecting Change in Your Own Practice

1. Evaluate your own practice patterns, and think about what you are doing as you do it. What are the patient-oriented outcomes of importance?
2. Open your mind to the idea of change.
3. Develop a systematic framework regularly for accessing high quality, relevant information. You will need: 1) a source to alert you to new information, 2) a rapid retrieval method to answer clinical questions, and 3) a prompting system to remind you of useful information that otherwise would get lost.
4. Identify the level of evidence for your common practices. Be ready to change if the level of evidence is weak.

thousands of unnecessary deaths from cardiovascular disease. Hydrochlorothiazide, costing pennies per month, is actually better at preventing stroke, myocardial infarction, and premature death, than much more expensive calcium-channel blockers.

We have all been trained to do what is best for each and every patient we encounter. This assumes that we can devote whatever money is necessary to the care of the person right now, and we will somehow come up with the money when they need care some time in the future. We have to remember that an individual patient has or will have health care needs in addition to his current one, and that unnecessary consumption of resources for the current problem drains resources that could be used for the same patient at some other time. As family physicians, we must care for the patient as well as the greater family—the community—to which this individual and his own family belong.

How do we do this? The first step is to learn about the benefits, harms, and costs of what we do. We must work to do it right the first time by finding the best approach to patient management based on the best available information. Family physicians will have a crucial role in this process. Using information mastery and POEMs as our guide to what services to offer and which to leave out can clearly help eliminate the waste in medicine. In so doing, we will improve the fairness of resource distribution.

CASE DISCUSSION

The single best question to screen for depression is "During the past month, have you been bothered by little interest or pleasure in doing things, or feeling down, depressed, or hopeless?" It is 90% sensitive (it will find most patients with depression) but only 56% specific (some who answer affirmatively will not have depression). The positive likelihood ratio is 5.6 (moderate evidence to rule in depression if positive), and the negative likelihood ratio 0.5 (weak evidence to rule out depression if negative) (16).

Ms. B answers yes to the screening question. Further questioning is a way to improve specificity, and it confirms a diagnosis of mild to moderate depression without suicidal intent. Because you know that your patient has previously expressed an interest in alternative health care, you ask her whether she would prefer to begin treatment with counseling, a medication, a supplement, or a combination of interventions.

She states that she would like to begin by taking a natural supplement, and asks for your opinion. Because you subscribe to an evidence-based monthly summary of recent research, you remember a recent well-designed randomized controlled trial that found St. John's wort to be as effective as SSRIs in primary care patients with mild to moderate depression (17). It is also safe as long as the patient is not taking an SSRI already. This helps you feel comfortable working with the patient to tailor her treatment to her values, knowing that it is supported by good evidence. Because supplements vary in content, you recommend that she use the brand and dose that was studied.

You also don't push counseling too hard, because you know that while it may have a benefit in mild to moderate depression, this benefit is relatively small, and it can always be added in a few weeks (18). Taking an evidence-based approach has increased, not limited, your treatment options, and enabled you to take a patient-centered approach to care.

REFERENCES

1. Hurwitz B. How does evidence based guidance influence determinations of medical negligence? BMJ. 2004;329:1024–1028
2. Covell DG, Uman GC, Manning PR. Information needs in office practice: are they being met? Ann Intern Med. 1985;103:596–599.
3. Slawson DC, Shaughnessy AF, Bennett JH. Becoming a medical information master: feeling good about not knowing everything. J Fam Pract. 1994 May;38(5):505–513.
4. Ebell MH, Barry HC, Slawson DC, Shaughnessy AF. Finding POEMs in the medical literature. J Fam Pract. 1999;48:350–355.
5. Sackett DL, Richardson WS, Rosenberg W, Haynes RB. Evidence-Based Medicine. How to Practice and Teach EBM. New York: Churchill Livingstone; 1997.
6. Rosser W, Slawson DC, Shaughnessy AF. Information mastery: Evidence Based Family Medicine, 2nd ed. Toronto: B.C. Decker, 2004.
7. Sox HC, Blatt MA, Higgins MC, Marton KI. Understanding new information: Bayes Theorem. Medical Decision Making. Boston, MA: Butterworth-Heinemann; 1988; 67–101.
8. Oxman AD, Guyatt GH. The science of reviewing research. Ann NY Acad Sci. 1993;703:125.
9. Shaughnessy AF, Slawson DC. What happened to the valid POEMs? A survey of review articles on the treatment of type 2 diabetes. BMJ. 2003;327:266–269.
10. Antman EM, Lau J, Kupelnick B, Mosteller F, Chalmers TC. A comparison of results of meta-analyses of randomized control trials and recommendations of clinical experts. Treatments for myocardial infarction. JAMA. 1992;268:240–248.
11. Yusuf S, Peto R, Lewis J, Collins R, Sleight P. Beta blockade during and after myocardial infarction: an overview of the randomized trials. Prog Cardiovasc Dis. 1985;27:335–371.
12. Davis DA, Thomson MA, Oxman AD, Haynes RB. Evidence for the effectiveness of CME: a review of 50 randomized controlled trials. JAMA. 1992;268:1111–1117.
13. Elmore JG, Wells CK, Lee CH, Howard DH, Feinstein AR. Variability in radiologists' interpretations of mammograms. N Engl J Med. 1994;331:1493–499.
14. Fleming KA. Evidence-based pathology. J Pathol. 1996;179:127–128.
15. Farmer ER, Gonin R, Hanna MP. Discordance in the histopathologic diagnosis of melanoma and melanocytic nevi between expert pathologists. Hum Pathol. 1996; 27:528–531.
16. Brady DS, Hahn SR, Spitzer RL, et al. Identifying patients with depression in the primary care setting: a more efficient method. Arch Intern Med. 1998;158:2469–2475.
17. Philipp M, Kohnen R, Hiller KO. Hypericum extract versus imipramine or placebo in patients with moderate depression: randomised multicentre study of treatment for eight weeks. BMJ. 1999;319:1534–539.
18. Depression in primary care vol 2. Treatment of Major Depression. Rockville, MD: US Dept of Health and Human Services; April 1993; 27–29, 109–113. AHCPR publication 93-0551.

Preventive Care

CHAPTER 4

Prenatal Care

Beth A. Choby

CASE

Mrs. L is a 37-year-old G2 P1001 who presents at 21 weeks' gestation with an uncertain last menstrual period. She has not been taking prenatal vitamins, and asks about whether she should. Her first pregnancy was delivered via emergency cesarean delivery secondary to preterm delivery at 36 weeks. The baby weighed 9 lbs at birth despite being premature. She asks about genetic screening, as her sister had a baby with Down syndrome, and she is worried that "it runs in the family." She thinks she may have had abnormal blood glucose during the first pregnancy, but cannot remember specific details.

CLINICAL QUESTIONS

1. What is the best means of accurately determining the gestational age of this patient's pregnancy?
2. When are prenatal vitamins indicated during pregnancy?
3. Does this patient require screening for gestational diabetes or Down syndrome?
4. How does a history of prior cesarean delivery influence delivery options for this pregnancy?

Prenatal care introduces many women into the medical system. It allows physicians to address non-obstetric issues such as baseline health status and immunization history. It may positively influence the treatment of certain obstetric conditions. Prenatal care likely benefits both maternal and infant health by encouraging long-term health maintenance, and increasing the likelihood that infants receive timely care.

Family physicians' knowledge, scope of practice and comprehensive training makes them uniquely suited to provide prenatal care for women and their families. Bonds formed during maternity care often translate into lifelong relationships with families. Prenatal care is a highly rewarding part of family medicine because of this special type of continuity.

Family physicians care for pregnant women in a variety of settings. Twenty-four percent of family physicians perform deliveries as a regular part of their practice, 18% perform vacuum extraction, 6.4% do forceps deliveries, and 6.5% offer trial of labor after cesarean delivery (TOLAC) (1). Although only 4.3% of family physicians perform cesarean deliveries, in rural areas of the upper Mountain and Midwest states, 23%–27% of family doctors perform cesareans (1). A large percentage of family physicians provide prenatal care or see pregnant women during routine office visits. This chapter explores evidence-based prenatal care, medical and psychosocial issues in pregnancy, and the role of family physicians as maternity care providers.

PRENATAL CARE IN PERSPECTIVE

The idea of organized prenatal care is attributed to Ballantyne at the University of Edinburgh. He suggested that the high maternal and perinatal mortality rates during the early 20th century resulted from limited care during pregnancy and inadequate management of labor. Improving education for maternity healthcare providers was given increased emphasis in the 1930s. Seeking out care during pregnancy and delivering in the hospital rather than at home became more common. Antibiotic use, improved blood transfusion technology, and safer anesthesia were increasingly available. Maternal and infant mortality significantly improved, and this was largely attributed to prenatal care. Prenatal care was also assumed to be cost-effective.

In 1985, the Institutes of Medicine (IOM) recognized prenatal care as a national policy issue. Congress later enacted legislation that expanded Medicaid coverage for pregnant women. The effect of these changes over the past 25 years is noticeable: 84% of U.S. women enter care in the first trimester, and 75% have care considered both early and adequate (2).

Despite the widespread use of prenatal care, evidence of its effectiveness is lacking. Rates of preterm delivery and low birth weight infants have not improved over the past decades. The United States has some of the highest per capita healthcare expenditures of industrialized nations. Yet, the U.S. maternal and infant mortality rates are significantly higher than rates in nations dedicating fewer resources to healthcare. Maternal mortality has declined drastically over the past century, but even in the 1990s, 12 per 100,000 women died annually of pregnancy-related causes in the United States. Major racial disparities continue to exist. Maternal mortality in African-American women is 12 per 100,000 compared with 8.1 per 100,000 in whites. African-American women have three to four times the risk of pregnancy-related death compared to whites. This striking difference has been observed over the past 60 years and continues as the largest disparity in the area of maternal and child health (3).

The United States currently ranks 36th worldwide in infant mortality. Congenital anomalies, low birth weight, and sudden infant death syndrome (SIDS) are the three leading causes of infant death in the United States and together account for 45% of total infant deaths. The 2002 US infant mortality rate was 7.0 per 1,000, an increase from the record low of 6.8 per 1,000 live births in 2001. Singapore, Sweden, and Hong Kong have the lowest infant mortality rates (less than 3 per 1,000) (4). Many nations with lower infant mortality rates provide universal access to prenatal care.

Initial cross-sectional studies on the effectiveness of prenatal care are affected by selection bias. Women who receive prenatal care or who choose early care are likely quite different from those who lack care. For example, women who deliver with no prenatal care tend to be less educated, multiparous, living with a child, uninsured, smokers, and have past histories of substance abuse (5). Risk factors for inadequate prenatal care include low educational achievement, age less than 20, high parity and being unmarried. Attributing improved outcomes to prenatal care without considering the influence of selection bias is unsound.

If disadvantaged women without prenatal care have increased risk of adverse birth outcomes, universal access to care for all pregnant women should improve both maternal and neonatal morbidity/ mortality. This is not supported by research though, because many American women with health coverage still do not seek prenatal care. Cultural issues, transportation, child care availability, and a limited number of providers willing to care for low-income women may better explain why American women do not seek prenatal care, independent of insurance coverage.

More recent descriptive and randomized controlled trials (RCTs) associate prenatal care with improved birth outcomes. Future research must explore whether enhanced prenatal care benefits certain groups of women, i.e. the young, the uninsured, and women in high-risk ethnic groups. Focusing additional resources on those at highest risk is more expensive than routine prenatal care, but is likely cost-effective when the resources necessary for caring for very low birth weight infants are considered.

What comprises "adequate" prenatal care also remains unclear. Although an increasing number of evidence-based recommendations for prenatal care are available through the Cochrane Database and other EBM collections, many topics still require study.

PLANNING THE PREGNANCY AND RISK ASSESSMENT

The preconception visit can be used to maximize the expectant parents' health and well-being prior to conception. The consultation ideally occurs 3 to 6 months prior to conception and covers health promotion, risk assessment, and medical intervention. It is likely the most important prenatal visit for the prevention of birth defects. Unfortunately, planned pregnancies are the exception rather than the rule in the United States. Approximately 50% of pregnancies in adult women and 95% of pregnancies in teens are unplanned (6). Opportunities for informal preconception guidance include well-woman exams, pap smears, visits for contraception or a negative pregnancy test, and follow-up visits after poor birth outcomes.

A recent survey of general practitioners indicates that 88% know about the concept of preconception care, and most provide some type of advice to patients. Ninety-three percent consider this counseling as part of their duties, but only 53%

feel sufficiently knowledgeable to give adequate advice (7). Additional factors hindering provision of preconception care include lack of resources, and training/protocols, and difficulty determining which patients are contemplating pregnancy. Although board-certified family physicians receive a great depth of training and are likely facile with preconception care, formal opportunities to provide it are fairly uncommon.

Post-conception days 17–56 represent the time of greatest fetal vulnerability to toxins and environmental insults (8). Many women may not realize that they are pregnant, and few women initiate prenatal care this early in gestation. The preconception period is the ideal time to address safety issues of early pregnancy.

OCCUPATIONAL RISKS

Specific occupational exposures affect pregnancy either in the preconception period or during the gestation. A temporal relationship is often present. Untoward effects are related to the gestational age of the fetus at the time of exposure. Environmental exposures that adversely affect the fetus include solvents (e.g. pesticides, paint thinner/strippers, fertilizers) and heavy metals such as lead, mercury or arsenic. Exposure to waste anesthetic gas may reduce fertility in settings where gas-scavenging equipment is not available. Women who work in a hospital setting should avoid exposure to ionizing radiation, chemotherapeutic agents, and misoprostol. Non-ionizing radiation found in microwaves, radio waves, and ultrasound are safe during pregnancy.

FOLIC ACID

Strong epidemiologic evidence demonstrates that increased preconception intake of folic acid reduces the risk of neural tube defects (NTDs). The Medical Research Council Vitamin Study found that mothers with a previous child with a neural tube defect reduced the risk of having another child with an NTD by 72% if 4mg of folic acid was taken daily prior to conception and during the first trimester (9). A Cochrane meta-analysis compares risk of NTD in women who take folic acid to those who do not. Women consuming folic acid have a threefold overall decrease in the risk of NTD, from 10.2/1000 in the control group to 2.4/1,000 in the folic acid group. The number needed to treat (NNT) is 847 to prevent one NTD (10). Current recommendations are that folic acid is best obtained through a diet rich in folic acid sources, combined with a daily vitamin supplement containing 400 mcg (0.4 mg) of folic acid. Leafy green vegetables and fortified whole grains are both good dietary sources of folic acid. Only one-third of women are estimated to take folic acid supplements prior to conception, probably because many pregnancies are unplanned. The preconception visit provides an opportunity to advise women about the benefits of folate supplementation starting at least 1 month prior to conception.

GENETIC SCREENING AND COUNSELING

Risk stratification of medical and genetic conditions is an integral part of preconception care. Certain heritable genetic diseases are best diagnosed in individuals prior to becoming pregnant.

The goal of preconception genetic counseling is twofold. Individuals who are at risk for a fetal anomaly or genetic disorder can be counseled about risk in a future pregnancy and couples can be informed about available screening tests. Specific questionnaires for genetic screening are available from the American College of Obstetricians and Gynecologists (ACOG) at *http://www.acog.org*. In patients with known familial disorders, genetic testing allows for carrier testing (i.e. sickle cell disease).

Certain ethnic groups are at increased risk for genetic disorders (see Table 4.1). Routine preconception screening with an enzyme assay for hexosaminidase is currently recommended by ACOG in those at risk of Tay-Sachs disease.

Women at risk for sickle cell disease should be screened using hemoglobin electrophoresis. Sickle cell solubility tests such as the Sickledex may not identify significant hemoglobin gene abnormalities and are not recommended. In women who are known carriers of sickle cell trait, screening of the partner is recommended to estimate risks for a planned pregnancy. When both partners are carriers, the fetus has a 50% chance of being affected with sickle cell disease.

Women at risk of thalessemia (those of Mediterranean or Asian descent) can be screened using the mean corpuscular volume (MCV). In women with a low MCV, no iron deficiency, and a normal hemoglobin electrophoresis, DNA testing for abnormal thalassemia hemoglobin types is indicated. Solubility testing is not useful for identifying carriers. Most variants of alpha-thalassemia are mild. Fetuses with the most severe form, Bart's hemoglobin, usually deliver stillborn at 28 to 30 weeks. Cases number 14,000 to 28,000 annually, and preconception screening in couples at risk may decrease the number of affected pregnancies (11).

Cystic fibrosis (CF) is an autosomal recessive genetic condition resulting from mutations in the CF transmembrane conductance regulator (CFTR). More than 1,000 mutations have been described in the CFTR gene. Whites of northern European descent have a carrier frequency of 1: 29 for cystic fibrosis. CF also affects individuals of other ethnic groups, including African-Americans, Hispanics, and Asians with carrier rates ranging from 1 in 46 to 1 in 90 (12). ACOG, the National Institutes of Health (NIH) and the American College of Medical Genetics (ACMG) recommend screening for CF in individuals at high risk (see Table 4.1).

DNA testing can determine if women or their partners are CF carriers. When both partners are carriers, there is a 25% chance that a pregnancy will result in a fetus with cystic fibrosis. Couples should also be counseled on the availability of chorionic villus sampling or amniocentesis to diagnose CF once they become pregnant.

Medical Conditions

Preconception care provides an opportunity for women with medical conditions to optimize their treatment and improve the likelihood of a healthy pregnancy.

DIABETES MELLITUS

Infants of mothers with diabetes mellitus are at a fourfold increased risk for congenital malformations like cardiac and neural tube defects. Congenital malformations occur during organogenesis. Elevated maternal blood glucose levels increase the likelihood of anomalies, especially during the first trimester. Since many women with diabetes do not realize that they are pregnant during this critical period, maximizing glycemic control before conception is essential.

Optimizing glycemic control prior to pregnancy is the main goal of preconception care in women with diabetes. Preprandial (fasting) blood glucose should range from 4 to 7 mmol/L and the hemoglobin A1c (HgA1c) ideally should be less than 6%. In a recent small, non-randomized prospective trial, investigators found a spontaneous abortion rate of 8.4% in women managed with intensive insulin therapy compared with 28% in women who received standard insulin therapy (13).

A recent metaanalysis of preconception care in diabetes described major and minor anomalies in 2.4% of infants of mothers with preconception care compared with 7.7% in mothers without this intervention (14). The glycosylated hemoglobin (HgA1c) was lower in the group with preconception care. Preconception care resulted in a net cost-savings of approximately $34,000 per pregnancy, probably due to a decreased incidence of fetal anomalies and attendant costs of care.

EPILEPSY

Women with epilepsy also benefit from preconception counseling. Women with epilepsy have higher baseline rates of infertility and miscarriage. Infants of women with epilepsy have increased risk of anomalies, especially cardiac and neural tube defects. Several medications used to treat epilepsy decrease the effectiveness of certain hormonal contraceptives, emphasizing the importance of proactive preconception care.

The majority of women with epilepsy have uncomplicated pregnancies and deliver healthy infants. Seizure activity during pregnancy poses a risk to the fetus, as do certain antiepileptic medications. Known adverse effects of specific antiepileptic drugs include intrauterine growth restriction, fetal malformation and dysmorphism, and developmental delay during infancy. It is not clear whether these abnormalities are caused by epilepsy, or the by the medications used to treat it. Most studies report a two- to threefold increase in major malformations in the offspring of women taking antiepileptic drugs (15). Older medications like valproic acid, carbamazepine, and phenytoin are more strongly associated with congenital anomalies; polytherapy further increases risk. Information on teratogen risk with newer generation antiepileptics (gabapentin, tiagabine, oxcarbazepine, topiramate) is scarce and mostly based on case series and uncontrolled studies.

One cohort study examined the effectiveness of preconception counseling in women with epilepsy. Women presenting to a preconception epilepsy clinic were compared with women seeking care when already pregnant. Women receiving preconception care were started on folic acid and changed to drug monotherapy when possible. Six percent of women were able to discontinue antiepileptic medications altogether. The group with preconception care had no major fetal malformations, compared with a rate of 18% in the control group. Higher dose folic acid supplementation (1–4 mg daily) is recommended for women with epilepsy who are trying to conceive, although this is based on expert opinion.

TOBACCO AND ALCOHOL

A review of tobacco, alcohol, and illicit substance use is important during the preconception visit. Cigarette smoking causes numerous preventable problems in both pregnancy and the neonatal period. Smoking is associated with placenta previa,

TABLE 4.1 Preconception Screening Recommendations for Specific Diseases

Disease	Cause	Heritability	Epidemiology	Screening Available	Recommendations for screening
Tay-Sachs	Deficiency of the enzyme hexosaminidase-A	Recessively inherited lysosomal storage disease	1:30 carrier risk in people of Ashkenazi Jewish heritage; Cajuns and French Canadians also carriers	Enzyme assay for hexosaminidase-A	Routine preconception screening for those at risk*
Sickle cell anemia	Amino acid substitution of valine for glutamic acid on the HBB gene of chromosome 11	Autosomal recessive	10% African-Americans are carriers; Indo-Pakistani and Arab ethnic groups	Hemoglobin electrophoresis	Preconception screening for women at risk; for women with sickle cell trait, partner screening recommended (50% chance of affected fetus when both partners carriers)*
Thalessemia Alpha and Beta type	Abnormality in hemoglobin production with inadequate oxygen carrying capability and anemia	Autosomal recessive	1:12 carrier rate in people of Asian or Mediterranean descent	DNA testing for abnormal thalessemia hemoglobin in women with low MCV, normal hemoglobin electrophoresis.	Preconception screening for women at risk and partners of women with abnormal hemoglobin genes; 25% risk of being affected if both parents carriers
Cystic Fibrosis (CF)	Mutations in the CF transmembrane conductance regulator (CFTR).	Autosomal recessive	1:29 carrier risk in whites of northern European heritage	DNA testing	Preconception screening of individuals with family history of CF, partners of women with CF, and couples where one/both are white. Make available to others not in these categories*†‡

*Recommended by ACOG.
†Recommended by American College of Medical Genetics.
‡Recommended by the National Institutes of Health (NIH).

placental abruption, preterm premature rupture of membranes (PPROM) and ectopic pregnancy. Sudden infant death syndrome (SIDS), intrauterine growth restriction, and stillbirth are also increased when women smoke during pregnancy. Estimates suggest that US infant deaths would decrease by 10% if women did not smoke during pregnancy (16).

Evidence-based recommendations for smoking cessation are available through the Cochrane Collaboration. Interventions that increase tobacco cessation in the general population include brief physician advice, telephone counseling, group therapy, nicotine replacement and drug therapy with buproprion or nortriptyline. Cigarette smoking is one of the most significant modifiable causes of adverse obstetric outcomes in the United States. Obtaining a history of tobacco use is essential during the preconception visit. Women who use tobacco and wish to conceive are strongly encouraged to set a quit date.

Discussing patterns of alcohol consumption is important during the preconception visit. Effects on the fetus depend on the amount of alcohol consumed, the duration of use and timing in gestation. Binge drinking involves consuming more than 5 drinks in one sitting and is more dangerous to fetal neurologic development than non-binge usage. While there is a general consensus that women should not drink excessively during pregnancy, it remains unclear what level of alcohol is harmful to a pregnant woman and her fetus. Many U.S. authorities recommend against the consumption of any alcohol before or during pregnancy.

The CAGE questionnaire listed in Table 4.2 is a quick and straightforward screening test for women who report current alcohol use during a preconception visit. Any positive response warrants further investigation. Written self-help manuals may improve cessation rates of women who are already pregnant. Although a recent metaanalysis of physician counseling for non-pregnant women with alcohol abuse did not show a beneficial effect on cessation (17), a project funded by the Centers for Disease Control on alcohol cessation and improving contraception for women at risk for both pregnancy and alcohol exposure resulted in nearly 70% of at-risk participants using effective birth control and not drinking at 6-month follow-up. (18) Medications helpful in promoting alcohol cessation include disulfiram and naltrexone. Disulfiram (Antabuse) is contraindicated during pregnancy because of an association with clubfoot, phocomelia of the lower extremities,

and VACTERL syndrome (congenital anomalies). VACTERL syndrome consists of vertebral anomalies, anal atresia, cardiac defects (especially ventricular septal defects), tracheo-sophageal (TE) fistula, renal anomalies, and limb abnormalities (generally radial dysplasia). Women who conceive while taking disulfiram should receive counseling before deciding to continue the pregnancy (19). A multidisciplinary approach may work best for women with alcoholism who become pregnant. Abstinence from alcohol is currently the safest policy in the preconception period.

MEDICATION HISTORY

Use of all prescription and over-the-counter drugs, herbal supplements, and vitamins should be reviewed and documented at the preconception visit. If a woman requires a drug with teratogenic potential, informed consent and a discussion about safer options is necessary. Switching to an alternative with a better-known safety profile is prudent, especially during organogenesis. Certain medications are unsafe in pregnancy, and should be discontinued in any woman attempting to conceive. Misoprostol, isoretinoin, warfarin and HMG-CoA reductase inhibitors are incompatible with pregnancy.

IMMUNIZATIONS

The preconception visit is a useful time to update immunization status. Screening all women for rubella susceptibility by history of previous vaccination or serology is recommended during the initial preconception encounter. Non-immune women should be immunized with the measles-mumps-rubella (MMR) vaccine. Persons born after 1956 who lack evidence of immunity to measles are also candidates for MMR. Vaccination on or after the first year of life, proof of immunity via serology, or physician-diagnosed measles implies immunity. While women have historically been counseled not to conceive within 3 months of MMR immunization, the likelihood of the fetus developing congenital rubella syndrome is largely theoretical. In one study, 683 women inadvertently given MMR within 3 months of conception or during pregnancy had no increased incidence of fetal anomalies or congenital rubella syndrome (20).

Immunity to varicella (chicken pox) should be documented during the preconception visit. Varicella is spread by respiratory droplets and has a high attack rate. Ninety percent of non-immune household contacts will contract varicella when exposed. Although uncommon during pregnancy, congenital varicella in the newborn and maternal varicella pneumonia causes significant morbidity and mortality. Eighty-five to ninety percent of adults who deny having had varicella are actually immune. A negative history of varicella can be confirmed through titers. Women who are not immune should receive immunization with varicella vaccine (Varivax®) prior to conception.

DIAGNOSING AND DATING THE PREGNANCY (CONFIRMATION OF PREGNANCY)

Amenorrhea, nausea, fatigue, and breast tenderness are the most common symptoms of early pregnancy. Amenorrhea in a sexually active female is 63% sensitive and 60% specific for the diagnosis of pregnancy. Nausea gravidarum, also known

---

TABLE 4.2 The CAGE Questionnaire

1. Have you ever felt the need to **Cut down** on your drinking?
2. Have you ever felt **Annoyed** by another's criticism of your drinking?
3. Have you ever felt **Guilty** about your drinking?
4. Have you ever used alcohol as an **Eye opener** (early morning drinking)?

Score of 2 to 3: high index of suspicion for alcohol dependence
Score of 4: definitive for alcohol dependence
From: Ewing JA. Detecting alcoholism: the CAGE questionnaire. JAMA 1984;252:1905–1907.

TABLE 4.6 Categorization of Drug Safety Classifications in Pregnancy and Lactation

Food and Drug Administration (FDA) Categories on Potential Fetal Risk

Class	Description	Examples
A	Controlled human studies show no fetal risk in first trimester; no evidence of risk in later pregnancy; fetal harm remote	
B	Animal studies show no risk/ there are no controlled studies in pregnant women; or animal studies show adverse affect not confirmed in first trimester human studies; no evidence of risk in later trimesters	Acetaminophen, diphenhydramine, azithromycin, cephalosporins, penicillin, low-molecular weight heparin, buproprion, methyldopa, loratadine, metochlopromide, sucralfate, H2 antagonists
C	Use only when benefit outweighs risk; animal studies with teratogenic or embryocidal effects and no controlled human studies available; or no research available	Tramadol, ibuprofen*, ketorolac, trimethoprim, clarithromycin, heparin, amitryptiline, venlafaxine, calcium channel blockers, clonidine, albuterol, promethazine, disulfuram, ethosuximide, gabapentin, lamotrigine, vancomycin
D	Documented human fetal risk; use only if benefit is clearly acceptable despite risk; no safer alternatives available	Most benzodiazepines, sulfonamides (third trimester), tetracyclines, most anticonvulsants, ACE inhibitors, ARBs, lithium, nicotine patches, spray and inhalers
X	Contraindicated in women who are or may become pregnant; fetal risk/known abnormalities in humans	Warfarin flurazepam, temazepam, HMG-CoA reductase inhibitors, isoretinoin, oral contraceptives, methotrexate, cytotec, ergotamines

*Risk category D in third trimester

ACOG Position on Antimicrobial Use in Pregnancy

Class	Description
A	Considered safe in pregnancy
B	Probably safe but use with caution
X	Contraindicated in pregnancy

American Academy of Pediatrics Safety in Lactation

Class	Description
A	Lactation compatible
B	Compatible with concerns
C	No available studies
D	Lactation strongly discouraged; hazards to mother or infant
TX	Discontinue lactation for specific number of hours listed
X	Contraindicated in lactation

weeks' gestation, with return visits monthly until 28 weeks. From 28–36 weeks, appointments are usually scheduled every 2 weeks. After 36 weeks, weekly visits ensue, with many providers scheduling biweekly visits after 40 to 41 weeks' gestation. The current visit schedule is more tradition-based than evidence-based. A recent Cochrane review shows that a model with fewer prenatal visits is not likely to increase maternal or fetal risk compared to the traditional model. A benefit of the abbreviated system is decreased cost, although women may be less satisfied with fewer visits (52).

Traditional components of the subsequent prenatal visit include measurement of weight, blood pressure, fundal height, fetal heart tones, and a urine dipstick for protein and glucose.

Different low-risk prenatal guidelines lack consensus as to which of these components are useful at follow-up visits. Most recommend routine measurement of maternal weight, blood pressure, fundal height and fetal heart tones. The evidence supporting the recommendations varies widely.

Inadequate weight gain may be associated with low birth weight, preterm delivery, and intrauterine growth restriction. A recent metaanalysis found that women with morbid obesity are more likely to develop gestational diabetes and hypertension, preeclampsia, and arrest of labor. Infants of these women are more likely to develop fetal distress, have meconium, and be delivered by cesarean. Whereas weight gain of more than 25 pounds is associated with large for gestation infants, poor weight gain is an inadequate correlate for low birthweight (53). For this reason, some recent guidelines recommend that routine weights at subsequent visits be discontinued. Because the information may not change clinical management and may create undue anxiety, measurements are needed only in women for whom nutrition is a concern (e.g. underweight, overweight or obese). Other guidelines recommend weights at every prenatal visit, but acknowledge that the supporting evidence is only fair.

Most guidelines recommend measuring blood pressure at every prenatal visit. Early detection of an elevated blood pressure trend that persists over time is the best screening strategy for gestational hypertensive disorders. The test is simple and inexpensive, and although no direct proof exists that blood pressure screening reduces maternal or fetal morbidity and mortality, it is indicated on an empiric basis.

When the patient presents for care in the second or third trimester, fundal height is a good estimate of uterine size and gestational age. Fundal height is measured as the distance in centimeters between the superior edge of the pubic symphysis and the top of the uterine fundus. At 20 weeks' gestation, the fundus should be at the level of the umbilicus. During each week between 20 and 36 weeks' gestation, the fundal height increases by 1 cm. Measurements deviating by more than 2 cm may indicate problems with fetal growth. Currently, there is not enough evidence to evaluate the use of fundal height measurement in low-risk prenatal care. However, it is inexpensive, noninvasive, and requires minimal training to assess, and most guidelines recommend that it be done at subsequent visits unless better evidence proves otherwise.

Auscultation of the fetal heart rate (FHR) is generally done at all follow-up visits. Normal fetal heart rate ranges from 110 to 160 beats per minute. Although hearing the fetal heart confirms that the fetus is alive, well-being is harder to evaluate because decelerations or poor variability are rarely noted during this rapid check. This part of the exam is likely reassuring for expectant parents, although this has not been studied. Guidelines differ in recommendations for FHR, with some recommending measuring FHR at every prenatal visit beginning at 10 to 12 weeks, and others recommending that FHR not be used based on currently available evidence. These guidelines do suggest measuring FHR upon patient request (31, 32).

Routine urine dipstick tests for protein and glucose are no longer recommended during prenatal visits. They are unreliable in detecting the moderate or variable elevations of albumin that occur with preeclampsia. The 1-hour glucola (below) should be used for the diagnosis of gestational diabetes.

Subsequent Laboratory Tests

As discussed in the section on genetic screening, the quadruple screen is recommended between 16 and 18 weeks' gestation.

DIABETES SCREENING

Gestational diabetes mellitus (GDM) is one of the most common obstetric complications, with incidence ranging from 3% to 10% in developed countries. There is currently a lack of consensus in the medical literature regarding screening for GDM. While observational research suggests an association between fetal macrosomia and GDM, the relationship to shoulder dystocia, birth trauma, and maternal-fetal morbidity

is less clear. No conclusive data demonstrate that universal screening for GDM benefits the population, although it is a currently accepted standard of care in the United States.

Selective screening exempts women considered at low-risk for GDM. To be considered low-risk, women must meet all of the following criteria: age less than 25, pre-pregnancy BMI less than 25, no family history of diabetes, no personal history of GDM or abnormal glucose tolerance, and not belonging to a high-risk ethnic group. High-risk ethnic groups include Native American, Hispanic, African-American, Asian, and Pacific Islander. ACOG states that although universal screening is the most sensitive means of detection, certain low-risk women may benefit from selective screening (SOR = C). The American Diabetes Association (ADA) also endorses selective screening for GDM.

Screening for GDM is generally performed at 24 to 28 weeks' gestation. The 1-hour test measures blood glucose 1 hour after oral ingestion of 50 g glucose in 150 ml fluid. The sensitivity and specificity of the test are 79% and 87%, with a LR+ of 6 and LR− of 0.24 respectively. Positive predictive value is 14%, while negative predictive value is 99.4 (54). The test is performed either fasting or non-fasting, although fasting may increase the chances of a false positive screen. The upper limit of normal for the 1-hour test is between 130 and 140 mg/dl. Women at higher risk for GDM can be screened at the initial prenatal visit, with follow-up testing done at 24 to 28 weeks if the first test is normal. High-risk groups include women with a history of GDM, history of a previous infant with birthweight over 9 lbs, women over age 35, women from certain ethnic groups, and BMI less than 19.8 or over 25.

If the 1-hour test is abnormal, a 3-hour glucose challenge test (GTT) should be administered. The test is performed after an overnight fast. A 100-g glucose load is given orally, with blood drawn prior to ingestion and hourly for three consecutive samples. A diet containing at least 150 g of carbohydrates must be consumed for 3 days prior to testing. Carbohydrate depletion causes spuriously high glucose levels on the GTT. A diagnosis of GDM is made when elevation occurs with either the fasting glucose alone or with two or more of the 3-hour measurements.

The first line of intervention for pregnant women diagnosed with GDM is diet. A recent metaanalysis, however, found no differences in birthweight over 4,000 g, cesarean rates, birth trauma, preterm birth, or gestational hypertension in women with GDM treated with diet compared to those who were not (55).

When diet alone is ineffective for controlling blood glucose, insulin is generally instituted. Use of oral diabetes medications is increasingly common, although insulin continues to be the therapy with the best-known safety profile. Sulfonylureas (glipizide and glyburide) and metformin (Glucophage®) are being used in women with preexisting type-2 diabetes, especially when polycystic ovarian disease is present.

RH SCREENING

An antibody screen for isoimmunization in women who are Rh negative is done at 28 weeks' gestation. Rho(D) immune globulin is given to Rh-negative women with a negative screen. Women with a positive antibody screen do not benefit from Rho(D) injection and should be evaluated for Rh hemolytic disease.

Screening for Anemia

Retesting for anemia with a hematocrit or hemoglobin at 28 weeks' gestation is appropriate because the maternal blood volume expands during the second trimester. Dietary counseling and supplements are prescribed for pregnant women found to be anemic.

Infectious Disease Screening

In the third trimester, both ACOG and USPSTF recommend repeat screening for hepatitis B, syphilis, gonorrhea, and chlamydia in high-risk populations. High-risk populations include women younger than age 25 with two or more sexual contacts, women who are prostitutes, and women with prior history of syphilis or gonorrhea.

Patients and their partners should be asked about a history of genital and orolabial herpes simplex infection (HSV). Herpes outbreaks are classified as primary, nonprimary (first infection with herpes simplex type 2 in a woman with previous type 1 outbreak) or recurrent. Rates of vertical transmission at delivery are 50% in primary HSV infections and 33% in nonprimary first episodes. Transmission risk for recurrent infection is 0% to 3% (56). Genital herpes infection during pregnancy does not increase the risk of neonatal HSV infection as long as seroconversion is complete before labor begins.

The manifestations of neonatal herpes vary in severity and morbidity. The infection is transmitted to the fetus as it passes through the birth canal, with localized disease causing lesions on the neonate's face, eyes and mouth. More severe infection involving the central nervous system carries 15% mortality, while disseminated HSV infection causes 57% mortality in neonates (57). ACOG recommends antiviral therapy (acyclovir) for women with primary HSV infections and those at risk for recurrent infections after 36 weeks' gestation (SOR = C). Delivery by cesarean is recommended for women who have active genital lesions present at the time of delivery. Pregnant women should avoid sexual contact if either partner has lesions.

Group B streptococcus (GBS), *Streptococcus agalacteie*, is a leading cause of neonatal morbidity and mortality. GBS exists in the genital and gastrointestinal tract of pregnant women, affecting 6.6% to 20% of mothers in the United States. The Centers for Disease Control (CDC), ACOG and the AAP all recommend that women be offered screening for GBS at 35 to 37 weeks' gestation. Specimens are collected using two swabs: one is collected from the lower vagina and posterior fourchette, and the second from the rectum. Studies show that women can collect their own specimens when given appropriate instructions. Self-collected specimens have similar sensitivities to those collected by physicians.

Women who are culture positive for GBS should receive antibiotic prophylaxis when in labor. The antibiotic of choice is intravenous penicillin G (PCN G) in non-allergic women. The dosage is 5 million units followed by 2.5 million units every 4 hours starting at rupture of membranes or active labor and continuing until delivery.

Intravenous ampicillin is a secondary choice because it has a less narrow spectrum of activity against GBS compared to PCN G. The dosage is 2 g IV and then 1g IV every 4 hours until delivery. Sensitivity testing of GBS isolates is recommended in women with a penicillin allergy. Erythromycin and clindamycin are indicated for susceptible isolates, with vancomycin given for resistant cultures. Women positive for GBS who have an elective cesarean delivery do not require antibiotic prophylaxis providing that surgery is done prior to onset of labor or rupture of membranes. Women with GBS urinary tract infections should be treated both when diagnosed and again at delivery because GBS bacteriuria indicates very heavy colonization.

Women who miss GBS screening because of no prenatal care or unavailable results should be managed according to a risk-based protocol when in labor. Women meeting any of the following criteria require antibiotic prophylaxis.

- Ruptured membranes for greater than 18 hours
- Fever
- Less than 37 weeks' gestation
- History of GBS bactiuria with the current pregnancy
- History of previous infant with invasive GBS disease

SUBSEQUENT COUNSELING

Subsequent visits are an appropriate time for talking with couples about issues related to normal pregnancy. Couples have numerous questions, including making plans for delivery. Anticipatory guidance in the second and third trimester helps reinforce that pregnancy is a natural life event.

Women experience numerous physiologic changes during normal pregnancies. Most are benign and resolve following delivery. Reassuring women that these changes are normal, common, and transient is important.

Heartburn is common because of relaxation of the lower esophageal sphincter due to increased progesterone. Women experience epigastric burning resulting from reflux of stomach acid into the esophagus. Progesterone also increases bowel transit time. Eating smaller meals and avoiding greasy foods often improves symptoms. Antacids containing calcium carbonate or magnesium hydroxide are indicated for severe heartburn.

Urinary frequency and incontinence occur commonly in the first and third trimesters. Stress incontinence, or urine loss after coughing, sneezing or laughing, is often confused with rupture of membranes. Urinary symptoms generally resolve after pregnancy and women are encouraged to do Kegel exercises while pregnant to strengthen the pelvic floor muscles.

Hemorrhoids worsen in pregnancy due to increased venous congestion in the rectal vascular plexus. Topical treatments, such as witch hazel pads and sitz baths, may help mild hemorrhoids. Several prenatal vitamins contain prophylactic stool softeners like docusate sodium (Colace®).

Backache is common in later pregnancy because of the compensatory lordosis from the enlarging uterus. Relaxins released in the second trimester cause loosening of ligaments in the pubic symphysis, back and pelvis. Wearing flat-heeled shoes and maintaining good posture can counter changes in the center of gravity.

Round ligament pain occurs because of spasm of the round ligaments. Pain is described as sharp, stabbing, sporadic, and located in the inguinal area. Pain is worse in multiparas and although uncomfortable for the mother, it is not harmful to the fetus. Exercise, warm baths, a pregnancy girdle, and acetaminophen (Tylenol®) sometimes help with symptoms.

Leukorrhea is the heavier, whitish vaginal discharge noted in pregnancy. It results from increased vaginal blood flow and high estrogen levels. Reassurance is helpful, because women often assume it is caused by infection.

Many expectant couples excitedly anticipate developing a birth plan. Large amounts of information are available during pregnancy through books, videos, and the internet. Many women have specific ideas about what they want during labor. Women desiring "natural childbirth" need to be questioned about what this means to them. Use of epidural, breastfeeding, infant rooming-in versus nursery care, pacifier use, and circumcision can all be addressed as part of the birth plan. Discussing the planned course early allows the physician flexibility in accommodating the couples' wishes while assuring the highest standards of maternity care.

The World Health Organization (WHO) recommends that all infants be fed with breast milk exclusively from birth to at least age 6 months. Babies who are breastfed are less likely to develop otitis media, gastroenteritis, upper respiratory infections, and urinary tract infections. A recent Cochrane review found that two to four short (10–15 minutes) breastfeeding education sessions with a lactation consultant provided to low income women 2–4 times during prenatal care resulted in a significant increase in the women's duration of breastfeeding (58).

Physicians often recommend structured educational programs for childbirth and parenting. Several observational studies demonstrate improved performance in labor in expectant women who attend childbirth classes. The research is limited due to selection bias. Knowing what to expect during labor helps parents play a more active and informed role. Most classes include a tour of the maternity care area, and introductions to topics like newborn care and breastfeeding. Larger randomized controlled trials will hopefully better describe the effect of classes on women's anxiety, need for analgesia, and length of labor.

Trial of Labor after Cesarean (TOLAC)

Discussing plans for delivery in women with a previous cesarean delivery is best done starting in the late second trimester. For many women, trial of labor after cesarean (TOLAC) is preferred over elective repeat cesarean delivery (ERCD). The total cesarean rate has increased from 5.5% in 1970 to 26.1% in 2002, with the primary cesarean rate at 18% in 2002 (59). In 2002, 12.4% of women elected to attempt TOLAC, down from a high of 28.3% of women in 1996.

Both ACOG and AAFP have issued guidelines for women considering TOLAC. Women with one previous cesarean delivery with a low transverse uterine incision are candidates for and should be offered a trial of labor. Several factors influence the likelihood of success of a vaginal birth after cesarean (VBAC). Positive factors include maternal age less than 40, having a prior vaginal delivery or VBAC, a favorable cervix, spontaneous labor, and a nonrecurrent indication that was the reason for the prior cesarean delivery (i.e., breech). Factors that decrease the likelihood of successful VBAC include a history of multiple surgical deliveries, gestational age over 40 weeks, fetal weight over 4,000 g and the need for labor augmentation or induction (60).

Prostoglandins (Prepidil, Cervidil) are not recommended for cervical ripening or induction as their use is associated with higher rates of uterine rupture. ACOG and AAFP differ on recommendations as to facilities in which TOLAC should be attempted. ACOG recommends that TOLAC be restricted to facilities in which surgical teams are physically present throughout labor. The AAFP states that there is not good evidence available that having a surgical team standing by results in improved outcomes, and that a clinically appropriate plan for uterine rupture or any emergency requiring rapid surgical delivery must be documented for any woman attempting TOLAC. Providers should discuss all issues pertinent to a woman's decision, including recovery time, safety and prior birth experiences. Unfortunately, no evidence-based recommendation is currently available regarding the best method for presenting risks and benefits of TOLAC to patients.

Postdates Pregnancy

One-tenth of pregnancies continue to at least 42 weeks' gestation and are considered post-dates. Maternal risks associated with post-dates pregnancy include dystocia, postpartum hemorrhage, emergent surgical delivery, and cephalopelvic disproportion. Fetal risks include asphyxia, meconium aspiration, septicemia, and death. The perinatal mortality rate (stillbirths and neonatal deaths) is 2 to 3 per 1,000 at term, doubles by 42 weeks, and is four to six times greater by 44 weeks' gestation (61).

Management of pregnancy beyond 40 weeks' gestation depends on the accurate assessment of gestational age. The most common cause of post-term pregnancy is inaccurate dating. Elective induction of pregnancies before 42 weeks is advocated to reduce risks of adverse maternal and fetal outcomes. A Cochrane review of 19 RCT's found that routine labor induction at 41 weeks resulted in lower perinatal mortality, but no change in rates of cesarean delivery. NNT was 500 women induced to prevent 1 perinatal death (62). No difference between groups was noted for meconium aspiration syndrome or other neonatal morbidity, but infants in the expectant management group more frequently had meconium stained amniotic fluid.

There is not a current consensus on the management of post-dates pregnancy. The Society of Obstetricians and Gynecologists of Canada (SOGC) recommends routine induction of labor at 41 weeks' gestation. ACOG does not define an upper gestational age at which induction is suggested, but does recommend fetal assessment beginning at 42 weeks' gestation. When a physician and patient elect to manage a post-term pregnancy expectantly, fetal monitoring is indicated. A combination of twice-weekly non-stress testing, amniotic fluid index (AFI) or biophysical profile (BPP) is used, although evidence of benefit is unclear and no single test is better than another (see Table 4.7). A reactive NST has a negative predictive value for stillbirth of 99.8%, and a positive predictive value of 10%. The BPP has a negative predictive rate of 99.9%, while an abnormal study has a PPV of 40% (63).

If gestational age is reliable, the risks and benefits of induction versus expectant management should be discussed at 41 weeks' gestation. If the patient desires induction and has a favorable cervix and vertex fetus, the procedure can be scheduled at this time. Women who wish to avoid induction may be monitored using biweekly NSTs, modified BPP (NST & AFI), or full BPP until 42 weeks. Induction should be done at 42 weeks. If oligohydramnios is present, expectant management is contraindicated. The fetus should be delivered

TABLE 4.7 Testing Methods for Post-Dates Pregnancy Surveillance

Nonstress Testing

Result	Criteria
Reactive (normal)	Two or more fetal heart rate accelerations over a 20 minute period; each acceleration must be at least 15 beats above the baseline heart rate and last at least 15 seconds; testing may be extended to 40 minutes to account for fetal sleep-wake cycles
Non-reactive (abnormal)	No accelerations seen over a 40-minute period

Biophysical Profile Parameters

Subsets	Score of 0	Score of 2
Fetal movement	Absent, abnormal or insufficient	Three or more discrete body or limb movements within 30 minutes
Fetal tone	Abnormal, absent or insufficient	At least one extension of extremity with return to flexion; opening or closing of hand
Fetal breathing	Abnormal, absent or insufficient	One episode of fetal breathing movements lasting 30 seconds or more within 30 minutes
Amniotic fluid volume	Largest vertical pocket 2 cm or less	Single vertical pocket greater than 2cm
Nonstress test	Non-reactive	Reactive

Adapted from: ACOG practice bulletin. Antepartum fetal surveillance. Number 9, October 1999. Clinical management guidelines for obstetrician-gynecologists. Int J Gynaecol Obstet 2000; 68:175–185.

promptly to avoid cord accidents or other adverse outcomes. Either management strategy depends on a frank discussion of risks and benefits preferably begun early in pregnancy.

FAMILY PHYSICIANS' APPROACH TO MATERNITY CARE

Family medicine is the only specialty that emphasizes longitudinal, comprehensive care for families without regard to age, sex, or disease condition. Family physicians view pregnancy as a normal, healthy life event rather than from a disease context. Providing prenatal and infant care as part of an ongoing family relationship allows for continuity that is so often lacking in the modern healthcare system. Family physicians who deliver babies are more likely to earn higher incomes, be more psychologically satisfied with work, perform more procedures, and have a younger practice than those who do not do obstetrics (64).

Family physicians who provide maternity care have a broad range of practice patterns. Some provide prenatal care only, while others perform cesarean deliveries and share call with obstetrician-gynecologists. Family physicians are well trained to provide independent, evidence-based maternity care for women and competently manage low-risk pregnancies. Family physicians with advanced fellowship training are capable of managing higher acuity pregnancy care.

FAMILY PHYSICIANS AND OBSTETRIC CONSULTANTS

Family physicians work closely with their obstetric consultants in caring for pregnant women who require higher acuity care.

When the consultation process works effectively, the patient benefits from a specialty opinion while maintaining the continuity relationship with the primary physician. The AAFP-ACOG liaison committee has published guidelines for consultations between family physicians and obstetrician-gynecologists (65). Family physicians are encouraged to request consults in a timely fashion, clearly discuss the reasons for consultation, and maintain collegial relationships with physicians who provide back-up. Physicians who provide back-up for family physicians should see the patient in a timely fashion, and be a collaborative part of the care team. Family physicians who act as consultants for obstetrician-gynecologists for medical referrals should also strive to provide timely and evidence-based care. Evidence-based recommendations for prenatal care are found in Table 4.8.

CASE DISCUSSION

Mrs. L presents with several risk factors, including unsure dates, late entry into care, possible history of abnormal glucose tolerance, previous operative delivery, previous preterm delivery, and history of a macrosomic infant.

An ultrasound for dating and organ survey is advisable. Establishing an accurate due date is important because of her previous cesarean delivery. A screening ultrasound with biometry at this gestational age accurately predicts gestational age within a 7- to 10-day margin. The fundal height on physical exam is expected to be 21 cm, measured 1 cm above the umbilicus. If both ultrasound and fundal height correlate, they can be used to establish the gestational age in lieu of the unknown last menstrual period.

Folate in prenatal vitamins is recommended prior to con-

TABLE 4.8 Summary of Evidence-Based Recommendations

Preconception Care

Recommendation	Strength of Recommendation*	Reference
Women considering becoming pregnant and pregnant women should be counseled that dietary supplementation with folic acid (400 mcg) before conception and during the first trimester decreases the risk of neural tube defects in the fetus.	A	9, 10
Intensive preconception glycemic control in women with diabetes prevents major congenital anomalies in offspring.	A	10
Women with epilepsy planning to conceive should be changed to monotherapy or less teratogenic medications when possible, and advised to take at least 1 mg of folic acid daily prior to conception	B	10
Smoking cessation should be advised for all women who anticipate becoming pregnant because of decreases in neonatal morbidity and mortality	A	32

Pregnancy Care

Recommendation	Strength of Recommendation*	References
The traditional visit schedule can be abbreviated without an increase in adverse maternal or neonatal outcomes. The abbreviated schedule is less expensive, but women may be less satisfied with the decreased number of visits.	A	24
Women with a continuity provider more likely attend prenatal education, discuss concerns, require less analgesia in labor, and feel prepared for delivery and infant care.	A	23
Maternal weight and height should be measured at the fist antenatal appointment in order to calculate the body mass index (BMI)	B	31, 32, 33
Blood pressure measurement is recommended at each prenatal visit.	C	33
Routine breast examination during antenatal care is not recommended for the promotion of postpartum breast feeding	A	32
Routine cervical examination is not effective for predicting preterm birth and should not be offered unless clinically indicated	A	32
Pregnant women should be offered fundal height measurements at each prenatal visit to detect small or large for gestation fetuses.	A	32
Routine ultrasound prior to 24 weeks allows for better estimation of gestational age and decreased need for labor induction for post-dates pregnancy. No significant difference in clinical outcomes is apparent.	A	42

Pregnant women over age 35 or with an abnormal screening test (triple screen, quadruple screen) should be offered screening for Down syndrome. The screening test should have a detection rate above 60% and a false positive rate less than 5%. These tests fulfill these criteria:
 	
• 11 to 14 weeks:
  ○ nuchal translucency (NT)
  ○ the combined test (NT, HCG and PAPP-A)
• 14–20 weeks:
  ○ the triple test (HCG, uE3, and AFP)
  ○ the quadruple test (HCG, uE3, AFP, and inhibin A)
	B	32

(continued)

TABLE 4.8 Summary of Evidence-Based Recommendations
Pregnancy Care (continued)

Healthy, pregnant women are encouraged to participate in mild to moderate exercise three or more times weekly.	A	33
Individualized exercise programs should consider each pregnant woman's pre-pregnancy activity and fitness levels.	B	33
Pregnant women should be counseled as to the proper use and positioning of seat belts (three-point restraints located across the hips and above the fundus).	B	32
Sexual intercourse during pregnancy is not associated with harmful effects in the absence of obstetric contraindications.	B	32

*A, consistent, good-quality patient-oriented evidence; B, inconsistent or limited-quality patient-oriented evidence; C, consensus, disease-oriented evidence, usual practice, expert opinion, or case series. For information about the SORT evidence rating system, see *http://www.aafp.org/afpsort.xml.*

ception and during the first trimester to prevent neural tube defects. If Mrs. L is found to have anemia, iron supplements may be useful. Although routine prenatal vitamin supplementation is not recommended during pregnancy, supplements may augment diets lacking in certain nutrients. The patient has several risks for gestational diabetes, including possible history in the first pregnancy and a previous macrosomic infant. She should be screened at this visit with a 1-hour glucose challenge with repeat testing at 24 to 28 weeks if the test is normal. Down syndrome screening is advisable secondary to maternal age and is best done between 16 and 21 weeks' gestation; Mrs. L may be too late by her LMP.

An early discussion of delivery plans is also indicated. With a history of an emergent operative delivery, the surgical records must be reviewed to make sure that she had a low-transverse uterine incision and not a classical cesarean. Her history of unsure dates and a macrosomic infant increased her risk if TOLAC is attempted. It is a good idea to involve either a family physician credentialed in cesarean delivery or obstetric consultant early regardless of whether she desires a repeat cesarean or TOLAC.

References

1. American Academy of Family Physicians; AAFP-ACOG Liaison Committee; 2005.
2. DATA 2010. The Healthy People 2010 Database–November, 2004 edition. Available at *http://wonder.cdc.gov/scripts/broker.exe.* Accessed 16, 2005
3. Centers for Disease Control. Pregnancy-Related Mortality Surveillance–United States 1991–1999. February 25, 2003. United States Department of Health and Human Services Centers for Disease Control and Prevention. Available at *http://www.cdc.gov/od/oc/media/pressrel/fs030220.htm;.* Accessed September 19, 2005.
4. US Deptartment of State and the CIA World Fact Book—2003. Available at *GeographyIQ.com.* Accessed September 19, 2005.
5. Maupin R, Lyman F, Fatsis J, et al. Characteristics of women who deliver with no prenatal care. J Matern Fetal Neonatal Med. 2004 Jul;16(1): 45–50.
6. Henshaw S. Unintended pregnancy in the United States. Family Planning Perspectives, 1998;30:24–29.
7. Gaytant MA, Cikot RJ, Branspenning JC, et al. Preconception counseling in family practice: a survey of 100 family physicians. Ned Tijdschr Geneeskd. 1998 May 23;142(21): 1206–1210.
8. Brundage S. Preconception health care. Am Fam Physician. 2002;65:2507–2514.
9. MRC Vitamin Study Research Group. Prevention of neural tube defects: results of the Medical Research Council Vitamin Study. Lancet 1991;338:131–137.
10. Lumley J, Watson L, Watson M, Bower C. Periconceptual supplementation with folate and/or multivitamins for preventing neural tube defects. Cochrane Database Systematic Reviews 2002; Issue 3.
11. Dugdale M. Anemia. Obstet Gynecol Clin North Am. 2001; 28:363–381.
12. Grody WW, Cutting G, Klinger K, et al. Laboratory standards and guidelines for population-based cystic fibrosis carrier screening. Genet Med. 2001;3:149–154.
13. Dicker D, Feldberg D, Samuel N, et al. Spontaneous abortion in patients with insulin-dependent diabetes mellitus: the effect of preconceptional diabetic control. Am J Obstet Gynecol. 1988;158:1161–1164.
14. Ray JG, O'Brien TE, Chan WS. Preconception care and the risk of congenital anomalies in the offspring of women with diabetes mellitus: a metaanalysis. QJM: Monthly Journal of the Association of Physicians. 2001;94(8):435–444.
15. Tomson T, Battino D. Teratogenicity of antiepileptic drugs: state of the art. Curr Opin Neurol. 2005;18:135–140.
16. U.S. Department of Health and Human Services. Women and Smoking: A Report of the Surgeon General. Atlanta: Department of Health and Human Services, Centers for Disease Control and Prevention, National Center for Chronic Disease Prevention and Health Promotion, Office on Smoking and Health, 2001. Available at *www.cdc.gov/tobacco/sgr_forwomen/index.htm.* Accessed November 2005.
17. Kahan M, Wilson L, Becker L. Effectiveness of physician-based interventions with problem drinkers: a review. CMAJ. 1995;152:851–859.
18. Floyd RL, Ebrahim SH, Boyle CA, Gould DW. Observations from the CDC. Preventing alcohol-exposed pregnancies among women of childbearing age: the necessity of a preconceptional approach. J Womens Health Gen Based Med. 1999;8:733–736.
19. Pregnant, Substance-Using Women Treatment Improvement Protocol (TIP) Series 2 Guideline 3—Medical Withdrawal From Alcohol; U.S. Department of Health and Human Services and SAMHSA's National Clearinghouse for Alcohol and Drug Information. Available at *http://*

ncadi.samhsa.gov/govpubs/bkd107/2d3.aspx. Accessed January 21, 2006.

20. American Academy of Pediatrics. Poliovirus infections. In: Pickering LK, ed. 2000 Red Book: Report of the Committee on Infectious Diseases, 25th ed. Elk Grove, Ill.: American Academy of Pediatrics, 2000;465–470.

21. Paul M, Schaff E, Nichols M. The roles of clinical assessment, human chorionic gonadotrophin assays, and ultrasonography in medical abortion practice. Am J Obstet Gynecol. 2000; 183(2 Supplement):S34–S43.

22. Taipale P, Hilesma V. Predicting delivery date by ultrasound and last menstrual period in early gestation. Obstet Gynecol. 2001;97:189–194.

23. Hodnett ED. Continuity of caregivers for care during pregnancy and childbirth (Cochrane Review). In : The Cochrane Library, Issue 2, 2004. Chichester, UK: John Wiley and Sons, Ltd.

24. Villar J, Carroli G, Khan-Neelofur D, Piaggio G, Gulmezoglu M. Patterns of routine antenatal care for low-risk pregnancy (Cochrane Review). In: The Cochrane Library, Issue 2, 2004. Chichester, UK: John Wiley and Sons, Ltd.

25. Melvin CL, Dolan-Mullen P, Windsor RA Jr, et al. Recommended cessation counseling for pregnant women who smoke: a review of the evidence. Tob Control. 2000;9(suppl 3):11180–11184.

26. ACOG Committee. Smoking cessation during pregnancy. Opinion No. 316. American College of Obstetricians and Gynecologists. Obstet Gynecol. 2005;106:883–888.

27. Treatment of periodontitis curbs preterm births. Fam Pract News. 2003;33:26.

28. National Collaborating Centre for Women's and Children's Health. Antenatal care: routine care for the healthy prenatal woman. Clinical Guideline October 2003; Royal College of Obstetricians and Gynecologists. Available at http://www.vcog.org.uk/resources/Public/Antenatal_care.pdf. Accessed August 2005.

29. Blackadar CS, Viera AJ. A retrospective review of performance and utility of routine clinical pelvimetry. Fam Med. 2004;36(7):505–507.

30. Pattison RC. Pelvimetry for fetal cephalic presentations at term. Cochrane Database Syst Rev. 2003; CD 00161.

31. Institute for Clinical Systems Improvement (ICSI). Routine prenatal care. Bloomington (MN): Institute for Clinical Systems Improvement (ICSI): 2004 Jul. 74 pages.

32. Veterans Health Administration, Department of Defense. DoD/VA clinical practice guideline for the management of uncomplicated pregnancy. Washington, DC: Department of Veteran Affairs; 2002 Oct.

33. Mollison PL, Engelfriet CR, Contreras M. Chapter 2: Transfusion in oligaemia. In Blood Transfusion in Clinical Medicine, 9th ed. Boston: Blackwell Scientific, 1987;48–75.

34. Dorfman DH, Glaser JH. Congenital syphilis presenting in infants after the newborn period. N Engl J Med. 1990;323: 1299–1302.

35. Graves JC, Sellers AD. Preconceptual and prenatal care. Clin Fam Pract. 2000; 2:467–483

36. Boucher M, Gruslin A. SOGC clinical practice guidelines: the reproductive care of women living with hepatitis C infection. Available at http://sogc.medical.org/sogcnet/sogcdocs/common/guide/pdfs/ps96.pdf. Accessed October 2005.

37. Goldenberg RL, Klebanoff MA, Nugent R, et al. Bacterial colonization of the vagina during pregnancy in four ethnic groups: vaginal infections and prematurity study group. Am J Obstet Gynecol. 1996;174:1618–1621.

38. McDonald H, Brocklehurst P, Parsons J. Antibiotics for treating bacterial vaginosis in pregnancy (Cochrane Review). In:

The Cochrane Library, Issue 1, 2005. Chichester, UK: John Wiley and Sons, Ltd.

39. Conner EM, Sperling RS, Gelber R, et al. Reduction of maternal-infant transmission of human immunodeficiency virus type 1 with zidovudine treatment. AIDS Clinical Trials Group Protocol 076 Study Group. N Engl J Med. 1994;331: 1173–1180.

40. Kotler DP. Human immunodeficiency virus and pregnancy. Gastroenterol Clin North Am. 2003;32:437–448.

41. Ewigman BG, Crane JP, Frigoletto FD, et al. Effect of prenatal ultrasound screening on perinatal outcome. RADIUS Study Group. N Engl J Med. 1993;329:821–827.

42. Neilson JP. Ultrasound for fetal assessment in early pregnancy. The Cochrane Database of Systematic Reviews 2005 Issue 3. The Cochrane Collaboration. Chichester, UK: John Wiley and Sons, Ltd.

43. American College of Obstetricians and Gynecologists; Nonmedical use of obstetric ultrasonography. ACOG Committee Opinion No. 297; 2004 Aug;104(2).

44. American College of Obstetricians and Gynecologists Committee on Practice Bulletins- Obstetrics. ACOG Practice Bulletin. Clinical Management Guidelines for Obstetrician-Gynecologists. Prenatal diagnosis of fetal chromosomal abnormalities. Obstet Gynecol. 2001; 97:suppl:1–12.

45. Kramer MS. High protein supplementation in pregnancy. Cochrane Database Systemic Reviews. 2000; CD 000105 [Review].

46. Bothwell T. Iron requirements in pregnancy and strategies to meet them Am J Clin Nutr. 2000;72:257–264.

47. Mahomed K. Iron and folate supplementation in pregnancy (Cochrane review). In: The Cochrane Library, Issue 1, 2005. Chichester, UK. John Wiley and Sons, Ltd.

48. Atallah AN, Hofmeyr GJ, Duley L. Calcium supplementation during pregnancy for preventing hypertensive disorders and related problems. The Cochrane Database of Systematic Reviews Issue 2, 2005. The Cochrane Collaboration. Published by John Wiley & Sons, Ltd.

49. U.S. Food and Drug Administration. Draft advice for women who are pregnant, or who might become pregnant, and nursing mothers, about avoiding harm to your baby or young child from mercury in fish and shellfish. Available at: http://www.cfsan.fda.gov/~dms/admehg.html. Accessed October 2005.

50. Signorello, L, McLaughlin J. Maternal caffeine consumption and spontaneous abortion: a review of the epidemiologic evidence. Epidemiology. 2004 Mar;15(2):229–239.

51. Tyroch, AH, Kaups KL, Rohan J, Song S, Beingesser K. Pregnant women and car restraints: belief and practices. J Trauma Infect Crit Care. 1999;46(2):241–245.

52. Carroli GC, Villar J, Piaggio G, et al. WHO systematic review of randomized controlled trials of routine antenatal care. Lancet. 2001;357:1565–70.

53. Bianco AT, Smilen SW, Davis Y, et al. Pregnancy outcome and weight gain recommendations for the morbidly obese woman. Obstet Gynecol. 1998;91:97–102.

54. Coustan D. Gestational diabetes: Chapter 35; accessed at http://www.hawaii.edu/hivandaids/Gestational%20Diabetes.pdf on January 26, 2006.

55. Walkinshaw SA. Dietary regulation for 'gestational diabetes.' Cochrane Database of Systematic Reviews. 2000;(2).

56. Kirkham C, Harris S, Grzybowksi S. Evidence-based prenatal care: Part II. Third-trimester care and prevention of infectious diseases. Am Fam Physician. 2005;71(8):1555–1560.

57. ACOG Practice Bulletin. Management of herpes in pregnancy. Number 8 October 1999. Clinical management guidelines for obstetrician-gynecologists. Int J Gynaecol Obstet. 2000;68:165–173.

58. Dyson L, McCormick F, Renfrew MJ. Interventions for promoting the initiation of breastfeeding. Cochrane Database of Systemic Reviews. 4, 2005.

59. Natl Vital Stat Rep 2003; 51:1–20. Available at http:/www.cdc.gov/nchs/nvss.htm

60. American Academy of Family Physicians. Trial of labor after cesarean (TOLAC), formerly trial of labor versus elective repeat cesarean section for the woman with a previous cesarean section. AAFP; March 2005.

61. Briscoe D, Nguyen H, Mencer M et al. Management of pregnancy beyond 40 weeks' gestation. Am Fam Physician. 2005; 71(10):1935–1939.

62. Crowley P. Interventions for preventing or improving the outcome of delivery at or beyond term. Cochrane Database Syst Rev. 2004;(3): CD000170.

63. ACOG Practice Bulletin. Anterpartum fetal surveillance. No 9, October 1999. Clinical management guidelines for obstetrician-gynecologists. Int J Gynaecol Obstet. 2000;68: 175–85.

64. Larimore W, Sapolsky B. Maternity care in family medicine: economics and malpractice. J Fam Pract. 1995;40:153–160.

65. The American Academy of Family Physicians and the American College of Obstetricians and Gynecologists. AAFP-ACOG Liaison Committee position statement on consultations and referrals. Available at *www.aafp.org*. Accessed December 2005.

CHAPTER 5

Well Child and Adolescent Care

Beat Steiner

KEY CLINICAL QUESTIONS

1. What screening tests are recommended for a 4-year-old child who comes for a well child visit?
2. What information should be provided to patients and parents when discussing the risks and benefits of the immunizations that are given to a 6-month-old child?
3. What health-related behavior can physicians expect to influence most when seeing adolescent patients in the office?

BACKGROUND

Despite the proven long- and short-term benefits of preventive efforts during childhood and adolescence, they are frequently not put into practice. Several studies have investigated why preventive services delivery rates are less than optimal. The most common barriers identified are lack of time during the office visit, inadequate insurance reimbursement, patient refusal to discuss or comply with recommendations, and lack of physician expertise in counseling techniques (1). To overcome these obstacles and provide effective well child care, clinicians should find efficient and innovative ways to incorporate prevention into the routine of a busy day. Some specific strategies to accomplish this are discussed below.

Improving Delivery of Preventive Services

Establish rapport with both the child and the parent early in the visit. Spend a minute interacting with the child as you enter the exam room. When the child is young, much of the communication will be with the parent. But unless trust is established with the child, the parent is less likely to trust your messages of prevention.

During the physical exam, do not approach the child too quickly. To build confidence and allay fears, the least invasive (or least painful) parts of the examination should be done first. Let the child touch the stethoscope. You might even listen to the parent's heart first. Attention to such details allows you to perform a more accurate physical exam.

In older children, seek an appropriate balance between the increased independence of the child and the role of the parent. With the parent present, a 6-year-old child can give much of the history. A 9- or 10-year-old child should be offered the opportunity to be alone with the physician for at least part of the visit. With adolescents, most of the visit will occur without the parent in the room, but the concerns of the parents should still be elicited. This progression allows young patients to gain ownership of their own health.

Incorporate small pieces of well child care into acute care visits. Many patients, especially adolescents, seek help only when there is a problem. Acute care visits may be the only opportunity for preventive care.

Methods that go beyond the physician-patient interaction must also be used if preventive services are to be implemented effectively. It has been estimated that a family physician caring for a typical panel of patients would need 7.4 hours a day just to provide the preventive services recommended by the United States Preventive Services Task Force (USPSTF) (1). Physicians must make more effective use of innovative practice models such as group visits and telephone consultations. Using electronic health records with preventive services prompts will make them more efficient. Physicians must also learn to take advantage of different forms of communication such as the internet and electronic mail. And perhaps most importantly, physicians must learn to work more effectively with the remainder of the health care team including nurses, health educators and others. Delivery of preventive services through new models of practice, new media, and other health professionals is an exciting challenge, but will require substantial changes in the way medicine is practiced including changes in the current system of reimbursement.

Preventive services, whether they are delivered in a well child visit, incorporated in an acute care visit, or delivered in an innovative new way, should address three major areas: screening, immunization, and counseling. This chapter examines each of these three areas as they apply to children and adolescents, emphasizing services that have been found to be effective. Unless otherwise referenced, evidence presented in this chapter comes from the USPTF. The latest version of these guidelines can be found at *http://www.ahrq.gov/clinic/uspstfix.htm*.

SCREENING

Recommended screening tests for children and adolescents are listed in Table 5.1. A clinician should also remain alert for conditions listed in Table 5.2, but realize that no effective screening tests exist to discover these conditions in asymptomatic individuals.

Screening Newborns

The profound, irreversible effects of unrecognized hypothyroidism and phenylketonuria, as well as the documented benefits of early treatment, have led states to require that all newborns be screened for these disorders before discharge from the hospital. Other conditions are included in mandatory new-

TABLE 5.1 Screening Recommendations for Children and Adolescents

Age	Screening Test	Comments	Level of Evidence for Effectiveness*
All children	Height, weight, head circumference, developmental screen	The optimal frequency has not been defined.	B
	Blood pressure, auscultation of heart (in children) and palpation of femoral pulses (in newborns)	The optimal frequency has not been defined; accurate blood pressure measurements are particularly difficult in children < 3 years of age	B
	Mantoux test (using PPD) for TB	Screen only high-risk groups†; start screening at 12–15 months of age	B
Newborn	Newborn screen content varies by state	Repeat TSH, PKU at 2 weeks of age if tested before 24 hours of life	A
	Red Reflex	Unknown test characteristics	
6–12 mo	Hemoglobin or hematocrit	Screen only high-risk groups*	B
	Blood-lead concentration	Screen only high-risk groups*	B
3–5 yr	Vision screening for amblyopia and strabismus	Use cover-uncover test or Random Dot E; screening before age 3	B
Adolescents	Gonorrhea, Syphilis	Screen high-risk group*	B
	HIV	All adolescents >13 y.o. if sexually active	B
	Pap smear, chlamydia (female only)	Screen if sexually active*	A

Data from US Preventive Services Task Force. Guide to Clinical Preventive Services. *http://www.ahrq.gov/clinic/uspstf/uspstopics.htm*
PKU, phenylketonuria; TSH, thyroid-stimulating hormone; PPD, purified protein derivative; HIV, human immunodeficiency virus.
*Level of evidence for effectiveness: A, strong or moderate research-based evidence (consistent across several studies, including at least two randomized controlled trials); B, limited research-based evidence (less consistent or extensive evidence, but preponderance of evidence supports use of treatment); C, common practice with little or no research-based evidence; X, moderate or strong evidence suggesting that this intervention is not effective.
†High risk for anemia: low income populations, immigrants from developing countries, premature and low birth-weight infants
High risk for lead: persons living in communities where prevalence of elevated lead levels is high, living in houses built before 1950 with dilapidated paint or undergoing recent renovation, or living with someone whose hobby involves lead exposure such as stained glass work or metal sculpture.
High risk for TB: persons infected with HIV, close contacts of persons with known or suspected tuberculosis, immigrants from countries with high tuberculosis prevalence, and medically underserved populations including the homeless
High Risk for STD: men who have had sex with men; men and women having unprotected sex with multiple partners; past or present injection drug users; men and women who exchange sex for money or drugs or have sex partners who do; individuals whose past or present sex partners were HIV-infected, bisexual, or injection drug users; persons being treated for sexually transmitted infections and persons requesting an HIV test

born screening on a state-by-state basis. You can read about these conditions at this Web site: *http://www.aboutnewborn screening.com/stats.htm*. Some states screen for as few as four disorders and others for as many as 36, so you should become familiar with the characteristics of the screening tests that are used in the state in which you practice. Almost all states provide education on their newborn screening program for parents and providers, but fewer than one-fourth inform parents of their option to obtain tests for additional disorders not included in the state's program. Also, most states do not require parental consent prior to screening, but do allow exemption for religious and other reasons (2). Infants discharged at less than 24 hours of age should have testing repeated by 2 weeks of age, because of the greater possibility of false-negative results in the immediate postpartum period.

Congenital heart disease has an incidence of approximately 1% of births and accounts for half of all deaths due to congenital defects. Most cases can be detected in the first 6 months of life. Although not specifically evaluated by the *Guide to Clinical Preventive Services* as a screening test, most clinicians advise auscultation of the heart and palpation of pulses (including femoral pulses) during the newborn period, and at least twice in the first 6 months to detect asymptomatic septal defects and aortic coarctation.

Screening Infants and Children
IRON DEFICIENCY ANEMIA (HEMOGLOBIN OR HEMATOCRIT)

Iron deficiency anemia in infancy and early childhood has been associated with delayed growth and development and is reversible with adequate supplementation (note that the criteria for anemia in children are age dependent). In children with significant iron deficiency anemia, the effects of treatment are dramatic. Screening for and treating milder iron deficiency anemia remains more controversial. Hemoglobin as a screening tool for detecting iron deficiency in toddlers in the United States seems to lack sensitivity and specificity, and treating anemia found with such screening may not be beneficial (3). Universal supplementation with multivitamins and iron for high risk infants (e.g., low-income populations, immigrants from developing countries, premature and low-birth-weight

TABLE 5.2	Conditions for Which Universal Screening Is Not Recommended but Clinicians Should Remain Alert
Age	**Condition**
All children	Evidence of early childhood caries Dental crowding or misalignment
Children less than 3 years of age	Symptoms and signs of hip instability or dislocation Congenital heart disease Undescended testes Signs of ocular misalignment Symptoms and signs of hearing impairment
Children and adolescents	Family violence Hyperlipidemia Exercise-induced asthma Visual acuity
Adolescents	Depressive symptoms Large spinal curvatures

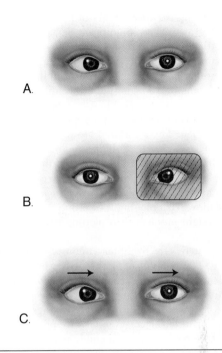

Figure 5.1 • Demonstration of cover-uncover test on child with nonparalytic right monoccular esotropia. **A.** Examiner shines light in child's eyes, asking child to focus on light. *Corneal reflections not symmetrical.* **B.** Examiner covers left eye while still asking child to focus on light. *Right eye (weaker eye) moves to fix on light.* **C.** Examiner uncovers left eye while still asking child to focus on light. *The left eye (good eye) is uncovered and "takes over" and fixes on light. Right eye moves inward again.* From Bickley LS, Szilagyi P. Bates' Guide to Physical Examination and History Taking, 8th ed. Philadelphia: Lippincott Williams & Wilkins, 2003.

infants), may turn out to be more effective (4). Primary preventive strategies require further studies and the USPSTF guidelines continue to recommend screening high risk infants with a hematocrit or hemoglobin between the ages of 6 to 12 months.

LEAD TOXICITY (BLOOD LEAD CONCENTRATION)

Low-level lead toxicity (serum levels of 10 to 25 mg/dL) can lead to subtle effects on behavior, cognition, sleep patterns, and growth rate and eliminating such elevations is one of the national health objectives of 2010 (5). Over the past decade, blood levels have decreased dramatically but it is still estimated that over 300,000 children aged 1–5 years remain at risk for exposure to harmful lead levels (6). Elevated levels remain more common in children living: 1. in communities where prevalence of elevated lead levels is high, 2. in houses built before 1950 with dilapidated paint or undergoing recent renovation, 3. with someone whose hobby involves lead exposure such as stained glass work or metal sculpture. Children given food supplements contaminated by lead or eating off pottery containing lead are also at risk. This is seen more commonly in recent immigrants, especially from Latin American countries. It remains controversial if reduction in blood lead levels leads to clinical improvement (behavior, cognition) in children with low to moderate levels of lead intoxication. Environmental lead abatement programs do reduce risk of exposure for other children. Thus, children belonging to high-risk subgroups should be screened at approximately 12 months of age.

VISION SCREENING

The eye examination of the newborn and infant less than 4 months of age screens for congenital cataracts and ocular tumors such as retinoblastoma. A normal red reflex test should reveal identical, simultaneous red images; asymmetry indi-

cates either a problem with light transmission through the eye or a retinal defect.

In children under the age of 5 years, the aim is to identify children with strabismus. Between ages 3 and 5 years, stereograms such as Random Dot E can be used (sensitivity of 54%–64% and specificity of 87%–90%). The cover-uncover test (Figure 5.1) can be more easily performed because no special equipment is needed, but its test characteristics remain unknown. Using these screening tools for children aged less than 3 years has generally been unsuccessful.

There appear to be no significant benefits of finding asymptomatic refractive errors with screening tests. As pointed out in Table 5.2, however, clinicians should ask parents and children if they have concerns about vision (e.g., trouble seeing letters on the board in class, reading billboards, reading or drawing).

Screening Children and Adolescents
GROWTH

Inadequate growth may be the presenting feature of a variety of disorders, such as endocrinopathies, cardiac diseases, and renal dysfunction but is more commonly a result of poor psychosocial support and family dysfunction. Height, weight, and head circumference should be measured during all routine office visits during the first 2 years of life and plotted on a standardized growth chart. Significant deviations are worrisome. After that, only height and weight need to be plotted, as head circumference is 90% completed by age 2.

On the other end of the spectrum, childhood obesity is rapidly developing into a major public health problem. Based on definitions by the Centers for Disease Control (CDC), 15% of children are overweight, a number more than three times as high as in 1980. These children are more likely to suffer socially, and have increased morbidity and mortality as adults. Unlike adult BMI, normal BMI varies with age and thus should be plotted on norm referenced charts at each visit. Such charts are available at *http://www.cdc.gov/growthcharts/*. A study has shown that plotting BMI prompted greater recognition of a weight problem than plotting height and weight (7).

Unfortunately, effective interventions continue to elude us. The USPSTF and a recent Cochrane Review found insufficient evidence for the effectiveness of behavioral counseling (or other preventive interventions with overweight children that can be conducted in primary care settings) (8). It may require broader societal changes in how we prepare and serve food and where we live (i.e., can children walk to school) to affect a significant change in obesity. But as with substance abuse, the scope of the problem makes it reasonable to address during office visits even in the absence of solid evidence.

DEVELOPMENT

Development can be monitored by documenting achievement of age-appropriate milestones for intellectual, motor, and social skills. Early intervention has been shown to be effective in children with developmental delays. Unfortunately, clinical assessment alone detects <30% of children with developmental disabilities. Standardized developmental screening instruments such as Denver-II screening test, Battelle Developmental Inventory, and others, are more sensitive. Parent report instruments, such as the Parents' Evaluation of Developmental Status and Child Development Inventories, can be similarly effective and require much less physician time (9).

Sexual development should also be assessed. A recent large cross-sectional study suggests that sexual development occurs earlier in girls than reported by many text books (10) (Table 5.3). Such a well-designed study does not exist for boys, but it is generally reported that the first physical manifestation

for boys is enlargement of testes, which occurs at about age 11. A pronounced growth spurt is also associated with onset of puberty (about 1 year after onset of breast bud development in girls, and 2 years after onset of genital enlargement in boys).

HYPERTENSION AND HEART DISEASE

Hypertension is rare in children. However, a relatively high proportion of children with hypertension have secondary, potentially curable forms. Thus, there is a general consensus that blood pressure should be measured periodically in children and adolescents. No good evidence exists for when measurement should first occur and at what intervals it should be repeated. Guided by how well children can cooperate and the tradition of the annual examination, many clinicians first check blood pressures when a child is 3 years old and repeat these measurements annually. Blood pressure measurements should be taken bilaterally using a cuff of correct width (two-thirds of upper arm length). An undersized cuff will give a falsely elevated reading. Criteria for childhood hypertension vary with age, but in general a blood pressure greater than the 95th percentile for that age group is diagnostic (Table 5.4). As in adults, elevated blood pressure should be confirmed on at least three separate occasions.

TUBERCULOSIS

The annual incidence of tuberculosis in children declined by nearly 50% in the United States between 1993 and 2001, to 1.5 cases/100,000. Certain subgroups, however, remain at much higher risk and should be screened as discussed below. Screening is performed with the Mantoux test in which purified protein derivative (PPD) is injected intradermally. When administered properly, the sensitivity of the test is between 90% and 95%. Induration of 10 mm constitutes a positive test for high-risk individuals and children less than 4 years of age. Induration of 15 mm for low-risk individuals is assumed to be specific for tuberculous infection (note that it is important to measure induration and not just erythema). If the test is positive, chemoprophylaxis is recommended to prevent subsequent development of active tuberculosis in an asymptomatic child (11). The true specificity of the test, however, remains poorly defined because there is no reliable gold standard for latent infection.

TABLE 5.3 Mean Age of Onset of Puberty in Girls

	Caucasian	African-American
Breast development	10 years	8.9 years
Growth of pubic hair	10.5 years	8.8 years
Onset of menses	12.9 years	12 years

Adapted from Herman-Giddens ME et al. Secondary sexual characteristics and menses in young girls seen in office practice: a study from the Pediatric Research In Office Setting network. Pediatrics. 1997;99(4):505–512.

TABLE 5.4 95th Percentile Cutoff for Blood Pressure by Age and Gender

Age	Male	Female
2 years	106/61	105/62
4 years	111/68	108/69
6 years	114/74	111/73
8 years	116/77	115/75
10 years	119/80	119/78
12 years	123/81	123/80
14 years	128/82	126/83
16 years	130/85	128/84

Cutoffs given for children at 50% for height. In general, add 3–4 points to systolic values and 2–3 points for diastolic values for children at 95% for height.

False-positive reactions do occur with atypical mycobacteria infection, previous bacille Calmette-Guérin (BCG) vaccination, and hypersensitivity reaction. Because of false-positive results and the cost, potential toxicity, and inconvenience of INH, screening is recommended only in high risk groups. This includes persons infected with human immunodeficiency virus (HIV), close contacts of persons with known or suspected tuberculosis, immigrants from countries with high tuberculosis prevalence, and medically underserved populations including the homeless. Screening should begin at 12–15 months of age and be repeated annually or biannually if the child or adolescent remains in a high-risk group. Any child or adolescent found to have active tuberculosis should also be tested for HIV infection.

Screening Adolescents
SEXUALLY TRANSMITTED INFECTIONS AND CERVICAL DYSPLASIA

Clinicians frequently forget to think about sexual activity in young adolescents but by ninth grade 37% of males and 29% of females are sexually active (12). These youth are disproportionately affected by chlamydia, *Neisseria gonorrhea*, and other sexually transmitted infections. Asymptomatic carrier states are common and associated morbidity is high. Infection may also be a cofactor in the heterosexual transmission of HIV.

A number of tests exist to screen for chlamydia and gonorrhea, including cultures, direct fluorescent antibody testing, unamplified nucleic acid hybridization, and enzyme immunoassay performed on endocervical, rectal or urethral sample. Urine can also be used as a more convenient but more expensive test using nucleic acid amplification.

All sexually active female adolescents should be screened annually for chlamydia and gonorrhea. There is insufficient evidence to recommend for or against screening asymptomatic males. High-risk adolescents of both sexes should also be screened for syphilis. High risk is defined using epidemiologic data and includes: men who have had sex with men, men and women having unprotected sex with multiple partners, past or present injection drug users, men and women who exchange sex for money or drugs or have sex partners who do, individuals whose past or present sex partners were HIV-infected, bisexual, or injection drug users, persons being treated for sexually transmitted infections, and persons requesting an HIV test. In 2006, the CDC revised its policy on HIV screening. Instead of screening only high-risk individuals, the CDC now recommends diagnostic HIV testing and opt-out HIV screening as a part of routine clinical care in all health-care settings for adolescents and adults age 13–64.

Finally, clinicians should also remember that adolescent females who are sexually active should have routine Papanicolaou (Pap) smears. This same group of patients is at risk for unintended pregnancy and should be counseled accordingly (see Chapter 33, Sexually Transmitted Infections).

SUBSTANCE ABUSE

Three-quarters of young adolescents have tried alcohol at least once. Furthermore, 19% of 9th graders and 37% of 12th graders reported binge drinking (five or more drinks on one occasion) in the past month (12). Alcohol is also involved in half of all adolescent deaths due to motor vehicle crashes, other unintentional injuries, suicides, and homicides. The burden of suffering of alcohol abuse, the sensitivity of simple screening questions such as the CAGE questionnaire, and the availability of alcohol abuse treatment resources makes this an important topic to address with all adolescents. While the USPSTF still finds insufficient evidence to recommend screening and counseling of adolescents on alcohol use, the magnitude of this problem and the associated serious health consequences make this a reasonable topic to discuss during the visit. Screening instruments such as the CAGE can also be incorporated into a standard review of systems form to be completed by the adolescents and then discussed at the visit. While there is even less evidence to support screening and counseling against use of other illegal drugs, once the physician begins to discuss alcohol use, it is relatively easy to transition the conversation to use of other illegal drugs.

SUICIDE AND YOUTH VIOLENCE

Seventeen percent of adolescents report having made a plan to commit suicide and it is the third leading cause of death in persons 15 to 24 years old. Unfortunately, we have not yet found screening tools that show clear benefits when used in asymptomatic adolescents. Youth violence is also increasingly recognized as a major health problem, but again the effectiveness of screening remains unproven. Clinicians should, however, remain keenly alert for signs and symptoms of depression, problems with drugs or alcohol, a history of violent or criminal behavior, and the availability of weapons in the home. Prevalence rates for these risk behaviors come in large part from the Youth Behavior Risk Survey. Updated results can be found online at *www.cdc.gov/nccdphp/dash/yrbs/*.

Screening Examinations and Laboratory Tests for Which Insufficient Evidence Exists

A number of screening procedures for which insufficient outcomes-based evidence exists have also been traditionally incorporated into well child checks. Because there are many components of the well child visit in which supporting evidence is much stronger, a case can be made that these traditional elements of the well child exam should be abandoned in favor of activities in which we know we can make a difference. However, because many of these exams are still considered standard of care in many communities, for medicolegal reasons, and because of patient expectations, some clinicians may opt to continue to perform them. Performing such exams may also be useful to strengthen the doctor-patient relationship through the laying on of hands.

The Ortolani-Barlow maneuver in the newborn period screens for developmental dysplasia of the hip (1.5 per thousand births). A testicular exam in the infants may identify cryptorchidism (1% of male toddlers) requiring surgical correction. A thorough abdominal exam in children less than 5 years of age may pick up occult abdominal tumors such as neuroblastomas (annual incidence: 7 to 10 cases per million) or Wilms' tumor (annual incidence: 7 cases per million). Examining the back in adolescents can identify large curvatures that require surgical treatment, although such severe scoliosis is rare and is usually brought to the attention of the clinician by the patient or the parent.

Routine urine dipstick testing of school-aged children is not supported by evidence because of the low prevalence of asymptomatic disease and the high proportion of false-positive tests. There is also insufficient evidence for routine cholesterol screening. The American Academy of Pediatrics (AAP) does suggest screening children with family histories of premature heart disease.

IMMUNIZATIONS

Immunization has probably saved more lives than any other public health intervention, with the possible exception of providing clean water (13). Although U.S. childhood immunization rates have risen over the past 2 decades, disparities continue, with lower rates among children living in poverty, among urban children, and among black and Hispanic children (14). Clinicians should withhold immunizations only for true contraindications (Table 5.5), implement office systems to effectively track immunization status of patients, obtain appropriate informed consent from the patient or the family, use every visit to provide indicated immunizations, and stay current on immunization recommendations.

The immunization schedule recommended by the CDC is shown in Table 5.6. and can be viewed online at *http://www.cdc.gov/nip/recs/child-schedule.htm.* Clinicians should be aware that this schedule has changed a number of times during the past decade and is likely to continue to change as new and more effective vaccines are introduced. Vaccines for certain high-risk populations are numerous (e.g., respiratory syncytial virus, rabies, Lyme disease, etc) and are not further discussed in this chapter. The remainder of this section addresses vaccine safety and specific commonly used vaccines; unless otherwise noted, the recommendations are consistent with those of the AAFP/AAP task forces above and the USPSTF.

Vaccine Safety

In recent years, an increasing number of articles in parent magazines and Web site postings have begun to question the safety of the vaccine programs. Do vaccines cause autism, sudden infant death syndrome (SIDS), seizures, encephalitis and other neurologic problems? The evidence-based answer is consistently no. While large and systematic analysis of the data have consistently found no links to such adverse effects, clinicians must take the time to address these questions and use available scientific knowledge to help parents make informed decisions.

The Institute of Medicine has released a comprehensive series of reports over the past 5 years that examine adverse effects of the major vaccines and may be used as an evidence-based reference when discussing this topic with concerned parents (15) (the full text can be found online at *http://www.iom.edu/*). Two other websites, one maintained by Johns Hopkins School of Public Health (*http://www.vaccinesafety.edu/*) and one maintained by the Immunization Action Coalition (*http://www.immunize.com*), provide regularly updated advice on how to answer many of these safety concerns. Highlights from these sources and from package inserts of individual vaccines are discussed in further detail below. Clinicians should not rely on these summaries alone, but should also read the inserts carefully.

Thiomeresol in particular has received much attention recently. This preservative has been used in vaccines since the 1930s and contains traces of mercury. In a review of all available data, the Institute of Medicine found that there are inadequate data to make a conclusion for or against any adverse side effects of thiomeresol. Nevertheless, a thiomeresol-free version of all vaccines given to children under 6 years of age is now available.

Individual Immunizations
DIPHTERIA, TETANUS, PERTUSSIS VACCINE (DTP)

Guillain-Barre syndrome, brachial neuritis, acute encephalopathy, and hyporesponive episodes have been weakly linked to the old pertussis vaccine. Cases were rare (on the order of 1–10 cases per 1 million vaccines) and most of the evidence comes from case reports and uncontrolled studies. To address these concerns, the acellular pertussis antigen (DTaP) is now being used. Even with the newer formulation, anaphylaxis has been reported, and patients with hypersensitivity reactions to components of the vaccine should avoid the vaccine. Minor

TABLE 5.5 Contraindications and Precautions for Childhood Immunizations

True Contraindications and Precautions	Not True Contraindications (Vaccines May Be Given)
Anaphylactic reaction to vaccine	Mild to moderate local reactions (soreness, redness, swelling) following a dose of injectable vaccine
Moderate or severe acute illness following a dose of an injectable vaccine	Mild acute illness with or without low-grade fever
Known hypersensitivity to component of vaccine	Current antimicrobial therapy
Moderate or severe acute illness as it may be difficult to identify subsequent reactions from immunization	Convalescent phase of illness
	Prematurity (same schedule and indications as full-term infants)
Pregnancy in vaccine recipient (certain vaccines only)	Recent exposure to an infectious agent
	History of penicillin or other nonspecific allergies in child or any allergy in a relative

Adapted from American Academy of Pediatrics. Guide to Contraindications and Precautions to Immunizations, 2003. Red Book. 2003:798–801.

TABLE 5.6 Recommended Childhood and Adolescent Immunization Schedule
(Based on 2007 CDC Recommendations)

Vaccine \ Age	Birth	1 month	2 months	4 months	6 months	12 months	15 months	18 months	24 months	4-6 years	11-12 years	13-14 years	15 years	16-18 years
Pediarix [1]			Pediarix*	Pediarix*	Pediarix*									
Hepatitis B [2]	HepB	HepB**	HepB**	HepB**[1]		HepB**								
Diphtheria, Tetanus, Pertussis [3]			DTaP**	DTaP**	DTaP**			DTaP		DTaP	Tdap			
Inactivated Poliovirus			IPV**	IPV**	IPV**		IPV**			IPV				
Haemophilus influenzae type b [4]			Hib	Hib	Hib [3]		Hib							
Measles, Mumps, Rubella [5]							MMR			MMR				
HPV [6]											HPV(1-3)			
Rotavirus [7]			Rota	Rota	Rota									
Varicella [8]						Varicella	Varicella			Varicella				
Meningococcal [9]									MPSV4		MCV4			MCV4
Pneumococcal [10]			PCV	PCV	PCV	PCV	PCV				PPV			
Influenza [11]						Influenza (Yearly)					Influenza (Yearly)			
Hepatitis A [12]										HepA Series				

** These vaccines should not be given if Pediarix is used.

Vaccines within broken line are for selected populations

Range of recommended ages

11-12 year old assessment

(continued)

TABLE 5.6 *(Continued)*

1. *Pediarix* includes DTaP, IPV, and HepB for 2, 4, and 6 months. If these shots are begun individually, Pediarix should not be given. HepB #1 is not included in Pediarix and should be given at the hospital.

2. *Hepatitis B vaccine (HepB).* (Minimum age: birth)
   At birth:
   • Administer monovalent HepB to all newborns before hospital discharge.
   • If mother is hepatitis surface antigen (HBsAg)-positive, administer HepB and 0.5 mL of hepatitis B immune globulin (HBIG) within 12 hours of birth.
   • If mother's HBsAg status is unknown, administer HepB within 12 hours of birth. Determine the HBsAg status as soon as possible and if HBsAg-positive, administer HBIG (no later than age 1 week).
   • If mother is HBsAg-negative, the birth dose can only be delayed with physician's order and mother's negative HBsAg laboratory report documented in the infant's medical record.
   After the birth dose:
   • The HepB series should be completed with either monovalent HepB or a combination vaccine containing HepB. The second dose should be administered at age 1–2 months. The final dose should be administered at age ≥24 weeks. Infants born to HBsAg-positive mothers should be tested for HBsAg and antibody to HBsAg after completion of ≥3 doses of a licensed HepB series, at age 9–18 months (generally at the next well-child visit).
   4-month dose:
   • It is permissible to administer 4 doses of HepB when combination vaccines are administered after the birth dose. If monovalent HepB is used for doses after the birth dose, a dose at age 4 months is not needed.

3. *Diphtheria and tetanus toxoids and acellular pertussis vaccine (DTaP).* The fourth dose of DTaP may be administered as early as age 12 months, provided 6 months have elapsed since the third dose and the child is unlikely to return at age 15–18 months. The final dose in the series should be given at age ≥4 years.   Tetanus and diphtheria toxoids and acellular pertussis vaccine (Tdap – adolescent preparation) is recommended at age 11–12 years for those who have completed the recommended childhood DTP/DTaP vaccination series and have not received a Td booster dose. Adolescents 13–18 years who missed the 11–12-year Td/Tdap booster dose should also receive a single dose of Tdap if they have completed the recommended childhood DTP/DTaP vaccination series. Subsequent tetanus and diphtheria toxoids (Td) are recommended every 10 years.

4. *Haemophilus influenzae type b conjugate vaccine (Hib).* Minimum age: 6 weeks)
   • If PRP-OMP (PedvaxHIB® or ComVax® [Merck]) is administered at ages 2 and 4 months, a dose at age 6 months is not required.
   • TriHiBit® (DTaP/Hib) combination products should not be used for primary immunization but can be used as boosters following any Hib vaccine in children aged ≥12 months.

5. *Measles, mumps, and rubella vaccine (MMR).* (Minimum age: 12 months)
   Administer the second dose of MMR at age 4–6 years. MMR may be administered before age 4–6 years, provided ≥4 weeks have elapsed since the first dose and both doses are administered at age ≥12 months.

6. *Human Papillomavirus (HPV).* Administer the first dose of the HPV vaccine series to females at age 11-12 years. Administer the second dose 2 months after the first dose and the third dose 6 months after the first dose. Administer the HPV vaccine series to females at age 13-18 years if not previously vaccinated.

7. *Rotavirus.* Administer the first dose at age 6-12 weeks. Do not start the series later than age 12 weeks. Administer the final dose in the series by age 32 weeks. Do not administer a dose later than age 32 weeks. Data on safety and efficacy outside of these age ranges are insufficient.

8. *Varicella.* Administer the second dose of varicella vaccine at age 4-6 years. Varicella vaccine may be administered before age 4-6 years, provided that 3 months or more have elapsed since the first dose and both doses are administered at or after age 12 months. If the second dose was administered more than 28 days following the first dose, the second dose does not need to be repeated.

9. *Meningococcal polysaccharide vaccine (MPSV4).* (Minimum age: 2 years) • Administer MPSV4 to children aged 2–10 years with terminal complement deficiencies or anatomic or functional asplenia and certain other highrisk groups. See MMWR 2005;54(No. RR-7):1–21.

10. *Pneumococcal vaccine.* (Minimum age: 6 weeks for pneumococcal conjugate vaccine [PCV]; 2 years for pneumococcal polysaccharide vaccine [PPV]) • Administer PCV at ages 24–59 months in certain high-risk groups. Administer PPV to children aged ≥2 years in certain high-risk groups. See MMWR 2000;49(No. RR-9):1–35.

11. *Influenza vaccine.* (Minimum age: 6 months for trivalent inactivated influenza vaccine [TIV]; 5 years for live, attenuated influenza vaccine [LAIV]) • All children aged 6–59 months and close contacts of all children aged 0–59 months are recommended to receive influenza vaccine. • Influenza vaccine is recommended annually for children aged ≥59 months with certain risk factors, health-care workers, and other persons (including household members) in close contact with persons in groups at high risk. See MMWR 2006;55(No. RR-10):1–41. • For healthy persons aged 5–49 years, LAIV may be used as an alternative to TIV. • Children receiving TIV should receive 0.25 mL if aged 6–35 months or 0.5 mL if aged ≥3 years. • Children aged <9 years who are receiving influenza vaccine for the first time should receive 2 doses (separated by ≥4 weeks for TIV and ≥6 weeks for LAIV).

12. *Hepatitis A vaccine (HepA).* (Minimum age: 12 months)
   • HepA is recommended for all children aged 1 year (i.e., aged 12–23 months). The 2 doses in the series should be administered at least 6 months apart.
   • Children not fully vaccinated by age 2 years can be vaccinated at subsequent visits.
   • HepA is recommended for certain other groups of children, including in areas where vaccination programs target older children. See MMWR 2006;55(No. RR-7):1–23.

Please access the CDC website (http://www.cdc.gov/hip/recs/child-schedule/htm) for complete and updated recommendations.

side effects are common and should be expected within the first 48 hours. Ten to twenty percent of children will have fever above 38°C but less than 2% will have fever above 39°C. Ten to twenty percent will be fretful or drowsy or have a decreased appetite.

POLIO VACCINE

The live oral polio vaccine (OPV) is highly effective against the poliovirus, but one of 2.5 million vaccinations results in a case of vaccine-induced paralytic poliomyelitis. This concern was allayed with the substitution of the inactivated poliovirus vaccine (IPV) which must be injected. Anaphylaxis has been reported, and patients with hypersensitivity to neomycin, streptomycin, and polymyxin B, as well as other components of the vaccine should avoid the vaccine. Minor adverse side effects are similar to DTaP.

HEPATITIS B

The vaccine is produced by recombinant DNA technology and to date no serious adverse effects have been documented in controlled studies. Anaphylaxis has been reported, and patients with hypersensitivity to yeast and other components of the vaccine should avoid the vaccine. Minor side effects are similar in frequency to DTaP, and IPV.

HAEMOPHILUS INFLUENZAE TYPE B (HiB)

The incidence and type of reactions reported with the combined HiB vaccine is no different from that when DTaP is administered alone. Anaphylaxis has been reported, and patients with hypersensitivity to components of the vaccine should avoid the vaccine.

MEASLES, MUMPS, AND RUBELLA (MMR)

In general, the use of live virus immunizations during pregnancy or in an immunocompromised host carries increased risk for causing clinical disease, and should be avoided. Women should be advised not to become pregnant for 3 months after vaccination. Susceptible immunocompromised hosts and pregnant women can also acquire these infections when a close contact is immunized with a live vaccine, although this risk is largely theoretical. Evidence favors a causal relationship with reversible thrombocytopenia on the order of 1 case per 30,000 to 40,000 vaccinated children. Anaphylaxis has been reported, and patients with hypersensitivity reactions to eggs, neomycin, and other components of the vaccine should avoid the vaccine. There have been reports of subacute sclerosing panencephalitis (SSPE) in patients who had no history of natural measles but who received the vaccine (1 case in 1 million vaccines). Because SSPE is believed to exist only after measles infections, these cases are either vaccine related or due to subclinical measles infection in the first year of life. Minor side effects from live vaccines occur later. Warn parents that the child is likely to experience mild rash, arthralgias, and a low-grade fever 8 to 12 days later.

VARICELLA

Like the MMR vaccine, this is a live vaccine and in general should be avoided in immunocompromised children. Although varicella infection is generally a mild illness, serious complications do occur. Before introduction of the vaccine, about 4 million cases were reported annually. Of these, 10,000

were hospitalized and 100 died. Since the introduction of the vaccine, varicella rates, hospitalizations, and deaths have declined sharply. Minor reactions are similar in frequency reported for other vaccines and similar to other live vaccines; they tend to occur later. Three to five percent of patients develop a mild varicella like rash 5–26 days after immunization. Vaccine-associated viral transmission is rare even with such rashes (three well-documented cases after 4 years and more than 14 million doses of varicella vaccine) (16). There is limited experience regarding the risk of developing herpes zoster after immunization compared with infection with wild strain of varicella, but preliminary studies suggest that the risk will be lower.

INFLUENZA VACCINE (IV)

The most common symptom associated with IV administration is soreness at the injection site. Fever after 6–24 hours occurs in about 10%–35%, especially in children less than 2 years. Nausea, lethargy, headache, muscle aches, and chills also are reported. Immunization of children with asthma does not increase bronchial hyperactivity. Some studies have expressed concern that in children with HIV infection, there might be a transient increase in HIV-1 replication. However, most experts believe that the benefits of influenza immunization outweigh the risks in children with HIV infection. Like MMR, influenza vaccine should not be given to children with allergic reactions to chicken or egg proteins.

MENINGOCOCCAL VACCINE (MCV4)

Side effects have been studied in two randomized controlled trials. Local reactions were common, but severe reactions were rare. Immunization with MCV4 is contraindicated among people known to have hypersensitivity to any component of the vaccine, including diphtheria toxoid, and to dry, natural rubber latex, which is used in the vial stopper.

HPV VACCINE

Released in 2006, Gardasil is the first vaccine developed to prevent cervical cancer, precancerous genital lesions, and genital warts caused by human papilloma virus (HPV). It targets HPV types that cause up to 70% of all cervical cancers and about 90% of genital warts. The series of three immunizations is recommended for girls age 9–26 with a focus on girls 11–12 years of age. At the time of publication, the vaccine is not recommended for boys. It does not contain thimerosal. To date, no serious side effects have been reported.

HEPATITIS A VACCINE

Added in 2006 to the list of vaccines recommended for all children, Hepatitis A vaccine is formalin inactivated. Side effects have been primarily limited to local reactions but anaphylaxis has been reported.

ROTAVIRUS VACCINE

In 2002, the Advisory Committee on Immunization Practices (ACIP) and the CDC recommend a newly licensed vaccine, RotaTeq™, to protect against rotavirus, a viral infection that can cause severe diarrhea, vomiting, fever and dehydration (gastroenteritis) in infants and young children. In 1999, RotaShield®, a different rotavirus vaccine, was withdrawn from the market because it was associated with an increased risk of intussusception. No such association was found with the current vaccine in a large scale trial of more than 70,000 children.

COUNSELING

Counseling, which is the third component of well child care, has a powerful potential for changing behavior and improving the long-term health of the patients. Unfortunately, counseling interventions are time intensive. When time is limited, clinicians should focus first on problems that present a large burden of suffering and where interventions exist that have been proven effective. A limitation to this recommendation is that for many topics we simply do not yet have the studies that examine effectiveness. But based on the most current evidence, a summary of recommended counseling topics is presented in Table 5.7.

A key principle of preventive counseling is patient centeredness. Use language and information that consider the age, educational level, cultural background, and values of the patient. An adolescent may see little relevance to the fact that cigarette smoking can cause lung cancer but may be very concerned that cigarettes are expensive and cause bad breath. The Readiness to Change Model developed by Prochaska and

TABLE 5.7 Counseling for Children and Adolescents

	Counseling Message	Does Health Improve if Behavior Is Changed?*	Does Counseling Help Change Behavior?*
Newborns	Counseling to prevent sudden infant death syndrome		
	Place infant on back to sleep	A	C
	Counseling to promote a healthy diet and breast-feeding	A	C
Children	Counseling to prevent household injuries		
	Smoke detectors	B	B
	Flame-retardant sleepwear	A	B
	Hot water heaters set, 120–130°F	A	B
	Childproof containers for medication	A	B
	Approved bicycle helmets	A	B
	Safe storage of firearms	B	C
	Counseling to prevent dental disease		
	Fluoride supplementation if inadequate in water	A	C
	Regular visits to dentist	B	C
	Regular brushing and flossing	B	C
	Counseling to prevent tobacco use		
	Effects of passive smoking	A	A
Children and adolescents	Counseling to prevent motor vehicle injuries		
	Use child safety seats, lap/shoulder belts	A	B
	Counseling to promote a healthy diet and physical activity		
	Limiting intake of dietary fat	A	C
	Emphasizing products containing fiber	B	C
	Regular physical exercise	A	C
Adolescents	Counseling to prevent tobacco use	A	C
	Counseling to prevent alcohol use	B	C
	Counseling to prevent drug use	B	C
	Counseling to prevent sexually transmitted diseases		
	Abstinence	A	C
	Regular use of condoms	A	C
	Regular use of female barrier methods	B	C
	Counseling to prevent unintended pregnancies		
	Abstinence or regular use of contraceptives	A	B
	Counseling to prevent youth violence		
	Acquisition of problem-solving skills	C	C
	Reduction of heavy or problem drinking	B	C

Data from US Preventive Services Task Force. Guide to Clinical Preventive Services, 3rd ed. Periodic updates at *http://www.ahrq.gov/clinic/gcpspu.htm*.
*Level of evidence for effectiveness: A. strong or moderate research-based evidence (consistent across several studies, including at least two randomized controlled trials); B. limited research- based evidence (less consistent or extensive evidence, but preponderance of evidence supports use of treatment); C, common practice with little or no research-based evidence; X. moderate or strong evidence suggesting that this treatment is not effective.

DiClemente will help you tailor your counseling message appropriately.

Recommended Counseling Measures
PREVENTION OF SUDDEN INFANT DEATH SYNDROME (SIDS)

Although the pathophysiology of SIDS remains largely unknown, a number of studies have helped clinicians provide advice on how to reduce the chance of this devastating event. An association modifiable between SIDS and the child's sleeping position has been found in repeated studies. Children who slept on their stomachs had roughly twice the incidence of SIDS, an association that has prompted multiple organizations to recommend putting healthy children to sleep on their backs (Back to Sleep Campaign) (17). The validity of this recommendation is supported by the decline in the incidence of SIDS since this new sleep position was first advocated.

INJURY PREVENTION

Injuries remain the leading cause of death in children. Motor vehicle injuries are the principal cause during most of childhood and adolescence, accounting for one-third of all deaths in persons between the ages of 15 and 24. Drowning, fires, asphyxiation, unintentional shootings, poisoning, and falls (in that order) cause many of the remaining deaths in youth ages 0 to 19. It remains unclear whether clinician counseling convinces parents to modify hazards that can lead to such injuries. However, the number of children injured by these hazards, the health benefits of such modifications, and the ease with which many of these hazards can be modified likely make brief counseling on these topics (e.g., gun safety, the use of car seats, and the use of bike helmets) an effective use of clinician time.

DENTAL HEALTH

Dental caries and periodontal disease are significant health problems for children. Evidence suggests that people of low socioeconomic status lack adequate knowledge of oral disease prevention. Daily brushing and flossing and frequent exposure to small amounts of fluoride has been proven to be effective. Brushing should start soon after the child has teeth, but toothpaste should not be added until the child is old enough to not swallow the toothpaste. Children living in an area with inadequate water fluoridation and exclusively breast-fed children older than 6 months of age should be supplemented with daily fluoride drops (Table 5.8). Fluoride varnish may prove to be an equally effective alternative option. Routine visits to a dentist have also been shown to improve dental health, although the optimal frequency remains unknown.

DIET AND EXERCISE

Although routine screening for iron deficiency anemia is not recommended, evidence shows that iron-enriched foods should be included in the diet of infants and young children. No restriction of fat and cholesterol is currently recommended for children under age 2. In children over age 2 and adolescents, counseling should focus on limiting dietary intake of fat (<30% of total calories) and cholesterol (<300 g/d), and increasing the intake of fruits, vegetables (>5 servings), and

TABLE 5.8 Daily Fluoride Dosage (mg) According to Age and Water Supply Content*

	Fluoride Concentration in Local Water Supply (ppm)		
Age	0.3	0.3–0.6	0.6
0–6 mo	0	0	0
6 mo–3 yr	0.25	0	0
3–6 yr	0.5	0.25	0
6–16 yr	1.0	0.5	0

Adapted from Centers for Disease Control and Prevention. Recommendations for using fluoride to prevent and control dental caries in the United States. MMWR 2001;50(No. RR-14):16.
ppm, parts per million.
*Water can often be tested for fluoride concentration by the local health department. Although canned or bottled fluids (i.e., ready-to-feed formula or sodas) are generally not fluoridated, fluoride supplementation should be adjusted according to other sources of fluoride that the child is receiving (i.e., drinking fluoridated water while out of the home, fluoride supplementation programs at school, and so forth). All breast-fed babies over the age of 6 months should receive supplementation as well, because fluoride does not enter breast milk in appreciable amounts.

grain products containing fiber (>6 servings). Children and adolescents should also be strongly encouraged to participate in regular physical exercise. These recommendations rest largely on the proven efficacy of dietary modifications and regular physical exercise, not on the proven efficacy of office-based counseling.

TOBACCO, ALCOHOL, AND DRUG USE

Strong evidence shows that brief counseling messages by clinicians can reduce tobacco use. Parents should be urged to stop smoking because of the documented ill effects on health of secondhand smoke. Clinicians should also give anti-tobacco messages to adolescents who smoke. Although the evidence is less strong for alcohol and other drugs, most guidelines urge clinicians to discuss these topics with adolescents. Although a discussion around drugs and alcohol may not change the adolescent's behavior on that visit, it encourages the adolescent to ask questions or raise concerns on that topic on future visits (18).

SEXUAL BEHAVIOR

Discussions should be based on a careful sexual history and tailored to the needs of individuals. As noted earlier, these conversations should take into account the early initiation of sexual activity by many teens. It is not unreasonable to begin these conversations between ages 10–12. Clinicians should discuss measures that can reduce risk, including abstaining from sex, maintaining a mutually faithful relationship with an uninfected partner, consistently using latex condoms, and avoiding sexual contact with casual partners. Other forms of contraception should also be discussed, but clinicians must emphasize that only latex condoms have been shown to effectively prevent transmission of most forms of sexually transmitted infections. Whereas these behavior changes are clearly effective, it remains less clear whether counseling adolescents in the office can bring about such changes.

Counseling for Which Evidence Is Less Available

Most of the evidence on counseling pertains to the behaviors discussed above. But clinicians also spend a large amount of time answering questions on topics that are not usually the subject of rigorous study. This occurs most often in the early years of a child's life and helps parents understand the wide range of normal development. Such counseling also teaches parents what is abnormal and what may require further evaluation. The most frequently raised topics during infancy involve routine care items such as infant stimulation, feeding, sleeping, crying, skin care, and bowel habits.

INFANT STIMULATION

Parents will agree intuitively that stimulation is important to develop an alert and curious infant. Clinicians can play a pivotal role in providing ideas and encouragement. Parents and caregivers can stimulate the infant by talking, reading, and singing. Other ideas include creating a brightly colored environment, periodically changing the location of the bed, rearranging the toys in the crib, hanging attractive mobiles over the crib, dancing, and taking frequent walks with the baby. As the infant grows, early introduction of books in the child's life may improve literacy. One nationwide program that provides children with books early in life is the Reach Out and Read Program. It provides doctors' offices with books at low cost. These books are given during well child visits to children with few books at home. More information about this program can be found at *http://www.reachoutandread.org/*.

FEEDING

There are well-proven benefits to breast-feeding, including improved absorption of calcium, lower risk of allergies, less susceptibility to infections, reduced cost, and quicker recovery from pregnancy. With some important exceptions (e.g., certain maternal infections such as HIV or medications), breast-feeding should be encouraged.

Breast milk or formula should remain the sole dietary source until age 4 to 6 months, when swallowing reflexes and digestive processes are developed enough to begin to handle simple non-liquids such as infant cereal and purified vegetables. Whole milk should not be introduced until age 12 months.

SLEEPING

Infant sleeping patterns vary, with the amount of sleep time generally decreasing from birth through the preschool years. To prevent dental caries, a baby should never be put to bed with a bottle of milk or juice. Sleep location (a crib versus the parents' bed, a separate room versus the parents' room) is controversial, with arguments in favor of all arrangements. Although cultural and personal preferences must be considered, there is evidence from observational studies that sleeping in the parent's bed in rare cases leads to inadvertent smothering when the patient rolls onto the child. The importance of

putting children to sleep on their backs was discussed earlier n the chapter.

CRYING

All babies cry as their primary way of communicating. Crying may signal hunger, a wet diaper, fever, frustration, anger, pain, or the desire for physical contact. Unusual patterns of crying and irritability can signify an illness that may require medical attention.

Repeated crying and irritability during much of the baby's waking hours is often referred to as colic. The cause of this syndrome is unknown, but family turmoil or stress, parental misinterpretation of the baby's crying pattern, heightened sensitivity to natural bowel distention, gastroesophageal reflux, and cow milk intolerance have all been incriminated in what is surely a multifactorial process. Hypoallergenic diets and formula, soy formula, herbal teas, and decreased infant stimulation have been somewhat effective. Dicyclomine (Bentyl) also has been shown to be somewhat effective, but should be avoided in children less than 6 months. Other treatments commonly used to treat colic have not been found to be effective. These include simethicone (Mylicon, Gas-X), scopolamine, lactase enzyme (Lactaid), fiber-enriched formula, increased carrying, car ride simulators, and sucrose (19). Large doses of clinician empathy and support, combined with a tincture of time, are usually sufficient in this self-limiting process. Colic usually resolves or improves by 4 months of age.

When the child is somewhat older, episodes of fussiness and crying are often attributed to teething. Teething usually begins from 5 to 8 months of age and may cause local discomfort and fussiness, especially when the molars are erupting. Local treatment of the gums with cool liquids, chilled teething rings, and acetaminophen for analgesia should be sufficient symptomatic care. Do not use paregoric for teething, because of its high toxic-to-therapeutic ratio. Fever above 101°F (38.3°C) and profuse diarrhea should not be attributed to teething.

SKIN CARE

If dry skin is a problem, bathing frequency should be decreased. Apply a moisturizer such as Eucerin cream after bathing. For cradle cap (seborrheic dermatitis) not responding to washing with non-medicated shampoo, ketoconazole shampoo or topical steroids twice a week may be considered. Diaper rash (also called diaper dermatitis) is another common skin condition and is most commonly a contact dermatitis or a yeast superinfection. Contact dermatitis may occur due to fragrances or chemicals in disposable diapers or residual ammonia or detergent in cloth diapers. Change diapers frequently and leave the perineum open to air if possible. Barrier creams such as zinc oxide may help, but parents should avoid oils and powders. Antifungal medication may be needed if yeast is suspected.

BOWEL HABITS

The most common concern regarding bowel habits is one of frequency and consistency. In most situations, reassurance will be appropriate. Frequencies in normal children can vary from one bowel movement every few days to several bowel movements per day. Consistency can vary from very loose and yellow in breast-fed babies to more well formed in bottle-fed infants. Further exploration may be warranted if the stool has a very foul odor or is very voluminous.

CASE

Travis is a 15-year-old boy who comes to the office complaining of a sore throat. He is accompanied by his mother who is concerned that he has strep throat. He has no significant medical history and in fact has not been seen in the office since he was 12 years old. A rapid strep test is positive, and he gets a prescription for penicillin.

QUESTION

1. How can you work prevention into this acute visit?

DISCUSSION

This is perhaps the only opportunity to address some important prevention issues with Travis. Although you may be tempted to save some time and address only the acute complaint, an important opportunity to affect Travis' future health may be lost. Take advantage of such visits to address one or two of the relevant screening and counseling topics discussed in this chapter. Make sure his immunizations are current.

You can use his chief complaint (sore throat) to naturally transition to topics of preventive health. For an example you might say "Because exposure to cigarette smoke can lead to sore throats, I am going to ask you some questions about smoking." This will help Travis understand the reason for subsequent questions and discussion. It may be more difficult to transition to topics that are less directly related to his sore throat but you can try introductory statements such as, "Generally, healthy people like yourself don't come to the doctor very often, so I like to take advantage of the times that you are here to talk about areas of health that are very important to adolescents . . . would that be OK with you?". Travis will be more receptive to these conversations if you have tactfully asked his mom to wait outside and have reassured him of the confidential nature of the conversation.

Try to engage Travis in a conversation, don't just talk at him. Find out how much he knows. We know that everyone (including Travis) learns much more effectively when they are engaged and the material is relevant. Sequencing questions from less to more private topics can help draw Travis into the conversation. For an example, if you decide that today your focus with Travis will be alcohol use, you might first ask, "Some people your age drink alcohol. Do you know any such people?" If the answer is "yes," the follow-up question might be, "Are any of them close friends of yours?", and finally, "Have you yourself tried alcohol?"

Depending on what you find out, you may respond with a short appropriately tailored counseling message, a more intensive acute intervention, or a follow-up visit. If

Travis does not disclose any health-risk behaviors, perhaps the most important component of the visit is to make it clear that these topics are a legitimate reason for seeking care in the future.

References

1. Yarnall KS, Pollak KI, Ostbyte T, Krause KM, Michner JL. Primary care: is there enough time for prevention? Am J Public Health. 2003;93(4):635–641.
2. United States General Accounting Office Report to Congressional Requesters. Newborn Screening: Characteristics of State Programs. 2003. Available at *http://www.gao.gov/new.items/d03449.pdf*. Accessed October 26, 2005.
3. White K. Anemia is a poor predictor or iron deficiency among toddlers in the Unites States. Pediatrics. 2005;115: 315–320.
4. Geltman PL, Meyers AF, Mehta SD, Brugnara C, Villon I, Wu YA, Bauchner H. Daily Multivitamins with iron to prevent anemia in high risk infants: a randomized clinical trial. Pediatrics. 2004;114:86–93.
5. Healthy People 2010 Objectives. Available at *http://www.healthypeople.gov/*. Accessed October 26, 2005.
6. Blood Lead Levels United States 1992–2002. MMWR. May 27, 2005;54(20);513–516
7. Perrin EM, Flower KB, Ammerman AS. Body mass index charts: useful yet underused. J Pediatr. 2004;144(4):455–460
8. Summerbell C, Waters E, Edmunds L, Kelly S, Brown T, Campbell K. Interventions for preventing obesity in children. Cochrane Database Systematic Review. 2005;July 20(3) CD001871.
9. American Academy of Pediatrics Policy Statement. Development surveillance and screening of infants and young children. Pediatrics. 2001;108(1):192–196.
10. Herman-Giddens ME, Slora EJ, Wasserman RC, et al. Secondary sexual characteristics and menses in young girls seen in office practice: a study from the Pediatric Research in Office Settings network. Pediatrics. 1997;99(4):505–512.
11. Controlling tuberculosis in the United States. Recommendations from the American Thoracic Society, CDC, and the Infectious Diseases Society of America. MMWR. 2005;54(No. RR-12).
12. Centers for Disease Control and Prevention. Surveillance summaries. MMWR. 2004 May 21;53(No.SS-2).
13. Plotkin SL, Plotkin SA. A short history of vaccination. In Plotkin SA, Orenstein WA, eds. Vaccines. Philadelphia: Saunders, 1999.
14. Szilagyi PG, Schaffer S, Shone L, Barth R, Humiston SG, Sandler M, Rodewal LE. Reducing geographical, racial, and ethnic disparities in childhood immunization rates by using reminder/recall interventions in urban primary care practices. Pediatrics. 2002;110(5):58.
15. Institute of Medicine. Immunization Safety Review Series. Washington, DC: National Academy Press. Released between 2001 and 2004.
16. AAP Committee on Infectious Diseases. Varicella vaccine update. Pediatrics. 2000; 105(1):136–141.
17. Creery D, Mikrogianakis A. Sudden infant death syndrome. Clin Evid. 2005;13:434–443.
18. Steiner B, Gest KL. Do adolescents want to hear preventive counseling messages in outpatient settings? J Fam Pract. 1996; 43(4):375–381.
19. Effective and ineffective interventions for infant colic. J Fam Pract. 2004;3(8):604, 606.

CHAPTER 6

Well Adult Care

Steven M. Schwartz and Marguerite Duane

CASE

A 44-year-old white man comes to your office requesting a "routine physical." The only remarkable item in his history is his father's myocardial infarction at age 50.

CLINICAL QUESTIONS

1. What is a well adult care plan?
2. How can a clinician implement a well adult care plan in a busy practice?
3. How can you customize population-based guidelines to suit individual patients?

RATIONALE FOR PREVENTIVE CARE

A major goal of prevention and health promotion is to reduce the burden of suffering for the major preventable diseases. This goal applies to the population as a whole as well as to individual patients. Another goal of prevention and health promotion is to control health care expenditures by reducing the need for costly intensive management of illness in its later stages. These two goals can be met by applying the principles of evidence-based medicine to providing preventive health services in clinical practice.

Preventive care includes three main services:

1) Immunization and chemoprophylaxis
2) Screening for early detection of disease.
3) Education and counseling of patients about behaviors that impact on their health

Family physicians are well suited to provide preventive health services since they provide both acute care as well as wellness care in a continuity setting. Family physicians emphasize health behaviors and counseling (1). Continuity of care facilitates implementation and tracking of screening tests and other services that should be repeated periodically. Continuity visits also provide opportunities to reinforce a message with repetition. For example a patient may come in for a blood pressure check and comment, "My pressure may be high; there was a lot of traffic today." This situation is an ideal time to remind the patient about seatbelt use. In fact, family physicians deliver preventive services in about one third of acute care visits (2).

Unfortunately, it is often challenging to provide preventive care in actual practice. In one study of more than 4,000 patients, only 55% of screenings, 24% of immunizations, and 9% of health habit counseling milestones were up to date (3).

Nationally, half the population does not receive key preventive services such as tobacco cessation counseling, vision screening, regular screening for colorectal cancer, and vaccination counseling (4). Every visit for upper respiratory infection provides an opportunity to advise a smoker to quit, or provide other counseling. Additionally, a strong doctor/patient relationship fosters a better understanding of the patient's wishes. This may allow counseling efforts to have a greater impact in affecting patient behavior change.

IMPLEMENTING PREVENTIVE CARE

There are many factors to consider when one plans for and offers well adult care services. Successful implementation requires using every teachable moment and documenting preventive health topics as they are addressed.

Construct a framework for providing well adult care that encompasses preventive health services. Consider what, when, how, and to whom various services should be provided. Use evidence of benefit as the guiding principle in offering services. As with making a clinical diagnosis, the history provides the most important factors needed to decide to whom which services should be offered. Be familiar with evidence-based guidelines for preventive services. Concentrate efforts on delivering the most valuable services, specifically services with the greatest health impact or value/cost effectiveness (4). Employ a system that will automatically provide you with guideline updates and allow access to or reminders of these guidelines at the point of care. The end of this chapter provides a list of some useful PDA and Web resources of preventive services.

Patients need to be educated about appropriate evidence-based wellness care and become active partners in their own care. It has been shown that patients who are more actively involved may be more likely to follow through with health advice, and be satisfied (5).

Where to Deliver Preventive Health Services

Though most of the interventions discussed in this chapter refer to preventive services in the office setting, other settings are well suited for these purposes. Some well adult care is perhaps better accomplished in non-office settings. The clinician may provide a talk to a community, school, or church group. She may participate in health fairs or community blood pressure screenings. She may write preventive health counseling advice in a published column. Public health initiatives such as seatbelt and bicycle helmet laws, public smoking bans, the addition of folate to the food supply, and public safety campaigns that encourage the creation of the "designated driver" are not initiated in the exam room but may be reinforced there.

The Periodic Health Evaluation

The periodic health evaluation (PHE) is an ideal time to provide evidence-based preventive health services. There is no consensus on the frequency and content of the PHE. Family physicians spend an average of 35% of their office time performing adult PHEs (6). However, clinicians often spend a disproportionate amount of time on an extensive screening physical exam and reviewing laboratory tests of unknown usefulness. Worse yet, they may even perform tests they know are not useful and may even be harmful, creating unnecessary discomfort, cost, waste, and potential harm. Table 6.1 lists several examples of ineffective tests, including tumor markers, coronary computed tomographic scans, routine stress tests, and Pap smears in women without a cervix; approximately 10 million women had unnecessary Pap smears performed from 1992–2002 in the United States (7). The money saved from these unnecessary Pap smears could pay for the 17 million women not currently screened for cervical cancer, often because of lack of access to health care (8). It may be confusing to patients when clinicians in the same office have very different practices regarding screening—for example, when one performs Pap smears in women who have had a hysterectomy and another does not. When developing your clinical office system, be sure to educate your patients, your colleagues, and your staff to encourage the use of effective services and discourage the use of ineffective ones.

Prevention is often forgotten while attending to more urgent clinical concerns, but given the right emphasis, preventive care can be done in the acute setting. For example, emergency departments generally do an excellent job of updating tetanus immunizations. Similarly, each history and physical examination for hospital admission should include a section on health maintenance issues.

Many resources are available for a physician or medical office wishing to implement a formal preventive health program. *Putting Prevention into Practice* (PPIP, *http://www.ahrq.gov/clinic/ppipix.htm*) is a program designed to increase the appropriate use of clinical preventive services based on the US Preventive Services Task Force recommendations. *The Clinician's Handbook of Preventive Services* (the guidebook behind PPIP) recommends 10 steps to implement an effective preventive program in the office setting. These steps are:

1. Assess the need for a new system
2. Assess readiness to make a systems change
3. Enlist staff support
4. Perform a chart audit to evaluate your baseline performance
5. Establish preventive care protocols
6. Analyze service delivery and patient flow
7. Use basic tools such as tracking flow sheets, postcard reminders, in-office visual prompts, patient materials
8. Use other helpful tools such as chart reminders and prevention prescriptions
9. Delegate staff roles
10. Perform follow-up evaluations to assess progress (9)

One needs first to make a commitment to provide quality preventive care. Begin by evaluating current practices. For example, a clinician could review her records and determine the pneumovax immunization rate among eligible patients.

Use as many resources as possible in the office; for example, posting adult screening schedules, sending mailed or emailed reminders, and offering vaccine to every patient who presents for a visit or PHE. If trying to educate patients about diet, provide patient education materials on wellness in the waiting area, and show examples of exercise programs or effective diets, such as the DASH diet (*http://www.nhlbi.nih.gov/health/public/heart/hbp/dash/*), with take home menus.

In the triage or exam rooms, the nurse, medical assistant, and physician each can make entries on preventive care flow sheets or appropriate templates in the electronic health record (EHR), tracking patient risks such as smoking status and services such as screening tests and vaccines. The receptionist can distribute health history questionnaires, which can be reviewed with the patient by the physician later in the visit. Office staff can manage a "tickler" file to send patients reminder cards for their preventive services.

As much as possible, preventive health services should become part of the office system and office routine rather than relying on physician memory and initiative. As the EHR becomes more commonplace, automated tracking and prompting can be implemented. Use of the EHR has been shown to increase the adherence to many types of preventive services (10, 11).

USING EVIDENCE-BASED GUIDELINES

The three components; clinical expertise, patient preferences, and evidence from research are germane to providing preventive health services. Expertise is required in taking the appropriate history to identify patient risk, to be familiar with both the harms and benefits of preventive services, and the conditions they prevent. The physician must be able to effectively communicate the value of the services and motivate the patients to accept appropriate services and dissuade from requests for inappropriate services. Incorporating patient preference, using shared decision-making becomes important when the evidence is lacking or if it is unclear whether the magnitude of potential benefit from a service outweighs the magnitude of potential harm. Weighing benefit to harm may depend on the value that an individual patient assigns to a service and may not be universal (e.g., is a patient willing to risk impotence or incontinence as an outcome of finding and treating prostate cancer, when mortality reduction from prostate-specific antigen screening is yet to be demonstrated) (12).

Specific recommendations in this chapter rely heavily on guidelines from the US Preventive Services Task Force (USPSTF). The USPSTF methodology is very rigorous for evaluation of effectiveness. Also, despite a lack of consensus about many recommendations from other bodies, nearly 90% of family physicians surveyed agreed with all of the USPSTF recommendations (13). The USPSTF has provided a standard recommendation language (rating system) based on the quality of evidence available. The current ratings are shown in a footnote to Table 6.6.

A very useful tool to identify recommendations of the USPSTF by age, sex, and pregnancy status is the Interactive Prevention Services Selector for Palm or Pocket PC handheld computers; it can be freely downloaded at *http://pda.ahrq.gov/index.html*.

TABLE 6.1 Well Adult—Preventive Services NOT Recommended in Asymptomatic Patients

Screen	Test	Potential Harms	Special considerations	Level of Evidence
Bacteriuria	Urinalysis, microscopy	Overuse of antibiotics	Level A recommendation in pregnant women between 12 and 16 weeks gestation	D
Bladder Cancer	Urinalysis, microscopy or urine cytology	Many false positives lead to unnecessary invasive procedures	Smokers at increased risk. Counsel on quitting smoking	D
Cornary Heart Disease in low risk adults	ECG, Exercise treadmill test, Electron beam CT	Unnecessary invasive testing, over treatment and labeling	Patient at high risk of CHD, no benefit over assessment of CHD risk factors.	D
Hepatitis B	Blood test	Labeling	Level A recommendation in pregnant women	D
Hepatitis C	Blood test	Unnecessary biopsies, Labeling	Insufficient evidence to recommend for patients at high risk for HCV–IV drug use, dialysis, transfusion before 1990	D
Genital Herpes–HSV	Serologic tests for HSV antibodies	False-positive test results, labeling, and anxiety	In symptomatic patients, antiretroviral therapy does improve outcomes	D
HRT for prevention of chronic conditions in post-menopausal women	Combined estrogen and progesterone or unopposed estrogen if pt had hysterectomy	Breast cancer, DVT, CHD, stroke, cholecystitis, dementia	Does reduce risk for fracture, but harms outweigh benefits	D
Ovarian Cancer	CA-125 or transvaginal ultrasound	Unnecessary surgery, anxiety	No evidence that early detection will reduce mortality	D
Pancreatic cancer	Abdominal palpation, US, serologic markers	Invasive diagnostic tests, poor tx outcomes		D
Peripheral arterial disease	Ankle Brachial index	False positive results, unnecessary work-ups		D
Testicular cancer	Clinical or self exam		No evidence that early detection will reduce mortality	D

The USPSTF recommends against routinely providing the service to asymptomatic patients. The USPSTF found at least fair evidence that [the service] is ineffective or that the harms outweigh benefits.

Many organizations have created evidence-based guidelines that model this rating system. Consider bias that may arise in guidelines from specialty organizations whose members may gain by delivering a particular service or disease advocacy groups or payers, who may have an agenda that includes screening as a way to increase disease awareness or cost saving priorities over demonstrated benefit to patients. Be aware of these standards when making recommendations to patients about services. Patient preference becomes particularly important in deciding on services with a C or I rating or when recommendations from different organizations vary significantly.

ORGANIZING YOUR THINKING ABOUT PREVENTIVE HEALTH SERVICES

The RISE mnemonic, using history and education as its cornerstone, is a useful tool to provide prevention services for individual patients. R is for risk identification; I is for immunizations or chemoprophylaxis; S is for screening (primary or secondary); and E is for education. Offer services based on specific guidelines or standards and revise the patient's program based on evolving evidence.

TABLE 6.2 Leading Causes of Death, 2003

Rank	All Races, 25–44	Number
	All Causes	130,761
1	Unintentional injuries	29,307
2	Malignant neoplasm	19,250
3	Diseases of the heart	16,850
4	Suicide	11,667
5	Homicide and legal intervention	7,626
6	HIV disease	6,928
7	Chronic liver disease and cirrhosis	3,378
8	Cerebrovascular disease	3,043
9	Diabetes Mellitus	2,706
10	Pneumonia and influenza	1,365
		15,225

Rank	All Races, 45–65	Number
	All Causes	439,300
1	Malignant neoplasm	145,535
2	Diseases of heart	102,792
3	Unintentional injuries	20,007
4	Diabetes mellitus	16,389
5	Cerebral vascular disease	16,073
6	Chronic lower respiratory disease	15,614
7	Chronic liver disease and cirrhosis	13,894
8	Suicide	10,324
9	HIV disease	5,959
10	Septicemia	5,808
		34,501

Rank	All Races, 65 and over	Number
	All Causes	1,804,373
1	Diseases of the heart	563,390
2	Malignant neoplasm	388,911
3	Cerebrovascular disease	138,134
4	Chronic lower respiratory disease	109,139
5	Alzheimer's disease	62,814
6	Pneumonia and influenza	57,670
7	Diabetes Mellitus	54,919
8	Nephritis, nephritic syndrome	35,254
9	Unintentional injuries	34,335
10	Septicemia	26,445

(Adapted from National Center for Health Statistics
Health, United States, 2005, With Chartbook on Trends in the Health of Americans
Hyattsville, Maryland: 2005, *http://www.cdc.gov/nchs/hus.htm*. Accessed March 26, 2006)

Risk Assessment

To develop a rational and efficient well adult care plan you must first have information on the leading causes of morbidity and mortality in the target population. Table 6.2 shows the leading causes of death by age in the US adult population. Many of the leading diseases causing mortality can be attributed to patient behaviors which are summarized in Table 6.3 (14, 15). Prevention of premature death is not our sole goal, though; preventing unnecessary morbidity and disability is important as well. Table 6.4 lists the leading causes of disability in the US adult population.

Tailor the history, exam, and interventions (immunization, screening, and counseling) to the individual based on the patient's age, sex, race, and history-specific risks. Although Table 6.2 provides information on leading causes of death for the general adult population, similarities and disparities of subpopulations by age, sex, and race can be found in additional tables from the Centers for Disease Control and Prevention (CDC) at *http://www.cdc.gov/nchs/fastats/lcod.htm*. We can learn from these tables, for example, that a 28-year-old black woman is most likely to die from HIV infection, unintentional injury, heart disease, malignant neoplasm, and assault (homicide) (16). A woman's lifetime risk of dying is greatest from heart disease, malignant neoplasm, cerebrovascular disease, chronic obstructive lung disease, and pneumonia. Therefore, her history and/or screening questionnaires should focus on gathering pertinent information regarding behaviors and family or genetic risk factors that increase her risk of these conditions. Standard surveys can be used to gather a general history and serve as an icebreaker on often-sensitive areas such as sexual history, exposure to violence, and depression. Specific screening instruments focus on diet, mental status, and depres-sion. Sample screening tools for depression and mental status are shown in Figures 6.1 and 6.2. A screening tool does not substitute for the history, physical, and evaluation performed by the physician. For our hypothetical 28-year-old patient, a history of depression, family history of completed suicide, and the presence of a gun in the home would place her at high risk of suicide in the future.

The USPSTF recognizes "high-risk" populations that may benefit from additional interventions beyond those recommended for the general population. Some of these risk groups include individuals with high-risk sexual behavior, intravenous drug use, the presence of certain chronic medical conditions, and several subpopulations who might benefit from additional vaccines or screening for tuberculosis. With the completion of the mapping of the human genome, the practicing clinician will soon have to start considering specific genetic risks for disease as well.

Immunizations and Chemoprophylaxis
IMMUNIZATIONS

Immunizations have cut the incidence of diseases such as measles, rubella, mumps, tetanus and polio by 100-fold to 1000-fold in some cases (17). Adults are less likely than children to be up-to-date with recommended vaccinations. For example, most adults do not know their tetanus immunization status, and most cases of tetanus now occur in inadequately immunized older adults. An invaluable tool for point-of-care information on immunization in adults and children is "Shots" from the Group on Immunization Education of the Society of Teachers of Family Medicine. Updated each year, this free application for handheld computers is downloadable from *http://www.immunizationed.org/default.aspx*

TABLE 6.3 Actual Causes of Death in the United States 1990–2000

Actual Cause	No. (%) in 1990*	No (%) in 2000†
Tobacco	400,000 (19)	435,000 (18.1)
Poor diet and physical inactivity	300,000 (14)	400,000 (16.6)
Alcohol consumption	100,000 (5)	85,000 (3.5)
Microbial agents	90,000 (4)	75,000 (3.1)
Toxic agents	60,000 (3)	55,000 (2.3)
Motor vehicle	25,000 (1)	43,000 (1.8)
Firearms	35,000 (2)	29,000 (1.2)
Sexual behavior	30,000 (1)	20,000 (0.8)
Illicit drug use	20,000 (<1)	17,000 (0.7)
Total	1,060,000 (50%)	1,159,000 (48.2)

Deaths from Medical Error 5,000‡–98,000§/year (unclear)

*Data from McGinnis and Foege, 1993.
†From Mokdad AH, Marks JS, Stroup DF, Gerberding JL, 2004.
The percentages are for all deaths.
‡From Hayward RA, Hofer TP, Estimating Hospital Deaths Due to Medical Errors: Preventability Is in the Eye of the Reviewer. JAMA. 286(4):415–420. July 25, 2001.
§From Brennan TA, Leape LL, Laird NM, et al. Incidence of adverse events and negligence in hospitalized patients: results of the Harvard Practice Study I. N Engl J Med. 1991; 324:370–376.

TABLE 6.4   Selected Chronic Health Conditions Causing Limitation of Activity

Type of chronic health condition	18–44 years		45–54 years		55–64 years	
	Rate	SE	Rate	SE	Rate	SE
	Number of persons with limitation of activity caused by selected chronic health conditions per 1,000 population					
Mental illness	12.9	0.5	23.1	1.1	24.1	1.4
Fractures or joint injury	7.0	0.4	15.5	0.9	20.6	1.2
Lung	5.0	0.3	12.6	0.8	25.6	1.3
Diabetes	2.5	0.2	13.4	0.8	33.4	1.5
Heart or other circulatory	5.9	0.3	28.4	1.2	74.3	2.4
Arthritis or other musculoskeletal	22.2	0.7	61.9	1.8	100.7	2.6

SE Standard error.
Notes: Data are for the civilian noninstitutionalized population. Conditions refer to response categories in the National Health Interview Survey; some conditions include several response categories. "Mental illness" includes depression, anxiety or emotional problem, and other mental conditions. "Heart or other circulatory" includes heart problem, stroke problem, hypertension or high blood pressure, and other circulatory system conditions. "Arthritis or other musculoskeletal" includes arthritis or rheumatism, back or neck problem, and other musculoskeletal system conditions. Persons may report more than one chronic health condition as the cause of their activity limitation. Starting with *Health, United States, 2005,* estimates for 2000 and later years use weights derived from the 2000 census. See related *Health, United States, 2005,* table 58. See Appendix II, Condition; Limitation of Activity.
Source: Centers for Disease Control and Prevention, National Center for Health Statistics, National Health Interview Survey.

Table 6.5 summarizes adult vaccine recommendations adapted from the Advisory Committee on Immunization Practices (ACIP) of the CDC. Two new tetanus-diphtheria-acellular pertussis (TdaP) vaccines were licensed in 2005 for adolescents and adults to age 65, adding protection against pertussis for adults. In 2006, the ACIP recommended administration of TdaP in place of Td for adolescents and adults up to age 65 every 10 years (18). Td should still be used for adults over age 65, although this recommendation may change with additional evidence of safety and efficacy. The influenza vaccine should be given annually to adults 50 years or older, persons with certain chronic medical conditions, nursing home residents, women in their second or third trimester of pregnancy, and household contacts or caregivers of high-risk individuals, including all health care workers. Pneumococcal polysaccaride vaccine (PPV) should be administered once to adults 65 and older, and to younger patients with chronic disease, immunosuppression, or asplenia. Alaskan natives and certain Native American populations should also receive PPV. Varicella vaccine is recommended for susceptible adults. Hepatitis B vaccine is recommended for all persons under 18 not previously immunized, and for all persons at high risk for infection. Hepatitis A vaccine is recommended for high-risk patients, such as travelers to endemic areas, residents of domestic areas of high hepatitis A prevalence, and possibly to food handlers. Patients with chronic hepatitis from other causes (hepatitis B, hepatitis C, alcohol, and other etiologies.) should also receive the vaccine. A single dose of zoster vaccine is recommended for adults 60 years of age and older, whether or not they report a prior episode of herpes zoster. Persons with chronic medical conditions may be vaccinated unless contraindicated or precaution exists for their condition (1).

Routine vaccination with three doses of quadrivalent HPV vaccine is recommended for females 11–12 years of age. The vaccination series can be started in females as young as 9 years of age. Catch-up vaccination is recommended for females 13-26 years of age who have not been vaccinated previously or who have not completed the full vaccine series. Ideally, vaccine should be administered before potential exposure to HPV through sexual contact. HPV vaccine can be given to females who have an equivalent or abnormal Pap test, a positive Hybrid Capture II® high risk test, or genital warts.

Document the completion of childhood vaccines, including measles, mumps, and rubella (MMR) and polio. Adults born after 1956 should receive at least one dose of MMR. Two doses are required for certain subgroups. Rubella immunity is especially important in a woman contemplating conception, though pregnancy should be avoided within 30 days of vaccination. Consider giving inactivated polio vaccine (IPV) to patients who have not completed their primary series, and members of certain high-risk groups.

International travel poses additional risks and unique preventive care needs. Travelers should be aware of local health risks. The most common risk of any travel is accidental injury, but there are preventable causes of morbidity as well. Know where to access information about communicable disease risk, immunization recommendations, food and water precautions, advice on the prevention and treatment of traveler's diarrhea, and other health information. Local health departments have immunization clinics that usually include overseas travel information. You can also access pertinent travel information from travel guidebooks and obtain the most current information from the CDC directly via Internet *http://www.cdc.gov/travel/*, or phone 404-332-4555 (19). The main

PATIENT NAME _____

AGE _____ **SEX** _____ **DATE** _____

Please check a response for each of the 20 items.	None OR a Little of the Time	Some of the Time	Good Part of the Time	Most OR All of the Time	
1. I FEEL DOWNHEARTED, BLUE, AND SAD	○ 1	○ 2	○ 3	○ 4	
2. MORNING IS WHEN I FEEL THE BEST	○ 4	○ 3	○ 2	○ 1	
3. I HAVE CRYING SPELLS OR FEEL LIKE CRYING	○ 1	○ 2	○ 3	○ 4	
4. I HAVE TROUBLE SLEEPING THROUGH THE NIGHT	○ 1	○ 2	○ 3	○ 4	
5. I EAT AS MUCH AS I USED TO	○ 4	○ 3	○ 2	○ 1	
6. I ENJOY LOOKING AT, TALKING TO, AND BEING WITH ATTRACTIVE WOMEN/MEN	○ 4	○ 3	○ 2	○ 1	
7. I NOTICE THAT I AM LOSING WEIGHT	○ 1	○ 2	○ 3	○ 4	
8. I HAVE TROUBLE WITH CONSTIPATION	○ 1	○ 2	○ 3	○ 4	
9. MY HEART BEATS FASTER THAN USUAL	○ 1	○ 2	○ 3	○ 4	
10. I GET TIRED FOR NO REASON	○ 1	○ 2	○ 3	○ 4	
11. MY MIND IS AS CLEAR AS IT USED TO BE	○ 4	○ 3	○ 2	○ 1	
12. I FIND IT EASY TO DO THE THINGS I USED TO DO	○ 4	○ 3	○ 2	○ 1	
13. I AM RESTLESS AND CAN'T KEEP STILL	○ 1	○ 2	○ 3	○ 4	
14. I FEEL HOPEFUL ABOUT THE FUTURE	○ 4	○ 3	○ 2	○ 1	
15. I AM MORE IRRITABLE THAN USUAL	○ 1	○ 2	○ 3	○ 4	
16. I FIND IT EASY TO MAKE DECISIONS	○ 4	○ 3	○ 2	○ 1	
17. I FEEL THAT I AM USEFUL AND NEEDED	○ 4	○ 3	○ 2	○ 1	
18. MY LIFE IS PRETTY FULL	○ 4	○ 3	○ 2	○ 1	
19. I FEEL THAT OTHERS WOULD BE BETTER OFF IF I WERE DEAD	○ 1	○ 2	○ 3	○ 4	
20. I STILL ENJOY THE THINGS I USED TO DO	○ 4	○ 3	○ 2	○ 1	
				RAW SCORE	
				SDS INDEX	

SDS Index	Equivalent Clinical Global Impressions
Below–50	Within normal range, no psychopathology
50–59	Presence of minimal to mild depression
60–69	Presence of moderate to marked depression
70 and over	Presence of severe to extreme depression

Conversion of Raw Scores to the SDS Index

Raw Score	SDS Index	Raw Score	SDS Index	Raw Score	SDS Index	Raw Score	SDS Index	Raw Score	SDS Index
20	25	32	40	44	55	56	70	68	85
21	26	33	41	45	56	57	71	69	86
22	28	34	43	46	58	58	73	70	88
23	29	35	44	47	59	59	74	71	89
24	30	36	45	48	60	60	75	72	90
25	31	37	46	49	61	61	76	73	91
26	33	38	48	50	63	62	78	74	92
27	34	39	49	51	64	63	79	75	94
28	35	40	50	52	65	64	80	76	95
29	36	41	51	53	66	65	81	77	96
30	38	42	53	54	68	66	83	78	98
31	39	43	54	55	69	67	84	79	99
								80	100

Figure 6.1 • Zung self-rating depression scale. (Reprinted with permission from Zung WWK. A self-rating depression scale. Arch Gen Psychiatry. 1965;12:63–70.)

prevention targets for travelers include water and foodborne illnesses, such as traveler's diarrhea from bacteria and parasites, hepatitis A, cholera and typhoid fever, and insect-borne illness, primarily malaria, dengue, and yellow fever. Most countries expect travelers to have received basic childhood immunizations, and a current Td or TdaP. Some countries or authorities recommend or require the following: hepatitis A or γ-globulin, hepatitis B, malaria chemoprophylaxis, cholera vaccine, yellow fever, or typhoid vaccine.

Patient education about prevention of food, water- and insect-borne illness is very important. Advise travelers to be extra cautious about new sexual contacts. With safe sex education, they may avoid acquiring sexually transmitted diseases (STDs) and HIV. Recommend taking along extra supplies of regular prescription medication and over-the-counter medications, as these may be unavailable at their destination. Consider prescribing medications for travelers' diarrhea or malaria prophylaxis if travel will be to endemic areas.

Short Blessed Cognitive Status Screen (BSCS)

Question	Maximum Error	Patient's # Errors	X	Weight Subscore
1. What year is it now?	1	_____	4	_____
2. What month is it now?	1	_____	3	_____
Repeat this phrase after me and remember it: John Brown, 42 Market Street, Chicago Number of trials to learning: _____ [Allow up to 5 trials]				
3. About what time is it without looking at your watch? [correct = within 1 hour]	1	_____	3	_____
4. Count backwards from 20 down to 1 [any incorrect response is an error; but score only first two errors]	2	_____	2	_____
5. Say the months of the year in reverse. [Any incorrect response is an error; but score only first 2 errors]	2	_____	2	_____
6. Repeat the name and address I asked you to remember. [Mark each incorrect word or phrase as noted below; you may score up to 5 errors]	5	_____	2	_____

John Brown 42 Market Street Chicago

___ ___ ___ __ _____ _____

TOTAL WEIGHTED ERROR SCORE   _____

Figure 6.2 • Modified short Blessed Cognitive Status Screen. This brief examination is particularly well suited for primary care. It takes much less time than the Mini-Mental Status Examination, is available in the public domain, and does not require any equipment or preprinted forms. Interpretation: 0–7 = normal or mild cognitive impairment; 8–19 = moderate cognitive impairment; 20+ = severe cognitive impairment. (Adapted from Katzman R, Brown T, Fuld P, Peck A, et al. Validation of a short orientation-memory-concentration test of cognitive impairment. Am J Psychiatry 1983;140:734–738; Fillenbaum GFG, Heyman A, Wilkinson WE, Haynes CS. Comparison of two screening tests in Alzheimer's disease: the correlation and reliability of the Mini-Mental Status Examination and the modified Blessed test. Arch Neurol. 1987;44:924–927; and Davis PB, Morris JC, Grant E. Brief screening tests versus clinical staging in senile dementia of the Alzheimer's type. J Am Ger Soc. 1990;38:129–135.

CHEMOPROPHYLAXIS

The USPSTF no longer recommends hormone replacement therapy (HRT) for chemoprophylaxis. Although the USPSTF found evidence that the use of combined estrogen and progestin results in both benefits and harms, they concluded that the harmful effects likely outweigh the chronic disease prevention benefits. The USPSTF also recommends against the routine use of unopposed estrogen for prevention of chronic conditions in women who have previously had a hysterectomy.

The USPSTF recommends consideration of aspirin chemoprophylaxis in adults at increased risk for coronary heart disease. Physicians should discuss the potential benefits and harms of aspirin therapy in men 40 years or older, postmenopausal women, and younger people with risk factors for coronary heart disease (e.g., diabetes, hypertension, and smoking). Given that there is good evidence that aspirin therapy decreases the incidence of coronary heart disease in patients at increased risk but increases the incidence of gastrointestinal

TABLE 6.5 Well Adult Care Recommendations—Immunizations

Immunization	Indication	Schedule	Contraindications/Special Concerns
Tetanus, diphtheria acellular pertussis (TdaP/Td)	All adults 18 age 65 (TdaP) 65 and over (Td)	Two doses at least 4 weeks apart, 3rd dose 6–12 months after 2nd dose Booster every 10 years	Give if wound present & >5 years since last dose Avoid if severe hypersensitivity
Measles, mumps, rubella vaccine	• Born after 1956, if no documentation • Healthcare personnel • Travelers to foreign countries • HIV without severe immunosuppression • Entering college	At least one dose. A second dose is recommended for healthcare workers, international travelers, and college students	Measles & rubella considered for separate indications, but given as MMR unless contraindicated. Measles: recent exposure Rubella: women of childbearing age who lack laboratory evidence of immunity. Do NOT give to pregnant women.
Varicella vaccine	• Absence of reliable history of disease or evidence of immunity • High-risk susceptible individuals*	Two doses at least 4–8 weeks apart	Avoid in active TB, immunosuppressed, immunodeficiency, pregnancy, recent immune globulin
Polio vaccine IPV—inactivated vaccine OPV—oral (live) vaccine	• Routine adult vaccine not necessary • Travelers to endemic areas • Community members if outbreak • Lab workers handling virus • Health care workers at risk of exposure	Primary series is 3 doses	OPV not recommended in the U.S. Complete primary or incomplete series with IPV. Select travelers should consider a booster even if primary series complete
Influenza vaccine	• 50 years and older • Nursing home/ institutional residents • Chronic disease† • Pregnancy, 2nd & 3rd trimester • Healthcare employees including those in long-term care or assisted-living facilities • Close contacts of high-risk persons	Annually each fall	Avoid if: Anaphylactic allergy to eggs Acute febrile illness
Pneumococcal polysaccharide vaccine (PPV)	• 65 years and older • Chronic disease‡ • Alaskan Natives/American Indian • Residents of nursing homes/long-term care	One dose needed if given after age 65 Consider 5-year booster if highest risk	Give 2 weeks before elective splenectomy. Give to patients with unknown vaccine status if indicated. Track long-term care residents' status
Hepatitis A vaccine	• Travelers to endemic areas • Chronic liver disease • Clotting factor disorder • Men who have sex with men • Illegal drug use • Lab exposure • Consider food handlers	Two doses given 6–12 months apart	Avoid if hypersensitivity to alum or 2-phenoxyethanol. Pregnancy class C

(continued)

TABLE 6.5 Well Adult Care Recommendations—Immunizations (*continued*)

Immunization	Indication	Schedule	Contraindications/Special Concerns
Hepatitis B vaccine	• Occupational risk of blood exposure • Clients/staff at institutions for Development disabled • Hemodyalysis • Clotting-factor recip. • Household/sex contacts of HBV patients • Certain international travel • IVDU • Men who have sex with men • Multiple sex partners or recent STD • Prison Inmates • Unvaccinated adolescents	Three doses: 2nd dose 1–2 months after 1st; 3rd dose 4–6 months after 1st. Alternate 2-dose schedule available for adolescent.	Special dosing needed in certain subgroups.
Meningococcal vaccine (MCV4, MPSV4)	• Asplenic adults • College students • Military recruits • International travel to hyperendemic countries	1 dose A 2nd dose may be indicated after 5 years for adults still at high risk previously vaccinated with MPSV4	Menigococcal conjugate vaccine (MCV4) is generally preferred an part of routine childhood vaccine series. MCV4 does not require booster dose
Zostavax® Zoster Vaccine	• Adults 60 and over	Once as a single dose	• History of anaphylaxis to gelatin, neomycin • Immunodeficiency including leukemia; lymphomas, AIDS • On immunosuppressive therapy • active untreated tuberculosis • may be pregnant
Gardasil® Human Papiloma Virus (HPV) Vaccine[2]	• Females 11–16 (may start at 9) • Prior abnormal pap, genital warts and positive HPV OK to give	Three doses: 2nd dose 2 months after first, 3rd dose 6 months after first	Pregnancy

Adapted from the recommendations of the ACIP.
Foreign travel and less commonly used vaccines such as typhoid, rabies, and meningococcal are not included.
*Preventing Tetanus Diphtheria, and Pertussin Among Adults: Use of Tetanus Toxoid, Reduced Diptheria Toxoid and Acellular Pertussin Vaccine, Recommendation of the ACIP, MMWR, Dec. 15, 2006/ 55(RR17);ZS1–33 http://www.cdc.govmmwr/preview/mmwrhtml/rr5517a1.htm?s_cid-rr5517ale accessed 2/14/2006.
†Chronic disease includes cardiovascular, pulmonary including asthma, metabolic including diabetes, renal dysfunction, hemaglobinopathies, immunosuppressive, or immunodeficiency disorders.
‡Same as above plus asplenic, CHF, chronic liver dysfunction, alcoholism, CSF leaks, hematologic malignancies, organ transplant.
[2]ACIP Provisional Recommendations for the Use of Zoster Vaccine posting of provisional recommendations: November 20, 2006. http://www.cdc-gov/nip/recs/provisional_Bcs,ster-11-20-06.pdf
[3]ACIP Provisional Recommendations for the Use of Quadrivalent HPV Vaccine, posting of provisional recommendations: August 14, 2006, http://www.cdc.gov/nip/recs/provisional__recs/hpv.pdf

bleeding, the USPSTF concluded that the balance of benefits and harms is most favorable in patients at high risk for coronary heart disease (5-year risk ≥3%).

Screening for Asymptomatic Disease

A large part of the public's perception of the "routine physical" is screening for disease that might be present but is not yet symptomatic. Many tests and examinations are available, with little agreement on who should receive which measures, and how often the screens should be done. The following five criteria are necessary to justify the general use of a screening intervention:

1. The prevalence of the disease and burden of suffering caused by the disease must be high enough to justify widespread screening.
2. The condition must have an asymptomatic period during which treatment will significantly reduce morbidity or mortality.
3. Acceptable methods of treatment must be available at a reasonable cost.
4. The screening test and interventions must be effective with few adverse effects.
5. The screening test must have a high sensitivity (20).

Consider that a screening test initiates a diagnostic algorithm that could have significant risk and cause harm as well as provide benefit. If a test has a low specificity but high sensitivity, the number of false positives increases. A positive screening test usually leads to a more expensive or more invasive test. In the case of colon cancer screening, for example, a positive fecal occult blood test (FOBT) usually leads to a colonoscopy with biopsies (21). The risks of this test, although fairly low, include bleeding, intestinal perforation, irritation, and adverse effects from sedatives. The most serious risk of colonoscopy, perforation of the colon, occurs in 0.2%–1% of procedures (22). If FOBT screening were conducted annually on persons between the ages of 50 and 75, an individual would have a 45% probability of a false positive result at some point, leading to another test, usually a colonoscopy. The preparation, anxiety, cost, and risk for one false positive adds up quickly in a population where the average risk of having colon cancer is about 5%–6%. As another example, over one-third of women age 40 to 50 years undergoing annual mammography will experience a "cancer scare." (23) Cancer scares can lead to long-term worry. Men who receive a false positive PSA test result report more worry about cancer and belief that their cancer risk is increased, despite negative biopsy (24).

Remember, screening tests are offered to patients who are asymptomatic. They are healthy and therefore the prevalence of disease in this population is low. When addressing cancer screening in elderly patients, one should first consider life expectancy, current and anticipated quality of life, the risk of cancer death, and the number needed to screen to prevent one death. There is considerable variability depending on the patient's life expectancy. Individuals with a shorter life expectancy (due to other illness or health status) are significantly less likely to benefit from screening than those with a longer life expectancy, regardless of age (25). From an ethical perspective, nonmaleficence (i.e., doing no harm) should be the dominating principle since the harm of a screening program (including both the screening test and any further investigations

that arise from it) falls on healthy persons. Consent needs to be more informed than for routine care, and apply to the screening program not just the test. The discussion must include both benefits and harm. Because screening is by "invitation," evidence for the effectiveness of a screening test should be better than that expected for routine care (26).

Although the recommendations for screening services are based on current data and expert opinion, many are still controversial. The target populations, screening intervals, and technical procedures for providing these services are unclear. Table 6.6 summarizes adult screening recommendations. Apply recommendations to individual patients with consideration of other priorities, such as your location, availability of testing, and the probability of disease in this patient (risk factor assessment), as well as patient wishes after informed consent.

Preventive care can be expensive. A major issue in screening is who pays the bill? Medicare, for example, covers mammography every two years, but pays for only a single preventive health exam on enrollment at 65. Many traditional third-party payers (insurance companies) do not pay for preventive care. One advantage of some prepaid (HMO, PPOs) health insurance plans is that preventive care may be a higher priority, and the patient might not be directly billed for these services. Several managed care plans also use performance of screening tests as a measure of physician quality.

Educating Patients

The last element of the RISE mnemonic is patient education. This aspect of prevention uses risk factor identification to tailor educational messages about lifestyle change. Patient education or counseling can be in the form of brief advice or more comprehensive counseling. For patients resistant or ambivalent to change, using techniques of motivational interviewing may be effective to move patients along the path to change (27). Continuity provided in family medicine and other primary care specialties provides the opportunity to reinforce a message, such as the importance of smoking cessation, as does hearing this message from each specialist a patient may encounter. Both public and one-to-one programs have been shown to be effective (17). For example, recent reductions in coronary artery disease mortality have at least in part resulted from public education and individual counseling about diet and exercise as well as from better control of hypertension (20). Likewise, declining HIV infection rates among gay men can be attributed to education and behavior change.

When educating patients, provide written materials, since the average patient retains only about 50% of what is said during the physician visit. A good source for patient information is *http://www.familydoctor.org* sponsored by the American Academy of Family Physicians and MedlinePlus *http://medlineplus.gov/* sponsored by the National Institutes of Health. The Agency for Health Care Research and Quality, the parent agency for the USPSTF and PPIP programs, has a personal health guide for patients, available at *http://www.ahrq.gov/ppip/adguide/*. This guide gives patients brief information about the various services, and allows for self-tracking.

The USPSTF makes specific recommendations regarding counseling and patient education. The most relevant for the family physician are summarized below.

TABLE 6.6 Well Adult—Recommended Preventive Services

Screen / Chemoprophylaxis	When to Begin / When to End	Interval	Tools / Special Concerns	Level of Evidence
Alcohol misuse screening and counseling interventions	Adulthood	Unknown	May use CAGE or Alcohol Use Disorders Identification Test to screen. May use 5 As—assess, advise, agree, assist, arrange—for behavioral counseling	B
Aspirin for primary prevention of cardiovascular events	Men older than 40 Postmenopausal women Younger people at risk for CHD	Every 5 years or when other CHD risk factors are detected	Address potential benefits and harms of aspirin therapy	A
Blood Pressure	First visit	Every 1–2 years, optimum not been determined. If on medication then 2–3X/year	Chart Record, flow sheet	A
Cholesterol	Men 35 & older Women 45 & older 20 & older if risk factors for coronary heart disease No established age to stop screening	Every 5 years More often if lipid levels close to needing therapy Less often if lipid levels low	Risk factors: -diabetes -FH of heart disease, male <50, female<60 -FH of high chol.—multiple risks for CHD (e.g., HTN, smoking)	A B
Colon Cancer screening	Age 50 average risk Age 40 increased risk End when age or co-morbid conditions limit life expectancy	Depends on test see next	All agree screening should be done, but how and how often varies	A
Fecal Occult Blood Test	As above	Annually	High false positive. Lowest cost and risk	
Sigmoidoscopy	As Above	Every 5 years	Some recommend use together with FOBT. Evidence for combined unclear. USPSTF recommends either FS or FOBT	
Colonoscopy	As above	Every 10 years	Highest Cost, highest risk, most accurate. Growing interest in general screen but no formal recommendation for general pop.	
Depression	Adulthood No established age to stop screening	Unknown	Should have systems in place to ensure accurate diagnosis effective treatment and follow-up.	B
Diabetes, Type 2	Adults with HTN or hyperlipidemia	1 to 3 years	ADA recommends Fasting plasma glucose(>126) for screening Insufficient evidence to recommend for or against screening asymptomatic adults	B

HIV	High risk patients; Pregnant women; *Universal screening recommendation expected summer 2006	High Risk *Intermediate and average risk groups may be included interval of testing expected to be revised.	All pregnant women, men who have had sex with men, hx prior STD, new or multiple partners, IV drug users; men and women who exchange sex for money or drugs or partners who do; individuals whose past or present partners were HIV-infected, bisexual, or injection drug users;	A
Obesity	First visit	Periodically	Use height/weight to calculate body mass index (BMI). May use waist circumference as measure of central adiposity	B
Syphillis	High risk adults; All pregnant women	Unknown	High risk adults include men who have sex with men, persons who exchange sex for drugs, commercial sex workers, adults in a correctional facility	A
Tobacco use and counseling to prevent tobacco caused disease	All adults	Unknown	Brief interventions–screening, counseling and/or pharmacotherapy have increased tobacco abstinence rates	A
Women Only				
Breast Cancer Screening	Age 40; No established age to stop screening	Every 1–2 years; Women with limited life expectancy unlikely to benefit	Screening mammography with or without clinical breast exam	A
Cervical Cancer	Three years after onset of sexual activity or age 21 whichever comes first	At least every 3 years (USPSTF, AAFP, ACPM, CTF); Annual(ACS, ACOG)	No need for routine pap after hysterectomy for benign reasons.	A
Chlamydia	All sexually active women <25; Asymptomatic women at increased risk for infection	Routine with pap (annual) or other pelvic until 25; Also women over 25 at increased risk; Pregnancy	Increase risk if prior STD, new or multiple partners, inconsistent use of condoms, African American, or unmarried,	A; C (>25 and low risk)
Gonorrhea	All sexually active women <25; Asymptomatic women at increased risk for infection; High risk pregnant patients	Non-pregnant women interval uncertain. In pregnancy–1st prenatal visit, then repeat in 3rd trimester	Increase risk if prior STD, new or multiple partners, inconsistent use of condoms, sex work, drug use or African American	B; D (if low risk)

(continued)

TABLE 6.6 Well Adult—Recommended Preventive Services (continued)

Screen / Chemoprophylaxis	When to Begin / When to End	Interval	Tools/ Special Concerns	Level of Evidence
Osteoporosis	Age 65 Age 60 high risk	Minimum 2 years to measure change in bone mineral density (BMD) Longer intervals ok for screening	DEXA scan of femoral neck best predictor of hip fracture (fx). Low body weight (<70kg) best predictor of low BMD, then not using estrogen. Other risks: White / Asian, history (hx) of fracture, Hx of osteoporotic fx, hx of falls, smoking, alcohol or caffeine use, limited physical activity	B
Men Only				
Abdominal Aortic Aneurysm	Age 65–75 with history of smoking	One time if initial screen negative If intermediate size AAA (4–5.4cm), periodic screening	Abdominal US has 95% sensitivity and 100% specificity in setting with adequate quality assurance	A
Prostate Cancer includes PSA testing and DRE	Age 50–70 Age 45 high risk	Unknown	Most authorities do not recommend screening High risk: African American or first degree relative with Prostate cancer	I
Chlamydia	First sex	Periodically	Urethral swab, urine tests being studied	I

Data are from The Guide to Clinical Preventive Services 2005. Recommendations of the U.S. Preventive Services Task Force.
Level of evidence for effectiveness: A, good evidence that [the service] improves important health outcomes and that benefits substantially outweigh harms; B, at least fair evidence that [the service] improves important health outcomes and that benefits outweigh harms; C, at least fair evidence that [the service] can important health outcomes but concludes that the balance of the benefits and harms is too close to justifying a general recommendation; D, at least fair evidence that [the service] is ineffective or that harm outweighs benefits; I, Evidence that [the service] is effective is lacking, of poor quality, or conflicting and the balance of benefit and harms cannot be determined. (Note this language has been modifies from the USPSTF 2nd edition to the 3rd edition.)

SMOKING

Physicians should systematically identify smokers and provide strong clear and personalized advice to quit. The first step is to assess readiness to quit. For patients who are ready, clinicians should provide smoking cessation counseling, consider drug therapy with nicotine products and/or buproprion, and offer referral as appropriate to in-person or telephone-based smoking cessation programs. Counseling should be done on a regular basis to smokers, as multiple messages are often needed; the harmful effect of smoking on children's health should be emphasized to smoking parents.

ALCOHOL AND OTHER DRUG ABUSE

The USPSTF recommends screening and behavioral counseling interventions to reduce alcohol misuse by adults, including pregnant women, although there is insufficient evidence to recommend for or against routine screening for drug abuse. Screening tools for harmful drinking and abuse include CAGE, AUDIT and other questionnaires. CAGE (representing key words Cut down, Annoyed, Guilt, Eye opener in a 4-question screening tool) and THE ALCOHOL USE DISORDERS IDENTIFICATION TEST (AUDIT), a 10-question tool are validated measures to detect patients at risk for problem drinking. All persons who use alcohol should be counseled about the dangers of operating a motor vehicle or performing other potentially dangerous activities after drinking alcohol. Pregnant women should be advised to limit or cease drinking during pregnancy. Minimal interventions by primary care clinicians, such as advice to modify current use patterns and warnings about adverse health consequences, can have beneficial effects, especially for patients in the early stages of addiction (28). Patients identified as drug abusers require appropriate treatment or referral.

DENTAL AND ORAL HEALTH

Patients should be advised to see a dentist regularly. They should also be encouraged to avoid sugary snacks and to brush regularly with toothpaste that has fluoride.

UNINTENTIONAL INJURY

Advise patients to use seatbelts. The American Academy of Family Physicians additionally advises counseling on the use of child safety seats, bicycle safety, motorcycle helmet use, smoke detectors, poison control center numbers, and driving while intoxicated. The USPSTF recommends counseling elderly patients on specific measures to reduce the risk of falling.

DOMESTIC VIOLENCE

The American College of Obstetrics and Gynecology (ACOG) recommends counseling on abuse and neglect to young women, teens, and the elderly. However, the USPSTF found insufficient evidence to recommend for or against routine screening of women for intimate partner violence, or of older adults or their caregivers for elder abuse.

NUTRITION

The USPSTF recommends that clinicians screen all adult patients for obesity and offer intensive counseling and behavioral interventions to promote sustained weight loss for obese adults. Most major authorities recommend counseling patients on nutrition though a clinician; a dietician also may do this counseling. Counseling should provide patients with basic information about managing a healthy diet. Use the food pyramid *http://www.mypyramid.gov/* or nutritional facts label as tools. The US Department of Agriculture and the US Department of Health and Human Services recommend the following in their publication, *Dietary Guidelines for Americans:*

- Eat a variety of foods.
- Balance the food you eat with physical activity; maintain or improve your weight.
- Choose a diet with plenty of grain products, vegetables, and fruits.
- Choose a diet low in fat (less than 30% of calories), saturated fat (less than 10% of calories), and cholesterol (300 mg or less per day).
- Choose a diet that is moderate in sugars.
- Choose a diet that is moderate in salt and sodium (less than 2400 mg per day).
- If you drink alcoholic beverages, do so only in moderation (no more than one drink daily for women or 2 drinks daily for men).
- One drink is 12 oz of regular beer, 5 oz of wine, or 1.5 oz of 80-proof distilled spirits.

Obese patients should be counseled to limit their calorie intake and increase activity to achieve a weight loss goal of 1\2 to 1 pound per week. Women of all ages should be educated on getting adequate calcium intake to prevent osteoporosis, and women of childbearing age should be counseled to have adequate folate intake to prevent neural tube defects.

PHYSICAL ACTIVITY

Assess and counsel all patients about regular physical activity. Exercise programs should be medically safe, gradual, enjoyable, convenient, realistic, and structured. Experts agree that physical activity that is at least of moderate intensity, for 30 minutes or longer, and performed on most days of the week is sufficient to confer health benefits. Patients who are not willing or able to reach these goals should be encouraged to increase the amount of physical activity in their daily lives, such as taking stairs or walking rather than driving when available. For those at risk and all women, adequate calcium intake should be coupled with weight-bearing exercise for adequate bone development and prevention of bone loss. Providers can and should be role models for physical fitness. Studies show that providers who exercise regularly are significantly better at providing exercise counseling to their patients than those who do not (9).

STDS, HIV, AND UNINTENDED PREGNANCY

All adolescents and adults should be counseled on the risks for acquiring STDs and HIV. Counseling should be tailored to each patient based on his or her risk factors, needs, and abilities. Unintended pregnancy is the responsibility of both partners and can be avoided with proper planning. The periodic health exam, a visit for an STD, or an acute ill visit may provide an opportunity to assess a patient's risk and provide information about birth control and STD prevention. Specific education materials or advice about abstinence, avoidance of high-risk behaviors, or high-risk partners, barrier methods including latex condom use, and other contraception including the emergency contraception the "morning after" pill may reduce the risk of STDs and unintended pregnancy. The clinician should also advise the patient that the use of drugs or alcohol increase risk of acquiring STDs or becoming pregnant unintentionally by increasing high-risk sexual behavior.

SKIN CANCER

Clinicians should advise patients to avoid excessive sun exposure. Recommending appropriate use of clothing and sunscreen especially to parents of young children and patients with history of sunburn or fair skin is appropriate.

Don't Give Up

Some students and practitioners develop a certain fatalism about patient education. This attitude results from seeing patients who do not make lifestyle changes that would obviously benefit their health. When this happens, remember that education is only one element needed to produce change. The crucial element is motivation, which comes largely from the individual, the family and the social support network. From this perspective, it is often better to be content with partial results and to be encouraged by the patients who do follow your recommendations.

SPECIAL CONSIDERATIONS IN PREVENTION

In several areas where the benefits of prevention seem intuitively obvious, there is insufficient evidence to recommend a specific intervention. Evidence is growing in these areas, and the USPSTF recommends that clinicians give special attention to them. These areas include skin lesions with malignant features, peripheral arterial disease, symptoms and signs of oral cancer and premalignancy, subtle or nonspecific symptoms and signs of thyroid dysfunction, changes in functional performance (with aging), depression, suicide risk, family violence, drug abuse, and poor oral hygiene. For these conditions, there may be a high burden of suffering. Case-finding and counseling have low propensity for harm, are low cost, and have potential for benefit. Two of these topics deserve further mention—issues of aging and family violence.

Older Adults

Aging affects not only the patient, but also the persons closest to him or her. Many older adults are active and continue to work, travel, and maintain a home for the remainder of their lives. For some, aging proves a challenge in day-to-day physical and cognitive activities. All older adults need routine care. The American College of Physicians recommends screening each older adult for functioning in basic activities of daily living and mental status (29). The Short Blessed Cognitive Status Screen is a tool that is useful for cognitive screening. It is important to remember that older adults can also be affected by alcoholism, depression, drug abuse, and violence. These problems may not be evident unless the questions are asked. Loneliness and depression can manifest as a dementia-like illness.

Family Violence

Family violence is a difficult and often avoided issue. The victims are generally women and children, but men and the elderly are also at risk in some settings. Persons encountering violence rarely reveal this to the physician as their chief complaint. Often, they present with symptoms of chronic pain, anxiety, insomnia, drug use, or depression (30,31). The patient may not be willing to bring up the subject, but may be relieved to be asked. The ACOG, American Medical Association, and American Academy of Family Physicians all have recently published statements stressing the importance of screening patents (women in particular) about violence (30–32). A set of questions known as the SAFE screen (33) has been advocated by some, even though its validity as a screen has not yet been proven. SAFE is a simple pneumonic representing a screening tool with 8 questions in 4 areas:

1. **S**tress and **S**afety; do you feel safe in your relationship?
2. **A**fraid or **A**bused; Has your partner ever threatened you or your children? Has your partner ever abused you or your children?
3. **F**riends and **F**amily; If you were hurt, would your friends or family know? Would they be able to help you?
4. **E**mergency Plan; Do you have a safe place to go in an emergency? Do you need help in locating a shelter? Would you like to talk to a counselor about this?

CHALLENGES IN PROVIDING PREVENTIVE CARE

There are several challenges in providing preventive care. The first is time constraint. In fact, to provide all the services recommended by the USPSTF using a theoretical model of a physician with a typical size patient panel representative of the US population, a physician would have to spend 7.4 hours per working day to provide these services (34)! Next, it can be difficult to motivate both patients and physicians. Often the patient and physician have different goals and expectations. Many patients, especially men, do not schedule well visits and even avoid the doctor. Patients may refuse available preventive measures because of different cultural beliefs about health. Some are unwilling to accept the risk of certain procedures. Though the value of prenatal, well baby, and well child care may be fairly well established in both the physicians' and patients' minds, well adult care is not. Neither the patient nor the physician may have a good understanding of what services should be offered, or what services are likely to be beneficial. Evidence supporting the usefulness of some common preventive health services may be lacking, or may not apply to an individual patient. Significant customization is required in well adult care. For example, there is widespread disagreement on the role of PSA testing to screen for prostate cancer. Despite the lack of evidence for its benefit, recommendations range from initiating screening in men at age 40 to recommendations against screening because of current evidence that the harm may outweigh the benefit. In this example, despite the majority of recommending bodies advising against routine screening or advising the performance of screening only after informed consent, there is significant use of this test in the community.

As with most of medicine, preventive care cannot be learned from one article, one chapter, or one chart; it takes practice. There is a growing body of evidence to support or refute a variety of traditional preventive clinical practices. Evidence-based guidelines are growing in number and are now readily available on the Internet at the point of care for laptop and PDA for both patients and physicians. They are becoming integrated with EHRs. These resources can support a good doctor/patent relationship and a well-organized office system to deliver preventive services.

Electronic Resources:
World Wide Web

- National Guidelines clearing house—*http://www.guidelines.gov*
- Agency for Healthcare Research and Policy/ U.S. Preventive Service Task Force—*http://www.ahrq.gov/clinic/prevenix.htm*
- American Academy of Family Physicians Recommendations for Clinical Preventive Services—*http://www.aafp.org/online/en/home/clinical/exam.html*
- Pocket Guide to Good Health for Americans—*http://www.ahrq.gov/ppip/adguide/*
- Putting Prevention Into Practice—*http://www.ahrq.gov/clinic/ppipix.htm*

PDA Applications

- USPSTF selector download—select appropriate services by age gender service type and level of evidence *http://pda2.ahrq.gov/ipss/ipss.htm*
- "Shots"—Updated each year includes adult and pediatric immunization schedules and information on each vaccine *http://www.immunizationed.org/default.aspx*
- American Cancer Society (ACS) C-Tools 2.0—ACS recommendations for cancer screening as well as tools to assist with smoking cessation and PSA decision making *http://www.cancer.org/docroot/COM/content/div_TX/COM_5_1x_The_C-Tools_20.asp?sitearea = COM*

CASE DISCUSSION

Using the RISE format, you can focus on each element of preventive care for this man.

R—Risk factors need to be identified. Does he abuse tobacco, alcohol, or drugs? Is there a family history of cancer or a personal history of problems, such as elevated cholesterol or blood pressure? Are there sexual or occupational risk factors?

I—Immunizations must be updated. When was his last TdaP vaccination? Is he in a special risk group that needs the hepatitis vaccine? Is he a frequent international traveler? Is he a candidate for the flu shot? He is likely due for TdaP and flu vaccine in season.

S—He can then be screened considering your assessment of risk factors by limited physical examination and laboratory tests, as indicated in Table 6.6. Appropriate tests would include height, weight, and blood pressure measurements. Limited evidence supports a detailed skin exam. If he has no other significant historical factors, additional exam has little yield and should only serve to strengthen the doctor patient relationship. Take time to discuss screening programs, such as when and how to start colon cancer screening and if PSA testing should be considered. One also may screen for depression.

E—A large part of this patient's encounter will focus on education, centered on his risk factors and what he can do to minimize them. The family history of early coronary artery disease is an indication and likely a motivator for learning about diet, exercise, and weight control. Other topics could include dental visits, accident prevention, and appropriate alcohol use.

Obviously this may be too much to discuss effectively in one office visit. In a family practice setting, these issues and others are usually covered over several visits, often over many years. Scheduling a visit to interpret laboratory data presents another opportunity to discuss preventive health issues.

References

1. Bertakis KD, et al. Physician practice styles and patient outcomes: differences between family practice and general internal medicine. Med Care. 1998;36(6):879–891.
2. Flocke SA, et al. Patient and visit characteristics associated with opportunistic preventive service delivery. J Fam Prac. 1998;47(3):202–208.
3. Stange KC, et al. Direct Observation of rates of preventive service delivery in community family practice. Prev Med. 2000;31(2 pt 1):167–176.
4. Maciosek MV, Coffield AB, Edwards NM, Goodman MJ, Flottemesch TJ, Solberg LI. Priorities among effective clinical preventive services: results of a systematic review and analysis. Am J Prev Med 2006;31(1): 52–61.
5. Speedling EJ, Rose DN. Building an effective doctor-patient relationship: from patient satisfaction to patient participation. Soc Sci Med. 1985;21(2):115–120.
6. Luckmann R, Melville SK. Periodic health evaluation of adults: a survey of family physicians. J. Fam Pract. 1995;40(6): 547–554.
7. Sirovich BE, Welch HG. Cervical cancer screening among women without a cervix. JAMA. 2004;291:2990–2993.
8. Saraiya M, et al. Observations from the CDC. An assessment of Pap smears and hysterectomies among women in the United States. J Womens Health Gend Based Med. 2002;11: 103–109.
9. US Preventive Service Task Force. The Clinicians Handbook of Preventive Services, 2nd ed. 1998. US Department of Health and Human Services General Printing Office. 1998. *http://www.ahrq.gov/clinic/ppiphand.htm.*
10. Garr DR, et al. The effect of routine use of computer-generated preventive reminders in a clinical practice. Am J Prev Med. 1993;9(1):55–61.
11. Ornstein SM, et al. Implementation and evaluation of a computer-based preventive service system. Fam Med. 1995;27(4): 260–266.
12. Sheridan SL, Harris RP, Woolf SH. The Shared Decision-making Workgroup, Third US Preventive Services Task Force. Current methods of the US Preventive Services Task Force: a review of the process. Am J Prev Med. 2004;26(1): 56–66.
13. Stange KC, et al. Physician agreement with US Preventive Services Task Force recommendations. J Fam Pract. 1992; 34(4):409–416.
14. McGinnis J, Foege W. Actual causes of death in the United States. JAMA. 1993;270(18):2207–2212.
15. Mokdad AH, Marks JS, Stroup DF, Gerberding JL. Actual causes of death in the United States, 2000. JAMA. 2004; 291(10):1238–1245.
16. National Vital Statistics Reports, Center for Disease Control, 53(17) March 2005, *http://www.cdc.gov/nchs/data/nvsr/nvsr53/nvsr53_17.pdf.* Accessed April 24, 2006.

Academy of Hospice and Palliative Medicine, "Palliative Care is the comprehensive management of physical, social, spiritual, and existential needs of patients, in particular those with incurable, progressive illnesses. . . . The goal of palliative care is to achieve the best possible quality of life through relief of suffering, control of symptoms, and restoration of functional capacity while remaining sensitive to personal, cultural, and religious values, beliefs, and practices." (6) According to the Institute of Medicine, the focus of palliative care is "to prevent, relieve, reduce or soothe the symptoms of disease without effecting a cure. . . . Palliative care in this broad sense is not restricted to those who are dying. . . . It attends closely to the emotional, spiritual, and practical needs and goals of patients and those close to them." (7) Obviously there is great overlap between hospice and palliative care. Palliative care, however, includes symptomatic care in hospitals and nursing homes, and may be offered in home care programs independent of hospice care. Leading hospitals now offer palliative care consulting services to assist in difficult symptom management, or to facilitate complex advance care planning discussions for patients who wish to retain the option for ongoing efforts to cure the disease. Clinical markers and patient satisfaction are both improved with access to such a service (8, 9).

The ideal system would seamlessly integrate palliative care from the acute, inpatient setting through hospice care at home, the nursing home, or a hospice residential facility. However, the current regulatory environment and reimbursement system, as well as physicians' and the public's attitudes and perceptions regarding hospice, create a powerful bias toward curative or disease-focused treatment. A false dichotomy results, where care is viewed as either curative or comfort care, missing the more holistic approach of palliation throughout the course of care. This dichotomy limits early palliation, with the symptom burden viewed as an inevitable consequence of aggressive treatment, and ultimately results in late referrals to hospice. Many hospices have addressed this concern by embracing the "open access" concept, where therapies once denied as incompatible with hospice philosophy are now allowed, removing the psychological and clinical barrier that hospice is "giving up." This approach will presumably expand the pool of eligible patients who elect earlier enrollment in hospice programs, but empirical data on the impact of the open access model are not yet available.

The National Consensus Project, an interdisciplinary coalition of professional organizations dedicated to hospice and palliative care, completed a comprehensive overview of the conceptual foundations of palliative care and established a set of clinical practice guidelines (10). The guidelines are described within eight domains of palliative care, as outlined in Table 7.1. In addition, the National Institutes for Health, under the auspices of the Agency for Healthcare Research and Quality (AHRQ) and the National Institute of Nursing Research, commissioned a "state of the science" conference in 2004 to establish evidence-based best practices, and to identify a future palliative medicine research agenda (11).

Public attention to end-of-life care also increases following high profile "media events," such as the Supreme Court case consideration of Oregon's legalization of physician-assisted suicide (PAS) or the Terri Schiavo right-to-die case. The highly divisive controversy over such cases generally obscures a more basic problem, which is that many patients—and far too many of their physicians—are unaware of the extent to which modern palliative care and hospice practices, or optimal advance care planning, could address the untreated symptoms or other concerns that led to the initial request for PAS, or the unresolved conflicts within families or between families and care providers that lead to litigation. Toward that end, extensive professional and public education efforts are underway to enhance understanding of the distinctions between palliative care and hospice as well as their areas of overlap, as shown in Table 7.2.

PREVENTION AND PREPARATION

Quality end-of-life care is hampered by American society's avoidance of frank discussions about death as a routine and expected part of human life. A number of difficulties can be averted by early and regular communication within families and between patients and their physicians. Family physicians, as proponents of continuity of care, have a special obligation to become skilled at these forms of communication.

Advance Directives

One trigger to helpful communication and reflection is completing an advance directive form before a person suffers a health care crisis or develops a terminal disease. Available types of advance directives range from the general, which state in broad terms the types of care a patient would or would not want, to the concrete, such as physician orders for life-sustaining treatment that are now accepted in many states. When the patient remains competent, this prior discussion helps pave the way for candid discussion of treatment options. Revisiting the conversation will promote an exploration of any values or desires that have changed since the advance directive was originally completed. If the patient becomes incompetent, families often take comfort knowing that they do not have to choose a course of treatment on their own, but can be guided by the patient's own previously expressed values. To secure these later benefits, the method of completing the advance directive ought to be one that stimulates the greatest possible degree of discussion among the patient, the family, and the physician. A paper form that meets legal requirements, and which is filled out in detail, but which the patient has never discussed with the physician or with family, may offer little aid when complex decisions need to be made.

Once noncontroversial from both ethical and legal standpoints, advance directives have recently come under fire. An empirical attack on "living wills" claims that they do not accomplish their goals (12). A more basic criticism is that allowing now-healthy people to refuse life-prolonging therapy at a later stage of their lives, when they may become incompetent to make decisions, offends some community values (13). However, even the most severe critics of advance directives are in favor of procedures that allow patients to specify *who* should make decisions on their behalf (durable power of attorney for health care), and focus most of their criticisms on forms that record *what* care the patients do or do not wish to receive ("living wills"). It remains to be seen whether the medical, ethical, and legal communities will be influenced by these recent criticisms.

TABLE 7.1 National Consensus Project Clinical Practice Guidelines for Quality Palliative Care

1. Structure and Processes of Care
   - Guideline 1.1: The plan of care is based on a comprehensive interdisciplinary assessment of the patient and family.
   - Guideline 1.2: The care plan is based on the identified and expressed values, goals, and needs of patient and family and is developed with professional guidance and support for decision making.
   - Guideline 1.3: An interdisciplinary team provides services to the patient and family, consistent with the care plan.
   - Guideline 1.4: The interdisciplinary team may include appropriately trained and supervised volunteers.
   - Guideline 1.5: Support for education and training is available to the interdisciplinary team.
   - Guideline 1.6: The palliative care program is committed to quality improvement in clinical and management practices.
   - Guideline 1.7: The palliative care program recognizes the emotional impact on the palliative care team of providing care to patients with life-threatening illnesses and their families.
   - Guideline 1.8: Palliative care programs should have a relationship with one or more hospices and other community resources to ensure continuity of the highest-quality palliative care across the illness trajectory.
   - Guideline 1.9: The physical environment in which care is provided should meet the preferences, needs, and circumstances of the patient and family to the extent possible.
2. Physical Aspects of Care
   - Guideline 2.1: Pain, other symptoms, and side effects are managed based on the best available evidence, which is skillfully and systematically applied.
3. Psychological and Psychiatric Aspects of Care
   - Guideline 3.1: Psychological and psychiatric issues are assessed and managed based on the best available evidence, which is skillfully and systematically applied.
   - Guideline 3.2: A grief and bereavement program is available to patients and families, based on the assessed need for services.
4. Social Aspects of Care
   - Guideline 4.1: Comprehensive interdisciplinary assessment identifies the social needs of patients and their families, and a care plan is developed to respond to these needs as effectively as possible.
5. Spiritual, Religious, and Existential Aspects of Care
   - Guideline 5.1: Spiritual and existential dimensions are assessed and responded to based on the best available evidence, which is skillfully and systematically applied.
6. Cultural Aspects of Care
   - Guideline 6.1: The palliative care program assesses and attempts to meet the culture-specific needs of the patient and family.
7. Care of the Imminently Dying Patient
   - Guideline 7.1: Signs and symptoms of impending death are recognized and communicated, and care appropriate for this phase of illness is provided to patient and family.
8. Ethical and Legal Aspects of Care
   - Guideline 8.1: The patient's goals, preferences, and choices are respected within the limits of applicable state and federal law, and form the basis for the care plan.
   - Guideline 8.2: The palliative care program is aware of and addresses the complex ethical issues arising in the care of persons with life-threatening debilitating illness.
   - Guideline 8.3: The palliative care program is knowledgeable about legal and regulatory aspects of palliative care.

TABLE 7.2 Explanation of Palliative Care

Palliative care is:
- Expert care of pain and symptoms throughout illness
- Communication and support for decision making, including advance directive planning
- Attention to practical support and continuity across settings
- Care that patients want at the same time as efforts to cure or prolong life
- Care that can ease the transition from life to death, even if the patient does not choose hospice care

Palliative care is *not*:
- "Giving up" on patients
- What we do when there is "nothing more that we can do"
- In place of life-supporting or curative treatment, although when life-sustaining treatment is no longer appropriate, it is a good alternative to "doing nothing"
- The same as hospice

From: Fine RL. The imperative for hospital based palliative care: patient, institutional, and societal benefits. Proc (Bayl Univ Med Cent). 2004;17(3):259–264. Used with permission.

Breaking Bad News

Consideration of hospice care is often delayed when the patient and family have not received clear communication about a poor prognosis or the rate at which a disease is progressing. This communication breakdown often occurs because physicians are loath to transmit bad news, or view worsening disease as a personal failure. Physicians who are skilled and comfortable at breaking bad news treat their patients more humanely and also facilitate timelier decision making. Buckman developed an easily learned protocol for breaking bad news that is particularly sensitive to each patient's individual needs and emotional reactions. This protocol is outlined in Table 7.3 (14, 15).

System Issues

Medicare, most Medicaid programs, and many private insurers provide a hospice benefit. Hospice eligibility criteria require the attending physician to certify that the patient's life expectancy is 6 months or less, if the disease runs its expected course. However, hospice patients may remain on service beyond the 6-month life expectancy provided there is adequate documentation that they met hospice eligibility criteria upon initiation of hospice services, and their condition remains hospice appropriate at the time of their recertification. Patients receiving the Medicare hospice benefit sign a statement choosing the Medicare hospice benefit in place of standard Medicare-covered benefits for their illness, and enroll in a Medicare-certified hospice program.

Unfortunately, many patients miss out on hospice care, or are referred very late in the course of their terminal illness, because physicians feel they must be able to predict a life expectancy of less than 6 months with relative certainty. The National Hospice and Palliative Care Organization has published guidelines for determining prognosis for a variety of noncancer diagnoses (16). However, prognosis is an inexact science, and the rate of error is high (17, 18). Rather than asking if a patient will die in 6 months or less, a more appropriate question might be: "Would you be surprised if this patient died in the next 6 months?" This approach has been demonstrated to more effectively engage hospice benefits earlier in a patient's decline (19). Medicare has approved a pre-election benefit, which provides a nominal professional fee for a hospice medical director to consult with a patient regarding their eligibility for hospice care and their treatment alternatives. Palliative care consultations also provide this function, and enable the palliative care physician or advance practice nurse to provide a higher level of ongoing service if medically appropriate. Palliative care programs facilitate the provision of expert care for severely ill and dying patients before they are eligible for hospice care, thus eliminating the need for the 6-month prognosis for death, which seems to be a barrier for many physicians and families to engage hospice services.

Forward-looking proponents of palliative care anticipate a day when our currently fragmented system of care will be replaced by a more integrated system that allows for a continuum of palliative care across the entire duration of a chronic illness. Rather than beginning with curative care and then discharging the patient to hospice when cure is deemed impossible, curative and palliative efforts would go hand in hand at each stage of the patient's treatment, with curative care predominating early in the illness and palliative care predominating near the end (see Figure 7.1). The exact relationship between these two modes of care at each intermediate stage of illness should ideally be determined by the individual patient's needs and values, not by arbitrary time limits or peculiarities of reimbursement.

Hospice programs use an interdisciplinary team, including nurses, home health aides, pastoral care, volunteers to assist the family and provide respite care, and bereavement programs for the family after the patient's death. Ideally, most end-of-life care is carried out in the patient's home setting (which may be a nursing home or assisted-living facility). Many hospices offer a residential facility for patients unable to remain at home. Hospitalization is occasionally indicated due to severe symptoms or patient/family preferences, and Medicare offers a General Inpatient benefit to cover these services as a part of the patient's hospice care plan. Regardless of location, the basic principles of end-of-life care can be carried out provided adequate institutional support and services are available.

SYMPTOM MANAGEMENT

Relief of suffering applies to all stages of life and is especially important in end-of-life care. Although end-of-life care is most effectively delivered by an interdisciplinary approach, effective symptom management requires strong physician leadership. Physicians ultimately make the final diagnostic judgments and write orders; physicians lacking symptom management skills can impede even outstanding advocacy by

TABLE 7.3   SPIKES Protocol for Breaking Bad News

<u>**SET** up the interview</u>
  Arrange to give potentially bad test results in person
  Arrange for privacy, adequate time, and no interruptions
  Involve significant others
  Sit down, establish rapport, allow for silence/tears
  Mentally rehearse and emotionally prepare for the interview
<u>Assess the patient's **PERCEPTION**</u>
  "Ask before you tell"—what does the patient know/understand
  Ask open-ended questions, tailor news to current understanding, correct misinformation,
  identify denial
<u>Obtain the patient's **INVITATION**</u>
  Most patients, but not all, want full disclosure
  Discuss information disclosure at the time of ordering tests and before giving results
<u>Give **KNOWLEDGE** (information) to the patient</u>
  Warn the patient bad news is coming, e.g., "I'm sorry, but I have bad news" or "I'm sorry to
  tell you that . . ."
  Target to the patient's vocabulary/comprehension
  Avoid euphemisms, technical jargon, and excess bluntness
  Ask the patient to repeat back what you've said
  Regardless of prognosis, identify goals—e.g., cure, pain and symptom relief, family issues
<u>Address the patient's **EMOTIONS** with empathic responses</u>
  Physicians are generally uncomfortable with patients' emotional reactions to bad news
  Four components of an empathetic response:
    Observe the patient's emotion
    Identify the emotion to yourself
    Identify the reason for that emotion
    Let the patient know that you have connected with that emotion
<u>**STRATEGIZE** and **SUMMARIZE**</u>
  A clear plan lessens the patient's anxiety and fosters patient self-determination
  Ask if the patient is ready to discuss a plan
  Use the patient's knowledge, expectations, and goals as a starting point; discuss fears; gently
  work past denial
  Arrange follow up meetings

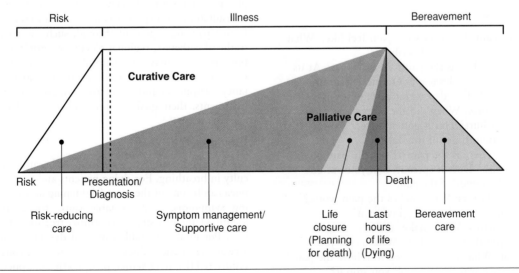

Palliative Medicine's Continuum of Care

Figure 7.1 • **Continuum of curative to palliative care.**

apy). Four different neurotransmitters mediate stimulation of the vomiting center in the medulla: serotonin, dopamine, histamine, and acetylcholine. Diagnostic evaluation should consider gastrointestinal, CNS, pharmacologic, metabolic, and psychological causes. If an underlying medical cause can be identified, appropriate treatments should be initiated. Palliative measures to alleviate nausea and vomiting include both nonpharmacologic and pharmacologic therapies. Prokinetic agents are especially useful and warrant first line therapy. Pharmacologic therapies are listed in Table 7.6.

Fatigue

Tiredness is one of the most distressing symptoms associated with end-of-life care (23). Treatable causes should be sought and corrected (e.g., anemia, medication adverse effects); however, persistent fatigue is often not treatable. In such situations, you can help by validating the patient's fatigue to family members, who may see the symptom as simply "mind over matter." Specific recommendations should focus on energy conservation and optimizing fluid and nutritional status, concordant with the patient's stage of illness and stated goals for therapy. Medical interventions are limited, but some patients will benefit from treatment with low-dose glucocorticoids (e.g., dexamethasone 2–8 mg by mouth daily) or psychostimulants (e.g., methylphenidate 2.5–5 mg each morning and noon initially, titrated to effect).

Constipation

Constipation is a frequent adverse effect of opioid analgesics, calcium channel blockers, and anticholinergic medications. Differential diagnosis includes: medication effect, decreased gastrointestinal motility, ileus, mechanical obstruction, metabolic abnormalities, spinal cord compression, dehydration, autonomic dysfunction, and malignancy. A common problem when treating constipation is the failure to titrate to an effective dose of a given agent, leading to the sense that "nothing works." Fecal impaction should also be ruled out for constipa-

tion that does not respond to standard treatments. Treatment alternatives are listed in Table 7.7.

Edema

Edema frequently occurs in advanced illness due to hypoalbuminemia, which leads to decreased oncotic pressure. Some edematous patients have lymphatic or venous obstruction because of compression by primary or metastatic tumors or from postsurgical changes. When edema has an identifiable cause (e.g., uncompensated CHF), treatment of the underlying process should be optimized. Physical measures such as compression stockings or positioning should be considered; skin care should receive careful attention.

Pressure Ulcers

A preventive approach is crucial. Skin should be kept clean and dry, with particular attention to challenges posed by incontinence. Protective techniques include padding and/or occlusive dressings for high-risk areas. Patients should be repositioned as frequently as possible, ideally every 2 hours. Appropriate mattresses and bed coverings should be used. Early detection and treatment of pressure ulcers is vital (24). Care of pressure ulcers in the terminally ill should have comfort, not healing, as the primary goal, and the relatively poor prognosis for healing should be discussed with the patient and family. Minimizing dressing changes, use of nonadherent dressings, and attention to odor management are ways to promote comfort.

ETHICAL AND LEGAL ISSUES

The issue of PAS emerged from the public's fears and frustrations over the medical community's inadequacies in caring for patients at the end of life. It would be naïve to assert that *all* requests for PAS would be obviated by excellent end-of-life care; some patients request PAS as a matter of control, or if they perceive intolerable suffering even with aggressive pallia-

TABLE 7.6 Pharmacologic Management of Nausea

Cause	Drug Class	Recommended Agents and Dosage
Movement-related nausea	Antihistamine	Meclizine 25–50 mg orally every 6 hours Hydroxyzine 25–50 mg orally every 6 hours
Tumor-related elevated intracranial pressure	Glucocorticoids	Dexamethasone 6–20 mg orally once daily
Gastric stasis	Prokinetic agent	Metoclopramide 10–15 mg orally every 6 hours, 30 minutes before meals/food and at bedtime
Stimulation of chemoreceptor trigger zone (drugs, uremia)	Dopamine antagonist	Prochlorperazine 5–20 mg orally every 6 hours, or 25 mg rectally every 12 hours, or 5–10 mg intravenously every 4 hours (maximum IV dose = 40 mg/day) Promethazine 25 mg orally or rectally, or 12.5–25 mg intravenously, every 4–6 hours Haloperidol 0.5–2 mg orally, intravenously, or subcutaneously every 6 hours, then titrate
	Serotonin antagonist	Ondansetron 4–8 mg orally three times per day
Constipation	Laxative	See Table 7.7

TABLE 7.7 Constipation Management

Treatment	Recommended Agent and Dosage	Comments
Stimulant laxatives	Prune juice 120–240 mL orally once or twice daily Senna 2 tablets or 5–10 mL of syrup orally at bedtime, titrate to effect Docusate 2 tablets orally at bedtime, titrate to effect Bisacodyl 5–15 mg orally or 10 mg suppository rectally at bedtime, titrate to effect	• Irritates the bowel and stimulates peristalsis. • Prolonged use can lead to laxative dependency and loss of normal bowel function.
Osmotic laxatives	Milk of magnesia 5–15 mL orally 1–3 times per day Lactulose 15–30 mL orally up to every 4–6 hours, then titrate to effect Magnesium citrate 1 (240mL) orally as needed	• Attracts water into the intestinal lumen, maintaining or increasing the moisture content and volume of the stool, distending the bowel, and inducing peristalsis. • Use caution with magnesium containing products in patients with renal insufficiency.
Detergent laxatives (stool softeners)	Docusate sodium 100 mg capsule orally daily, titrate to effect Docusate calcium 1–4 orally once daily, titrate to effect	• Promotes water retention in stool. Most effective for hard stools. • Onset of effect can take 3 days. For opiate-related constipation that does not respond to the above, use in combination with a stimulant laxative.
Prokinetic agents	Metoclopramide 10–20 mg orally every 6 hours	Stimulates the bowel's myenteric plexus, increasing peristalsis.
Lubricant laxatives	Mineral oil 5–30 mL at bedtime Glycerin suppositories	Lubricates intestinal mucosa and softens stool.
Large-volume enemas	Tap water enemas Soap suds enemas	• Softens the stool and distend the bowel, inducing peristalsis. • Soap suds function like a stimulant laxative.

tive care. However, most requests for PAS have more to do with fear of abandonment, or fear that their suffering will not be effectively treated, than from an actual desire to end life. A compassionate and sensitive response to a request for PAS may lead to the discovery of concerns that have not been adequately addressed, and may deepen the relationship between the physician and patient (25).

A related ethical issue is physicians' fear that providing adequate analgesia will hasten death and is tantamount to euthanasia. The concept of *double effect* counters this misperception by asserting that the hastening of death from adequate symptom relief is an unfortunate but acceptable consequence of appropriately managing the patient's symptoms. In this scenario, the intent is not to shorten the patient's life, but to provide comfort; the hastened death is deemed less undesirable than intense suffering from symptoms that can be medically relieved. The underlying intent in administering the medication is the crux of this notion: the medication is administered to alleviate pain or other symptoms that are causing undue suffering, *not* to end the patient's life.

Physicians who are unwilling to administer high-dose opioids to terminal patients out of ethical qualms that they would be committing euthanasia make two errors—an ethical and a scientific error. The ethical error, as noted, is to confuse the intent (relief of suffering, which only opioids can provide) with the consequence (the risk that the patient will die sooner). The scientific error is the belief that the risk of hastening death via respiratory depression is a significant risk in this group of patients. The assumption that opioids, titrated to the patient's pain level, hasten a patient's death is not supported by medical evidence and instead is more likely an outgrowth of the long-standing phobia of opioids in 20th century medicine and nursing.

PSYCHOSOCIAL ISSUES

Anxiety

Anxiety is a common response to the uncertainty associated with confronting one's impending death. However, anxiety also may result from inadequate control of symptoms, such as pain or dyspnea, or it may be a primary psychiatric condition. Nonpharmacologic therapy includes counseling (both psychological and spiritual), social services consultation, and family support. With chronic use, short-acting agents (e.g., alprazolam), may not provide smooth symptom relief and may also induce withdrawal symptoms if a dose is missed. Short or intermediate acting benzodiazepines are the drug of choice for medical management of acute anxiety (e.g., lorazepam 0.25–2 mg every 6 hours orally, sublingually, subcutaneously, or intravenously). Chronic anxiety often responds well to selective serotonin reuptake inhibitors (SSRIs) or tricyclics. Anxiolytics should be started at low doses and titrated to effect. Remain vigilant for adverse effects of sedation, confusion, or memory disturbance. Benzodiazepines can also trigger paradoxical agitation, particularly in the frail elderly.

Depression

The notion that terminally ill patients are inherently depressed or desire a prompt death is a misconception (26). Most patients with a terminal diagnosis will experience feelings of sadness, anger, and helplessness that are either temporary, or moderate and intermittent. However, clinical depression may indeed be associated with terminal illness. In patients with depression, early diagnosis and intervention improves the likelihood that treatment will be helpful. Risk factors for depression include refractory pain, comorbid conditions or significant physical limitations, medication adverse effects (e.g., corticosteroids, benzodiazepines), family dysfunction, substance abuse, and history of depression.

Diagnosis of depression in end-of-life care is made more difficult by the fact that many somatic symptoms used as markers for depression in physically healthy adults (such as sleep disturbance, loss of appetite, or fatigue) may be caused by the underlying disease in the terminally ill, rather than by depression. Therefore, psychological criteria for depression (i.e., dysphoria, anhedonia, and feelings of worthlessness or guilt) become more important in end-of-life care.

Treatment alternatives for depression include counseling, spiritual support, and medication. Medical management may include SSRI or tricyclic antidepressants. In general, start with low dosages and titrate upward to effect. Psychostimulants are a useful alternative for patients with severe depression or those very close to death, where the time needed to reach antidepressant effect is an issue.

Delirium

Delirium may develop rapidly, and is characterized by disorientation, cognitive impairment, and/or fluctuating levels of consciousness. Causes may include infection, medication adverse effects or withdrawal, and metabolic or hypoxic encephalopathy. If a reversible cause is identified (e.g., hypoxemia or opioid toxicity), it should be addressed specifically. If medical treatment is needed to relieve agitation, short-acting neuroleptics or benzodiazepines are indicated. Patients nearing death may experience terminal delirium, which includes day/night reversals, agitation, restlessness, and moaning/groaning. At this time, the goal of management is to relieve distress for both patient and family, and longer-acting, more sedating agents may be used.

Spiritual Issues

When aware that the end of life is approaching, most patients develop a heightened sense of the transcendent. Spiritual concerns are most commonly addressed via religious traditions, but many patients address spiritual concerns independent of organized or formal religion. The extent to which individual physicians wish to engage spiritual issues will depend on the comfort with which they can communicate with the patient on this topic. This can range from simple inquiries into the patient's spiritual needs and support system to actually praying with patients.

Patients generally want their physicians to address spiritual issues during serious illness (27), but this does not mean that physicians should go beyond their own comfort or expertise, nor is it a license to evangelize or proselytize. Often, consultation with a spiritual or pastoral care advisor will be helpful. Hospitals and hospice programs have trained chaplains who are generally quite skilled at working with patients from diverse backgrounds on the patient's terms.

Communication

Physicians should address the support and communication needs of terminally ill patients and their families. Patients' needs range from simple information (e.g., prognosis or what symptoms to expect) to complex issues of unresolved family conflicts or making final arrangements. Appropriate consultation and collaboration with social workers, counselors, or chaplains are often the most effective means of addressing more complex needs.

Family Issues

Caring for a loved one during his or her final days can present a substantial burden for families, but can also be very rewarding. Family needs can be basic, such as coordinating chores and supporting activities of daily living. They can also be quite complex, such as bathing a dying parent when the family has cultural prohibitions against seeing a parent's nakedness, or navigating the emotional minefield of adult children who had been physically or sexually abused by the dying parent. Families often need outside help, including respite care (often provided by hospice volunteers under the Medicare hospice benefit), financial support, spiritual and psychological counseling, and arrangements for disposition of the body after death.

THE ACTIVE DYING PROCESS

Managing the death itself is often a matter of preparation: laying out the expected time frame (while acknowledging its variability and unpredictability); having medications and equipment available to manage symptoms; and establishing lines of communication and coverage for the final hours. As death approaches, the family should be prepared, as best able, for terminal symptoms, and the anticipated course of decline and demise. These conversations should be frequently revisited and modified based on the patient's actual clinical course. Symptoms that should be expected include progressive weakness and fatigue, loss of appetite, changes in breathing, and cognitive dysfunction. If not anticipated, these symptoms may be quite disconcerting to family members and may lead to inappropriate calls for emergency interventions (e.g., 911).

Family members and caregivers may wonder whether supplemental fluids or nutrition are necessary. Physician guidance should include instruction that intravenous fluids may actually worsen symptoms and prolong the uncomfortable terminal stage (28). Most hospices have family handouts that review the signs and symptoms of impending death, and experienced hospice nurses are skilled at preparing families for anticipated symptoms of the active dying process.

IMMEDIATELY AFTER DEATH

Regulations regarding death pronouncements vary from state to state, so family physicians should be familiar with the regulations in their state. Typically, the primary physician is notified of the death, but a hospice nurse actually makes the death pronouncement. The absence of vital signs and the lack of response to noxious stimuli establish death.

Previous discussions should have established the patient's wishes regarding organ donation and final disposition of the body. Preparations are particularly important if special religious or cultural considerations need to be taken into account. After the death, consulting physicians and other health professionals involved in the patient's care should be notified. The attending physician of record is responsible for completing the death certificate and declaring the official cause of death, and noting any contributing medical conditions.

GRIEF AND BEREAVEMENT

Supportive preparation before the death will ease the family's burden and facilitate grieving. However, even with excellent preparation, a prolonged death can be physically and emotionally draining for the family and caregivers. "Tasks" of grieving include accepting the loss, experiencing the pain of the loss, adjusting to one's environment after the loss, and building a new life. Normal grief does not require medical intervention. When agitated grieving impairs basic functions of daily living (e.g., unremitting crying, not eating or sleeping), a brief and carefully monitored course of benzodiazepines may be helpful. Later on, the judicious use of antidepressants is indicated if grief is accompanied by prolonged or incapacitating depression. It bears repeating that pharmacologic management is *not* indicated for "normal" grieving, but should be reserved for situations when basic functions of daily living are impaired, or protracted grieving appears to have evolved into a clinical depression.

The extent of involvement with the family will vary based on your relationship with the family. Personal expressions of condolence range from a phone call or card, to visiting the family at their home, to attending the formal visitation or funeral. Primary care physicians often care for other family members and should offer professional follow up to assess grief and personal issues following the death of their loved one. Additional resources may be available through the multidisciplinary hospice team.

CONCLUSION

The amazing technological progress of modern medicine comes with an unfortunate drawback: the desire to cure disease often overshadows the obligation to care for the patient.

Eric Cassell observed, "The relief of suffering and the cure of disease must be seen as twin obligations of a medical profession that is truly dedicated to the care of the sick. Physicians' failure to understand the nature of suffering can result in medical intervention that (though technically adequate) not only fails to relieve suffering but becomes a source of suffering itself" (29).

Physicians active in hospice and palliative care are often asked if their work is depressing. Most respond that the opposite is true: the work itself is very gratifying, because the prospect of patients not receiving the best available care at their time of greatest need is what is truly depressing. Caring for patients and families through the entire spectrum of the natural life cycle, including the time of bereavement following the death of a loved one, is an integral role for the family physician. Hospice and palliative care are not the last resort when medicine fails, but the completion of whole person care.

REFERENCES

1. Sullivan AM, Lakoma MD, Block SD. The status of medical education in end-of-life care: a national report. J Gen Intern Med. 2003;18(9):685–695.
2. Sullivan AM, Warren AG, Lakoma MD, Liaw KR, Hwang D, Block SD. End-of-life care in the curriculum: a national study of medical education deans. Acad Med. 2004;79(8): 760–768.
3. Rabow MW, Hardie GE, Fair FM, McPhee SJ. End-of-life care content in 50 textbooks from multiple specialties. JAMA. 2000;283:771–778.
4. Ross DD, Shpritz D, Hull MM, Goloubeva O. Long-term evaluation of required coursework in palliative and end-of-life care for medical students. J Palliat Med. 2005;8(5): 962–974.
5. Pan CX, Carmody S, Leipzig RM, Granieri E, Sullivan A, Block SD, Arnold RM. There is hope for the future: national survey results reveal that geriatric medicine fellows are well-educated in end-of-life care. J Am Geriatr Soc. 2005;53(4): 705–710.
6. Storey P, Knight CF, Schonwetter RS. Pocket Guide to Hospice/Palliative Medicine. Glenview, IL: American Academy of Hospice and Palliative Medicine, 2003.
7. Field MJ, Cassel CK, eds. Approaching Death: Improving Care at the End of Life. Washington, DC: National Academy Press, 1997.
8. O'Mahony S, Blank AE, Zallman L, Selwyn PA. The benefits of a hospital-based inpatient palliative care consultation service: preliminary outcome data. J Palliat Med. 2005;8(5): 1033–1039.
9. Manfredi PL, Morrison RS, Morris J, Goldhirsch SL, Carter JM, Meier DE. Palliative care consultations: how do they impact the care of hospitalized patients? J Pain Symptom Manage. 2000;20(3):166–173.
10. National Consensus Project for Quality Palliative Care (2004). Clinical Practice Guidelines for Quality Palliative Care. *http://www.nationalconsensusproject.org*. Accessed Feb. 12, 2007.
11. Lorenz K, Lynn J, Morton SC, Dy S, Mularski R, Shugarman L, et al. End-of-Life Care and Outcomes. Summary, Evidence Report/Technology Assessment No. 110. (Prepared by the Southern California Evidence-based Practice Center, under Contract No. 290-02-0003.) AHRQ Publication No. 05-E004-1. Rockville, MD: Agency for Healthcare Research and Quality. December 2004.
12. Fagerlin A, Schneider CE. Enough: the failure of the living will. Hastings Center Report 2004;34(2):30–42.

13. President's Council on Bioethics. Taking Care: Ethical Caregiving in our Aging Society. Washington, DC, 2005; *www.bioethics.gov*. Accessed Feb. 12, 2007

14. Buckman R. How to Break Bad News: A Guide for Health Care Professionals. Baltimore: Johns Hopkins University Press, 1992.

15. Baile WF, Buckman R, Lenzi R, et al. SPIKES-A Six-step Protocol for Delivering Bad News: Application to the Patient With Cancer. Oncologist. 2000;5(4):302–311.

16. Stuart B, et al. Medical Guidelines for Determining Prognosis in Selected Non-Cancer Diseases, 2nd ed. Arlington, VA: National Hospice Organization, 1996.

17. Christakis NA, Lamont EB. Extent and determinants of error in doctors' prognoses in terminally ill patients: prospective cohort study. BMJ. 2000;320:469–473.

18. Christakis NA. Timing of referral of terminally ill patients to an outpatient hospice. J Gen Intern Med. 1994;9:314–320.

19. Lynn J, Schuster JL, Kabcenell A. Improving Care for the End of Life: A Sourcebook for Clinicians and Managers. New York: Oxford University Press, 2000.

20. Cancer Pain Relief and Palliative Care. Technical Report Series 804. Geneva: World Health Organization, 1990.

21. Jacox A, Carr DB, Payne R, et al. Management of Cancer Pain. Clinical Practice Guideline no. 9. AHCPR Publication No. 94-0592. Rockville, MD. Agency for Health Care Policy and Research, US Department of Health and Human Services, Public Health Service, 1994.

22. Curt GA, Breitbart W, Cella D, et al. Impact of cancer-related fatigue on the lives of patient: New findings from the fatigue coalition. Oncologist. 2000;5:353–360.

23. Chandler S. Nebulized opioids to treat dyspnea. Am J Hosp Palliat Care. 1999;16(1):418–422.

24. Bergstrom N, et al. Pressure Ulcers in Adult: Prediction and Prevention. Clinical Practice Guideline No. 3. AHCPR Publication No. 92-0047. Rockville, MD. Agency for Health Care Policy and Research, US Department of Health and Human Services, Public Health Service, 1992.

25. Emanuel LL. Facing requests for physician-assisted suicide: toward a practical and principled clinical skill set. JAMA. 1998;280:643–647.

26. Chochinov HM, Wilson KG, Enns M. Desire for death in the terminally ill. Am J Psychiatry. 1995;152(8):1185.

27. Ehman JW, Ott BB, Short TH. Do patients want physicians to inquire about their spiritual or religious beliefs if they become gravely ill? Arch Int Med. 1999;159:1803–1806.

28. McCann RM, Hall WJ, Groth-Juncker A. Comfort care for terminally ill patients: the appropriate use of nutrition and hydration. JAMA. 1994;272(16):1263–1266.

29. Cassell EJ. The nature of suffering and the goals of medicine. N Engl J Med. 1982;306:639–645.

Common Problems

CHAPTER 8

Introduction to Common Problems

Philip D. Sloane and Mark H. Ebell

CLINICAL QUESTIONS

1. What are the most common symptoms and diagnoses seen in family medicine practice?
2. What are the common decision-making approaches used by family physicians? How can decision support tools, evidence-based practice guidelines, and electronic health records (EHRs) be used to improve decision making?
3. How should a family physician approach the following issues: dealing with clinical uncertainty, identifying hidden agendas, and deciding how far to pursue rare diagnoses?

The "bread and butter" of family medicine is the outpatient management of medical problems. These problems come in all shapes, sizes, and presentations. Not surprisingly, different problems are approached quite differently. Basic principles discussed earlier in the book, such as understanding the family, the community context, and prevention, are incorporated to varying extents into all problem visits.

The remaining chapters of this book discuss the most common problems seen in family practice. This chapter provides a brief overview of these problems, and a general approach to their management. We will begin by discussing what we mean by common problems.

WHY PATIENTS COME TO THE DOCTOR

Every patient who comes into a physician's office does so for a purpose. We usually refer to this purpose as the reason for visit. Table 8.1 lists the most common reasons patients visit family physicians, according to the National Ambulatory Medical Care Survey (1). As you review Table 8.1, note that:

- Family practice is broad and complex. The majority of visits involve complaints that are relatively rare, occurring in fewer than 1 in 50 patients. In contrast, physicians in many medical or surgical specialties spend the majority of their time regularly treating only a handful of diseases.
- Preventive care is the most common single reason for visiting. However, the majority of patients want help with specific medical problems.
- Most of the common reasons for visiting a family physician are symptoms (noted in boldface type in Table 8.1). Symptoms can be thought of as mysteries that need to be solved before the family physician can come up with a treatment plan.

Also note that no psychological conditions are listed among the 20 most common reasons for visiting although as many as half of family practice visits involve issues such as stress, adjustment problems, depression, and anxiety. The explanation for this apparent contradiction is that the stated reason for a visit is often not the patient's actual reason for coming to see their family physician. Often, people who are in psychological distress either consciously or unconsciously use symptoms as their "admission ticket" to a medical office. At other times the patient's psychological distress is interwoven with medical and often social issues. Thus, the family physician must not only address the patient's presenting complaint, but also be vigilant for less obvious issues that may constitute the patient's underlying reason for coming.

The broad training of family physicians means that addressing multiple problems during a single visit is common. In fact, a study that directly observed a large group of family physicians found that they addressed an average of 2.8 problems during each visit and took an average of eight clinical actions (i.e., ordering a test or prescribing a drug) (2). Juggling diverse problems and making good decisions during a 15-minute visit is part of the challenge of being a good family physician.

MAKING A DIAGNOSIS

Because most patients present with one or more symptoms, the physician's first task is to arrive at a diagnosis. Once the diagnosis is established, a management plan can be developed. Thus, the process that occurs in the examining room could be diagrammed like this:

$$Symptom \rightarrow Diagnosis \rightarrow Management$$

Often, the family physician's diagnosis is a provisional one, and the management plan is designed to both treat the symptoms and confirm the diagnosis.

Table 8.2 lists the most common diagnoses coded by family physicians. Note that:

- Family physicians see patients with a wide diversity of diagnoses, and no single diagnosis predominates.
- The most common diagnoses are chronic diseases (e.g., hypertension, diabetes, and asthma) and acute respiratory problems (e.g., upper respiratory infections, bronchitis, and pharyngitis).
- Several of the common diagnoses are outside of the traditional realm of internal medicine— for example, strains/sprains, depression, and contact dermatitis. These exemplify why family practice training extends into a variety of specialty fields.

TABLE 8.1 Reasons for Visits Making Up at Least 1% of a Typical Family Physician's Practice*

Reason for Visit	Total	Percent
General medical examination	18,421,885	10.0%
Throat symptoms	**8,813,215**	**4.8%**
Cough	**7,334,876**	**4.0%**
Follow-up visit, not otherwise specified	4,848,549	2.6%
Medication refill	4,652,357	2.5%
Back symptoms	**4,195,140**	**2.3%**
Earache or ear infection	**3,895,772**	**2.1%**
Stomach and abdominal pain, cramps and spasms	**3,602,115**	**2.0%**
Hypertension	3,550,581	1.9%
To review test results	3,452,875	1.9%
Physical examination required for school or employment	3,489,396	1.9%
Skin rash	**3,355,396**	**1.8%**
Headache or pain in head	**3,158,733**	**1.7%**
Blood pressure test	3,206,089	1.7%
Congestion or coryza	**2,803,792**	**1.5%**
Diabetes mellitus	2,766,687	1.5%
Vertigo or dizziness	**2,308,424**	**1.3%**
Sinus problems	**2,478,782**	**1.3%**
Chest pain and related symptoms	**2,137,976**	**1.2%**
Nasal congestion	**2,269,546**	**1.2%**
Well baby examination	2,199,212	1.2%
Foot and toe symptoms	**1,988,928**	**1.1%**
Prenatal examination	2,017,484	1.1%
General ill feeling	**1,819,460**	**1.0%**
Anxiety and nervousness	1,881,967	1.0%
Knee symptoms	**1,883,499**	**1.0%**
Total	184,439,549	100.0%

*Symptoms are noted in boldface type.
Data source: National Ambulatory Medical Care Survey, 2000: *http://www.cdc.gov/nchs/about/major/ahcd/ahcd1.htm*

Clinical Decision Making

Medical students often feel quite confused as they begin to observe a busy private medical practice. Many patients have problems that seem to defy classification, and the causes of illness are often multifactorial. Patient management proceeds often at an unfamiliar fast pace, and seemingly without need of detailed histories or comprehensive examinations. The physician seems to be cutting corners much of the time. Decisions are made that often have a social rather than medical context. Outcomes of care are mostly good, and the patients seem satisfied. Why and how is this done?

The answer is, partly, because the physician is experienced and well trained. However, just as important is the fact that decision making in primary care differs in certain respects from what students have been taught in hospital settings. Traditional medical education, which focuses on mechanisms of disease, teaches that symptoms result from disease, and that treatment of the disease heals the symptoms. In primary care, this concept is often reversed. Symptoms are often quite likely to get better on their own; making a specific diagnosis may not be necessary or even beneficial to the patient. Thus, the clinical reasoning and decision-making styles learned in medical schools often are not appropriate in the primary care setting.

Decision making develops from three main activities: gathering information (the history, physical examination findings, and test results), analyzing the information (the reasoning process), and making judgments about the data. It is enriched by previous knowledge of the patient, and the patient's environment—the context of the decision. Throughout the process, the family physician directs the encounter to efficiently obtain specific information. The result is a working

TABLE 8.2 Diagnoses Making Up at Least 1% of a Typical Family Physician's Practice*

Diagnosis	ICD9†	Total	Percent
Hypertension	401	10,914,623	5.9%
Diabetes mellitus	250	7,609,110	4.1%
Acute upper respiratory infection	465	5,921,349	3.2%
Sinusitis	473	4,522,162	2.5%
Acute pharyngitis	462	4,325,443	2.3%
Otitis media	382	4,209,868	2.3%
Bronchitis	490	3,427,114	1.9%
Back problems	724	3,308,000	1.8%
Hyperlipidemia	272	3,092,575	1.7%
Urinary tract disorders	599	2,951,909	1.6%
Allergic rhinitis	477	2,297,409	1.2%
Back pain	847	2,244,799	1.2%
Abdominal or pelvic symptoms	789	2,087,897	1.1%
Join pain	719	2,078,852	1.1%
Depression or anxiety	300	2,007,297	1.1%
Asthma	493	1,973,222	1.1%
Chest pain or shortness of breath	786	1,944,114	1.1%
Soft tissue problems	729	1,884,148	1.0%
Acute bronchitis and bronchiolitis	466	1,868,160	1.0%
Skin problems	782	1,830,356	1.0%
Tendinitis	726	1,786,904	1.0%
Total		184,439,549	100.0%

Data Source: National Ambulatory Medical Care Survey, 2000: *http://www.cdc.gov/nchs/about/major/ahcd/ahcd1.htm*
*Excludes preventive diagnoses such as "general medical examination," "prenatal care," and "well child care."
†International Classification of Diseases, 9th Edition. This is a common system used to code diagnoses for reimbursement and research purposes.

diagnosis and management strategy. This is communicated to the patient, and the decision is confirmed or rethought, with the patient generally being a partner in management decisions.

This flow of information is shown in Figure 8.1. Considerable time and effort goes into managing this flow of information, and family physicians are increasingly using sophisticated EHRs and clinical decision support tools to assist them with this process.

Primary care physicians use four distinct clinical reasoning styles to develop working diagnoses: hypothesis generation and testing, pattern recognition, algorithmic reasoning, and exhaustive methods. Each has its place in primary care. Furthermore, they are not mutually exclusive; a particular patient encounter may involve more than one of the styles. The four methods are briefly discussed below.

HYPOTHESIS GENERATION AND TESTING

Hypothesis generation and testing is the method most commonly used in primary care. In this method the physician begins generating diagnostic hypotheses within seconds after meeting the patient (sometimes beforehand, if the nurse has

already gathered the chief complaint). The initial hypothesis is often quite general, such as "this child has something serious." The physician directs the interview to obtain information that will test and refine this hypothesis (in the case of a sick child, asking about fever, vomiting, appetite, and activity). While testing and refining hypotheses, the physician remains open to information that would suggest other hypotheses, because the biggest danger in using this diagnostic method is making too hasty a decision and missing or ignoring key information. In a typical clinical encounter, expert clinicians generate likely diagnoses, on average, within 30 seconds and correct hypotheses within 6 minutes. This is an efficient and low-cost reasoning process, widely applied in office practice. Examples of problems effectively addressed with this reasoning style are fatigue, abdominal pain, and dizziness.

PATTERN RECOGNITION

Pattern recognition is a method in which the physician rapidly arrives at a diagnosis (or a very limited differential diagnosis) because the clinical picture looks exactly like something he or she has seen before. The pattern itself could be any combina-

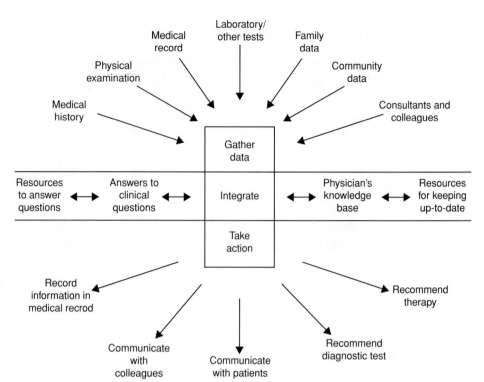

Figure 8.1 • The flow of information in primary care practice. (Reprinted from Ebell MH, Frame P. What can technology do to, and for, family medicine? Fam Med. 2001;33: 311–319. Used with permission.)

tion of data from the history and examination. This method is quick, efficient, and inexpensive, but it requires considerable clinical experience to be successful. It is used extensively by office-based clinicians, but one drawback is that some visits may be closed prematurely, missing important problems or cues. Conditions that are often diagnosed using this method include conditions whose diagnosis relies largely on physical findings, such as rashes, arthritis, or bursitis, and common diseases with distinctive clinical patterns, such as otitis media, depression, and cystitis.

ALGORITHMIC REASONING

Algorithmic reasoning involves following a consistent, logical method that does not vary from patient to patient. The physician's decision-making process can be diagrammed as a flowchart with branching decision points, in which objective data from the history, examination, or laboratory allow the physician to choose one pathway or another. This method is most useful when the data required are relatively discrete (i.e., black-and-white choices), the diagnostic possibilities are few, and the data required are modest. Because so many primary care problems are vague and/or have many diagnostic possibilities, algorithmic decision making is used for a minority of visits. Problems often approached algorithmically include anemia, hyperlipidemia, vaginal discharge, and dysuria. Practice guidelines often use algorithms, and the best ones are flexible enough to allow for the possibility of missing or inaccurate data.

EXHAUSTIVE METHODS

Exhaustive methods involve gathering comprehensive history and physical examination data and pursuing intensive laboratory testing to cover all possibilities. The data are then sifted for abnormal findings. This reasoning style is often the model taught and used in medical schools for inpatient care. It is too inefficient, time-consuming, and expensive for most problems seen in the office. More importantly, this method may be hazardous for patients because it poses real risks of laboratory errors and adverse effects of invasive tests. Therefore, this method is reserved for unusual and complex medical problems. One legitimate use of this method might be the assessment of a new elderly patient, with multisystem disease.

In making a diagnosis, the language we use moves from the words of the patient to those of the doctor. This reflects the significant responsibility that rests with the physician—to interpret the patient's problem in medical terms. The diagnostic label we supply will help us communicate with other health professionals and plan treatment. It also helps the patient understand his or her problems in the broader context of health care and health information. Not surprisingly, however, patients are less interested in diagnosis than they are in the prognosis and the treatment plan.

Pitfalls in the Diagnostic Process

Among the many pitfalls to accurate diagnosis are premature closure, hidden agendas, zebras, "I got burned once" (IGBOs), and the rare disease rule. Each of these is discussed briefly below; your goal as a clinician is to be aware of them and to keep them from steering you off course as you evaluate patients in the office.

PREMATURE CLOSURE

Premature closure occurs when the physician settles on a diagnosis before all of the information is in, or sticks with a diagnosis despite compelling information to the contrary. In studies of diagnostic reasoning, this was the most common reason for misdiagnosis (3). It is related to our general tendency as human beings to ignore nonconfirmatory data—for example, the man who complains about a "typical woman driver" but ignores all of the excellent women drivers that he encounters every day as he drives around town. Because primary care always involves a certain element of uncertainty—even as the patient walks out the door—the important thing is to remain receptive to unexpected information and be willing to alter or amend your diagnosis.

HIDDEN AGENDA

Hidden agendas occur when the actual reason for coming is not initially stated. This is very common, particularly when a psychosocial concern underlies the patient's complaint. For example, why does one patient with a cold schedule an appointment when another does not? Usually, there is a hidden agenda. Perhaps the patient is concerned that it might develop into pneumonia, because this happened in the past. Or perhaps it is because he is a smoker and wants reassurance that he does not have cancer or because he is going out of town in a few days and believes that an antibiotic will help him get better quicker. Or perhaps his son was killed in an auto accident 1 year ago, and he is having an anniversary reaction, is feeling depressed, and wants to talk. Thus, it is the family physician's job to discover the underlying issues behind the visit so the patient can receive the treatment, education, or reassurance that he or she needs. Useful strategies include asking the patient "Is there any reason you are especially concerned about this symptom?" and asking early in the interview: "Is there anything else you want to discuss today?" It is better to identify hidden agendas early in the visit rather than waste the visit on the pretext for the encounter and not learn about the true reason until your hand is on the doorknob.

ZEBRAS

"Think horses, not zebras" is familiar advice. In practical terms, this means that you should first consider the diseases that are most common in a given clinical situation. Within the United States, certain diseases, although rare in many areas, are relatively common in others. Examples include Rocky Mountain spotted fever in North Carolina (fever and headache); lead poisoning in the inner cities (exhaustion, muscle cramps); and Lyme disease in New England (fever, rash, arthritis). You must, therefore, be aware of the incidence and prevalence of illness in your community when making diagnostic and treatment decisions. Remembering the frequency of a disease is also important when interpreting diagnostic tests, as a positive test with a rare disease is likely to represent a false positive, while a positive test with a common disease is probably a true positive.

IGBO

"I got burned once" is a kind of personal zebra. It occurs when a physician's practice style is too heavily influenced by an unusual, often recent, patient. Although we all need to learn from experience, IGBOs can steer the unwary physician into inappropriate tests, referrals, or therapies. For example, the physician who misses a pulmonary embolism may subsequently order too many helical computed tomography scans on future patients. The best antidote to an IGBO is for physicians to discuss problem cases and process the implications of the experience. Formal groups, such as morbidity and mortality conferences, are excellent settings for working through an IGBO.

RARE DISEASE RULE

The rare disease rule reminds us that zebras exist. It states that "if you don't think of it, you won't make the diagnosis." It acknowledges that, although common things occur commonly, rare diagnoses cannot be forgotten. It reminds you that when the pieces do not fit together, you may have to do some thinking and/or research. Strategies include leaving the patient's room to reflect on the case (long hallways in group practices are great for this), consulting an electronic reference or textbook, or presenting a problem case to a colleague or consultant (in person, by phone, or even online). Good physicians use these strategies daily.

Diagnostic Tests

While you may think of a diagnostic test as a blood test or imaging study, it is useful to think more broadly. For example, the following single question was developed by a family medicine researcher as a diagnostic test: "When was the last time you had more than five drinks in one day (more than four drinks for women)?" If the patient responds that they have done so in the past 3 months, this positive response is 86% sensitive and specific for problem drinking (4). In the original study, 77% responding in the affirmative were problem drinkers compared with 7% who responded "more than 3 months ago" and 1% who responded "never." (See Chapter 3, Information Mastery: Basing Care on the Best Available Evidence, for more on use of diagnostic tests.)

Physical examination maneuvers are also diagnostic tests. An increasing body of literature is examining their actual diagnostic accuracy. Some widely used maneuvers are actually very inaccurate (e.g., Homan's sign for deep vein thrombosis [DVT], epigastric tenderness for peptic ulcer disease, and Tinel's sign for carpal tunnel syndrome). Conversely, some little-used maneuvers are actually quite accurate (e.g., square wrist sign for carpal tunnel and spider angiomas for serious hepatic disease).

Individual elements of the history and physical examination are rarely accurate enough to rule in or rule out a diagnosis. Instead, physicians use combinations of findings. An increasing area of research, much of it by primary care physicians, identifies the best individual predictors of a disease from the history and physical examination, combines them into a simple score, and then tests or "validates" that score in a separate group of patients. These scores are often called clinical decision rules or clinical decision guides. Well-known examples include the Ottawa ankle rules, the strap score, the Wells score for DVT, and the Simple Cardiac Risk Index for preoperative evaluation.

A clinical decision rule is often used to place the patient in a low-, intermediate-, or high-risk group. This information then informs the decision to order (or not order) further diagnostic tests, and even the interpretation of their results. It is useful to think in terms of two thresholds, the "no test/test" threshold and the "test/treat" threshold. When the probability of disease goes below the "no test/test" threshold, the physician has at least provisionally ruled out the diagnosis in question. When the probability exceeds the "test/treat" threshold, the physician is comfortable enough with the diagnosis to initiate

Figure 8.2 • The starting point is a 20% estimate of the overall risk of strep throat among patients in your practice presenting with a complaint of sore throat. Your "no test/test" threshold is 3% (e.g., if the probability is less than 3%, you consider that strep is effectively ruled out, remembering that you can never achieve perfect diagnostic certainty), and the "test/treat" threshold is 50% (e.g., if probability of strep is greater than 50%, you would initiate antibiotics).[15]

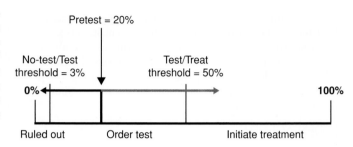

treatment (although further confirmatory diagnostic testing may still be considered). When the probability of a disease lies between these thresholds, further diagnostic evaluation (i.e., questions, examination, or testing) is required.

Although there are formal methods for setting these thresholds, physicians generally establish them implicitly based on their values, and those of their patient. When tests are inexpensive and noninvasive, the "no test/test" threshold tends to move lower; when they are noxious, costly, or dangerous, it moves higher or may even merge with the "test/treat" threshold (e.g., brain biopsy for Alzheimer's disease). Similarly, the "test/treat" threshold is lower when treatment is benign, cheap and effective and higher when there are potential dangers to treatment (e.g., anticoagulants for DVT). A fully worked out example of using a validated clinical decision rule to risk stratify a patient with a common problem, and then use that information to guide diagnostic and treatment decisions, is shown in Figures 8.2 through 8.4. (See Chapter 21, Sore Throat, for the full clinical decision rule.)

The patient's risk of disease should also guide the interpretation of subsequent tests. Figure 8.5 provides a general framework for linking clinical decision rules that stratify risk using the history and physical examination with subsequent diagnostic tests. For example, DVT can be ruled out on the basis of a low risk on the Wells score and a normal D-dimer or venous ultrasound. On the other hand, patients with moderate or high DVT risk based on the Wells score who have a negative D-dimer or ultrasound, require further testing or close follow-up, as they still have a high "post-test" probability of DVT, since their "pre-test" probability was so high.

This approach to clinical decision making is widely used for important conditions like DVT, heart disease, pulmonary embolism, and pneumonia. It makes the best possible use of the provider's history and physical examination skills and customizes the diagnostic evaluation to the patient rather than using a wasteful and potentially inaccurate "one-size-fits-all" approach.

CHRONIC DISEASE MANAGEMENT

There are two types of patient visits in family practice in which the doctor does not have to make a diagnosis. The first—preventive care—is discussed in Part II of this book. The other is the care of people with chronic conditions for which a diagnosis has been established before the office visit. Examples include hypertension, congestive heart failure, asthma, and arthritis. As you can see from Table 8.2, this type of office visit is very common in family medicine.

In chronic disease management visits, the primary care process can be diagrammed like this:

Established diagnosis → Review since last visit → Management

The visit involves addressing both the patient's concerns and the status of the identified disease. The visit typically begins by finding out what issues the patient is concerned about. These may be completely unrelated to the disease, but if they are foremost in the patient's mind, they should be addressed early in the visit.

Effective chronic disease management is an important and growing element of family medicine. It often requires the patient to make and maintain lifestyle changes, such as dietary modification, exercise, administration of medication, and self-monitoring. These lifestyle modifications affect the patient's personal and family life; therefore, addressing psychosocial issues is an important element of chronic disease visits.

In addition to helping the patient make and maintain the necessary lifestyle changes, chronic disease care involves

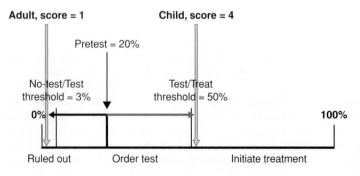

Figure 8.3 • Using the validated clinical decision rule for strep pharyngitis (Chapter 21, Sore Throat), a 50-year-old patient with sore throat and fever, but no tonsillar findings, no adenopathy, and with a cough, would get 1 point (1% probability of strep). A 10-year-old with sore throat, fever, adenopathy, no exudates, and no cough would get 4 points (_% probability of strep). Their probability of strep, revised after using the clinical decision rule, is shown above. Note that for these patients the probability of strep either dropped below the no-test/test threshold (adult) or exceeded the test/treat threshold (child) using the clinical examination alone.[5]

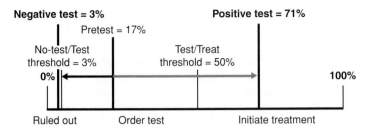

Negative test = 3%   **Positive test = 71%**

Pretest = 17%

No-test/Test threshold = 3%

Test/Treat threshold = 50%

0%   100%

Ruled out   Order test   Initiate treatment

Figure 8.4 • A 20-year-old with sore throat, fever, adenopathy, no exudates, and who is coughing, would receive 2 points and have an intermediate risk of strep. This becomes the starting point when interpreting the result of a rapid strep test. Further testing with the rapid strep test moves the probability above or below the two thresholds (to 71% if positive or 3% if negative).[5]

periodically assessing the patient's status through history-taking, examination, and selected laboratory tests. These periodic evaluations require considerable skill and organization on the part of the physician. Often, optimal chronic disease management involves a team approach in which other professionals, such as nurses, pharmacists, podiatrists, physical therapists, and other medical specialists (e.g., ophthalmology for patients with diabetes), regularly participate in patient management.

For patients with one or more chronic diseases, it is imperative that the medical record be well organized and that communication with other health care professionals is clear and frequent. This is facilitated by use of an EHR, ideally one that includes evidence-based guideline recommendations and flowcharts for monitoring chronic diseases. For example, physicians can be reminded with an EHR if a diabetic patient has not seen the ophthalmologist in more than a year or is overdue for a foot exam.

Deciding on a Management Plan

After analyzing the data and developing a working diagnosis, you often need to make a judgment about whether to order a test, initiate a treatment, or refer the patient. This decision should be based on recommendations from evidence-based guidelines (see Chapter 3, Information Mastery, for more on choosing a good guideline). Good guidelines provide flexibility for patients and physicians and recognize that patients may have different degrees of tolerance for risk and different financial resources. For example, some patients may choose not to have a mammogram until age 50, because the evidence is less compelling for its use between the ages of 40 and 50 years.

Thus, cost, time, convenience for the patient, and any potential adverse effects of testing or therapy may all impact clinical decisions. Finally, and most importantly, the patient's personality, anxieties, and social situation may all influence your clinical decision. Is this patient well known in the practice for "crying wolf" over minor symptoms? Is the patient the family breadwinner who will lose income while submitting to hospital tests? How high is the patient's need for reassurance that he or she is not seriously ill? How far does he or she trust the doctor (unaided by laboratory tests) to provide this reassurance?

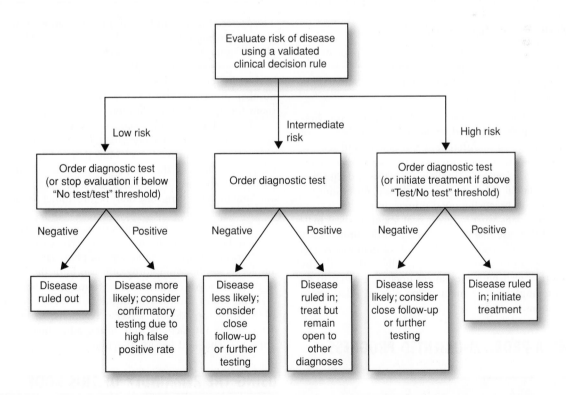

Figure 8.5 • **A general approach to diagnostic test interpretation that makes use of the history and physical examination.**

Knowledge of the patient is relevant data accumulated from past experience. Long-term continuity with an individual and family helps the physician learn how they deal with stress, what they believe about their health, how they take their medications, and how responsible they are in managing their own problems. All of these factors enter the melting pot of clinical decision making.

Clinical Uncertainty

In primary care practice, uncertainty goes with the territory (6). Diagnostic uncertainty comes from three sources:

- Cognitive uncertainty, which is related to the physician's perception of the clinical problem
- The emotional state (anxiety, usually) of the physician
- The variability of the patient's response to communication and therapy

In many cases, you will not be able to make a specific diagnosis or will need to wait a period of time before the diagnosis becomes clear or the patient gets better. It is not uncommon for physicians to identify and treat symptoms, realizing that they may resolve spontaneously before a diagnosis is made; examples include diarrhea and abdominal pain, both of which typically resolve without a specific laboratory-confirmed diagnosis.

In resolving uncertainty, time is a very powerful diagnostic tool. Its effective use requires considerable skill, however. The physician who is too anxious to await the evolution of a symptom may order unnecessary tests and have the patient return too frequently, at considerable cost. On the other hand, the physician who does not consider more than one hypothesis or who does not ask the patient to return may miss an important diagnosis.

Methods of managing uncertainty include:

- Sharing your uncertainty with colleagues and patients
- Educating patients about possible outcomes
- Reassuring patients that you will continue to observe them for diagnostic clues

The degree of uncertainty faced by primary care clinicians is greater than that faced by other providers because of the larger numbers of undifferentiated problems and relative lack of research data about primary care conditions. As a result, good communication and follow-up between doctor and patient are essential. Management of clinical uncertainty is one of the keys to practicing good primary care.

Some physicians worry a great deal about medical malpractice, and they use that as an excuse to order unnecessary tests or questionable treatments. The risk of malpractice can be reduced by documenting visits carefully and clearly, by communicating well with the patient (including what to do if not improving), and by maintaining a good relationship with the patient.

WRITING A PROBLEM-ORIENTED PROGRESS NOTE

When you record patient visits in the family practice office, it is recommended that you write problem-oriented progress notes. Each problem should be written up as follows:

Problem 1: (here name the primary problem addressed—for example, fever and cough, or well person examination)

S: (for *subjective*—all relevant historical data)
O: (for *objective*—physical examination and laboratory data)
A: (for *assessment*—your clinical impression)
P: (for *plans*—plans for therapy, additional testing, and patient education)

Organize the next portion of the note the same way:
Problem 2: (name the second problem)

S:
O:
A:
P:

As you proceed through your training, you will likely adopt a shorthand approach that combines the above into a more concise, unified SOAP format:

S: (all relevant historical data for all problems)
O: (all physical examination and laboratory data for all problems)
A/P: 1) Assessment and plan for problem #1
2) Assessment and plan for problem #2
3) Assessment and plan for problem #3

This approach maintains the basic SOAP format but is more efficient and concise than a separate SOAP note for each problem.

PRESCRIPTION WRITING

The prescription is your formal communication of therapeutic plans regarding a medication. It should be legible and complete. Figure 8.6 provides a model prescription, with labels discussing its components. Prescription forms with the name of the physician and his or her (DEA) Enforcement Agency number preprinted are commonly used, as are forms with room for up to three medications per prescription.

Use of Latin abbreviations, such as prn or qd, is discouraged, as they may be misunderstood. For example, it is easy for qid to be mistakenly read as qd. More detailed descriptions that tell the patient why they are taking a medicine, and exactly when to take it, are also helpful. For example, you should write out "omeprazole 20 mg once daily before dinner for heartburn" instead of the more cryptic "omeprazole 20 mg po qd."

Electronic prescribing software is increasingly becoming the standard of care. Its use reduces errors caused by poor handwriting or misdosing because of physician error. For example, these prescribing programs can limit the list of drugs to those on a patient's insurance formulary, and only show available doses for each medication. If integrated with an EHR, they can identify adverse reactions, drug-drug and drug-disease interactions, and dosing adjustments caused by impaired renal and hepatic function.

USING THE REMAINDER OF THIS BOOK

The rest of this book consists of chapters devoted to common problems. Many are organized around a symptom, such as

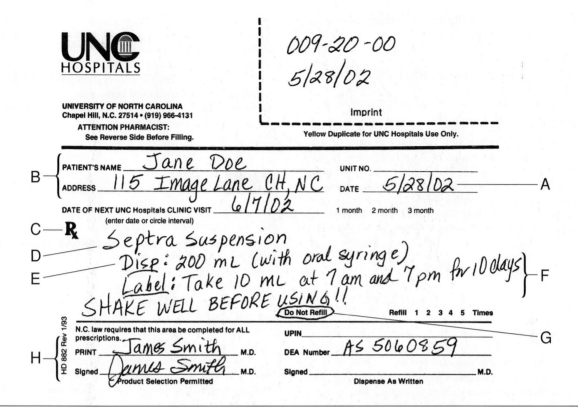

Figure 8.6 • *Standard prescription form.* A. **Date:** schedule II medication prescriptions must be filled within 72 hours after writing. Schedule III and IV prescriptions cannot be filled or refilled 6 months after writing. B. **Patient's name and address:** required on schedule II prescriptions. C. **Superscription:** designated as the symbol *Rx*, the abbreviation for recipe (Latin for "take thou"). D. **Inscription:** the body of the prescription, containing the name and strength of the drug. E. **Subscription:** the direction(s) to the pharmacist, detailing the amount of the drug to be dispensed, such as "dispense 30 tablets," "dispense 3 months (of oral contraceptives)," or "dispense 120 mL with an oral syringe." F. **Transcription:** the directions for the patient. Latin abbreviations (e.g., BID, AC, QHS) should not be used. The directions cover the amount of drug to be taken, timing and frequency of dosing, route of administration, and duration of therapy. Directions for use should always begin with a verb, such as "take," "apply," or "insert." Use directions that remind the patient of the purpose of the prescription, such as "for pain relief" or "to relieve itching." G. **Refill information:** schedule II drugs cannot be refilled and schedule III and IV prescriptions cannot be refilled more than 5 times within the 6-month duration. Unless refills are specified, always circle or write "do not refill" to prevent forgeries for extra refills. H. **Signature:** the physician's personal signature, DEA registry number, and practice address.

abdominal pain, back pain, or dizziness. Others are devoted to a specific chronic disease, such as hypertension, obesity, and asthma. A few discuss clusters of diseases whose presentation, pathophysiology, and approach overlap, e.g., upper respiratory infections and sexually transmitted diseases.

In choosing what to put in each chapter, we have tried to focus on the issues that are most important to good patient management. Thus, some chapters focus on diagnosis, others on treatment, and others on both. When appropriate, we have tried to include easy-to-use tables and algorithms, detailed information about the accuracy of diagnostic tests, evidence-based treatment recommendations, dosages for commonly used drugs, and the general approach to management.

CASE 1

A 54-year-old man returns to the office sooner than his first scheduled appointment after hospitalization. In the

hospital 2 weeks before, he was treated for an acute myocardial infarction and congestive heart failure. Now he comes to the office complaining of headache and backache, but these symptoms are vague and have no obvious medical diagnosis. Therefore the physician asks directly, "How do you think we can help you today?"

"Well, I was hoping you could tell me whether being on all of these pills means that I had an especially bad attack or whether everyone gets treated like this," says the man, who was discharged with prescriptions for a β-adrenergic blocker, an angiotensin-converting enzyme inhibitor, and aspirin. "I never took so much as an aspirin in my life, and now I'm eating pills day and night. And at work I used to carry heavy boxes around, and now I'm not even allowed to walk to the corner for the paper."

The physician points out that the patient is still wearing his plastic identification bracelet from the hospitalization. "They forgot to cut it off me," the patient replies, "and I didn't get around to cutting it off. Besides, maybe

I'll flop over again, and with the bracelet they'll know to bring me right here."

CLINICAL QUESTIONS

1. What are the major problems that have been identified in this scenario?
2. How would you manage this patient?

DISCUSSION

In this example, the patient has used somatic complaints—headache and backache—to gain entry to the physician's office. However, his actual reason for coming involved fears of death and disability; therefore, appropriate management involves allowing the patient to further express his fears, providing information about prognosis, and reassuring him that he is expected to make a full recovery.

CASE 2

A 29-year-old school librarian has a several-week history of fatigue and lack of energy. She was seen 2 weeks earlier for a sore throat, which was believed to be viral. At that time several psychosocial issues were elicited. She had broken up with her boyfriend 5 months earlier and spent a couple of months in counseling because she was quite "low" after the breakup; she also had recently changed jobs because of a conflict with her boss at work. She felt isolated and did not spend much time with friends. Her chart is rather thick and includes a number of visits for minor medical complaints.

Physical examination findings are normal. After the examination, the physician draws blood "to check for anemia and mono." Because the test results will not be immediately available, the physician sends the patient home, telling her that her symptoms seem psychologically based, caused by the separation from her boyfriend. The patient seems upset, requires extensive explanation, and leaves unconvinced.

CLINICAL QUESTIONS

1. What went wrong in this visit?
2. What should the physician have done differently?

DISCUSSION

After the visit, the results of a mononucleosis test drawn at the visit come back positive. The physician calls the patient, informing her of the diagnosis and apologizing for assuming that her symptoms were purely psychological. The patient returns twice in the next 3 weeks, and is allowed to vent her frustration with the misdiagnosis.

In this case the physician made a premature declaration of the symptom etiology. He should have emphasized that the diagnosis was tentative, and that he was considering other possibilities. Fortunately, he had ordered the appropriate test and was able to correct his error. Although overtesting can be as harmful as undertesting, patients often need to be told that a diagnosis is tentative and that only with time will it become certain.

Dealing with mistakes in clinical diagnosis can be difficult. A simple apology without extensive explanation is always helpful. Identifying and verbalizing to the patient his or her emotion can be helpful, such as "you seem angry" or "this must have been frustrating for you," and then just listening. Most patients need permission to express negative feelings to their doctor. These lessons are some of our most important educational experiences.

CASE 3

Dr. Hoehm, a family physician in a small town, is preparing for bed at 10 PM when the answering service calls about Sarah, a 9-month-old child with a fever. Dr. Hoehm knows that Sarah lives with her mother and 5-year-old brother in a trailer.

Dr. Hoehm telephones the mother and learns that Sarah has had a cold for several days. Earlier this evening she ate most of her dinner, but as the evening progressed she became increasingly irritable and felt warm. The mother took her axillary temperature and it was 101°F. Sarah has been healthy except for an ear infection 3 months ago. She has no dyspnea and is currently asleep. Her mother thinks that she may have been fussing with her right ear.

Dr. Hoehm asks Sarah's mother if she wants Sarah to be seen right away. The mother hesitates. "I finally got her to sleep," the mother says. Dr. Hoehm then suggests that they meet the next morning in the office, and that the mother give Tylenol if Sarah becomes fussier during the night. Dr. Hoehm then reminds Sarah's mother of the answering service number and instructs her to call if Sarah's temperature gets above 104°F or if she notices anything unusual about the child.

CLINICAL QUESTIONS

1. Was the doctor correct in not advising the mother to bring Sarah in?
2. Is it possible that Sarah could have meningitis? If so, how can Dr. Hoehm justify not seeing the patient now?

DISCUSSION

Dr. Hoehm's decision not to see Sarah was based on the following:

- The child did not sound very sick.
- The most likely diagnosis, given her previous episode and history, is an ear infection, which is not generally life threatening and for which antibiotics are only marginally better than no treatment.
- It would have been inconvenient for the patient to be seen emergently.
- The mother is reliable and can monitor Sarah and call back if she acutely worsens.

Dr. Hoehm does not know the diagnosis; that will wait until morning.

A number of other diagnoses are possible, including early meningitis. However, these are zebras in this clinical scenario, and it is, therefore, good medical practice not to see Sarah. It is important, however, to make sure the mother knows to observe the patient carefully and call if any signs of clinical deterioration develop.

REFERENCES

1. National Ambulatory Medical Care Survey, 1997. American Academy of Family Physicians Web site. Available at: *http://www.aafp.org/facts*. Accessed May 8, 2001.

2. Flocke SA, Frank SH, Wenger DA. Addressing multiple problems in the family practice office visit. J Fam Pract. 2001; 50(3):211–216.

3. Elstein AS, Shulman LS, Sprafka SA. In: Medical Problem Solving: An Analysis of Clinical Reasoning. Cambridge, MA: Harvard University Press, 1978.

4. Williams R, Vinson DC. Validation of a single screening question for problem drinking. J Fam Pract. 2001;50:307–312.

5. McIsaac WJ, Goel V, To T, Low DE. The validity of a sore throat score in family practice. CMAJ. 2000; 163:811–815

6. Mushlin AI. Uncertain decision making in primary care: causes and solutions. Primary Care Research: Theory and Methods Conference. Washington, DC: US Department of Health and Human Services, Agency for Health Care Policy and Research; September 1991:153–166.

chest pain is essential to their proper evaluation and management.

ACUTE CORONARY SYNDROMES

The pain of ACS reflects hypoperfusion and consequent lack of oxygenation of the myocardium, usually from occlusion of a coronary artery. The currently dominant pathophysiologic model involves instability of an atherosclerotic plaque, leading either to leakage of its prothrombotic contents or frank plaque rupture. Thrombus then forms on the disrupted endothelium, occluding the artery and producing ischemia in the area of myocardium supplied by the artery if collateral circulation is not adequate. The afflicted myocardium begins to progress through a well-defined series of ischemic changes. If perfusion is not restored within 3 to 6 hours, loss of cell integrity as evidenced by leaking of cardiac troponins, myoglobin, and later creatine kinase occurs. Cell death in the affected area is the final stage, at which point acute ischemia becomes myocardial infarction.

UA is defined as rest pain for 20 minutes or more that is likely to be associated with an unstable vessel occlusion and resulting hypoperfusion. However, unstable angina also includes new-onset, effort-dependent angina and a recent (within 2 months) clinically significant increase in chronic angina symptoms. Such accelerations of angina may represent rupture or other acute changes in a plaque, formation of a thrombus not fully occluding an artery, or simple progression of atheroma. Although it is generally not possible to differentiate among these mechanisms at the time of symptom presentation, they have very different prognostic implications for the patient.

Whereas the long-term mortality of unstable angina is substantial and not much less than that of myocardial infarction (1, 2), it is important to distinguish one from another as their acute management strategies do differ. Unfortunately, such a distinction can often be made only in retrospect, well after critical initial treatment decisions have been made.

Variant angina, also known as vasospastic or Prinzmetal angina, is a diagnosis commonly considered when a patient with chest pain is evaluated and has normal coronary arteries. In the case of variant angina, ischemic pain is produced by smooth muscle spasm narrowing the artery acutely rather than by thrombotic occlusion. Despite the frequency with which it is considered, careful study shows that very few chest pain patients without coronary occlusions actually have coronary vasospasm (3).

Less common but potentially important causes of ACS include non-atherosclerotic coronary artery inflammation or dissection, as well as systemic conditions that either severely limit oxygen delivery to the heart (severe anemia, hypotension) or dramatically increase consumption (sepsis, thyrotoxicosis). Pre-existing CAD increases the risk for ischemia in the setting of these and other extraordinary physiologic stressors.

STABLE ANGINA

Stable angina, also known as chronic effort-dependent angina, is the result of an imbalance between myocardial oxygen needs and oxygen delivery to the myocardium at increasing levels of activity. The imbalance is caused by decreased blood flow past the hallmark atherosclerotic plaques of CAD. When the myocardium demands additional oxygen during physical activity and perfusion cannot increase commensurately, the afflicted region becomes ischemic. Energy metabolism in the cardiac muscle cell becomes impaired, producing the characteristic electrical changes on electrocardiogram (ECG) (ischemic muscle conducts electricity differently) and wall motion abnormalities on echocardiography (ischemic muscle does not contract normally).

PANIC DISORDER

It is not known why a panic attack can cause chest pain. The origins of panic attacks are also unknown and remain a subject of active controversy and research (4). The debate is between the theory of a primary psychological cause with secondary physical response and a primary physiologic or autonomic cause with secondary psychological consequences. Panic attacks may occur in isolation, as part of panic disorder, or as part of other anxiety disorders. Even in referral settings, panic disorder is present in more than 30% of chest pain patients and may coexist with CAD (5).

GASTROESOPHAGEAL REFLUX DISEASE (GERD) AND ESOPHAGEAL SPASM

Reflux of gastric acid contents into the distal esophagus is common. The acid irritates the mucosa, causing inflammatory infiltrates and sloughing of epithelium. Smooth muscle spasm in reaction to this irritation can cause additional pain. Reflux occurring severely and frequently enough is called GERD. Although about 10% of the adult population experience this degree of symptoms, less than 1% seek medical attention for it (6, 7). Reflux can be exacerbated by triggers that relax the lower esophageal sphincter, most notably caffeine, alcohol, and fatty foods.

MUSCULOSKELETAL PAIN

Although often attributed to inflammation of the costal cartilage, costochondral joints, or intercostal muscles, the actual mechanism of musculoskeletal chest pain remains unproven. Musculoskeletal chest pains are common, and most people who have them do not present for medical evaluation.

MITRAL VALVE PROLAPSE

Mitral valve prolapse (MVP) is often blamed for chest pain among young people (especially young women) on the basis of retrospective findings of MVP in patients with noncardiac pain. However, MVP is also common in the general asymptomatic population, and prospective studies have failed to show that MVP is more common in chest pain patients. In fact, there is evidence that reflux may be the actual cause of most pain attributed to MVP (8).

PLEURAL AND PULMONARY PAIN

Pulmonary embolism may produce pain, usually pleuritic in nature. The clinical manifestations of pulmonary embolism are notoriously variable and entirely absent in at least half of cases. Shortness of breath and tachypnea are the most frequent manifestations. Pleuritic pain can also be produced by inflammation from an infectious process or by neoplasm. Spontaneous pneumothorax is uncommon and is associated with vigorous exercise, primarily (by a ratio of 5:1) in men in their 20s.

RARE CAUSES

Chest pain can rarely result from dissection of the thoracic aorta (almost exclusively found among hypertensive patients; Marfan's syndrome and syphilis are very rare causes), vertebral or rib metastases from any of several different malignancies (and enlarged mediastinal nodes owing to lymphoma), sarcoidosis, and collagen vascular diseases.

Differential Diagnosis

Perhaps nowhere in medicine is the clinical epidemiology of a problem as varied, or as important in diagnosis, as in the case of chest pain. The four most common and important causes of chest pain in primary care are ischemic heart disease, panic, reflux, and musculoskeletal pain. Musculoskeletal pain is the most common, followed by reflux and other gastrointestinal sources. Heart disease is the most life-threatening, although panic causes substantial morbidity that is often inadequately recognized. Pulmonary embolism and aortic dissection are also associated with substantial morbidity and mortality, although both occur rarely in the outpatient setting.

The probabilities of the various causes differ sharply across the clinical settings in which chest pain is commonly encountered. Research and teaching regarding chest pain have traditionally centered on emergency departments and referral centers, where the prevalence of serious pathology is high. For example, acute chest pain in emergency departments represents acute cardiac ischemia in one-quarter to one-third of cases (9). The prior probability of acute ischemia in the primary care office setting, however, is only 1.5% (10), and decisions appropriate in the emergency department may not be valid in the office.

Table 9.1 presents the final diagnoses of cases of chest pain from a network of family physicians' offices (10). Gastroesophageal reflux alone accounts for at least 13% of all patients. Most of the psychosocial category, and likely many of the nonspecific cases as well, represent panic attacks, either isolated or in the setting of panic disorder. Pulmonary causes were pleuritic for the most part. Causes such as aortic dissection and pneumothorax are very rare in family practice, and

were not observed at all in the 399 cases used to construct Table 9.1. By contrast, typically about 30% of patients seen in the emergency department with chest pain will have an acute coronary syndrome, and 15% or more will actually suffer MI (9).

Acute chest pain that is present while the patient is being seen or occurring just prior to being seen is very different from chronic or recurrent pain, in which the patient schedules an appointment for evaluation, and must be approached with a different diagnostic mindset. Unfortunately, although good diagnostic research has been done on the detection of ACS, few objective data are available regarding the predictive values or key differentiating cues for nonacute pain.

CLINICAL EVALUATION

Because the causes of chest pain vary so much, proper evaluation involves a complete medical history and physical examination, which is time consuming. However, time can be critical: prompt reperfusion with thrombolysis or early percutaneous coronary intervention (PCI) can improve outcomes for properly selected patients with acute coronary syndromes, if those patients are identified quickly. Therefore, the evaluation of the chest pain patient proceeds in two steps: 1) rapid evaluation using a few key predictors of ACS, followed by immediate initiation of treatment if indicated (ideally within 10 to 20 minutes of initial presentation); and 2) a complete evaluation once an ACS has either been excluded or properly triaged. Treatment for ACS or other life threatening conditions should never be delayed while the complete evaluation phase is being performed unless serious doubt of the presence of an ACS exists and information from the complete evaluation is crucial to resolving it.

In the nonacute situation, when a patient has scheduled an appointment for the evaluation of chest pain but is not acutely ill, the focus shifts to detection of stable CAD, GERD, panic disorder, and musculoskeletal causes. A thorough evaluation typically precedes initiation of therapy. For both acute and nonacute cases of chest pain, intelligent evaluation of chest pain depends on a sound understanding of prior probabilities and how findings on history and examination modify them.

Decision-making tools have identified a small set of factors that are of genuine predictive utility for the diagnosis of ACS in the primary care setting (9, 11). Although published data do not include individual likelihood ratios for these findings, their weights in regression models do allow estimates for which findings are the most important. Table 9.2 presents these validated diagnostic cues in approximate order of importance for both rapid and detailed evaluation.

The Acute Cardiac Ischemia Time-Insensitive Predictive Instrument (ACI-TIPI) is a well-validated clinical prediction rule for estimating the likelihood of an ACS in patients with chest pain in the emergency department. The ACI-TIPI can be used in primary care settings, although its positive predictive value is lower because of the lower incidence of an ACS in that setting. A second well-validated tool has been developed for patients with acute chest pain and a normal or nonspecific ECG (see Table 9.3).

TABLE 9.1 Differential Diagnosis in Patients with Chest Pain

Diagnostic Category	% of Episodes in Family Practice Settings
Musculoskeletal pain	36
Gastrointestinal pain	19
Nonspecific chest pain	16
Stable angina	11
Psychosocial pain	7
Pulmonary pain	5
Nonischemic cardiac pain	4
Acute cardiac ischemia	2

Reprinted with permission from Klinkman MS, Stevens D, Gorenflo DW. Episodes of care for chest pain. J Fam Pract. 1994;38:344–352.

TABLE 9.5 Characteristics of Diagnostic Tests Useful in Patients with Chest Pain

Test	Sensitivity	Specificity	LR+	LR−
Coronary artery disease				
Nonsloping ECG ST segment depression during ECG stress (21)				
>2.5 mm			39	
2–2.5 mm			11	
1.5–1.99 mm			4.2	
1–1.49 mm			2.1	
0.05–0.99 mm			0.9	
Reversible perfusion defect on thallium scintigraphy (19)	71	94	11.8	0.31
Reversible wall motion abnormality on stress echocardiography (20)	81	89	7.4	0.21
Acute coronary ischemia				
ECG findings for ruling in ACI (21)				
New ST segment elevation >1 mm			6–54	
New left bundle-branch block			6.3	
Q wave			3.9	
T wave hyperacuity			3.1	
Serum markers for ruling out ACI (22)				
Myoglobin in normal range and not doubling over 2 h within 6 h of presentation	86	95	17	0.1
CK-MB normal, single test	34	88	2.8	0.75
CK-MB normal, serial measurements				0.04
Total CK normal, single test				0.85
Total CK normal, serial measurements				0.11
Serial troponin T <0.18 ng/ml with normal ECG (23)				0.003
Serial troponin T <0.18 ng/ml with ST-depression or T-wave inversion				0.013

Abbreviations: ACI, acute cardiac ischemia; CK-MB, creatinine kinase myocardial bands; ECG, electrocardiogram; LR, likelihood ratio

amplitude) or inversion in at least two leads (excluding aV$_R$, in which the T wave is normally inverted) is also important. A finding of new Q waves of ≥1 mm in at least two leads is strongly associated with acute injury, but may not be present for 24 to 36 hours after infarction. ST segment elevation during chest pain is useful for ruling in acute MI (LR+, 5.1; LR−, 0.59) (24). ST segment depression is associated with ischemia but less specifically with infarction.

The ECG changes associated with pulmonary embolism are far less specific. In the approximate order of positive predictive value (none have substantial negative predictive value) they are sinus tachycardia, S$_1$Q$_3$T$_3$ pattern, rightward axis deviation, right bundle-branch block, ST depression in the right precordial leads, p pulmonale, and ST elevation in lead III (25). None of these findings are very good at ruling out PE when absent.

COMPLETE EVALUATION

Chest radiographs will show widening of the mediastinum in half of the patients with aortic dissection (26). Other useful findings include consolidation in patients with pneumonia; the boot-shaped shadow of a fluid-filled pericardium; a tumor producing pleural irritation; a pneumothorax; or rarely, the wedge-shaped shadows of pulmonary infarcts from emboli. Although unnecessary for pain that is clearly panic or reflux on clinical evaluation, a chest film is recommended for most other situations.

Several laboratory tests are used to confirm MI, including serum measurements of creatine kinase (CK) and its MB isoenzyme (CK-MB), myoglobin, and cardiac-specific troponin I and troponin T. A normal CK level without elevation of MB fraction at 24 hours from onset of symptoms essentially excludes MI. However, patients with chest pain who do not have elevated CK-MB may have elevated troponins, and are thus considered to have had a myocardial infarction (27). Serum myoglobin levels can be helpful in rapidly "ruling out" myocardial infarction, particularly when serial measurements remain with the normal range and do not double over 2 hours' time, within 6 hours of symptom onset. Only 3% of such patients in the ED without change in myoglobin will have an MI (28). In the primary care office, where the likelihood of MI is much lower, the likelihood that a patient with normal, stable myoglobin levels does not have MI is at least 99%.

Cardiac troponins have become the marker of choice in

many centers because of their high sensitivity and particularly high specificity for cardiac injury. Normal serial troponin measurements at 10 hours after symptom onset can essentially exclude myocardial infarction. Furthermore, normal troponins can help to inform short term prognosis: only 1 in 300 patients with a normal ECG and a normal troponin I level 6 hours after chest pain onset will have an adverse cardiac outcome in the next 30 days (29). This can be particularly helpful when deciding where and how quickly to proceed with a diagnostic workup.

Significant troponin elevations in patients with characteristic chest pain—even with a normal ECG and normal or borderline CK-MB—yields a diagnosis of myocardial infarction. Troponin elevation also has prognostic significance, carrying a 2%–6% risk for further cardiac injury (MI or sudden cardiac death) within 6 months. These patients are candidates for intensive medical therapy or percutanous coronary intervention (PCI) (30, 31). Troponins T and I are similar in accuracy, and either may be used; individual laboratories should be consulted for their preference and reference ranges.

When working with a patient who has more chronic symptoms, testing for CAD may be done by exercise ECG, exercise echocardiography, or gated blood pool scanning. For any of these tests, pharmacologic stress testing can be substituted for exercise. The addition of thallium or 99m-technetium (sometimes referred to as sestamibi, the pharmaceutical to which the radionuclide is bound) imaging improves the specificity of these tests. Graded exercise ECG using the Bruce or equivalent graduated protocols is the usual test of choice for men with suspected CAD (32). Pharmacologic stress testing should be reserved for patients whose orthopedic or other conditions preclude adequate levels of exertion, as it does not provide the prognostic information on exercise duration offered by physiological stress testing.

Simultaneous nuclear imaging can reveal areas of reversible ischemic myocardium and is recommended for patients with baseline ECG abnormalities such as bundle-branch block, preexcitation syndrome (i.e., Wolff-Parkinson-White) baseline ST depression >1 mm, mechanical pacing, or digoxin therapy. In addition, selective thallium or technetium-sestamibi use may add sensitivity and specificity for symptomatic women and elders, two groups in whom ECG stress results are often less reliable. The American College of Cardiology/ American Heart Association (ACC/AHA) Guidelines for Exercise Testing suggest that women and patients over 65-years-old at risk for CAD because of symptoms be considered for initial radionuclide imaging. Stress echocardiography also reveals areas of wall motion abnormality induced by ischemia, and has seen increased use in centers staffed by experienced interpreters, on whom much of its utility rests. The accuracy of stress ECG, stress radionuclide, and echocardiogram testing is summarized in Table 9.5.

Five-year mortality prognosis can also be estimated for outpatients from exercise ECG data (33). Angina is scored 0 for none, 1 for angina induced by but not limiting the treadmill test, and 2 for angina that limits the test. The score is (exercise in minutes) − (5 × maximal ST deviation) − (4 × angina score). Patients with scores of 5 or greater have a 5-year survival rate of 99%; those with scores of −10 to +4 have a 5-year survival rate of 95%; and those with scores of −11 or lower have a 5-year survival rate of only 79%.

Suspected dissection of the aorta can be evaluated with angiography, transesophageal echocardiography, helical CT, or MRI. Although all perform well in high-risk groups and effectively rule out the diagnosis when normal (34), angiography performs surprisingly poorly as the likelihood of disease decreases. Only MRI appears to offer better than a 50% positive predictive value when the risk of aortic dissection is low (<1%) (35).

It is important to evaluate the possibility of pulmonary embolism in patients with chest pain. The recommended diagnostic strategy is described in detail in Chapter 12, Venous Thromboembolism.

MANAGEMENT

Recommended Diagnostic Strategy for Chest Pain

Management of the patient with chest pain is very different for each of the many causes previously discussed. Key elements in managing chest pain are listed in Table 9.6. Figure 9.2 illustrates the approach to the patient. The basic principles of therapy for the most important causes of chest pain in primary care are summarized below. Table 9.7 summarizes the pharmacotherapy for chest pain. Management of GERD (Chapter 24) and pulmonary embolism (Chapter 12) are discussed elsewhere in this text.

Acute Coronary Syndromes
ANTI-PLATELET THERAPY

All patients with suspected ACS should receive aspirin, 325 mg swallowed or chewed, immediately and then continued daily indefinitely. Aspirin therapy prevents 3 to 10 deaths or MIs per 100 ACS patients, making it the most effective medical intervention available (36–39). It should only be withheld for true absolute contraindications, such as anaphylaxis, other major allergic reaction, or current active gastrointestinal bleed (not merely positive occult blood or a history of bleed). Patients with true contraindications should receive clopidogrel 300 mg as a loading dose as soon as an ACS is diagnosed and 75 mg daily thereafter (40, 41). The duration of therapy is guided by subsequent evaluation and intervention.

REPERFUSION THERAPY

The patient with ST segment elevation greater than 1 mm in two or more contiguous leads, new LBBB, or perhaps ST depression in anterior V leads suggesting posterior MI, should be considered for immediate reperfusion. Restoring coronary blood flow limits infarct size, preserves LV function, and enables myocardial remodeling, all of which contribute to substantial decreases in short- and long-term mortality. Both thrombolytic therapy and emergent PCI provide these benefits: treatment choice depends on characteristics of both the patient and the treating institution.

Indications for thrombolytic administration are very narrow: characteristic pain onset within 6 hours of presentation (perhaps up to 12 hours, but with lesser benefit) plus either ST segment elevation in >2 contiguous leads or new LBBB. Thrombolysis is contraindicated for patients who do not meet

TABLE 9.6 Key Elements in Management of Chest Pain, by Cause

Target Disorder	Intervention	SORT Rating*	Comments
ACS, CAD	Aspirin	A	Withhold only for absolute contraindications
	β-blockers	A	Withhold only for absolute contraindications; oral administration only
	Nitroglycerin	B	Pain relief and improvement of hemodynamic indices; unclear if improves survival
CAD	Coronary revascularization (bypass or angioplasty)	A	For patients meeting very specific selection criteria
	Lipid lowering	A	Reduce LDL cholesterol to <100 mg/dl; <70 mg/dl for patients with history of ACS
	Smoking cessation	B	Largest absolute risk reduction of any treatment if patient successfully quits
ACS	Clopidogrel	A	For ASA contraindicated patients suspected of UA/NSTEMI; duration of therapy depends on diagnosis
	Unfractionated or low-molecular weight heparin	A	Usually reserved for ongoing symptoms of pain or instability
	Morphine sulfate	C	Clearly effective for pain and anxiety relief, although not formally studied; inadequate dosing is common and inexcusable
MI	ACE inhibitors	A	Improve survival post-MI in anterior infarcts with ejection fraction <40%
	Emergent reperfusion (thrombolysis or PCI) for STEMI patients	A	Target time to thrombolysis: <30 min Target time to PCI: <60 min
PE	Unfractionated or low-molecular weight heparin	A	Treatment should not be delayed while confirming a strong clinical suspicion of PE
GERD	H$_2$-receptor antagonists	A	
	Proton pump inhibitors	A	
	Elevation of head of bed	B	
	Decreased fat intake	B	
	Avoidance of chocolate, onions, peppermint, and garlic	B	
Panic	Benzodiazepines	A	High rate of placebo response, and much better short-term than long-term efficacy
	Tricyclic antidepressants	A	
	Cognitive therapy	A	
	Combined drug and cognitive therapy	A	
Musculoskeletal pain	NSAIDs	C	

Abbreviations: ACS, acute coronary syndromes; CAD, coronary artery disease; GERD, gastroesophageal reflux disease; LDL, low-density lipoprotein; MI, myocardial infarction; NSAIDs, nonsteroidal anti-inflammatory drugs; PE, pulmonary embolism.
*Strength-of-Recommendation Taxonomy (SORT): A, Consistent, good quality patient-oriented evidence; B, Inconsistent or limited-quality patient-oriented evidence; C, Consensus, disease-oriented evidence, usulay practice, expert opinion or case series for studies of diagnosis, treatment prevention, or screening; X, moderate or strong evidence suggesting that this treatment is not effective.

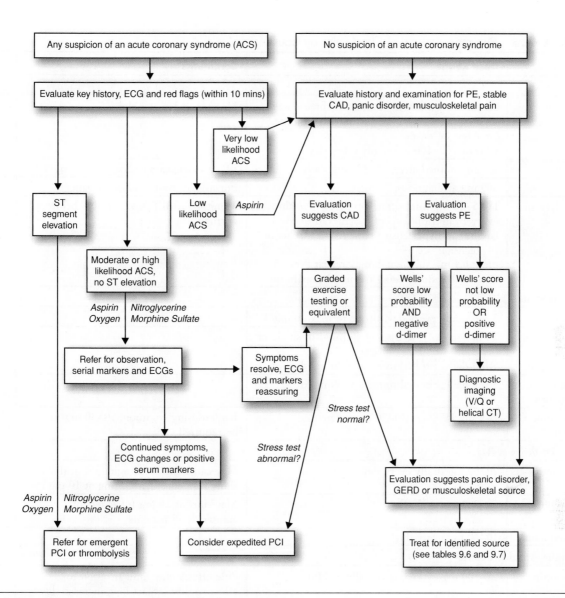

Figure 9.2 • Approach to the patient with chest pain. CAD, coronary artery disease; ECG, electrocardiogram, GERD, gastroesophageal reflux disease; PCI, percutaneous coronary intervention

these criteria (32, 34). Other contraindications include active gastrointestinal and genitourinary bleeding (not menses), abdominal or thoracic surgery within 1 month, head trauma, recent stroke, hypertensive crisis, aortic dissection, and pancreatitis. Although age is not an absolute contraindication to thrombolytic therapy, patients over the age of 75 are at greater risk for bleeding complications from thrombolysis, and may be better served by emergent PCI (42).

Evaluation and administration of thrombolysis should occur within 30 minutes of presentation to an equipped facility (usually an emergency department). For properly screened patients, thrombolysis reduces in-hospital and 1-year mortality by approximately 6 per 100 patients treated, although it probably does not improve 3-year outcomes (43). Hospitals typically administer thrombolytic agents (usually streptokinase or recombinant tissue plasminogen activator—rtPA) under specific protocols; see your institution's policy for details.

The term percutaneous coronary intervention (PCI) refers primarily to percutaneous transluminal coronary angioplasty (PTCA) with or without intracoronary stenting. Rotary atherectomy, laser ablation, and endoluminal radiation are also emerging percutaneous interventions, but long-term data from large studies of their performance are not yet available. Emergent PCI yields better outcomes than thrombolysis in centers suitably staffed, equipped, and experienced to provide it without delay (44, 45) but only where these stringent conditions are met. PCI is not superior in hospitals with lower volumes, and if a door-to-balloon time of 90 minutes cannot be achieved, delaying thrombolysis to seek PCI can worsen outcomes (46).

There is emerging evidence that early PCI may also lower rates of vessel reocclusion (10% after PCI, up to 30% after thrombolysis) as well as overall short- and long-term survival (47). The advent of intracoronary stenting has contributed

TABLE 9.7 Pharmacotherapy of Chest Pain, by Cause

Drug	Dose Range	Comments	Cost*
ACS			
Metoprolol	Acute: 5 mg IV every 2 min for three doses, then 50 mg orally BID starting 15–60 min after last IV dose Chronic: 50–100 mg orally every day	Monitor as for atenolol	$$
Aspirin	325 mg immediately, 81–325 mg daily	Effect disappears at doses >325 mg/d	$
Clopidogrel	300 mg at diagnosis, 75 mg daily	For aspirin contraindicated patients	$$$
Nitroglycerin	IV: 5–10 mg/min, titrate up by 10 mg/min every 10 min until relief is achieved or until baseline in hypertensive patients, headache, or hypotension occurs Oral: 0.4 mg sublingual; may repeat every 5 min, with 3 doses being the usual maximum	Monitor for SBP <90, or 30% below normal	$
ACE Inhibitors			
Lisinopril	5 mg orally every day, titrate to max 20 mg/d		$
Enalapril	2.5–5 mg daily, to max of 40 mg/d in single or divided dose		$
Benazepril	2 mg daily, titrated to max of 20 mg/d		$$
Fosinopril, quinapril	5 mg daily, titrated to max of 30 mg/d		$$
Morphine sulfate	2–4 mg IV every 10–20 min as needed	Underdosing common; 10–30 mg may be required	$
Panic Disorder SSRIs			
Paroxetine	20–50 mg orally every day	May cause increased agitation in the short run; consider starting at 10 mg	$$
Sertraline	50–200 mg every day	May start at 25 mg for elders or complexly ill patients	$$
Citalopram	10–60 mg every day		$$
Tricyclic Antidepressants			
Desipramine	25–300 mg every day (usually at HS)	Side effects may limit titration to effective doses. Start low, increase slowly once weekly	$$
Nortryptiline	10–150 mg	May be more well tolerated than other tricyclics	$
Benzodiazepines			
Diazepam	2.5–5 mg TID	Many other benzodiazepines are available and probably equally effective	$$
Alprazolam	0.25 mg TID, titrated to max of 4 mg/d	Some antidepressant effect; may require careful dose adjustment for panic	$
Clonazepam	0.5 mg TID, titrated to maximum of 20 mg/d		$$
Buspirone	Start with 7.5 mg BID; increase by 5 mg every day for 3 days to a max dose of 15–30 mg/d divided BID–TID	See text	$$$

Abbreviations: BID, twice daily; GERD, gastroesophageal reflux disease; HR, heart rate; IV, intravenously; SBP, systolic blood pressure; SSRI, selective serotonin reuptake inhibitor; TID, three times a day.
* Relative cost: $ = <$33.00; $$ = $34.00–$66.00; $$$ = >$67.00

significantly to these improvements, although stenting has yet to show improved overall mortality benefit compared with PTCA alone. Likewise, platelet inhibition with intravenous glycoprotein IIb/IIIa receptor antagonists (abciximab, eptifibatide, or tirofiban) seems to improve early survival, primarily for patients with NSTEMI and UA who are at particularly high risk for complications (48). Early PCI may also be considered for high-risk ACI patients (e.g., UA or NSTEMI with recurrent ischemia after stabilization, prior MI with baseline depressed LV function) who either do not meet criteria for thrombolysis, or are at relatively higher risk for thrombolytic complications (e.g., elders). Whether ultimately treated with thrombolysis or PCI, the patient with chest pain caused by an acute coronary syndrome benefits greatly from prompt diagnosis and early reperfusion when indicated.

MEDICAL THERAPY

Until very recently, intravenous beta blocker administration has been considered first line anti-ischemic therapy for patients with acute coronary syndromes. New evidence shows, however, that IV beta-blockade in patients suffering myocardial infarction increases absolute risk for cardiogenic shock without improving rates of arrhythmia, reinfarction or survival (49). As a result, IV beta blockers are now contraindicated in MI treatment, and should only be reserved for patients with specific and urgent indications like tachyarrythmias and hypertensive crises *without* evidence of uncompensated CHF or low cardiac output (SBP <120, pulse <60, flash pulmonary edema, clinical evidence of hypoperfusion, etc.).

Oral beta-blockers, on the other hand, remain strongly recommended to reduce death and reinfarction rates in patients with ACS, and should be initiated within 24 hours of diagnosis for patients without signs of CHF or low cardiac output. Oral metoprolol has been studied at 200 mg daily in either BID regular- or QD long-acting dose preparations, and is preferred in many institutions. Atenolol is now disfavored based meta-analyses that show it to be substantially less effective than other agents in its class (50).

Nitroglycerin provides some favorable hemodynamic effects (preload and afterload reduction) and significant relief of chest pain for ACI. MI patients commonly receive it intravenously, but most chest pain patients initially receive up to three sublingual tablets over 15 minutes. It should not be given to hypotensive (systolic blood pressure <90 mm Hg), bradycardic, or tachycardic patients, and it is dangerous in right ventricular infarction.

Heparin administration has become standard therapy for higher risk UA/NSTEMI patients as it decreases infarction and PCI rates (51). Recently, low-molecular-weight heparin (LMWH) has gained a small but definite advantage over unfractionated heparin (UFH) both in efficacy and safety (52). ACE inhibitors are indicated within 24 hours of onset for patients who sustain MI, but not for ACS patients in general. For patients with large anterior infarcts, ejection fractions below 40%, or transient LV dysfunction, ACE inhibitors provide an approximately 0.5% absolute risk reduction for mortality (1 fewer death for every 200 patients treated) (53, 54). Benefit for other MI patients is unclear, and ACE inhibitors should be held for patients with hypotension, hyperkalemia, or rising creatinine.

Oxygen (usually 2 L/min by nasal prongs) and bed rest are traditionally prescribed for ACI patients. These are not of proven benefit, although some physiologic rationales support oxygen. Morphine has an important role in the control of pain and anxiety, and is commonly underused both in dose and frequency because of an exaggerated fear of respiratory depression. Doses of 2 to 4 mg intravenously repeated every 20 to 30 minutes as needed are appropriate.

Calcium channel blockers do not generally improve outcomes and may increase mortality among patients with LV dysfunction or pulmonary edema (34). They should generally not be used in acute treatment of ACS, except for specific indications such as atrial arrhythmias and genuine variant angina (which is rare). Prophylactic administration of lidocaine is contraindicated because it increases mortality (55). Antiarrhythmic therapy should be reserved for sustained, symptomatic ventricular arrhythmias (32).

When the acute coronary syndrome is managed, patients should be treated for their CAD, as discussed in the next section.

Coronary Artery Disease

Therapy for CAD is aimed at controlling symptoms that interfere with the patient's function and reducing the risk of death or infarction. Aspirin, 81 to 325 mg taken orally daily, is a mainstay and should be given to all patients who do not have absolute contraindications (see those listed previously) (56). Beta-blockers, because of their proven mortality-reducing effect, are the first-choice antianginal drugs.

Smoking cessation, although challenging to accomplish, is essential. Smokers with CAD who quit reduce their absolute risk of death over the ensuing decade by 11% to 16%, making smoking cessation the single most important intervention in this group (57, 58). Smoking cessation also reduces the risk of disability and hospitalization.

In patients with known CAD and baseline low-density lipoprotein levels ≥130 mg/dl on diet alone, reduction in LDL cholesterol to below 100 mg/dl can prevent 4 deaths in 100 patients treated for 5 years (59). HMG-CoA reductase inhibitors (statins) used in combination with diet are the preferred agents because they are the only agents shown to achieve this level of benefit. Very aggressive lipid lowering with statins, to target LDLs <70, can further reduce subsequent ACS events among patients with recent ACS (60).

Nitrates are used for additional symptomatic relief. Sublingual or spray forms are used for acute symptoms, and long-acting oral agents or transdermal patches are used for daily prevention. If patches are used, they should be removed at night to prevent disappearance of effect due to tachyphylaxis. Calcium channel blockers (CCBs) are also useful for symptomatic relief, and long-acting agents seem to be safe, but the short-acting agents should be avoided because case-control studies suggest a nearly four-fold increase in odds ratio for cardiovascular mortality among hypertensive patients (61). CCBs can supplement, but should not replace, survival-enhancing β-blockers in patients' antianginal regimens.

Revascularization reduces mortality for patients with 50% or greater left main coronary artery stenosis, three-vessel disease and diminished LV function, or two-vessel disease involving the left anterior descending artery (32, 34). Symptom improvement may be achieved for patients with any degree of CAD who suffer lifestyle-limiting anginal symptoms not adequately controlled by medical therapy. In general, the debate between coronary artery bypass graft (CABG) and angioplasty is beyond the scope of this chapter, but it should be noted that diabetic patients requiring insulin or oral agents seem to have a lower mortality rate with CABG (62).

NSAIDs and Coronary Artery Disease Risk

Non-steroidal anti-inflammatory drugs (NSAIDs) act primarily to inhibit two key enzymes in the arachidonic acid pathway, cyclooxygenase 1 (COX-1) and cyclooxygenase 2 (COX-2). Each NSAID has a specific mix of COX-1 and COX-2 activity which influences both its behavior as an analgesic and its potential for adverse events. It is now clear that all NSAIDs increase risk for MI and cardiac death for patients with CAD, in direct proportion to their degree of COX-2 inhibition (63). Higher risk NSAIDs include not only those marketed as 'COX-2 selective inhibitors' like rofecoxib, celecoxib and valdecoxib, but also relatively COX-2 selective drugs like diclofenac and nabumetone—all should be avoided in patients with CAD.

First-line analgesic medications for CAD patients should include acetaminophen, non-acetylated salicylates (e.g. salsalate) and aspirin. Should these be insufficient or not well-tolerated, a trial of NSAIDs with lower COX-2 selectivity (e.g. naproxen or piroxicam) could be considered. Patient with CAD needing high, daily doses of even these NSAIDs for pain management may be good candidates for a trial of low-dose opioids or adjuvant medications.

Panic Disorder

The two primary approaches to treatment of panic disorder are cognitive therapy and pharmacotherapy. The best results are obtained by combining the two modalities because they have been shown to be mutually potentiating in the few trials in which they were combined (64).

Cognitive therapy teaches the patient to interpret the somatic sensations that accompany an attack as something other than evidence of serious illness. Panic patients have been shown to interpret such sensations in much more alarming ways than nonpanic patients. Cognitive therapy has been shown both to change those interpretations successfully and to provide improvement similar to that from pharmacotherapy (65).

Pharmacotherapeutic management with either antidepressants or anxiolytics is often necessary for more than 6 months. Treatment with either class of agent is more effective than placebo among patients in blinded trials willing to maintain treatment (66).

Tricyclic antidepressants are the most thoroughly studied antidepressants for panic disorder. Therapy should be initiated at low doses, and physicians should be careful to explain the expected adverse effects as normal so that panic patients do not interpret them as serious. Benzodiazepines are the primary anxiolytic class; buspirone may be useful but is not well studied yet. Alprazolam and lorazepam are often used for panic disorder, but it is likely that all members of the class are effective. Although tolerance is common with long-term use and tapering may be necessary to prevent withdrawal, addiction (increasing dose requirements, behavioral "drug seeking," concealment of multiple sources, etc.) is generally uncommon. Care should be taken, however, in prescribing these medications for patients with a significant history of addiction, personality disorder or complex chronic pain, as rates of overuse rise in these groups. Benzodiazepines should be used on a fixed schedule, never as needed, for panic disorder treatment.

Because of their tolerability and safety profile, selective serotonin reuptake inhibitors (SSRIs) have become first line pharmacologic treatment for panic disorder. SSRIs have been shown to be better than placebo in a meta-analysis of randomized controlled trials (67) and are equivalent in effect to tricyclics and benzodiazepines. Patients should be warned that they can cause increased agitation in the first few weeks of use; a short-term prescription for benzodiazepines is often prescribed during these initial weeks to counter this adverse effect.

Relaxation therapy has been shown to improve patients' ability to tolerate anxiety, but has not been shown to reduce the frequency or severity of panic attacks. It is therefore not a primary treatment recommendation for panic disorder, although it may be for other anxiety disorders.

Musculoskeletal Pain

Musculoskeletal chest pain is traditionally treated with nonsteroidal anti-inflammatory drugs or acetaminophen. It is unclear what fraction of patients derive symptomatic improvement from this therapy. Considerable attention to the patient's worry about heart disease, with appropriate reassurance, is an important part of management.

CASE DISCUSSION

MANAGEMENT QUESTIONS

1. Should you admit Mr. S to the hospital to rule out infarction?
2. How should you advise Mr. S today?
3. What diagnostic workup should you pursue?

DISCUSSION

Mr. S's pain is consistent with myocardial ischemia, although it occurred at rest. Unstable angina (UA) is a possibility, but MI is very unlikely given his short duration of pain and normal ECG. Because he has no high-risk features (remember that long-term risk factors contribute little here; it is MI in male relatives before age 55 or in female relatives before age 65 that confers increased risk), outpatient management is appropriate if his 6-hour troponin level is normal. Because outpatient management depends on his adherence to advice and close follow-up, if these are in doubt, he should be admitted until CAD has been detected or excluded. A rule-out-MI protocol is not indicated because, if admission is required, it would be for evaluation for CAD rather than to rule out infarction. You contact your hospital's emergency department, discuss his case, and send him there to have his troponin level checked and to be observed in the holding area until the result is known. If the result indicates him to be at risk, he will be admitted.

Before he leaves your office, Mr. S should know that you are concerned about possible CAD, and that there are other possibilities that require evaluation as well. He should remain on daily aspirin until the matter is settled. You will have to emphasize to him that aspirin could be very important to his survival (he believes it to be "just aspirin," after all!). Mr. S should also be instructed to go directly to the emergency room, without calling for advice first, if he has pain lasting 20 minutes or more.

The emergency department physician contacts you at home 7 hours later, informing you that Mr. S's troponin I level was normal. Mr. S has no indications for imaging nor contraindications to exercise testing. Therefore, you ask the emergency department to release him, after scheduling him for exercise treadmill testing on Monday and a follow-up in your office Tuesday morning.

OUTCOME

Mr. S returns to your office on Tuesday, having had no more pains. He does bring with him a copy of the treadmill report. He reached 11 mets (metabolic equivalents) and had 1 mm of ST segment depression. This is reported as an equivocal result, and the cardiologist reading it recommends cardiac catheterization. Mr. S is very worried about the report, so you proceed with the referral.

His catheterization shows an isolated 40% occlusion of his left anterior descending coronary artery with a smooth surface. Unconvinced that this explains his pain, you schedule him for a longer visit and take a very detailed history. He describes several episodes from his early twenties to the present wherein he would have spells of "feeling unreal," accompanied by palpitations and shortness of breath with brief aching chest pains, once or twice per week. These episodes lasted a few weeks to 2 months each, and resolved spontaneously. You schedule him to meet with your practice's psychologist partner and, in the meantime, start him on paroxetine 10 mg daily, to be increased as necessary under your guidance.

REFERENCES

1. White L, Lee T, Cook E, et al. Comparison of the natural history of new onset and exacerbated chronic ischemic heart disease. The Chest Pain Study Group. J Am Coll Cardiol. 1990;16:304–310.
2. Karlson B, Herlitz J, Pettersson P, et al. A one-year prognosis in patients hospitalized with a history of unstable angina pectoris. Clin Cardiol. 1993;16:397–402.
3. Beitman BD, Mukerji V, Russell JL, Grafting M. Panic disorder in cardiology patients: a review of the Missouri Panic/Cardiology Project. J Psychiatr Res. 1993; 27(Suppl)1:35–46.
4. Ballenger JC. Overview of panic disorder. Trans Am Clin Climatol Assoc. 1993;105:36–51.
5. Fleet RP, Dupuis G, Marchand A, Burelle D, Beitman BD. Panic disorder, chest pain, and coronary artery disease: literature review. Can J Cardiol. 1994;10:827–834.
6. Isolauri J, Laippala P. Prevalence of symptoms suggestive of gastro-oesophageal reflux disease in an adult population. Ann Med. 1995;27:67–70.
7. Petersen H. The prevalence of gastro-oesophageal reflux disease. Scand J Gastroenterol. 1995;211(Suppl):5–6.
8. Woolf PK, Gewitz MH, Berezin S, et al. Noncardiac chest pain in adolescents and children with mitral valve prolapse. J Adolesc Health. 1991;12:247–250.
9. Selker H, Griffith J, D'Agostino R. A tool for judging coronary care unit admission appropriateness, valid for both real-time and retrospective use. Med Care. 1991;29:610–627.
10. Klinkman MS. Episodes of care for chest pain. J Fam Pract. 1994;38:345.
11. Goldman L, Weinberg M, Weisberg M. A computer-derived protocol to aid in the diagnosis of emergency room patients with acute chest pain. N Engl J Med. 1982;307:588–596.
12. Everts B, Karlson BW, Wahrborg P, Hedner T, Herlitz J. Localization of pain in suspected acute myocardial infarction in relation to final diagnosis, age and sex, and site and type of infarction. Heart Lung. 1996;25:430–437.
13. Weaver WD, Litwin PE, Martin JS, et al. Effect of age on use of thrombolytic therapy and mortality in acute myocardial infarction: the MITI Project Group. J Am Coll Cardiol. 1991; 18:657–662.
14. Diamond G, Forrester J. Analysis of probability as an aid in the clinical diagnosis of coronary-artery disease. N Engl J Med. 1979;300:1350–1358.
15. Green LA, Yates JF. Influence of pseudodiagnostic information on the evaluation of ischemic coronary disease. Ann Emerg Med. 1995;25:451–457.
16. Jayes RLJ, Beshansky JR, D'Agostino RB, Selker HP. Do patients' coronary risk factor reports predict acute cardiac ischemia in the emergency department? A multicenter study. J Clin Epidemiol. 1992;45:621–626.
17. Moraes D, McCormack P, Tyrrell J, Feely J. Earlobe crease and coronary heart disease. Ir Med J. 1992;85:131–132.
18. Tranchesi B Jr, Barbosa V, de Albuquerque CP, et al. Diagonal earlobe crease as a marker of the presence and extent of coronary atherosclerosis. Am J Cardiol. 1992;70:1417–1420.
19. Diamond G, Forrester J. Analysis of probability as an aid in the clinical diagnosis of coronary-artery disease. N Engl J Med. 1979;300:1350–1358.
20. O'Keefe JH. Comparison of stress echocardiography and stress myocardial perfusion scintigraphy for diagnosing coronary disease and assessing its severity. Am J Cardiol. 1995; 75:25D-34D.
21. Panju AA, Hemmelgarn BR, Guyatt GH, Simel DL. Is this patient having a myocardial infarction? JAMA. 1998;280(14): 1256–1263.
22. Zimmerman J, Fromm R, Meyer D, et al. Diagnostic marker cooperative study for the diagnosis of myocardial infarction. Circulation. 1999;99:1671–1677.
23. Hamm CW, Goldmann B, Heeschen C, Kreymann G, Berger J, Meinertz T. Emergency room triage of patients with acute chest pain by means of rapid testing for cardiac troponin T or troponin I. N Engl J Med. 1997;337:1648–1653.
24. Rude RE, Poole WK, Muller JE, et al. Electrocardiographic and clinical criteria for recognition of acute myocardial infarction based on analysis of 3,697 patients. Am J Cardiol. 1983;52:936–942.
25. University of Michigan VTE Evidence-Based Guideline Panel. Venous thromboembolism (2004 update). Available at National Guidelines Clearinghouse, *http://www.guidelines.gov*. Accessed June 2006.
26. Luker GD, Glazer HS, Eagar G, Gutierrez FR, Sagel SS. Aortic dissection: effect of prospective chest radiographic diagnosis on delay to definitive diagnosis. Radiology. 1994;193: 813–819.
27. Ravkilde J, Nissen H, Horder M, Thygesen K. Independent prognostic value of serum creatine kinase isoenzyme MB mass, cardiac troponin T, and myosin light chain levels in suspected acute myocardial infarction. Analysis of 28 months of follow-up in 196 patients. J Am Coll Cardiol. 1995;25: 574–581.
28. Tucker JF, Collins RA, Anderson AJ, et al. Value of serial myoglobin levels in the early diagnosis of patients admitted for acute myocardial infarction. Ann Emerg Med. 1994;24: 704–708.
29. Hamm CW, Goldmann B, Heeschen C, Kreymann G, Berger J, Meinertz T. Emergency room triage of patients with

acute chest pain by means of rapid testing for cardiac troponin T or troponin I. N Engl J Med. 1997;337:1648–1653.

30. Ebell MH, White LL, Weismantel D. A systematic review of troponin T and I values as a prognostic tool for patients with chest pain. J Fam Pract. 2000;49:746–753.

31. Ebell MH, Flewelling D, Flynn CA. A systematic review of troponin T and I for diagnosing acute myocardial infarction. J Fam Pract. 2000;49:550–556.

32. Ryan TJ, Anderson JL, Antman EM, et al. ACC/AHA guidelines for the management of patients with acute myocardial infarction: a report of the American College of Cardiology/ American Heart Association Task Force on Practice Guidelines (Committee on Management of Acute Myocardial Infarction). J Am Coll Cardiol. 1996;28:1328–1428.

33. Mark DB, Shaw L, Harrell FE Jr, et al. Prognostic value of a treadmill exercise score in outpatients with suspected coronary artery disease [see comments]. N Engl J Med. 1991; 325:849–853.

34. Braunwald E, Mark DB, Jones RH, et al. Unstable Angina: Clinical Practice Guideline No. 10. Washington, DC: Agency for Health Care Policy and Research; 1994.

35. Barbant SD, Eisenberg MJ, Schiller NB. The diagnostic value of imaging techniques for aortic dissection. Am Heart J. 1992; 124:541–543.

36. ISIS-2 (Second International Study of Infarct Survival) Collaborative Group. Randomised trial of intravenous streptokinase, oral aspirin, both, or neither among 17,187 cases of suspected acute myocardial infarction: ISIS-2. Lancet. 1988; 2:349–360.

37. Lewis HD Jr, Davis JW, Archibald DG, et al. Protective effects of aspirin against acute myocardial infarction and death in men with unstable angina. Results of a Veterans Administration Cooperative Study. N Engl J Med. 1983;309: 396–403.

38. Wallentin LC. Aspirin (75 mg/day) after an episode of unstable coronary artery disease: long-term effects on the risk for myocardial infarction, occurrence of severe angina, and the need for revascularization. Research Group on Instability in Coronary Artery Disease in Southeast Sweden [comments]. J Am Coll Cardiol. 1991;18:1587–1593.

39. Cairns JA, Gent M, Singer J, et al. Aspirin, sulfinpyrazone, or both in unstable angina. Results of a Canadian multicenter trial. N Engl J Med. 1985;313:1369–1375.

40. The CURE Trial Investigators. The effect of clopidogrel in addition to aspirin in patients with acute coronary syndromes without ST-segment elevation. N Engl J Med. 2001;345: 494–502.

41. Yusuf S, Wittes J, Friedman L. Overview of results of randomized clinical trials in heart disease. II. Unstable angina, heart failure, primary prevention with aspirin, and risk factor modification. JAMA. 1988;260:2259–2263.

42. Cerqueira MD, Maynard C, Ritchie JL, Davis KB, Kennedy JW. Long-term survival in 618 patients from the Western Washington Streptokinase in Myocardial Infarction trials. J Am Coll Cardiol. 1992;20:1452–1459.

43. Thiemann DR, Coresh J, Schulman SP, et al. Lack of benefit for thrombolysis in patients with myocardial infarction who are older than 75 years. Circulation. 2000;101:2239–2246.

44. Keeley EC, Boura JA, Grines CL. Primary angioplasty versus intravenous thrombolytic therapy for acute myocardial infarction: a quantitative review of 23 randomized trials. Lancet 2003;361:13–20.

45. Cucherat M, Bonnefoy E, Tremeau G. Primary angioplasty versus intravenous thrombolysis for acute myocardial infarction. Cochrane Database Syst Rev 2004:CD001560.

46. Van de Werf F, Gore JM, Avezum A, et al., for the GRACE Investigators. Access to catheterisation facilities in patients admitted with acute coronary syndrome: multinational registry study. BMJ. 2005; 330:441–444.

47. Zijlstra F, Hoorntje JCA, de Boer M-J, et al. Long-term benefit of primary angioplasty as compared with thrombolytic therapy for acute myocardial infarction. N Engl J Med. 1999;341:1413–1419.

48. The PURSUIT Trial Investigators. Inhibition of glycoprotein IIb/IIIa with eptifibatide patients with acute coronary syndromes. N Engl J Med. 1998;339:436–443.

49. COMMIT Investigators. Early intravenous then oral metoprolol in 45,852 patients with acute myocardial infarction: randomized placebo-controlled trial. Lancet 2005;366: 1622–3162.

50. Khan N, McAlister FA. Re-examining the efficacy of B-blockers for the treatment of hypertension: a meta-analysis. CMAJ 2006;174:1737–1742.

51. Braunwald E, Antman EM, Theroux P, et al. ACC/AHA 2002 guideline update for the management of patients with unstable angina and non-ST-segment elevation myocardial infarction: a report of the American College of Cardiology/ American Heart Association Task Force on Practice Guidelines (Committee on the Management of Patients With Unstable Angina). 2002. Available at *http://www.acc.org/clinical/ guidelines/unstable/incorporated/index.htm*.

52. Magee KD, Sevcik W, Moher D, Rowe BH. Low molecular weight heparins vs. unfractionated heparin for acute coronary syndromes. Cochrane Database; last update Feb 2005.

53. Ball SG, Hall AS, Murray GD. Angiotensin-converting enzyme inhibitors after myocardial infarction: indications and timing. J Am Coll Cardiol. 1995;25:42S–46S.

54. LeJemtel TH, Hochman JS, Sonnenblick EH. Indications for immediate angiotensin-converting enzyme inhibition in patients with acute myocardial infarction. J Am Coll Cardiol. 1995;25:47S–51S.

55. Hine LK, Laird N, Hewitt P, Chalmers TC. Meta-analytic evidence against prophylactic use of lidocaine in acute myocardial infarction. Arch Intern Med. 1989;149:2694–2698.

56. Antiplatelet Trialists' Collaboration. Collaborative over-view of randomised trials of antiplatelet therapy—I: Prevention of death, myocardial infarction, and stroke by prolonged antiplatelet therapy in various categories of patients. BMJ. 1994; 308:81–106.

57. Cavender JB, Rogers WJ, Fisher LD, Gersh BJ, Coggin CJ, Myers WO. Effects of smoking on survival and morbidity in patients randomized to medical or surgical therapy in the Coronary Artery Surgery Study (CASS): 10-year follow-up. CASS Investigators. J Am Coll Cardiol. 1992;20:287–294.

58. Daly LE, Mulcahy R, Graham IM, Hickey N. Long-term effect on mortality of stopping smoking after unstable angina and myocardial infarction. BMJ. 1983;287:324–326.

59. Scandinavian Simvastatin Survival Study Investigators. Randomised trial of cholesterol lowering in 4444 patients with coronary heart disease: the Scandinavian Simvastatin Survival Study (4S). Lancet. 1994;344:1383–1389.

60. Ridker PM. Morrow DA. Rose LM. Rifai N. Cannon CP. Braunwald E. Relative efficacy of atorvastatin 80 mg and pravastatin 40 mg in achieving the dual goals of low-density lipoprotein cholesterol <70 mg/dl and C-reactive protein <2 mg/l: an analysis of the PROVE-IT TIMI-22 trial. J Am Coll Cardiol. 2005;45:1644–1648.

61. Alderman MH, Cohen H, Roque R, Madhavan S. Effect of long-acting and short-acting calcium antagonists on cardiovascular outcomes in hypertensive patients. Lancet. 1997;349: 594–598.

62. Clinical Alert. Washington, DC: National Heart, Lung, and Blood Institute; September 21, 1995.

63. Antman EA, Bennett JS, Daugherty A, et al. American Heart Association (AHA) Scientific Statement on the Use of Non-steroidal Anti-Inflammatory Drugs (NSAIDS)—An Update for Clinicians. American Heart Association, *in press*.

64. Mavissakalian M. Combined behavioral therapy and pharmacotherapy of agoraphobia. J Psychiatr Res. 1993;27(Suppl)1: 179–191.

64. Gelder MG, Clark DM, Salkovskis P. Cognitive treatment for panic disorder. J Psychiatr Res. 1993; 27(Suppl)1:171–178.

64. Curtis GC, Massana J, Udina C, Ayuso JL, Cassano GB, Perugi G. Maintenance drug therapy of panic disorder. J Psychiatr Res. 1993;27(Suppl)1:127–142.

67. Otto MW, Tuby KS, Gould RA, McLean RY, Pollack MH. An effect-size analysis of the relative efficacy and tolerability of serotonin selective reuptake inhibitors for panic disorder. Am J Psychiatry. 2001;158(12):1989–1992.

CHAPTER 10

Chronic Cardiac Disease

Douglas R. Smucker and Philip M. Diller

CASE

Mr. Jones, who is 62 years old, comes to see you for the first time. He was feeling fine until the past few months when he experienced increasing shortness of breath with activity. Five years ago, he had experienced chest pains and was diagnosed with coronary artery disease. Angiography was performed at that time and he recalls that "I have just a mild blockage in one of the arteries but didn't need the balloon treatment." Over the past year, he has experienced episodes of central chest pain once or twice a week, usually when he is at rest, and promptly relieved by taking one sublingual nitroglycerin tablet.

The shortness of breath is exertional, particularly when he is working in his garden. He needs to stop once in a while during daily activities to catch his breath. Sometimes he has palpitations when he works hard. He occasionally wakes up short of breath at night, but has solved that by sleeping on two or three pillows. Over the past few months his weight has increased about 8 lbs and he has had some swelling around his ankles. His only medication is one aspirin per day. He smokes a half pack of cigarettes per day and was told his cholesterol is "OK."

On physical examination he is a mildly obese male, his blood pressure is 160/92, his heart rate is 90 with frequent premature beats, and respirations are 18. He is comfortable at rest. His head and neck examination reveal no abnormalities. Lung exam reveals bilateral rales extending about 10 cm up from the bases. Heart exam shows a normal PMI location, a regular rate with 10–20 single premature beats per minute, and a II/VI mid-systolic murmur at the aortic area without radiation to the neck. His abdomen is normal, and he has 2 + pitting edema around his ankles.

CLINICAL QUESTIONS

- What is the role of prevention in the management of coronary artery disease and chronic stable angina?
- What is the best approach to evaluation and management of different types of heart failure?
- What are the principal goals of managing atrial fibrillation, and what advice should family physicians give regarding anticoagulation?
- When is a cardiac murmur significant?

Chronic heart disease has a tremendous impact on clinical care, public health, and national resources. Heart disease is the leading cause of mortality in the United States. On average, 2,500 Americans die each day from cardiovascular disease (1). This chapter will review three of the most common chronic cardiac conditions encountered in family practice.

Patients with chronic stable angina pectoris due to coronary artery disease (CAD) are routinely cared for by family physicians (2). Angina affects greater than 6 million Americans, and CAD is responsible for 1 in every 5 deaths (1). Heart failure is the most common cause of hospitalization for individuals over the age of 65. Each year 400,000 new cases develop and 250,000 deaths occur from heart failure (1, 3). The family physician will also encounter many patients with cardiac arrhythmias in clinical practice, of which atrial fibrillation is the most common serious arrhythmia (4). For each of these three conditions, we will review evidence regarding initial evaluation, management, and long-term monitoring. In addition, the chapter includes a brief introduction to other cardiac arrhythmias and common valvular diseases.

The general approach to patients with any chronic cardiac condition includes two overarching goals: 1) to prevent further disability or death from chronic cardiac disease, and 2) to help patients cope with their condition by treating symptoms and improving physical capacity. These goals can best be achieved in the context of a continuity doctor-patient partnership using a combination of approaches including lifestyle changes, modification of cardiac risk factors, medications, diagnostic testing, and specialty consultation or referral when appropriate.

CHRONIC STABLE ANGINA

For patients who survive an acute myocardial infarction (MI) and have known CAD, family physicians are often closely involved in managing and preventing further complications (5). Angina pectoris is a symptom complex resulting from atherosclerotic coronary vessels that cannot supply adequate oxygen to meet myocardial demand. The primary tasks in the management of stable angina due to chronic ischemic heart disease include (5–8):

- Characterizing the chest pain pattern
- Reducing risk factors to prevent progression of coronary artery disease
- Prescribing medications to decrease mortality from CAD
- Treating the symptoms of angina
- Detecting changes in the pattern and severity of angina symptoms
- Preventing myocardial infarction and death

The evaluation of a patient with chronic stable angina who presents with chest pain is shown in Figure 10.1 and discussed in more detail below.

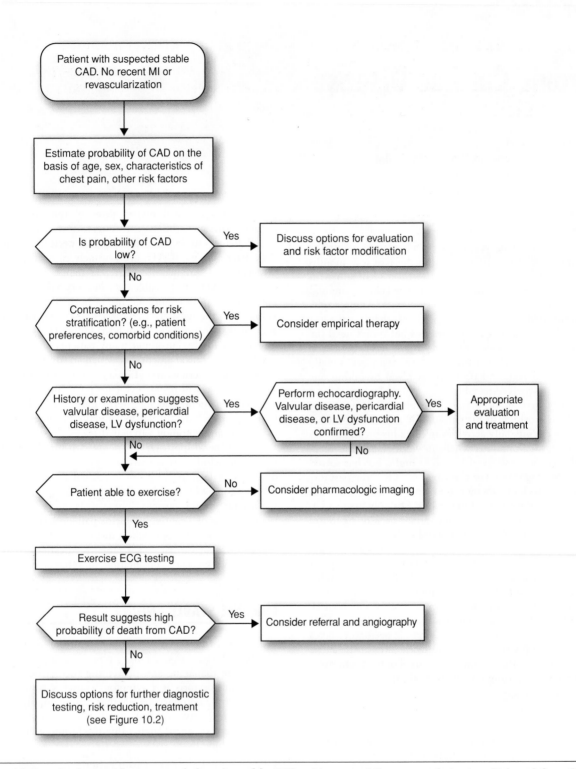

Figure 10.1 • Patient with suspected chronic stable CAD. No recent MI or revascularization. (Adapted from Snow V, Barry P, Fihn SD, et al. Evaluation of primary care patients with chronic stable angina guidelines from the American College of Physicians. Ann Intern Med. 2004;141:57–64. Used with permission.)

TABLE 10.1 Protest Likelihood of Coronary Artery Disease in Symptomatic Patients, According to Age and Sex*

Age	Nonanginal Chest Pain		Atypical Angina		Typical Angina	
	Men	Women	Men	Women	Men	Women
y	◄——————————————— % ———————————————►					
30–39	4	2	34	12	76	26
40–49	13	3	51	22	87	55
50–59	20	7	65	31	93	73
60–69	27	14	72	51	94	86

*Each value represents the percentage of patients with significant coronary artery disease on catheterization. (Adapted from Snow V, Barry P, Fihn SD, et al. Evaluation of primary care patients with chronic stable angina guidelines from the American College of Physicians. Ann Intern Med. 2004;141:57–64. Used with permission.)

Diagnosis
HISTORY AND PHYSICAL EXAMINATION

Characterizing the quality, pattern, and frequency of chest pain is a crucial task in evaluating patients with known coronary artery disease (2). Chest pain can be categorized as typical angina, atypical angina, or non-cardiac chest pain. Typical angina is defined as having all three of the following characteristics: 1) Substernal chest discomfort or pressure, 2) discomfort/pressure that is provoked by exertion or emotional stress, and 3) discomfort/pressure that is relieved by rest or by taking nitroglycerin.

If only two of those three characteristics are present, the patient is said to have atypical angina. For example, a patient with substernal pain or pressure that occurs at rest, but is relieved by nitroglycerin has atypical angina. The third category is non-cardiac chest pain in which a patient has only one of the three characteristics listed above (2, 6). The type of chest pain and the patient's age and gender help determine the likelihood of CAD (see Table 10.1).

You should ask patients about the quality, location, and duration of that pain, and about associated symptoms such as diaphoresis, shortness of breath, nausea, and palpitations. It is also important to identify factors that worsen or relieve pain. Patients with a fairly predictable pattern of chest pain with exertion are categorized as having stable angina. Patients who have new onset angina or a worsening pattern of pain have unstable angina. Unstable angina is associated with a much higher short-term risk for an acute myocardial infarction or other cardiac event, and calls for prompt evaluation and often requires immediate hospitalization (5, 6).

The family physician should regularly assess the impact of CAD on the patient's physical functioning. The New York Heart Association (NYHA) classification scale is widely used for this purpose (see Table 10.2). Efforts to control cardiovascular risk factors such as smoking, hyperlipidemia, diabetes mellitus, and hypertension should also be reviewed regularly (2). In patients with diabetes, it is particularly important to assess lipids and hypertension because a combination of these risk factors is strongly associated with worsening CAD over time. The metabolic syndrome, a constellation of lipid and non-lipid risk factors, puts patients at significantly increased risk for worsening CAD and acute MI. Detecting metabolic syndrome should prompt additional efforts to reduce cardiac risk factors (10).

During an initial physical examination the physician should also search for signs of vascular disease (abnormal fundi, decreased peripheral pulses, bruits), end-organ damage caused by hypertension (abnormal fundi, bruit), aortic valve stenosis (systolic murmur, abnormal pulses), left heart failure (third heart sound, displaced apical pulse, basilar rales), and right heart failure (jugular venous distension, ascites, pedal edema).

DIAGNOSTIC TESTING

In a patient with known CAD, exercise testing with imaging remains an important clinical tool (2, 5, 6). Stress imaging can

TABLE 10.2 New York Heart Association Functional Classification

Class I	No limitation of activity. Ordinary activity does not cause undue fatigue, palpitation, dyspnea, or anginal pain.
Class II	Slight limitations of physical activity. Patient is comfortable at rest. Ordinary activity results in fatigue, palpitation, dyspnea, or anginal pain.
Class III	Marked limitation of physical activity. Patient is comfortable at rest, but less than ordinary activity causes fatigue, palpitation, dyspnea, or anginal pain.
Class IV	Inability to carry out physical activity without symptoms. Fatigue, palpation, dyspnea, or anginal pain at rest. Increased symptoms or discomfort with even minor physical activity.

Adapted from Criteria Committee, New York Heart Association: Nomenclature and Criteria for Diagnosis of Diseases of the Heart and Great Vessels, 9th ed. Boston: Little, Brown; 1994: 253–256. Used with permission.

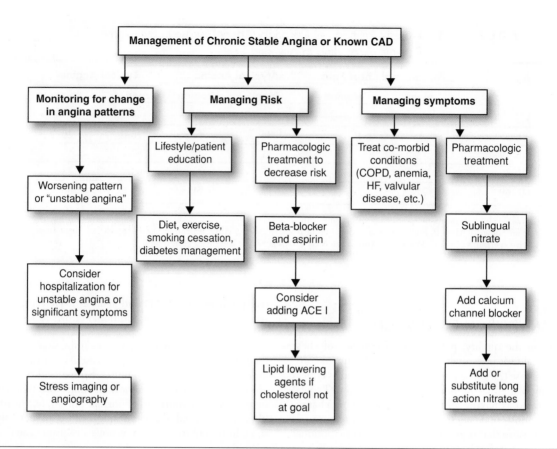

Figure 10.2 • Management of chronic stable angina or known CAD.

be used to stratify CAD patients based on their level of risk, to evaluate changes in anginal patterns, or to assess exercise capacity. For any patient with known coronary artery disease, thallium or technetium imaging should be completed before and after stressing the myocardium with exercise. Echocardiography before and after cardiac stress is another imaging option, but it has been less well studied as a tool for risk stratification in patients with known CAD (2).

For CAD patients who are unable to exercise, who have left bundle branch block, or who have an electronically paced ventricular rhythm on baseline ECG, stress imaging using a pharmacologic agent is recommended (2). Dobutamine, dipyriadamole, and adenosine can be used to stress the cardiac muscle while the patient is at rest, causing differences in perfusion and wall motion in the areas with coronary artery obstruction.

The "gold standard" for evaluation of coronary artery disease is coronary angiography. Indications for coronary angiography include (2, 5, 6):

- High pretest probability of left main or 3-vessel CAD
- Patients who cannot undergo noninvasive testing due to disability, illness, or morbid obesity
- Uncertain diagnosis after noninvasive testing where the benefits of diagnosis outweighs the risks of angiography
- Occupational requirement for definitive diagnosis (pilots, police, etc.)
- Coronary artery spasm is suspected and provocative testing may be necessary

A suggested approach to diagnostic testing is shown in Figure 10.1.

Treatment of Stable Angina

There are two primary goals in the management of patients with known CAD, particularly those with angina. The first, and highest priority, is to prevent further coronary artery obstruction, MI, and death from cardiac events. The second goal is to improve quality of life by limiting the occurrence of angina and other symptoms of cardiac ischemia that can be distressing and impair exercise capacity (5). These goals are accomplished primarily by using a combination of lifestyle changes and medications to modify cardiac risk factors and treat angina symptoms, as outlined in Figure 10.2.

LIFESTYLE CHANGES

The modification of risk factors associated with CAD is an important goal in the management of angina pectoris. Common risk factors for CAD include: age, male sex, family history of early CAD, smoking, hypertension, hyperlipidemia, diabetes mellitus, obesity, sedentary life style, and being postmenopausal for women. General non-pharmacologic interventions for CAD include smoking cessation, diet modification, weight loss, exercise, and stress management (5–7). The family physician should encourage the patient and family to stop smoking and should provide counseling, nicotine replacement, and cessation programs. It is never too late to gain an advantage over chronic cardiac disease by cessation of smoking (11).

TABLE 10.3 Effectiveness of Treatment for Coronary Artery Disease

Treatment Strategy	Strength of Recommendation*	Recommendations/Comments
Pharmacologic treatment		
Sublingual nitroglycerin	C	For immediate relief of angina
Beta-blockers	B	Initial Therapy in absence of contraindications
Calcium channel blockers and long-acting nitrates	B	In combination with β-blockers or when β-blockers are ineffective or contraindicated
Risk factor modification		
Aspirin	A	If contraindicated consider clopidogrel
Smoking cessation therapy	B	Provide counseling, nicotine replacement, formal programs
Cholesterol reduction	A	When LDL≥ 130 and target LDL < 100 mg/dl
Cholesterol reduction	B	When LDL= 100 to 129 and target LDL < 100 mg/dl
Blood pressure control	A	Goal ≤ 130/85 (Joint National Conference VI Guidelines)
Weight reduction	C	In patients > 120% ideal body weight
Exercise program	B	Moderate intensity activity 30 minutes 3 to 4 times per week
Diabetes management	C	Data are lacking on control of diabetes and risk reduction for CAD
Revascularization		
Coronary artery bypass grafting	A	Significant left main coronary disease, three-vessel coronary disease, or two-vessel CAD including significant proximal LAD disease
Percutaneous transcutaneous angioplasty	B	Anatomy suitable for catheter treatment and normal LV function
CABG or PTCA	B	Patients who failed medical therapy

*A = consistent, good-quality patient-oriented evidence; B = inconsistent or limited-quality patient-oriented evidence; C = consensus, disease-oriented evidence, usual practice, expert opinion, or case series. For information about the SORT evidence rating system, see *http://www.aafp.org/afpsort.xml*.

Common dietary goals in patients with CAD include reducing saturated fats (if hyperlipidemic), reducing sodium intake (if hypertensive), and controlling blood sugar (if diabetic). All patients with hyperlipidemia should start an American Heart Association (AHA) Step II Diet consisting of less than 30% total fat (9). Motivated patients should be encouraged to go even further with dietary changes to prevent further cardiac disease. The Mediterranean diet emphasizes increased intake of vegetables, legumes, fruits, cereal, fish, reduced intake of meat and dairy, and moderate consumption of alcohol. There is evidence from a well-designed prospective cohort study that a Mediterranean-style diet is associated with reduced cardiovascular mortality in patients with known CAD (12). An intensive program to change multiple lifestyle risk factors designed by Dean Ornish, MD (stress management, smoking cessation, exercise, psychosocial support) includes a very low-fat vegetarian diet (13). A small study with 5-year follow-up showed that in patients who could adhere to the Ornish program it could stabilize or even reverse coronary artery obstruction and reduce the number of subsequent cardiovascular events (13).

MEDICATIONS THAT DECREASE CAD MORTALITY

Interventions that have the greatest evidence for preventing infarction or death remain underused in appropriate patients

with known CAD (Table 10.3) (5, 6). Medications with evidence for CAD mortality reduction in patients with known CAD include: 1) antiplatelet medications, 2) β-blockers, 3) lipid-lowering agents, and 4) angiotensin-converting enzyme inhibitors (see Table 10.3) (5).

Antiplatelet Agents

Aspirin should be taken routinely by all patients with known CAD, particularly higher risk patients with chronic stable angina. For patients who do not tolerate aspirin, who have experienced worsening CAD while taking aspirin, or for patients who have had recent angioplasty with stenting, clopidogrel (Plavix) is another option (2). Apart from these circumstances, there is no evidence to routinely prescribe clopidogrel for all patients with CAD (14). In the past, dipyridamole, which causes a vasodilatory effect on coronary vessels and has some antiplatelet activity, was widely used as alternative to aspirin. Recent evidence has shown that usual doses of dipyridamole can worsen exercise-induced myocardial ischemia in patients with stable angina and therefore should not be used as an antiplatelet agent in these patients. It still may have a role in prevention of stroke, though (5).

β-Blockers

Beta-blockers have been repeatedly shown to reduce the risk of myocardial infarction (MI) and other adverse cardiac events in patients with CAD, particularly in patients who have had a previous MI. Beta-blockers reduce heart rate, decrease myocardial contractile force, and block deleterious sympathetic tone on coronary arteries (5, 6). No one β-blocker has shown superiority over others in reducing angina or adverse outcomes. Some β-blockers are cardio-selective (atenolol, metoprolol) and affect primarily β1 receptors. Propranolol is a common nonselective β-blocker that demonstrates β2 (pulmonary smooth muscle) and β1 effects. Nonselective β-blockers may induce bronchospasm in patients with asthma or chronic obstructive pulmonary disease (COPD). Other potential side effects of β-blockers are bradycardia, impaired glucose control in diabetes, exercise intolerance, depression, and impotence (although depression and impotence are much less common than previously supposed) (15). Physicians should ensure that all eligible patients with known CAD, particularly those who have had an MI, are taking a β-blocker. While diabetes mellitus has traditionally been considered a relative contraindication to β-blocker therapy, a number of randomized trials have shown that β-blockers improve morbidity and mortality in hypertensive patients with diabetes mellitus (16).

Lipid-lowering Agents
Patients with known CAD should have close attention paid to their lipids and an aggressive approach to lowering levels of low-density lipoproteins (LDL). For patients with CAD, the National Cholesterol Education Program (NCEP) recommends that LDL cholesterol be maintained at less than 100 mg/dl, high-density lipoproteins (HDL) at greater than 35 mg/dl, and serum triglycerides at less than 200 mg/dl (9). More recent randomized trials suggest that an even lower goal for LDL to less than 70 mg/dl may be beneficial for patients with CAD and multiple other risk factors for an acute cardiac event, most importantly diabetes mellitus (17). If diet and exercise do not achieve these goals, drugs that lower cholesterol should be prescribed, beginning for most patients with a statin (9).

Angiotensin-converting Enzyme (ACE) Inhibitors
Several studies have shown that ACE inhibitors reduce the risk of cardiovascular death, MI, and stroke in patients who have vascular disease (18). Even small doses of ACE inhibitors with only a small change in blood pressure may have a vasoprotective effect in preventing adverse events among patients with coronary artery disease. In addition to aspirin, a β-blocker, and close attention to lipids, the addition of ACE inhibitors should be considered for every patient who has known CAD. This is especially important in patients with diabetes who will also gain protection of renal function from an ACE inhibiror.

MEDICATION TO TREAT ANGINA SYMPTOMS

For patients with symptoms of angina, the second major goal is to limit symptoms and improve quality of life (5–8). The two agents primarily used to limit symptoms are nitrates and calcium antagonists. Neither of these agents has been shown to reduce mortality in patients with known CAD but their use can reduce the frequency and distress caused by angina. Nitrates decrease venous return, reduce left ventricular wall stress, and dilate stenotic coronary arteries. They exist in sev-

eral forms of administration (sublingual, oral, spray, transdermal, and intravenous) that are similarly effective in relieving ischemic episodes. All patients with CAD should have a rapid acting nitroglycerin for rescue from acute anginal episodes. A long-acting nitrate, such as isosorbide dinitrate (ISDN) or isosorbide mononitrate (ISMN), can be used for individuals with frequent angina. Hypotension and headache are common side effects of nitrates.

Calcium channel blockers are often added or substituted for long-acting nitrates to control angina symptoms (5, 6). They function by blocking movement of calcium into myocardial and smooth muscle cells, resulting in muscular and vascular relaxation. Two classes of calcium channel blockers exist: non-dihydropyridines (i.e., verapamil, diltiazem), and dihydropyridines (i.e., nifedipine, amlodipine). The dihydropyridines produce significant peripheral vasodilatation and may produce a reflex tachycardia. Verapamil and diltiazem modestly reduce peripheral resistance, decrease heart rate, reduce contractility, and slow electrical conduction. A potentially unsafe anti-anginal drug combination is dihydropyridine calcium channel blockers and a nitrate, which may produce profound hypotension. Another is diltiazem or verapamil combined with a β-blocker, which can cause significant bradycardia or conduction defects.

Long-term Monitoring
The ACC/AHA guidelines suggest five questions that should be answered regularly during the follow-up of a patient with chronic stable angina (see Table 10.4). In addition to a follow-up history, a brief focused physical exam covering the cardiovascular and pulmonary systems should be performed at each visit. Laboratory assessments should be directed by the history, physical exam, and clinical course of the patient with particular attention to meeting recommended goals for blood lipids. An electrocardiogram (ECG) is indicated when there is a change in the patient's anginal pattern, symptoms of dysrhythmia, or syncope. Cardiac stress imaging should be considered

---

TABLE 10.4 History Questions to Monitor Symptoms in Patients with Chronic Stable Angina

- Has the patient's level of physical activity decreased since the last visit?
- Have the patient's anginal symptoms increased in frequency or become more severe since the last visit?
- How well is the patient tolerating therapy?
- How successful has the patient been in modifying risk factors and improving knowledge about ischemic heart disease?
- Has the patient developed any knew co-morbid illness or has the severity of treatment of known co-morbid illnesses worsened the patient's angina?

Adapted from Snow V, Barry P, Fihn S, et al. Primary care management of chronic stable angina and asymptomatic suspected or known coronary artery disease: a clinical practice guideline from the American College of Physicians. Ann Intern Med. 2004;141:562–567. Used with permission.

for any CAD patient with a change in the pattern of angina symptoms (5–8).

Revascularization

A challenge for the clinician caring for patients with chronic stable angina is knowing when revascularization is indicated as opposed to medical management (5, 19). Decisions regarding revascularization should generally be made in consulation with a cardiologist or cardiovascular surgeon. The presence of any of the following factors indicates that revascularization with coronary artery bypass grafts (CABG) may be beneficial (20):

- Significant left main coronary disease
- Significant stenosis of the proximal left anterior descending and left circumflex arteries.
- The presence of three-vessel coronary artery disease (or two-vessel disease and significant proximal left anterior descending stenosis)
- Disabling angina despite maximal medical therapy
- Significant CAD in the presence of left ventricular dysfunction (ejection fraction < 50%)

Percutaneous transcutaneous coronary angioplasty (PTCA) should be considered as an option to CABG in patients with one-, two-, or three-vessel disease who have anatomy suitable for catheter therapy and who have normal left ventricular function.

HEART FAILURE

Heart failure (HF) is a heterogeneous condition caused by impaired function of the left ventricle either during systole, diastole, or both (3, 18). Subsequent signs and symptoms are due to the body's maladaptive response to impaired left ventricular (LV) function. In the United States, CAD is the most common etiology of HF. CAD leads to myocardial injury and infarction, with the eventual development of systolic HF, in which the left ventricular ejection fraction (LVEF) is reduced (LVEF <40%). Other etiologies of systolic HF include hypertension, valvular heart disease, alcohol abuse, congenital abnormalities, viral infections, and idiopathic cardiomyopathy.

Not all HF is systolic, however; an estimated 40% of HF arises in patients with normal LV systolic function (21). These patients have diastolic HF, in which the left ventricle is stiff, fails to relax, and does not fill adequately at normal diastolic pressures. Aging, hypertension, and CAD are the most common causes of diastolic HF.

The pathophysiology of HF is a complex interplay of hemodynamic and neurohormonal mechanisms as the body attempts to compensate for ventricular dysfunction. Reduced renal perfusion stimulates the renin-angiotensin-aldosterone system (RAAS) and the sympathetic nervous system. Heightened activity of these two neurohormonal systems leads to myocardial toxicity, peripheral vasoconstriction, and renal salt and water retention. In systolic failure, the left ventricle dilates and loses contractility. In diastolic dysfunction, the neurohormonal systems are also activated but to a lesser degree.

Initial Evaluation

Four tasks are important in the clinical evaluation of HF patients (3, 21–23): 1) Establish HF as the patient's diagnosis, 2) determine the type of HF (systolic or diastolic), 3) assess the presence of fluid retention (euvolemic or hypervolemic), and 4) determine the severity of a patient's functional limitation.

HISTORY AND PHYSICAL EXAMINATION

A complete history is important in order to elicit symptoms of chronic HF and search for clues regarding its etiology (3). The classic symptoms are fatigue, dyspnea, and edema. In HF, dyspnea on exertion often progresses to paroxysmal nocturnal dyspnea, orthopnea, and dyspnea at rest. Peripheral edema, typically of the feet and legs, is the result of fluid overload and poor cardiac function. Other symptoms of HF include nocturia, anorexia, abdominal bloating, cachexia, and mental confusion. Asking about previous chest pain or MI is important in determining the cause of and planning treatment of HF. Other risk factors for HF include hypertension, diabetes mellitus, dyslipidemia, obesity, alcoholism, smoking, viral infections, valvular heart disease, and congenital heart disease. Attention to risk factors and symptoms that suggest underlying CAD is also important in the initial evaluation of heart failure.

The physical examination helps establish the diagnosis of HF, assess the fluid retention status, and provides clues to the etiology and type of the HF. The physical findings that best rule in systolic HF are gallop rhythm (positive likelihood ratio [LR+] = 24), displaced point of maximum impulse or PMI (LR+ 16), and jugular venous distention (LR+ 9). All of these signs are very specific but not very sensitive, meaning that when present they are strong evidence in favor of HF but when absent do not rule it out. Other useful signs and symptoms include dyspnea on exertion or at night when recumbent (paroxysmal nocturnal dyspnea [PND]), unexpected weight gain, wheezing or rales, and presacral or leg edema (3). Tachycardia may be a compensatory response for a low cardiac output, and a reduction in heart rate in response to medical treatment is an indicator of treatment efficacy. Low BP (systolic BP <90 mm Hg) indicates poor cardiac output and is a predictor of poor outcome. A weight gain of 1 to 2 kg over 1 to 3 days suggests fluid retention, although some patients may initially present with much greater weight gains (5 to 10 kg or more). Pulmonary congestion is suggested by wheezes on auscultation, whereas rales suggest frank pulmonary edema.

DIAGNOSTIC TESTING

Patients should undergo diagnostic testing to confirm the diagnosis and determine whether the HF is systolic or diastolic (3, 23). A transthoracic two-dimensional echocardiogram with Doppler flow studies is the most important initial diagnostic study because it defines the type(s) and severity of LV impairment. It allows measurement of the ejection fraction (EF), ventricular mass, chamber dimensions, and wall motion in addition to evaluation of valvular, pericardial, and vascular structures. It also allows measurement of flow across the mitral valve, categorizing patients into normal (E > A), delayed relaxation (E < A), and restrictive (E >> A) filling patterns. An abnormal E:A ratio is associated with diastolic HF (24).

In the acutely dyspneic patients, the B-natriuretic peptide (BNP) level can be helpful in ruling out HF in a dyspneic patient. A BNP level > 100 pcg/dl is 90% sensitive and 76%

specific for the diagnosis of systolic HF in acutely dyspneic patients presenting to the emergency department (LR + 3.8, LR − 0.13) (25). Routine studies for all patients with suspected HF include complete blood count, urinalysis, comprehensive metabolic profile (including serum magnesium, phosphorus, and calcium), thyroid stimulating hormone (TSH), chest radiograph, and electrocardiogram (ECG). Radionuclide angiography or cardiac catheterization with LV angiography also provides reliable measurement of LVEF and regional wall motion. The latter also permits confirmation of diastolic HF by the measurement of ventricular filling pressures and indices of LV diastolic relaxation. However, because it is more invasive than other studies, it is not part of the routine evaluation of all patients with suspected HF.

All HF patients with CAD as the suspected cause of heart failure should undergo an exercise or dipyridamole stress test with follow-up angiography as indicated. Ongoing assessment of functional status also plays an important role in the management of HF patients (3). Functional status is an indicator of disease severity and treatment success and is strongly associated with long-term HF outcomes. Evaluation of functional status includes measurement of physical capacity, emotional status, social function, and cognitive abilities. Just as with chronic stable angina, the NYHA classification of heart disease is a useful functional assessment tool (Table 10.2). A validated prediction model is also available online (*www.ccort.ca/CHFRiskModel.asp*) (26).

Treatment of Heart Failure

Treatment of HF depends on its cause and type. Patients with HF caused by valvular heart disease need surgical repair, whereas those with hypertension require effective blood pressure control. Systolic and diastolic HF are physiologically different and require different management (see Figure 10.3 and Table 10.5)

Nonetheless, certain general principles apply to the management of all HF patients (3):

- The prevention of coronary insufficiency and MI that may lead to HF is essential. Interventions include the cessation of smoking, weight reduction, and the control of hypertension, hyperlipidemia, and diabetes. In patients with MI, coronary reperfusion (thrombolysis, angioplasty, or revascularization) should be considered. After an MI, treatment with ACE inhibitors and β-blockers decreases the incidence of HF and improves survival. Effective lipid lowering also has been shown to prevent HF.
- Fluid retention should be monitored by measuring daily body weight and controlled by restricting daily salt intake to less than 2 g.
- Daily aerobic activity improves physical capacity in HF patients.
- Atrial fibrillation with rapid ventricular response should be controlled to avoid cardiac decompensation.
- Certain medications should be avoided in HF. Nonsteroidal anti-inflammatory agents inhibit the effects of diuretics and ACE inhibitors. Most calcium antagonists are ineffective in systolic HF, although they may be appropriate in patients with diastolic HF. Antiarrhythmic agents used to suppress asymptomatic ventricular arrhythmias have proarrhythmic

and cardio-suppressant effects and are generally not recommended.
- All HF patients should have regular clinic follow-up or close case management to detect any decline in their clinical condition.

Successful management of HF requires a partnership between patient, family, and the physician. This is accomplished by educating the patient and family regarding HF. A patient's responsibilities include home monitoring of weight and HF symptoms, following a low-sodium diet, taking medication as prescribed, daily aerobic exercising, avoiding alcohol and the use of NSAIDs, and keeping medical appointments (11). Physicians must encourage patients to participate in their own care.

SYSTOLIC HEART FAILURE

Angiotensin-converting enzyme inhibitors (ACEIs) such as enalapril, captopril, and lisinopril, are the cornerstone of treatment for chronic systolic HF (3, 27) (see Table 10.5). Many large clinical trials have shown that ACEIs improve symptoms, reduce mortality, decrease hospitalizations, and improve quality of life in all NYHA classes of HF. All HF patients who do not have contraindications should receive an ACEI. Contraindications include pregnancy, bilateral renal artery stenosis, hypotension (systolic blood pressure <90), worsening renal, potassium retention (K+ >5.5), angioedema, and chronic cough. Treatment with ACEIs should be initiated at low doses and increased by doubling the dose every 3 to 7 days until recommended target doses are achieved. Serum blood urea nitrogen (BUN), creatinine, potassium, and blood pressure should be measured before initiating therapy, again at 2 weeks, and with any change in dose. Angiotensin receptor blockers (ARBs such as losartan, valsartan, and candesartan) are alternatives for those who are intolerant of ACEIs (28). ARBs have been shown to be equivalent to ACEIs in reducing mortality; but the evidence is inconsistent that adding ARBs confers a mortality benefit beyond optimal therapy with an ACEI and a β-blocker. The combination of hydralazine and isosorbide dinitrate may be a particularly effective treatment for black patients, either as an addition or an alternative to ACEI to decrease afterload (29).

All patients with stable NYHA class II and III HF should receive a β-blocker unless there is a contraindication (3, 30). Beta-blockers (i.e., carvedilol, bisoprolol, and extended-release metoprolol) are usually taken together with ACEIs. Studies have shown that they delay clinical progression of HF and reduce mortality. They also should be initiated at low levels and titrated to target doses. Contraindications include hypotension, fluid retention, worsening HF, bradycardia, and heart block.

Diuretics are an important component of successful HF therapy, primarily to improve symptoms. They act rapidly to reduce fluid retention, and complement treatment with ACEIs and β-blockers (3, 27). Measuring daily body weight is helpful in assessing the response to diuretic therapy and for defining when increased dosing is needed. Diuretic resistance, often seen in severe failure, can be overcome by using a combination of two diuretics (i.e., furosemide and metazolone). Spironolactone or eplerenone, potassium-sparing diuretics that block aldosterone receptors, reduces the risk of morbidity and

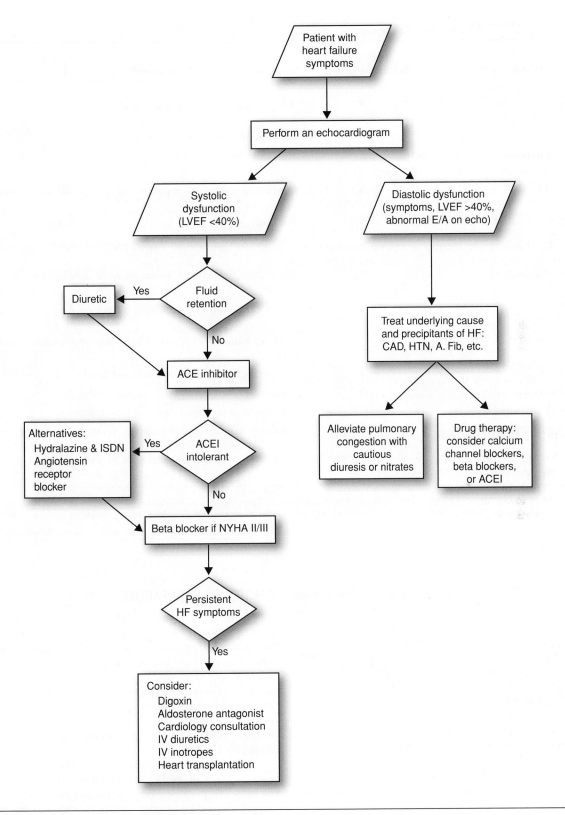

Figure 10.3 • Patient with heart failure symptoms.

TABLE 10.5 Effectiveness of Pharmacologic Treatment for Heart Failure

Treatment Strategy	Strength of Recommendation*	Recommendations/Comments
Systolic Dysfunction		
Angiotensin converting enzyme inhibitors	A	All patients unless contraindicated
Diuretics	A	All patients with fluid overload
Beta adrenergic receptor blockers	A	All NYHA class II or III patients
Digoxin	A	In selected symptomatic patients despite ACEI and diuretics; caution in women
Anticoagulants & warfarin	A	For patients with atrial fibrillation or previous embolic event
Hydralazine & isosorbide dinitrate	B	Alternative for patients intolerant to ACE inhibitors
Angiotensin receptor blockers	A	Alternative for patients intolerant to ACE inhibitors
Spironolactone	B	For NYHA class III or IV patients taking ACEI
Diastolic dysfunction		
Anticoagulants & warfarin	A	Only for patients with atrial fibrillation or previous embolic event
Digoxin	A	For ventricular rate control in atrial fibrillation
Diuretics & nitrates	C	Cautiously, for symptomatic improvement
Calcium channel blockers	C	May improve symptoms and exercise tolerance
Beta adrenergic receptor blockers	C	Improves left ventricular filling by reducing heart rate
Angiotensin converting enzyme inhibitors	C	Appears to reverse left ventricular hypertrophy

*A = consistent, good-quality patient-oriented evidence; B = inconsistent or limited-quality patient-oriented evidence; C = consensus, disease-oriented evidence, usual practice, expert opinion, or case series. For information about the SORT evidence rating system, see *http://www.aafp.org/afpsort.xml*.

mortality in class III and IV HF patients. In conjunction with ACEIs and a loop diuretic, one of the potassium-sparing diuretics should be considered for use in all advanced HF patients (3, 31). The risks of treatment with diuretics include electrolyte depletion, activation of the RAAS, hypotension, and azotemia. It is important to monitor closely for hyperkalemia if potassium-sparing diuretics are used; research trials measured potassium as often as once each month, after the initiation phase (3).

Digitalis glycosides have long been used for HF and are also used to control the ventricular response rate in patients with atrial fibrillation (AF) (3, 27). Their benefit for selected patients includes the alleviation of symptoms and reduction in hospitalizations. Digitalis has no effect on mortality, and may even increase mortality in women (32). Treatment is initiated with a dose of 0.125 to 0.25 mg daily with an optimal serum digoxin range of 0.5 to 0.8 ng/ml (33). It is important to monitor serum levels of digoxin to detect toxicity, but serum levels do not correlate with therapeutic effects. Risks of digoxin include arrhythmias, gastrointestinal symptoms, and neurologic complaints.

DIASTOLIC HEART FAILURE

Approximately one-third of HF patients have normal or near-normal systolic function. They have diastolic HF, in which the ventricles are stiff, cannot fill without high end-diastolic pressures, and have impaired capacity to change filling with varying activity levels. The clinical diagnosis is made when patients have typical symptoms of HF, only mildly reduced or normal LVEF, and changes on echocardiography suggesting poor diastolic filling of the left ventricle. Distinguishing diastolic and systolic HF is important because their treatment strategies are different.

There have been no randomized controlled trials of intervention for diastolic HF (17, 21). Thus, the management of diastolic HF must be guided by limited clinical trials, clinical experience, and knowledge of pathophysiology. Initially, treatment should be directed at treating underlying causes of diastolic HF such as CAD, hypertension, arrhythmias, severe anemia, thyrotoxicosis, hemochromatosis, and constrictive pericarditis. The next management goal is to reduce symptoms of fluid overload and elevated ventricular filling pressure (3, 21). Careful use of loop diuretics and nitrates can reduce fluid

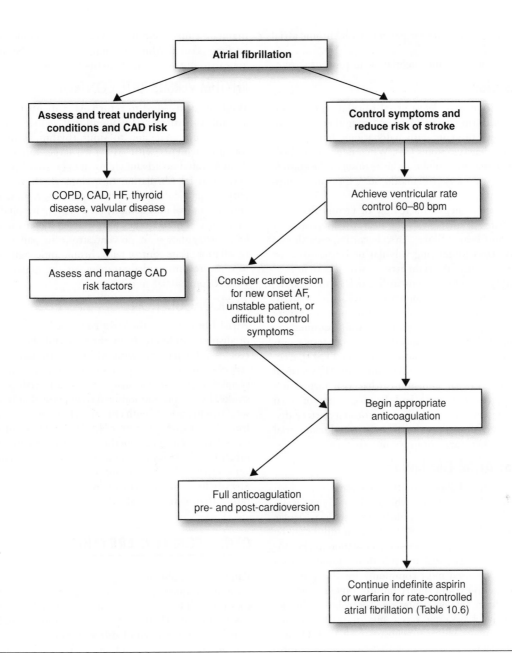

Figure 10.4 • Atrial fibrillation.

volume and pulmonary artery pressure. However, even small reductions in vascular volume may significantly reduce ventricular filling, lower cardiac output, and worsen symptoms. Non-dihydropyridines calcium channel blockers, β-blockers, and ACE inhibitors have properties that may improve diastolic failure. Calcium channel blockers have been shown to improve symptoms and exercise tolerance in clinical trials. Beta-blockers act by slowing heart rate and thereby enhancing ventricular filling. ACEIs, over time, may reverse left ventricular hypertrophy in diastolic failure.

ATRIAL FIBRILLATION

Atrial fibrillation (AF) is the most common chronic cardiac rhythm disturbance that causes significant morbidity and

mortality in the general population (1, 4). It is characterized by an irregularly, irregular cardiac rhythm. Whereas many patients with AF are asymptomatic, those with rapid ventricular response and resultant low cardiac output often present with symptoms of palpitations, dizziness, angina, dyspnea, or heart failure. Atrial fibrillation can be classified as paroxysmal, persistent, or chronic. Figure 10.4 outlines a general approach to the evaluation and management of patients with chronic atrial fibrillation. Key tasks for the physician include (4):

• Detecting underlying causes for atrial fibrillation and co-existing cardiovascular disease
• Determining whether to attempt cardioversion to sinus rhythm

- Controlling ventricular rate for patients with chronic atrial fibrillation
- Determining a plan for anticoagulation to prevent stroke

Initial Evaluation

The family physician may detect atrial fibrillation (AF) initially in a patient during an ECG done for another reason or because the patient presents with palpitations, fatigue, dyspnea, or other cardiac symptoms (34). When new atrial fibrillation is detected, the amount of time since onset of the episode may be uncertain as many patients do not experience symptoms.

Initial evaluation includes a review of factors that may cause or exacerbate AF such as valvular heart disease, coronary artery disease, and heart failure. An echocardiogram should be included to detect underlying valvular or cardiac disease, and to evaluate the size of the right atrium, which is an indicator of reversibility. Significant non-cardiac risk factors for AF are diabetes, hypertension, pulmonary disease, anemia, thyrotoxicosis, alcohol abuse (especially binge drinking), and severe infections. A complete history and physical examination, screening for alcohol abuse, and specific laboratory tests (complete blood count, thyroid-stimulating hormone [TSH], electrolyte panel) will rule out non-cardiac causes of AF. Optimal treatment of these cardiac and non-cardiac risk factors has the potential to prevent the onset and the progression of atrial fibrillation. Patients who have coexisting coronary artery disease may experience more episodes of chest pain during atrial fibrillation than when they are in a sinus rhythm.

Treatment of Atrial Fibrillation

Ventricular rate control should be the first therapeutic goal in newly diagnosed AF patients who are hemodynamically stable (see Figure 10.4) (34). The reduction of the ventricular response rate to between 60 and 80 beats per minute may be accomplished with drugs that decrease conduction at the AV node. Digoxin, β-blockers, and non-dihydropyridine calcium channel blockers are used most commonly for this purpose. For patients with co-existing heart failure, digoxin may be most beneficial choice for ventricular rate control. Beta-blockers are effective and have rapid onset, but are relatively contraindicated in patients with bronchospasm or COPD, and must be initiated slowly in patients with systolic heart failure. Calcium channel blockers such as verapamil or diltiazem may be the safest, most effective drugs for ventricular rate control in most AF patients without co-morbidities.

Two-thirds of patients admitted to the hospital with acute atrial fibrillation will spontaneously convert to a sinus rhythm (35). For patients with new onset atrial fibrillation, who are unstable, or who have difficult to control symptoms, electrical or pharmacologic conversion should be considered. Electrical cardioversion is about 90% successful in the short term, while the success of pharmacologic cardioversion varies between 60% and 90%. Medications used to convert AF include class Ia (e.g., procainamide), class Ic (e.g., flecamide), and class III (e.g., amiodarone) antiarrhythmic drugs. Warfarin therapy for 3 weeks before and 4 weeks after cardioversion is crucial, as cardioversion is accompanied by a 3% risk of stroke. For patients successfully converted to sinus rhythm from atrial fibrillation, some will benefit from short-term use of medications such as amiodarone, disopyramide, propafanone, or sotalol to maintain sinus rhythm. However, most should not be placed on long-term rhythm maintenance therapy because the risks appear to outweigh the benefits (34, 35).

RHYTHM VERSUS RATE CONTROL

While it seems ideal to return AF patients to sinus rhythm, a number of studies have found that ventricular rate control, rather than conversion to sinus rhythm, is the best choice for most patients with AF. Two large, randomized studies demonstrated no advantage to an aggressive approach of converting atrial fibrillation to a sinus rhythm (34). For some patients, particularly for elderly patients, repeated attempts at rhythm control may actually lead to more hospitalizations and morbidity. These studies also showed a consistent advantage of anticoagulation to prevent stroke in patients with atrial fibrillation. Rate control with chronic anticoagulation is therefore the recommended strategy for the majority of patients with chronic atrial fibrillation.

ANTICOAGULATION

Atrial fibrillation is the most common cardiac condition that predisposes individuals to thromboembolic stroke (relative risk = 7 for patients with AF) (1, 4). In paroxysmal AF the risk of stroke is 2% per year. Fortunately, treatment with antiplatelet agents or warfarin significantly reduces the risk of stroke. Data from randomized trials show that treatment with warfarin in patients with chronic AF reduces the risk of stroke from 4.5% to 1.4% per year (4, 34). A number of randomized trials have examined whether low-risk patients may have as much benefit from aspirin as from warfarin, with fewer adverse effects. Table 10.6 outlines a practical decision rule to identify low-risk AF patients who can be treated with aspirin rather than warfarin (31).

OTHER COMMON ARRYTHMIAS

Palpitations, light-headedness, syncope, chest pain, and dyspnea are frequent presenting complaints of patients with arrhythmias. The clinician should inquire about the perceived onset, rate, and rhythm of these symptoms in addition to the frequency and pattern of different episodes. Information regarding medications, emotions, caffeine, alcohol, and recreational drug use is important because these factors may cause arrhythmia. The patient's past medical history should be searched for hypertension, heart disease, pulmonary, and thyroid disease as potential etiologies. A general physical exam should be performed; however, it contributes relatively little to understanding the nature of an arrhythmia. Appropriate laboratory evaluation consists of electrolytes (including potassium, calcium, and magnesium), thyroid functions studies, pulse oxymetry, serum medication levels, a 12-lead ECG, and screening for drug and alcohol use. Twenty-four-hour electrocardiographic monitoring (Holter monitor) and longer-term event monitoring are helpful to capture transient arrhythmias. A stress test to detect coronary artery disease or an echocardiogram may be helpful to evaluate cardiac anatomy and function and to understand the etiology of abnormal rhythms.

Classification of arrhythmias is based primarily on electrocardiographic information. In general, they can be classified based on location (supraventricular or ventricular), morphol-

TABLE 10.6 Decision-Making Tool for Choosing Between Warfarin (Coumadin) and Aspirin Therapy in Patients with Nonvalvular Atrial Fibrillation

Step 1. Determine the patient's annual risk of stroke using the two clinical decision rules shown below:

ACCP Rule

Definition	Risk Group	Annual Stroke Rate, % (95% CI)
History of stroke or TIA; hypertension; heart failure; age older than 75 years; or at least two moderate risk factors	High	3.0 (2.5 to 3.8)
Age 65 to 75 years, DM or coronary artery disease; not high risk	Moderate	1.0 (0.4 to 2.2)
Not moderate or high risk	Low	0.5 (0.1 to 2.2)

CHADS$_2$ Rule

Risk Factor	Points	Point Totals	Risk Group	Annual Stroke Rate, % (95% CI)
			Risk Score Interpretation	
Congestive heart failure	1	3 or more	High	5.3 (3.3 to 8.4)
Hypertension	1	1 or 2	Moderate	2.7 (2.2 to 3.4)
Age older than 75 years	1	0	Low	0.8 (0.4 to 1.7)
Diabetes mellitus	1			
Stroke or TIA	2			

Total points: _____

Step 2. If patient is high or low risk under both rules, select the most appropriate treatment:

Low or moderate risk by ACCP and moderate or high risk by CHADS$_2$: oral anticoagulation with warfarin recommended

Step 3. If patient is moderate risk, estimate bleeding risk and weigh risks and benefits with patient.

Outpatient Bleeding Risk Index

Risk Factor	Points	Point Total	Risk Group	Major Bleeds per Total Number of Patients
			Risk Score Information	
Age at least 65 years	1	0	Low	0 per 128
History of GI tract bleeding	1	1 or more	High	5 per 92
History of stroke	1			
Recent MI, hematocrit lower than 30 percent, creatinine higher than 1.5, or DM	1			

Total points: _____

ACCP = American College of Chest Physicians; CI = confidence interval; TIA = transischemic attack; DM = diabetes mellitus; CHADS = congestive heart failure, hypertension, age greater than 75 years, diabetes and history of stroke or TIA; GI = gastrointestinal; MI = myocardial infarction. (Adapted from Ebell M. Choosing between warfarin (coumadin) and aspirin therapy for patients with atrial fibrillation. Am Fam Physician. 2005;71:2348–2351. Used with permission.)

ogy (width of QRS complex), rate (tachycardia or bradycardia), and regularity. Supraventricular rhythms that originate in the SA node, atria, or AV node generally have a narrow QRS complex (<0.12 ms). A complete discussion of acute arrhythmias is beyond the scope of this chapter. The following section briefly describes a few common chronic arrhythmias that family physicians encounter in office practice (37).

Premature Beats

Premature atrial contractions (PACs) or premature ventricular contractions (PVCs) may be asymptomatic and discovered incidentally on ECG or may be symptomatic when a patient experiences palpitations or fluttering. In the case of PACs, the resulting ECG has abnormal shaped P waves with normal appearing QRS complexes. With each PAC there is a pause before the normal rhythm resumes. This pause allows time for extra ventricular filling that results in a subsequent forceful contraction or "kick" often felt by the patient. PACs are a normal finding in patients of all ages, and they rarely require treatment. For symptomatic patients, decreasing caffeine intake, smoking cessation, and stress reduction techniques may decrease symptomatic PACs.

PVCs appear on ECG as wide QRS complexes without P waves and are typically followed by a compensatory pause. Two PVCs in a row are called couplet, while three or more are termed ventricular tachycardia (VT). Potential structural causes of PVCs include coronary artery disease with ischemic episodes, myocardial infarction, valvular heart disease, and cardiomyopathy. As with PACs, there are many extrinsic causes of PVCs. The clinician should investigate serum electrolytes, oxygenation, acid-base status, medication related effects, hyperthyroidism, cocaine, caffeine, alcohol, etc. Any underlying abnormality should be treated or the offending agent withdrawn.

In patients not found to have an underlying cause for PVCs and who don't experience syncope or other significant symptoms, management consists of reassurance only. Studies indicate that in patients without known heart disease, drug treatment for PVCs has no impact on survival and may increase all-cause mortality (38). Even in the case of patients with episodes of non-sustained ventricular tachycardia, asymptomatic individuals without structural heart disease may be managed without medication. On the other hand, those patients with CAD, HF, and cardiomyopathy need optimal therapy for their underlying condition. If these patients are symptomatic with PVCs they should be referred to a cardiologist for electrophysiologic testing and, potentially, arrhythmia suppression therapy. High-risk patients are treated with implantable defibrillators.

Sinus Rhythms

Sinus tachycardia and sinus bradycardia are rhythms that originate in the sinoatrial node and are usually of no clinical significance unless a patient is symptomatic. Sinus tachycardia (a heart rate greater than 100 beats per minute) is most often a response to stress, exercise, or emotion. It may also be produced by pathologic causes such as fever, infection, dehydration, anemia, hyperthyroidism, heart failure, shock, and hypoxia.

The definition of sinus bradycardia is a heart rate less than 50 beats per minute or less than 60 beats per minute in symptomatic patients. Frequently, normal athletic individuals have heart rates less than 50 beats per minute and are asymptomatic. Treatment is directed at underlying disorders including hypothyroidism, hypothermia, and intracranial lesions. Sick sinus syndrome (SSS), a combination of bradycardia and tachycardia most often found in elderly patients, is caused by sinus node dysfunction secondary to ischemia, inflammation, or scarring (39). Significant bradycardia or SSS that is accompanied by syncope or other symptoms may require placement of a pacemaker (40).

Supraventricular Tachycardia

Supraventricular tachycardias (SVTs) are rapid heart rhythms with rates between 120 and 250 beats per minute that originate above the level of the ventricles. They typically have narrow QRS complexes on electrocardiogram unless there is preexisting bundle branch block or an intraventricular conduction defect. Patients with SVT may experience palpitations, chest pain, lightheadedness, diaphoresis, or anxiety. Reversible underlying causes of SVTs include electrolyte imbalance, hypoxia, hypercapnea, caffeine intake, and other sympathomimetic drugs. Often SVT is well tolerated and occurs

intermittently. Patients who are relatively asymptomatic are best treated conservatively with observation. For patients with a severe initial episode or frequent episodes, therapy should be provided (41).

In symptomatic patients with intermittent, stable, but symptomatic episodes of SVT, pharmacologic treatment is appropriate. Non-dihydropyridine calcium channel blockers, β-blockers, or digoxin may be useful for long-term suppression of SVT. Patients who experience syncope or other difficult symptoms related to SVT should be referred for more extensive evaluation including electrophysiologic testing.

VALVULAR HEART DISEASE

The first clues to valvular heart disease are often cardiac murmurs found during routine physical examination. Most of these murmurs are clinically insignificant. Yet in each case, the family physician must answer three questions (42):

- Is this murmur significant to the patient's health?
- Is therapeutic intervention warranted?
- When is medical or surgical therapy is indicated?

A simplified approach to decide which murmurs are significant would be to assume that the following murmurs are pathological until further testing proves otherwise (43):

- Diastolic or continuous murmurs
- Holosystolic or late systolic murmurs
- Grade 3 or higher murmurs
- Grade 1 and 2 murmurs with other cardiac signs and symptoms

Each of these murmurs should be evaluated with a 2-D ECG and Doppler flow study. This is an important noninvasive means to determine the significance of cardiac murmurs by imaging cardiac structures and function and by assessing the velocity of flow through cardiac valves and chambers. Chest x-ray and ECG are also commonly ordered to evaluate cardiac murmurs. The chest radiograph provides qualitative information about chamber size, pulmonary vascular redistribution, and calcification of cardiac structures. An ECG may detect ventricular hypertrophy, atrial enlargement, arrhythmia, evidence of coronary artery disease, and previous myocardial infarction. These findings help identify the etiology and significance of cardiac murmurs. Definitive evaluation of valvular heart disease is by cardiac catheterization and coronary angiography usually in anticipation of surgery.

Aortic Stenosis

Aortic stenosis (AS) is the most common primary and acquired valvular heart disease (42, 43). It commonly results from the degeneration and calcification of aortic valve leaflets especially in persons born with bicuspid aortic valves. On physical examination, one notes a systolic crescendo-decrescendo (diamond-shaped) cardiac murmur heard in the aortic area that radiates to the neck. Once symptoms are present, aortic valve replacement surgery may be indicated. Except for prophylaxis against endocarditis, no medical therapy is of proven benefit for AS.

Aortic Regurgitation

Aortic regurgitation (AR) is the result of age-associated changes of the aortic root or injury to the valve leaflets that is most often produced by infective endocarditis or rheumatic fever (42). The left ventricular stroke volume is much increased by the regurgitation, which produces a hyperdynamic circulation. Classic signs of AR are a "water-hammer" bounding pulse, systolic hypertension, and a blowing murmur at the left sternal border. The patient often presents with signs of left heart failure (dyspnea, orthopnea, and PND). Medical therapy for asymptomatic patients consists of dihydropyridine calcium channel blockers (e.g., nifedipine or amlodipine) or an ACE inhibitor with prophylaxis for endocarditis. When a patient becomes symptomatic, aortic valve replacement is the best course of action.

Mitral Stenosis

Mitral stenosis (MS) is rare since it is typically a sequela of rheumatic heart disease, the incidence of which has declined in developing countries (42). The presenting symptoms of MS are initially dyspnea on exertion, orthopnea, and paroxysmal nocturnal dyspnea. As pulmonary hypertension develops, patients may present with hemoptysis. On cardiac auscultation MS has a classic diastolic rumble that follows an opening snap. Medical treatment for mild MS symptoms includes diuretics and antibiotic prophylaxis for bacterial endocarditis. Advanced mitral disease may require mitral valve replacement.

Mitral Regurgitation

The etiology of mitral regurgitation (MR) is myxomatous valve degeneration, ischemic heart disease, endocarditis, or chordal rupture (42). Patients often present with signs of left heart failure and have a holosystolic apical murmur that radiates to the axilla. Acute mitral regurgitation is a medical emergency requiring vasodilators or intraaortic balloon counterpulsation to improve forward cardiac output. Chronic MR benefits little from vasodilators, and surgical valve correction is standard therapy for mitral regurgitation. Asymptomatic individuals may be followed until left ventricular ejection fraction falls below 60% or end-systolic dimension exceeds 45 mm when surgery is recommended. Endocarditis prophylaxis is indicated in MR.

Mitral Valve Prolapse

Mitral valve prolapse (MVP) most commonly occurs in the absence of other illness (42). It is a condition during systole when the mitral leaflets move past the point of coaptation into the left atrium. On auscultation a mid-systolic click and a late systolic murmur may be heard. MVP frequently presents in young, healthy, and asymptomatic women. However, some MVP is associated with palpitations, chest pain, or postural syncope. Beta-blockers, diltiazem, or verapamil may be useful for these symptoms. Endocarditis prophylaxis is only indicated for those with frank mitral regurgitation on echocardiogram.

CASE DISCUSSION

Based only on the history and physical examination, you can determine a number of potential causes for Mr. Jones' symptoms and issues to be addressed. They include the possibility of coronary artery disease progression, the consideration of heart failure as a diagnosis, concerns about possible significant arrhythmias, the evaluation of his heart murmur, and atten-

tion to cardiac risk factors including smoking, hypertension, and obesity. Although he has not experienced chest pain recently, the fact that Mr. Jones had at least early CAD on a previous coronary angiogram should prioritize an evaluation of the potential role of CAD as a cause of his symptoms. A 12-lead ECG should be completed during this first visit. A treadmill stress ECG with imaging should be scheduled to determine if ischemia occurs with exertion.

Mr. Jones meets the criteria for a diagnosis of heart failure based on your findings of paroxysmal nocturnal dyspnea, rales, and ankle edema on examination with symptom severity that corresponds with NYHA class II. A chest x-ray and blood work to detect other underlying causes of his symptoms should be completed at this visit. An echocardiogram should be scheduled to evaluate left ventricular function and determine whether valvular disease is contributing to his heart failure.

Treatment with an ACEI has the best supporting evidence for positive benefit in Mr. Jones' case and can be started at low dose at this first visit. The ACEI also will improve his blood pressure, improve heart failure outcomes, and help prevent acute ischemic events. Mr. Jones should return to the office within a few weeks to review the results of the treadmill ECG and his blood work, and to evaluate the effects of the ACEI on his symptoms, fluid retention status, blood pressure, and potassium level. The primary goals of subsequent visits will be to increase the ACEI dose, start additional medications for heart failure in a stepwise fashion, monitor for adverse drug effects, and assist Mr. Jones with smoking cessation and other lifestyle changes.

REFERENCES

1. Thom T, Haase N, Rosamond W, et al. Heart disease and stroke statistics—2006 update. A report from the American Heart Association statistics committee and stroke statistics subcommittee. Circulation. 2006;e85.
2. Snow V, Barry P, Fihn SD, et al. Evaluation of primary care patients with chronic stable angina guidelines from the American College of Physicians. Ann Intern Med. 2004;141:57–64.
3. ACC/AHA Task Force on Practice Guidelines. ACC/AHA 2005 guideline update for the diagnosis and management of chronic heart failure in the adult. J Am Coll Cardiol. 2005;46:e1–e82.
4. ACC/AHA/ESC Task Force on Practice Guidelines. ACC/AHA/ESC guidelines for the management of patients with atrial fibrillation: executive summary. J Am Coll Cardiol. 2001;38:1231–1265.
5. Snow V, Barry P, Fihn S, et al. Primary care management of chronic stable angina and asymptomatic suspected or known coronary artery disease: a clinical practice guideline from the American College of Physicians. Ann Intern Med. 2004;141:562–567.
6. Abrams J. Chronic stable angina. N Engl J Med. 2005;352:2524–2533.
7. Kuritzky L. Atherosclerotic vascular disease: management of angina in the office setting. Primary Care. 2005;27:615–629.
8. Sanger DR, Solomon AG, Gersh BJ. Contemporary management of angina: part II. Medical management of chronic stable angina. Am Fam Physician. 2000;61:129–138.
9. National Cholesterol Education Project Expert Panel. Detection, evaluation, and treatment of high blood cholesterol in adults (adult treatment panel III). National Institutes of Health 2001. NIH Publication no. 01-3670.
10. Grundy SM, Cleeman JI, Daniels SR, et al. Diagnosis and management of the metabolic syndrome. An American

Heart Association/National Heart, Lung, and Blood Institute scientific statement. Circulation. 2005;112:2735–2752.

11. Critchley J, Capewell S. Smoking cessation for the secondary prevention of coronary heart disease (Cochrane Review). In: The Cochrane Library, Issue 1, 2005. Chichester, UK: John Wiley and Sons, Ltd.

12. Trichopoulou A, Bamia C, Trichopoulos D. Mediterranean diet and survival among patients with coronary heart disease in Greece. Arch Intern Med. 2005;165:929–933.

13. Ornish D, Scherwitz LW, Billings JH, et al. Intensive lifestyle changes for reversal of coronary heart disease. JAMA. 1998; 280:2001–2007.

14. Bhatt DL, Fox KAA, Hacke W, et al. Clopidogrel and aspirin versus aspirin alone for the prevention of atherothrombotic events. N Engl J Med. 2006;354:1706–1717.

15. Ko DT, Hebert PR, Coffey CS, Sedrakyan A, Curtis JP, Krumholz HM. Beta-blocker therapy and symptoms of depression, fatigue, and sexual dysfunction. JAMA. 2002 Jul 17;288(3):351–357.

16. UK Prospective Diabetes Study Group. Tight blood pressure control and risk of macrovascular and microvascular complications in type 2 diabetes: UKPDS 38. BMJ. 1998; 317: 703–712.

17. Grundy SM, Cleeeman JI, Merz CNB, et al. Implications of recent clinical trials for the national cholesterol education program adult treatment panel III guidelines. Circulation. 2004;110:227–239.

18. The heart outcomes prevention evaluation study investigators. Effects of an angiotensin-converting—enzyme inhibitor, ramipril, on cardiovascular events in high-risk patients. N Engl J Med. 2000; 342:145–153.

19. Davie AP, Francis CM, Caruana L, Sutherland GR, McMurray JJ. Assessing diagnosis in heart failure: which features are any use? QJM. 1997 May;90(5):335–339.

20. Antman EM, Smith SC, Alpert JS, et al. ACC/AHA 2004 guideline update for coronary bypass graft surgery: summary article. J Am Acad Cardiol. 2004;44:1146–1154.

21. Satpathy C, Mishra TK, Satpathy R, Satpathy HK, Barone E. Diagnosis and management of diastolic dysfunction and heart failure. Am Fam Physician. 2006;73:841–846

22. Shamsham F, Mitchell J. Essentials of the diagnosis of heart failure. Am Fam Physician. 2000;61:1319–1328.

23. Caruana L, Petrie MC, Davie AP, McMurray JJV. Do patients with suspected heart failure and preserved lift ventricular systolic function suffer from "diastolic heart failure of from misdiagnosis?" BMJ. 2000;321:215–229.

24. Mandinov L, Eberli FR, Seiler C, Hess OM. Diastolic heart failure. Cardiovasc Res. 2000 Mar;45(4):813–825.

25. Mueller C. Scholer A, Laule-Kilian K, et al. Use of B-type natriuretic peptide in the evaluation and management of acute dypnea. N Engl J Med. 2004;350:647–654.

26. Lee DS, Austin PC, Rouleau JL, Liu PP, Naimark D, Tu JV. Predicting mortality among patients hospitalized for heart failure: derivation and validation of a clinical model. JAMA. 2003 Nov 19;290(19):2581–2587.

27. McConaghy JR, Smith SR. Outpatient treatment of systolic heart failure. Am Fam Physician. 2004;70:2157–2164, 2171–2172.

28. Granger CB, McMurray JJV, Yusuf S, et al. Effedcts of candesartan in patients with chronic heart failure and reduced left-ventricular systolic function intolerant to angiotensin-converting enzyme inhibitors: the CHARM-Alternative trial. Lancet. 2003;362:772–776.

29. Taylor AL, Siesche S, Yancy C, et al. Combination of isosorbide dinitrate and hydralazine in blacks with heart failure. N Engl J Med. 2004;351:2049–2057.

30. Foody JM, Farrell MH, Krumholz HM. Beta-blocker therapy in heart failure. Scientific review. JAMA. 2002;287:883–889.

31. Pitt B, Zannad F, Remme WJ, et al. The effect of spironolactone on morbidity and mortality in patients with severe heart failure. N Engl J Med. 1999;34:709–717.

32. Rathore SS, Wang Y, and Krumholz HM. Sex-based differences in the effect of digoxin for the treatment of heart failure. N Engl J Med. 2002;347:1403–1411.

33. Rathore SS, Curtis JP, Want Y, Bristow MR, Krumholz HM. Association of serum digoxin concentration and outcomes in patients with heart failure. JAMA. 2003;289:871–878.

34. Snow V, Weiss KB, LeFevre M, et al. Management of newly detected atrial fibrillation. A clinical practice guideline from the American Acamy of Family Physicinas and the American College of Physicians. Ann Intern Med. 2003;139:1009–1017.

35. Danias PG, Caulfield TA, Weigner MJ, et al. Likelihood of spontaneous conversion of atrial fibrillation to sinus rhythm. J Am Coll Cardiol. 1998;31:588–592.

36. Ebell M. Choosing between warfarin (coumadin) and aspirin therapy for patients with atrial fibrillation. Am Fam Physician. 2005;71:2348–2351.

37. The Cardiac Arrhythmia Suppression Trial (CAST) Investigators. Effect of encainide and flecainide on mortality in a randomized trial of arrhythmia suppression after MI. N Engl J Med. 1989;321:406–412.

38. Roden DM. Antiarrhythmic drugs: from mechanisms to clinical practice. Heart. 2000; 84:339–346

39. Adan V, Crown LA. Diagnosis and treatment of sick sinus syndrome. Am Fam Physician. 2003;67:1725–1732, 1738

40. Gregoratos G. Indications and recommendations for pacemaker therapy. Am Fam Physician. 2005;71:1563–1570.

41. Delacretaz E. Suprventricular tachycardia. N Engl J Med. 2006;354:1039–1051.

42. ACC/AHA Task Force on Practice Guidelines. ACC/AHA guidelines of the management of patients with valvular heart disease. J Am Coll Cardiol. 1998;32:1486–1588.

43. Hara JH. Valvular heart disease. Primary Care. 2000;27: 725–740.

CHAPTER 11

Hypertension

Anthony J. Viera and Warren P. Newton

CASE 1

L.J. is a 48-year-old woman who works in an animal laboratory. She sustained a laceration at work; at the visits for the laceration repair and suture removal, you note that her blood pressure (BP) has been elevated, 168/96 and 156/98, respectively. She has no history of hypertension and is not on any medications.

CLINICAL QUESTIONS

1. Would you diagnose hypertension now? If not, what would you do to establish the diagnosis?
2. Once the diagnosis has been established, what would your initial evaluation be?
3. Assuming that the initial evaluation is unremarkable, what should be your initial management of this patient?

CASE 2

R.T. is a 56-year-old construction worker whom you have diagnosed with hypertension because his usual BP is approximately 175/105. His serum potassium, blood urea nitrogen, creatinine, and glucose levels are normal; his total cholesterol is 243 mg/dL; and urinalysis does not show protein. He has no symptoms or signs of end-organ disease. A 6-month trial of exercise and weight loss has been partially successful, with a reduction in BP to approximately 165/100.

CLINICAL QUESTIONS

1. Should you start medication? If so, which one, at what dose, and why?
2. If R.T. had a previous myocardial infarction, what antihypertensive medication would you start and why?
3. If R.T. had diabetes, what medication would you consider?

Hypertension—defined as having a sustained systolic BP (SBP) greater than 140 mm Hg and/or a sustained diastolic BP (DBP) greater than 90 mm Hg, and/or being on antihypertensive treatment—is a chronic condition that currently affects more than 65 million Americans, or about 31% of the US adult population (1, 2). Its prevalence greatly increases with age, affecting approximately 6% of 18- to 34-year-old individuals but over 77% of those 75 years or older (1). The

estimated lifetime risk of developing hypertension in the United States is 90% (3).

Hypertension is responsible for 35% of all myocardial infarctions (MIs) and strokes as well as half of all episodes of congestive heart failure (CHF) (4). Hypertension is also a major contributor to peripheral vascular disease, end-stage renal disease, aortic aneurysm, and retinopathy (5–8). Nearly one out of four premature deaths is caused by hypertension, making it the single most important cause of premature death in developed countries (7, 9). Hypertension is the most common primary diagnosis in the United States, and annual costs associated with its treatment are estimated to be nearly $56 billion (8, 10).

Treatment of hypertension dramatically lowers the incidence of end-organ complications and patient-oriented outcomes. For example, lowering the SBP to 150 mm Hg decreases the incidence of strokes of all types (11). Lowering DBP by 10 mm Hg reduces the number of strokes by up to 56% and the incidence of coronary heart disease by 37% (12). Overall, antihypertensive therapy leads to a 35% to 40% mean reduction in stroke incidence, 20% to 25% mean reduction in MIs, and greater than 50% reduction in incidence of CHF (8). In patients with SBP between 140–159 mm Hg and additional cardiovascular disease risk factors, it is estimated that a sustained reduction of 12 mm Hg in the SBP for 10 years prevents 1 death for every 11 patients treated. In the setting of preexisting cardiovascular disease or target-organ damage, only 9 patients need to be treated to prevent 1 death (13).

Nationally, the death rate from stroke has dropped by 60% in the last 3 decades, and mortality from coronary heart disease has declined by 53%. Both changes are in part attributable to better detection and control of hypertension (14). Yet, despite what is known about the benefits of treatment, 42% of patients with hypertension are not being treated, and 69%–75% do not have their hypertension under control (15, 16). Over 30% of people with hypertension are not even aware of their problem (15). Although lack of access to medical care might explain some of this quality gap, much of the undiagnosed and uncontrolled hypertension occurs in patients who have health insurance and access to a physician (17).

The major responsibility for detecting and treating hypertension does not rest with special hypertension clinics or programs, but rather with family physicians and other primary care clinicians. This chapter focuses on what you should know about adult hypertension, such as making the diagnosis, the initial evaluation, recommending lifestyle modification and drug therapy, and planning long-term management. Hypertensive emergencies and hypertension in children and pregnant women are special topics and are not addressed in this chapter.

SCREENING

The first step in treating hypertension is finding it. Every family physician should have a strategy for detecting hypertension in his or her patient population. Based on substantial indirect evidence that benefits outweigh harms, the US Preventive Services Task Force strongly recommends that clinicians screen adults 18 years and older for hypertension, but makes no recommendation regarding the interval at which screening should take place (Strength of Recommendation A) (7). Most screening for hypertension occurs opportunistically, in that patients presenting to a clinic for any reason will have their BP measured. This approach works well for those patients who come to the physician several times per year. Some groups, however, such as younger to middle-aged men and underserved populations do not regularly seek medical care and may require special contact via mailings, health fairs, or work-site screening (18). When physicians have defined panels of patients, such as in HMOs or small communities, it is easier to identify and target these people for screening. Quality improvement efforts for hypertension care might include development of office-based systems that allow better identification and tracking of patients with hypertension. For example, electronic health records, patient registries, reminder systems, and other practice-based approaches may help identify people with elevated BP who remain undiagnosed or undertreated (19).

MEASUREMENT OF BLOOD PRESSURE

Whereas measurement of BP is one of the most commonly performed tasks in clinical medicine, it is also fraught with error. The gold standard for noninvasive measurement of BP is the auscultatory method using a mercury sphygmomanometer with an appropriately sized cuff. However, concerns over potential environmental hazards posed by mercury have led to phasing out of mercury instruments (20). Aneroid sphygmomanometers use a column of air rather than a column of mercury and can easily lose calibration (21). With either type of sphygmomanometry, several sources of error are introduced by the person obtaining the measurement. These include errors of technique (e.g., improper patient positioning, improper cuff size or placement), and terminal digit bias (the tendency to record 5 or 0 as the last digit). Further, different observers may use different Korotkoff sounds in their interpretation of BP. Increasingly, clinical settings are relying on automatic devices to obtain BP measurements. These devices obviously eliminate some of the observer factors (e.g., digit bias), but their limitations include not being able to accurately assess BP in people with arrhythmias (e.g., atrial fibrillation) or severe atherosclerosis (due to poor compliance of arteries). Finally, automatic devices should be periodically calibrated against a gold standard, i.e., a mercury manometer.

Because BP may be elevated by worry or previous activity, patients should be relaxed and seated for at least 5 minutes before the measurement is taken. A distended bladder or the recent use of tobacco or caffeine may give spuriously high readings. The patient should be seated, with the arm bare and supported. The cuff should be centered with the air bladder portion of the cuff encircling 80% of the arm. A wider cuff should be used on obese or thick arms. A small cuff or the presence of clothing under the cuff will falsely elevate the readings by as much as 10 to 15 mm Hg. With the auscultatory method, the ipsilateral radial pulse should be palpated during inflation to be certain that systolic pressure has been exceeded. The pulse should disappear when the cuff is adequately pressurized; otherwise, the presence of an auscultatory gap will confuse the systolic reading. Listen with the bell of the stethoscope to hear the low-frequency Korotkoff sounds. The first repetitive sound corresponds to the systolic pressure. Diastolic pressure should be noted at the disappearance of the sounds, not muffling, because disappearance is a more reliable criterion for diagnosis, and most studies of treatment have used it. Finally, on the initial measurement, BP should be checked in both arms (21, 22).

Some patients have BP that is elevated when measured in the office setting but not when measured out of the office setting using either self-BP monitoring or 24-hour ambulatory BP monitoring. Sometimes, this "white-coat hypertension" will be suspected because the patient will tell you that his/her BP is always "normal" when checked elsewhere. However, automatic blood pressure devices in grocery stores and pharmacies are likely to be inaccurate and should not be relied upon (23). Home (or self) BP monitoring may be extremely useful as an adjunct to diagnosis or management (24). There are numerous automatic BP devices suitable for home or self-BP monitoring, but not all have been independently validated. A Web site listing automatic devices that have been validated is maintained at: *www.dableducational.com* (25). In patients who seem to have an elevated BP in the office setting, but in whom you suspect white-coat hypertension based on no evidence of target organ damage, a 24-hour ambulatory BP monitor measurement may be useful (8, 26). Keep in mind, however, that white-coat hypertension, while conferring less risk than sustained hypertension, may not be entirely benign (27–29). A diagnostic algorithm is shown in Figure 11.1, and the different cut-offs for what is considered an elevated BP are shown in Table 11.1. Note that "normal" out-of-office BP is about 5 mm Hg lower than "normal" office BP (24).

CLINICAL ASSESSMENT

Making the Diagnosis

Once you have identified a patient with an elevated BP, remember that the final diagnosis of hypertension is a clinical one—a function of the actual blood pressure, risk factors, and the effect of the diagnosis on the patient (30, 31). Be wary of prematurely labeling the patient as hypertensive. Having the diagnosis of hypertension has been shown to increase absenteeism from work by 80% and may dramatically affect access to, or cost of, life insurance (30). A single greatly elevated BP reading in the office setting (SBP >200 mm Hg and/or DBP >120) is adequate to make the diagnosis of hypertension in the absence of a recognized cause of secondary elevation. For most patients with somewhat elevated blood pressure (SBP >140 mm Hg and/or DBP >90), an average of three readings

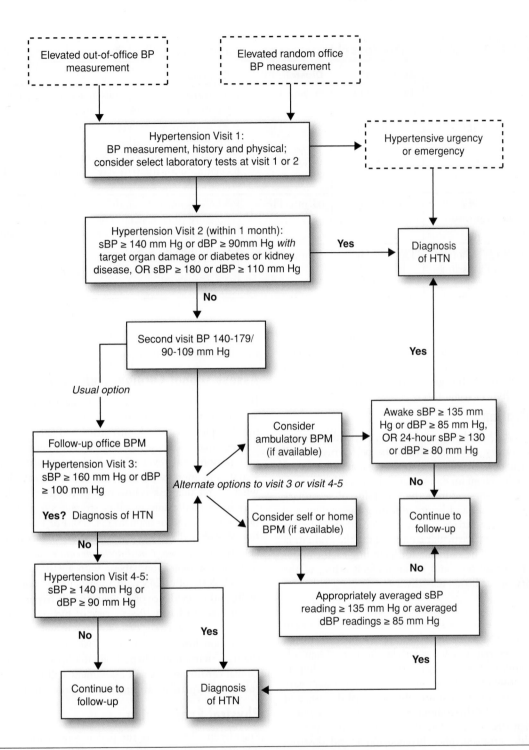

Figure 11.1 • Algorithm for expedited diagnosis of hypertension (HTN). BP = blood pressure; BPM = blood pressure measurement; SBP = systolic blood pressure; DBP = diastolic blood pressure. (Adapted from Myers MG, Tobe SW, McKay DW, et al. New algorithm for the diagnosis of hypertension. Am J Hypertens. 2005;18:1369–74. Used with permission.)

over at least 6 weeks should be used. If the average SBP is >140 mm Hg and/or the average DBP is >90, the diagnosis is confirmed. If uncertainty remains, base your assessment on additional readings.

The term "isolated systolic hypertension" refers to a SBP >140 mm Hg when the DBP is <90 mm Hg. Isolated systolic

hypertension is common in the elderly. Historically, DBP was used to classify the severity of hypertension. However, longitudinal studies have demonstrated that SBP is a better predictor of future morbidity and mortality, especially for middle-aged and older individuals (8, 32). Patients are thus classified based on whichever level of BP (systolic or diastolic) is in the higher

TABLE 11.1 Cut-offs for Diagnosis of Hypertension Based on Type of Blood Pressure Measurements

Setting	Systolic BP	Diastolic BP	Comment
Office measurements	140 mm Hg	90 mm Hg	Two readings, 5 minutes apart, sitting in chair. Confirm reading in other arm.
Home or self blood pressure measurements	135 mm Hg	85 mm Hg	At minimum use average of measurements taken on three consecutive days, two measurements taken in the morning and two measurements taken in the evening with the first day's measurements discarded (24).
Awake average of 24-hour ambulatory blood pressure measurements	135 mm Hg	85 mm Hg	There is normally a 10%–20% decrease of blood pressure during sleep. Patients that do not have this decrease ("non-dippers") may be at increased cardiovascular disease risk (26).
Entire average of 24-hour ambulatory blood pressure measurements	130 mm Hg	80 mm Hg	

range (8). Those in whom the SBP is between 140 and 159 or the DBP is between 90 and 99 mm Hg are said to have stage 1 hypertension, whereas those in whom SBP is greater than 159 mm Hg or DBP is greater than 99 mm Hg are said to have stage 2 hypertension (8).

Initial Evaluation

Table 11.2 lists the key elements of history, physical examination, and laboratory tests that should be performed on all patients with a new diagnosis of hypertension. The initial evaluation should screen for end-organ damage and other cardiovascular risk factors, address the possibility of secondary causes of hypertension, and begin educating the patient and family. There is very little scientific evidence that addresses whether including any particular component of the evaluation improves outcomes. The rationale for including each component is based on tradition, and on an understanding of the natural history of cardiovascular disease.

History

As a first step, make note of symptoms suggesting end-organ disease, such as chest pain, orthopnea, paroxysmal nocturnal dyspnea, lower extremity edema, or claudication. Then address the possibility of secondary or treatable causes of hypertension. The most common secondary causes in primary care settings are significant alcohol use, chronic renal disease, and drugs (including over-the-counter agents such as decongestants and illicit drugs); also consider renovascular hypertension, hyperaldosteronism, pheochromocytoma, and obstructive sleep apnea (OSA). More than 50% of patients with OSA have hypertension, and treatment of OSA reduces BP in these patients (33). A useful mnemonic to help think about the secondary causes of hypertension is shown in Table 11.3 (33). Ask about specific symptoms that suggest secondary causes, such as sweating, palpitations, or flushing.

Keep in mind that in primary care settings at least 90%–95% of newly diagnosed hypertensives will not have a secondary cause. More extensive work-up is indicated only for patients under age 25, and for those in whom a secondary disease is suspected on clinical grounds, such as severity of hypertension, malignant course, a lack of response to therapy,

or physical findings of secondary disease, such as a renal bruit or a Cushingoid appearance.

Assess Global Cardiovascular Risk

It is important to identify other cardiac risk factors that interact with hypertension to increase risk such as smoking, diabetes, dyslipidemia, or a family history of early cardiac disease. Cardiovascular disease risk calculators can provide an estimate of a person's risk over a specified time frame (e.g., next 10 years), and more sophisticated calculators can determine to what degree that risk is lowered by treatment with an antihypertensive medication or other strategies (e.g., tobacco cessation, a statin, and/or aspirin) (34, 35). For example, using the free Web-based or personal digital assistant calculator available from *http://www.med-decisions.com/cvtool/*, a 56-year-old male non-smoker, nondiabetic with a SBP of 175 mm Hg, a total cholesterol of 243 with high-density lipoprotein (HDL) of 30, and no evidence of left ventricular hypertrophy on electrocardiogram has a 10-year risk of having a cardiovascular event of approximately 29%. Treatment with a blood pressure medication lowers the 10-year risk to 21%. (Treating both the hypertension and hyperlipidema lowers the risk to 15%.) Global cardiovascular risk assessment will likely play a larger role in how patients are managed in the future.

Physical Examination

Start by making note of the patient's body mass index (BMI). To assess end-organ damage, cardiovascular examination should note cardiac size and rhythm, the presence of a third heart sound (S3), peripheral edema or other signs of cardiac failure; decreased pulses; or carotid bruits. Focal weakness, abnormal gait, or other abnormalities on neurologic testing may suggest a prior cerebrovascular accident. Ophthalmoscopic examination may disclose hypertensive retinopathy. Physical features that suggest a secondary cause of hypertension include Cushingoid features such as moon facies and central adiposity, a diastolic abdominal bruit suggestive of renovascular hypertension, or the diminished femoral pulses with hypertension in the arms that suggest coarctation of the aorta.

TABLE 11.2 Key Features of Evaluation of Hypertension

History
Features suggesting secondary disease
Age<25
Malignant course
Lack of response to therapy
End-organ disease
Chest pain
Orthopnea
Claudication
Other cardiovascular risk factors
Diabetes
Smoking
Family history of early coronary artery disease
History of elevated cholesterol level
Physical examination
Pulse
Weight
Height
Cardiac: size, rhythm, S3, JVD, edema
Vascular: carotids, peripheral pulses
Back: renal bruits
Fundus
Neurologic
Laboratory tests
Urinalysis
Urine microalbumin
BUN/creatinine
Potassium and sodium
Glucose
Fasting lipid panel (HDL, LDL, triglycerides)
Electrocardiogram

BUN, blood urea nitrogen; HDL, high-density lipoprotein; LDL, low-density lipoprotein; JVD, jugular venous distention.

Laboratory or Other Diagnostic Tests

Laboratory tests should include urinalysis to identify proteinuria and hematuria, as well as serum blood urea nitrogen (BUN) and creatinine to assess renal function. In those in whom the urinalysis shows no protein, consider a urinary microalbumin to screen for early nephropathy. Obtain an electrocardiogram (ECG) to check for left ventricular hypertrophy (see Table 11.4), arrhythmia, and baseline ST segment changes or signs of previous MI. An echocardiogram may be indicated if left ventricular hypertrophy is suspected based on the ECG or physical examination. Obtain a fasting blood glucose level and a full cholesterol panel (including low-density lipoprotein,

HDL, and triglycerides) to detect silent diabetes mellitus and hyperlipidemia. There are no firm rules regarding additional tests. Most physicians screen for hyperaldosteronism by checking serum potassium and sodium levels.

Patient Education

Patients may find it difficult to understand hypertension (36). There are no symptoms, and for most patients, the major issue is a risk of stroke or heart attack 15 to 20 years later, far removed from their current experience. They may also have fears and negative images about blood pressure medications (36). By taking time for a thorough history and physical examination, you underscore the importance of hypertension, and begin to teach the patient how lifestyle influences the problem. Over the long term, your effectiveness in managing the hypertensive patient depends on your ability to educate both your patient and the family. Ultimately, it is the patient who decides what recommendations to follow, including whether or not to take a medication for the rest of his/her life.

MANAGEMENT

General Approach

After the initial evaluation, take time to develop an individualized treatment plan that contains elements of lifestyle modifications and, if appropriate, pharmacotherapy. Figure 11.2 provides an algorithm describing initial management. The overall goal of treatment is to improve long-term survival and quality of life rather than quickly lowering the BP to a normal range. Indeed, if blood pressures are only mildly elevated, a 3- to 6-month period of lifestyle modifications without pharmacotherapy may be sufficient to bring a patient's BP to goal. Left unaddressed, however, approximately 20% of patients with stage 1 hypertension will progress to stage 2 over a 4-year period (37).

Evidence for treatment of SBP ≥160 mm Hg is strong, and there is strong observational evidence that the risk reduction achieved with lowering SBP is a graded continuous phenomenon—the lower the SBP, the lower the rate of complications. Note, however, that lowering the blood pressure too much is associated with increased mortality. Also, those with the highest blood pressure have the greatest benefit from treatment, while, as discussed below, the benefit of normalizing mild elevations in BP is much more modest. The target BP should be <140/90 mm Hg for most patients and <130/80 for patients with diabetes mellitus, renal disease, or known cardiovascular disease.

Although lifestyle modifications should never be abandoned, to achieve this goal, most patients with hypertension will require drug therapy. Indeed, almost all patients with stage 2 hypertension benefit from pharmacotherapy. Using data from the Hypertension Detection and Follow-up Program (HDFP), only three patients with DBPs between 115 and 129 mm Hg would have to be treated for 5 years to prevent one death, stroke, or MI (number needed to treat [NNT] = 3) (38). For patients with mild hypertension, however, the benefit of treatment is less clear. The data from HDFP patients with diastolic pressures between 90 and 94 mm Hg show an NNT of 345 to prevent one death over a

TABLE 11.3 'ABCDE' Mnemonic for Secondary Causes of Hypertension (33)

Mnemonic	Think About	Comment
A	Accuracy Alcohol Apnea Aldosteronism	Are the blood pressure readings accurate? Could chronic alcohol use be playing a role? Does the patient have obstructive sleep apnea? Does the patient have hypokalemia or other suggestions of primary hyperaldosteronism?
B	Bruits Bad kidneys	Is there an abdominal bruit suggestive of renovascular hypertension? Does the patient have renal parenchymal disease (which can be cause or a consequence of hypertension)?
C	Catecholamines Coarctation Cushing's	Is the patient having palpitations, tachycardia, diaphoresis, headaches, and/or paroxysmal hypertension suggestive of pheochromocytoma? Are there decreased or delayed femoral pulses, or rib notching on chest x-ray suggestive of coarctation of the aorta? Any weight gain, hirstuism, amenorrhea, striae, or moon facies suggestive of Cushing's syndrome?
D	Drugs Diet	Any use of sympathomimetics, corticosteroids, NSAIDs, oral contraceptive pills, MAOIs, or other drugs that can elevate blood pressure? Are excess dietary sodium or obesity contributing?
E	Endocrine Erythropoietin	Is there untreated thyroid disease or hyperparathyroidism? Is there another disorder (COPD) leading to increased erythropoietin levels?

NSAID, non-steroidal anti-inflammatory drug; MAOI, monoamine oxidase inhibitor; COPD, chronic obstructive pulmonary disease

1-year period, and those from other trials have yielded an NNT as high as 5,000 for mildly hypertensive patients (39). What seems clear is that patients with any degree of hypertension do have an increased risk of stroke and other sequelae of hypertension. Patients with a greater baseline risk because they have other cardiac risk factors such as diabetes, smoking, or end-organ disease benefit most substantially from treatment with medication (40–43). Treating isolated systolic hypertension in the elderly patient can reduce the incidence of strokes, although the adverse effects of some medications may be greater in this population (44). Lifestyle changes may be a reasonable place to start.

Lifestyle Modifications

Consider lifestyle modifications for every patient. Table 11.5 lists individual strategies, with an approximation of their BP-

lowering efficacy. There is good evidence that certain individual and combined strategies improve blood pressure—a disease-oriented outcome—and there is also some evidence that these strategies reduce key long-term patient-oriented outcomes, such as stroke (45). Lifestyle modifications offer additional health benefits, fewer adverse effects, and are cheaper, but they are not a panacea for hypertension treatment from a clinical standpoint. In most cases, the proper use of lifestyle modifications, such as an exercise prescription or a weight loss program, requires a great deal of commitment by both physician and patient. Furthermore, some therapies, such as biofeedback, may be very expensive and offer relatively little in terms of efficacy (46). The lifestyle modifications that are recommended are exercise, weight loss, diet, moderation of alcohol intake, and reduction of sodium intake. Of course, tobacco cessation should be strongly encouraged for anyone who smokes.

Exercise

A number of different trials have found that an exercise regimen lowers BP in patients with both normal and high initial BPs and may decrease the number and dosage of medications needed to control BP (47, 48). The effect of exercise on lowering BP is even more pronounced in those with hypertension (47). Other benefits of an exercise program include reducing life stress through improved psychological health, facilitating weight loss, increasing serum HDL levels, and lowering overall mortality (49). Exercise is an appropriate first step for most hypertensive patients. An example of an initial, minimal exercise regimen would be walking briskly for 30 minutes three to five times per week.

Weight Loss

For overweight (BMI ≥25) and obese (BMI ≥30) patients—who currently constitute over 65% of the US adult

TABLE 11.4 Simplified Criteria for Left Ventricular Hypertrophy on Electrocardiogram

Deepest S wave in lead V_1 or V_2 plus tallest R wave in lead V_5 or V_6 ≥ 35 mm   and/or   R wave in lead aVL ≥ 12 mm

Age ≥ 35 years

Left ventricular "strain" pattern (asymmetric ST segment depression and T wave inversion, usually seen in leads I, aVL, V_4-V_6)

(Adapted from Goldberger AL. Clinical Electrocardiography: A Simplified Approach, 6th ed. St. Louis, MO: CV Mosby; 1999; and Grauer K. 12-Lead ECGs: A "Pocket Brain" for Easy Interpretation, 2nd ed. Gainesville, FL: KG/EKG Press; 2001.)

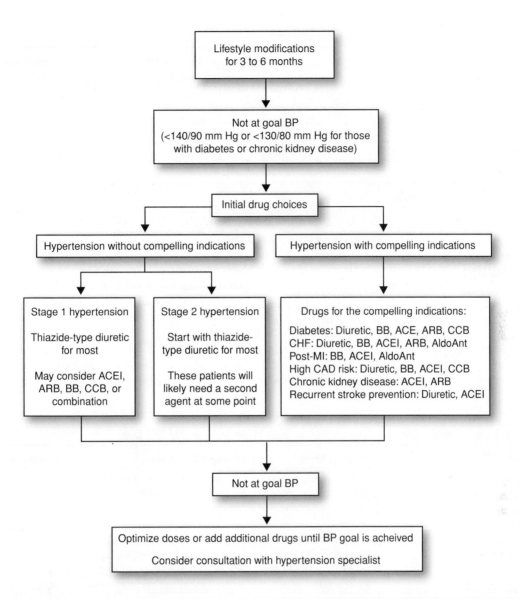

Figure 11.2 • Management of hypertension. BP, blood pressure; ACEI, angiotensin converting enzyme inhibitor; ARB, angiotensin receptor blocker; AldoAnt, aldosterone antagonist; BB, β-blocker; CCB, calcium channel blocker; CAD, coronary artery disease; MI, myocardial infarction. (Adapted from Chobanian AV, Bakris GL, Black HR, et al. The seventh report of the joint national committee on prevention, detection, evaluation, and treatment of high blood pressure: the JNC 7 report. JAMA. 2003;289: 2560–72. Used with permission.)

population (50)—weight reduction should be an essential part of the management plan. There is a strong correlation between obesity and hypertension, especially in people with centrally distributed body fat. Clinical trials of weight loss, often combined with exercise, have resulted in lowered blood pressure, and increased the impact of pharmacotherapy (51, 52). If a weight loss program is prescribed, a simple instruction such as "you should try to lose some weight" is insufficient. The physician should specify a target weight, coordinate a dietary intervention (such as a 1,500-calorie diet), give an exercise prescription, and use frequent follow-up office visits (such as every 4 to 6 weeks) or local community groups, such as Weight Watchers, to help the patient lose weight. Patients do not need to attain ideal body weight

to benefit. Weight loss of as little as 10 pounds may result in substantial reductions in BP, perhaps eliminating the need for medication (or a second medication). Further, weight loss has numerous additional health benefits.

DASH Diet

The Dietary Approaches to Stop Hypertension (DASH) diet is an eating plan rich in potassium, magnesium, and calcium obtained from fruits, vegetables, and low-fat dairy products (53, 54). An example of a DASH eating plan based on a 2,000-calorie diet is shown in Table 11.6. Randomized trials have demonstrated a significant decrease in both SBP and DBP for as long as 18 months in patients adhering to the DASH diet (55).

TABLE 11.5 Effectiveness of Lifestyle Measures

Therapy	Average Systolic BP Lowering (mm Hg)	Average Diastolic BP Lowering (mm Hg)
Regular aerobic exercise	−5	−4
Weight loss of 3% to 9% in overweight patients	−3	−5.5
DASH diet	−11	−5.5
Alcohol moderation	−4	−2.5
Sodium restriction	−5	−3

BP, blood pressure; DASH, Dietary Approaches to Stop Hypertension.
(Adapted from Lochner J, Rugge B, Judkins D. How effective are lifestyle changes for controlling hypertension? J Fam Pract. 2005;55:73–74.)

Sodium Restriction

Population studies show a consistent correlation between salt intake and hypertension. Recent clinical trials have demonstrated that reducing sodium intake can lower BP (56, 57). However, sodium restriction is probably best thought of as a population approach rather than a clinical approach. Whereas not all patients are "salt-sensitive," it is recommended that all patients with hypertension reduce their sodium intake to less than 2.4 grams per day (8). On a population level, such a reduction can lower BP and could reduce strokes, MIs, and CHF (57). Today's salt substitutes offer improved palatability and can help your patients reduce their sodium intake.

Alcohol Reduction

Alcohol acts as a vasopressor, and meta-analysis of randomized controlled trials has shown that reduction of heavy alco-

TABLE 11.6 Sample Dietary Approaches to Stop Hypertension (DASH) Diet

Food Group	Daily Servings	Serving Sizes	Examples and Notes	Significance
Grains & grain products	7 to 8	1 slice bread, ½ cup dry cereal, ½ cup cooked rice, pasta, or cereal	Whole wheat bread, English muffin, pita bread, bagel, cereals, grits, oatmeal	Major sources of energy and fiber
Vegetables	4 to 5	1 cup raw, leafy vegetable, ½ cup cooked vegetable, 6 oz vegetable juice	Tomatoes, potatoes, carrots, peas, squash, broccoli, turnip greens, collards, kale, spinach, artichokes, sweet potatoes, beans	Rich sources of potassium, magnesium, and fiber
Fruits	4 to 5	6 oz fruit juice, 1 medium fruit, ¼ cup dried fruit, ½ cup fresh, frozen, or canned fruit	Apricots, bananas, dates, oranges, orange juice, grapefruit, mangoes, melons, peaches, pineapples, prunes, raisins, strawberries, tangerines	Important sources of potassium, magnesium, and fiber
Low fat or nonfat dairy foods	2 to 3	8 oz milk, 1 cup yogurt, 1.5 oz cheese	Skim or 1% milk, skim or low-fat buttermilk, nonfat or low-fat yogurt, part skim mozzarella cheese, nonfat cheese	Major sources of calcium and protein
Meats, poultry, and fish	2 or less	3 oz cooked meats, poultry, or fish	Select only lean; trim away fat; broil, roast, or boil, instead of frying; remove skin from poultry	Rich sources of protein and magnesium
Nuts, seeds, and legumes	4 to 5 per week	1 ½ oz or ⅓ cup nuts, ½ oz or 2 Tbs seeds, ½ cup cooked legumes	Almonds, filberts, mixed nuts, peanuts, walnuts, sunflower seeds, kidney beans, lentils	Rich sources of energy, magnesium, potassium, protein, and fiber

Table is based on 2,000 cal diet; oz, ounces; Tb, tablespoon. (From National Heart, Lung, and Blood Institute, "Your Guide to Lowering Your Blood Pressure with DASH," *http://www.nhlbi.nih.gov/health/public/heart/hbp/dash/*, accessed June 29, 2006.)

hol use can lower blood pressure (58). Intake of alcohol should be limited to no more than 1 oz of ethanol per day for men and 0.5 oz per day for women (8). This amounts to no more than 24 oz beer, 10 oz wine, or 3 oz of 80-proof whiskey per day for men (2 drinks) and half that amount (1 drink) for women.

Comprehensive Lifestyle Modification

A multicenter, randomized trial demonstrated that patients with hypertension can sustain multiple lifestyle changes over a period of 18 months, and such changes improve control of their blood pressure (55). Of course, volunteers for this trial were obviously motivated individuals, thereby limiting its generalizability. However, it seems clear that multiple lifestyle modifications (e.g., weight loss, exercise, and DASH diet) are more effective than a single modification (e.g., diet alone). In fact, a low-sodium (1,600 mg) DASH diet is as effective as single drug therapy (59). The challenge with any of the lifestyle modification recommendations is to actually get the patient to adopt them.

ANTIHYPERTENSIVE MEDICATIONS

Because of their low cost, once-daily dosing, and tremendous amount of favorable patient-oriented evidence for treatment of hypertension, a thiazide diuretic (e.g., hydrochlorothiazide [HCTZ] or chlorthalidone) should be considered first-line in uncomplicated hypertension (60). Low doses are sufficient (e.g., no more than 25 mg HCTZ per day) and will minimize side effects. If an alternate initial agent is chosen because of a compelling indication (e.g., angiotensin-converting enzyme [ACE] inhibitor because of CHF with systolic dysfunction or because of diabetes), and a second agent is needed, a thiazide diuretic should be prescribed for most patients unless contraindicated or precluded by side effects. Table 11.7 lists characteristics for antihypertensive medications.

The evidence for the benefit of the low-dose diuretics as well as the agents recommended for compelling indications (Figure 11.2) comes from many randomized clinical trials (8). A special research method called network meta-analysis allows comparison of many treatments across many studies, both directly and indirectly. A study using this method with data from 42 clinical trials (192,478 patients), demonstrated that low-dose diuretics, β-blockers, ACE inhibitors, calcium channel blockers, and angiotensin receptor blockers (but not α-blockers) are all superior to placebo in reducing most cardiovascular disease outcomes (including cardiovascular disease mortality and total mortality) (60). However, no particular class of drug is superior to low-dose diuretics in reducing these outcomes (see Table 11.8) (60). Low-dose thiazide diuretics should not only be the first-line medication for most hypertensive patients, but they should be the gold-standard to which newer antihypertensive drugs are compared in randomized controlled trials (60).

Coexistent Medical Problems

Think about a patient's coexistent medical problems ("compelling indications") and how an antihypertensive medication might help. Diuretics improve symptoms of CHF. Beta-blockers have been shown to reduce long-term mortality in post-

MI patients and in patients with CHF. ACE inhibitors provide a substantial benefit for CHF patients with systolic dysfunction. In patients with diabetes, there is excellent evidence that an aggressive approach to BP control will improve outcomes. Setting a target of 155/85, the United Kingdom Prospective Diabetes Study Group (UKPDS) showed a reduction of diabetic complications (NNT = 6) and deaths from diabetes (NNT = 15) (61). In fact, in the UKPDS study, "tight" glucose control did not reduce mortality while "tight" BP control with a β-blocker or ACE inhibitor reduced both diabetes-related complications and mortality (61). Given this dramatic finding, some authorities have set target blood pressures for patients with diabetes as low as 130/80, but this recommendation is not yet supported by trial evidence (8). Both thiazide diuretics and β-blockers may worsen glycemic control mildly, but these effects are less important than the demonstrated improvement in patient-oriented outcomes in diabetic hypertensives given these drugs. An ACE inhibitor may be preferred in diabetic patients to reduce the rate of progression of nephropathy. Patients who cannot tolerate ACE inhibitors (e.g., develop cough or angioedema) may benefit from an angiotensin receptor blocker (ARB).

Adverse Effects

In a 5-year period, at least 9% of patients taking an antihypertensive medication will have side effects severe enough to have to stop the medication (62). Many patients will require more than one medication to achieve control (8), and additional medications will multiply this effect. Therefore, consider an antihypertensive medication's side effect profile as you plan pharmacotherapy. Hypokalemia induced by thiazide diuretics and hyperkalemia caused by ACE inhibitors may lead to serious arrhythmias, especially in patients with cardiac arrhythmias or in patients who are receiving digitalis. Whereas it has been conventional wisdom that β-blockers are contraindicated in patients with asthma or chronic obstructive lung disease because they might trigger bronchospasm, cardioselective β-blockers have proven to be safe in these patients and should be prescribed when indicated (63, 64). Cardiac conduction delay may be worsened by β-blockers or calcium channel blockers. Patients with depression or sleep disorders may be adversely affected by all adrenergic blocking agents, including clonidine, β-blockers, methyldopa, and reserpine.

Sexual dysfunction has been ascribed to all of the antihypertensive medications, particularly β-blockers, thiazide diuretics, and centrally acting agents such as clonidine and methyldopa. You need to be able to talk openly to your patient about this adverse effect. Whether any of these adverse effects forces a change in the drug regimen depends on the severity of symptoms and the patient's priorities.

Clonidine or methyldopa may cause sedation and impair the manual coordination required at work. Similarly, β-blockers can make aerobic conditioning more difficult and may be less attractive for patients with occupations that require strenuous physical activity or those in athletic training. Patients on β-blockers sometimes complain of fatigue and difficulty concentrating, other potential side effects to keep in mind. However, it is important to note that β-blockers have a much better tolerability profile than previously thought. A meta-analysis of 15 trials involving 35,000 patients found no significant increase in the risk of depression and only small

TABLE 11.7 Characteristics of Some Antihypertensive Medications/Medication Classes

Drug	Major Disadvantages	Dosing Regimen	Generic Available	Comment	Average Cost per Month[a]
Thiazide diuretics (e.g., HCTZ)	Hypokalemia, hyperuricemia, hyperglycemia, elevation of low-density lipoprotein	QD	Yes	Consider first-line for most patients	HCTZ = $9.00
Beta-blockers (e.g., atenolol, metoprolol, ropranolol)	Fatigue, heart block, nightmares and sleep disturbances, increased bronchospasm, decreased cardiac output/tolerance to exercise	QD to BID	Yes (for some agents)	Indicated for post myocardial infarction (regardless of BP); improve survival in patients with CHF	Atenolol = $11.00 Metoprolol = $14.00
ACE inhibitors (e.g. enalapril, fosinopril, lisinopril)	Hyperkalemia, rash, transient loss of taste, drug fever, proteinuria, cough, angioedema	QD to TID	Yes	Renal protection in diabetes; patients with CHF should be on higher doses than that typically used for hypertension	Lisinopril = $19.00
Angiotensin-2 receptor blockers (ARBs; e.g., candesartan, irbesartan, losartan)	Fatigue, dizziness, back pain, dyspepsia, hyperkalemia, angioedema	QD to BID	No	Usually reserve for when ACE inhibitor desired but not tolerated	Candesartan = $50.00
Calcium channel blockers (e.g., amlodipine, diltiazem, nifedipine, verapamil)	Constipation, dizziness, edema	QD to TID	Yes (for some agents)	Long-acting dihydropyridine agent preferred	Amlodopine = $46.00
Alpha1-blockers (e.g., doxazosin, prazosin, terazosin)	Dizziness, headache, lethargy, syncope. Not well proven to improve patient oriented outcomes.	BID to TID	Yes (for some agents)	Best use probably for men with hypertension and benign prostatic hyperplasia	Prazosin = $20.00
Clonidine (available in both oral tablets and transdermal patches)	Mood changes/depression, sedation, dry mouth, hypertensive crisis with rapid withdrawal	QD to BID (q week for patch)	Yes	Can help reduce hot flashes in post-menopausal women	Clonidine = $13.00 (tablet), $100.00 (patch)
Reserpine (Serpasil)	Mood changes/depression, sexual dysfunction (both male and female), nasal stuffiness, peptic ulceration	QD	Yes	Not commonly used	Reserpine = $12.00

ACE, angiotensin-converting enzyme; BID, twice daily; HCTZ, hydrochlorothiazide; QD, every day; TID, three times daily.
[a]Prices for average monthly dose were obtained from www.drugstore.com June 28, 2006. Actual prices will vary depending on dose, formulation, local conditions, co-pays, and other factors.

TABLE 11.8 Comparison of First-line Medications for Hypertension

Low-dose Diuretic vs.	Relative Risk (95% Confidence Interval) of Outcome					
	CHD	**CHF**	**Stroke**	**CVD Events**	**CVD Mortality**	**Total Mortality**
Placebo	0.79 (0.69–0.92)	0.51 (0.42–0.62)	0.71 (0.63–0.81)	0.76 (0.69–0.83)	0.81 (0.73–0.92)	0.90 (0.84–0.96)
Beta-blockers	0.87 (0.74–1.03)	0.83 (0.68–1.01)	0.90 (0.76–1.06)	0.89 (0.80–0.98)	0.93 (0.81–1.07)	0.99 (0.91–1.07)
ACE inhibitors	1.00 (0.88–1.14)	0.88 (0.80–0.96)	0.86 (0.77–0.97)	0.94 (0.89–1.00)	0.93 (0.85–1.02)	1.00 (0.95–1.05)
CCBs	0.89 (0.76–1.01)	0.74 (0.67–0.81)	1.02 (0.91–1.14)	0.94 (0.89–1.00)	0.95 (0.87–1.04)	1.03 (0.98–1.08)
ARBs	0.83 (0.59–1.16)	0.88 (0.66–1.16)	1.20 (0.93–1.55)	1.00 (0.85–1.18)	1.07 (0.85–1.36)	1.09 (0.96–1.22)
Alpha-blockers[a]	0.99 (0.75–1.31)	0.51 (0.43–0.60)	0.85 (0.66–1.10)	0.84 (0.75–0.93)	1.00 (0.75–1.34)	0.98 (0.88–1.10)

Adapted from references (60) and (67)

[a]Alpha-blockers were no more effective than placebo for prevention of CHD, stroke, CVD mortality, or total mortality.
CCB, calcium channel blocker; ARB, angiotensin receptor blocker; CHD, coronary heart disease; CHF, congestive heart failure; CVD, cardiovascular disease; ACE, angiotensin-converting enzyme.
Example of how to interpret this table: Compared to patients receiving ACE inhibitors, patients receiving low-dose diuretics had a relative risk of 0.93 for CVD mortality, with a 95% confidence interval of 0.85 to 1.02. Because this confidence interval crosses the null (1.00), this difference is not statistically significant.

increases in the risk of sexual dysfunction (NNH = 200 per year) and fatigue (NNH = 57 per year) (65).

Dosing

Therapeutic regimens should be as simple as possible to enhance adherence. Dosing frequency is more important than the total number of medications used. If possible, prescribe a medication that is taken once daily (e.g., thiazides, atenolol, some ACE inhibitors). Some older medications have been reformulated to allow daily dosing. Remember that improvements in formulation may also incur an added cost to the patient for these agents. Products consisting of a combination of antihypertensive agents, usually prescribed after titrating individual agents to achieve BP control, may allow smaller doses of each drug to be used. This may decrease the overall drug cost, although caution must be exercised. Patients should be asked about insurance coverage for medications.

Cost

Think in terms of monthly cost of the medication to the patient. Newer agents such as ARBs are currently much more expensive than older agents, primarily because of the lack of generic products available for substitution. Generic products, if available and of adequate quality, can save the patient up to 20-fold (e.g., $5.00 versus $100.00 a month).

After you have chosen a medication and started treatment, take care to bring BP down slowly, aiming for 5 to 10 mm Hg/week. Lowering the BP too rapidly can result in deleterious effects, such as postural hypotension, syncope, or other cardiac events, and is a common cause of nonadherence and therapeutic failure. Treatment is usually not urgent, and the overall goal is to prevent long-term complications such as strokes. If control is not achieved after an adequate trial of a

particular medication (i.e., 4 weeks), three options are available: increase the daily dosage, substitute another agent, or add a second agent. It is usually preferable to maximize one agent first.

LONG-TERM MANAGEMENT

Initially, the patient should be seen every 1 to 2 weeks until the BP is stabilized. Then, gradually decrease the frequency of visits to every 3 months for 1 year, and finally, to every 6 to 12 months. Patients should be told to bring their medications with them to each visit. Ideally, patients should have their BPs checked occasionally between visits, either at work or at home. Reliable home BP monitoring devices are readily available, but even when a patient obtains a monitor that has been independently validated and recommended for use (check the *www.dableeducational.com* Web site), you should make sure the cuff size is appropriate and check that the device is measuring BP accurately (e.g., against your calibrated office sphygmomanometer) for that particular patient. Finger monitors and most wrist monitors should be avoided (25). Home monitoring has been shown to increase BP control and the proportion of people who get to goal BP, perhaps by improving medication adherence and self-efficacy in hypertension management (66). Patients who perform BP monitoring on their own should be told to bring a record of their BP readings to each visit. Some monitors have small printers that facilitate such recordings.

In addition to a review of all medications and possible adverse effects, each visit should include a review of cardiac symptoms, BP, heart rate, rhythm, new murmurs, S3, jugular venous distention (JVD), edema, and rales. A more detailed examination should be performed annually to detect evidence of end-organ damage, such as left ventricular hypertrophy, stroke, or vascular disease. Urinalysis, BUN, and creatinine levels should be checked annually, along with serum potassium if the patient is taking a diuretic or an ACE inhibitor. A flowsheet in the patient's chart or the electronic health record will allow you to easily follow the patient's BP, physical findings, laboratory study results, and prescribed treatments over time.

Sometimes you will find that a patient's BP seems to be more difficult to control than expected. There are several ways to assess patient adherence with the treatment plan. Asking family members about the actual usage of pills may be useful, as is counting the remaining pills that the patient brings to the office visit. Other tests of adherence include checking the serum uric acid level, which is almost always elevated in patients taking diuretics, or monitoring the pulse rate of patients, which is often reduced in patients taking β-blockers. Finally, if you are still concerned, calling the patient's pharmacy will reveal the frequency of refills. Consider 24-hour continuous ambulatory monitoring for patients whose blood pressure is labile or difficult to control (8, 26).

Over time, the key issues in the management of hypertension are patient education and patient involvement in his/her own care. Because hypertension is a "silent" disease, treatment does not usually make the patient feel better. In fact, the patient may actually feel worse because of the effects of medication. The physician's task is to diagnose hypertension and then to educate the patient and family about its importance. Often the physician must persuade the patient to make major lifestyle changes or take medication for the rest of his or her life that may be expensive or have long-term unpleasant adverse effects. Therefore, it is important to encourage the patient's sense of responsibility for monitoring and treatment. Regular BP measurements at home or work provide direct reinforcement for continuing a diet, exercise, or medication program. How well the physician educates and helps the patient maintain a normal blood pressure determines the success of the treatment plan at 5, 10, and 15 years. Key recommendations are summarized in Table 11.9.

Keeping up to date with advances in hypertension is also a challenge for the physician. Because of the scope of the problem, there are thousands of studies and scores of clinical guidelines from a variety of different perspectives published yearly; reviewing the primary literature completely is impossible for practicing clinicians. Fortunately, however, the number of well-designed studies that report long-term outcomes is small. Clinicians should look for practice guidelines that have explicit descriptions of how the literature was reviewed and summarized, and that emphasize long-term patient-oriented outcomes. The best source of summary information is the report of the Joint National Committee on Prevention, Detection, Evaluation, and Treatment of High Blood Pressure (the most recent, the seventh report, can be found at *http://www.nhlbi.nih.gov/guidelines/hypertension/*).

CASE DISCUSSIONS

CASE 1: L.J.

Diagnosis requires three separate readings unless the level is markedly elevated; therefore, the appropriate action is to have the patient return for follow up. A third similar BP would establish the diagnosis. If she tells you that her BP is always normal at the animal lab, you might consider a 24-hour ambulatory BP monitor to evaluate for white-coat hypertension. Once you make a diagnosis of hypertension, the initial evaluation should consist of considering whether a work-up should be done for a secondary cause, looking for signs and symptoms of end-organ disease, and exploring other cardiac risk factors. Initial management should be lifestyle modification.

CASE 2: R.T.

Lifestyle modification has had a partial effect. The decrease of blood pressure is clinically significant, but a further decrease of blood pressure to below 140/90 would further reduce the risk of stroke and heart attack. Medication is therefore indicated. A diuretic (such as hydrochlorothiazide 25 mg each day) is the best first choice. A β-blocker or ACE inhibitor might be added later, if needed. These

TABLE 11.9 Key Recommendations

Recommendation	Strength of Recommendation*
Adults age 18 years and older should be screened for hypertension (7).	A
In patients with newly diagnosed hypertension, perform a urinalysis, BUN/creatinine, potassium, sodium, glucose, fasting lipid panel, and an electrocardiogram (8).	C
Recommend lifestyle modifications (Table 11.5) for all patients with hypertension (8).	B
For patients with uncomplicated hypertension in whom pharmacotherapy is needed, prescribe a low-dose thiazide diuretic as first-line (8, 60).	A
For hypertensive patients who have a compelling indication, prescribe antihypertensive medication(s) based on the compelling indication(s) (8).	A

*A = consistent, good-quality patient-oriented evidence; B = inconsistent or limited-quality patient-oriented evidence; C = consensus, disease-oriented evidence, usual practice, expert opinion, or case series. For information about the Strength of Recommendation Taxonomy evidence rating system, see *http://www.aafp.org/afpsort.xml*.

agents have been proven to reduce long-term cardiovascular disease outcomes, are inexpensive, need to be taken only once per day, and are generally well tolerated. For a patient with hypertension and a previous MI, a β-blocker would be absolutely indicated. For patients with diabetes and hypertension, it is important to recognize that BP control should be tighter, and the ACE inhibitors are attractive because of their renal protective effects.

REFERENCES

1. Fields LE, Burt VL, Cutler JA, Hughes J, Roccella EJ, Sorlie P. The burden of adult hypertension in the United States 1999 to 2000: a rising tide. Hypertension. 2004;44(4):398–404.
2. Wang Y, Wang QJ. The prevalence of prehypertension and hypertension among US adults according to the new joint national committee guidelines: new challenges of the old problem. Arch Intern Med. 2004;164(19):2126–2134.
3. Vasan RS, Beiser A, Seshadri S, et al. Residual lifetime risk for developing hypertension in middle-aged women and men: the Framingham Heart Study. JAMA. 2002;287(8):1003–1010.
4. Padwal R, Straus SE, McAlister FA. Evidence based management of hypertension. Cardiovascular risk factors and their effects on the decision to treat hypertension: evidence based review. BMJ. 2001;322(7292):977–980.
5. Klein R, Klein BE, Moss SE. The relation of systemic hypertension to changes in the retinal vasculature: the Beaver Dam Eye Study. Trans Am Ophthalmol Soc. 1997;95:329–348; discussion 348–350.
6. Lederle FA, Johnson GR, Wilson SE, et al. Prevalence and associations of abdominal aortic aneurysm detected through screening. Aneurysm Detection and Management (ADAM) Veterans Affairs Cooperative Study Group. Ann Intern Med. 1997;126(6):441–449.
7. Sheridan S, Pignone M, Donahue K. Screening for high blood pressure: a review of the evidence for the U.S. Preventive Services Task Force. Am J Prev Med. 2003;25(2):151–158.
8. Chobanian AV, Bakris GL, Black HR, et al. The seventh report of the Joint National Committee on Prevention, Detection, Evaluation, and Treatment of High Blood Pressure: (JNC VII). JAMA. 2003;289(19):25601–2572.
9. Ezzati M, Lopez AD, Rodgers A, Vander Hoorn S, Murray CJ. Selected major risk factors and global and regional burden of disease. Lancet. 2002;360(9343):1347–1360.
10. American Heart Association. Heart Disease and Stroke Statistics—2004 Update. Dallas, TX: American Heart Association; 2003.
11. Perry HM, Jr., Davis BR, Price TR, et al. Effect of treating isolated systolic hypertension on the risk of developing various types and subtypes of stroke: the Systolic Hypertension in the Elderly Program (SHEP). JAMA. 2000;284(4):465–471.
12. MacMahon S, Peto R, Cutler J, et al. Blood pressure, stroke, and coronary heart disease. Part 1, Prolonged differences in blood pressure: prospective observational studies corrected for the regression dilution bias. Lancet. 1990;335(8692):765–774.
13. Moser M. Update on the management of hypertension: recent clinical trials and the JNC 7. J Clin Hypertens (Greenwich). 2004;6(10 Suppl 2):4–13.
14. The Joint Committee on Detection, Evaluation, and Treatment of High Blood Pressure. The sixth report of the Joint National Committee on Prevention, Detection, Evaluation, and Treatment of High Blood Pressure (JNC VI). Arch Intern Med. 1997;157(21):2413–2446.
15. Hajjar I, Kotchen TA. Trends in prevalence, awareness, treatment, and control of hypertension in the United States, 1988–2000. JAMA. 2003;290(2):199–206.
16. Spranger CB, Ries AJ, Berge CA, Radford NB, Victor RG. Identifying gaps between guidelines and clinical practice in the evaluation and treatment of patients with hypertension. Am J Med. 2004;117(1):14–18.
17. Hyman DJ, Pavlik VN. Characteristics of patients with uncontrolled hypertension in the United States. N Engl J Med. 2001;345(7):479–486.
18. Viera AJ, Thorpe JM, Garrett JM. Effects of sex, age, and visits on receipt of preventive healthcare services: a secondary analysis of national data. BMC Health Serv Res. 2006;6:15.
19. Walsh J, McDonald KM, Shojania KG, et al. Closing the Quality Gap: A Critical Analysis of Quality Improvement Strategies. Technical Review 9. AHRQ Publication No. 04-0051-3. January 2005.
20. Jones DW, Appel LJ, Sheps SG, Roccella EJ, Lenfant C. Measuring blood pressure accurately: new and persistent challenges. JAMA. 2003;289(8):1027–1030.
21. Pickering TG, Hall JE, Appel LJ, et al. Recommendations for blood pressure measurement in humans and experimental animals: Part 1: blood pressure measurement in humans: a statement for professionals from the Subcommittee of Professional and Public Education of the American Heart Association Council on High Blood Pressure Research. Hypertension. 2005;45(1):142–161.
22. Reeves RA. The rational clinical examination. Does this patient have hypertension? How to measure blood pressure. JAMA. 1995;273(15):1211–1218.
23. Van Durme DJ, Goldstein M, Pal N, Roetzheim RG, Gonzalez EC. The accuracy of community-based automated blood pressure machines. J Fam Pract. 2000;49(5):449–452.
24. Verberk WJ, Kroon AA, Kessels AG, de Leeuw PW. Home blood pressure measurement: a systematic review. J Am Coll Cardiol. 2005;46(5):743–751.
25. O'Brien E. A website for blood pressure measuring devices: dableducational.com. Blood Press Monit. 2003;8(4):177–180.
26. Pickering TG, Shimbo D, Haas D. Ambulatory blood-pressure monitoring. N Engl J Med. 2006;354(22):2368–2374.
27. Angeli F, Verdecchia P, Gattobigio R, Sardone M, Reboldi G. White-coat hypertension in adults. Blood Press Monit. 2005;10(6):301–305.
28. Sega R, Trocino G, Lanzarotti A, et al. Alterations of cardiac structure in patients with isolated office, ambulatory, or home hypertension: Data from the general population (Pressione Arteriose Monitorate E Loro Associazioni [PAMELA] Study). Circulation. 2001;104(12):1385–1392.
29. Ohkubo T, Kikuya M, Metoki H, et al. Prognosis of "masked" hypertension and "white-coat" hypertension detected by 24-h ambulatory blood pressure monitoring 10-year follow-up from the Ohasama study. J Am Coll Cardiol. 2005;46(3):508–515.
30. Haynes RB, Sackett DL, Taylor DW, Gibson ES, Johnson AL. Increased absenteeism from work after detection and labeling of hypertensive patients. N Engl J Med. 1978;299(14):741–744.
31. Kannel WB. Blood pressure as a cardiovascular risk factor: prevention and treatment. JAMA. 1996;275(20):1571–1576.
32. Stamler J, Stamler R, Neaton JD. Blood pressure, systolic and diastolic, and cardiovascular risks. US population data. Arch Intern Med. 1993;153(5):598–615.
33. Onusko E. Diagnosing secondary hypertension. Am Fam Physician. 2003;67(1):67–74.
34. Sheridan S, Pignone M, Mulrow C. Framingham-based tools to calculate the global risk of coronary heart disease: a systematic review of tools for clinicians. J Gen Intern Med. 2003;18(12):1039–1052.
35. Pignone M, Sheridan SL, Lee YZ, et al. Heart to Heart: a computerized decision aid for assessment of coronary heart

disease risk and the impact of risk-reduction interventions for primary prevention. Prev Cardiol. 2004;7(1):26–33.

36. Gascon JJ, Sanchez-Ortuno M, Llor B, Skidmore D, Saturno PJ. Why hypertensive patients do not comply with the treatment: results from a qualitative study. Fam Pract. 2004;21(2): 125–130.

37. Vasan RS, Larson MG, Leip EP, Kannel WB, Levy D. Assessment of frequency of progression to hypertension in non-hypertensive participants in the Framingham Heart Study: a cohort study. Lancet. 2001;358(9294):1682–1686.

38. Laupacis A, Sackett DL, Roberts RS. An assessment of clinically useful measures of the consequences of treatment. N Engl J Med. 1988;318(26):1728–1733.

39. Hoes AW, Grobbee DE, Lubsen J. Does drug treatment improve survival? Reconciling the trials in mild-to-moderate hypertension. J Hypertens. 1995;13(7):805–811.

40. Effects of treatment on morbidity in hypertension. II. Results in patients with diastolic blood pressure averaging 90 through 114 mm Hg. JAMA. 1970;213(7):1143–1152.

41. Langford HG, Stamler J, Wassertheil-Smoller S, Prineas RJ. All-cause mortality in the Hypertension Detection and Follow-up Program: findings for the whole cohort and for persons with less severe hypertension, with and without other traits related to risk of mortality. Prog Cardiovasc Dis. 1986; 29(3 Suppl 1):29–54.

42. MRC trial of treatment of mild hypertension: principal results. Medical Research Council Working Party. BMJ (Clin Res Ed). 1985;291(6488):97–104.

43. Taguchi J, Freis ED. Partial reduction of blood pressure and prevention of complications in hypertension. N Engl J Med. 1974;291(7):329–331.

44. SHEP Cooperative Research Group.Prevention of stroke by antihypertensive drug treatment in older persons with isolated systolic hypertension. Final results of the Systolic Hypertension in the Elderly Program (SHEP). JAMA. 1991; 265(24):3255–3264.

45. He FJ, Nowson CA, MacGregor GA. Fruit and vegetable consumption and stroke: meta-analysis of cohort studies. Lancet. 2006;367(9507):320–326.

46. Eisenberg DM, Delbanco TL, Berkey CS, et al. Cognitive behavioral techniques for hypertension: are they effective? Ann Intern Med. 1993;118(12):964–972.

47. Fagard RH. Effects of exercise, diet and their combination on blood pressure. J Hum Hypertens. 2005;19(Suppl 3):S20–24.

48. Whelton SP, Chin A, Xin X, He J. Effect of aerobic exercise on blood pressure: a meta-analysis of randomized, controlled trials. Ann Intern Med. 2002;136(7):493–503.

49. Leon AS, Connett J, Jacobs DR, Jr., Rauramaa R. Leisure-time physical activity levels and risk of coronary heart disease and death. The Multiple Risk Factor Intervention Trial. JAMA. 1987;258(17):2388–2395.

50. Hedley AA, Ogden CL, Johnson CL, Carroll MD, Curtin LR, Flegal KM. Prevalence of overweight and obesity among US children, adolescents, and adults, 1999–2002. JAMA. 2004;291(23):2847–2850.

51. Leiter LA, Abbott D, Campbell NR, Mendelson R, Ogilvie RI, Chockalingam A. Lifestyle modifications to prevent and

control hypertension. Recommendations on obesity and weight loss. CMAJ. 1999;160(Suppl 9):S7–12.

52. Mulrow CD, Chiquette E, Angel L, et al. Dieting to reduce body weight for controlling hypertension in adults. Cochrane Database Syst Rev. 2000(2):CD000484.

53. Getchell WS, Svetkey LP, Appel LJ, Moore TJ, Bray GA, Obarzanek E. Summary of the Dietary Approaches to Stop Hypertension (DASH) randomized clinical trial. Curr Treat Options Cardiovasc Med. Dec 1999;1(4):295–300.

54. Appel LJ, Moore TJ, Obarzanek E, et al. A clinical trial of the effects of dietary patterns on blood pressure. DASH Collaborative Research Group. N Engl J Med. 1997;336(16): 1117–1124.

55. Elmer PJ, Obarzanek E, Vollmer WM, et al. Effects of comprehensive lifestyle modification on diet, weight, physical fitness, and blood pressure control: 18-month results of a randomized trial. Ann Intern Med. 2006;144(7):485–495.

56. Obarzanek E, Proschan MA, Vollmer WM, et al. Individual blood pressure responses to changes in salt intake: results from the DASH-Sodium trial. Hypertension. 2003;42(4): 459–467.

57. He FJ, MacGregor GA. Effect of longer-term modest salt reduction on blood pressure. Cochrane Database Syst Rev. 2004(3):CD004937.

58. Xin X, He J, Frontini MG, Ogden LG, Motsamai OI, Whelton PK. Effects of alcohol reduction on blood pressure: a meta-analysis of randomized controlled trials. Hypertension. 2001;38(5):1112–1117.

59. Sacks FM, Svetkey LP, Vollmer WM, et al. Effects on blood pressure of reduced dietary sodium and the Dietary Approaches to Stop Hypertension (DASH) diet. DASH-Sodium Collaborative Research Group. N Engl J Med. 2001;344(1): 3–10.

60. Psaty BM, Lumley T, Furberg CD, et al. Health outcomes associated with various antihypertensive therapies used as first-line agents: a network meta-analysis. JAMA. May 21 2003;289(19):2534–2544.

61. UK Prospective Diabetes Study Group. Tight blood pressure control and risk of macrovascular and microvascular complications in type 2 diabetes: BMJ. 1998;317(7160):703–713.

62. Curb JD, Schneider K, Taylor JO, Maxwell M, Shulman N. Antihypertensive drug side effects in the Hypertension Detection and Follow-up Program. Hypertension. 1988;11(3 Pt 2):II51–55.

63. Salpeter S, Ormiston T, Salpeter E. Cardioselective beta-blockers for chronic obstructive pulmonary disease. Cochrane Database Syst Rev. 2005(4):CD003566.

64. Salpeter S, Ormiston T, Salpeter E. Cardioselective beta-blocker use in patients with reversible airway disease. Cochrane Database Syst Rev. 2001(2):CD002992.

65. Ko DT, Hebert PR, Coffey CS, Sedrakyan A, Curtis JP, Krumholz HM. Beta-blocker therapy and symptoms of depression, fatigue, and sexual dysfunction. JAMA. 2002; 288(3):351–357.

66. Cappuccio FP, Kerry SM, Forbes L, Donald A. Blood pressure control by home monitoring: meta-analysis of randomised trials. BMJ. 2004;329(7458):145.

67. Saseen JJ, Turner C, Russell RG. Clinical inquiries. What is the best regimen for newly diagnosed hypertension? J Fam Pract. 2005;54(3):281–282.

CHAPTER 12

Venous Thromboembolism

David Weismantel

David Weismantel

CASE 1

B.T. is a 32-year-old woman who presents with a 3-day history of gradually progressive left leg discomfort and swelling. Her symptoms began soon after her return from a vacation in Europe; initially she thought she had strained a muscle. She describes a dull ache from the posterior thigh to the foot. It has been difficult for her to find a shoe that will now fit her swollen foot. She has experienced no fever, chills, or shortness of breath. She is in excellent health, and her only current medication is a combined oral contraceptive.

On examination, she is moderately overweight with normal vital signs. Her left leg has pitting edema from the mid-thigh to the foot; the left calf has a 5-cm greater circumference than the right as measured 10 cm below the tibial tuberosity. Prominent superficial veins are noted about the left thigh and calf, and there is only minimal erythema and tenderness of the extremity.

CLINICAL QUESTIONS

1. What is the probability that B.T. has an acute deep venous thrombosis (DVT)?
2. What would be the most efficient diagnostic strategy at this time?
3. If a diagnosis of DVT is confirmed, what is your recommendation for duration of oral anticoagulant therapy?

CASE 2

P.G. is a 56-year-old man who presents with a 1-day history of rather acute onset of cough, left-sided pleuritic chest pain, and shortness of breath. It has become very difficult for him to climb even a single flight of stairs. He describes his health as excellent and denies any recent travel, immobilization, or trauma. His only medications are atenolol and hydrochlorothiazide. His past medical history is most remarkable for hypertension and an episode of deep venous thrombosis, which occurred after surgery to repair a traumatic femur fracture almost 30 years ago.

On examination, he appears anxious with heart rate 112, respirations 24, and blood pressure 136/88. Pulse oximetry reveals an SpO_2 of 90%. The lungs are clear to auscultation, heart with a regular rhythm without murmur, and lower extremities are without swelling, erythema, or tenderness. A stat electrocardiogram reveals tachycardia without acute or ischemic changes.

CLINICAL QUESTIONS

1. What is the probability that P.G. has an acute pulmonary embolism (PE)?
2. What would be the most efficient diagnostic strategy at this time?
3. If a diagnosis of PE is confirmed, what is your recommendation for duration of oral anticoagulant therapy?

INTRODUCTION

Venous thromboembolism (VTE) describes clinical diagnoses that include deep venous thrombosis (DVT) and pulmonary embolism (PE). DVT is defined as a partial or complete occlusion of a deep vein by thrombus; PE is the blocking of a pulmonary artery or one of its branches by a thrombus or foreign material. Most pulmonary emboli originate from thrombi within the deep vessels of the lower extremities and pelvis—the popliteal, femoral, or iliac veins (1). Upper extremity DVT is less common but may also lead to PE, especially in the presence of a venous catheter.

The age- and sex-adjusted annual incidence of VT is 117 cases per 100,000 persons (DVT is 48 per 100,000; PE is 69 per 100,000). The incidence increases steadily with advancing age and reaches 900 episodes per 100,000 by the age of 85 years (2, 3). PE is diagnosed in more than 500,000 patients in the United States each year and results in approximately 200,000 deaths (4–6). These numbers certainly underestimate the true incidence of PE as it is thought that half of all patients remain undiagnosed. In addition to age, other risk factors for the development of VTE include previous thromboembolism, obesity, pregnancy, the postpartum period, malignancy, inherited thrombophilias, oral contraceptive use, and exogenous estrogen therapy. Environmental risk factors include immobility, trauma, and surgery. The classic Virchow triad of stasis, vascular damage, and hypercoagulability describes the basic pathophysiologic factors that alone, or more commonly in combination, promote the development of thrombosis.

Leg pain and swelling are relatively common presenting complaints in primary care practice. In the 1995 National Ambulatory Medical Care Survey, 1.3% of patients presenting to family physicians had a complaint of leg pain or leg swelling (7). Although these symptoms may be caused by a number of vascular, musculoskeletal, infectious, or dermatologic causes, DVT must always be a primary consideration. Yet when evaluating a patient with suspected DVT, it is important to appreciate that only a small fraction of patients actually have the disease. For this reason, noninvasive testing is required to minimize the likelihood of inappropriate invasive testing or anticoagulation. Considering the risks of postphlebitic syndrome, PE, and death associated with a delayed or missed diagnosis of DVT, and the potential risk of chronic anticoagulation in a patient who does not have a DVT, accurate diagnosis is essential. Likewise, since the most common symptoms (dyspnea, pleuritic pain, cough) and signs (tachypnea, rales, tachycardia) of PE are also extremely common among patients without PE, additional testing is needed to confirm or exclude the diagnosis of PE (8, 9).

This chapter describes an effective diagnostic approach to patients with suspected DVT or PE, making the best possible use of the history and physical examination in validated clinical decision rules. Subsequently, an evidence-based and efficient approach to the treatment of VTE will be outlined.

INITIAL EVALUATION OF THE PATIENT WITH SUSPECTED DEEP VENOUS THROMBOSIS

Pathophysiology and Differential Diagnosis

Leg pain and swelling are typically caused by an imbalance of the oncotic and fluid pressures between the intravascular and extravascular spaces. Acute causes of leg pain and swelling include superficial thrombophlebitis, trauma, cellulitis, and dermatitis. Superficial thrombophlebitis often presents with erythema, induration, and tenderness of a superficial vein caused by thrombus and inflammation; the long saphenous vein is most commonly involved. Twenty-three percent of all patients with superficial thrombophlebitis have simultaneous DVT by duplex ultrasound evaluation (10). Trauma from fractures, muscle tears, and hematomas may also cause pain or swelling in a lower extremity. Symptoms will typically be unilateral with a specific time of injury noted; however, trivial

or occult injuries may at times present as a painful and swollen extremity. Cellulitis is a bacterial infection of the dermis and subcutaneous tissues most often caused by group A β-hemolytic *Streptococcus* or *Staphylococcus aureus*; chronic lower-extremity edema, minor trauma, or a dermatosis may predispose the patient to this problem by damaging the skin. A dermatitis can also cause diffuse tenderness and swelling of a leg; local histamine action causes pruritus and discomfort, with secondary edema of the dermis and subcutaneous tissues.

Chronic causes of leg pain and swelling include chronic venous insufficiency, postphlebitic syndrome, congestive heart failure, pretibial myxedema, and hypoalbuminemia. Often bilateral in nature, chronic venous insufficiency is a result of incompetent valves in the greater or lesser saphenous veins. There is a hereditary predisposition, and women are more commonly affected. DVT and venous hypertension can cause valvular damage and incompetence resulting in postphlebitic syndrome, which in turn can cause chronic lower extremity discomfort, edema, and ulceration. Decreased cardiac output from congestive heart failure may result in systemic venous congestion and lower-extremity edema. Nonpitting pretibial myxedema is a characteristic finding among patients with hypothyroidism; other accompanying symptoms often include weakness, fatigue, weight gain, and cold intolerance. Decreased intravenous oncotic pressure secondary to hypoalbuminemia may cause a chronic, bilateral, lower-extremity pitting edema. Primary etiologies include malnutrition, hepatocellular failure, or excess renal or gastrointestinal loss of albumin. The decrease in intravascular volume stimulates salt retention and leads to further edema formation because the underlying oncotic deficit remains.

A concise differential diagnosis of the painful and swollen lower extremity is shown in Table 12.1. Specific historical and physical examination findings that would suggest a progressive or life-threatening illness are listed in Table 12.2.

TABLE 12.1 Differential Diagnosis of Leg Pain and Swelling

Diagnosis	Frequency in Primary Care Practice
Vascular	
Superficial thrombophlebitis	Very common
Chronic venous insufficiency	Very common
Congestive heart failure	Common
Deep venous thrombosis	Uncommon
Postphlebitic syndrome	Uncommon
Lymphedema	Uncommon
Dermatologic	
Cellulitis	Very common
Dermatitis	Very common
Endocrine and metabolic	
Lymphedema	Uncommon
Hypoalbuminemia	Rare
Traumatic	
Fracture, muscle tear, hematoma	Very common

TABLE 12.2 Red Flags Suggesting Progressive or Life-Threatening Disease in the Patient Suspected of DVT

History and Physical Examination Finding	Diagnoses Suggested
Dyspnea, tachypnea	Pulmonary embolism, congestive heart failure, dysrhythmia
Chest pain	Pulmonary embolism, congestive heart failure, dysrhythmia
Syncope	Pulmonary embolism, dysrhythmia
Hypotension, pulmonary edema, cyanosis	Pulmonary embolism, congestive heart failure, dysrhythmia
Fever	Pulmonary embolism, systemic infection

DVT, deep venous thrombosis.

Clinical Evaluation
HISTORY AND PHYSICAL EXAMINATION

The patient presenting with an acutely painful and swollen leg is at risk for DVT and requires rapid assessment through a focused history and physical examination. Individual historical elements and physical examination findings are of limited value in the diagnosis of DVT. Larger and better-designed studies (11, 12) generally find lower sensitivities and specificities for physical examination findings than poorly designed studies (13). The historical elements with the greatest positive predictive values for DVT are recent surgery and immobilization for more than 3 days in the past 4 weeks (14). The test characteristics of individual historical elements and physical examination findings from the highest-quality studies are outlined in Table 12.3. Note that Homan's sign is of no value in the diagnosis of DVT and should be omitted from the examination.

CLINICAL DECISION RULE

Although the individual elements of the history and physical examination have limited value, groups of these signs and symptoms can be very useful. A clinical decision rule combining the results of nine carefully defined signs and symptoms was developed by Wells et al (14). Later validation of this rule in different groups of patients found that it effectively stratified patients into groups according to their risk of having DVT (15, 16). Patients stratified to the low-, moderate-, and high-risk groups based on this rule had a 3%, 17%, and 75% risk of DVT, respectively. The ability to sort these patients by risk with a clinical decision rule will significantly influence the interpretation of subsequent noninvasive tests. The decision rule is found in Table 12.4.

LABORATORY TESTING

Diagnostic tests for DVT include impedance plethysmography (IPG), duplex venous ultrasound, magnetic resonance imaging (MRI), helical computed tomography, D-dimer, and contrast venography. The latter is an invasive test and is considered to be the reference standard. The accuracy of noninvasive tests varies with the study population (symptomatic versus asymptomatic), and the type of DVT being diagnosed (proximal, distal, or both). The tests are generally much less accurate in asymptomatic patients, and less accurate for diagnosis of distal DVT than for proximal DVT. Table 12.5 summarizes the risk-stratified performance of the various tests for the diagnosis of DVT in symptomatic patients (17–21). Impedance plethysmography and duplex venous ultrasound have excellent positive predictive values to rule in DVT in the high-

TABLE 12.3 Key Elements of the History and Physical Examination for Leg Pain and Swelling

History and Physical Examination Maneuver	Sensitivity (%)	Specificity (%)	LR+	LR−
Immobilization (>3 d in past 4 wk) (14)	24	90	2.4[a]	0.8
Venous dilatation (13)	25	89	2.3	0.8
Recent surgery (14)	9	94	1.5	1.0
Swelling (12)	84	44	1.5	0.4
Temperature difference (11)	72	48	1.4	0.6
Edema (11)	97	33	1.4	0.1[a]
Calf pain (11)	86	19	1.1	0.7
Homan sign (12)	56	39	0.9	1.1
Local tenderness (12)	76	11	0.9	2.2
Erythema (12)	24	62	0.6	1.2

[a]Best individual signs and symptoms for ruling in (immobilization) and ruling out (no edema) DVT in symptomatic patients.

TABLE 12.4 Wells Clinical Decision Rule to Evaluate the Probability of DVT Using the History and Physical Examination

1. Count the number of risk factors for your patient and calculate the risk score:

Risk Factor	Points
Active cancer (treatment ongoing or within previous 6 months or palliative)	1
Paralysis, paresis, or recent plaster immobilization of the lower extremities	1
Recently bedridden for >3 days or major surgery within 4 weeks	1
Localized tenderness along the distribution of the deep venous system	1
Entire leg swelling	1
Calf swelling by >3 cm when compared with the asymptomatic leg (measured 10 cm below the tibial tuberosity)	1
Pitting edema (greater in the symptomatic leg)	1
Collateral superficial veins (nonvaricose)	1
Alternative diagnosis as likely or greater than that of deep vein thrombosis	−2
Total (range, −2 to 8)	

2. Determine the pretest likelihood of DVT:

Risk Score	Risk Category	Probability of DVT
≤0	Low	3% (95% CI, 2%–6%)
1–2	Moderate	17% (95% CI, 12%–23%)
>2	High	75% (95% CI, 63%–84%)

CI, confidence interval; DVT, deep venous thrombosis.
(Adapted from Wells PS, Anderson DR, Bormanis J, et al. Value of assessment of pretest probability of deep-vein thrombosis in clinical management. Lancet. 1997;350:1795–1798.)

risk patient, while D-dimer testing has an excellent negative predictive value to rule out the diagnosis in the low-risk patient.

IPG is a noninvasive modality that has historically proved useful in the evaluation of patients with suspected DVT. Serial IPG is less sensitive than previously thought, however, and it may not detect clinically important proximal thrombi (22). Although IPG remains popular in some countries, it is highly operator-dependent and relatively unavailable in the United States.

Duplex venous ultrasound is the most widely used modality for evaluating patients with suspected DVT. Ultrasound assessment is operator-dependent, unable to distinguish between acute and chronic thrombus, inaccurate in detection of pelvic and calf DVT, and less reliable in the presence of significant edema or obesity. False-positive examinations may be caused by superficial phlebitis, popliteal cysts, and abscess.

Yet when used in combination with a clinical prediction rule, ultrasound examination is accurate in predicting the need for anticoagulation. However, a normal ultrasound study in a moderate- to high-probability patient requires additional investigation (D-dimer or repeat ultrasound) before DVT can be ruled out. If suspicion for DVT persists despite an initial negative duplex ultrasound result, you should repeat the test 4 to 7 days later and educate the patient about warning signs of pulmonary embolism or worsening DVT. Two studies with

a total of 2,107 patients repeated the ultrasound 5 to 7 days later if the first ultrasound result was normal and did not anticoagulate patients with two normal ultrasound results (23, 24). Only 0.6% of these patients had a thromboembolic complication (DVT or PE) during the next 3 months, and only one of these occurred during the week between ultrasounds. A third study repeated the ultrasound 1 day and again 6 days later in patients with a normal initial ultrasound result (25). Of 390 patients with three normal ultrasound results, only 6 had a thromboembolic complication during the next 3 months. Thus, in patients with two normal ultrasound results a week apart, the risk of a thromboembolic complication during the next 3 months is only about 1%.

Although there is considerable interest in MRI for the diagnosis of DVT, the studies to date have been small (26–28) or methodologically flawed, with limitations ranging from a failure to blind, to a retrospective design, to a poor-quality reference standard (29–31). When compared with contrast venography, MRI sensitivity ranges from 80% to 100%, and specificity from 93% to 100%. Use of MRI to diagnose DVT should currently be limited to cases in which there is considerable local experience with the technique and in which contrast venography may be indicated but there are relative contraindications to the use of intravenous contrast agents (32, 33). Likewise, there is insufficient evidence to support the routine use of helical computed tomographic (CT) venography for the

TABLE 12.5   Risk-Stratified Characteristics of Diagnostic Tests for Venous Thromboembolism in Symptomatic Patients

Test	Sensitivity (%)	Specificity (%)	Pretest Probability by Wells Clinical Decision Rule (%)					
			High Risk: 75%		Moderate: 17%		Low Risk: 3%	
			PPV	NPV	PPV	NPV	PPV	NPV
Deep Venous Thrombosis								
Impedence plethysmography (17)	77 to 98	83 to 97	93 to 99	55 to 94	48 to 87	95 to 100	12 to 50	99 to 100
Duplex ultrasonography (17)	88 to 97	80 to 96	93 to 99	69 to 91	47 to 83	97 to 99	12 to 42	99 to 100
Helical computed tomography (18)	71	93	97	52	68	94	24	99
Magnetic resonance imaging (19)	56 to 100	88 to 100	93	40	49	91	13	99
D-dimer (20)	89	77	39	89	—	—	14	99
Pulmonary Embolism			High Risk: 78.4%		Moderate: 27.8%		Low Risk: 3.4%	
Helical computed tomography (42)	77	89	96	52	73	91	20	99
Magnetic resonance imaging (42)	77	87	96	51	70	91	17	99
Transthoracic echocardiography (42)	68	89	96	43	70	88	18	99
Transesophageal echocardiography (42)	70	81	93	43	59	88	12	99
D-dimer erythrocyte agglutination (SimpliRed) (42)	89	59	89	60	46	93	7	99
Ventilation-perfusion scanning (43)	98	10	80	58	30	93	3	99

NPV, negative predictive value, PPV; positive predictive value.
(Adapted from Ramzi DW, Leeper KV. DVT and pulmonary embolism: Part I. Diagnosis. Am Fam Physician. 2004;69:2829–36.)

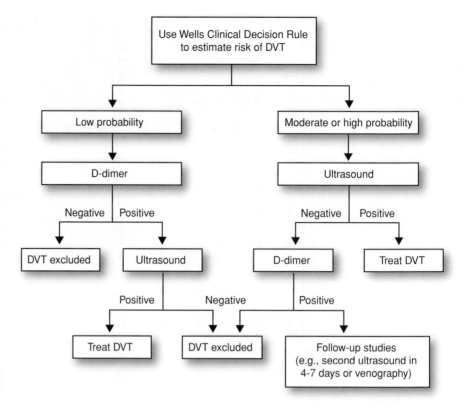

Figure 12.1 • Algorithm for evaluation of DVT using a combination of the Wells Clinical Decision Rule and diagnostic testing. Abbreviations: DVT, deep venous thrombosis. (Adapted from Institute for Clinical Systems Improvement. Healthcare guidelines. Venous thromboembolism. *http://www.icsi.org/knowledge/detail.asp?catID=29&itemID=202.* Accessed June 1, 2006).

diagnosis of DVT (34). Both MRI and CT venography are relatively expensive compared to duplex venous ultrasound.

Elevated levels of D-dimer, a fibrin degradation product, are associated with an increased risk of DVT. Different D-dimer assays vary considerably in their performance. Latex agglutination assays are quick and inexpensive but are not recommended because they are less accurate. Microplate enzyme-linked immunosorbent assays (ELISAs) are accurate but expensive; membrane ELISAs are less expensive and almost as accurate. Note that a negative D-dimer test alone does not rule out DVT; 2% to 5% of patients with suspected DVT and a negative D-dimer test result actually have a DVT. This is similar to the performance of ultrasound alone in unselected patients with suspected DVT. The D-dimer test is most useful in patients with a moderate risk of DVT, and a normal duplex venous ultrasound result. In one study, only 1 of 598 patients with a normal duplex ultrasound and a normal D-dimer test result developed a DVT during the next 3 months. Of 88 patients with a normal duplex ultrasound result but an elevated D-dimer test result, 5 had a DVT detected 1 week later with a repeat ultrasound, and an additional 2 patients had a venous thromboembolic complication during the next 3 months (35).

Another recent study found that the combination of a low-risk assessment by a validated clinical prediction rule and a negative D-dimer test effectively ruled out DVT (36). Finally it has been demonstrated that patients with a Wells clinical prediction rule score of less than 2 points and a negative D-dimer test were less likely to have VTE during follow up than were patients with a negative ultrasound examination (0.4% versus 1.4%) (37). It is important to note that a positive

D-dimer test does not raise the likelihood of DVT appreciably and is therefore of limited diagnostic value.

Approach to the Patient

The indiscriminate application of diagnostic testing to all patients with suspected DVT would risk the overtreatment of low-risk patients and the undertreatment of high-risk patients. Initial use of the Wells DVT Clinical Decision Rule will stratify patients into low-, moderate-, or high-risk groups. The rule was developed and validated in nonpregnant patients with a first episode of DVT; pregnant patients and those with a history of previous DVT should be evaluated more aggressively, as they have an increased risk of DVT.

Once a patient has been placed in the low-, moderate-, or high-risk group, the algorithm in Figure 12.1 should guide further evaluation. This algorithm was developed by the Institute for Clinical Systems Improvement (ICSI) and incorporates evidence-based recommendations for the use of pretest clinical probability with prediction rules, D-dimer testing, and imaging in the diagnosis of DVT (38). The diagnosis may be considered ruled out in low-risk patients with a negative duplex venous ultrasound and in moderate-risk patients with a normal D-dimer and negative ultrasound. Moderate- and high-risk patients with a normal initial ultrasound but an abnormal D-dimer should undergo a repeat ultrasound in 1 week or proceed to contrast venography. Moderate- and high-risk patients with an abnormal ultrasound should be treated for DVT. It is important that this algorithm not be used inflexibly. Patients with new or progressive symptoms, such as a patient with suspected DVT who then develops signs and symptoms of PE, should be evaluated immediately.

INITIAL EVALUATION OF THE PATIENT WITH SUSPECTED PE

Although acute PE is an important diagnostic possibility in the patient presenting with chest pain and shortness of breath, many other cardiac, pulmonary, gastroenterologic, and musculoskeletal etiologies are possible and should always be considered in the evaluation. Table 12.6 presents a concise differential diagnosis of chest pain.

Clinical Evaluation
HISTORY AND PHYSICAL EXAMINATION

The patient presenting with chest pain and shortness of breath is at risk for PE and requires rapid assessment through a focused history and physical examination. Individual historical elements and physical examination findings are of limited value in the diagnosis of PE. The classic triad of signs and symptoms (chest pain, dyspnea, hemoptysis) are neither sensitive nor specific. They occur in fewer than 20% of patients in whom the diagnosis of PE is made, and most patients with these symptoms are found to have another diagnosis to account for them. The most common symptoms and signs are summarized in Table 12.7 (39, 40).

CLINICAL DECISION RULE

A clinical decision rule combining the results of seven carefully defined signs and symptoms was developed and validated by Wells and colleagues (41). Patients stratified to the low-, moderate-, and high-risk groups based on this rule had a 3%, 28%, and 78% risk of PE, respectively. The ability to sort these patients by risk with a clinical decision rule will again significantly influence the interpretation of subsequent noninvasive tests. The decision rule is found in Table 12.8.

TABLE 12.7 Symptoms and Signs in Acute Pulmonary Embolism

Symptom	Frequency
Dyspnea	73%
Pleuritic chest pain	66%
Cough	37%
Hemoptysis	13%
Sign	
Tachypnea	70%
Rales	51%
Tachycardia	30%
Fourth heart sound	24%
Accentuated pulmonic component of second heart sound	23%
Circulatory collapse	8%

LABORATORY TESTING

Diagnostic tests for PE include ventilation-perfusion (V/Q) scanning, helical computed tomography, D-dimer testing, and pulmonary angiography. The latter is an invasive test and is considered to be the reference standard. Table 12.5 summarizes the risk-stratified performance of the various tests for the diagnosis of PE in symptomatic patients (42, 43). Helical computed tomography has an excellent positive predictive value to rule in PE in the high-risk patient, while D-dimer testing has an excellent negative predictive value to rule out the diagnosis in the low-risk patient.

The V/Q scan has historically been the standard diagnostic study in patients with suspected PE. Defects in radio-

TABLE 12.6 Differential Diagnosis of Chest Pain and Shortness of Breath

Diagnosis	Frequency in Primary Care Practice
Cardiac	
Coronary artery disease	Common
Aortic dissection	Uncommon
Pericarditis	Uncommon
Pulmonary	
Pneumonia	Very common
Pulmonary embolism	Uncommon
Pneumothorax	Uncommon
Gastroenterologic	
Gastroesophageal reflux disease	Very common
Esophageal spasm	Uncommon
Musculoskeletal	
Trauma	Very common
Costochondritis	Very common

TABLE 12.8 Wells Clinical Decision Rule to Evaluate the Probability of PE Using the History and Physical Examination

1. Count the number of risk factors for your patient and calculate the risk score:

Risk Factor	Points
Clinical signs or symptoms of DVT (leg swelling, pain with palpation of deep veins)	3
Alternative diagnosis less likely than PE	3
Heart rate greater than 100 beats per minute	1.5
Immobilization or surgery within past 4 weeks	1.5
Previous DVT or PE	1.5
Hemoptysis	1
Malignancy	1
Total (range, 0 to 12.5)	

2. Determine the pretest likelihood of DVT:

Risk Score	Risk Category	Probability of DVT
<2	Low	3.3% (95% CI, 1.7%–4.8%)
2–6	Moderate	20.2% (95% CI, 17.1%–23.3%)
>6	High	62.9% (95% CI, 52.9%–73.0%)

CI, confidence interval; DVT, deep venous thrombosis; PE, pulmonary embolism.
(Adapted from Wells PS, Anderson DR, Rodger M, et al. Derivation of a simple clinical model to categorize patients' probability of pulmonary embolism: increasing the model utility with the SimpliRED D-dimer. Thromb Haemost. 2000; 83:418.)

active tracer uptake from ventilated and perfused areas of the lungs are reported as normal, nearly normal, or indicating a low, intermediate, or high probability of embolus. A high-probability V/Q scan provides sufficient evidence and specificity for the initiation of treatment for PE. Likewise, a normal or near-normal scan should be considered sufficiently sensitive to rule out the diagnosis. Unfortunately, at least half of scans are indeterminate (low or intermediate probability). In the Prospective Investigation of Pulmonary Embolism Diagnosis (PIOPED) study, 40% of patients with confirmed PE had a high-probability V/Q scan, 40% had an intermediate-probability scan, and 14% had a low-probability scan (43).

Helical CT scanning has a sensitivity and specificity of nearly 90% to detect large main and lobar emboli, yet is typically unable to detect smaller subsegmental involvement (44). Current use of helical CT scanning is determined by its availability. This imaging modality is often used to supplement other diagnostic tests (V/Q scanning and D-dimer) when such tests are nondiagnostic. As CT technology improves and resolution increases to the point that reliable evaluation of subsegmental vessels is possible, helical CT scanning may replace pulmonary angiography as the gold standard in the diagnosis of PE. It has been suggested that helical CT scanning may be safe to use for ruling out PE, at least in patients with a low or moderate clinical probability of embolism (45, 46). In summary, the diagnostic accuracy of helical CT scanning appears to vary widely from institution to institution due to differences in image quality and interpreter experience (47, 48).

D-dimer testing in combination with the Wells Clinical Prediction Rule has been shown to be effective in ruling out PE in patients presenting to the emergency department (49). Use of D-dimer for the diagnosis of PE has been extensively studied and is best characterized as having good sensitivity and negative predictive value, but poor specificity. It is for this reason that D-dimer testing is typically used in coordination with other testing modalities in the evaluation of the moderate- to high-risk patient.

Approach to the Patient

As with DVT, the indiscriminate application of diagnostic testing to all patients with suspected PE would risk the overtreatment of low-risk patients and the undertreatment of high-risk patients. Initial use of the Wells PE Clinical Decision Rule will again stratify patients into risk groups. Once a patient has been placed in the low-, moderate-, or high-risk group, the algorithms in Figures 12.2 and 12.3 should guide further evaluation with helical CT and V/Q scanning respectively. These algorithms were also developed by the ICSI and incorporate evidence-based recommendations for the use of pretest clinical probability with prediction rules, D-dimer testing, and imaging in the diagnosis of PE (38). The diagnosis may be considered ruled out in low-risk patients with a normal D-dimer. Moderate- and high-risk patients require imaging by helical CT or V/Q scan. It should again be stressed that these algorithms not be used inflexibly.

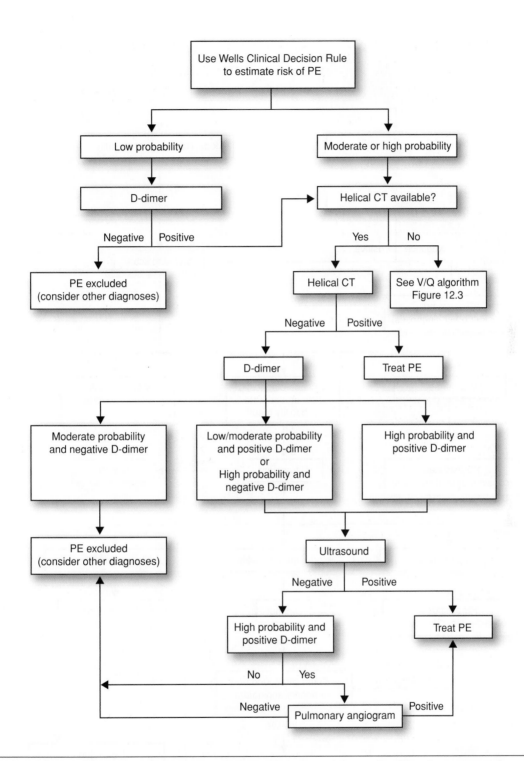

Figure 12.2 • Algorithm for Evaluation of PE using a combination of the Wells Clinical Decision Rule and Helical CT Scan.   CT, computed tomography; PE, pulmonary embolism. (Adapted from Institute for Clinical Systems Improvement. Healthcare guidelines. Venous thromboembolism. *http://www.icsi.org/knowledge/detail.asp?catID = 29&itemID = 202.* Accessed June 1, 2006.)

MANAGEMENT

The algorithm in Figure 12.4 outlines a basic, evidence-based approach to the treatment of VTE, including initial heparin anticoagulation, oral warfarin therapy, and other supportive measures. It emphasizes interventions that have been shown to minimize the likelihood of acute or long-term complications. Because DVT and PE are clinical manifestations of the same pathophysiologic process, the standard anticoagulation protocols are identical.

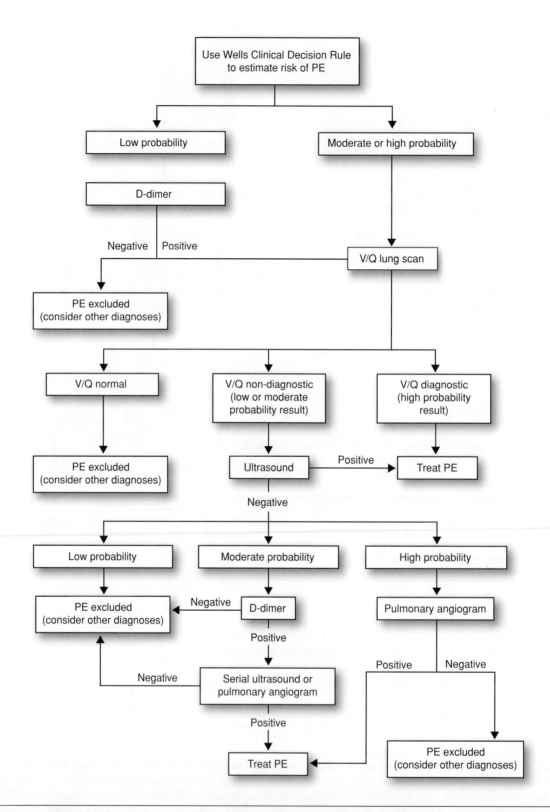

Figure 12.3 • Algorithm for Evaluation of PE using a combination of the Wells Clinical Decision Rule and Ventilation-Perfusion Lung Scan. PE, pulmonary embolism; V/Q, ventilation-perfusion. (Adapted from Institute for Clinical Systems Improvement. Healthcare guidelines. Venous thromboembolism. *http://www.icsi.org/knowledge/detail.asp?catID = 29&itemID = 202.* Accessed June 1, 2006.)

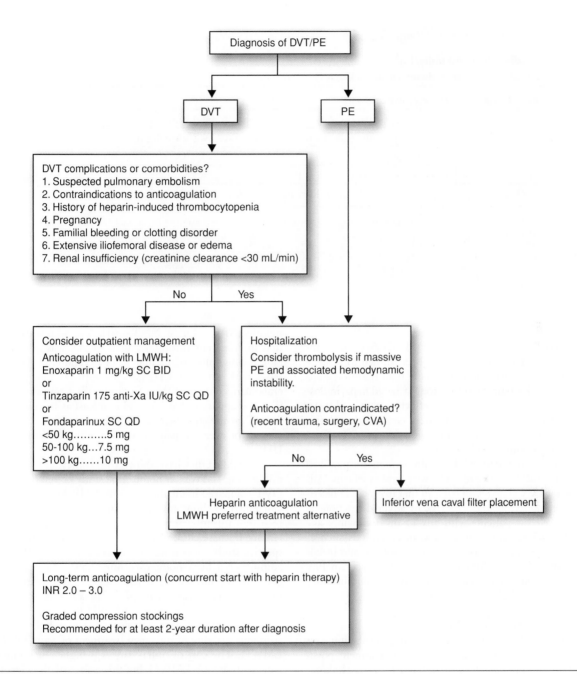

Figure 12.4 • Algorithm for treatment of VTE. BID, twice daily; DVT, deep venous thrombosis; LMWH; low-molecular-weight heparin; PE, pulmonary embolism; QD, every day; SC, subcutaneously; VTE, venous thromboembolism.

Initial Management of VTE

Prompt anticoagulation with heparin is the first priority in treating the patient with VTE; this prevents the local extension, embolization, and recurrence of venous thromboembolic disease. Oral warfarin is started simultaneously. Heparin acts immediately to catalyze the inhibition of several activated coagulation factors and leads to the stabilization of the intravascular thrombus. Heparinization is typically continued for 5 days and until a stable and therapeutic international normalized ratio (INR) is established with oral warfarin therapy. There are three approved approaches to the initial anticoagu-

lant treatment of a patient with acute VTE: intravenous unfractionated heparin (UH), subcutaneous low-molecular-weight heparin (LMWH), and subcutaneous fondaparinux, a factor Xa inhibitor.

UNFRACTIONATED HEPARIN

The traditional treatment of VTE has been anticoagulation with intravenous UH; the goal of this therapy is the prompt establishment of an activated partial thromboplastin time (APTT) of 1.5 to 2.5 times the control (50). Successfully achieving a therapeutic APTT within 24 hours has been associated with a decreased likelihood of recurrent thromboembo-

TABLE 12.9 Weight-Based Intravenous Heparin Nomogram

Loading dose: 80 units/kg
Initial maintenance dose: 18 units/kg/h

APTT Level	Dosage Adjustment
<35 sec	80 units/kg bolus, then increase infusion rate by 4 units/kg/h
35–45 sec	40 units/kg bolus, then increase infusion rate by 2 units/kg/h
46–75 sec	No change
71–90 sec	Decrease infusion rate by 2 units/kg/h
>90 sec	Hold infusion 1 h, then decrease infusion rate by 3 units/kg/h

APTT levels are drawn 6 hours after any dosage change and should be ordered every 24 hours until two consecutive APTT levels are therapeutic.
APTT, activated partial thromboplastin time.
(Reprinted from Raschke RA, Reilly BM, Guidry JR, et al. The weight-based heparin dosing nomogram compared with a "standard care" nomogram. Ann Intern Med. 1993;119:874–881.)

lism (5% versus 23%; absolute risk reduction [ARR]—18%; number needed to treat [NNT]—5.5) (51, 52). Several protocols for managing UH therapy have been shown to achieve therapeutic anticoagulation more rapidly than traditional approaches. Table 12.9 summarizes a weight-based heparin dosing nomogram that has been proven effective, safe, and superior to standard therapy in a randomized controlled trial; this protocol achieved therapeutic anticoagulation in 97% of patients within 24 hours (53).

Patients treated with UH should remain hospitalized until therapeutically anticoagulated with oral warfarin. Adverse reactions associated with heparin therapy include bleeding and thrombocytopenia. The risk of adverse reactions is most increased for patients with any of the following: age greater than 65 years, recent surgery, or conditions such as peptic ulcer disease, liver disease, occult neoplasia, and bleeding diathesis. Transient thrombocytopenia may occur in 10% to 20% of patients, but major hemorrhagic complications occur in fewer than 2% of patients (54).

LMWHS AND FONDAPARINUX

The advantages of LMWHs are fixed dosing, a subcutaneous route of administration (making outpatient treatment possible), and a more predictable anticoagulant response. Laboratory monitoring is typically unnecessary as a result of better bioavailability, a longer half-life, and dose-independent clearance. If monitoring of LMWH is necessary, an anti-Xa level of 0.4 to 0.7 U/mL is the goal of therapy (55). The only LMWHs currently approved and labeled by the US Food and Drug Administration for the treatment of acute VTE are enoxaparin at a dosage of 1 mg/kg administered subcutaneously twice daily (outpatient or inpatient therapy) or 1.5 mg/kg once daily (inpatient therapy only), tinzaparin at a dosage of 175 anti-Xa IU/kg administered subcutaneously once daily, and fondaparinux (<50 kg, 5 mg; 50–100 kg, 7.5 mg; >100 kg, 10 mg) administered subcutaneously once daily.

A meta-analysis of 11 randomized controlled trials with a total of 3,674 patients demonstrated the safety and effectiveness of LMWH therapy for acute DVT. Compared with UH, LMWH significantly reduced the risk of death over 3 to 6

months (ARR—1.65%; NNT—61). A trend toward a reduction in recurrent thromboembolic events was also observed (56). A subsequent meta-analysis of 13 randomized controlled trials, with a total of 4,447 patients with DVT or pulmonary embolism, confirmed these findings (57). From this information, it is apparent that LMWH is at least as safe and effective as UH for the treatment of DVT, and that one death is prevented for every 60 patients treated with LMWH instead of UH.

Several studies have shown the efficacy and safety of administering LMWH at home. One study of 400 patients with DVT compared home therapy with LMWH to inpatient UH and failed to show any significant difference in the risk of recurrent thromboembolism or major bleeding (58). No difference in these clinical outcomes was found in another prospective study comparing patient self-injection with injection administered by a home-care nurse (59). Most patients are both capable and willing to participate in this treatment regimen; 91% were pleased with home therapy and 70% felt comfortable with self-injection of LMWH (60).

A cost-effectiveness analysis published in 1999 studied the economic viability of universal treatment of acute DVT with LMWH. The cost of initial care was higher in hospitalized patients receiving LMWH, but this was partially offset by the reduced costs for early complications. Treatment with LMWH cost $7,820 for each quality-adjusted year of life gained. Further analysis showed that LMWH saved money when at least 8% of patients were treated at home or if late complications were assumed to occur 25% less frequently in patients receiving LMWH. Thus, LMWH is highly cost-effective and is the preferred treatment of DVT (61).

Several organizations have published recommendations or guidelines suggesting an outpatient treatment for uncomplicated DVT (38, 50, 62). It is generally agreed that patients with an uncomplicated DVT, good cardiopulmonary reserve, no excessive bleeding risk, and normal renal function can be safely treated with LMWH at home. Those with the comorbidities or possible contraindications to anticoagulation noted in Figure 12.4 should typically be hospitalized for initial management. Also, the home therapy patient will require education regarding the correct dosage and administration of LMWH, recognition of adverse events, and available resources for addressing questions and problems during the treatment course. Whether patients are treated in the hospital or at home, LMWH should be considered the primary standard treatment for VTE. The relative safety, tolerability, efficacy, and cost-effectiveness of LMWH make it the obvious and preferred therapeutic alternative. Because of the risks of hypoxemia and hemodynamic instability, initial outpatient treatment of PE is not currently advised, although clinical trial evidence for its safety in carefully selected patients is building.

THROMBOLYSIS

Although thrombolytic therapy is not typically recommended for the treatment of DVT, it is clearly indicated in patients with massive PE and associated hemodynamic instability. However, the role of thrombolysis in the treatment of patients with submassive PE remains controversial. In the largest study to date, improved survival was observed in patients treated with alteplase plus heparin compared with heparin alone. Using death and major complications as the end point, the number needed to treat was 7.3 for patients with PE and pulmonary hypertension or right ventricular dysfunction but without arterial hypotension or shock. One fewer death was observed for every 82 patients treated with this combination therapy (63). In patients with PE, the usual dose of 100 mg of alteplase is given by intravenous infusion over a period of 2 hours. Streptokinase is given in a 250,000 IU loading dose, followed by 100,000 IU per hour for 24 hours. Delivery of thrombolytics directly into the thrombus by catheter has not been shown to be superior to peripheral infusion.

VENA CAVA FILTER PLACEMENT

Placement of an inferior vena cava filter is reserved for patients with a contraindication to anticoagulation, a serious complication of anticoagulation, or recurrent thromboembolism despite adequate anticoagulation. To date there have been no randomized trials or cohort studies directly comparing inferior vena cava interruption with standard anticoagulation therapy. However, a recent clinical trial studied the effect of vena cava filter placement in 400 anticoagulated patients and showed a significant decrease in PE assessed at day 12 of therapy (ARR—3.7%; NNT—27) but a significant increase in the rate of recurrent symptomatic DVT over the next 2 years (absolute risk increase [ARI]—9.2%; number needed to harm [NNH]—11) (64). The available evidence does not support the use of a vena cava filter in patients with an initial and uncomplicated DVT.

ACTIVITY

Although patients with acute DVT have traditionally been confined to bed rest for 3 to 7 days, there is no evidence that this practice improves clinical outcomes. An observational study of 638 patients with DVT who were allowed to ambulate with compression stockings showed a low incidence of V/Q lung scan—documented PE as compared with that in the literature (65). A more recent randomized trial of 126 patients with acute proximal vein thrombosis compared 8 days of strict bed rest with early mobilization; there was no statistically significant difference in the incidence of scintigraphically

detectable PE (66). These studies do not support the previous recommendation of bed rest for the acute treatment of DVT.

Long-Term Management
EXTENDED ORAL ANTICOAGULATION

After the initial evaluation, stabilization, and treatment of the patient with VTE, subsequent long-term therapy will minimize the risk of recurrent thromboembolism and chronic postphlebitic complications. Although unsupported by specific evidence, most recommendations include discontinuing and avoiding any exogenous estrogen therapy. Oral anticoagulation with warfarin decreases the incidence of recurrent thromboembolic events. Because warfarin therapy is contraindicated during pregnancy, long-term treatment with LMWH should be substituted when VTE occurs in a pregnant woman (62).

For a patient presenting with VTE, oral anticoagulation with warfarin should be started on the first day of treatment, after heparin loading is complete. Adequacy of therapy is monitored by measurement of the INR, a standardization of the prothrombin time ratio now used to correct for the variance between laboratories resulting from the use of different thromboplastin reagents. The full antithrombotic effect of warfarin requires 3 to 5 days to establish; therefore, heparin is overlapped with warfarin for at least the first 5 days of therapy.

Both 5 mg and 10 mg algorithms have been proposed and validated for initiation of warfarin. Two studies in hospitalized patients receiving heparin found that the 5 mg algorithm was preferable (67, 68) while a larger, more recent study in outpatients receiving LMWH supports a 10 mg algorithm (69). Unless new data demonstrate that one or the other of these algorithms is definitely better, both should be considered reasonable options for the initiation of warfarin (70); the algorithms are shown in Tables 12.10a and 12.10b. For older patients, an even lower 2.5 mg dose is sometimes used. The heparin may be discontinued after 5 days if the INR is within the therapeutic range of 2.0 to 3.0 (62).

The optimal duration of oral anticoagulant therapy for a first episode of VTE varies and depends on whether risk factors are transient or persistent. In general, patients with a clear risk factor for an initial DVT or PE, such as a long plane flight or being postoperative, only require 3 months of treatment. A comparison of 3 months anticoagulation with extended oral anticoagulation of approximately 10 months for patients with DVT or PE found a reduction in the risk of recurrent VTE (ARR—26%; NNT—4), but an increased risk of major bleeding (ARI—3.8%; NNH,—26) in the extended therapy group over a period of 2 years (71). In general, longer durations of oral anticoagulant therapy are associated with a decreased risk of venous thromboembolic recurrence, yet an increased risk of bleeding complications. A recent Cochrane review of 2,994 patients with DVT or PE in eight studies similarly found a decreased risk of recurrent VTE with prolonged warfarin therapy (0.9% versus 7.8%; ARR—6.9%; NNT—14) but an increased incidence of major bleeding (2.0% versus 0.2%; ARR—1.8%; NNH—56) (72).

In the case of recurrent VTE, lifetime anticoagulant therapy should be considered in the absence of risk factors for bleeding. The specific recommendations for duration of oral

TABLE 12.10a	Algorithm for Initiation of Warfarin Using 5 mg Initial Dose	
Day	**INR**	**Dosage**
1		5.0 mg
2	< 1.5	5.0 mg
	1.5–1.9	2.5 mg
	2.0–2.5	1.0–2.5 mg
	> 2.5	0.0 mg
3	< 1.5	5–10 mg
	1.5–1.9	2.5–5.0 mg
	2.0–3.0	0.0–2.5 mg
	> 3.0	0.0 mg
4	< 1.5	10 mg
	1.5–1.9	5.0–7.5 mg
	2.0–3.0	0.0–5.0 mg
	> 3.0	0.0 mg
5	< 1.5	10 mg
	1.5–1.9	7.5–10.0 mg
	2.0–3.0	0.0–5.0 mg
	> 3.0	0.0 mg
6	< 1.5	7.5–12.5 mg
	1.5–1.9	7.5–10.0 mg
	2.0–3.0	0.0–7.5 mg
	> 3.0	0.0 mg

anticoagulation have been adapted from the American College of Chest Physicians and are included in Table 12.11 (62).

The incidence of recurrent VTE is increased in patients with cancer, and these patients also are more likely to have complications from long-term warfarin therapy. A large multicenter trial in patients with cancer and VTE found that the likelihood of recurrent thrombosis was lower in the patients who received long-term treatment with LMWH than in those who received warfarin. In this trial, 13 patients needed to be treated with LMWH instead of warfarin to avoid one episode of recurrent DVT (73). However, 6 months of treatment costs over $10,000, making the cost of preventing one recurrent DVT in excess of $100,000.

COMPRESSION STOCKINGS

The addition of compression stockings to standard oral anticoagulant therapy is supported by a study of 194 patients. Those using knee-high 30- to 40-mm Hg custom-fitted graded compression stockings for 2 years had a lower risk of developing mild-moderate postphlebitic syndrome (ARR—27.1%; NNT—4), and the incidence of severe postphlebitic syndrome was also decreased (ARR—12%; NNT—8). Although there was no reduction in the rate of recurrent VTE, extended use of compression stockings improved the long-term clinical course and should be considered a valuable addition in the management of DVT (74).

INVESTIGATION FOR POSSIBLE MALIGNANCY OR INHERITED THROMBOPHILIA

Although there is an increased incidence of cancer at the time of presentation in patients with idiopathic VTE (i.e., no clear

TABLE 12.10b Algorithm for the Initiation of Warfarin Using 10 mg Initial Dose

Patients are given 10 mg of warfarin on days 1 and 2.

Day 3 INR	Warfarin Dose in mg on Days 3 and 4		Day 5 INR	Warfarin Dose in mg on Days 5, 6, and 7
			<2.0	15.0, 15.0, 15.0
			2.0 to 3.0	7.5, 5.0, 7.5
<1.3	15.0, 15.0		3.1 to 3.5	0.0, 5.0, 5.0
1.3 to 1.4	10.0, 10.0	→	>3.5	0.0, 0.0, 2.5
			<2.0	7.5, 7.5, 7.5
1.5 to 1.6	10.0, 5.0		2.0 to 3.0	5.0, 5.0, 5.0
1.7 to 1.9	5.0, 5.0	→	3.1 to 3.5	2.5, 2.5, 2.5
			>3.5	0.0, 2.5, 2.5
			<2.0	5.0, 5.0, 5.0
			2.0 to 3.0	2.5, 5.0, 2.5
2.0 to 2.2	2.5, 2.5		3.1 to 3.5	0.0, 2.5, 0.0
2.3 to 3.0	0.0, 2.5	→	>3.5	0.0, 0.0, 2.5
			<2.0	2.5, 2.5, 2.5
>3.0	0.0, 0.0		2.0 to 3.0	2.5, 0.0, 2.5
		→	3.1 to 4.0	0.0, 2.5, 0.0
			>4.0	0.0, 0.0, 2.5

INR, international normalized ratio.
(Adapted from Kovacs MJ, Rodger M, Anderson DR, et al. Comparison of 10-mg and 5-mg warfarin initiation nomograms together with low-molecular-weight heparin for outpatient treatment of acute venous thromboembolism. A randomized, double-blind, controlled trial. Ann Intern Med. 2003;138:716.)

TABLE 12.11 ACCP Recommendations for Long-Term Anticoagulation in Patients with DVT or PE
(INR goal: 2.0 to 3.0)

Thromboembolism	Anticoagulation	Duration	SOR
First episode of VTE with a reversible or time-limited risk factor (e.g., trauma, surgery)	Warfarin	3 months	A
First episode symptomatic thrombosis confined to deep veins of calf	Warfarin	3 months	A
First episode of idiopathic VTE	Warfarin	6–12 months, consider indefinite therapy	A
First episode of VTE with a single documented thrombophilic condition	Warfarin	6–12 months, consider indefinite therapy	A
First episode of VTE with documented antiphospholipid antibodies or two or more thrombophilic conditions	Warfarin	12 months, consider indefinite therapy	A
Recurrent VTE	Warfarin	Indefinitely	B
Any episode VTE with cancer	LMWH	Indefinitely, or until cancer is resolved	A

ACCP, American College of Chest Physicians; DVT, deep venous thrombosis; PE, pulmonary embolism; VTE, venous thromboembolism.
(Adapted from Buller HR, Agnelli G, Hull RD, et al. Antithrombotic Therapy for Venous Thromboembolic Disease: The Seventh ACCP Conference on Antithrombotic and Thrombolytic Therapy. Chest. 2004;126: 401S–428S.)

predisposing cause such as bed rest), a complete medical evaluation including history, physical examination, and basic laboratory studies, and further evaluation as indicated based on these findings, has been shown to adequately detect malignancy in this setting. A retrospective study with 986 consecutive patients (142 with DVT and 844 with DVT ruled out) found no difference in the incidence of cancer over the next 34 months (75). A study of 260 patients with DVT followed for 2 years of regular visits found that all subsequent cancers were diagnosed because the patient became symptomatic and sought care from a family physician (76). Beyond initial and age-appropriate cancer screening, there is no evidence that an aggressive search for an underlying malignancy is warranted.

The inherited thrombophilias are associated with an increased risk for VTE, yet the diagnosis of one of these defects does not substantially change the clinical management of initial or recurrent VTE. Likewise, counseling regarding the increased risk associated with prolonged immobilization, surgery, pregnancy, and exogenous estrogen therapy would be unchanged. A sensible approach may be to screen for hereditary thrombophilias (factor V Leiden, prothrombin G20210A mutation, protein C deficiency, protein S deficiency, antithrombin III deficiency, anti-phospholipid antibodies, and hyperhomo-cysteinemia) in the case of recurrent VTE, a younger patient, or a patient with a family history of thromboembolic disease. If an inherited thrombophilia is diagnosed, further screening and possible identification of other family members could lead to avoidance of known secondary risk factors and subsequent thromboembolic events. The typical patient with an initial episode of VTE will not benefit from the investigation for an inherited coagulation defect.

PATIENT EDUCATION

Patients with VTE should be instructed about the importance of an extended course of oral anticoagulation in decreasing

the likelihood of recurrent thromboembolism. Oral anticoagulation therapy requires regular evaluation of the INR and adjustment of the warfarin dosage. The patient should also avoid periods of prolonged immobilization and exogenous estrogen therapy in the future. Most importantly, each patient should learn to recognize the symptoms of a recurrent VTE so that therapy may be started in a timely fashion.

CASE 1

Historical elements that predispose B.T. to DVT are her recent prolonged immobilization while traveling on her European vacation, and her current use of oral contraceptives. The physical examination identifies the following specific risks per the Wells Clinical Decision Rule: 1) entire leg swelling; 2) calf swelling by more than 3 cm when compared with the asymptomatic leg; 3) pitting edema; and 4) collateral superficial veins. The total score is four, which places B.T. in the high-risk category, with a 75% probability of DVT prior to any diagnostic imaging.

The next diagnostic step would be a venous duplex ultrasound. A positive test would confirm the diagnosis of DVT, and a negative test should be followed by a D-dimer. A negative D-dimer would effectively rule out DVT, while a positive test would require further follow-up testing with venography or a repeat ultrasound in 3–7 days. The high pretest probability mandates a highly sensitive test to rule out this potentially serious diagnosis.

If a diagnosis of DVT is confirmed, B.T. should complete at least a 3-month course of oral warfarin anticoagulant therapy for a first-time occurrence of DVT, with reversible risk factors of exogenous estrogen therapy (oral contraceptive) and immobilization. This should be an informed decision made after a careful review of the decreased risk of recurrent thromboembolism and increased risk of bleeding complications with longer courses of oral anticoagulant therapy. B.T. should also be encouraged to discontinue her oral contraceptive as this will increase the likelihood of recurrent thromboembolic disease.

CASE 2

The only historical element that predisposes M.G. to PE is the past history of an episode of VTE. The physical examination identifies tachycardia with a heart rate greater than 100 beats per minute as a specific risk per the Wells Clinical Decision Rule. The total score is 3 points, which places M.G. in the moderate-risk category with a 20% probability of PE prior to any diagnostic imaging. Based on the algorithms in Figures 12.2 and 12.3, the next diagnostic step would be a helical CT scan or a V/Q lung scan. A positive imaging test would confirm the diagnosis of PE, and a negative CT or nondiagnostic V/Q scan should be followed by further risk stratification and testing with D-dimer or venous duplex ultrasound per the diagnostic algorithms.

If a diagnosis of PE is confirmed, M.G. should remain on oral warfarin anticoagulant therapy indefinitely for a recurrent episode of VTE. This should be an informed decision made after a careful review of the decreased risk of recurrent thromboembolism and increased risk of bleeding complications with longer courses of oral anticoagulant therapy.

REFERENCES

1. Moser KM, LeMoine JR. Is embolic risk conditioned by location of deep venous thrombosis? Ann Intern Med. 1981;94(4 pt 1):439–444.
2. Anderson FA, Wheeler HB, Goldberg RJ, et al. A population-based perspective of the hospital incidence and case-fatality rates of deep vein thrombosis and pulmonary embolism: the Worcester DVT study. Arch Intern Med. 1991;151:933–938.
3. Silverstein MD, Heit JA, Mohr DN, et al. Trends in the incidence of deep vein thrombosis and pulmonary embolism. A 25-year population-based study. Arch Intern Med. 1998;158:585–593.
4. Horlander KT, Mannino DM, Leeper KV. Pulmonary embolism mortality in the United States, 1979–1998: an analysis using multiple-cause mortality data. Arch Intern Med. 2003;163:1711.
5. Dismuke SE, Wagner EH. Pulmonary embolism as a cause of death. The changing mortality in hospitalized patients. JAMA. 1986;255:2039.
6. Dalen JE, Alpert JS. Natural history of pulmonary embolism. Prog Cardiovasc Dis. 1975;17:257.
7. US Department of Health and Human Services. National Ambulatory Medical Care Survey (1995). NCHS CD-ROM Series 13, No. 11, SETS Version 1.221. Washington, DC: US Department of Health and Human Services; 1997.
8. Stein PD, Terrin ML, Hales CA, et al. Clinical, laboratory, roentgenographic and electrocardiographic findings in patients with acute pulmonary embolism and no pre-existing cardiac or pulmonary disease. Chest. 1991;100:598.
9. Stein PD, Saltzman HA, Weg JG. Clinical characteristics of patients with acute pulmonary embolism. Am J Cardiol. 1991;68:1723.
10. Jorgensen JO, Hanel KC, Morgan AM, et al. The incidence of deep venous thrombosis in patients with superficial thrombophlebitis of the lower limbs. J Vasc Surg. 1993;18:70–73.
11. Sandler DA, Duncan JS, Ward P, et al. Diagnosis of deep-vein thrombosis: comparison of clinical evaluation, ultrasound, plethysmography, and venoscan with x-ray venogram. Lancet. 1984;2:716–718.
12. O'Donnell TF Jr, Abbott WM, Athanasoulis CA, et al. Diagnosis of deep venous thrombosis in the outpatient by venography. Surg Gynecol Obstet. 1980;150:69–74.
13. McLachlan J, Richards T, Paterson JC. An evaluation of clinical signs in the diagnosis of venous thrombosis. Arch Surg. 1962;85:738–744.
14. Wells PS, Hirsh J, Anderson DR, et al. Accuracy of clinical assessment of deep-vein thrombosis. Lancet. 1995;345:1326–1330.
15. Wells PS, Anderson DR, Bormanis J, et al. Value of assessment of pretest probability of deep-vein thrombosis in clinical management. Lancet. 1997;350:1795–1798.
16. Wells PS, Hirsh J, Anderson DR, et al. A simple clinical model for the diagnosis of deep-vein thrombosis combined with impedance plethysmography: potential for an improvement in the diagnostic process. J Intern Med. 1998;243:15–23.
17. Peterson DA, Kazerooni EA, Wakefield TW, Knipp BS, Forauer AR, Bailey BJ, et al. Computed tomographic venography is specific but not sensitive for diagnosis of acute lower-extremity deep venous thrombosis in patients with suspected pulmonary embolus. J Vasc Surg. 2001;34:798–804.
18. Gottschalk A, Stein PD, Goodman LR, Sostman HD. Overview of prospective investigation of pulmonary embolism diagnosis II. Semin Nucl Med. 2002;32:173–182.
19. Fraser DG, Moody AR, Morgan PS, Martel AL, Davidson I. Diagnosis of lower-limb deep venous thrombosis: a prospective blinded study of magnetic resonance direct thrombus imaging. Ann Intern Med. 2002;136:89–98.
20. Wells PS, Anderson DR, Rodger M, Forgie M, Kearon C, Dreyer J, et al. Evaluation of D-dimer in the diagnosis of suspected deep-vein thrombosis. N Engl J Med. 2003;349:1227–1235.
21. Ramzi DW, Leeper KV. DVT and pulmonary embolism. Part I. Diagnosis. Am Fam Physician. 2004;69:2829–2836.
22. Cogo A, Prandoni P, Villalta S, Polistena P, Bernardi E, Simioni P, et al. Changing features of proximal vein thrombosis over time. Angiology. 1994;45:377–382.
23. Cogo A, Lensing AW, Koopman MW, et al. Compression ultrasonography for diagnostic management of patients with clinically suspected deep vein thrombosis: prospective cohort study. BMJ. 1998;316:17–20.
24. Birdwell BG, Raskob GE, Whitsett TL, et al. The clinical validity of normal compression ultrasonography in outpatients suspected of having deep venous thrombosis. Ann Intern Med. 1998;128:1–7.
25. Heijboer H, Buller HR, Lensing AW, et al. A comparison of real-time compression ultrasonography with impedance plethysmography for the diagnosis of deep-vein thrombosis in symptomatic outpatients. N Engl J Med. 1993;329:1365–1369.
26. Spritzer CE, Sostman HD, Wilkes DC, Coleman RE. Deep venous thrombosis: experience with gradient-echo MR imaging in 66 patients. Radiology. 1990;177:235–241.
27. Moody AR, Pollock JG, O'Connor AR, Bagnall M. Lower-limb deep venous thrombosis: direct MR imaging of the thrombus. Radiology. 1998;209:349–355.

28. Vukov LF, Berquist TH, King BF. Magnetic resonance imaging for calf deep venous thrombophlebitis. Ann Emerg Med. 1991;20:497–499.

29. Laissy JP, Cinqualbre A, Loshkajian A, et al. Assessment of deep venous thrombosis in the lower limbs and pelvis: MR venography versus duplex Doppler sonography. Am J Roentgenol. 1996;167:971–975.

30. Erdman WA, Jayson HT, Redman HC, et al. Deep venous thrombosis of extremities: role of MR imaging in the diagnosis. Radiology. 1990;174:425–431.

31. Spritzer CE, Norconk JJ, Sostman HD, Coleman RE. Detection of deep venous thrombosis by magnetic resonance imaging. Chest. 1993;104:54–60.

32. ACCP Consensus Committee on Pulmonary Embolism. Opinions regarding the diagnosis and management of venous thromboembolic disease. Chest. 1998;113:499–504.

33. Tapson VF, Carroll BA, Davidson BL, et al. The diagnostic approach to acute venous thromboembolism. Clinical practice guideline. American Thoracic Society. Am J Respir Crit Care Med. 1999;160:1043–1066.

34. Peterson DA, Kazerooni EA, Wakefield TW, Knipp BS, Forauer AR, Bailey BJ, et al. Computed tomographic venography is specific but not sensitive for diagnosis of acute lower-extremity deep venous thrombosis in patients with suspected pulmonary embolus. J Vasc Surg. 2001;34:798–804.

35. Bernardi F, Prandoni P, Lensing AWA, et al. D-dimer testing as an adjunct to ultrasonography in patients with clinically suspected deep vein thrombosis: prospective cohort study. BMJ. 1998;317:1037–1040.

36. Bates SM, Kearon C, Crowther M, Linkins L, O'Donnell M, Douketis J, et al. A diagnostic strategy involving a quantitative latex D-dimer assay reliably excludes deep venous thrombosis. Ann Intern Med. 2003;138:787–94.

37. Wells PS, Anderson DR, Rodger M, Forgie M, Kearon C, Dreyer J, et al. Evaluation of D-dimer in the diagnosis of suspected deep-vein thrombosis. N Engl J Med. 2003;349:1227–1235.

38. Institute for Clinical Systems Improvement. Healthcare guidelines. Venous thromboembolism. *http://www.icsi.org/knowledge/detail.asp?catID = 29&itemID = 202.* Accessed June 1, 2006.

39. Stein, PD, Terrin, ML, Hales, CA, et al. Clinical, laboratory, roentgenographic and electrocardiographic findings in patients with acute pulmonary embolism and no pre-existing cardiac or pulmonary disease. Chest. 1991;100:598.

40. Stein, PD, Saltzman, HA, Weg, JG. Clinical characteristics of patients with acute pulmonary embolism. Am J Cardiol. 1991;68:1723.

41. Wells PS, Anderson DR, Rodger M, et al. Derivation of a simple clinical model to categorize patients' probability of pulmonary embolism: increasing the model utility with the SimpliRED D-dimer. Thromb Haemost. 2000;83:418.

42. Kline JA, Johns KL, Colucciello SA, Israel EG. New diagnostic tests for pulmonary embolism. Ann Emerg Med. 2000;35:168–180.

43. The PIOPED Investigators. Value of the ventilation/perfusion scan in acute pulmonary embolism. Results of the Prospective Investigation of Pulmonary Embolism Diagnosis (PIOPED). JAMA. 1990;263:2753–2759.

44. Mullins MD, Becker DM, Hagspiel KD, Philbrick JT. The role of spiral volumetric computed tomography in the diagnosis of pulmonary embolism. Arch Intern Med. 2000;160:293–298.

45. Van Strijen MJ, de Monye W, Schiereck J, Kieft GJ, Prins MH, Huisman MV, et al. Single-detector helical computed tomography as the primary diagnostic test in suspected pulmonary embolism: a multicenter clinical management study of 510 patients. Ann Intern Med. 2003;138:307–314.

46. Musset D, Parent F, Meyer G, Maitre S, Girard P, Leroyer C, et al. Diagnostic strategy for patients with suspected pulmonary embolism: a prospective multicentre outcome study. Lancet. 2002;360:1914–1920.

47. Eng J, Krishnan JA, Segal JB, et al. Accuracy of CT in the diagnosis of pulmonary embolism: a systematic literature review. AJR Am J Roentgenol. 2004;183:1819.

48. Rathbun SW, Raskob GE, Whitsett TL. Sensitivity and specificity of helical computed tomography in the diagnosis of pulmonary embolism: a systematic review. Ann Intern Med. 2000;132:227.

49. Wells PS, Anderson DR, Rodger M, Stiell I, Dreyer JF, Barnes D, et al. Excluding pulmonary embolism at the bedside without diagnostic imaging: management of patients with suspected pulmonary embolism presenting to the emergency department by using a simple clinical model and D-dimer. Ann Intern Med. 2001;135:98–107.

50. Hirsh J, Hoak J. Management of deep vein thrombosis and pulmonary embolism. A statement for healthcare professionals. Council on Thrombosis (in consultation with the Council on Cardiovascular Radiology), American Heart Association. Circulation. 1996;93:2212–2245.

51. Hull RD, Raskob GE, Hirsh J, et al. Continuous intravenous heparin compared with intermittent subcutaneous heparin in the initial treatment of proximal vein thrombosis. N Engl J Med. 1986;315:1109–1114.

52. Hull RD, Raskob GE, Brant RF, et al. Relation between the time to achieve the lower limit of the APTT therapeutic range and recurrent venous thromboembolism during heparin treatment for deep vein thrombosis. Arch Intern Med. 1997;157:2562–2568.

53. Raschke RA, Reilly BM, Guidry JR, et al. The weight-based heparin dosing nomogram compared with a "standard care" nomogram. Ann Intern Med. 1993; 119:874–881.

54. Juergens CP, Semsarian C, Keech AC, Beller EM, Harris PJ. Hemorrhagic complications of intravenous heparin use. Am J Cardiol. 1997;80:150–154.

55. Weitz JI. Low-molecular-weight heparins. N Engl J Med. 1997;337:688–698.

56. Gould MK, Dembitzer AD, Doyle RL, et al. Low-molecular-weight heparins compared with unfractionated heparin for treatment of acute deep venous thrombosis. A meta-analysis of randomized, controlled trials. Ann Intern Med. 1999;130:800–809.

57. Dolovich LR, Ginsberg JS, Douketis JD, et al. A meta-analysis comparing low-molecular-weight heparins with unfractionated heparin in the treatment of venous thromboembolism. Arch Intern Med. 2000;160:181–188.

58. Koopman MMW, Prandoni P, Piovella F, et al. Treatment of venous thrombosis with intravenous unfractionated heparin administered in the hospital as compared with subcutaneous low-molecular-weight heparin administered at home. N Engl J Med. 1996;334:682–687.

59. Wells PS, Kovacs MJ, Bormanis J, et al. Expanding eligibility for outpatient treatment of deep venous thrombosis and pulmonary embolism with low-molecular-weight heparin: a comparison of patient self-injection with homecare injection. Arch Intern Med. 1998;158:1809–1811.

60. Harrison L, McGinnis J, Crowther M, et al. Assessment of outpatient treatment of deep-vein thrombosis with low-molecular-weight heparin. Arch Intern Med. 1998;158:2001–2003.

61. Gould MK, Dembitzer AD, Sanders GD, et al. Low-molecular-weight heparins compared with unfractionated heparin

TABLE 13.1 Developmental Screening Tools (87)

Name	Age Range	Scoring	Sensitivity Specificity	Time	Number of Items	Cost
Tools with information obtained from parents						
Ages and Stages Questionnaire (ASQ)	0–60 months	Pass/fail	70–90% 76–91%	10–15 minutes	30	~$4.60
Parents' Evaluations of Developmental Status (PEDS)	0–8 years	Low, medium, or high risk	74–79% 70–80%	2 minutes	10	~$1.19
Infant-Toddler Checklist for Language and Communication	6–24 months	Manual table of cutoff scores	78% 74%	5–10 minutes	24	~$3.60
Tools requiring direct examination of children						
Bayley Infant Neurodevelopmental Screener (BINS)	3–24 months	Low, medium, or high risk	Accuracy 75–86%	10–15 minutes	10–13	~$10.45
Brigance Screens	0–90 months	Cutoffs, age equivalents, percentiles, and quotients	70–82%	10 minutes		~$11.68
Battelle Developmental Inventory Screening Test (BDIST)	12–96 months	Cutoffs	70–80% 70–80%	15–35 minutes		~$20.55

(From Glascoe FP. Commonly Used Screening Tools. In: *http://www.dbpeds.org/articles/detail.cfm?textid=539*: Developmental and Behavioral Pediatrics Online (*dbpeds.org*); Accessed 11/22/2005. Used with permission.)

screening tests are normal, referral for further evaluation should be considered if parents remain concerned.

There are three types of screening tests (see Table 13.1). Structured parent interviews and general checklists both rely on parental report of the child's skills and behaviors. Multiple studies have shown that parental report is accurate and can be used successfully for screening (15–17). The third type of screening test is direct examination screening. Direct examination testing should only be used if a parent cannot give a report. This may be the case in situations of foster care or adoption, when the parent or caregiver does not yet know the child well. In addition, it may occur when a parent is significantly impaired.

MANAGEMENT

The Individuals with Disabilities Education Act (IDEA) Amendments of 1997 require early intervention for individuals with developmental disabilities through the development of community-based systems (18). Children younger than 3 years of age may receive services through the state's early intervention program. Those older than 3 years of age receive services through the local school district. The family physician will often need to put together an interdisciplinary team to optimize management. Table 13.2 lists key recommendations for practice.

TABLE 13.2 Key Recommendations for Practice

Recommendation	Strength of Recommendation*	References
Developmental screening should be performed at all well child checks, infancy through school age	A	4, 8
Early treatment of developmental delays should be achieved, ideally in the preschool years, because it significantly improves outcomes	A	2, 3
Parental concern about behavior or development should always trigger screening	A	11–14

*A = consistent, good-quality patient-oriented evidence; B = inconsistent or limited-quality patient-oriented evidence; C = consensus, disease-oriented evidence, usual practice, expert opinion, or case series. For information about the SORT evidence rating system, see *http://www.aafp.org/afpsort.xml*.

FAILURE TO THRIVE

Growth is one of the most fundamental tasks of childhood. When growth is interrupted, failure to thrive occurs. Causes may be medical, nutritional, behavioral, psychological, or environmental. Whatever the underlying causes, the immediate cause of failure to thrive is malnutrition. This malnutrition may result because insufficient calories are offered, because of a child's inability to take or to retain sufficient calories, or because of increased caloric need secondary to increased metabolism (19). The diagnosis of failure to thrive should prompt an investigation of the underlying causes. Appropriate investigation may lead to the earlier diagnosis of medical or psychosocial problems.

Traditionally failure to thrive has been considered to be organic in about 30% of cases and nonorganic in about 70% of cases. Instead, it is now understood that the causes of failure to thrive are usually intermixed and multifactorial. For example, an infant with gastrointestinal reflux disease may have decreased caloric intake due to discomfort. The infant may also have a decreased ability to retain sufficient calories secondary to emesis. As the parents watch their infant eating less, and possibly showing a growth disturbance, they will become anxious. The parents then coax or even force feed their infant. This can lead to a power struggle with further decreased intake by the child, and increasing frustration of the parent. The malnourished child will then become irritable and lethargic, escalating mealtime conflicts. Once the diagnosis of failure to thrive is made the parent may feel a sense of failure, further complicating the parent-child relationship (19, 20). As in this example, with any cause of failure to thrive behavioral complications related to feeding will usually develop and will often persist after the underlying disturbance has been corrected (21).

Failure to thrive is usually diagnosed by the primary care physician during well child visits (22). Parents are often unaware of a growth disturbance until it is pointed out during a visit. Eighty percent of children who will have failure to thrive are diagnosed by 18 months of age (23). The single greatest risk factor for failure to thrive is poverty. For children living in poverty inadequate food availability, homelessness, and stress can all lead to malnutrition (24, 25). Children living in poverty are also less likely to receive early diagnosis and intervention for medical and psychosocial problems, which are precursors for failure to thrive.

Initial Evaluation

There is no single definition, measurement, or set of criteria that best diagnose failure to thrive (26). Most clinicians will look for children without weight gain in 2 months or children who have dropped 2 percentile curves in less than 6 months (23). The most common cause of an abnormal growth curve, however, is measurement or plotting error; this should always be considered and ruled out before other action is taken.

Growth failure will initially be evident in weight alone, followed by height, and then head circumference. Once height has been affected the malnutrition has become chronic. By the time head circumference is affected the child will be at increased risk for long-term neurological complications.

Failure to thrive must also be distinguished from other causes of growth disturbance. In congenital, constitutional, familial, and endocrine causes of growth disturbance, length will decline before weight, or proportionately to weight. Children with constitutional growth delay will be both short and thin. Those with endocrine related delays will be short and heavy. In familial short stature, growth will remain parallel to the growth curve.

Once the diagnosis of failure to thrive is established, the cause must be pursued. History is generally the most important diagnostic tool in finding the underlying cause of failure to thrive (23). Often several visits will be needed to obtain the full history. A thorough physical exam is also important. History and physical should be complete before any laboratory studies or radiographs are considered. There is no routine panel of tests for children with failure to thrive. History and physical should guide the choice of any diagnostic studies. Often, no diagnostic studies will be needed.

Almost any medical problem can lead to failure to thrive in young children. Inadequate intake of calories can occur due to dysphagia, nausea, anorexia, or altered taste secondary to problems like dental caries, enlarged adenoids, or medication side effects (21, 27). A choking episode may result in food phobia. Cardiac or pulmonary disease may cause fatigue that interferes with intake. Malabsorption of calories can occur in diseases like cystic fibrosis, inflammatory bowel disease, and diarrhea. Increased caloric need can result from tumors, recurrent infections, or endocrine disorders.

Psychosocial factors leading to failure to thrive can be broken down into three categories—interactions between the child and caregiver, psychosocial health of the caregiver, and infant characteristics (23). A caregiver suffering from an affective disorder or substance abuse may be unable to recognize a child's cues. This may lead to over- or underfeeding. An infant with special needs, prematurity, or a difficult temperament may be unable to adequately communicate their needs. Difficulty may arise from poor fit between the temperament of the child and the caregiver. For example, a baby that needs a firm, regular schedule may not do well with a caregiver who prefers an irregular schedule. Similarly, a calm caregiver may have difficulty with an energetic, crying baby.

Management

The management of children with failure to thrive must focus on the antecedents to the growth problem. Because the cause is usually multifactorial, the child may require nutritional, medical, psychological, and developmental treatment (28).

Even when the underlying cause of the malnutrition isn't curable, nutrition can be optimized by working with the child and the family. The family should be educated in how to make mealtimes pleasant, and minimize mealtime conflict. Parents can be taught how to recognize infant cues and educated about normal toddler behavior.

Hospitalization is rarely needed for the child with failure to thrive. However, hospitalization should be considered in cases of severe malnutrition, hypothermia, bradycardia, or hypertension. Hospitalization is also appropriate in the face of abuse or neglect, when there is an impaired caregiver, when there has been a lack of catch-up growth with outpatient treatment, or when there is a need to observe parent-child feeding interactions.

Long-Term Monitoring

Whether or not there are long-term sequelae from failure to thrive depends on the cause and the severity of the problem. When there are significant psychosocial problems involved, children seem to have more long-term disturbances. This is likely related to the underlying cause of the failure to thrive, rather than the malnutrition itself. In addition, failure to thrive in the first year of life, particularly the first 6 months, is more likely to impact brain development. Under nutrition at this time may cause persistent fine and gross motor problems and speech and language delay.

AUTISTIC SPECTRUM DISORDER

Autistic spectrum disorder (ASD) refers to a continuum of disorders of brain development involving impaired communication skills, impaired social interactions, and restricted, repetitive, or stereotypical patterns of behavior (29). The etiology of ASD remains poorly understood, although there is clearly a strong genetic component which seems to be modulated by the child's environment. Each symptom of ASD may range from mild to severe in the individual child.

ASD, also referred to as pervasive developmental disorder (PDD), includes 5 subtypes, including autistic disorder, Aspergers' syndrome, pervasive developmental disorder not otherwise specified (PDD-NOS), Rett's syndrome, and childhood disintegrative disorder. On the severe end of the spectrum is autistic disorder, with higher functioning children having the milder Asperger's syndrome. Children with Asperger's syndrome exhibit poor peer relationships, lack of empathy, and a tendency to over focus on specific topics. They often have normal intelligence and normal language skills. PDD-NOS refers to children who don't meet the criteria for autistic disorder but who have severe impairments.

Rett's syndrome and childhood disintegrative disorder are very rare and very severe autistic spectrum disorders. Rett's syndrome is a neurodegenerative disorder that affects girls ages 1–3 years, following a period of normal development. Patient's experience a loss of hand skills, gross motor and coordination skills, language and cognitive skills, and social interaction skills. Childhood disintegrative disorder occurs after age 24 months, following a period of normal development. It results in profound losses in play, language, social, and motor skills.

The prevalence of autistic disorder is thought to be about 1 in 1,000 children. Studies have found that at least 2 in 1,000 children, and possibly more, suffer from ASD (30, 31). Prevalence rates are increasing. This may represent changing inclusion criteria, increased awareness, or a true increase in prevalence (32, 33). Recurrence rates in siblings are 3%–7%, emphasizing the importance of genetic counseling for families that have a child with ASD (34).

Initial Evaluation

Early diagnosis and intervention is critical for optimal outcomes for children with ASD. Unfortunately, fewer than 50% are diagnosed before kindergarten. Parental concern about the develop-ment of social skills is fairly rare. Therefore, when it occurs it should be taken very seriously (35).

Concern should be raised when a child exhibits aberrant social skills, abnormal eye contact, aloofness, failure to orient to name, failure to use gestures to point or show, lack of interactive play, or lack of interest in peers (35). Several screening tools are available for use in the primary care of fice including the Checklist for Autism in Toddlers (CHAT) for 18 month olds, and the Pervasive Developmental Disorder Screening Test. When ASD is suspected based on history, clinical findings, or screening tests, referral should be made to a specialist who can confirm the diagnosis.

Management

There are no widely accepted guidelines or protocols for treatment of ASD. However, there is agreement that early and sustained intervention greatly improves outcomes. The effectiveness of most specific interventions remains unknown. For most children treatment should include parental education and support, community services, occupational therapy, physical therapy, structured play, behavior management, and, in some cases, medication.

CEREBRAL PALSY

CP is a disorder of movement and posture caused by injury to the motor areas of the brain. Motor abnormalities must be static, not progressive over time. Because of rapid developmental changes in the first year of life, a definitive diagnosis of CP should not be made until after one year of age. In most cases, muscle tone will be decreased in early infancy, with increased tone occurring by 12–18 months of age.

CP has many different etiologies, all involving injury to the developing brain. The insult may occur during the prenatal period, during labor and delivery, or in the first few years of life. In 20%–30% of cases, no etiology is found despite a thorough work-up. Congenital CP is present from birth, but may not be identified until later. Major causes of congenital CP include prenatal infection, particularly by rubella, cytomegalovirus, or toxoplasmosis, and Rh histoimmuno incompatibility syndrome. When CP occurs during labor and delivery, it is usually caused by severe asphyxia leading to hypoxic-ischemic encephalopathy. This type of CP is much less common than previously believed, accounting for only about 6% of cases. Postnatal CP may occur secondary to central nervous system infection, such as bacterial meningitis or viral encephalitis, injury, such as motor vehicle accidents, falls, child abuse, or stroke as a result of prematurity or coagulation disorders.

Initial Evaluation

The diagnosis of CP should be suspected if the child is over 1 year of age, and abnormalities occur in several of the following areas: posture, oropharyngeal problems (tongue thrusts, swallowing), strabismus, increased or decreased muscle tone, abnormal evolution of primitive reflexes, or abnormal deep tendon reflexes. Other conditions that often occur with CP include seizures, refractive errors, hearing loss, MR, failure to thrive, learning disabilities, attention problems, and behavior problems.

There are four subtypes of CP—spastic, athetoid, ataxic, or mixed. For each type severity can range from extremely mild to debilitating. Spastic CP is the most common, occurring in 70%–80% of cases. It may occur as a diplegia involving only the bilateral lower extremities, a quadriplegia, or a hemiplegia. Muscles will often become stiffly contracted. Often legs will rotate inward and cross at the knees resulting in a scissors gait. Athetoid or dyskinetic CP occurs in 10%–20% of cases and involves uncontrolled, slow, writhing movements. Dysarthria, drooling, and grimacing may also occur. Ataxic CP accounts for an additional 5%–10% of cases and involves abnormalities of balance and depth perception. Children with ataxic CP will often have poor coordination, a wide-based gait, and an intention tremor.

Management

The prognosis for children with CP is extremely variable depending upon the type and severity of the neurologic insult. Best outcomes will occur when an interdisciplinary team is involved early on in treatment. This should include the primary care physician; a social worker and psychologist; occupational, physical, and speech therapists; a communication therapist, and educational and vocational specialists.

MENTAL RETARDATION

MR refers to cognitive ability that is markedly below average for chronological age with a decreased ability to adapt to the environment. The diagnosis of decreased cognitive ability must be made via standardized testing. Because standardized testing is less predictive in young children, the term developmental delay is usually used for children under age 3.

MR occurs at four levels of severity. Mild MR refers to individuals with IQs of 50–70. They are able to attain math and reading skills at a 3rd- to 6th-grade level. Individuals with mild MR can conform socially, can maintain employment, and can integrate quite well in society. Individuals with moderate MR have IQs of 35–49. They can perform simple activities and basic self-care. Individuals with severe MR have IQs of 20–34. They require supervision and support, but may participate in simple, repetitive self-care activities. Those with profound MR have IQs less than 20 and are not capable of self-care (29).

MR occurs in 2%–3% of the general population. In 50%–70% of cases, an etiology can be found with adequate work-up. Acquired MR may occur in children from near-drowning, traumatic brain injury, central nervous system malignancy, or lead exposure. Prenatal MR can occur from infection, first trimester maternal fever, intrauterine alcohol or anticonvulsant exposure, or untreated maternal phenylketonuria. MR is more common in premature infants with very low birth weights. MR can also result from metabolic diseases (e.g., hypothyroidism), single-gene mutations (e.g., Fragile X syndrome or neurofibromatosis), or chromosomal abnormalities, such as in Down's syndrome, Klinefelter's syndrome, or Prader-Willi syndrome (36, 37).

ATTENTION DEFICIT — HYPERACTIVITY DISORDER

ADHD is the most common neurodevelopmental disorder of childhood and is characterized by inattention, hyperactivity, and impulsivity (29). Most studies on the prevalence of ADHD report between 4%–8% of children in community-based samples have symptoms impairing function. Prevalence data are largely limited to children between 6 and 12 years old (38). The cost of treating a child with ADHD ranges between $1,000 and $8,000 per year (39). ADHD can lead to depression, low self-esteem, increased risk of injury, school failure, early school dropout, substance abuse, and increased risk of criminality. ADHD has been traditionally thought of as a disease of childhood; however, recent studies demonstrate that 60%–80% of children with ADHD have symptoms with functional impairment into adulthood (40).

The AAP recommends that primary care clinicians initiate an evaluation for ADHD in all children between 6 and 12 years old presenting with symptoms of hyperactivity, inattention, impulsivity, academic underachievement, or behavior problems. The reliable diagnosis of ADHD requires the use of the *Diagnostic and Statistical Manual of Mental Disorders, 4th Edition* (DSM IV) diagnostic criteria (Table 13.3), collection of information from multiple sources, and a thorough clinical evaluation (41). Successful treatment requires the following: 1) establishing a management program, 2) setting appropriate, behaviorally oriented treatment goals, 3) the use of stimulant and/or behavior therapy, and 4) reassessment and monitoring (42).

Initial Evaluation

The evaluation should begin with the chief complaint. Why are the parents bringing the problem to the clinician's attention? Is this a routine exam? How is school? Has the teacher raised concerns with learning? Can the child complete tasks such as homework? Do the parents or caregivers have problems with behavior at home or school? In setting the tone for the evaluation of ADHD, approach the parent as a partner. Recognize that many parents present with an agenda or opinion (often well-informed), particularly with regard to medication. Describe the course, time frame, and contents of the evaluation.

DSM IV criteria should guide history taking (see Table 13.3 for diagnostic criteria). Symptoms must be present for 6 months. There are three subtypes of ADHD—inattentive, hyperactive, and mixed type. A child must have six symptoms of inattention or six symptoms of hyperactivity and/or impulsivity as listed in the diagnostic criteria. Many children will meet criteria for both inattentive type- and hyperactive-impulsive type-ADHD (combined type). Symptoms of ADHD must be present prior to age 7 and must be present in two or more settings (e.g., school and home). There must be clear impairment in functioning (social, academic, or occupational). Other disorders must be ruled out as the sole cause of symptoms (pervasive developmental disorder, schizophrenia, mood disorders, personality disorders, etc.) (29).

Many disorders co-occur with ADHD. The presence of these disorders does not preclude the effective evaluation or treatment of ADHD, but special attention to comorbid disease should be paid in the initial evaluation of patients for ADHD as the presence these co-occuring diseases may complicate diagnosis, and affect management plans. Co-occurrence rates with ADHD in community-based samples are as follows: oppositional defiant disorder—35%; conduct disorder (CD)—26%; anxiety disorders—26%; and depressive disor-

TABLE 13.3 DSM-IV Criteria for ADHD

I. Either A or B:

A. Six or more of the following symptoms of inattention have been present for at least 6 months to a point that is disruptive and inappropriate for developmental level:

Inattention

1. Often does not give close attention to details or makes careless mistakes in schoolwork, work, or other activities.

2. Often has trouble keeping attention on tasks or play activities.

3. Often does not seem to listen when spoken to directly.

4. Often does not follow instructions and fails to finish schoolwork, chores, or duties in the workplace (not due to oppositional behavior or failure to understand instructions).

5. Often has trouble organizing activities.

6. Often avoids, dislikes, or doesn't want to do things that take a lot of mental effort for a long period of time (such as schoolwork or homework).

7. Often loses things needed for tasks and activities (e.g., toys, school assignments, pencils, books, or tools).

8. Is often easily distracted.

9. Is often forgetful in daily activities.

B. Six or more of the following symptoms of hyperactivity-impulsivity have been present for at least 6 months to an extent that is disruptive and inappropriate for developmental level:

Hyperactivity

1. Often fidgets with hands or feet or squirms in seat.

2. Often gets up from seat when remaining in seat is expected.

3. Often runs about or climbs when and where it is not appropriate (adolescents or adults may feel very restless).

4. Often has trouble playing or enjoying leisure activities quietly.

5. Is often "on the go" or often acts as if "driven by a motor."

6. Often talks excessively.

Impulsivity

1. Often blurts out answers before questions have been finished.

2. Often has trouble waiting one's turn.

3. Often interrupts or intrudes on others (e.g., butts into conversations or games).

II. Some symptoms that cause impairment were present before age 7 years.

III. Some impairment from the symptoms is present in two or more settings (e.g., at school/work and at home).

IV. There must be clear evidence of significant impairment in social, school, or work functioning.

V. The symptoms do not happen only during the course of a Pervasive Developmental Disorder, Schizophrenia, or other Psychotic Disorder. The symptoms are not better accounted for by another mental disorder (e.g., Mood Disorder, Anxiety Disorder, Dissociative Disorder, or a Personality Disorder).

Based on these criteria, three types of ADHD are identified:

1. ADHD, *Combined Type*: if both criteria 1A and 1B are met for the past 6 months

2. ADHD, *Predominantly Inattentive Type*: if criterion 1A is met but criterion 1B is not met for the past 6 months

3. ADHD, *Predominantly Hyperactive-Impulsive Type*: if criterion 1B is met but criterion 1A is not met for the past 6 months.

(Reprinted with permission from the Diagnostic and Statistical Manual of Mental Disorders, 4th Edition, Text Revision. (Copyright 2000). American Psychiatric Association.)

ders—18% (41). Children with more severe psychiatric disease (e.g., CDs and major depression) may be more appropriate for specialized care settings (42).

The AAP published evidenced-based guidelines in 2000 on the diagnosis of ADHD. In addition to the use of DSM IV criteria, the guidelines recommend that information about the core symptoms of ADHD, and the degree of impairment, be obtained directly from both parents and teachers (or others responsible for the care of the child) (41). An interview with the parents should also include detailed information about pregnancy, birth, development, current or prior illnesses, injuries, or hospitalizations. A detailed family history of a child with ADHD will often reveal parents with ADHD, substance abuse, or job or marital instability. The AAP supports the use of ADHD specific checklists as one way of obtaining information from multiple settings (and multiple parents) in a time efficient and consistent manner (41, 43). These checklists are not intended to be used as diagnostic or screening tests, and lack the sensitivity for a good screening test and the specificity for a good diagnostic test. They do, however, facilitate the collection of information from multiple sources. Some of available specific checklists include Conners': Swanson, Nolan, and Pelham IV (SNAP IV); ADHD IV; and ADD Comprehensive Teacher Rating Scale (ACTERS) (43). The AAP generally does not support the routine use of broad-band checklists for the evaluation of a child with suspected ADHD. These longer tests (such as Child Behavior Checklist (CBCL), Conners' long form, and Devereux Scales of Mental Disorders (DSMD)) lack the sensitivity and specificity to be clinically useful in most settings. However, in the case of a child with a complex presentation, broad-band checklists may help the clinician by supporting other diagnostic possibilities and helping to collect broader information from the child's teacher. Other school testing, such as psychological testing and minutes from individualized education plan (IEP) meetings should be obtained and reviewed when available (41).

Many diagnostic tests have been evaluated for routine or selected use during the evaluation of a child with suspected ADHD. These include thyroid testing, lead level, blood count, neuroimaging, electroencephalography, and continuous performance tests (computer administered test of attention). None of these tests have been shown to have sufficient sensitivity or specificity for routine use in the evaluation of a child with suspected ADHD. However, some of these tests are appropriate in the right clinical context (41).

A complete history and physical is essential. Has the child had recent hearing and vision tests? A child with moderate sensory impairment is likely to have difficulty attending to task. Has there been a recent change in family structure (marriage, divorce, death, or serious illness)? Are there undiagnosed or undertreated medical conditions that affect a child's ability to pay attention? The initial visits for ADHD are also opportunities to observe the child as well as the parents' response to the child. Is the child able to engage in a sustained conversion? Can he complete tasks? Is she fidgety? Does he respond appropriately to feedback? Do the parents have appropriate expectations? Are they firm and consistent, yet fair? Many children struggling behaviorally at school and home are criticized frequently by parents. This often becomes the dominant or exclusive form of attention. These clues may or may not affect your diagnosis but often help lead treatment.

Management

The cornerstone of successful management of ADHD is the clinician's relationship with the child and family. At the time of diagnosis, it is important to set realistic treatment goals and to define these goals in behavioral terms (42). Attention to the specific behaviors that prompted the initial evaluation will ensure addressing the needs of the whole family. If the parent was concerned that the child was having trouble focusing on homework for 15 minutes each night, then using that as an initial, achievable, and measurable parameter will help the parent and child to understand the impact of the treatment.

ADHD is increasingly thought of as a chronic condition and as such a treatment plan should resemble that of a chronic disease. This should include a management plan with goals, as well as a plan for follow up. Flowsheets can be helpful in monitoring progress (42).

There are essentially two distinct management strategies for ADHD—medication and behavior therapy. Both have proven successful in treating the core symptoms of ADHD. The AAP guidelines on treatment recommend initiating treatment with a stimulant medicine and/or behavior therapy. Stimulants are well tolerated, inexpensive, and effective. Any given stimulant results in improvement in 70% of children with ADHD. Approximately 80%–85% of children with ADHD will respond to at least one available stimulant. The AAP recommends that if a stimulant trial fails (inadequate improvement or intolerable side effects), another stimulant should be attempted. The mainstay of therapy for many years was short-acting methylphenidate. Short-acting dextroamphetamine also has also been widely used and studied (42, 44, 45). There has been a recent proliferation of novel drug delivery systems, which have improved the once daily dosing of methylphenidate, dextroamphetamine, and amphetamine-dextroamphetamine. These are usually about twice as expensive as short-acting generic products, and more difficult to titrate. However, they eliminate the need for in-school dosing and may eliminate some of the highs and lows of stimulant treatment (46, 47). Generally speaking, stimulants should be titrated to the highest tolerated dose, with added gains in control of core symptoms and without intolerable side effects. In practice, this often means frequent visits, with feedback from parents and teachers to establish a dose. After initial success, the dose should usually be titrated upwards. If there are no additional gains in symptom control or intolerable side effects occur, the dose should be lowered to the previous dose. Patients with hyperactive/impulsive type and combined type ADHD will often require higher doses of stimulants for symptom control (47–49).

The tricyclic antidepressants, particularly desipramine and imipramine, have been used extensively for the treatment of ADHD. They have been subject to fewer, smaller, and shorter duration randomized controlled trials than the stimulants; however, they show similar efficacy. They have a different side effect profile and may be more difficult to tolerate with adequate doses. However, in children with intolerable weight loss or insomnia on stimulants, they are an excellent second choice (44).

Other antidepressants, especially the noradrenergic agonists buproprion and venlafaxine, have been used for the treatment of ADHD. Similarly, atomoxetine, a selective norepinephrine re-uptake inhibitor, was recently developed and approved for the treatment of ADHD. Atomoxetine has been shown to improve the symptoms of ADHD, but has not been compared in direct trials against stimulants. In special cases, a variety of other drugs have been used in children with ADHD, including centrally acting alpha 2 blockers (clonidine and guafacine), β-blockers, anti-seizure medicines (e.g., carbamazepine and valproic acid), and antipsychotics (e.g., risperidone) (see Table 13.4).

Behavior therapy is best delivered as a broad set of specific interventions with application to the home and school environment by parents and teachers. This therapy emphasizes techniques such as positive and negative reinforcement, and token economies (e.g., child gets a star for each good day, and after three good days gets a special reward). Behavior therapy is distinct from psychological therapy directed at insight into problems and thought patterns. Psychological therapy has not been shown to be helpful in the treatment of ADHD. Several studies have shown that behavior therapy is effective at managing the core symptoms of ADHD; studies usually involve extensive and expensive programs, however. Treatment effects of behavior therapy alone are slightly less impressive than a structured medication program alone. However, the combination of a structured medication program and a behavior therapy program leads to lower doses of medicines and higher parent satisfaction (44, 49) (see Table 13.5).

Long-Term Monitoring

After stabilizing treatment, it is appropriate that children with ADHD should be seen at regular intervals to monitor contin-ued response to therapy, meeting of behavioral goals, academic progress, and side effects. The exact interval needed for each child is variable. In many states, this may be influenced by laws for prescribing controlled substances. Linear height and weight should be monitored every 3 to 6 months. Direct input from teachers should be solicited at least yearly. This can be easily accomplished by the repeat administration of ADHD-specific checklists. Blood testing is not indicated in monitoring ADHD or treatment, with the exception of pemoline. With significant weight loss, a clinician may also choose to screen for anemia periodically.

DISRUPTIVE BEHAVIOR

Disruptive behavior is the most common behavioral complaint presenting to a family physician. Disruptive behaviors represent a spectrum from normal disobedience and risk taking to severe CD. Oppositional defiant disorder (ODD) is characterized by negativistic, defiant, and hostile behavior toward authority figures. CD is the persistent violation of the rights of others and societal, age-appropriate norms. Both disorders must persist over time and cause significant impairment in function (29).

The family physician's role in the evaluation of behavior disorders is to normalize age-appropriate behavior (e.g., tantrums in toddlers, lying in preschoolers), offer appropriate parenting advice and resources in supportive and nonjudgmental ways, and refer children with more severe disorders or unclear diagnoses early for evaluation and treatment (50).

TABLE 13.4 Commonly Prescribed Medications for ADHD

Drug	Contraindications/Cautions/Adverse Effects	Dosage	Relative Cost *
Methylphenidate (immediate release)	Anorexia, stomachache, headache, weight loss, insomnia	5–20 mg BID to TID	$$
Methylphenidate (sustained release)	Anorexia, stomachache, headache, weight loss, insomnia	20–60 mg daily	$$$
Dextroamphetamine (immediate release)	Anorexia, stomachache, headache, weight loss, insomnia	2.5–10 mg BID	$$
Dextroamphetamine (sustained release)	Anorexia, stomachache, headache, weight loss, insomnia	10–40 mg daily	$$$
Amphetamine/ Dextroamphetamine (immediate release)	Anorexia, stomachache, headache, weight loss, insomnia	2.5–10 mg daily to BID	$$
Amphetamine/ Dextroamphetamine (sustained release)	Anorexia, stomachache, headache, weight loss, insomnia	10–30 mg daily	$$$
Atomoxetine	Nausea, vomiting, constipation, fatigue, dry eyes and mouth, potential in blood pressure	40–100 mg daily; max. in children/ adolescents ≤70 kg = the lesser of ¼ mg/kg or 100 mg	$$$
Triclyclics (desipramine and imipramine)	Sedation, constipation. dry eyes and mouth	10–50 mg BID (in children ≤12 years of age, max daily dose 5 mg/kg)	$

* $ = inexpensive; $$ = moderate; = $$$ expensive.

TABLE 13.5   Key Recommendations for Practice

Recommendation	Strength of Recommendation*	References
In children presenting with behavior/school problems, initiate evaluation for ADHD	B	(38, 41)
To diagnose ADHD, a child must meet DSM IV criteria	B	(38, 41)
Direct information on the core symptoms of ADHD must be gathered from parents and caregivers in multiple settings	B	(38, 41)
Evaluation should include assessment for co-existing conditions	A	(38, 41)
Establish a management program treating ADHD as a chronic disease	B	(42, 44)
Set goals with parents and teachers that are realistic and measurable	B	(42, 44)
Recommend stimulant medicine and/or behavior therapy as first line treatment	A (stimulant) B (behavior)	(42, 44, 49)

*A = consistent, good-quality patient-oriented evidence; B = inconsistent or limited-quality patient-oriented evidence; C = consensus, disease-oriented evidence, usual practice, expert opinion, or case series. For information about the SORT evidence rating system, see *http://www.aafp.org/afpsort.xml*.

Particularly with CD, referral for treatment should be made early in the course of disease.

The estimated prevalence of CD ranges from 1.5%–3.4%; boys are three to five times more likely to be affected (51). ODD is more common than CD, but estimates vary widely (52). CD is very common among children in contact with the juvenile justice system. Forty percent of children with CD will develop antisocial personality disorder (51).

Risk and causal factors for CD have been the subject of significant epidemiologic, genetic, and environmental research. Genetics clearly play a role but has been difficult to disentangle from the family environment. Poverty, male gender, increasing age (through adolescence), chronic illness, and disability have been consistent risk factors. Temperament, hyperactivity, and early aggressive behavior are constitutional risk factors for later CD. The most important risk factors for CD are in the domain of the family, including: poor family functioning, substance abuse, psychiatric disease in a parent, marital discord, child abuse and neglect, and poor parenting. Child abuse is the strongest and most consistent risk factor for CD (51).

Initial Evaluation

With any behavior complaint, the family physician should listen to the parent in a supportive manner. What is the problem? In what settings does the problem occur? What has been tried to modify the behavior? What has worked? A comprehensive developmental, family, and social history is invaluable in the assessment of behavior problems. Acute stress, grief, acute disease, and chronic disease can cause and aggravate behavior problems. Specific evaluation of the level of impairment is important in helping develop an initial management plan. Has the child been arrested, in fights, or using weapons? Is the child taking risks that are extreme for his or her age? How is he doing in school? Does she get along with peers (50)?

As with ADHD, comorbid disease is extremely common with CD and ODD. The family physician should consider both alternative and comorbid disorders, including ADHD, depression, anxiety, personality disorders, learning disabilities, and substance abuse (51, 52). Some clinicians find that broadband behavior rating scales such as the Child Behavior Checklist can help identify likely alternative or comorbid conditions (53). These scales lack sufficient sensitivity or specificity to be used for screening or diagnosis.

Management

The general approach to management will depend on the symptoms, severity, and differential diagnosis. The family physician is in an excellent position to offer supportive parenting advice and anticipatory guidance in a developmentally appropriate context from an early age. Parents should be reminded that the purpose of discipline is to teach a child to change, eliminate, or add a behavior. The parents should set the goals. A few simple principles can curb problem behaviors before they escalate to true disorders. Parents should be consistent, set limits, reward positive behavior, and use negative reinforcements, time-outs, and selective inattention for negative behaviors.

Children often act out in an effort to get attention. Parents can shift the balance of positive and negative attention by selectively ignoring "less" bad behaviors, such as whining (selective inattention). Time-in is a principle in which parents use minimal physical contact to frequently reward positive behavior. This could be a pat on the head for patiently waiting for adults to finish a conversation. Positive reinforcement should include the lavish use of praise, small rewards, and special time with parents or loved ones. Time-out should involve a short (1 minute per year age) quiet time and space. This is less of a punishment and more of a way to defer negative attention giving in response to a behavior; time-outs also allow a child to calm down. Token economies are a commonly used form of behavior modification in which a child will get a token (sticker, star, or chip) for a behavior. When the child gets a certain number of tokens (e.g., 1–5), the child gets a deferred reward. Tokens are given for desirable behaviors and taken away for undesirable behaviors. The child should be clear on the rules of any set of behavior change

TABLE 13.6 Key Recommendations for Practice

Target Disorder	Intervention	Strength of Recommendation*	Comment
ODD	Parent training programs	A	Several systematic reviews of RCTs
CD	Family and parenting interventions	A	Meta-analysis of RCTs
CD	Child skill training	A	Most effective in addition to above

RCTs, random controlled trials.

*A = consistent, good-quality patient-oriented evidence; B = inconsistent or limited-quality patient-oriented evidence; C = consensus, disease-oriented evidence, usual practice, expert opinion, or case series. For information about the SORT evidence rating system, see *http://www.aafp.org/afpsort.xml*.

efforts so that they understand the rewards and consequences of behavior. Parents should be consistent with one another and other caregivers, firm with rules, and frequently re-evaluate problems and solutions. Parents should select a limited number of behaviors to modify at any one time, and employ intermittent reinforcement to maintain new gains (50).

Children with more severe disorders often require referral for diagnosis and management. The treatment of comorbid disease is very important in behavior disorders. A child with ADHD and CD will be more frustrated if he or she is having trouble staying on task. Adequate treatment of comorbid diseases will often result in improvement in symptoms of ODD and CD (51, 52).

Family and parenting interventions have been consistently shown to reduce symptoms and morbidity from CD. Specifically, among delinquent youths with CD, a recent meta-analysis of randomized controlled trials showed that family and parenting interventions reduced the average number of days in an institution and future re-arrests for 1 to 3 years (54). Skill training for children is also helpful, but most helpful in the context of family or parenting interventions (51). Parent training programs have also consistently shown decreased target behaviors in ODD (55). Parent and family training programs for both disorders focus on the same themes discussed above, including positive and negative reinforcement, selective inattention, time-out, time-in, and token economies. These programs often combine group and family sessions, child age-appropriate instruction, and didactic and hands-on role playing or video examples (see Table 13.6).

Drug therapy has not been shown to be helpful in well-designed trials for ODD or CD, except when these disorders are present with comorbid ADHD. Most experts recommend treatment for other comorbid disorders to maximize success in the treatment of ODD or CD, especially depression and anxiety. A variety of drugs are commonly used for CD, including alpha blockers (e.g., clonidine), mood stabilizers (lithium, carbamazepine, valproic acid), antipsychotics, and antidepressants (51, 52, 56).

LANGUAGE AND LEARNING DISORDERS

Language and learning disorders (LLD) very often co-occur with ADHD and disorders of conduct, and should be considered in the differential diagnosis of any child with learning, behavior, or attention problems. Diagnosing disorders of ex-

pressive (speaking) or receptive (understanding) language requires delays in these areas not due to sensory or motor deficit or environmental deprivation. These delays must be in excess of those expected by nonverbal intelligence scores. Learning disorders (specific to reading or math) also require an IQ-achievement discrepancy (29). A child with average intelligence, who is reading several years behind grade level, may have a reading disability, for example. The diagnosis of any LLD requires significant impairment in school functioning. As with disorders of behavior, learning styles exist along a continuum. All people have learning strengths and weaknesses. Children not meeting criteria for disabilities often fail to receive the individualized attention required to meet their potential in school. Family physicians should encourage parents and children to understand a child's learning style, seek positive reinforcement for strengths, and help with weaknesses. Children at all levels of educational success can benefit from private tutoring and enrichment programs that meet the child's needs and strengths.

Children with LLD not only struggle to meet their academic potential, but may also have disorders of behavior, low self-esteem, and axis I psychiatric disorders. Fifty percent of children with LLD have axis I disorders, most commonly ADHD, anxiety, and depression (57). Seventy-five percent of children with learning disabilities have social skill deficits (58). In the classroom, they have less on-task behavior, more off-task behavior, more CD, more distractibility, and more withdrawn behavior (59). Ten to twenty percent of children have a LLD, with 10.3% of U.S. children receiving special education services—more than half are for learning disabilities and a quarter are for language disabilities (57).

More than other disorders in this chapter, the diagnosis of LLD often requires specialized testing not commonly performed by a family physician. However, the family physician may be the first to question the possibility of an LLD. The family physician may be in the best position to make a referral or advocate for school-based testing and also may manage other comorbid conditions (like ADHD) and coordinate the overall mental health treatment plan for the child. Family physicians can assist families by teaching them about their rights under IDEA. Family physicians may also assist families by attending IEP meetings. Lastly, the diagnosis of all LLDs requires that the condition occur in excess of any sensory or motor impairment. For example, a child with hearing loss may have either an expressive or receptive delay in language caused by the hearing condition alone. Correction of the hearing condition may improve the language disorder.

Initial Evaluation

In the context of school difficulty, the family physician should inquire about onset, severity, and context. What are the parents' concerns? Have they discussed these with the child's teacher? Teachers are often the first to notice and diagnose a specific disorder of learning. Records from school (report cards) and any prior psychological testing should be obtained. A thorough developmental, educational, social, and family history is important. A physical exam, with attention to sensory systems, and a general neurologic exam should be performed. Hearing and vision screening can identify sensory disorders early. Is there is a particular subject of difficulty (e.g., reading)? If a child is inattentive, and the physician is considering a diagnosis of ADHD, asking about multiple settings is essential. LLDs often affect attention and behavior at school only.

The diagnosis of LLDs is done predominantly through specialized testing by a speech pathologist and/or psychologist. Tests are normalized for age and include IQ tests and specialized testing of reading, mathematics, receptive, and expressive language. Tests must be culturally and linguistically appropriate.

Management

Children with a diagnosis of LLD qualify for specialized services in public schools, including an individualized education plan; parents and physicians may need to advocate for these services, however. Most treatment occurs in the school setting. There is an increasing evidence base about effective treatment strategies, including reading programs, summer school, one-on-one instruction, and self-concept interventions (60–64). The family physician can help parents identify local community resources to optimize the educational environment for a child.

EATING DISORDERS

Eating disorders are a group of conditions that involve dysfunctional eating habits, body image disturbance, and change in weight (65). The pathogenesis of eating disorders remains unclear. Environmental factors, social factors, psychological predisposition, and biological vulnerability may all play a role (66). Aggregation of eating disorders in families points to the possibility of a genetic predisposition as well (66). Eating disorders remain more common in industrialized countries, where there is a cultural value placed on thinness. However, they are being seen in increasing rates in developing countries as well. Within the United States, there are increasing rates of eating disorders among very young patients, male patients, patients of color, and patients of low socioeconomic status.

Eating disorders include anorexia nervosa (AN), bulimia nervosa (BN), eating disorder not otherwise specified (EDNOS), and binge eating disorder. The disorder AN describes an individual who refuses to maintain even a minimally normal body weight, who has an intense fear of gaining weight or becoming fat despite being underweight, and who exhibits a disturbance in the perception of the shape or size

or his or her body (29). By definition, amenorrhea is present in postmenarchal women. A minimally normal body weight is generally considered to be less than 85% of the normal body weight for age and height. Weight loss is generally accomplished via restricted caloric intake. Some patients will also lose weight by exercising excessively or using purging behaviors (29).

Patients with BN exhibit recurrent episodes of binge eating, with recurrent inappropriate compensatory behaviors to prevent weight gain. Patients with BN feel a sense of lack of control over their binge eating. Compensatory behaviors include vomiting, use of laxatives, diuretics, enemas or diet pills, fasting, and excessive exercise. To meet diagnostic criteria for BN, the binge eating and compensatory behaviors must occur at least twice a week for at least 3 months. Patients' self-esteem must be excessively influenced by their body image (29).

EDNOS occurs when a patient has many eating disorder symptoms but does not meet criteria for classic AN or BN. This may occur when a patient meets criteria for AN but does not have amenorrhea (29). Similarly, a patient may meet criteria for AN but be above 85% of normal body weight if they started at a very high weight. Other individuals with EDNOS may meet criteria for BN, but with binge eating and compensatory behaviors occurring less than twice a week for 3 months; others with EDNOS may perform compensatory behaviors after eating only small amounts of food. EDNOS should be considered a serious disorder, which causes significant suffering and is potentially life-threatening.

Binge eating disorder is a form of EDNOS that involves binge eating without regular compensatory behaviors: this disorder will result in varying degrees of obesity. Patients may report that their eating or weight has negatively affected their relationships, their work, and their self-esteem. Binge eating disorder is a newly recognized distinct entity without widely accepted diagnostic criteria.

The lifetime risk for AN is 0.3% to 1% for women (67); the rate of AN in men is about one-tenth of that seen in women. Eating disorders are most common in the adolescent age group, with 40% occurring between age 15 and 19 (68). Prevalence of BN is about 1% for females and 0.1% for males. The prevalence of binge eating disorder is estimated to be about 1% for both females and males. Because there are no clear diagnostic standards for EDNOS, and there is a wide heterogeneity of symptoms, the prevalence remains unknown.

Initial Evaluation

A patient with disordered eating may present with symptoms related to almost any organ system. Occasionally, the patient or a family member may express concern about weight loss, weight gain, disordered eating, or purging. More often, presenting complaints are physical, such as abdominal pain or syncope, or psychological, such as irritability, depression, or sleep disturbance. Often the patient will have already seen multiple providers and may have had significant medical work-ups to try to find a cause for their symptoms.

History and physical is the cornerstone to making an eating disorder diagnosis. An appropriate history and physical exam can often spare the patient a potentially invasive work-up for his or her medical complaints. There is no routine laboratory panel that will help to diagnose an eating disorder.

TABLE 13.7 Laboratory Abnormalities Commonly Seen with Disordered Eating

Weight Loss

- Decreased white blood cell count
- Decreased red blood cell count
- Increased aspartate aminotransferase or alanine aminotransferase
- Hypercholesterolemia
- Hypernatremia
- Increased blood urea nitrogen and creatinine
- Normal albumin and protein

Purging

Vomiting

- Hypochloremic, hypokalemic, metabolic alkalosis
- Increased amylase

Laxatives

- Metabolic acidosis
- Hypocalcemia

Diuretics

- Hyponatremia
- Hypomagnesemia
- Increased or decreased potassium

In healthy young people, laboratory studies often remain normal until disease is advanced. Nevertheless, there are laboratory abnormalities that are often seen in the presence of disordered eating or purging behaviors, as shown in Table 13.7.

Gastrointestinal symptoms are often severe and may be an area of intense focus by the patient. Food restriction and/or purging can lead to gastroparesis, gastroesophageal reflux disease, severe constipation, cathartic colon syndrome, gallstone disease, and ruptured esophagus. Cardiovascular complications can include arrhythmia, prolonged QT interval, mitral valve prolapse, bradycardia, hypotension, and heart failure. Neurologic changes can be seen on magnetic resonance imaging with enlarged ventricles and decreased cortical substance. Although both white and gray matter decreases during severe weight loss, only white matter returns to premorbid levels following weight gain. Loss of gray matter can persist (69).

Disordered eating can affect the endocrine system in several ways. Hypothalamic activation occurs due to a high stress state. Levels of Adronocorticotropic hormone (ACTH), cortisol, growth hormone, prolactin, epinephrine, norepinephrine, interleukin-1, interleukin-2, and tumor necrosis factor all increase, and hypothalamic abnormalities in thermoregulation occur. As bone remodeling decreases, the risk of osteoporosis increases. The role of oral contraceptives in restoring bone density in patients with disordered eating remains unclear. Dual-energy x-ray absorptiometry of bone is generally recommended. Documentation of osteopenia may be helpful to motivate patients in their recovery (70).

Decreased gonadotropin-releasing hormone leads to a decrease in leutinizing hormone and follicle stimulating hormone to prepubertal levels. Because these hormonal changes occur because of stress, up to 70% of patients with amenorrhea secondary to disordered eating lose their menstrual cycles prior to significant weight loss.

Management

Initial management of the patient with disordered eating should focus on correcting any immediate health risks. An electrocardiogram should be done to rule out prolonged QT interval. The remainder of the initial work-up should be tailored to the findings in the history and physical exam. Once the patient is stabilized, treatment should focus on weight restoration. Refeeding with electrolyte replacement is often indicated. Hospitalization is indicated for refeeding in the face of severe malnutrition, as well as in the presence of any significant hemodynamic compromise or electrolyte abnormality. Hospitalization may also be necessary for patients with poor motivation, suicidal ideation, severe psychiatric disease, or a difficult home environment, especially if abuse is present (70).

Once initial stabilization has occurred, a treatment team can be established. This will often involve a therapist, nutritionist, and the primary care physician. Treatment requires the establishment of a trusting long-term relationship with the patient. Often the family needs to be involved, particularly for patients under 18 years of age.

There may be some role for psychopharmacology in the treatment of eating disorders. Selective serotonin reuptake inhibitors (SSRIs) may help to decrease binging behavior, particularly in high doses, although SSRIs have not been shown to improve or hasten weight gain in starved patients (71, 72). Psychiatric symptoms often improve with weight gain, as the psychological effects of malnutrition decline. Thus, once some weight gain has occurred, it may be useful to treat remaining symptoms with psychotropic medications. Treatment of residual psychiatric symptoms may help to prevent relapse. Several small, open-label studies have shown that low-dose atypical antipsychotic agents may improve weight gain and depression in patients with eating disorders (73–75).

Long-Term Monitoring

For many individuals eating disorders will be long-term, chronic diseases. Mortality rates are 5%–6% for both AN and BN. When death occurs, it is usually due to frank starvation, purge-related arrhythmia, or suicide. In patients with AN, about half will recover and do well over time in regard to their body weight and nutritional status. Another 30% will do quite well but continue to have symptoms, with the remaining 20% doing poorly. With BN, 50% of patients achieve full recovery within 2 years. However, 20%–46% will continue to have symptoms after 6 years of treatment (76).

CHILD MALTREATMENT

Child maltreatment includes physical abuse, sexual abuse, psychological abuse, and neglect. Child maltreatment often presents with symptoms of inattention, school failure, disruptive symptoms, anxiety, depression, failure to thrive, and a broad range of somatic symptoms (ranging from the physical pain of a broken bone to psychogenic symptoms, such as recurrent abdominal pain).

Estimates of child maltreatment rates vary widely by methodology. The most widely used method to estimate the incidence of child abuse is official reporting statistics. These are biased because they only include those reports that come to the attention of protective services. Most public health and social service agencies count only substantiated reports, further undercounting real cases of abuse. In 2003 (the most recent year for which data are available), 906,000 children were found to be victims of abuse or neglect (12.4/1000) (77). An alternative method of ascertaining estimates of abuse is used in a periodic national incidence study (last completed in 1993). This study asks sentinel professionals who have regular involvement with children how many children they have seen in the last week who were harmed from abuse or neglect (harm standard). This counts only children subjected to abuse or neglect that is known about by another adult, who regularly and professionally has contact with children. In 1993, 1,553,800 children were abused or neglected using this methodology (78). The true incidence of child maltreatment may be much higher (79). In many cases of abuse or neglect, only the victim and the perpetrator are privy to the abuse.

All states, districts, and territories in the United States have child abuse reporting statutes that include physicians as mandated reporters for suspected child abuse and neglect. These laws include immunity from lawsuits for reports made in good faith. It is important for the parent or caregiver involved to understand that the reporter is not placing blame or making judgment, but carrying out a legal responsibility. This helps to absolve some of the guilt that a physician may feel in making a report to child protective services. A reporter is not required by law to inform the parent of the report being made; this can, however, set the stage for an open dialog and continued support of the family. How this is framed will depend on the nature of the suspected maltreatment, and the suspected perpetrator.

Physical Abuse

The family physician should suspect physical abuse in cases of childhood injury that are: 1) unexplained, 2) not plausible by the explanation offered, 3) in a pattern suspicious for inflicted injury, 4) developmentally inconsistent, or 5) caused by punishment with excessive force (80). In 2003 there were 148,877 substantiated cases of physical abuse according to social services (77); there were 338,900 victims of physical abuse in 1993 according to the National Incidence Study (78).

In considering an injury for suspicion of abuse, many physicians use the practical 24 hour rule. That is, if a mark lasts 24 hours, it is considered a significant injury. In most jurisdictions, red marks from spanking (with open hand, paddle, or switch) that resolve in less than 24 hours are usually not considered physical abuse by protective services (80). In evaluating any injury to a child, a detailed history should be obtained and carefully documented. In the case of suspicious injuries, detailed drawings or photographs can be helpful. The injury should be carefully matched to the reported mechanism. Does the skin mark resemble a known pattern of injury? Loops, teeth marks, and linear welts (from belts or switches) are common patterns in abusive injuries. Studies have shown that premobile children rarely bruise (<1% of children not yet cruising have bruises thought to be caused by unintentional injury) (81). Certain skeletal injuries are highly suggestive of abuse. Children less than 2 years old with rib fractures (in the absence of a high-impact trauma history or metabolic bone disease) are nearly always caused by abuse (82). Likewise, metaphyseal corner fractures of the long bones in children less than 2 years old are usually from abuse. Inflicted head injury is the most common cause of death due to child physical abuse. Children under 2 years old, with other significant abusive injuries, should be evaluated with brain imaging (CT or MR) to identify occult brain injury (83).

The most important consideration in identifying physical abuse is a high index of suspicion. Clinicians with special training or experience in child abuse can be helpful in clarifying mechanisms in ambiguous injuries. These clinicians will also help search for alternative explanations for disease and injury patterns (e.g., coagulopathy, metabolic bone disease). Detailed documentation of history and physical exam is essential for protective service and legal investigation.

Sexual Abuse

Sexual abuse includes all forms of sexual contact (oral-genital, genital, anal) by or to a child, in which there is age or developmental discordance between the child and the perpetrator. It also includes noncontact abuse, such as exhibitionism, voyeurism, and use of a child to produce pornography (84). In 2003 there were 78,188 substantiated cases of sexual abuse according to social services (77). There were 217,700 victims of child sexual abuse in 1993 according to the National Incidence Study (78).

Child sexual abuse usually presents with child disclosure. However, presentations may vary and include acute sexual trauma, sexually transmitted diseases, pregnancy, extremes of sexualized behavior, and somatic symptoms, such as dysuria and enuresis. Interviewing children for evidence of sexual abuse requires special skill and training. That does not preclude the family physician from taking a thorough medical history of a child, including open-ended and nonleading questions about various types of trauma, and the etiology of specific findings. In this nonthreatening and familiar setting, a child may disclose abuse. These disclosures are admissible in court. When possible, medical history documentation of a disclosure should include direct quotations of questions asked by the provider, and the responses of the victim.

The physical examination for child sexual abuse should include visual inspection of the genitals and anus in supine frog-leg and knee-chest positions. This exam may be aided by the use of specialized instruments such a lighting devices and a colposcope for magnification. Photodocumention can be helpful for legal reference, but accurate pen and paper diagrams can be used when photocolposcopy is unavailable. Routine cultures for sexually transmitted diseases are not necessary in the absence of symptoms. Clinicians unskilled in the physical exam for sexual abuse should seek expert consultation. In the case of uncertain findings, photodocumentation or expert consultation can clarify equivocal findings.

Neglect

Child neglect accounts for the vast majority of protective service cases with 497,512 substantiated cases in 2003 (77) and 551,700 children in 1993 according to the National Incidence

Study (78). Neglect accounts for nearly half of the annual 1,500 child maltreatment fatalities (77). Primary care physicians need to understand the symptoms of neglect, be willing to report suspected neglect, and help families meet the needs of their children.

Neglect can be thought of as failing to meet the basic needs of a child. These needs include adequate supervision, food, clothing, shelter, medical care, education, and love. Neglect, unlike physical and sexual abuse, often manifests as a pattern of chronic unmet needs, sometimes along one domain, but often along multiple domains. Some states exclude situations due to poverty from reporting laws. However, the family physician should avoid this judgment if she recognizes inadequate care that may jeopardize the health or development of a child. The cause of neglect may not be malevolent, but the risk to the child remains the same. For example, a poor single father may leave his 2-year old home alone sleeping at night to work a second shift job. Even though his circumstances drove him to this omission of care, the child is still at risk of significant harm.

Neglect may come to the family physician's attention in the form of medical non-adherence, failure or delay in seeking medical care, failure to thrive, unmanaged obesity, behavior problems, school failure, poor hygiene, or homelessness (85). The identification and management of neglect requires vigilance on the part of the family physician. In identifying a child suspected of being neglected, asking nonjudgmental questions about resources can help identify sources of problems and potential solutions. As neglect often manifests as a chronic pattern, the physician must have a way to follow children over time. If a child failing to thrive does not return as scheduled, the physician should have a system in place to call the patient, re-schedule the appointment, and identify barriers to follow through. When a pattern of omission in care (or a single egregious episode) rises to the level of harm or significant risk of harm, the physician is obligated to report the case to protective services.

Psychological Abuse

Psychological abuse of children is common; however, it is the least often substantiated type of abuse. This is due to social norms and the challenges of proving both intent of the parent and harm to the child. In 2003, there were 38,603 children with substantiated reports for psychological maltreatment (77). The National Incidence Study reported 212,800 cases of emotional neglect in 1993 (78). Some states include emotional neglect as a type of neglect, while others include a separate category of psychological maltreatment, which may or may not include both commissions of abuse and omissions of love and nurturing care. Despite the low number of psychological abuse cases, a population-based survey of parents reveals that this type of behavior is far more common. In North and South Carolina in 2003, 12.8% of parents surveyed endorsed one or more of the following in the past year: 1) threatening to leave or abandon a child, 2) threatening to kick a child out of the home, 3) locking a child out of the house, or 4) calling a child a name such as stupid, ugly, or useless (86). It is difficult to determine when such behavior is abusive as it is common, often chronic, and harm is difficult to measure or prove.

The diagnosis of psychological abuse is often made only through long-term observation of parent-child interaction.

This can be facilitated by querying other adults involved in the life of the child (e.g., teachers, coaches). Symptoms of psychological abuse include many of the behavior symptoms reviewed in this chapter: aggressiveness, impulsivity, depression, hyperactivity, school failure, inattention, disturbances of conduct, anxiety, eating disorders, and somatic symptoms. In evaluating children with behavior and development disorders, we often witness parents belittling children in cruel ways ("he's stupid just like his daddy" or "she drives me crazy"). Discussing destructive behavior and role modeling positive behavior can help ameliorate a difficult visit and begin to help a parent identify problem parenting. However, in this type of abusive behavior setting, a child struggling at home or school will be very difficult to treat with any measure of success. When such behavior is observed over time or seems to be correlated with behavioral symptoms, the treating physician should consider a referral for family therapy or to protective services.

CASE DISCUSSION

During the initial interview with the mother and child, you observe that the child is wild in the exam room. The mother responds with escalating threats without follow through. At one point she looks at you with frustration, and says "See what I mean? He is just bad, doesn't listen. I don't know if I can take it anymore." Social history reveals that the boy's parents separated 3 months ago, and they are in a difficult fight for custody. You ask the mother how she is dealing with the stress. She replies, "I do what I have to do." When asked about substance abuse or alcohol, she looks away and doesn't respond. Family history, social history, and physical exam are otherwise noncontributory. You tell the mother that you never make a judgment or treatment plan at a first visit, but you are concerned that the boy needs help. You provide her with ADHD rating scales for her, the boy's dad, and his two teachers.

At 2-week follow up, you score the rating scales before seeing the patient. Along the domain of attention, he scores average at school and below average from his father and mother. This indicates that his parents perceive that he has a problem with tending to task, but his teachers do not share this concern. Along the domains of hyperactivity and impulsivity, he scores slightly below average at school, moderately below average from his father, and in the severe range from his mother. In the comments area on the scale, a note from one teacher states that he is smart and good natured but has been more restless over the past few months.

It is clear from your careful evaluation that the boy is struggling with behavior primarily at home (with mom more than with dad). Mom is stressed, and you suspect that she is using alcohol or drugs; she displays ineffective parenting skills in your office. The child does not meet criteria for a specific disorder of conduct, but you are concerned that he may progress to ODD or CD if current patterns continue. The specific actions witnessed (calling the child bad, stating that she can't take it anymore) border on psychological abuse. You consider a report to child protective services, but decide at this time that it would be more productive to support the mother and foster a relationship with the family. This will allow you to monitor progress over time. If the mother fails at follow through or the child's condition worsens, you will report to protective services. You point out that the escalating behavior seems temporally related to the home situation. In a supportive manner you review some of the principles of effective discipline (firm limits, consistency, use of selective inattention, time in). You recommend that the mother take a parenting class offered by the local health department. Lastly, since you are the mother's doctor as well, you ask her to follow up with you in 2 weeks for her own appointment without her son present. At this session, you can be more open about the mother's own signs and symptoms, discuss depression and substance abuse, and offer support. If the mother fails to follow though and doesn't return for follow-up, a report to protective services would be appropriate after explaining your concern to the mother.

REFERENCES

1. Shonkoff JP, Phillips D. From Neurons to Neighborhoods. Washington, DC: National Academies Press; 2000.
2. Reynolds AJ, Temple JA, Robertson DL, Mann EA. Long-term effects of an early childhood intervention on educational achievement and juvenile arrest: A 15-year follow-up of low-income children in public schools. JAMA. 2001;285(18):2339–2346.
3. Gomby DS, Larner MB, Stevenson CS, Lewit EM, Behrman RE. Long-term outcomes of early childhood programs: analysis and recommendations. Future Child. 1995;5(3):6–24.
4. Roberts G, Palfrey JS, Bridgemohan C. Medical Evaluation of a child with developmental delay. Contemp Pediatr. 2004; 21:76.
5. Glascoe FP. Early detection of developmental and behavioral problems. Pediatr Rev. 2000;21(8):272–279; quiz 280.
6. Lavigne JV, Binns HJ, Christoffel KK, Rosenbaum D, Arend R, Smith K, et al. Behavioral and emotional problems among preschool children in pediatric primary care: prevalence and pediatricians' recognition. Pediatric Practice Research Group. Pediatrics. 1993;91(3):649–655.
7. Palfrey JS, Singer JD, Walker DK, Butler JA. Early identification of children's special needs: a study in five metropolitan communities. J Pediatr. 1987;111(5):651–659.
8. Glascoe FP. Developmental Screening. In: Wolraich ML, ed. Disorders of Development and Learning: A Practical Guide to Assessment and Management. St Louis, MO: Mosby; 1996.
9. Developmental surveillance and screening of infants and young children. Pediatrics. 2001;108(1):192–196.
10. Zuckerman BS, Parker S. Teachable moments: assessment as intervention. Contemporary Pediatrics. 1997;14:41–53.
11. Diamond K. Predicting school problems from preschool developmental screening. J Div Early Childhood. 1987;11:247–253.
12. Glascoe FP, Altemeier WA, MacLean WE. The importance of parents' concerns about their child's development. Am J Dis Child. 1989;143(8):955–958.
13. Mulhern S, Dworkin PH, Bernstein B. Do parental concerns predict a diagnosis of attention-deficit hyperactivity disorder? J Dev Behav Pediatr. 1994;15(5):348–352.
14. Thompson MD, Thompson G. Early identification of hearing loss: listen to parents. Clin Pediatr (Phila). 1991;30(2):77–80.
15. Diamond KE. The role of parents' observations and concerns in screening for developmental delays in young children. Top Early Child Spec Ed. 1993;13:68–81.
16. Doig KB, Macias MM, Saylor CF, Craver JR, Ingram PE. The Child Development Inventory: a developmental outcome measure for follow-up of the high-risk infant. J Pediatr. 1999;135(3):358–362.
17. Bricker D, Squires J. The effectiveness of parental screening of at risk infants: the infant monitoring questionnaires. Top Early Child Spec Ed. 1989;9:67–85.
18. Individuals with Disabilities Education Act Amendments. In: PL 105–17; 1997.
19. Bauchner J. Failure to Thrive. In: Behrman RE, Kliegman RM, Jenson HB, eds. Nelson Textbook of Pediatrics, 16th ed. Philadelphia, PA: W.B. Saunders; 2000.
20. Kane ML. Pediatric failure to thrive. Clin Fam Pract. 2003; 5(2):293–311.
21. Manikam R, Perman JA. Pediatric feeding disorders. J Clin Gastroenterol. 2000;30(1):34–46.
22. Careaga MG, Kerner JA, Jr. A gastroenterologist's approach to failure to thrive. Pediatr Ann. 2000;29(9):558–567.
23. Gahagan S, Holmes R. A stepwise approach to evaluation of undernutrition and failure to thrive. Pediatr Clin North Am. 1998;45(1):169–187.
24. Casey PH. Failure to Thrive. In: Levine MD, Carey WB, Crocker AC, eds. Developmental-Behavioral Pediatrics. Philadelphia, PA: W.B. Saunders; 1992.
25. Bithoney WG, Dubowitz H, Egan H. Failure to thrive/growth deficiency. Pediatr Rev. 1992;13(12):453–460.
26. Raynor P, Rudolf MC. Anthropometric indices of failure to thrive. Arch Dis Child. 2000;82(5):364–365.
27. Acs G, Lodolini G, Kaminsky S, Cisneros GJ. Effect of nursing caries on body weight in a pediatric population. Pediatr Dent. 1992;14(5):302–305.
28. Frank DA, Zeisel SH. Failure to thrive. Pediatr Clin North Am. 1988;35(6):1187–1206.
29. American Psychological Association. Diagnostic and Statistical Manual of Mental Disorders, 4th ed, Text Revision. Washington, DC: American Psychiatric Association; 2000.
30. Gillberg C, Wing L. Autism: not an extremely rare disorder. Acta Psychiatr Scand. 1999;99(6):399–406.
31. Fombonne E. The epidemiology of autism: a review. Psychol Med. 1999;29(4):769–786.
32. Filipek PA, Accardo PJ, Baranek GT, Cook EH, Jr., Dawson G, Gordon B, et al. The screening and diagnosis of autistic spectrum disorders. J Autism Dev Disord. 1999;29(6):439–484.
33. Filipek PA, Accardo PJ, Ashwal S, Baranek GT, Cook EH, Jr., Dawson G, et al. Practice parameter: screening and diagnosis of autism: report of the Quality Standards Subcommittee of the American Academy of Neurology and the Child Neurology Society. Neurology. 2000;55(4):468–479.
34. Simonoff E. Genetic counseling in autism and pervasive developmental disorders. J Autism Dev Disord. 1998;28(5):447–456.
35. American Academy of Pediatrics: The pediatrician's role in the diagnosis and management of autistic spectrum disorder in children. Pediatrics. 2001;107(5):1221–1226.
36. Jones KL, Smith DW. Smith's Recognizable Patterns of Human Malformations, 5th ed. Philadelphia: Saunders; 1997.
37. Daily DK, Ardinger HH, Holmes GE. Identification and evaluation of mental retardation. Am Fam Physician. 2000; 62(5):961–963.
38. Brown RT, Freeman WS, Perrin JM, Stein MT, Amler RW, Feldman HM, et al. Prevalence and assessment of attention-deficit/hyperactivity disorder in primary care settings. Pediatrics. 2001;107(3):E43.
39. Jensen PS, Garcia JA, Glied S, Crowe M, Foster M, Schlander M, et al. Cost-Effectiveness of ADHD Treatments: Findings From the Multimodal Treatment Study of Children With ADHD. Am J Psychiatry. 2005;162(9):1628–1636.

40. Wolraich ML, Wibbelsman CJ, Brown TE, Evans SW, Gotlieb EM, Knight JR, et al. Attention-deficit/hyperactivity disorder among adolescents: a review of the diagnosis, treatment, and clinical implications. Pediatrics. 2005;115(6):1734–1746.

41. Clinical practice guideline: diagnosis and evaluation of the child with attention-deficit/hyperactivity disorder. American Academy of Pediatrics. Pediatrics. 2000;105(5):1158–1170.

42. Clinical practice guideline: treatment of the school-aged child with attention-deficit/hyperactivity disorder. Pediatrics. 2001;108(4):1033–1044.

43. Zolotor A, Mayer J, Hill J. Clinical inquiries. Does a short symptom checklist accurately diagnose ADHD? J Fam Pract. 2004;53(5):412–416.

44. Brown RT, Amler RW, Freeman WS, Perrin JM, Stein MT, Feldman HM, et al. Treatment of attention-deficit/hyperactivity disorder: overview of the evidence. Pediatrics. 2005;115(6):e749–757.

45. Johnson LA, Safranek S, Friemoth J. Clinical inquiries. What is the most effective treatment for ADHD in children? J Fam Pract. 2005;54(2):166–168.

46. Szymanski ML, Zolotor A. Attention-deficit/hyperactivity disorder: management. Am Fam Physician. 2001;64(8):1355–1362.

47. Stein MA, Sarampote CS, Waldman ID, Robb AS, Conlon C, Pearl PL, et al. A dose-response study of OROS methylphenidate in children with attention-deficit/hyperactivity disorder. Pediatrics. 2003;112(5):e404.

48. Ibay AD, Bascelli LM, Graves RS, Hill J. Clinical inquiries. Does increasing methylphenidate dose aid symptom control in ADHD? J Fam Pract. 2003;52(5):400, 403.

49. A 14-month randomized clinical trial of treatment strategies for attention-deficit/hyperactivity disorder. The MTA Cooperative Group. Multimodal Treatment Study of Children with ADHD. Arch Gen Psychiatry. 1999;56(12):1073–1086.

50. Mortweet SL, Christophersen ER. Behavior Problems in a Pediatric Context. In: Roberts MC, ed. Handbook of Pediatric Psyhcology. New York, NY: Guildford Press; 2003.

51. Steiner H. Practice parameters for the assessment and treatment of children and adolescents with conduct disorder. American Academy of Child and Adolescent Psychiatry. J Am Acad Child Adolesc Psychiatry. 1997;36(10 Suppl):122S–139S.

52. Loeber R, Burke JD, Lahey BB, Winters A, Zera M. Oppositional defiant and conduct disorder: a review of the past 10 years, part I. J Am Acad Child Adolesc Psychiatry. 2000;39(12):1468–1484.

53. Achenbach TM. Manual for the Child Behavior Checklist/4–18 and 1991 Profile. Burlington: University of Vermont; 1991.

54. Woolfenden SR, Williams K, Peat JK. Family and parenting interventions for conduct disorder and delinquency: a meta-analysis of randomised controlled trials. Arch Dis Child. 2002;86(4):251–256.

55. Farley SE, Adams JS, Lutton ME, Scoville C, Fulkerson RC, Webb AR. Clinical inquiries. What are effective treatments for oppositional and defiant behaviors in preadolescents? J Fam Pract. 2005;54(2):162, 164–165.

56. Burke JD, Loeber R, Birmaher B. Oppositional defiant disorder and conduct disorder: a review of the past 10 years, part II. J Am Acad Child Adolesc Psychiatry. 2002;41(11):1275–1293.

57. Practice parameters for the assessment and treatment of children and adolescents with language and learning disorders. American Academy of Child and Adolescent Psychiatry. J Am Acad Child Adolesc Psychiatry 1998;37(10 Suppl):46S–62S.

58. Kavale KA, Forness SR. Social skill deficits and learning disabilities: a meta-analysis. J Learn Disabil. 1996;29(3):226–237.

59. Bender WN, Smith JK. Classroom behavior of children and adolescents with learning disabilities: a meta-analysis. J Learn Disabil. 1990;23(5):298–305.

60. Swanson HL, Sachse-Lee C. A meta-analysis of single-subject-design intervention research for students with LD. J Learn Disabil. 2000;33(2):114–136.

61. Summary of the practice parameters for the assessment and treatment of children and adolescents with language and learning disorders. American Academy of Child and Adolescent Psychiatry. J Am Acad Child Adolesc Psychiatry. 1998;37(10):1117–1119.

62. Elbaum B, Vaughn S. For which students with learning disabilities are self-concept interventions effective? J Learn Disabil. 2003;36(2):101–108; discussion 149–150.

63. Swanson HL. Reading research for students with LD: a meta-analysis of intervention outcomes. J Learn Disabil. 1999;32(6):504–532.

64. Cooper H, Charlton K, Valentine JC, Muhlenbruck L. Making the most of summer school: a meta-analytic and narrative review. Monogr Soc Res Child Dev. 2000;65(1):i–v, 1–118; discussion 119–127.

65. Kreipe RE, Yussman SM. The role of the primary care practitioner in the treatment of eating disorders. Adolesc Med. 2003;14(1):133–147.

66. Rome ES, Ammerman S. Medical complications of eating disorders: an update. J Adolesc Health. 2003;33(6):418–426.

67. Hoek HW, van Hoeken D. Review of the prevalence and incidence of eating disorders. Int J Eat Disord. 2003;34(4):383–396.

68. Lucas AR, Melton LJ, III, Crowson CS, O'Fallon WM. Long-term fracture risk among women with anorexia nervosa: a population-based cohort study. Mayo Clin Proc. 1999;74(10):972–977.

69. Lambe EK, Katzman DK, Mikulis DJ, Kennedy SH, Zipursky RB. Cerebral gray matter volume deficits after weight recovery from anorexia nervosa. Arch Gen Psychiatry. 1997;54(6):537–542.

70. Yager J, Andersen AE. Clinical practice. Anorexia nervosa. N Engl J Med. 2005;353(14):1481–1488.

71. Attia E, Haiman C, Walsh BT, Flater SR. Does fluoxetine augment the inpatient treatment of anorexia nervosa? Am J Psychiatry. 1998;155(4):548–551.

72. Strober M, Pataki C, Freeman R, DeAntonio M. No effect of adjunctive fluoxetine on eating behavior or weight phobia during the inpatient treatment of anorexia nervosa: an historical case-control study. J Child Adolesc Psychopharmacol. 1999;9(3):195–201.

73. Barbarich NC, McConaha CW, Gaskill J, La Via M, Frank GK, Achenbach S, et al. An open trial of olanzapine in anorexia nervosa. J Clin Psychiatry. 2004;65(11):1480–1482.

74. Malina A, Gaskill J, McConaha C, Frank GK, LaVia M, Scholar L, et al. Olanzapine treatment of anorexia nervosa: a retrospective study. Int J Eat Disord. 2003;33(2):234–237.

75. Powers PS, Santana CA, Bannon YS. Olanzapine in the treatment of anorexia nervosa: an open label trial. Int J Eat Disord. 2002;32(2):146–154.

76. Fisher M. The course and outcome of eating disorders in adults and in adolescents: a review. Adolesc Med. 2003;14(1):149–158.

77. Child Maltreatment 2003. Washington, DC: US Depart-

ment of Health and Human Services Administration on Children, Youth, and Families, US Government Printing Office; 2005.

78. Sedlak AJ, Broadhurst DD. Third National Incidence Study of Child Abuse and Neglect. Washington, DC: US Department of Health and Human Services, Administration on Children, Youth, and Families; 1996.

79. Zolotor AJ, Motsinger BM, Runyan DK, Sanford C. Building an effective child maltreatment surveillance system in North Carolina. NC Med J. 2005;66(5):360–363.

80. When inflicted skin injuries constitute child abuse. Pediatrics. 2002;110(3):644–645.

81. Maguire S, Mann MK, Sibert J, Kemp A. Are there patterns of bruising in childhood which are diagnostic or suggestive of abuse? A systematic review. Arch Dis Child. 2005;90(2):182–186.

82. Bulloch B, Schubert CJ, Brophy PD, Johnson N, Reed MH, Shapiro RA. Cause and clinical characteristics of rib fractures in infants. Pediatrics. 2000;105(4):E48.

83. Rubin DM, Christian CW, Bilaniuk LT, Zazyczny KA, Durbin DR. Occult head injury in high-risk abused children. Pediatrics. 2003;111(6 Pt 1):1382–1386.

84. Kellogg N. The evaluation of sexual abuse in children. Pediatrics. 2005;116(2):506–512.

85. Dubowitz H, Giardino A, Gustavson E. Child neglect: guidance for pediatricians. Pediatr Rev. 2000;21(4):111–1116.

86. Zolotor AJ, Runyan DK. Social Capital, Family Violence, and Neglect. Pediatrics. 2006;117(16):e1224–31.

87. Glascoe FP. Commonly Used Screening Tools. In: *http://www.dbpeds.org/articles/detail.cfm?textid=539*: Developmental and Behavioral Pediatrics Online (*dbpeds.org*); Accessed 11/22/2005.

CHAPTER 14

Fever in Infants and Preschool Children

Vince WinklerPrins and William C. Wadland

CASE 1

Friday at 4 PM, Mr. B brings his 10-week-old son, Alex, to see you because he has felt warm the last few hours and is not breastfeeding as eagerly. He has had no other symptoms. Alex was born healthy at term via spontaneous vaginal delivery in an otherwise unremarkable pregnancy. He and his mother were discharged after a 24-hour stay. He has not been previously ill. He received his routine immunizations 10 days ago. Physical examination reveals a temperature of 38.6°C (101.5°F) rectally. He is alert and appears well. No localizing signs of illness are noted on comprehensive examination.

CLINICAL QUESTIONS

1. What are the most important diagnostic considerations to be assessed in the evaluation of fever without obvious cause in an ill child?
2. How should you evaluate fever without obvious cause in an ill child?
3. How should you counsel Alex's father in regard to his son's care and follow-up?

CASE 2

Alice is a 10-month-old who was previously well and presents with a fever of 39.2°C (102.4°F) rectally. Her mother reports poor fluid intake, and the child appears lethargic, has a weak cry, and is poorly responsive to stimulation. Additional clinical findings include very dry mucous membranes, diminished skin turgor, a bulging anterior fontanelle, and cyanotic skin with peripheral pallor. Vital signs include a pulse of 180 beats/min and a respiratory rate of 40 breaths/min, but no retractions or cough. There is no nuchal rigidity; in fact, the child seems flaccid with decreased muscle tone. Chest examination is clear with no cardiac murmur. Otoscopy reveals acute otitis media bilaterally.

CLINICAL QUESTIONS

1. Is the presentation attributable to acute otitis media alone, or should a serious bacterial illness (SBI) be considered?
2. What should be the clinical and diagnostic evaluation?
3. Should Alice be admitted to the hospital or is outpatient care sufficient?

The assessment of fever of uncertain origin in infants and preschool children is diagnostically challenging and anxiety provoking to all physicians who care for children. Fever in infants and young children is the primary cause of unscheduled visits to family physicians, pediatricians, and emergency departments (1). At least two-thirds of all children visit a physician for an acute illness with fever before they are three, and while most have an identifiable source of infection, 14%–20% of these children have no obvious source (1, 2).

It is essential to be able to discriminate between children with benign disease from those with SBIs. SBIs are usually defined as bacteremia, urinary tract infections or meningitis, but may also encompass serious skin and bone infections. This task is complicated by the challenges in evaluating the very young child who is not only at greater risk for SBI but who often does not manifest the usual signs and symptoms of illness as distinctly (3).

The major challenge for all providers is to plan an expeditious evaluation that also avoids doing unnecessary harm. Parents are very willing to accept approaches that inflict less discomfort and avoid unnecessary antibiotics (4, 5) but because physicians are fearful of missing potential serious infections, they often opt for more aggressive investigations and greater use of antibiotics than necessary (4).

This chapter is not about the management of common childhood febrile diseases. Instead we will review the challenges faced in the assessment of the infant and young child who has fever without obvious source and suggest a means to understand, evaluate, and treat the ill child using the best available evidence. The successful care of the febrile child is not just an exercise in the application of guidelines. Excellent care will rely as much on effective communication, rapport building, and follow-up as on good clinical assessment and decision-making.

DIFFERENTIAL DIAGNOSIS AND PATHOPHYSIOLOGY

Definition and Assessment of Fever

Most clinicians and researchers define fever as a rectal temperature above 38.0°C (100.4°F). Temperatures above 41.1°C (106°F) are referred to as hyperpyrexia. Rectal temperatures are traditionally considered the most accurate means of detecting fever, but are also the most inconvenient to obtain. Although tympanic membrane and axillary thermometers are used frequently in the outpatient setting, their reliability, especially in children less than 36 months old, is questionable. Several studies report poor correlations between oral, axillary, and rectal temperatures (6–8).

TABLE 14.1 Risks for Serious Bacterial Infection by Age and Clinical Appearance of the Febrile Child

	Age <3 Months		Age 3–36 Months	
	Toxic Appearance	**Nontoxic Appearance**	**Toxic Appearance**	**Nontoxic Appearance**
Serious bacterial infection (%)	17.3 (8.0–30)	8.6 (3.7–15.6)	10.0 (5.0–90)	4.3 (3.0–11.0)*
Bacteremia (%)	10.7 (6.7–15.7)	2.0 (0.8–3.8)	—	—
Meningitis (%)	3.9 (1.7–7.1)	1.0 (0.2–2.4)	—	—

*Nontoxic-appearing children ages 3–36 months with a temperature of >39.0°C (102.2°F) rectally have a slightly higher risk of bacteremia of 6.8% (4.6%–9.4%).

The sensitivity to detect a temperature greater than 37.4°C (99.4°F) by oral or axillary thermometers is less than 50%, resulting in a high false-negative rate and many undetected fevers (6). Several studies have found that the younger the child, the less accurate the tympanic thermometer, with reports of sensitivities ranging between 66% and 80% (7–10). The accuracy of tympanic thermometers appears to vary with the age of the child, the operator's experience, and appropriate positioning of the thermometer tip in the ear canal. A systematic review of the utility of ear temperatures in the assessment of ill children suggested that the range of temperatures measured via ear thermometry was too wide to be a reliable measure of fever (11). A similar systematic review comparing axillary with rectal temperatures reached a similar conclusion (12).

When talking to a patient by telephone, physicians often ask the parent to measure the child's temperature. However, only 10% of the mothers in one study were able to correctly read three preset thermometers, despite 67% stating that they knew how to read them (13). Maternal reports of detecting a fever by tactile assessment are fairly accurate, with 84% sensitivity and 76% specificity (LR +, 3.5; LR −, 0.21) (14). Therefore a history of fever even without measurement is usually accurate.

Differential Diagnosis

Children can be stratified for risk of SBI by various means including age, whether or not they appear toxic (severe lethargy, poor tone, inability to drink fluids) at the time of presentation, height of fever, and other risk factors. The risk of SBI is greater in younger children, those who appear toxic, and those with rectal temperatures greater than 39°C. This is particularly so in the very young infant 28 days or younger. Such febrile (39°C or 102.2°F) infants, whether they appear toxic or not, have a relatively high incidence of SBIs (4% to 20%) (15, 16) with a more recent review suggesting 12% (17). Febrile children less than 3 months old who appear toxic have a 17% probability of SBI, more specifically an 11% probability of bacteremia, and a 4% probability of meningitis (1, 18, 19). The risk of occult bacteremia in febrile children (≥39°C or 102.2°F) between 3 months and 36 months who are nontoxic-appearing is approximately 7% (range, 5% to 9%) (15). Table 14.1 summarizes the risks for SBI by age and clinical appearance of the febrile child. The differential diagnosis of fever in children is summarized in Table 14.2.

TABLE 14.2 Most Frequent Diagnoses in Infants with Fever

Age ≤2 Months		Age ≤1 Year	
Diagnosis	**% of Cases**	**Diagnosis**	**% of Cases**
Nonspecific viral illness	36.7	Upper respiratory infection	38.6
Upper respiratory infection	24.8	Otitis media	32.9
Viral gastroenteritis	9.4	Nonspecific viral illness	15.9
Aseptic meningitis	8.5	Gastroenteritis	11.4
Otitis media	6.7	Pneumonia	1.6
Pneumonia	3.1	Bronchiolitis	1.2
Sepsis/meningitis	2.7	Croup	1.2
Bacterial gastroenteritis	2.7	Chickenpox	1.2
Other bacterial infection	2.7	Roseola	1.2
Urinary tract infection	1.7	Streptococcal pharyngitis	1.2

(Data from Kimmel SR, Gemill DW. The young child with fever. Am Fam Physician. 1988;37(6)196–206, and Hoekelman RA. Infectious illness during the first year of life. Pediatrics. 1977;59:119–21.)

VIRAL INFECTIONS

Uncomplicated upper respiratory infections (URIs) are by far the most common cause of fever in preschool children. More than 300 types of viruses have been implicated with rhinoviruses, the most common cause. Children have a higher incidence of URIs than adults because immunity occurs only after exposure. Preschool children commonly have 6–10 or more URIs per year, while adults usually have only two to three. The spread of URIs is likely by droplet as well as hand-to-face transmission (20, 21). Influenza is a frequent cause of fever in the winter months. The risk of SBIs in those identified as having influenza A may be less than in those who test negative for this virus, suggesting that the work-up for SBIs in those who test positive for influenza may not need to be as extensive (22, 23).

Herpes simplex virus (HSV) infections should also be considered in febrile infants less than 1 month old. Empiric acyclovir should be considered for ill infants at this age if they are not improving with appropriate antibiotic therapy, or there is significant reason to suspect this illness (primary maternal HSV infection at delivery is greatest risk) after sending appropriate viral skin cultures from vesicles and spinal fluid for culture and polymerase chain reaction (PCR) studies (24).

Infants with fever without known cause may have an enteroviral infection, especially between August and October, when the incidence is up to 50% (25). Human herpes virus 6 (HHV-6) may cause 10% of febrile illnesses in infants ≤90 days old (26).

OTITIS MEDIA

Otitis media (OM) usually occurs in children who have had a URI for several days. Most causes are felt to be viral, with the predominant bacterial causes being *Streptococcus pneumoniae* and *Haemophilus influenza*. A minority of children over 2 years old require antibiotics; however, adequate pain management is essential. Otitis media alone in a child less than 3 months does not increase or decrease the likelihood of SBI (27).

GASTROENTERITIS

Gastroenteritis is a common source of fever in children (see Table 14.2), and most resolve without concern. Mild diarrhea may also be a nonspecific marker of illness. If diarrhea predominates in an ill child, stool testing for white blood count (WBC) and culture are warranted, with special concern for salmonella, with its risk for meningitis and other sequelae.

ACUTE CHEST INFECTIONS: BRONCHITIS, BRONCHIOLITIS, AND PNEUMONIA

Chest infections can affect either the upper airways (bronchi and bronchioles), as with bronchitis and bronchiolitis, or the lung parenchyma, as with pneumonia. Bronchitis is characterized by rhonchi and bronchiolitis by wheezing, although the accuracy of these symptoms is low. Children with upper airway infections are usually not seriously ill and can be managed as outpatients. Respiratory syncytial virus (RSV) is an exception and can cause relatively severe lower respiratory infections (bronchiolitis) in infants. The likelihood of SBIs with RSV seems to be low (28, 29) and supports the need to discontinue antibiotics in the young with RSV if bacterial cultures are negative, although the frequently found infiltrates on x-ray with bronchiolitis often lead providers to prescribe antibiotics.

OTHER SERIOUS BACTERIAL INFECTIONS

Of the most commonly considered serious bacterial infections, UTIs are more common than bacteremia, which in turn is more common than meningitis. A retrospective review of the bacterial pathogens (n = 367) responsible for SBIs in infants <2 months of age presenting to an urban emergency department over a 4-year period revealed that 78% of SBIs were urine only, 13% blood only, and 3% CSF only. Seventy-nine percent were gram-negative rods, 12% group B strep, 6% enterococcus, 3% *S. pneumoniae*, and 1% *Neisseria meningitidis* (30). The incidence of *Listeria* as a neonatal pathogen seems to be diminishing.

UTIs have been reported in up to 4% of children age 3 to 24 months with fever and no diagnosed source (31, 32). A retrospective review of 354 hospitalized children under the age of 2 with UTIs showed that 9% had concomitant bacteremia, but all of these were less than 6 months of age, and the risk was inversely correlated with the age of the infant (33).

Bacteremia is more common in children under 2, and in those who appear toxic. Typical organisms include *S. pneumoniae* (65% to 70%), *Haemophilus influenzae* (20% to 25%), *N. meningitidis* (3% to 5%), and others (5% to 15%) (31). These patterns are changing, however, with use of the *H. influenzae* B vaccine nearly eliminating *H. influenzae* bacteremia. It remains to be seen what the effect of universal pneumococcal vaccination in children and improved efforts at screening and treating for group B strep in pregnant women will have on bacteremia and meningitis.

Typical symptoms of meningitis such as high fever, irritability, photophobia, vomiting, lethargy, and neck stiffness are often absent in infants. Meningitis can develop in children who present with only a mild respiratory infection and low-grade fever. You should carefully follow up (see Figs. 14.1 and 14.2) infants with fever and no clear etiology to ensure lack of progression to serious illness.

Pneumonia, which in most research studies is not categorized as an SBI (most are viral) should be considered in children with fever. A history of cough should increase suspicion for this diagnosis and consideration for a chest x-ray. In the very young, irregular breathing, tachypnea, or grunting may also be associated with SBI.

CLINICAL EVALUATION AND PROTOCOLS

The evaluation of fever in infants and preschool children requires a comprehensive history, a physical exam to include vitals, skin, ear, nose, and throat (ENT), lungs, an assessment of activity level and level of alertness, rational use of laboratory studies, and excellent communication and follow-up with parents to assess any changes and, in particular, exacerbations in clinical status. Frequently, the complaint of fever in children originates from a telephone call by parents seeking advice. If the child has constitutional symptoms such as malaise, poor fluid intake, rapid respirations, or lethargy, then the physician must see the child to complete an adequate evaluation.

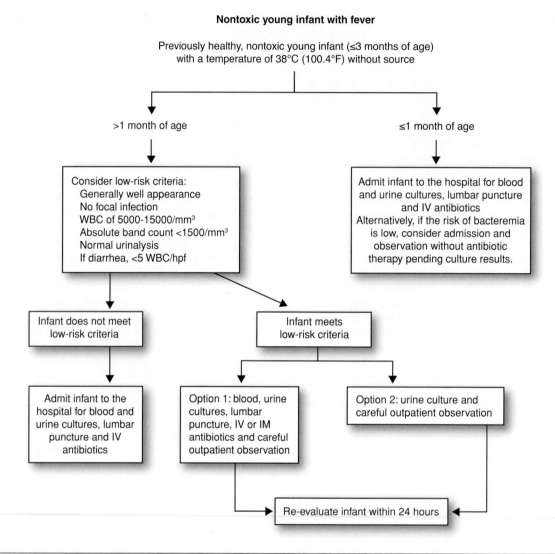

Nontoxic young infant with fever

Previously healthy, nontoxic young infant (≤3 months of age) with a temperature of 38°C (100.4°F) without source

>1 month of age

≤1 month of age

Consider low-risk criteria:
Generally well appearance
No focal infection
WBC of 5000-15000/mm³
Absolute band count <1500/mm³
Normal urinalysis
If diarrhea, <5 WBC/hpf

Admit infant to the hospital for blood and urine cultures, lumbar puncture and IV antibiotics
Alternatively, if the risk of bacteremia is low, consider admission and observation without antibiotic therapy pending culture results.

Infant does not meet low-risk criteria

Infant meets low-risk criteria

Admit infant to the hospital for blood and urine cultures, lumbar puncture and IV antibiotics

Option 1: blood, urine cultures, lumbar puncture, IV or IM antibiotics and careful outpatient observation

Option 2: urine culture and careful outpatient observation

Re-evaluate infant within 24 hours

Figure 14.1 • Algorithm for the management of nontoxic young infants with a temperature of 38.0°C (100.4°F) without source under three months of age. Reprinted with permission from Luszczak M. Evaluation and management of infants and young children with fever. Am Fam Physician. 2001;64:1219–1226.

History

A guide to the key elements of the history and physical in the evaluation of ill infants and children is seen in Table 14.3. Clinicians should inquire about the exact age of the child in months, the degree of temperature elevation, the route and reliability of reading the temperature, and the child's current health status including chronic medical conditions that may increase risk, including HIV positivity. He or she should also ask about immunization status, birth history (such as prematurity), previous hospitalizations, focal signs of infection (skin, bone, ears, etc.), feeding and drinking status, general activity level, and recent antibiotic use.

Because history is a less reliable marker of illness in the very young and the risk of SBI is higher, infants less than 1 month old with a rectal temperature ≥38°C (100.4°F) or with significant report of fever generally merit a full clinical evaluation, including laboratory studies and probable hospitalization (15).

There are conflicting reports in the literature regarding whether the height of fever is important (16, 34–36). While it appears that the height of the fever correlates somewhat with the likelihood of SBI, its discriminating ability does not have enough power alone to alter the approach to the evaluation of the ill or febrile child. Also, a positive response to antipyretics does not necessarily rule out SBI (37, 38).

Physical Examination

Age-specific vital signs should be evaluated and assessed. Signs suggestive of SBI include irregular respirations, stridor, retractions, cyanosis, altered consciousness, nasal flaring, poor muscle tone, and skin pallor (16, 34). Petechiae should prompt a more rigorous consideration of meningitis.

In children under 2 months of age, the presence of rales (positive likelihood ratio [LR +], 15), retractions (LR +, 13), rhonchi (LR +, 13), and/or a respiratory rate ≥60 (LR +, 8.3) help rule in pneumonia if present. However, their absence does not rule out pneumonia (negative likelihood ratio

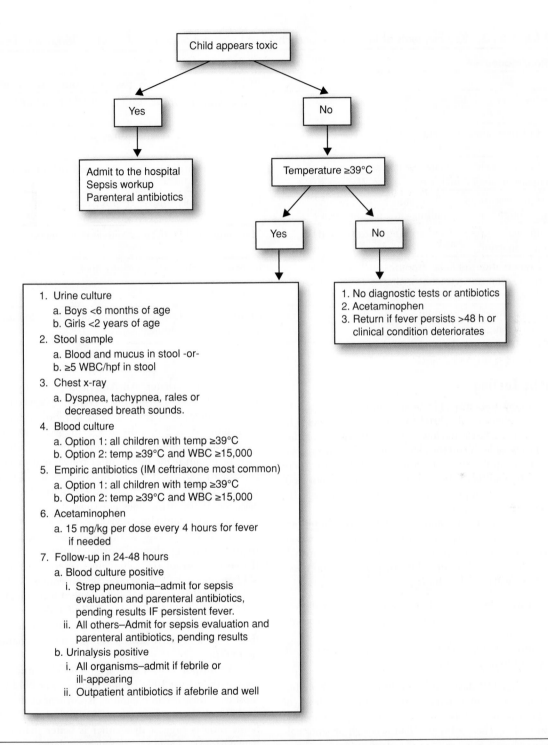

Figure 14.2 • Algorithm for the management of the previously healthy child three months to three years of age.
Adapted with permission from Baraff LJ, Bass JW, Fleisher GR, et al. Practice guidelines for the management of infants and children 0–36 months of age with fever without source. Ann Emerg Med. 1993;22(7):1198–1210.

[LR −], 0.5 to 0.9) (39). Pulse oximetry may be a more sensitive indicator of pneumonia than respiratory rate although this is still debated.

The Yale Observation Scale has been developed to identify febrile infants with SBI based on their clinical appearance. It includes factors such as quality of cry, reaction to parent stimulation, state variation, color, hydration, and response to social overtures. A score of 10 or above (out of a maximum of 30 points) is predictive of serious illness in toxic-appearing children (LR + 3.0, LR − 0.4). This scale is, however, of limited use in ruling out serious illness in children who do not appear toxic (LR − 0.9) (40).

TABLE 14.3 Key Elements of the History and Physical Examination in Infants and Children with Fever

Question/Maneuver	Purpose
Age	Risk of serious illness is greater if patient is <1 month old
Degree of fever	Rectal temperature ≥38.0°C (100.4°F) is defined as true fever
Method of fever measurement	Axillary and oral temperatures are unreliable in young children
Comorbidities such as concurrent illness, previous hospitalizations, or prematurity	These can contribute to an increased risk of serious illness
Focal signs of infection such as skin lesions, joint swelling, cough, redness, pulling on ears, diarrhea	Indicate possible sources of infection
Constitutional symptoms and feeding status (lethargy, irritability, inactivity)	May indicate dehydration and serious illness
Clinical observation for toxic findings such as rapid respirations, cyanosis, retractions, altered consciousness, skin pallor, decreased activity, and responsiveness	Increased likelihood of serious illness
Inquire about parents' capability to measure temperature, observe for changes, and return for follow-up	Ensures timely follow-up in case of progression and deterioration of clinical status

Diagnostic Testing

There are many tests available to the clinician that can be used in the evaluation of febrile infants and children. The utility of any single test is too low (low sensitivity and predictive value) to be able to comfortably assign a child into a low or high-risk group based on one test alone. While aspects of individual tests will be discussed below, it is combinations of signs and tests that improve our diagnostic accuracy sufficiently to be of use to the clinician.

While most infants and children with fever do not require laboratory investigations, specific groups of children in whom laboratory investigation (complete blood count [CBC], urinalysis, urine culture, blood cultures, lumbar puncture, and possibly others) are warranted include:

- Temperature >38°C rectal (100.4°F) and age <28 days
- Temperature >38°C rectal (100.4°F), age 28 to 90 days, and toxic-appearing
- Temperature >39°C rectal (102.2°F), age 91 days to 36 months, and toxic-appearing

Children aged 91 days to 36 months who are febrile but not toxic appearing may require an intermediate level of workup, guided by the CBC and targeted symptom specific evaluation such as chest x-ray (CXR) for cough or stool cultures for diarrhea.

The risk of SBI increases with a WBC >15,000 cells/mm^3, although the prevalence of bacteremia may still be as low as 2% to 4%. Most children with a WBC result in this range do not have a serious illness (41). Extreme elevations of WBCs (35,000 to 50,000 cells/mm^3) are associated with a 19% to 50% probability of SBI (42, 43).

Because urinary tract infections are the most common SBI in infants and young children, the single most useful diagnostic test is an evaluation of the urine. Girls and young uncircumcised boys are at greater risk for UTIs. In children less than 2 months of age, urine should be obtained suprapu-

bically or via catheter. An American Academy of Pediatrics (AAP) policy report from 1999 (44) that reviewed the approach to the evaluation of possible UTI in febrile infants and children older than 2 months of age suggested two options for evaluation: obtain urine for culture suprapubically or via catheter, or obtain urine by the most convenient means and perform a urinalysis. If the urine suggests a UTI, obtain and culture a urine specimen by either suprapubic aspiration or catheter. If the urine does not suggest UTI, it is reasonable to follow the child clinically.

In girls under age 2, the following criteria can be used to predict which girls need a urine culture. The rule is positive if two or more of the following five criteria are present: 1) <12 months old; 2) white race; 3) temperature >39°C; 4) fever ≥2 days; and 5) absence of any source of fever on examination. Given an overall likelihood of UTI of 4.3%, girls with a positive score have 6.4% chance of a positive urine culture, and those with a negative score have only a 0.8% chance of infection (45).

An unspun urine examined under oil immersion microscopy with at least 10 WBC per high-power field (hpf) is the most used measure in the initial assessment of the febrile child for UTI. A spun urine with ≥5 WBC/hpf may be better still. Some reports suggest that either is better than the standard urinalysis (31). Table 14.4 reveals the relative utility of various urine tests as noted in a practice parameter developed by the AAP (44).

Bacteremia is assessed via a single blood culture. As previously mentioned, the likelihood of a positive culture is correlated with the degree of fever and toxicity of the child but these are imperfect associations. Blood cultures have a very low yield in children with uncomplicated croup, bronchitis, varicella, or stomatitis and are generally not to be ordered routinely in these patients (46).

Spinal fluid analysis results will be positive for meningitis in only 8% of patients with indications for lumbar puncture,

TABLE 14.4 Sensitivity and Specificity of Components of the Urinalysis, Alone and in Combination (44)

Test	Sensitivity % (Range)	Specificity % (Range)
Leukocyte esterase	83 (67–94)	78 (64–92)
Nitrite	53 (15–82)	98 (90–100)
Leukocyte esterase *or* nitrite positive	93 (90–100)	72 (58–91)
Microscopy: WBCs	73 (32–100)	81 (45–98)
Microscopy: bacteria	81 (16–99)	83 (11–100)
Leukocyte esterase *or* nitrite *or* microscopy positive	99.8 (99–100)	70 (60–92)

especially in toxic-appearing infants less than 28 days of age. The numbers are even lower for nontoxic appearing children. Many children with indications for lumbar puncture, even with negative meningitis, have associated higher risks for bacteremia (3.2%), bacteriuria (5.4%), and stool pathogen (14%) (47).

A prospective study of the utility of CXR in the evaluation of the febrile child under 5 years of age in an emergency room with a fever >39°C and WBC>20,000 revealed that of the 81% of the 278 children in the study who did receive a CXR as part of their evaluation, 26% had radiologic findings of pneumonia (48). A CXR (indicated for cough with retractions, tachypnea, rales, and/or marked rhonchi) is actually more accurate if read by a radiologist blinded to the examining clinician's diagnosis (49). Although a positive chest radiograph is helpful at ruling in pneumonia (LR +, 4.0), a negative chest radiograph does not rule out the diagnosis (LR −, 0.4). Children without an obvious source of fever and elevated WBC should also be considered for a CXR (48).

Fecal leukocytes and occult blood are not reliable predictors of enteric pathogens in children with diarrhea (50); however, they are often incorporated into assessment criteria. Stool cultures should routinely be assessed in the ill child with significant diarrhea. A systematic review of the literature to ascertain the utility of other potential biomarkers of serious disease including interleukins, tumor necrosis factor and fibronectin yielded no particularly helpful new tests (51).

MANAGEMENT

Various groups have developed protocols that are frequently used in the initial assessment of febrile infants and children and to guide initial therapy. The most commonly cited protocols are the Boston (52), Philadelphia (53), and Rochester (54). These protocols are applied to the evaluation of the infant between birth and 3 months. Details of these criteria are listed in Table 14.5. Of these, the most commonly referenced is the Rochester protocol.

The University of Rochester criteria are to be applied to the evaluation of low-risk infants less than 60 days of age with a rectal temperature ≥38°C. The criteria have a sensitivity of 92%, specificity of 54%, positive predictive value (PPV) of 12.3, and negative predictive value (NPV) of 98.9 for identification of children with SBI. Children who meet all of these low-risk criteria are unlikely to have a SBI. Only 1% of the low-risk infants had a bacteremia, compared with 10% in

the high-risk group. Other than careful history and physical examination, only a CBC, urinalysis and stool testing (if indicated) are needed in these low-risk infants.

Evidence-based algorithms for the evaluation and management of febrile infants have been developed to assist the clinician. Figure 14.1 shows a strategy for evaluating the febrile infant 3 months of age or younger and Figure 14.2 for the evaluation of infants and children ages 3 months to 3 years.

Although following these protocols may not improve outcomes and may in fact increase hospitalizations and tests without improving care (55), they are widely cited as standards to be followed. There is no absolute standard however in the assessment and management of infants and children with fever. These guidelines should be used as suggestions for clinicians who must make judgments based on individual clinical findings and circumstances (15). Most practitioners are willing to accept that the majority of infants and children who are at higher risk will NOT have a SBI (low PPV) in exchange for protocols that rarely miss any children with an SBI (high NPV).

Age Less Than 28 Days

Conceptually, the very young appear to be at greater risk for SBI, seem to manifest signs of serious illness less distinctly, and are at risk for slightly different organisms than older children are. Most studies of febrile infants have broken down age assessment categories by day and/or month age groups for this reason.

Children less than 28 days of age with fever (38°C or 101.4°F or greater) should be admitted to the hospital for a full sepsis evaluation (CBC, blood culture, and lumbar puncture, urine culture), close observation, and initiation of parenteral antibiotics with ampicillin and either a third generation cephalosporin (ceftriaxone or cefotaxime) or gentamicin while awaiting culture results. Table 14.6 gives dosing instructions for referenced antibiotics. CXR, viral studies, and stool testing can also be considered if clinically appropriate. An alternative in nontoxic-appearing infants is to withhold antibiotics pending laboratory results (15). One investigator proposes close observation alone without antibiotic interventions in very-low-risk infants who have WBC <15,000, normal urinalysis, and normal stool screen results, because the likelihood of serious disease is low and intervention can be initiated with progression of clinical findings (56). However, low-risk criteria for older children may not be applicable for febrile infants aged 1 to 28 days (57, 58). A Cochrane review on the use of

TABLE 14.5 The Three Most Common Strategies for Managing Febrile Infants

	Rochester (54)	Philadelphia (53)	Boston (52)
Age	≤60 d	29–60 d	28–89 d
Temperature	≥38.0°C	≥38.2°C	≥38.0°C
History	• Term infant	• Not specified	• No immunizations within preceding 48 hrs
	• No perinatal antibiotics		• No antibiotics within 48 hrs
	• No underlying disease		• Not dehydrated
	• Not hospitalized longer than the mother		
Physical exam.	• Well appearing	• Well appearing	• Well appearing
	• No ear, soft tissue, or bone infection	• Unremarkable examination	• No ear, soft tissue, or bone infection
Laboratory	• WBC >5000 and <15,000/ mm^3	• WBC <15,000/mm^3	• WBC <20,000/mm^3
	• Absolute band count <1500/mm^3	• Band-neutrophil ratio <0.2	
	• UA ≤10 WBC/hpf	• UA<10 WBC/hpf	• UA<10 WBC/hpf
		• Urine gram stain negative	
		• CSF <8 WBC/mm^3	• CSF<10 WBC/mm^3
		• CSF gram stain negative	
		• CXR negative*	• CXR negative*
	• ≤5 WBC/hpf stool smear[b]	• Stool: no blood, few or no WBCs on smear[†]	
Statistics	Sensitivity 92% (83–97%)	Sensitivity 98% (92–100%)	Sensitivity not available
	Specificity 50% (47–53%)	Specificity 42% (38–46%)	Specificity 94.6%
	PPV 12.3% (10–16%)	PPV 14% (11–17%)	PPV not available
	NPV 98.9% (97–100%)	NPV 99.7% (98–100%)	NPV not available

* If obtained
[†] If indicated

intravenous immunoglobulin in the care of suspected or proven bacterial or fungal infection in infants less than 1 month of age showed no benefit (59).

Age 28 to 90 Days

Any febrile infant in this age group at high risk (see Figure 14.1) should be hospitalized for full sepsis evaluation and initial parenteral antibiotics with a third generation cephalosporin—ceftriaxone or cefotaxime. Low-risk infants in this age group can be managed in one of two ways: a full sepsis evaluation, parenteral therapy, and return to be reevaluated in 24 hours, or a urine culture, careful observation, and follow-up in 24 hours.

Age 3 to 36 Months

Children between the ages of 3 months and 36 months who appear toxic should be admitted for a full sepsis workup and parenteral antibiotics (see Figure 14.2). If there are no signs

of toxicity, these children can be evaluated as outpatients with studies based on specific symptoms and follow-up visits within 24–48 hours. One option is to obtain blood cultures on all children in this category, and another is to obtain blood cultures only on children with WBC ≥15,000. Using a cutoff of 15,000 to guide empiric treatment would result in 19 children without bacteremia receiving antibiotics for each child with bacteremia treated (60). Children who appear nontoxic, have a temperature <39°C (102.2°F), and have no clear source of infection require no additional diagnostic tests. They can be given antipyretic medication alone and should be followed up within 24–48 hours.

Reducing Fever

Antipyretic therapy with either acetaminophen or ibuprofen effectively controls fever with few adverse effects (58). A meta-analysis of safety and efficacy of acetaminophen versus ibuprofen showed comparable pain relief but slightly better fever control with ibuprofen after a single dose (61) (see Table 14.7).

TABLE 14.6 Common Medications Used in the Care of the Febrile Infant

Drug	Contraindications/Cautions/Adverse Effects	Dosage	Relative Cost
Acetaminophen	Hepatotoxicity with overdose, contraindicated in G6PD deficiency. Check concentration	12.5–15 mg/kg orally every 4–6 h prn, not to exceed 5 doses in 24 h	$
Ibuprofen	GI distress, granulocytopenia, anemia, inhibits platelet aggregation	5–10 mg/kg orally every 6–8 h prn, maximum daily dose: 40 mg/kg	$
Ampicillin	Known allergy	100–200 mg/kg/day IV every 6 h if weight > 2000 g (50–100 mg/ kg if <7 d of age)	$
Gentamicin	Renal toxicity. Monitor peak and trough levels and possibly auditory function	<7 d old 2.5 mg/kg/d every 12 h >7 d old 5 mg/kg/day every 8 h	$
Ceftriaxone	Caution with penicillin allergy, caution with jaundice	50–75 mg/kg/d given IV or IM (max 2 g)	$$
Cefotaxime	Caution with penicillin allergy	<7 d old 100 mg/kg/d every 12 h >7 d old 150 mg/kg/d given every 8 h	$$

Prn, as needed; IV, intravenously; IM, intramuscularly.

Parents frequently underdose antipyretics, using partial doses rather than full doses (62, 63) although overuse of acetaminophen and its availability in many products leaves increasing concern of overuse. Variable concentrations of commonly used acetaminophen products for infants and children complicate this (64). Inquiry about dosages and routes of administration (65, 66) is essential. Rectal administration may lead to variable absorption and subtherapeutic plasma levels (67). There is no proven efficacy in alternating acetaminophen and ibuprofen, although many physicians persist in recommending the practice (68). A Cochrane review of physical methods to assist in fever control revealed that sponging by tepid water is benefi-cial but may lead to more shivering and goose bumps (69). Other sources suggest differently (70, 71). Do not given aspirin because of risk of Reye's syndrome.

Antibiotic Selection

Details of the antibiotic prescribing for common infectious diseases will not be detailed here. A STEPS approach (Safety, Tolerability, Effectiveness, Price, Simplicity) to antibiotic prescribing in the febrile child is necessary. Neonates less than 1 month of age are still at risk for perinatal infections including *Listeria*. Combinations of ampicillin and a third generation cephalosporin (cefotaxine) or gentimicin are still the preferred

TABLE 14.7 Therapeutic Options Available for Management of Infants and Preschool Children with Fever

Treatment Strategy	Strength of Recommendation*	Recommendation/Comments
Antipyretic medication (acetaminophen or ibuprofen)	A	Advise giving appropriate doses per kilogram and review med concentration if suspect toxicity
Oral antibiotics for appropriate infections	B	Some reports of failure to prevent *H. influenza* in unimmunized infants
Parenteral antibiotics (IM/IV)	A	See text and figures
Oral hydration	A	Child must be nontoxic and tolerate oral fluids to prevent dehydration
Intravenous hydration	A	Hospitalize/infusion center/ER
Sponging for fever control	B	May be helpful
Aspirin	A	Do not use because of Reye's syndrome risk

*A = consistent, good-quality patient-oriented evidence; B = inconsistent or limited-quality patient-oriented evidence; C = consensus, disease-oriented evidence, usual practice, expert opinion, or case series. For information about the SORT evidence rating system, see *http://www.aafp.org/afpsort.xml*

medications in the under one month old group (see Table 14.6) with a third generation cephalosporin (cefotaxime) alone used after the first month.

FOLLOW-UP

Decisions to treat patients in the hospital or as outpatients rarely rely exclusively on illness characteristics of the patient. They also need to take into consideration social factors that include access (phone/transportation/financial/language) and assessment of reliability for follow-through. You must follow all patients managed as outpatients. Parents should be advised to check their child every 4 hours for activity, rectal temperature, skin color changes, and adequate fluid intake, and parents should call immediately if they have any concerns. Arrangements for timely follow-up in 24 to 48 hours should be made before leaving the office or emergency department (see protocols for details). Children who are still febrile at follow-up visits and have worsening symptoms should have a complete sepsis evaluation and be admitted to the hospital.

PREVENTION

H. influenza type B immunization has virtually eliminated this as an invasive organism for the immunized child. Universal pneumococcal as well as influenza A immunizations may also reduce illness in children but this is not entirely clear yet. A well-designed trial showed no reduction in illness in homes where bacterial home cleaning and hand washing practices were performed (72). Intravenous immunoglobulin does not warrant a place in the prevention of severe illness when preventatively given to preterm or low-birth-weight infants in a recent Cochrane review (73).

CASE DISCUSSION

CASE 1

Following the algorithm in Figure 14.1, this child should have a CBC with differential and urine testing. If these can be done in your office and are normal then you have two options: one is a culture of the blood, urine and CSF with an injection of ceftriaxone, or the other is a urine culture. With either choice, follow-up in 24 hours is necessary or sooner if the clinical situation is deteriorating. The physician assessment of the logistical challenges for families in assessing and monitoring their infant or child and careful communication will be important here.

CASE 2

Although the patient is older than 90 days and there is a definite focus of infection (OM), the toxic appearance suggests serious illness. Therefore, the child should have a full sepsis evaluation, empiric antibiotics, and hospitalization.

The relative dehydration merits intravenous fluids. This patient had meningitis caused by *S. pneumoniae* and responded well to intravenous antibiotics and hydration without residual sequelae.

REFERENCES

1. Baraff LJ. Management of infants and children 3 to 36 months of age with fever without source. Pediatr Ann. 1993; 22:497–498, 501–504.
2. Nelson DS, Walsh K, Fleisher GR. Spectrum and frequency of pediatric illness presenting to a general community hospital emergency department. Pediatrics. 1992;90:5–10.
3. Telle DW, Pelton SE, Grant MJ, et al. Bacteremia in febrile children under 2 years of age: results of cultures of blood of 600 consecutive febrile children seen in "walk-in" clinics. J Pediatr. 1975;87:227–230.
4. Kramer MS, Etezadi-Amoli J, Ciampi A, et al. Parents' versus physicians' values for clinical outcomes in young febrile children. Pediatrics. 1994; 93:697–702.
5. Oppenheim PI, Sotiropolous G, Baraff LJ. Incorporating patient preferences into patient guidelines: management of children with fever without source. Ann Emerg Med. 1994;24: 836–841.
6. Ogren JM. The inaccuracy of axillary temperatures measured with an electronic thermometer. Am J Dis Child. 1990;144: 109–111.
7. Hooker EA. Use of tympanic thermometers to screen for fever in patients in a pediatric emergency department. South Med J. 1993;86:855–858.
8. Peterson-Smith A, Barber N, Coody DK, West MS, Yetman RJ. Comparison of aural infrared with traditional rectal temperatures in children from birth to age 3 years. J Pediatr. 1994;125:83–85.
9. Terndrup TE, Milewski A. The performance of two tympanic thermometers in pediatric emergency departments. Clin Pediatr. 1991;30:18–23.
10. Terndrup TE, Rajk J. Impact of operator technique and device on infrared emission detection tympanic thermometry. J Emerg Med. 1992;10:683–687.
11. Craig JV, Lancaster GA, Taylor S, Williamson PR, Smyth RL. Infrared ear thermometry compared with rectal thermometry in children: a systematic review. Lancet. 2002;360: 603–609.
12. Craig JV, Lancaster GA, Williamson PR, Smyth RL. Temperature measured at the axilla compared with rectum in children and young people: systematic review. Br Med J. 2000; 320:1174–1178.
13. Banco L, Jayashekaramurthy S. The ability of mothers to read a thermometer. Clin Pediatr. 1990;29:343–345.
14. Graneto JW, Soglin DF. Maternal screening of childhood fever by palpation. Pediatr Emerg Care. 1996;12:183–184.
15. Baraff LJ, Bass JW, Fleisher GR, et al. Practice guidelines for the management of infants and children 0–36 months of age with fever without source. Ann Emerg Med. 1993;22(7): 1198–1210.
16. Nocicka A. Evaluation of the febrile infant younger than 3 months of age with no source of infection. Am J Emerg Med. 1995;13:215–218.
17. Teague JA, Harper, MB, Bachur R, et al. Epidemiology of febrile infants 14–28 days of age. Pediatr Res. 2003;53:214.
18. Baraff LJ, Oslund SA, Schreger DC, Stephen ML. Probability of bacterial infections in febrile infants less than three months of age: a meta-analysis. Pediatr Infect Dis J. 1992;11:257–264.

19. Bachur RG, Harper MB. Predictive model for serious bacterial infections among infants younger than 3 months of age. Pediatrics. 2001;108:311–316.
20. Hendley JO, Wenzel RP, Gwaltney JM Jr. Transmission of rhinovirus colds by self-inoculation. N Engl J Med. 1973;288: 1361–1364.
21. Dick EC, Jennings LC, Mink KA, Wartgow CD, Inhorn SL. Aerosol transmission of rhinovirus colds. J Infect Dis. 1987; 156:442–448.
22. Smitherman HF, Caviness C, Macias CG. Retrospective review of serious bacterial infections in infants who are 0 to 36 months of age and have influenza A infection. Pediatrics. 2005;115:710–718.
23. Sharma V, Dowd MD, Slaughter AJ, Simon SD. Effect of rapid diagnosis of influenza virus type A on the emergency department management of febrile infants and toddlers. Arch Ped Adol Med. 2002;156:41–43.
24. Harper MB. Update on the management of the febrile infant. Clin Ped Emerg Med. 2004;5:5–12.
25. Byington CL, Taggart EW, Carroll KC, Hillyard DR. A polymerase chain reaction-based epidemiologic investigation of the incidence of nonpolio enteroviral infections in febrile and afebrile infants 90 days and younger. Pediatrics. 1999; 103(3):E27.
26. Byington CL, Zerr DM, Taggart EW, et al. Human herpesvirus 6 infection in febrile infants ninety days of age and younger. Pediatr Infect Dis J. 2002;21(11):996–999.
27. Turner D, Leibovitz E, Aran A, et al. Acute otitis media in infants younger than two months of age: microbiology, clinical presentation and therapeutic approach. Pediatr Infect Dis J. 2002;21(7):669–674.
28. Purcell K, Fergie J. Concurrent serious bacterial infections in 2396 infants and children hospitalized with respiratory syncytial virus lower respiratory tract infections. Arch Ped Adol Med. 2002;156:322–324.
29. Levine DA, Platt SL, Dayan PS, et al. Multicenter RSV-SBI study group of the Pediatric Emergency Medicine Collaborative Research Committee of the American Academy of Pediatrics. Risk of serious bacterial infection in young febrile infants with respiratory syncytial virus infections. Pediatrics. 2004;13(6):1728–1734.
30. Berger Sadow K, Derr R, Teach SJ. Bacterial infections in infants 60 days and younger: epidemiology, resistance, and implications for treatment. Arch Ped Adol Med. 1999;153: 611–614.
31. Kramer MS, Tange SM, Drummond KN, Mills EL. Urine testing in young febrile children: a risk-benefit analysis. J Pediatr. 1994;125:6–13.
32. Marild S, Hellstrom M, Jodal U, Eden CS. Fever, bacteriuria, and concomitant disease in children with urinary tract infection. Pediatr Infect Dis J. 1989;8:36–41.
33. Bachur R, Caputo GL. Bacteremia and meningitis among infants with urinary tract infections. Pediatr Emerg Care. 1995;11(5):280–284.
34. Baraff LJ, Oslund SA, Schreger DC, Stephen ML. Probability of bacterial infections in febrile infants less than three months of age: a meta-analysis. Pediatr Infect Dis J. 1992;11:257–264.
35. Alpert G, Hibbert E, Fleisher GR. Case-control study of hyperpyrexia in children. Pediatr Infect Dis J. 1990;9:161–163.
36. Bonadio WA, Grunske L, Smith DS. Systemic bacterial infections in children with fever greater than 41 degrees. Pediatr Infect Dis J. 1989;8:120–122.
37. Baker MD, Fosarelli PD, Carpenter RO. Childhood fever: correlation of diagnosis with temperature response to acetaminophen. Pediatrics. 1987;80:315–318.
38. Baker RC, Tiller T, Bausher JC, et al. Severity of disease correlated with fever reduction in febrile infants. Pediatrics. 1989;83:1016–1019.
39. Crain EF, Bulas D, Bijur P, Goldman H. Is a chest radiograph necessary in the evaluation of every febrile infant less than 8 weeks of age. Pediatrics. 1991;88:821–824.
40. Mazur LJ, Kozinetz CA. Diagnostic tests for occult bacteremia: temperature response to acetaminophen versus WBC count. Am J Emerg Med. 1994;12:403–406.
41. Haddon RA, Barnett PL, Grimwood K, Hogg GG. Bacteraemia in febrile children presenting to a paediatric emergency department. Med J Australia. 1999;170:475.
42. Kramer MS, Tange SM, Mills EL, Ciampi A, Bernstein ML, Drummond KN. Role of the complete blood count in detecting occult focal bacterial infection in the young febrile child. J Clin Epidemiol. 1993;46:349–395.
43. Mazur LJ, Kline MW, Lorin MI. Extreme leukocytosis in patients presenting to a pediatric emergency department. Pediatr Emerg Care. 1991;7:215–218.
44. Bergman DA et al. Practice parameter: the diagnosis, treatment and evaluation of the initial urinary tract infection in febrile infants and young children. American Academy of Pediatrics. Committee on quality improvement. Subcommittee on urinary tract infection. Pediatrics. 1999;103:843–852.
45. Gorelick MH, Shaw KN. Screening tests for urinary tract infection in children: a meta-analysis. Pediatrics. 1999;104(5): 1.
46. Greenes DS, Harper MB. Low risk of bacteremia in febrile children with recognizable viral syndromes. Pediatr Infect Dis J. 1999;18(3):258.
47. Barnett ED, Bauchner H, Teele DW, Klein JO. Serious bacterial infections in febrile infants and children selected for lumbar puncture. Pediatr Infect Dis J. 1994;13:950–953.
48. Bachur R, Perry H, Harper MB. Occult pneumonias: Empiric chest radiographs in febrile children with leukocytosis. Ann Emerg Med. 1999;33:166–173.
49. Kramer MS, Roberts-Brauer R, Williams RL. Bias and "overcall" in interpreting chest radiographs in young febrile children. Pediatrics. 1992;90:11–13.
50. Huicho L, Sanchez D, Contreras M, et al. Occult blood and fecal leukocytes as screening tests in childhood infectious diarrhea: an old problem revisited. Pediatr Infect Dis J. 1993; 12:474–477.
51. Malik A, Hui CPS, Pennie RA, Kirpalani H. Beyond the complete blood count and c-reactive protein: a systematic review of modern diagnostic tests for neonatal sepsis. Arc Ped Adol Med. 2003;157:511–516.
52. Baskin MN, O'Rourke EJ, Fleisher GR. Outpatient treatment of febrile infants 28–89 days of age with intramuscular administration of ceftriaxone. J Pediatr. 1992;120:22–27.
53. Baker MD, Bell LM, Avner JR. Outpatient management without antibiotics of fever in selected infants. N Engl J Med. 1993;329:1437–1441.
54. Jaskiewicz JA, McCarthy CA, Richardson AC, et al. Febrile infants at low risk for SBIs—an appraisal of the Rochester criteria and implications for management. Pediatrics. 1994; 94:390–396.
55. Pantell RH, Newman TB, Bernzweig J, et al. Management and outcomes of care of fever in early infancy. JAMA 2004; 291:1203–1212.
56. McCarthy PL. The febrile infant. Pediatrics. 1994;94: 397–399.
57. Kadish HA, Loveridge B, Tobey J, Bolte RG, Corneli HM. Applying outpatient protocols in febrile infants 1–28 days of age: can the threshold be lowered? Clin Pediatr. 2000;39(2): 81.
58. Vauzelle-Kervroedan F, d'Athis P, Pariente-Khayat A, Debregeas S, Olive G, Pons G. Equivalent antipyretic activity

of ibuprofen and paracetamol in febrile children. J Pediatr. 1997;131(5):683.

59. Ohlsson A, Lacy JB. Intravenous immunoglobulin for suspected or subsequently proven infection in neonates (Cochrane Review). In: The Cochrane Library, Issue 1, 2005. Chichester, UK: John Wiley and Sons, Ltd.

60. Lee GM, Harper MB. Risk of bacteremia for febrile young children in the post-*Haemophilus influenzae* type B era. Arch Pediatr Adolesc Med. 1998;152(7):624.

61. Perrott DA, Piira T, Goodenough B, Champion GD. Efficacy and safety of acetaminophen vs ibuprofen for treating children's pain or fever: a meta-analysis. Arch Pediatr Adolesc Med. 2004;158:521–526.

62. Hyam E, Brawer M, Herman J, Zvieli S. What's in a teaspoon? Underdosing with acetaminophen in family practice. Fam Pract. 1989;6:221–223.

63. Simon HK, Weinkle DA. Over-the-counter medications: do parents give what they intend to give? Arch Pediatr Adolesc Med. 1997;151(7):654.

64. Barrett TW, Norton VC. Parental knowledge of different acetaminophen concentrations for infants and children. Acad Emerg Med. 2000;7:718–721.

65. Autret E, Breart G, Jonville AP, Courcier S, Lassale C, Goehrs JM. Comparative efficacy and tolerance of ibuprofen syrup and acetaminophen syrup in children with pyrexia-associated infectious diseases and treated with antibiotics. Eur J Clin Pharmacol. 1994;46:197–201.

66. Lesko SM, Mitchell AA. An assessment of the safety of pediatric ibuprofen: a practitioner-based randomized clinical trial. JAMA. 1995;273:929–933.

67. Hansen TG, O'Brien K, Morton NS, Rasmussen SN. Plasma paracetamol concentrations and pharmacokinetics following rectal administration in neonates and young infants. Acta Anaesth Scand. 1999;43(8):855.

68. Mayoral CE, Marino RV, Rosenfeld W, Greensher J. Alternating antipyretics: is this an alternative? Pediatrics. 2000; 105(5):1009.

69. Meremikwu M, Oyo-Ita A. Physical methods for treating fever in children (Cochrane Review). In: The Cochrane Library, Issue 1, 2005. Chichester, UK: John Wiley and Sons, Ltd.

70. Newman J. Evaluation of sponging to reduce body temperature. J Can Med Assoc. 1985;132:641–642.

71. Plaisance KI, Mackowiak PA. Antipyretic therapy: physiologic rationale, diagnostic implications, and clinical consequences. Arch Intern Med. 2000;160(4):449.

72. Larson EL, Lin SX, Gomez-Pichardo C, Della-Latta P. Effect of antibacterial home cleaning and handwashing products on infectious disease symptoms: a randomized, double-blind trial. Ann Intern Med. 2004;140:321–329.

73. Ohlsson A, Lacy JB. Intravenous immunoglobulin for preventing infection in preterm and/or low-birth-weight infants (Cochrane Review). In: The Cochrane Library, Issue 1, 2005. Chichester, UK: John Wiley and Sons, Ltd.

74. Luszczak M. Evaluation and management of infants and young children with fever. Am Fam Physician. 2001;64: 1219–1226.

CHAPTER 15

Diabetes

Sam Weir, Katrina Donahue, and Mary Roederer

CASE , PART 1

Mrs. S is a 47-year-old woman who presents to her family physician complaining of recurrent yeast infections over the past 2 months. On further questioning she admits to feeling thirsty all of the time and frequent urination. On exam, she is 5 feet 4 inches tall and weighs 160 lbs (body mass index [BMI] 27.5). Her initial blood pressure (BP) is 135/85. Her random capillary glucose is 140 mg/dl.

CLINICAL QUESTIONS

1. What clinical situations should prompt evaluation for possible diabetes?
2. How would you make the diagnosis of diabetes in this patient?
3. How would you initially evaluate this patient?
4. How do you tell a patient that they have diabetes? What recommendations would you make to this patient for initial management of their disease?
5. What components of care are necessary to manage diabetes over time?

Diabetes mellitus (DM) is a chronic disease which is rapidly increasing in prevalence and is associated with many serious micro- and macrovascular complications. It encompasses several disorders that are characterized by hyperglycemia due to defects in insulin secretion, insulin action, or both (1). Education and support of patient self-management, a comprehensive approach to care, and continuous health care are the cornerstones of successful treatment.

Diabetes is one of the five most common illness-related diagnoses in primary care (2). An estimated 20.8 million people in the United States have diabetes, of whom 14.6 million are diagnosed and 6.2 million are undiagnosed (3). Five percent to ten percent of diagnosed cases are type 1 diabetes; thus, type 2 diabetes accounts for the vast majority of cases. Estimated costs attributed to diabetes in the United States are $132 billion, including direct medical care costs and indirect costs of disability, work loss, and premature mortality (4, 5).

Type 1 diabetes is characterized by the autoimmune destruction of pancreatic beta cells. This silent destructive process occurs over weeks or months and usually presents with acute hyperglycemia, with or without ketoacidosis.

The development of type 2 diabetes is more insidious. It begins as a genetic trait of insulin resistance that, when combined with overeating and a sedentary lifestyle, contributes to central adiposity. Central adiposity exacerbates insulin resistance, eventually outstripping the pancreas' ability to produce insulin, resulting in hyperglycemia. Hyperglycemia is itself toxic to the pancreas and contributes to the gradual loss of pancreatic beta cell function. Thus, type 2 diabetes progresses from glucose intolerance (prediabetes), to elevated fasting glucose, to overt diabetes. Because the classic symptoms of diabetes (polyuria, polydipsia, polyphagia, weight loss) do not develop until fasting blood sugars are far above the threshold for diagnosis, persons with type 2 diabetes may be asymptomatic for many years before they are diagnosed (6).

Diabetes causes multiple complications and often leads to premature death (4). Adults with diabetes are between two and four times more likely to die from heart disease or have a stroke. Diabetes is the leading cause of blindness among adults and the leading cause of kidney failure. More than 60% of people with diabetes have neuropathy, and more than 60% of nontraumatic limb amputations are for complications of diabetes. Periodontal (gum) disease is also more common. Poorly controlled diabetes can also cause major birth defects and excessively large infants.

Diabetes is a lifelong disease that requires a multi-faceted approach to prevent complications. This approach must include behavior change, self management, and negotiation of behavior goals, in addition to the treatment of glycemia and addressing micro- and macrovascular risks.

CLINICAL PRESENTATION

Diabetes can range from obvious to subtle to asymptomatic. Classically, severe hyperglycemia generates symptoms of fatigue, weight loss, polydipsia (excessive thirst), polyphagia (frequent eating), and polyuria (excessive urination). More subtle presentations of diabetes require the physician to look at combinations of signs and symptoms consistent with the disease and deserving of further evaluation. These include:

- obesity
- recurrent infections (especially yeast vaginitis, skin infections, and periodontal infections)
- slow healing wounds
- neurological syndromes (especially focal limb neuropathies presenting with paresthesias, burning, and tingling in the extremities)
- visual changes and blurry vision
- abdominal pain from non alcoholic fatty liver or chronic pancreatitis (often from chronic excessive alcohol consumption)

- heart disease or stroke, especially among persons who have not had consistent medical care in the past
- in women, menstrual irregularity and obesity, polycystic ovarian syndrome (PCOS), an obstetric history of gestational diabetes or giving birth to an infant weighing more than 10 pounds (7).

Hyperglycemic Crises

Diabetes can also present acutely as either diabetic ketoacidosis (DKA), which is common in patients with type 1 diabetes, or hyperosmolar hyperglycemic state (HHS), which is more likely to occur in type 2 diabetes. These conditions are jointly referred to as hyperglycemic crises to emphasize their seriousness and the need for rapid and intensive management. Table 15.1 lists the common presenting signs and symptoms that constitute "red flags" suggesting these states.

The hallmark of DKA is the triad of hyperglycemia, ketosis, and acidosis. Common clinical settings include previously undiagnosed diabetes (20%) and precipitating conditions in diagnosed diabetics (80%), such as omission of previously prescribed insulin dose, pneumonia, urinary tract infection, alcohol abuse, trauma, pulmonary embolus, or myocardial infarction. Symptoms suggestive of diabetic ketoacidosis include a fairly rapid course (< 24 hours), nausea, vomiting, and abdominal pain. Signs of DKA include rapid, deep respirations (Kussmaul breathing), fruity smell to the breath, signs of dehydration, and mental status changes.

HHS can present with more extreme levels of hyperglycemia (more than 1,000 mg/dl) than does DKA, but without ketosis or acidosis. The hyperglycemia causes profound dehydration that leads to hyperosmolality. The typical presentation is an insidious onset over days to weeks, with increasing thirst, polydipsia, polyuria, weight loss, and mental status changes. Physical examination reveals signs of dehydration and often includes mental status changes, obtundation, or coma. HHS may also present as seizures or with focal neurologic signs, such as hemiparesis or visual loss. Although HHS is more

common in older adults, it can present in adolescents with previously undiagnosed type 2 diabetes. Signs and symptoms of hyperglycemic crises are summarized in Table 15.1 (8).

Diagnosing Diabetes

Table 15.2 lists the diagnostic criteria for diabetes. The best test to obtain depends on the clinical presentation. In the presence of classic symptoms (polyuria, polydipsia, weight loss) or if there is a concern of hyperglycemic crises, a random glucose is the appropriate test. Values greater than or equal to 200 mg/dl are diagnostic of diabetes. In the absence of these classic symptoms, patients should be asked to return for a fasting plasma glucose (i.e., after at least 8 hours without any calories). Any fasting glucose result greater than 125 mg/dl is strongly suggestive of diabetes and should be repeated; two results above 125 mg/dl from different days are needed to make the diagnosis. If either fasting plasma glucose is greater than 100, the patient is said to have impaired fasting glucose or prediabetes (1). The 2-hour oral glucose tolerance test (OGTT) is no longer recommended for routine clinical use.

CASE DISCUSSION

Mrs. S's family physician opted to test her with a fasting glucose. The result was 135 mg/dl. Her doctor asked her to return 2 weeks later, and her repeat fasting glucose was 130. On the basis of two fasting glucoses greater than 125, Mrs. S met criteria for the diagnosis of diabetes.

Evaluating the Newly Diagnosed Diabetic

The initial evaluation should include a history, physical exam, laboratory evaluation and referrals for specialized evaluation. The evaluation should classify the patient into diabetes type, identify any current diabetes complications, and help develop the patient's diabetes continuity care plan (1).

The patient's past medical history, social history, health

TABLE 15.1 Clinical Red Flags Suggesting a Hyperglycemic Crisis

Red Flags		Suggest a Diagnosis of:
Symptoms	**Signs**	
Rapid onset (< 24 hours) Nausea and vomiting Abdominal pain Malaise	Mild dehydration Rapid, deep breathing Fruity smelling breath	Diabetic ketoacidosis (DKA)
Gradual onset (days to a week or more) Nausea and vomiting Abdominal pain Headache Thirst Polydipsia Polyuria Weight loss Lethargy Dizziness Headaches	More severe dehydration Mental status changes Obtundation Coma Focal neurologic signs (hemiparesis, visual field deficits) Seizures	Hyperglycemic hyperosmolar state (HHS)

TABLE 15.2   Diagnostic Criteria for Diabetes, Impaired Fasting Glucose, and Impaired Glucose Tolerance*

Glucose Disorder	Criteria
Diabetes	1. Symptomatic and a random plasma glucose ≥200 mg/dl OR 2. Fasting plasma glucoses ≥126[†] OR 3. 2-hour (75 g) glucose tolerance test ≥200 mg/dl[†]
Impaired fasting glucose (IFG)	Fasting plasma glucose 100–125 mg/dl
Impaired glucose tolerance (IGT)	2-hour (75 g) glucose tolerance test 140–199 mg/dl

*Based on the 2006 American Diabetes Association recommendations.
[†]Two separate readings needed to make the diagnosis of diabetes.
The two hour glucose tolerance test is rarely needed to make the diagnosis of diabetes.

habits, and family history can provide information regarding current status and future risk of complications. Given the increased risk of heart disease, a high priority is to inquire about other cardiovascular risk factors, especially hypertension, dyslipidemia, and smoking. Symptoms to ask about include eye problems, periodontal disease, skin symptoms, symptoms of thyroid disease, sexual dysfunction, menstrual irregularities, and peripheral neuropathy (1). Within the family history, one should also ask about family history of diabetes and premature cardiovascular disease. If there is a family history of diabetes, inquire about any complications of diabetes in family members. For women who have had children, a history of gestational diabetes or having a baby weighing more than 9 pounds are important evidence of prior insulin resistance. In addition to current and past use of alcohol and tobacco, the social history should include current dietary habits (especially sweets, snacks, and regular soft drinks) and current physical activity.

The physical examination (see Table 15.3) should pay close attention to organ systems and physical findings that indicate possible complications. BMI should be calculated from height and weight. Blood pressure is critical; borderline readings should be repeated, and orthostatic blood pressures are indicated in patients who present with a history of weight loss, weakness, or lightheadedness. A funduscopic examination will assess for cataracts and retinopathy. The oral cavity should be thoroughly examined for periodontal disease. Palpation of the thyroid and examination of the skin can give clues about possible co-existing hypothyroidism. The cardiovascular exam should include palpation of peripheral pulses and auscultation for bruits over the carotid, renal, and femoral arteries. The abdominal exam should include percussion of the

TABLE 15.3   Components of the Initial Assessment Physical Examination of a Newly Diagnosed Diabetic

Exam Component	Why
Height, weight, and BMI	Comparison to norms, identify/document obesity
Blood pressure	Comparison to norms, identify hypertension. Perform orthostatics if indicated
Funduscopic evaluation	Screen for retinopathy, cataracts
Oral exam	Screen for periodontal disease
Thyroid palpation	Increased risk of concomitant thyroid disease in diabetics
Cardiac exam	Screen for cardiovascular disease (e.g., CHF, murmurs)
Abdominal exam	Look for hepatomegaly (usually due to fatty liver)
Evaluation of pulses	Screen for peripheral vascular disease
Hand/finger exam	Look for infections, evaluate sites for self glucose monitoring
Foot exam	Look for lesions, infections; screen for peripheral neuropathy by performing monofilament sensation
Skin exam	Look for signs of glucose intolerance, such as acanthosis nigricans, infections; evaluate potential injection sites
Neurologic exam	Evaluate for peripheral neuropathy; focus on vibratory sensation, touch (with monofilament), proprioception

liver span and description of any right upper quadrant tenderness. The skin should be carefully inspected for signs of infection or rashes.

Because they are a common site of neurological, vascular, and cutaneous manifestations of diabetes, the lower extremities should be a major focus of the physical examination. The skin should be inspected and palpated for skin color, temperature, and dryness, nail thickness, and hair distribution on the lower extremities and feet. Corns, calluses, and any bony deformities deserve a thorough description. Neurologic examination should include vibratory sensation, light touch, and proprioception of the feet; light touch can best be assessed with the use of a monofilament. The posterior tibial pulse should be palpated. If there is any concern of peripheral arterial disease, a Doppler evaluation of the ankle/brachial index can be performed in most medical offices. To do so, use a hand-held doppler and a blood pressure cuff to measure lower and upper extremity blood pressures; an ankle blood pressure that is less than 0.90 of the brachial blood pressure is abnormal and indicates peripheral vascular disease.

In addition to confirming the diagnosis of diabetes, the laboratory should be used to obtain several baseline measures:

- Obtain hemoglobin A1c to examine blood glucose control over the previous 3 months.
- Obtain a fasting lipid profile for cardiac risk stratification.
- Order an electrocardiogram if the patient has co-existing hypertension. (Diabetes is associated with left ventricular hypertrophy.)
- Order a urinalysis to test for ketones, protein, and sediment.
- Screen all type 2 diabetics with a microalbumin/creatinine test to determine future risk of renal disease. (Type 1 patients begin after having had diabetes for at least 5 years) (6).
- Obtain a serum creatinine in all adults and in children in whom proteinuria is present.
- Order thyroid stimulating hormone (TSH) in all patients with type 1 and if clinically indicated, in type 2 diabetes.

An initial referral for dilated eye exam is indicated for all patients with type 2 diabetes. Podiatry referral may also be indicated depending on the findings on the foot exam. Diabetes education and medical nutrition referrals are also indicated, to help support self management. For women of reproductive age, contraception until excellent glycemic control has been achieved is important to minimize risk of fetal abnormalities.

CASE, PART 2

Mrs. S's physician took a good history and comprehensive exam, focusing on the exam components in Table 15.2. Labs were ordered including a hemoglobin A1c, chemistry panel including serum creatinine, urine microalbumin/creatinine ratio and fasting lipids. An appointment was set up for diabetes education and medical nutrition therapy.

CLINICAL QUESTIONS

1. How would you tell this patient that she has diabetes?
2. What recommendations would you make to Mrs. S regarding her initial management?

Conveying the Diagnosis

The first task of the physician who has made a diagnosis of diabetes is to convey this news to the patient. When doing so, the single most important thing is to listen to the patient. It's appropriate to give the news quickly and clearly and then use open-ended questions and reflective listening to explore the patient's reaction to the diagnosis. Remember to listen on at least two tracks: content and affect. One effective strategy to build rapport with the patient is to summarize what they have just told you. Initially this may seem clumsy or obvious; however, summarizing back to the patient is powerful evidence that you have listened to them; it also gives them an opportunity to restate or reframe the patient's views. As part of the summary, you can ask if you "got it all" or if you "got it right."

There are three key facts related to diabetes that Mrs. S. needs to hear from her physician: (A) diabetes is a serious, chronic disease; (B) despite the fact that there is no cure, there are effective treatments for diabetes; and (C) successful treatment of diabetes will require the patient to be involved in his or her own care and to make changes in dietary and exercise habits. The third fact is crucial to laying the groundwork for self management of the disease.

This initial discussion is an important opportunity to assess the patient's understanding of diabetes and attitudes toward living with the disease. A good way of introducing this topic is to ask the patient, "What is your reaction to the news that you have diabetes?" You may need to be patient, and to lead the discussion carefully so as to understand the patient's reactions. Here is an example of wording in which the provider summarizes what she has heard and then probes further: "So, you're really not too surprised to hear that you have diabetes. You had suspected it because of your symptoms and your family history. It sounds like you're a little sad about having diabetes, is that right?"

As part of learning of a patient's reaction to diabetes, find out his or her personal and family experience with the disease. You can introduce the topic by saying something like, "Diabetes is very common, I'm sure that you know people who are living with the disease. Tell me about the people you know with diabetes and what you know about the disease?" After the patient has had an opportunity to discuss this topic, you can then summarize and introduce issues of disease severity and the potential for treatment. An example of what you might say would be: "It sounds like your grandmother had many of the problems that are related to diabetes and died after being on dialysis from kidney failure related to diabetes. Your mother has had a heart attack and some visual problems related to her diabetes. The good news is that we know so much more about the treatment of diabetes now then we did even a few years ago. I want to work with you to reduce your chances of developing the problems that your grandmother had, and that your mother is living with now."

At this point you are ready to begin discussing management of the disease, and to begin to assess the patient's motivation for making behavioral changes to manage the disease. While going from learning the diagnosis to making a solid commitment for longstanding behavior change will often take more than one visit, you will want to touch on the key issues of behavior change and self-management as part of this initial discussion. A way to introduce this topic is to build upon what you have already discussed. Here is an example: "I see that you have considerable firsthand experience with diabetes, and already know that diabetes is a serious disease that can affect everything from your eyesight to your feet. Unfortunately there is no cure for diabetes at this time. Once you have diabetes you will always have diabetes." (Pause, see if she has anything to say.) "Even though there is no cure, there are very effective treatments for diabetes, many of which are new and were not available to your mother or grandmother. One thing has remained the same, however: All successful treatments for diabetes require that you be an active part of the treatment and make decisions to change your own health habits—especially your eating habits and your level of exercise."

MANAGEMENT

Comprehensive management of diabetes must deal with both the metabolic problems and the increased risk of cardiovascular disease. It requires ongoing attention to cardiovascular risk factors, education, and support in self-management of the disease, and a focus on metabolic goals of therapy. To meet these goals, patients and their physicians need to combine behavioral strategies with pharmacologic interventions. Table 15.4 summarizes the components of comprehensive management of diabetes. Within the table and in the subsequent discussion, different management strategies are prioritized by the number needed to treat to prevent morbidity or mortality.

Management of Hypertension

Recent evidence from well done clinical trials demonstrates the primacy of blood pressure management in the comprehen-

sive care of people with diabetes. Tight management of blood pressure to goals of a systolic blood pressure <130 and a diastolic blood pressure <80 lowers the risk of both macrovascular and microvascular complications. In one large randomized trial, tight control of BP to a goal of <130/85 reduced diabetes-related endpoints by 24%, compared to a BP goal of <150/105. In contrast, tight blood glucose control reduced the same endpoints by only 12% (9). In another randomized trial, the NNT for 10 years to a diastolic goal of 80 (compared to a DBP goal of 90) to prevent one cardiovascular death was 14 (10).

Here are some tips on managing hypertenstion in diabetes:

- Initial management is behavioral—dietary change and increased physical activity.
- The Dietary Approaches to Stop Hypertension (DASH) eating plan (*http://www.nhlbi.nih.gov/health/public/heart/hbp/dash/*) is a low fat, low cholesterol dietary plan with high levels of fruits, vegetables, and low-fat dairy products. Several randomized controlled trials have established the efficacy of this diet on blood pressure in persons with diabetes and metabolic syndrome; the effect of lower sodium is additive to the positive effect of the DASH diet itself (11–13).
- In addition to diet and activity, many patients will require medications to reach blood pressure targets. Anti-hypertensives which have been shown to reduce cardiovascular events in diabetic patients include angiotensin converting enzyme (ACE) inhibitors, angiotensin receptor blockers (ARBs), β-blockers, diuretics, and calcium channel blockers (18). While all of these drug classes have proven efficacy against macrovascular complications in patients with diabe-

TABLE 15.4 Components of Comprehensive Diabetes Management

Component	Goal of Therapy	Number Needed to Treat (NNT)	Summary of Benefits	Strength of Recommendation*
Hypertension	SBP <130; DBP <80	NNT for 10 years to prevent 1 diabetes-related endpoint: 6	Decreased mortality, CVD, renal failure, amputation, blindness	A
Tobacco use	Smoking cessation	NNT for 10 years to save 1 life: 11	Decreased mortality (primarily from heart disease, stroke) and morbidity (lowers risk of nephropathy, neuropathy)	B
Endothelial dysfunction	Daily low-dose aspirin	NNT for 10 years to prevent death, MI, or stroke: 15	Decreased mortality and cardiovascular disease	A
Hypercholesterolemia	LDL <100	NNT for 10 years to prevent 1 major CHD event: 15	Decreased CVD events	A
Hyperglycemia	HbA1c <7.0	NNT for 10 years to prevent 1 diabetes related endpoint: 17; NNT for 10 years to prevent 1 CVD event (death, MI, CVD, angina, revascularization): 47	Decreased mortality, CVD, renal failure, amputation, blindness	A

*A = consistent, good-quality patient-oriented evidence; B = inconsistent or limited-quality patient-oriented evidence; C = consensus, disease-oriented evidence, usual practice, expert opinion, or case series. For information about the SORT evidence rating system, see *http://www.aafp.org/afpsort.xml*.

tes, the ACE inhibitors (e.g., enalapril) and angiotensin receptor blockers (e.g., losartan) have particular benefit in reducing the risk of microalbuminuria and the progression to nephropathy. With ACE inhibitors and ARBs, renal function and serum potassium require monitoring (14).

- Drug therapy for hypertension in diabetes mellitus should include an ACE inhibitor or ARB with the addition of a thiazide diuretic to achieve blood pressure targets. The most recent evidence is that low doses of ACE inhibitors prevent the development of microalbuminuria in people with diabetes who have normal blood pressures and no evidence of microalbuminuria. This is a particular effect of the ACE inhibitors and has not yet been shown for any other classes of anti-hypertensives. In patients with any degree of albuminuria or nephropathy who are unable to tolerate ACE inhibitors or ARBs, blood pressure management with β-blockers, diuretics, or non-dihydropyridine calcium channel blockers (DCCBs) is indicated (15).

Management of Tobacco Use

One of the most important things that a smoker with diabetes can do to improve his or her health is to quit smoking (16). Smoking is not only causally related to macrovascular complications of diabetes, such as heart disease, but also with the nephropathic and neuropathic complications of poorly controlled diabetes. The effectiveness of counseling to quit smoking varies depending on the length and the number of counseling sessions. Smoking cessation counseling from a physician is particularly effective. The number needed to counsel for one smoker to quit varies between 8 and 13 depending on the length of the counseling and the number of counseling sessions (16). Ideally, counseling should be given by multiple members of a diabetes care team at multiple visits over 6–8 weeks. Quit lines (e.g., 1-800-QUIT-NOW) can assist busy physicians by providing follow-up phone counseling to smokers who are ready to quit. See Chapter 46: Addictions for further information on smoking cessation.

Management of Endothelial Dysfunction with Aspirin

In diabetes, both hyperglycemia and insulin resistance trigger a cascade of events resulting in a constricted, inflamed, hypercoaguable vascular system (17). Management of hypertension deals with the vasoconstriction, aspirin (75–162 mg/day) is the key intervention to mitigate the inflamed and hypercoaguable arteries. However, these benefits of aspirin have to be weighted against the risks of gastrointestinal bleeding and hemorrhagic stroke. The US Preventive Services Task Force (USPSTF) has synthesized the available evidence and modeled that aspirin's benefits as primary prevention outweigh its risks for any person with diabetes and a 10 year risk of coronary heart disease (CHD) greater than 6%. At this level of risk, aspirin will prevent 4–12 CHD events, but cause 0–2 hemorrhagic strokes and 2–4 major gastrointestinal bleeds. There would be no effect in overall mortality (18).

In practice, the 10-year risk of CHD is easy to calculate using internet based tools that can be downloaded on to a PDA *(http://www.statcoder.com/cholesterol.htm)*. The majority of patients with diabetes over age 40 have a 10-year CHD risk greater than or equal to 6% and would therefore benefit from aspirin prophylaxis. In this population, aspirin lowers

the risk of macrovascular complications by 25%–30% (19). Adolescents and most young adults with diabetes will have a 10-year CHD risk less than 6%, and aspirin has more risks than benefits in this population. Other patient populations who may not be candidates for aspirin therapy include patients with aspirin allergy, clinically active hepatic disease, bleeding tendency, history of gastrointestinal bleeding, or current anticoagulant therapy (19). In people with these co-morbidities, the risks and significant benefits of aspirin therapy must be individually weighed.

Even in those with a history of gastrointestinal bleeding, the benefit of aspirin is still possible. Two equivalent management strategies are available for such patients. One is to prescribe a proton pump inhibitor with the aspirin; the second is to test for *Helicobacter pylori* and eradicate this stomach infection prior to initiation of low dose aspirin (20). Both of these strategies are associated with an endoscopy-proven risk of recurrent gastrointestinal bleeding of around 1% per year. For patients with an absolute contraindication to aspirin therapy, other antiplatelet therapy may be an option (19).

Management of Dyslipidemia

Diabetes is associated with multiple lipid abnormalities, including increased total cholesterol, triglycerides, and low-density lipoprotein (LDL) cholesterol, and a decreased high-density lipoprotein (HDL) cholesterol. Behavioral management with the DASH diet and exercise improves all of these abnormalities (13). Use of statins to lower LDL cholesterol to levels as low as 70 mg/dl has been proven to reduce CVD in diabetics with a 10-year cardiovascular disease (CVD) risk of 12% or greater (21, 22). In this group of diabetics, the number needed to treat (NNT) for 1 year to prevent 1 CHD event is 150. Current guidelines from the National Cholesterol Education Project (NCEP) have recommended an LDL target for all adults with diabetes of 100 mg/dl (and perhaps 70 mg/dl) by considering diabetes as a "CHD risk equivalent" (18).

In addition to lowering LDLs, the American Diabetes Association (ADA) advocates reducing triglycerides to less than 150 mg/dL and increasing HDLs to greater than 40 mg/dl in men or greater than 50 mg/dl in women. Meeting these targets may require medication in addition to lifestyle modification. Benefits of intervening to raise HDL cholesterol in those with an LDL cholesterol less than 140 mg/dl have been shown in a secondary prevention trial. Although historically there have been concerns of worsening glucose levels in persons treated with niacin to improve HDL, recent evidence has shown that the negative effect on blood glucose is minimal (23). A re-analysis of the Coronary Drug Trial documents a benefit of niacin for those with diabetes. Among the participants of this trial who had diabetes, the NNT for 10 years to prevent one death was 23 (24). Taken together, this evidence proves that using niacin or a fibrate to reduce triglyceride levels and raise HDL levels is associated with a reduction in cardiovascular events, particularly in patients with clinical CVD, low HDL and near-normal levels of LDL.

Combination therapy of a statin with niacin or a fibrate is often required to achieve lipid management goals. The combination of statins and niacin has been tested in a small randomized controlled trial that included patients with diabetes. In this secondary prevention trial, patients with preexisting heart disease and LDL cholesterol levels <130 were randomized to placebo or a combination of simvastatin and niacin. At the end of 38 months of follow-up, there was a 21% absolute reduction in the clinical endpoint of cardiovascular death, non-fatal myocardial infarction (MI), or revascularization. In this high-risk group, the NNT for 10 years to prevent one of these endpoints is two. The combination of statins and niacin has been evaluated more thoroughly than the combination of statins and fibrates (25).

Management of Hyperglycemia

Newly diagnosed patients with diabetes naturally focus on their blood sugar levels. Long-term successful management of blood glucose to a goal of HbA1c below 7.0 clearly lowers the risk of microvascular complications. This has been shown for both type 1 (26) and type 2 (27) diabetes. The relationship between management of hyperglycemia and risk of macrovascular complications has historically been less clear. However, recent analysis of the 17-year follow-up from the Diabetes Care and Complications trial indicates that successful management of blood glucose to a goal of HBA1c of 7.0 early in the course of type 1 diabetes is associated with a 3.6% statistically significant reduction in absolute risk of coronary artery disease (CAD). Thus, the NNT to a HBA1c target of 7.0 to prevent one patient from developing CHD (heart disease death, nonfatal MI, angina, coronary revascularization) is 47 (28). The relationship between glycemic control and subsequent complications is more logarithmic than linear. Clinically, this means that there is a greater reduction in subsequent risk of complications from lowering a HbA1c from 10 to 8 than there is from lowering the HbA1c from 8 to 6. As one might expect, the risk of hypoglycemic complications goes up as the HbA1c value gets closer to normal. Management of hyperglycemia begins with behavioral management.

Behavioral Management

Initial self management of hyperglycemia asks the patient to substitute some carbohydrates for others. Carbohydrates to be avoided include concentrated forms of sugar, such as soft drinks, sweetened coffee or iced tea, cookies, candy, cakes, pies, and pastries. In place of these carbohydrates, patients with diabetes are encouraged to eat whole grains, fruits, vegetables, and low-fat dairy products (29). Once the patient is successful in achieving acceptable levels of blood sugar, some of the carbohydrates that were previously eliminated may be added back in moderation as long as there is a plan for managing the subsequent hyperglycemic load (27). One eating plan that is consistent with these principles is the eating plan evaluated in the DASH studies. For more information on the DASH diet, see the discussion under management of blood pressure in diabetes. Dietary changes can lower HbA1c by an average of 1.9% over 6 months (30).

Patients with newly diagnosed diabetes should be encouraged to exercise. In one trial, a combined strength and aerobic exercise program can improve quality of life and HbA1c levels by an average of 0.6 within 1 month and 0.8 after 16 weeks of training. The program involved 2 days a week of 75 minutes of aerobic exercise (15 minutes of warm up and stretching, followed by 60 minutes of aerobic walking or cycling), and 2 days of weight lifting (15 minutes of warm up and stretching, followed by three sets of 12 repetitions of bench press, seated row, leg extension, pull down, pec-deck, and leg curl, and cool down) (31, 32).

Some of the most compelling evidence for diet and exercise as behavioral management of type 2 diabetes comes from the Diabetes Prevention Program's randomized controlled trial. In a population at high risk for type 2 diabetes (adult, overweight or obese, and pre-diabetes) intensive lifestyle modification reduced the incidence of type 2 diabetes by 58% over 3 years and was more effective than metformin (31% effective) (33). Unfortunately, attempts to prevent type 1 diabetes have been less successful (34).

Pharmacologic Management

For those patients who do not reach a HBA1c goal of 7.0 with behavioral management, drug therapy is recommended. There are three major classes of oral agents available for treatment of type 2 diabetes: metformin, the sulfonylureas, and the thiazolidinediones. Table 15.5 summarizes the common medications and their use.

The United Kingdom Preventive Diabetes Study (UKPDS) provides the best evidence to guide the initial choice of medication to control hyperglycemia. The major findings of this 10-year study can be summarized as follows:

- Sulfonylureas, metformin, and insulin were equally effective as initial therapy at reaching the intensive goal of a HbA1c of 7.0.
- Over the 10 years of follow-up, glycemic control deteriorated equally in all groups, requiring dosage increases and/ or additional agents to reach glycemic goals.
- The risk of a major hypoglycemic episodes was lower for metformin (0.6% per year) than for sulfonylureas (1% per year) or insulin (2% per year).
- Patients randomized to metformin had fewer deaths than patients randomized to other forms of intensive therapy or to conventional therapy (NNT for 1 year to prevent one death = 141).

Because of these findings, metformin is recommended as initial pharmacologic therapy for persons with type 2 diabetes when behavioral management is unsuccessful in meeting glycemic management goals (35). It was the only glycemic therapy in the UKPDS trial to show a positive impact on mortality, and was also associated with the lowest risk of hypoglycemia.

Metformin

As discussed above, metformin is recommended as initial pharmacologic therapy for type 2 diabetes. It acts primarily by reducing hepatic glucose production and increasing peripheral glucose utilization. It commonly lowers HbA1c by 1.5–2.0%. In addition to its beneficial effects on blood glucose, metformin also positively affects other important physiologic processes in patients with diabetes, including blood lipids, blood pressure, and clotting activity. It is eliminated by the kidneys and, therefore, is to be avoided when the serum creatinine is 1.5 or greater in men or 1.4 or greater in women.

The most common side effects of metformin are gastrointestinal; they include nausea, vomiting, anorexia, and diarrhea. These effects tend to be transient for 2–4 weeks after initiation or dosage increases, and are dose-related. To minimize these effects, start at 500 mg once a day (with the evening meal) and increase the dose slowly, titrating upward on a weekly

TABLE 15.5 Medications Commonly Used for the Treatment of Diabetes Mellitus

Medication	Medication Brand Name	Dosage Forms Available	Starting Dose	Maximum Dose	Elimination Route/ Dosage Adjustments	Cost
Biguanides						
Metformin	Glucophage, Glucophage XR	500, 850, 1,000 mg tablets 500 mg/5 ml oral solution 500, 750, 1,000 mg XR tablets	500 mg BID or 850 mg once daily with meals 500 mg XR once daily with evening meal	2,550 mg/d 2,000 mg/d for the XR	Renal excretion (avoid in men with SCr > 1.5 mg/ dl or women with SCr > 1.4 mg/dl)	$
Sulfonylureas						
Glimepiride	Amaryl	1, 2, 4 mg tablets	1–2 mg with the first meal	8 mg/d	60% renal excretion Titrate dose to effect	$
Glipizide, Glipizide extended release (ER)	Glucotrol, Glucotrol XL	5, 10 mg tablets 2.5, 5, 10 mg ER tablets	5 mg/d 2.5 mg/d in geriatric or hepatic disease before the first main meal	40 mg/d	80%–85% renal excretion Titrate dose to effect	$
Glyburide	Diabeta, Miconase, Glynase	1.25, 2.5, 5 mg tablets	2.5 mg given before the first main meal	20 mg/d	50% renal excretion	$
Micronized Glyburide	Glynase Prestab	1.5, 3, 4.5, 6 mg tablets	1.5–3 mg/d given before the first main meal	12 mg/d	50% renal excretion	$
Thiazolidine-diones						
Pioglitazone	Actos	15, 30, 45 mg tablets	15–30 mg/d	45 mg/d	Hepatic metabolism with renal and fecal excretion Hepatic elimination Monitor LFTs	$$$
Rosiglitazone	Avandia	2, 4, 8 mg tablets	4 mg/d QD or divided BID	8 mg/d		$$$
Oral Combination Products						
Glipizide-metformin	Metaglip	2.5/250, 2.5/500, 5/500 mg tablets	2.5/250 mg per day with a meal	10/1,000 mg/d	See individual medication section for specific recommendations	$$$
Glyburide-metformin	Glucovance	1.25/500, 2.5/500, 5/500 mg tablets	1.25/250 mg QD or BID with meals	20/2,000 mg/d		$$$
Rosiglitazone-metformin	Avandamet	1/500, 2/500, 2/1,000, 4/500, 4/1,000 mg tablets	Based on original requirements of medications	8/2,000 mg per day		$$$

BID, twice daily; QD, every day.

basis. The maximum dose is 2,500 mg daily given in divided doses with meals. If side effects occur, the dose can be reduced for a period of time or the drug can be stopped temporarily. Metformin alone rarely causes hypoglycemia; however hypoglycemia can occur with strenuous exercise without caloric intake or concomitant intake of alcohol or other hypoglycemic medications.

Metformin inhibits lactate metabolism, and the biggest risk of metformin is lactic acidosis, occurring at a rate of 3–5 cases per 100,000 patient-years (36). Risk factors include age >80, concurrent diuretic therapy, recent radiographic contrast, and dehydration (e.g., due to acute diarrhea or vomiting, septicemia, impaired hepatic function, acute renal failure, hypoxemia, or alcohol abuse). To minimize this risk:

- Metformin should not be used in persons with renal insufficiency (creatinine level ≥1.5 in men, 1.4 in women).
- The drug should be discontinued prior to and for 48 hours after radiographic studies with IV contrast that may transiently effect renal function.

Other contraindications include pregnancy and lactation and active liver disease (liver function tests greater than 1.5 times normal), chronic obstructive pulmonary disease (COPD), and active alcoholism. Education for patients prescribed metformin should include temporarily stopping it's use around any radiographic procedure involving IV contrast and during any acute gastrointestinal illness with vomiting and/or diarrhea.

The monthly cost of generic metformin is approximately $35.00–$55.00 depending on dose. The only advantage of the more expensive extended release form is that the maximum dose can be taken once a day (37, 38).

Sulfonylureas

Sulfonylureas lower blood glucose by stimulating pancreatic insulin secretion and increasing tissue sensitivity to insulin. Sulfonylureas commonly lower HbA1c 1.5%–2.0%. Although there are seven sulfonylureas, only the three second-generation drugs (glipizide, glyburide, and glimepiride) are commonly used. Several general principles guide the use of these agents:

- Choose an agent with a relatively short half-life to minimize the risk of hypoglycemia (glipizide has the lowest rate).
- Start with a low dose given with the morning meal.
- Increase the dose every 5 to 7 days, as needed to reach glycemic goal.
- Divide doses above 50% of the maximum—the second dose given with the evening meal.
- Do not switch back and forth between agents. There are no major differences their efficacy, and switching from one to another is rarely helpful.

The biggest risk of sulfonylureas is hypoglycemia, occurring in about 1% of patients per year. This risk is higher in drugs that have a longer half life and in patients with impaired renal function. For this reason, education for patients prescribed sulfonylureas should include reducing the dose if they are going to skip a meal or are not eating due to an acute gastrointestinal illness. All of the sulfonylureas are now available generically; the monthly cost is approximately $10.00–$15.00 depending on dose. There is no advantage to the long-acting forms except that they can be given once a day (37, 38).

Thiazolidinediones

The two thiazolidinediones, pioglitazone and rosiglitazone, act primarily by decreasing peripheral insulin resistance in skeletal muscle and adipose tissue. These drugs lower HbA1c by 1.0 to 1.5%. In addition to lowering glucose values, they also lower triglycerides slightly and increase both LDL and HDL cholesterol. They are used alone or in combination therapy with metformin, sulfonylureas, or insulin.

These agents are extensively metabolized in the liver. Therefore, thiazolidinediones are contraindicated in patients with active liver disease or liver enzymes greater than 2.5 times normal. Elevations in liver enzymes and liver failure can occur due to these agents; so liver transaminases (aspartate aminotransferase or alanine aminotransferase) should be monitored prior to beginning these drugs and every 2 months during the first year of therapy. Signs and symptoms of liver disease at any time require immediate testing of liver function, and the development of jaundice should prompt immediate drug discontinuation while further evaluation is pending.

These drugs can cause fluid retention, which can lead to weight gain, edema, and new or worsening congestive heart failure (CHF). Therefore, preexisting New York Heart Association Class III or Class IV CHF is a contraindication to their use. These drugs have not been evaluated in pregnant or lactating women and should not, therefore, be used during pregnancy or breastfeeding. They can occasionally induce ovulation in premenopausal women who are anovulatory; therefore, women of childbearing age taking these drugs need to use effective contraception.

Education for patients taking one of these drugs should include the need to seek prompt medical attention for any unexplained anorexia, fatigue, nausea, vomiting, abdominal pain or dark urine, which might represent liver toxicity. Patients should also be encouraged to report potential symptoms of CHF, such as rapid weight gain, orthopnea, paroxysmal nocturnal dyspnea, or worsening dyspnea on exertion. The average monthly cost of these medications varies from $80 to $160 depending on the dosage (37, 38).

Insulin

Rational therapy with exogenous insulin is based on knowledge of the physiology of endogenous insulin secretion. The pancreatic beta cell constantly secretes insulin even in a fasting state. This *basal* insulin secretion is supplemented with *bolus* insulin secretion following a meal, in response to rising levels of glucose. In type 2 diabetes insulin therapy is usually begun as a basal insulin strategy with once a day long-acting insulin injections. The pancreas, assisted by oral agents, continues to deal with post-prandial bolus insulin secretion. Pancreatic failure is progressive in type 2 diabetes, however; so many patients end up requiring a twice-a-day or more intensive insulin regimen. These regimens are designed to meet both basal and bolus insulin requirements.

Insulin therapy requires significant preparatory patient education in self blood glucose monitoring, adjustment of insulin dosing, insulin storage, and insulin injection technique before or while initiating insulin therapy. Most patients are anxious about using insulin, especially about having to do self-injections. Appropriate education for the patient and involved family members can help dispel anxiety, correct misconceptions, and overcome resistance.

Self blood glucose monitoring during insulin therapy is crucial, because patients will need to adjust their dose to avoid hypoglycemia and to adequately control hyperglycemia. Well done randomized controlled trials have found that patients adjusting their own insulin will tend to have better HbA1c levels than patients who only get their insulin adjusted by their physicians (39). Patient education prior to initiation of insulin is also an important time to review dietary and exercise habits and encourage continued changes in these crucial behaviors.

Nighttime Basal Insulin Therapy for Type 2 Diabetes

A recent Cochrane review has summarized the evidence of 20 randomized trials related to insulin therapy in type 2 diabetes (40). The following conclusions can be made from this review:

- Slightly better glucose control and reduced weight gain occur if oral metformin, alone or in combination with other agents, is continued when initiating basal insulin therapy.
- Insulin can be initiated at a dosage of 0.1 units/kg or at a dose that is the same as the fasting plasma glucose in mmol/L units. This number is easy to derive from the more commonly reported units by dividing the glucose value (in mg/dl) by 18.
- Basal insulin is given at bedtime. In most studies, no change was made in the dosages of oral agents when the insulin was initiated. However, if hypoglycemia is encountered, it is appropriate to reduce the dose of a sulfonylurea by 50%.
- Dosage adjustment after initial dosing of insulin is crucial for success of any insulin regimen. A commonly used algorithm is to ask patients to adjust their insulin dose every 3 days, as follows: If the mean fasting plasma glucose is greater than 100 mg/dl for the preceding 3 days, the patient is asked to increase their bedtime insulin dose by 2 units. Table 15.6 summarizes these recommendations.

There are two insulin preparations available for nighttime insulin therapy (Table 15.7). Neutral Protamine Hagedorn (NPH) insulin is the older, now generic, preparation. Glargine insulin is the newer insulin analog. Both are equally effective at lowering HbA1c and fasting plasma glucose when added to oral therapy in patients with type 2 diabetes. However, there is a significantly lower rate of hypoglycemia with glargine insulin than with NPH insulin; the NNT with glargine insulin for 1 year to prevent one severe hypoglycemic event is 71 (41). Hypoglycemic events with NPH were more likely to occur during the night; hypoglycemic events from glargine were more likely to occur between 9:00 AM and 1:00 PM. The average cost of a vial of NPH is $30.00; a vial of glargine insulin is $60.00.

TWICE-DAILY BASAL-BOLUS INSULIN THERAPY FOR TYPE 2 DIABETES

As type 2 diabetes progresses, bedtime insulin and oral agents may not be adequate, and the patient may once again exceed their HbA1c goal. In this situation, twice-daily insulin injections are indicated. A logical next step is to initiate a combined form of insulin, usually a 70/30 mix of a rapid and intermediate duration form of insulin—either 70/30 regular/NPH ($33.00/vial) or 70/30 aspart/protamine aspart ($77.00/vial). Here are some principles of these twice-daily insulin regimens (see Tables 15.5 and 15.6):

- Total insulin dose and risk of weight gain are lower if metformin is continued.
- Thiazolidinediones may be continued.
- The risk of hypoglycemia is greater with the rapid forms of insulin. To minimize this risk, discontinue any sulfonylurea when twice-daily insulin is begun.
- The evening dose of NPH or glargine insulin should be divided, with half given in the morning before breakfast and half given before the evening meal. The 70/30 dose (regular/NPH) is best given 30 minutes before a meal; 70/30 (aspart/protamine aspart) can be given 15 minutes before eating.

INSULIN THERAPY IN TYPE 1 DIABETES

All patients with type 1 diabetes require insulin therapy to avoid hyperglycemia and diabetic ketoacidosis. Given the insulin deficiency that accompanies type 1 diabetes, all of these regimens will need to replace both basal and bolus insulin requirements. Thus, patients will require at least two injections a day, often with mixtures of short- and long-acting insulin preparations. More recent regimens include three or four injections a day or continuous infusion insulin pumps; a common regimen would be the use of glargine insulin to replace basal needs (either once a day or equal injections twice a day) and multiple injections of lispro or aspart insulin solution 15 minutes before meals. The short-acting insulin analogs have shown to have a modest 0.1% greater reduction in HbA1c when compared with regular insulin in patients with type 1 diabetes (42). They also have a lower rate of hypoglycemia than traditional insulin therapy. These insulin analogues seem to offer more of an advantage when used with an insulin pump in continuous subcutaneous insulin infusion.

For patients using basal bolus regimens with injections (as opposed to an infusion pump), basal insulin adjustments are made every 3 to 5 days in the same way as in the nighttime regimen for type 2 diabetes described above. Adjustments in bolus insulin dosing is based both on the results of pre-prandial blood glucose and on the amount of carbohydrates that will be consumed at the impending meal. The need for frequent, precisely calculated injections of varying doses of insulin has created a need for more convenient and accurate dosing than traditional vial and needle injection techniques. This need has been filled with insulin injection devices that use pre-filled cartridges rather than a vial.

STRATEGY FOR USE OF HYPOGLYCEMIC MEDICATIONS IN TYPE 2 DIABETES

Figure 15.1 illustrates an overall strategy for the management of hyperglycemia in patients with type 2 diabetes. Initial evaluation includes the development of an individualized HbA1c goal. For most patients this will be <7.0%; it may be higher in patients who are diagnosed after 60 years of age or in whom some other disease is likely to shorten their life expectancy (43).

- Behavioral management is the cornerstone of hyperglycemic management of diabetes and deserves to be reemphasized at every visit. Initial treatment with behavioral management alone may be indicated for up to 3 months depending on the initial severity of the hyperglycemia and the initial response to behavior change (43).

- Many patients will require the addition of drug therapy;

metformin is the initial choice for patients who can take it (27).
- On the basis of their safety, efficacy, and relative cost, sulfonylureas are an appropriate choice for a second agent if one is needed.
- A thiazolidinedione may be considered if a third agent is

TABLE 15.6   Insulin Therapy Guidelines (49, 50)

Visit	Goals of Visit	Details
I. Starting a Patient on Nighttime Basal Insulin		
Prior to initiating insulin	Review behavioral management Teach or review self blood glucose monitoring Teach adjustment of insulin dose based on SBGM results Teach injection technique Review signs, symptoms, and treatment of hypoglycemia	Best done by a certified diabetes educator (CDE) Follow-up in 1 week
Visit at which insulin is initiated	Calculate initial insulin dose Review patient's injection technique Review SBGM, adjustment algorithm and hypoglycemia instructions	Initial dose = FPG (mg/dL)/18 Dosage adjustment: If mean of previous 3 FPG measurements is > 100 mg/dl and no PG measurement is less than 70 mg/dl, increase bedtime insulin dose by 2 units Rx for daytime hypoglycemia: • Mild hypoglycemia (can be managed by patient) during the day, reduce sulfonylurea dose by 25% • Severe (requires assistance from someone else) hypoglycemia during the day, reduce sulfonylurea dose by 50% Rx for nighttime hypoglycemia: • For any documented hypoglycemic episode at night, reduce insulin dose by 2 units, wait 1 week before any dose increases F/U (phone or visit) in 1 week
Subsequent visits	Consider non-visit review of SBGM (fax, email, electronic transmission from glucose meter)	Initial monitoring is daily, can become less frequent once patient has reached goals
II. Initiating and Adjusting BID Insulin		
Before starting BID regimen	Discontinue sulfonylurea; continue metformin, TZD agent Review SBGM, new insulin adjustment algorithm, diet and exercise plans; if not already SBGM BID, begin BID monitoring (fasting, before evening meal)	
Starting dose	AM: 50% of previous nighttime insulin dose	PM: 50% of previous nighttime insulin dose
Dose adjustment	AM dose adjustments based on before-evening meal SBGM readings	PM dose adjustments based on fasting before-breakfast SBGM readings
Dose adjustment frequency	Make dose *reductions* based on a reading <70 mg/dl the very next day	Make dose *increases* based on the average glucose reading from the previous 3 days every 3 days

(continued)

TABLE 15.6 Insulin Therapy Guidelines (49, 50) (*continued*)

Visit	Goals of Visit	Details
Dose decrease details	If any before supper PG measurement is <70 mg/dl, reduce the before-breakfast insulin dose by 2 units beginning the next morning	If any FPG measurements is <70 mg/dl, reduce the before-supper insulin dose by 2 units beginning that afternoon
Dose adjustment details	If average of the 3 previous before-supper measurements is between 80 and 100 and none of the 3 previous before-supper measurements is <70 mg/dl, make no change in the before-breakfast insulin dose	If average of the 3 previous FPG measurements is between 80 and 100 and none of the 3 previous before-supper measurements is <70 mg/dl, make no change in the before-supper insulin dose
	If average of the 3 previous before-supper measurements is between 100 and 140 and none of the 3 previous before supper measurements is <70 mg/dl, increase before-supper insulin dose by 2 units	If average of the 3 previous FPG measurements is between 100 and 140 and none of the 3 previous FPG measurements is <70 mg/dl, increase before-supper insulin dose by 2 units
	If average of the 3 previous before-supper measurements is >140 and none of the 3 previous before-supper measurements is <70 mg/dl, increase before-supper insulin dose by 4 units	If average of the 3 previous FPG measurements is >140 and none of the 3 previous FPG measurements is <70 mg/dl, increase before-supper insulin dose by 4 units

needed, although in patients who pay for their own prescriptions, cost issues may favor the addition of bedtime insulin at this point.

- If HbA1c goals have not been met with multiple oral agents, bedtime basal insulin therapy is indicated.
- Failure of bedtime basal insulin therapy justifies the change to a bid insulin regimen and the discontinuation of sulfonylureas.

A primary care-based team approach improves outcomes and patient satisfaction (44). Comprehensive management of diabetes may require several visits with different members of a diabetes care team, including a family physician and a diabetes case manager (dietician, nurse practitioner, pharmacist, etc). Initial management needs to focus on engaging the patient in self management to achieve specific goals for blood pressure, HbA1c, and LDL cholesterol.

CASE, PART 3

Six months have passed. Mrs. S has had monthly visits with either her family physician or a nurse practitioner trained to support self-management of patients with chronic disease. Medications include enteric coated aspirin 81 mg daily, metformin 500 mg twice a day, and lovastatin 20 mg daily. Fasting labs were drawn earlier this week and documented a fasting plasma glucose of 98 mg/dl and an LDL of 94 mg/dl. Her blood pressure (BP) today is 128/76.

CLINICAL QUESTION

1. What components of care are necessary to manage diabetes over time?

MANAGEMENT OF DIABETES OVER TIME

One of the greatest challenges for patients with diabetes and the physicians caring for them is the chronicity of the disease. It doesn't go away. Patients grow tired of the behavioral changes that living with the disease has led them to make. It is, therefore, imperative to reassess the status of the disease over time through regular monitoring. This includes behavior monitoring, periodic physical examinations, and serial laboratory testing (see Table 15.8). A second great challenge in caring for patients with diabetes over time is the progressive nature of the disease. Therapies often need to be adjusted based on the results of monitoring. In the UKPDS, 50% of patients initially managed with one drug for hyperglycemia required a second drug after 3 years; this rose to 66% after 6 years (45). A third component of ongoing diabetes care is screening for complications. Early identification of complications allows for interventions that can slow their development. Three key principles of ongoing care of diabetes are: monitor, adjust, and screen.

Monitoring

Monitoring of diabetes begins with monitoring the behavioral management of the disease. Providers can explore in a nonjudgmental, caring way the challenges and successes that their patients are having living. They can support their patient's efforts at self management through assessment of current behaviors, assessment of readiness to change, and appropriate self management counseling to adjust behavioral management.

Open-ended questions about a patient's recent experience of living with diabetes are a good way to begin an assessment of self management. For example, the provider could say:

TABLE 15.7 Pharmacology and Use of Insulin Preparations

	Insulin	Onset (hours)	Peak (hours)	Duration (hours)	Compatibilities*	Practical Use
Rapid-acting	Lispro insulin solution (analog); *Brand: Humalog*	0.25	0.5–1.5	2–5	NPH, ultralente	Rapid-acting insulin analogs are used with meals to decrease post-prandial rise in BG
	Insulin aspart solution (analog); *Brand: NovoLog*	0.25	1–3	3–5	NPH	
	Insulin glulisine solution; *Brand: Apidra*	0.25	1–1.5	3–5	NPH	
Short-acting	Insulin (regular); *Brand: Humulin R; Novolin R*	0.5–1	2–5	8–12	all except glargine	Regular human insulin used with meals to decrease post-prandial rise in BG Less expensive than rapid acting insulin analogs
Intermediate-acting	Isophane insulin suspension (NPH); *Brand: Humulin N; Novolin N*	1–1.5	4–12	24	regular, aspart, lispro	Used with regular insulin to manage total daily insulin requirements Usually administered twice daily
	Insulin zinc suspension (lente); *Brand: Humulin L*	1–2.5	7–15	24	regular, semilente, ultralente	Infrequent use
	Extended insulin zinc suspension (ultralente); *Brand: Humulin U*	4.8	10–30	20–36	regular, lente, semilente, lispro	Infrequent use
Long-acting	Insulin glargine solution (analog); *Brand: Lantus*	1.1	No real peak	24	none	Used as once daily long-acting insulin
	Insulin detemir solution; *Brand: Levemir*	Data not available	6–8	Dose-dependent	none	Can be used once or twice daily

* Compatabilities are important for mixing insulins to minimize the total number of subcutaneous injections daily.

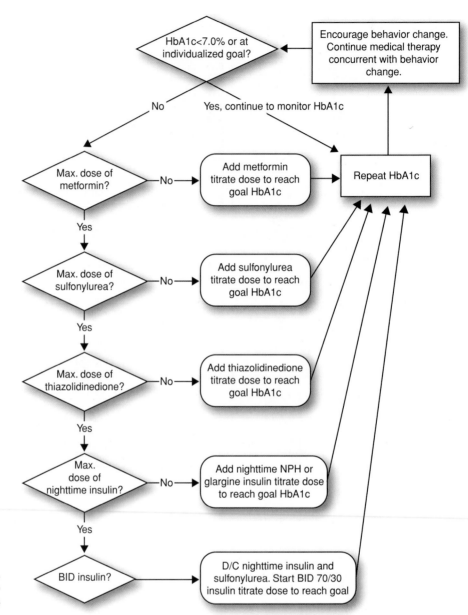

Figure 15.1 • Algorithm for hypoglycemic management of type 2 diabetes.

"Mrs. S, it was about 6 months ago that we discovered your diabetes. Thinking back over the last 6 months, what has been the hardest thing for you about living with diabetes?"

In addition to a global, open-ended inquiry, it is important to get more detailed data about self management. One broadly studied inventory of diabetes self management is the summary of diabetes self care activities measure shown in Figure 15.2 (46). Although originally developed as a research instrument, it is easily adopted into primary care clinical practice. The last question about readiness to change was added to the summary to help busy practitioners know how to approach the discussion of self management. An answer of 7 or greater indicates readiness to make additional behavioral changes. Less than 7 indicates that a patient is either ambivalent about making any changes (score of 3–6) or is not even considering lifestyle change at this time (score of 1–2). In

either case, brief encouragement to continue considering behavioral changes is indicated.

If a patient is ready to pursue behavior change, the next step is to determine what domain of behavior he or she would like to change. For patients who are ready to change a specific behavior relating to their diabetes, negotiation of a specific behavioral goal is appropriate. These behavioral goals need to be as specific as possible. For example, "I will walk at least 20 minutes a day after dinner with the dog at least 4 days each week. When it gets cold, I'll go to the mall and walk indoors." To be successful with this aspect of patient care, it is essential to work with patients to help them solve their problems, and not to try to solve their problems for them. The provider's role, therefore, is to clarify goals that the patient makes, helping him to specify a goal that will require effort but that is realistic. It is good practice to present the

TABLE 15.8 Recommended Monitoring Activities during Ongoing Diabetes Care

Category of Monitoring	What to Monitor	Frequency	Comments
Health behaviors and self-care	Eating habits	At each visit	
	Activity level	At each visit	
	Medications (including aspirin)	At each visit	
	Blood glucose self-monitoring	At each visit	
	Tobacco use	At each visit	
	Readiness to change	At each visit	
Physical examination	Height, weight, BMI	At each visit	
	Blood pressure	At each visit	
	Foot exam and foot care instruction	Annually	If high risk (hx of ulcer, foot deformity, loss of protective sensation), exams should be every 3 months
Laboratory	Hemoglobin A1c	At least every 6 months	More frequently if ≥7.0
	Fasting lipids	Annually	More frequently if hypercholesterolemic
	Retinal exams	Annually	Begin within months of diagnosis of type 2, within 5 years of diagnosis for type 1. If low risk, eye professional may recommend 2-year interval
	Urine microalb/creatinine ratio	Annually	Begin within months of diagnosis of type 2, within 5 years of diagnosis for type 1. Two positive screens within 6 months required to diagnose microalbuminuria

patient with a written hard copy of any goals that she has set for her to review later.

Other aspects of periodic monitoring involve the physical examination and laboratory. BMI monitoring is an important aspect of longitudinal diabetes care. Insulin resistance increases as BMI rises, and weight loss improves blood glucose, lipids, and blood pressure. Blood pressure should also be monitored at each office visit. In patients with labile blood pressure or in those with "white coat" hypertension, home blood pressure monitoring may be appropriate. Other key parts of the interval physical exam for patients with diabetes are the foot exam and the retinal exam.

Review of glucose monitoring data is another element of periodic visits. For patients taking insulin, the results of self blood glucose monitoring are used to adjust subsequent insulin doses, and this does lead to improved levels of HbA1c. For patients with type 2 diabetes who are not taking insulin, there is not enough scientific evidence to know whether review of glucose values improves management or not. HbA1c monitoring definitely improves glycemic control in patients with type 1 diabetes (47). Again, direct evidence is lacking for type 2 disease; however, HbA1c monitoring is recommended (43). Fasting lipid monitoring is also recommended. ADA guidelines call for glucose monitoring every 6 months and lipid monitoring annually in stable patients (43).

Screening for Early Signs of Complications

Retinopathy screening with either retinal photography or a retinal exam by an eye professional is an essential strategy to reducing the burden of blindness caused by diabetes. Improved blood pressure and glucose control, laser photocoagulation, vitrectomy, and other interventions can help preserve sight if retinopathy is identified in a timely fashion (43). The ADA recommends annual retinal exams soon after the discovery of type 2 diabetes and within 5 years of the diagnosis of type 1 diabetes.

The earliest sign of what may become diabetic kidney disease is microalbuminuria. The gold-standard test is a 24-hour urine specimen analyzed for albumin. Although there are false positives and occasional false negatives, the spot albumin/creatinine ratio on a random urine specimen is much more practical and is now the preferred test. To minimize the false positives, two positive results within 6 months are needed before a patient is diagnosed as having microalbuminuria. If the second specimen is negative after an initial positive, a third test is recommended. Microalbuminuria is defined as an albumin:creatinine ratio of between 30 and 300 mg/g; values greater than 300 represent frank proteinuria, and values of less than 30 are normal. False positives can occur in the setting of a urinary tract infection, CHF, gross hematuria, or fever. The ADA recommends annual screening (43).

Screening to prevent foot ulcers and amputation is done

Diabetes Self-Care Questionnaire

The questions below ask you about your diabetes self-care activities during the past 7 days. If you were sick during the past 7 days, please think back to the last 7 days that you were not sick. For each item, circle the number that best represents what actually happened.

Eating Habits

1. On how many of the last SEVEN DAYS have you followed a healthful eating plan?

       0   1   2   3   4   5   6   7

2. On how many of the last SEVEN DAYS did you eat five or more serving of fruits and vegetables?

       0   1   2   3   4   5   6   7

3. On how many of the last SEVEN DAYS did you eat high-fat foods such as red meat or full-fat dairy products?

       0   1   2   3   4   5   6   7

Exercise Habits

4. On how many of the last SEVEN DAYS did you participate in at least 30 minutes of physical activity?

       0   1   2   3   4   5   6   7

5. On how many of the last SEVEN DAYS did you participate in a specific exercise session (such as swimming, walking, biking) other than what you do around the house or as part of your work?

       0   1   2   3   4   5   6   7

Blood Sugar Testing

6. On how many of the last SEVEN DAYS did you test your blood sugar the number of times recommended by your health care practitioner?

       0   1   2   3   4   5   6   7

Medications

7. If you take aspirin, on how many of the last SEVEN DAYS did you take your recommended aspirin pills?

       0   1   2   3   4   5   6   7   Not applicable

8. If you take diabetes pills, on how many of the last SEVEN DAYS did you take your recommended diabetes pills?

       0   1   2   3   4   5   6   7   Not applicable

9. If you take insulin, on how many of the last SEVEN DAYS did you take your recommended insulin injections?

       0   1   2   3   4   5   6   7   Not applicable

Foot Care

10. On how many of the last SEVEN DAYS did you check your feet?

       0   1   2   3   4   5   6   7

11. On how many of the last SEVEN DAYS did you inspect the inside of your shoes?

       0   1   2   3   4   5   6   7

Smoking

12. Have you smoked a cigarette—even one puff—during the past SEVEN DAYS?

   0   No

   1   Yes. *If* yes, how many cigarettes did you smoke on an average day?

             Number of cigarettes: _____

Readiness to Change

13. On a scale of 1 to 10, how ready are you to make changes in your lifestyle to improve your diabetes care?

Not ready   Very ready

      0   1   2   3   4   5   6   7   8   9   10

Thank you for completing this survey.

Figure 15.2 • A version of the summary of diabetes self care activities adapted for primary care practice.

TABLE 15.9 Management of Diabetes: Key Recommendations for Practice

Area / Topic	Recommendation	Strength of Recommendation*
Treatment of hypertension	Maintain BP below 130/80	A
	Advise patients to use DASH diet	C
	If pt is on ACE inhibitors or ARBs, monitor renal function and serum potassium	C
	If any microalbuminuria is present, treat with ACE inhibitors or ARBs	C
	If diabetes, hypertension, microalbuminuria, and renal insufficiency, treat with ARBs to slow nephropathy	A
Smoking cessation	Counseling on smoking cessation	A
Management of endothelial dysfunction	If 10 year CAD risk ≥6%, prescribe aspirin prophylaxis (75–162 mg/day)	A
	If absolute contraindication to aspirin, use other antiplatelet therapy	C
Management of dyslipidemia	Prescribe DASH diet plus exercise	C
	For all diabetics: reduce LDL to ≤100 mg/dl, keep triglycerides <150 mg/dl, and maintain HDL >40 mg/dl in men or >50 mg/dl in women	C
	If 10 year CAD risk > or equal to 12%, prescribe statins to lower LDL-cholesterol to 70 mg/dl	A
Management of hyperglycemia	A team approach to care (e.g., physician, nurse, pharmacist, diabetes educator) improves outcomes and patient satisfaction	A
	Long-term HbA1c below 7.0 lowers risk of microvascular and macrovascular complications	A
	Behavioral management with diet and exercise is the cornerstone of hyperglycemic management and should be reemphasized at every visit	B
	Patients who do not reach a HbA1c goal of 7.0 with diet and exercise should receive drug therapy	A
	Metformin is the initial drug of choice for patients who can take it	B
	When insulin is started, oral agents should be continued, to reduce total insulin needs and weight gain	A
	Glucose self-monitoring improves overall management of hyperglycemia	C
	Monitor HbA1c every 6 months and fasting lipid values at least annually; monitor each more frequently if target levels have not been reached	C
Screening for and management of complications	In patients with retinopathy, control of blood pressure and glucose, laser photocoagulation, vitrectomy, and other interventions can help preserve sight	A
	Screen for nephropathy annually using the albumin/creatinine ratio (<30 mg/g is normal)	C
	Screen annually for peripheral neuropathy; monofilament testing is a better screen than vibratory sensation testing	B
	All diabetics should have an annual foot exam	C

*A = consistent, good-quality patient-oriented evidence; B = inconsistent or limited-quality patient-oriented evidence; C = consensus, disease-oriented evidence, usual practice, expert opinion, or case series. For information about the SORT evidence rating system, see *http://www.aafp.org/afpsort.xml*.

CHAPTER 16

Hyperlipidemia

Allen R. Last and Jonathan D. Ference

CASE, PART 1

Maria Ramirez is a healthy 47-year-old woman. Her husband was recently diagnosed with high blood pressure and elevated cholesterol levels. She is worried about her cholesterol and wonders if she should be tested. She is asymptomatic and has never had a lipid profile. Her medical history is benign. Her medications include only a daily multivitamin plus two fish oil capsules a day. She smokes half a pack of cigarrettes daily and does not drink alcohol. Her father died of a heart attack at age 65.

Her physical examination is normal. She is 65 inches tall, weighs 180 pounds, has a body mass index (BMI) of 30, and has a blood pressure of 125/75.

CLINICAL QUESTIONS

1. At what age should you screen asymptomatic people for dyslipidemia?
2. What tests should be used for lipid screening?

Dyslipidemia refers to abnormally high levels of total cholesterol, triglycerides (TG), low-density lipoprotein cholesterol (LDL-C), or an abnormally low amount of high-density lipoprotein cholesterol (HDL-C) in the serum (see Table 16.1). The link between dyslipidemia and coronary heart disease (CHD) has been well established. International studies have clearly demonstrated that CHD risk is significantly lower in areas of the world with low cholesterol levels, in spite of high rates of tobacco abuse and hypertension (1). The typical American diet (high in saturated fat and cholesterol) has been implicated as a major reason for the widespread dyslipidemia in this country. Transplanted people from low-risk areas of the world rapidly acquire the same risk as the native population, reinforcing the central role of behavioral factors such as diet and physical activity (1).

CHD is the leading cause of mortality in the United States. Nearly 70 million Americans have cardiovascular disease, and it is estimated that $394 billion was spent in 2005 to care for these people (2). Approximately 17%–30% of adults in the United States have elevated cholesterol levels, one of the major risk factors for CHD (3, 4). Primary care physicians commonly see patients with dyslipidemia in the outpatient setting and, therefore, should be adept at management of this common and treatable problem.

SCREENING

The Third Report of the National Cholesterol Education Program Adult Treatment Panel (NCEP ATP III), a report updated periodically from the National Institutes for Health (NIH), has identified LDL-C as the primary target for therapy, as it constitutes the majority of circulating total cholesterol and has been directly linked to atherosclerotic disease. Recent studies have demonstrated a 1% decrease in CHD risk for each 1 mg/dl drop on LDL-C. Achieving cholesterol control earlier in life is associated with an improved long-term prognosis. A 10% reduction in total cholesterol starting at age 40 results in a lifetime risk reduction of CHD of 50%, whereas the same 10% reduction starting at age 70 results in only a 20% risk reduction (1). The vascular changes that lead to CHD begin early in life. In fact, on autopsy fatty streaks were seen in 17% of white adolescents and 37% of black adolescents and their presence was strongly correlated with their LDL-C levels (5).

On the basis of this information, NCEP ATP III recommends screening all people every 5 years starting at age 20 with a full lipid panel (total cholesterol, LDL-C, HDL-C, and triglycerides). The United States Preventive Services Task Force (USPSTF), however, recommends screening every 5 years in men staring at age 35 and women at age 45 with a total cholesterol and HDL-C, arguing that the benefits of treatment are modest before middle age (6). The American Diabetes Association (ADA) recommends screening all diabetics for dyslipidemia yearly due to their increased risk for cardiovascular complications (7). The results of these blood tests are then used in conjunction with risk factor analysis to determine a treatment plan.

INITIAL EVALUATION

Most patients with lipid abnormalities are asymptomatic. The majority are diagnosed based on screening blood tests. Historical features are useful for identifying comorbidities, assessing CHD risk, and looking for secondary causes and medications that may alter lipids. Review of current and past medical problems is essential, as there are many secondary causes of dyslipidemia (Table 16.2), although they are present only in a minority of patients with abnormal cholesterol values. Obtaining a thyroid stimulating hormone (TSH) level is generally considered to be cost-effective. Carefully evaluate a patient's medications, as several medications, including some used to treat hypertension, can alter lipid levels (Table 16.3). Family history

TABLE 16.1 NCEP ATP III Lipid Classification System

	Value (mg/dl)	Classification
Total cholesterol		
	<200	Desirable
	200–239	Borderline high
	≥240	High
LDL cholesterol		
	<100	Optimal
	100–129	Near or above optimal
	130–159	Borderline high
	160–189	High
	≥190	Very high
HDL		
	<40	Low
	≥60	High
Triglycerides		
	<150	Normal
	150–199	Borderline high
	200–499	High
	≥500	Very high

NCEP ATP III, National Cholesterol Education Program Adult Treatment Panel III; LDL, low density lipoprotein, HDL, high density lipoprotein.
(Adapted from the Third Report of the National Cholesterol Education Program [NCEP] Expert Panel on Detection, Evaluation, and Treatment of High Blood Cholesterol in Adults [Adult Treatment Panel III] Final Report. NIH Publication No. 02-5215, September 2002.)

may indicate inherited hyperlipidemia, which will require earlier and more aggressive therapy. Tobacco abuse is another risk factor for CHD and should be assessed and addressed.

Dyslipidemia only rarely results in abnormal physical findings. Patients with very high triglycerides may develop eruptive xanthomas, which are yellow-red papules often seen on the buttocks. Lipemia retinalis may occur in patients with extremely high triglyceride levels (>2,000 mg/dl) and appears as opaque white blood vessels on funduscopic exam. High triglycerides have also been linked to acute and chronic pancreatitis. Tendinous xanthomas form on tendons (patella, Achilles, and dorsum of the hand) in the presence of very high LDL-C levels. These conditions are rare.

Standard laboratory assessment of lipids involves directly measuring total cholesterol, HDL-C and triglycerides and then calculating the LDL-C values using the Freewald equation:

LDL-C (mg/dl) = [total cholesterol] −
　　　　　　　　　[HDL-C] − [triglycerides / 5]

Because triglycerides significantly impact LDL-C calculation, high triglyceride levels make calculated LDL-C values increasingly less reliable, and at levels >400 mg/dL, LDL-C calculation becomes meaningless. Triglycerides levels are influenced by food intake, so patients should be fasting for at least 12 hours before blood is drawn. Total cholesterol and HDL-C levels are still valid in a non-fasting patient. Direct measurement of LDL-C is now possible and can be done on non-fasting patients and those with high triglyceride levels, but is more costly.

MANAGEMENT

CASE, PART 2

Mrs. Ramirez' lipid panel shows that her total cholesterol is 225 mg/dl, her LDL-C is 165 mg/dl, her HDL-C is 35 mg/dl, and her serum triglycerides (TG) are 125 mg/dl.

CLINICAL QUESTIONS
1. Should this patient be treated with pharmacotherapy, therapeutic lifestyle modification or both?
2. What interventions are available for treating her low HDL-C?
3. Are there alternative therapies that might be useful for this patient?

General Approach to Treatment

The general approach to addressing hyperlipidemias is as follows:

TABLE 16.2 Secondary Causes of Dyslipidemia

Cause	LDL-C	HDL-C	Triglycerides
	Lipids Affected		
Hypothyroidism	X		
Nephrotic syndrome	X		
Cholestasis	X		
Acute intermittent porphyria	X		
Anorexia nervosa	X		
Hepatoma	X		
Tobacco abuse		X	
Type 2 diabetes		X	X
Obesity		X	X
Gaucher disease		X	
Malnutrition		X	
Glycogen storage disease			X
Hepatitis			X
Alcohol use			X
Renal failure			X
Sepsis			X
Stress			X
Cushing syndrome			X
Pregnancy			X
Acromegally			X
Systemic lupus erythematosus			X

TABLE 16.3 Medications that Negatively Impact Lipids

Medication	LDL-C	HDL-C	Triglycerides
	Lipids Affected		
Steroids			
Glucocorticoids			X
Estrogen			X
Anabolic steroids		X	
Antihypertensives			
Thiazide diuretics	X		
Beta blockers		X	X
Furosemide			X
Atypical antipsychotics			
Clozapine			X
Olanzapine			X
Other			
Tegretol	X		
Cyclosporine	X		
HIV protease inhibitors			X
Retinoic acid			X

1. Dietary changes and weight loss form the cornerstone of all treatment options. Medications are used if cholesterol levels are particularly high, if the patient is at high risk for atherosclerotic disease, or if dietary modification and exercise insufficiently lower a patient's cholesterol. In practice, this means that mild cholesterol elevations can be treated initially with lifestyle modifications, such as lowering dietary fat and cholesterol, increasing physical activity, and weight loss. More severe elevations require pharmacological intervention in addition to therapeutic lifestyle changes, and in persons with very high lipid levels, drug treatment and lifestyle changes can be introduced simultaneously.

2. The top priority is to reduce LDL-C. This is because the link to cardiovascular disease is much stronger for LDL-C than for other lipid fractions, and the strongest clinical trial evidence for drug intervention is for agents that lower LDL-C. In general, HMG-CoA reductase inhibitors (statins) are first-line agents for lowering LDL-C, and bile acid sequestrants are second-line agents.

3. The target LDL-C level should be determined systematically (see Figure 16.1). In setting a LDL-C goal, one must take into account the 10-year risk of having a cardiovascular event. The higher the risk, the more aggressive the therapy should be. Here are the steps to take in assessing cardiovascular disease (CVD) risk:

   A. Review the patient's history to determine if he or she has already had a cardiovascular event. By this we mean CHD or a CHD equivalent (peripheral vascular disease, abdominal aortic aneurysm, symptomatic carotid artery disease, or diabetes). Patients in this category should have aggressive lipid-lowering therapy, with a target LDL-C of <100 mg/dl (some say <70 mg/dl) (8).

   B. For persons without CHD or a CHD equivalent, determine how many of the following risk factors the patient has: current cigarette smoking, hypertension (BP >140/90 mm Hg or those taking antihypertensive medications), low HDL-C (< 40 mg/dl), older age (≥45 for men, ≥55 for women), and family history of early CHD in a first degree relative (<55 for men, <65 for women). An HDL-C level greater than 60 mg/dl is considered a protective factor and reduces the total number of risk factors by one. If the patient has 0 or 1 risk factors, the target LDL-C should be ≤160 mg/dl.

   C. If the patient has 2 or more risk factors, the target LDL-C is determined based on their 10-year CHD risk, which is estimated using Framingham data (see Figure 16.2). The degree to which a patient has each of the above risk factors is represented by a certain number of points. The points derived from each risk factor are added and compared to a summary chart to determine the 10-year risk.

4. The exception to the above is if the serum triglyceride level is above 500 mg/dl. In such cases the risk of pancreatitis is high, and lowering the triglycerides becomes the first priority. In these situations, nicotinic acid and fibrates become the agents of choice. Once TG reduction below 500 mg/dl has been achieved, the LDL once again becomes the primary target of therapy because of its direct relationship to CHD.

5. Once the patient has achieved their LDL goal, the next step is to address lowering non-HDL cholesterol if their triglycerides are ≥200 mg/dl. This is calculated as: Total cholesterol − HDL cholesterol. The non-HDL is essentially a marker of LDL and TG, and its goal level is set at 30 mg/dL above that of the LDL-C goal. Nicotinic acid or a fibric acid derivative may be utilized as pharmacologic interventions to achieve this goal along with dietary changes and weight loss.

Therapeutic Lifestyle Changes

The foundation for treating any lipid disorder is dietary modification, exercise, and weight loss. These changes should be emphasized for all risk groups, whether pharmacotherapy is initiated or not.

The essential features of a lipid-lowering diet include:

- reducing intake of saturated fats to <7% of the total calories
- reducing cholesterol intake to <200 mg/day)
- increasing soluble fiber intake to 10–25 g/day, with consideration of adding plant sterols/stanols to 2 g/day

Reducing dietary saturated fats and cholesterol intake as above has been shown to reduce total cholesterol by 13% and LDL-C by 16% (9). Patients consuming a low-fat diet may actually lower their HDL-C by as much as 7%. Adding soluble fiber in the form of psyllium reduces total cholesterol by 4%–5% and LDL-C by 6%–7% (10, 11).

Moderate consumption of alcohol (less than 30 g or 1 oz per day) increases HDL-C by 4 mg/dl and may decrease CHD risk by almost 25% (12). Tobacco cessation should also be recommended for all patients and is also associated with a 4-mg/dl increase in HDL-C (13). A recent systematic review demonstrated that smoking cessation reduces total mortality in patients with established CHD (14). The Mediterranean diet, being high in vegetables, legumes, nuts, fruits, cereals, olive oil, fish, and alcohol, combines both fiber and alcohol and has been shown to reduce CHD, stroke, and death with a number needed to treat (NNT) of 11 over 4 years (15).

The addition of exercise to a low-fat diet can prevent diet-related decreases in HDL-C (9). The benefit of exercise on HDL-C can be slow to materialize, and can take as long as 2 years to develop (16). Formalized diet recommendations are beneficial in the primary prevention of CHD and should be given to all patients with dyslipidemia (17).

A treatment algorithm for therapeutic lifestyle changes is presented in Figure 16.3. Therapeutic lifestyle changes are initiated, including addressing fat and cholesterol in the diet and encouraging physical activity. The patient's lipid panel is re-evaluated after 6 weeks. If further reductions are needed, dietary interventions are intensified including the addition of fiber and plant stanols/sterols, followed by a repeat lipid profile 6 weeks later. If goals are not being met, consider adding medications to the treatment plan. Patients with lipid values suggesting drug therapy can be started on medications immediately, but lifestyle changes still should be emphasized.

Pharmacotherapy

Currently there are 6 classes of prescription medications aimed at lowering cholesterol: HMG-CoA reductase inhibitors (stat-

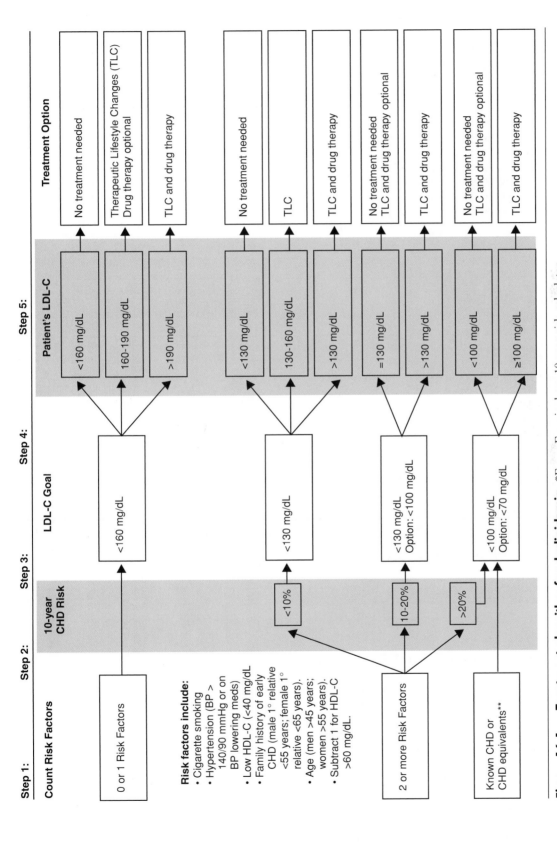

Figure 16.1 • Treatment algorithm for dyslipidemia. *From Framingham 10-year risk calculator.
**CHD equivalents include: peripheral vascular disease, abdominal aortic aneurysm, symptomatic carotid artery disease, diabetes. (Adapted from Grundy SM, Cleeman JI, Merz CNB, et al. Implications of recent clinical trials for the national Cholesterol Education Program Adult Treatment Panel III guidelines. Circulation. 2004;110:227–239.)

Directions: Add points from steps 1-5, then use step 6 to determine 10-year CHD risk

1. Points for age by gender

Age	Points Men	Women
20-34	-9	-7
35-39	-4	-3
40-44	0	0
45-49	3	3
50-54	6	6
55-59	8	8
60-64	10	10
65-69	11	12
70-74	12	14
75-79	13	16

2. Points for Systolic Blood Pressure by treatment & gender

Systolic BP	If untreated Men	Women	If treated Men	Women
<120	0	0	0	0
120-129	0	1	1	3
130-139	1	2	2	4
140-159	1	3	2	5
≥160	2	4	3	6

3. Points for HDL cholesterol by gender

HDL	Points Male	Female
≥60	-1	-1
50-59	0	0
40-49	1	1
<40	2	2

4. Points for total cholesterol by age and gender

Total cholesterol	Age: 20-39 Male	Female	40-49 Male	Female	50-59 Male	Female	60-69 Male	Female	70-79 Male	Female
<160	0	0	0	0	0	0	0	0	0	0
160-199	4	4	3	3	2	2	1	1	0	1
200-239	7	8	5	6	3	4	1	2	0	1
240-279	9	11	6	8	4	5	2	3	1	2
≥280	11	13	8	10	5	7	3	4	1	2

5. Points for tobacco use by age and gender

Tobacco use	Age: 20-39 Male	Female	10-49 Male	Female	50-59 Male	Female	60-69 Male	Female	70-79 Male	Female
Nonsmoker	0	0	0	0	0	0	0	0	0	0
Smoker	8	9	5	7	3	4	1	2	1	1

6. Summary chart

Men

Point total	10-year CHD risk
<0	<1%
0	1%
1	1%
2	1%
3	1%
4	1%
5	2%
6	2%
7	3%
8	4%
9	5%
10	6%
11	8%
12	10%
13	12%
14	16%
15	20%
16	25%
≥17	≥30%

Women

Point total	10-year CHD risk
<9	<1%
9	1%
10	1%
11	1%
12	1%
13	2%
14	2%
15	3%
16	4%
17	5%
18	6%
19	8%
20	11%
21	14%
22	17%
23	22%
24	27%
≥25	≥30%

Figure 16.2 • Method of estimating 10-year cardiovascular risk.
(Adapted from the Third Report of the National Cholesterol Education Program (NCEP) Expert Panel on Detection, Evaluation, and Treatment of High Blood Cholesterol in Adults [Adult Treatment Panel III] Final Report NIH Publication No. 02–5215, September 2002.)

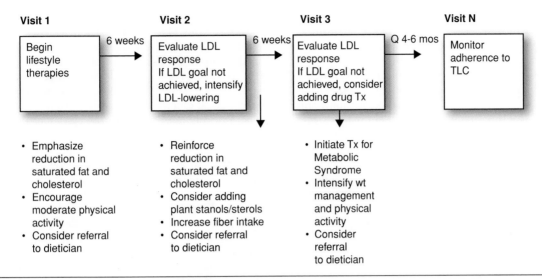

Figure 16.3 • Algorithm for therapeutic lifestyle changes (TLC).
(Adapted from Third report of the National Cholesterol Education Program (NCEP) Expert Panel on Detection, Evaluation, and Treatment of High Blood Cholesterol in Adults (Adult Treatment Panel III) Final Report. Circulation 2002. 106(25):3143–3421.

ins), bile acid sequestrants, nicotinic acid, fibric acid derivatives, intestinal brush boarder inhibitors, and omega-3 fatty acids. These agents can be used alone or in combination, and each class affects the lipid profile differently. Therapy should be tailored to the patient based on specific factors such as lipoprotein disorder, renal or hepatic function, co-morbid disorders, and cost. Medication therapy should begin with a single agent, titrated to the maximum dose. If the LDL-C goal

is not achieved with maximum recommended and/or tolerable dose of the first drug, then a second agent should be added. An algorithm for the general approach to medication therapy is provided in Figure 16.4.

HMG-COA REDUCTASE INHIBITORS (STATINS)

Generally, the 3-hydroxy-3-methylglutaryl coenzyme A (HMG-CoA) reductase inhibitors, or statins, are considered

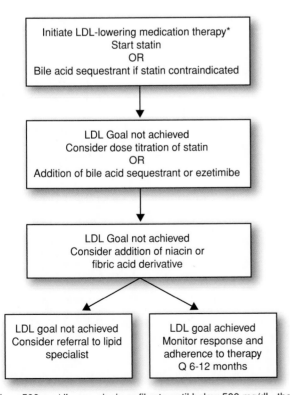

*If triglycerides >500 mg/dL, use niacin or fibrate until below 500 mg/dL, then reasses.

Figure 16.4 • Algorithm for lipid lowering medication therapy.

the agents of choice for treating primary hypercholesterolemia because they are the most potent LDL-C—lowering medications. Although differences exist with respect to each statin's ability to lower LDL-C, all have been shown to both slow the progression of coronary atherosclerosis and prevent primary and secondary coronary heart disease in randomized controlled trials (18–28). However, in a trial comparing statin therapy with usual care, statin therapy did not reduce CHD or all-cause mortality in older patients with well controlled hypertension and moderately elevated LDL-C (29). Rosuvastatin, the newest agent, seems to be the most potent, but lacks patient-oriented outcome data. Tables 16.4 and 16.5 summarize primary and secondary prevention trials with lipid-lowering medications. Statins have also been shown to be beneficial in the primary and secondary prevention of CHD in multiple meta-analysis and systematic reviews (30–32).

Statins exert their effect on LDL-C by inhibiting the enzyme, HMG-CoA reductase, responsible for the conversion of HMG-CoA to mevalonate, which is the rate-limiting step in cholesterol synthesis. They also enhance clearance of LDL-C through upregulation of hepatic LDL-C receptors. Statins may also enhance the degradation of apolipoprotein B, thus reducing hepatic production and secretion of very low-density lipoproteins (VLDL). Statins have been shown to reduce LDL-C by 18%–55%, increase HDL by 5%–15%, and decrease triglycerides by 7%–30% (1). Statins exhibit the majority of their LDL-C lowering effect at the starting dose; doubling the dose only produces a 6% further reduction (1).

Because of relatively short plasma half-lives, statins (except atorvastatin and rosuvastatin) should be taken at bedtime so peak concentrations occur in the early morning hours, when cholesterol production is at its greatest. Atorvastatin and rosuvastatin may be administered at any time of day. Table 16.6 summarizes important prescribing information for medications used in the treatment of hyperlipidemia.

Overall, statins are well tolerated, with a low frequency of adverse events (33). Of clinical importance, statins have been shown to cause liver transaminase elevations (greater than three times the upper limit of normal) in up to 2% to 3% of patients. Transaminase elevations usually occur in the first 12 weeks of therapy or after a dose titration and are reversible with dose reduction or discontinuation. If a statin has been discontinued, transaminase elevations do not often recur with rechallenge of the same agent or selection of another statin (1). Progression to severe hepatotoxicity is rare. It is recommended that transaminase levels be monitored more frequently at the beginning of therapy, or after an upward dose titration, at 6 or 12 weeks, and periodically thereafter (every 6 to 12 months).

Myopathies associated with statin therapy are their most publicized adverse effect (34). Elevations in creatine kinase (CK) are the best indicator of statin-induced myopathy, however 5% of patients with myopathy symptoms will have normal CK levels (33). Myopathies are more likely to occur in patients with multiple co-morbidities or in those patients taking concurrent medications that increase statin concentrations. The major metabolic pathway for the metabolism of lovastatin, simvastatin, and atorvastatin is via the CYP 3A4 isoform and inhibitors of this enzyme, such as erythromycin, azole antifungals, cyclosporine, amiodarone, and terbinafine, may increase statin concentrations. Routine measurement of CK is not warranted, but patients should be instructed to immediately report any muscle pain or weakness (34). If myopathies or rhababdomyolysis is strongly suspected, patients should immediately discontinue statin use and a serum CK should be drawn.

BILE ACID SEQUESTRANTS

There are three bile acid sequestrants (BAS) available in the United States (Table 16.6). These agents are not absorbed

TABLE 16.4 Summary of Key Primary Prevention Trials for Coronary Heart Disease Involving Lipid-Lowering Therapies

Name of Trial	Treatment	Control Group Event Rate	Treatment Group Event Rate	p Value	NNT
AFCAPS/TexCAPS	Lovastatin 20–40 mg	5.5%	3.5%	<0.001	50
ALLHAT-LLT	Usual care Pravastatin 40 mg	10.4%	9.3%	0.16	91
CARDS	Atorvastatin 10 mg	9.0%	5.8%	0.001	32
Helsinki	Gemfibrozil 1200 mg	4.1%	7.7%	<0.02	71
LRC-CPPT	Cholestyramine 24 g	9.8%	8.1%	<0.05	59
Oslo	Diet + smoking cessation	4.2	2.5	0.03	59
WSCOPS	Pravastatin 40 mg	7.9%	5.5%	<0.001	43

AFCAPS/TexCAPS, Air Force/Texas Coronary Atherosclerosis Prevention Study (Downs et al., 1998); ALLHAT-LLT, Antihypertensive and Lipid-Lowering Treatment to Prevent Heart Attack Trial; approximately 13–15% of patients had a history of coronary heart disease (events are CHD only); CARDS, Collaborative Atorvastatin Diabetes Study (Colhoun et al., 2004); Helsinki, The Helsinki Heart Study (Frick et al., 1987); LRC-CPPT, The Lipid Research Clinics Coronary Primary Prevention Trial (Insull et al., 1984); Oslo, The Oslo Study (Hjermann et al., 1988); WSCOPS, The West of Scotland Coronary Prevention Study (Shepherd et al., 1995)

NNT, number needed to treat

(Adapted from Talbert RL. Hyperlipidemia. In: DiPiro JT, Talbert RL, Yee GC, Matzke GR, Wells BG, Posey LM. Pharmacotherapy: A Pathophysiologic Approach. New York: McGraw-Hill; 2005. p. 446. Used with permission.)

TABLE 16.5 Key Secondary Prevention Trials for Coronary Heart Disease Involving Lipid-Lowering Agents

Name of Trial	Treatment	Control Group Event Rate	Treatment Group Event Rate	p Value	NNT
4S	Simvastatin 20 mg	11.5%	8.2%	0.0003	30
AVERT	Atrovastatin 80 mg	21%	13%	0.048	12
CARE	Pravastatin 40 mg	13.2%	10.2%	0.003	33
CDP	Niacin 3 g + Clofibrate 1.8 g	20.9%	20.6%	NS *	333
HPS	Simvastatin 40 mg	14.7%	12.9%	0.003	56
LIPID	Pravastatin 40 mg	9.8%	8.1%	<0.05	59
MIRACL	Atorvastatin 80 mg	17.4%	14.8%	0.048	39
PROSPER	Pravastatin 40 mg	16.2%	14.1%	0.014	48
PROVE-IT	Pravastatin 40 mg Atorvastatin 80 mg	26.3% (P)	22.4% (A)	0.005	26
VA-HIT	Gemfibrozil 1200 mg	21.7%	17.3%	0.006	23
WHO	Clofibrate 1.6 g	3.9%	3.1%	<0.005	125

4S, Scandinavian simvastatin Survival Study (Pederson et al, 1994); AVERT, The Atorvastatin Versus Revascularization Treatments; CARE, Cholesterol and Recurrent Events (Melendez et al., 1996); CDP, Coronary Drug Project (Berge et al., 1975); HPS, Heart Protection Study; results expressed as all-cause mortality (HPS Collaborative Group 2002); LIPID, Long-Term Intervention with Pravastatin in Ischaemic Disease Study (MacMahon et al., 1995); MIRACL, Myocardial Ischemia Reduction with Aggressive Cholesterol Lowering (Schwartz et al., 2001); PROSPER, PROspective Study of Pravastatin in the Elderly at Risk (Shepherd J et al., 2002); PROVE-IT, Intensive versus moderate lipid lowering with statins after acute coronary syndromes (Cannon et al., 2004); VA-HIT, Veterans Administration-High-Density Lipoprotein Cholesterol (HDL-C) Intervention Trial (Bloomfield et al, 1999). NNT, number needed to treat; NS, Not significant
(Adapted from Talbert RL. Hyperlipidemia. In DiPiro JT, Talbert RL, Yee GC, Matzke GR, Wells BG, Posey LM. Pharmacotherapy: A Pathophysiologic Approach. New York: McGraw-Hill; 2005. p. 447. Used with permission.)

systemically; they work by binding bile acids in the intestine, reducing resorption. Bile acid sequestrants produce a 5%–25% reduction in LDL-C and 3%–5% increase in HDL-C (1). They may actually increase triglyceride levels; so, they should be used with caution when triglyceride levels are >200 mg/dl and are contraindicated when triglycerides exceed 400 mg/dl. These agents are second-line agents as monotherapy for patients with moderately elevated LDL-C levels. They may be added to statin therapy for further LDL-C reduction when LDL-C goals are not met (35–37). Cholestyramine has been demonstrated to reduced the risk of CHD (Table 16.4), and colestipol to improve coronary atherosclerosis when combined with niacin and lovastatin (38–41). A recent meta-analysis found a benefit from bile acid sequestrants in terms of cardiac mortality, but not overall mortality (32).

Because these medications remain unabsorbed in the gastrointestinal tract, they lack systemic toxicity. However, gastrointestinal side effects are common. Cholestyramine and colestipol, due to their bulk and local action, are associated with constipation, abdominal pain, bloating, and flatulence (1). Forty percent of patients will discontinue use within 1 year because of these symptoms (42). Gastrointestinal side effects are seen less frequently with colesevelam, the only BAS available in tablet form. Side effects may be managed with patient education, increasing dietary fiber and fluid intake or stool softeners.

Clinical use of cholestyramine and colestipol is also limited by their number of drug interactions. These agents may decrease absorption of certain medications that are adminis-

tered concomitantly, such as levothyroxine, propanolol, warfarin, amiodarone, and digoxin. This interaction may be avoided by administering other medications 1 hour before or 4 hours after administration of the BAS.

NICOTINIC ACID (NIACIN)

Nicotinic acid, or niacin, is the most effective agent for increasing HDL-C, raising levels by as much as 15%–35% (1). It also produces a moderate degree of LDL-C and triglyceride lowering. Because of its primary effect on HDL-C, nicotinic acid is generally utilized when non-HDL cholesterol (total cholesterol − HDL cholesterol) is the target of therapy or when triglycerides are very high (>500 mg/dl). The NCEP ATP III guidelines recommend that after the LDL-C goal has been achieved, non-HDL cholesterol (total cholesterol minus HDL-C) should be calculated and a non-HDL goal of 30 mg/dl greater than the LDL-C goal should be set. Non-HDL cholesterol becomes the primary target of therapy when triglycerides are >500 mg/dl, bcause of the risk of pancreatitis. In this case nicotinic acid or a fibric acid derivative, discussed later, are the medications of choice, in addition to a very low-fat diet, weight management, and increased physical activity. Once triglycerides levels have been lowered to less than 500 mg/dl, LDL-C once again becomes the target of therapy.

Clinical trials evaluating nicotinic acid for the prevention of CHD are sparse. Older trials, which studied the effects of niacin for secondary prevention, failed to demonstrate a benefit from treatment in terms of both cardiac and overall mortality, and there are no trials evaluating the use of niacin as a means of primary prevention (32).

TABLE 16.6 Prescribing Information for Lipid Lowering Medications

Medication	Contraindications/Cautions/Adverse Effects	Dosage	Relative Cost *
Elevated LDL-C			
Atorvastatin (Lipitor)	Contraindicated in pregnancy or lactation; serious adverse effects include LFT elevations and myopathies; available in combination with amlodipine	10–80 mg/day	$$$
Fluvastatin (Lescol)	Same as above	20–80 mg at bedtime	$$
Lovastatin (Mevacor)	Same as above; available in combination with niacin	20–80 mg with evening meal	$
Pravastatin (Pravachol)	Same as above	10–40 mg at bedtime	$$$
Rosuvastatin (Crestor)	Same as above	5–20 mg daily	$$$
Simvastatin (Zocor)	Same as above	10–80 mg at bedtime	$$$
Simvastatin/ Ezetimibe (Zetia)	Same as above	20/10 mg–40/10 mg	$$$
Cholestyramine (Questran)	Contraindicated when triglycerides >400 mg/dl and biliary obstruction; consitpation, GI distress common; multiple drug interactions	8–32 mg daily in divided doses	$$
Colesvelam (Welchol)	Same as above; no drug interactions	1,875–4,375 mg daily in divided doses	$$
Low HDL-C			
Extended-release niacin (Niaspan)	Contraindicated in active liver disease or peptic ulcer disease; flushing common adverse effect; LFT elevations	500–2,000 mg at bedtime	$$
OTC Niacin (Various)	Same as above; may cause more flushing and LFT elevations	2–4.5 g daily in divided doses	$
High Triglycerides			
Fenofibrate (TriCor, Lofibra, Antara, Triglide)	Contraindicated in gall bladder disease; adverse effects include myopathies, gall stone formation and GI distress	TriCor 48–145 mg/day	$$$
		Lofibra 67–200 mg/day Antara 43–130 mg/day Triglide 50–160 mg/ day	
Omega-3 acid ethyl esters (Omacor)	Use with caution with fish allergy; may cause taste perversion or body odor	4 g/day	$$

*Relative cost: $ = <$33.00; $$ = $34.00 - $66.00; $$$ = >$67.00

Nicotinic acid may be added to statin therapy to further improve lipoprotein levels (43, 44). The addition of once daily extended-release niacin added to statin therapy has been shown to slow the progression of atherosclerosis in patients with moderately low HDL-C levels (45). The combination of a statin and niacin is safe and generally well tolerated (33). A regimen aimed at increasing HDL-C levels, consisting of short-acting niacin, gemfibrozil, and cholestyramine, slows or prevents progression of coronary stenosis (40, 41, 46) but does not reduce the risk of cardiovascular events when compared with conventional therapy (47).

Nicotinic acid reduces hepatic uptake of free fatty acids and synthesis of very-low-density-lipoprotein (VLDL) and enhances clearance of plasma chylomicrons and VLDL. Although its mechanism is not entirely understood, this increase in VLDL catabolism results in decreased LDL-C and triglycerides and an increase in HDL-C. Nicotinic acid is available as several over-the-counter (OTC) immediate-release and sustained release formulations. Extended-release niacin, Niaspan, is the only prescription formulation available (Table 16.6). Variations exist among the different OTC sustained-release formulations, so patients should be advised not to switch from one preparation to another without contacting their physician.

Nicotinic acid is associated with many adverse reactions.

Most of these can be appropriately managed and do not require discontinuation of the agent. They include:

- Cutaneous flushing and itching. These are the most common side effects and can be reduced by pretreating with aspirin 325 mg 1 half-hour before nicotinic acid administration and by taking the medication during or after meals (1). Extended-release niacin may be associated with fewer cutaneous reactions than other formulations (1).
- Headaches and gastrointestinal distress, including activation of peptic ulcer disease. There appears to be no difference in the frequency of these side effects between OTC immediate and sustained release products.
- Hepatotoxicity. This occurs rarely. Sustained-release formulations have been associated with severe cases; extended release niacin, on the other hand, appears to cause fewer transaminase elevations (33).
- Hyperuricemia. This occurs occasionally, and nicotinic acid may even precipitate an attack of gout. Routine monitoring of uric acid levels is not necessary, but patients should be educated to recognize the symptoms of an acute gout attack and report these to their physician if they occur, especially if there is a history of gout.
- Hyperglycemia. This occurs because nicotinic acid decreases insulin sensitivity. Therefore, blood glucose levels should be monitored carefully in diabetics taking nicotinic acid. Diabetes is no, however, considered to be a contraindication to their use. Glycemic control is not significantly altered in well-controlled type 2 diabetics taking extended-release niacin <2 g/day (48).

All side effects occur more frequently in doses of 2 g or higher, regardless of formulation.

FIBRIC ACID DERIVATIVES

Fibric acid derivatives, or fibrates, are primarily used for lowering triglycerides and may lower them by 25%–50% (1). They produce moderate HDL-C elevations and only slight LDL-C lowering. In some patients with severe hypertriglyceridemia, fibrates may actually cause a rise in LDL-C. There are two fibrates available in the United States: gemfibrozil, and fenofibrate (Table 16.6). Clofibrate, once available, has been discontinued by the manufacturer.

Gemfibrozil and clofibrate have been shown to reduce the risk in first fatal and nonfatal myocardial infarctions in clinical trials (49, 50). Gemfibrozil also reduced death due to CHD and non-fatal myocardial infarction in men with documented CHD and low levels of HDL-C (51). These results have not, however, been consistent, and a meta-analysis of cholesterol-lowering medications on mortality showed that fibrates did not reduce the risk of cardiac or overall mortality and that non-cardiovascular mortality was increased (32). These conflicting results should not discourage their use for lowering triglycerides to prevent pancreatitis. They do suggest, however, that fibrates may not be as effective as other available agents.

Fibrates may also be utilized in addition to statin therapy to improve lipoprotein levels. However, gemfibrozil and statin combinations have been associated with increased occurrence of myopathy; so, if combination therapy is initiated, fenofibrate should be used (52). When combination therapy is used, clinicians should be sure the patient has normal renal function

and low doses should be used initially. Patients should also be counseled to recognize the symptoms suggestive of myopathy and discontinue use and contact their physician if they occur. Although the combination of a fibrate and niacin has not been studied extensively, one trial did find that the combination of clofibrate and niacin was not beneficial in the secondary prevention of CHD (53).

Although the mechanism of action for the fibrates is not clearly understood, it is thought that they alter gene transcription ultimately causing reduced secretion of VLDL by the liver and increased VLDL clearance. They are generally well tolerated; the most common side effects are gastrointestinal symptoms, fatigue, and headache. Myopathy has also been reported with fibrate monotherapy. Fibrates also increase biliary cholesterol excretion and can increase the risk of cholesterol gallstone development; so they should not be used in patients with active gallbladder disease. Gemfibrozil is administered twice daily and should be taken 30 minutes before morning and evening meals. Fenofibrate is formulated either as micronized capsules to be taken with food or as tablets which may be taken anytime.

EZETIMIBE

Ezetimibe works by inhibiting the intestinal absorption of cholesterol and phytoesterols at the brush border. It may be used alone or in combination with statins to alter lipoprotein levels. There are no trials evaluating ezetimibe, alone or in combination, for the prevention of CHD. It has, however, been shown to reduce LDL-C levels by 19% as monotherapy. When combined with statins, it reduces LDL-C more than a statin alone (54–57). Ezetimibe is available as a tablet as well as in combination with simvastatin (Table 16.6). In combination, ezetimibe is a therapeutic option for patients who have not achieved their LDL-C goal and cannot tolerate high-dose statin therapy. It may also be used as monotherapy in patients who are intolerant to a statin or BAS.

Ezetimibe has few systemic adverse effects and drug interactions. It is recommended, however, that transaminase levels be monitored periodically, especially when combined with statins. Also, patients taking cyclosporine may have increased levels of ezetimibe and should be monitored carefully.

OMEGA-3 FATTY ACIDS

Until recently, the only available sources of omega-3 fatty acids were OTC fish oil supplements or in a diet rich in fatty fish. Omacor (omega-3 acid ethyl esters) is now approved to treat hypertriglyceridemia (see Table 16.6). Omacor, as with most OTC fish oil supplements, is a combination of marine-derived, purified eiosapentaenoic acid (EPA) and docosahexaenoic acid (DHA). Omega-3 fatty acids are used primarily to reduce triglycerides and have been shown to reduce serum levels by 30% when administered as 3–4 g/day (58). In a large, open-label, secondary prevention trial comparing a fixed combination of EPA and DHA alone, vitamin E alone, EPA/DHA plus vitamin E, or no supplement, the omega-3 fatty acid combination produced a statistically significant reduction in rates of all-cause death, nonfatal myocardial infarctions, and nonfatal stroke (59). However, after 3.5 years approximately 50% of study participants were also receiving statin therapy. Clinical trials providing a clear benefit for cardioprotection of omega-3 fatty acid supplementation are lacking. A systematic review of dietary or supplemental omega-3 fatty acids provided no clear evidence that either treatment altered total mortality or cardiovascular events (60).

Omega-3 fatty acids are generally safe and well tolerated, but serious bleeding disorders and thrombocytopenia have been observed with high doses. The current role for omega-3 fatty acid supplementation for primary or secondary prevention is, therefore, not well defined and well-controlled clinical trials are needed before they may be recommended for general use. It is reasonable to recommend omega-3 fatty acid use for patients that require a reduction in triglycerides levels and cannot tolerate fibric acid derivatives or nicotinic acid.

ALTERNATIVE AND COMPLEMENTARY THERAPIES

The use of OTC herbal products is becoming increasingly popular. The most common reasons for use of herbals are a desire to avoid adverse reactions of prescription therapy, failure of conventional therapy to cure a problem, and recommendations from a friend (61). Several herbal remedies are promoted for hyperlipidemia. Some of the more popular remedies

TABLE 16.7 Summary of Recommendations

Treatment Goal and Intervention	Efficacy	Strength of Recommendation*	Comment
Primary coronary heart disease prevention			
HMG-CoA reductase inhibitors	14% reduction in mortality over 3 years	A	Meta-analysis
Secondary coronary heart disease prevention			
HMG-CoA reductase inhibitors	22% reduction in mortality over 2.5 years	A	Meta-analysis
Smoking cessation	36% reduction in mortality	B	Systematic review
Cardiac mortality			
Bile acid sequestrants	30% reduction	A	Meta-analysis
Elevated total cholesterol			
Low fat diet (dietary fat 25%–35%, saturated fat <7% of total calories, cholesterol <200 mg/day)	13% reduction in total cholesterol	C	Disease-oriented outcome, but high-quality evidence
Elevated LDL-C			
Low-fat diet (as above)	16% reduction in LDL-C	C	Disease-oriented outcome, but high-quality evidence
HMG-CoA reductase inhibitors	18%–55% reduction in LDL-C	C	Disease-oriented outcome, but high-quality evidence
Bile acid sequestrants	15%–30% reduction	C	Disease-oriented outcome, but high-quality evidence
Low HDL-C			
Moderate alcohol consumption (30 g/day)	4 mg/dl increase	C	Disease-oriented outcome, but high-quality evidence
Tobacco cessation	4 mg/dl increase	C	Disease-oriented outcome, but high-quality evidence
Nicotinic acid	15%–35% increase	C	Disease-oriented outcome, but high-quality evidence
Elevated triglycerides			
Fibric acid derivatives	25%–50% reduction	C	Disease-oriented outcome, but high-quality evidence
Omega-3 fatty acid supplements	30% reduction	C	Disease-oriented outcome, but high-quality evidence

*A = consistent, good-quality patient-oriented evidence; B = inconsistent or limited-quality patient-oriented evidence; C = consensus, disease-oriented evidence, usual practice, expert opinion, or case series. For information about the SORT evidence rating system, see *http://www.aafp.org/afpsort.xml*.

include garlic, guggul, fenugreek, red yeast rice, and Asian ginseng. Despite their popularity with the public, many medical professionals caution against their routine use, citing their modest effect on surrogate markers, such as cholesterol, versus placebo, and the lack of evidence that they improve clinical outcomes. Garlic, red yeast rice, artichoke, and guggul may provide slight reductions in cholesterol; however, most studies are of poor methodological quality and of short duration (62, 63). A double-blind random controlled trial comparing standard and high-dose guggulipid tablets to placebo found that guggulipid actually increased LDL-C significantly more than placebo and may have been associated with a cutaneous hypersensitivity reaction (64). Patients should be aware, therefore, that, although these herbal remedies may be effective versus placebo in altering the lipid profiles, they have not been shown to impact outcomes such as morbidity or mortality. Therefore, they may be cautiously supplemented to proven cholesterol lowering medications but should not be routinely used as monotherapy for primary or secondary prevention.

LONG-TERM MONITORING

Most patients being treated for hyperlipidemia are asymptomatic, and, therefore, monitoring their response to treatment is based on lab values or clinical outcomes. Enough time should be allowed to observe a response to therapy, whether lifestyle modification or lifestyle changes in conjunction with pharmacotherapy, before a treatment is deemed a failure or a decision is made to increase a dose. In most cases a fasting lipid panel every 6 to 12 weeks is appropriate. Clinical manifestations such as eruptive xanthomas may improve but often take considerable time. Once the patient is stable on therapy, a lipid profile every 6 months to 1 year is necessary. Adherence to therapy should be evaluated at each visit and can be accomplished through the use of a dietary diary, a pill count, or prescription records.

Education and support should also be provided on an ongoing basis regarding management of modifiable risk factors such as weight management, exercise, smoking cessation, and blood pressure control. For patients receiving cholesterol lowering medications, subjective and objective adverse effects should be monitored, as discussed previously.

SUMMARY

Reducing elevated serum lipids is one of the most effective preventive tools available to the family physician. Table 16.7 summarizes the indications for, and the evidence supporting, the various recommended uses of lipid-lowering therapies. Lifestyle modification should always be the cornerstone of treatment, and all primary care physicians need to be well versed in methods of encouraging and aiding patients in modifying lifestyles to lower cardiovascular risk. Potent medications are available as well, which in combination with lifestyle changes can markedly improve the prognosis of patients with hyperlipidemias and multiple additional CVD risk factors.

CASE DISCUSSION

Mrs. Ramirez' LDL-C and total cholesterol are significantly elevated, to moderate levels. In determining her therapeutic goal, we note that Maria has no CHD equivalents, is a tobacco user, does not have hypertension, has no significant family history of early CHD, is younger than 55 years old, and has an HDL-C of 35. Thus, she has one risk factor. According to Figure 16.1, her LDL-C goal should be <160.

Therapeutic lifestyle changes should be initiated, such as tobacco cessation, reduced dietary fat, weight loss, and exercise. The addition of medications to help lower her LDL-C is optional at this time and could await trial of lifestyle alterations. If a medication were added, a low-dose statin would be the preferred choice because she has no contraindications to their use. Maria is currently using fish oil, which may have a beneficial effect on her triglycerides. Hers are in the normal range (125 mg/dl), so, assuming that she is not experiencing any significant side effects, she can be reassured about continued use if she so desires.

REFERENCES

1. National Cholesterol Education Program (NCEP) Expert Panel on Detection, Evaluation, and Treatment of High Blood cholesterol in Adults (Adult Treatment Panel III). Third Report of the National Cholesterol Education Program (NCEP) Expert Panel on detection, evaluation, and treatment of high blood cholesterol in adults (Adult Treatment Panel III: Final Report.) Circulation. 2002;106:3143–3421.
2. Strategies for a Heart-Healthy and Stroke-Free America. *http://www.cdc.gov/nccdphp/publications/aag/cvh.htm.* Accessed December 6, 2005.
3. McGovern PG, et al. Recent trends in acute coronary heart disease. Mortality, morbidity, medical care, and risk factors. N Engl J Med. 1996;334:884–890.
4. Szklo M, et al. Trends in cholesterol levels in the atherosclerosis risk in communities (ARIC) study. Prev Med. 2000;30:252–259.
5. Newman WP, et al. Relation of serum lipoprotein levels and systolic blood pressure to early atherosclerosis. The Bogalusa Heart Study. N Engl J Med. 1986;314:138–144.
6. *http://www.ahrq.gov/clinic/ajpmsuppl/lipidrr.htm* accessed December 6, 2005.
7. Standards of Medical Care in Diabetes—2006. American Diabetes Association. Diabetes Care. 2006;29:S4–S42.
8. Grundy SM, Cleeman JI, Merz CNB, et al. Implications of recent clinical trials for the national Cholesterol Education Program Adult Treatment Panel III guidelines. Circulation. 2004;110:227–239.
9. Yu-Poth S, et al. Effects of the National Cholesterol Education Program's Step I and Step II dietary intervention programs on cardiovascular disease risk factors: a meta-analysis. Am J Clin Nutr. 1999;69:632–646.
10. Anderson JW, et al. Long-term cholesterol-lowering effects of psyllium as an adjunct to diet therapy in the treatment of hypercholesterolemia. Am J Clin Nutr. 2000;71:1433–1438.
11. Anderson JW, et al. Cholesterol-lowering effects of psyllium intake adjunctive to diet therapy in men and women with hypercholesterolemia: meta-analysis of 8 controlled trials. Am J Clin Nutr. 2000;71:472–479.
12. Rimm EB, et al. Moderate alcohol intake and lower risk of coronary heart disease: meta-analysis of effects on lipids and haemostatic factors. BMJ. 1999;319:1523–1528.
13. Maeda K, Noguchi Y, Fukui T. The effects of cessation from

smoking on the lipid and lipoprotein profiles: a meta-analysis. Prev Med. 2003;37:283–290.

14. Critchley J, Capewell S. Smoking cessation for the secondary prevention of coronary heart disease. Cochrane Database Syst Rev. 2004;(1):CD003041.

15. De Lorgeril M, et al. Mediterranean diet, traditional risk factors, and the rate of cardiovascular complications after myocardial infarction: final report of the Lyon diet heart study. Circulation. 1999;99:779–785.

16. King AC, et al. Long-term effects of varying intensities and formats of physical activity on participation rates, fitness, and lipoproteins in men and women aged 50 to 65 years. Circulation. 1995;91:2596–2604.

17. Hjermann I. Strategies for dietary and anti-smoking advice: practical experiences from the Oslo study. Drugs. 1988; 36(Suppl 3):105–109.

18. Waters D, Higginson L, Gladstone P, et al. Effects of monotherapy with an HMG-CoA reductase inhibitor on the progression of coronary atherosclerosis as assessed by serial quantitative arteriography. Circulation. 1994;89:959–968.

19. Jukema JW, Bruschke AVG, van Boven AJ, et al. Effects of lipid lowering by pravastatin on progression and regression of coronary artery disease in symptomatic men with normal to moderately elevated serum cholesterol levels. Circulation. 1995;91:2528–2540.

20. Oliver MF, de Feyter PJ, Lubsen J, et al. Effect of simvastatin on coronary atheroma: the multicentre anti-atheroma study. Lancet. 1994;344:633–638.

21. Herd JA, Ballantyne CM, Farmer JA, et al. Effects of fluvastatin on coronary atherosclerosis in patients with mild to moderate cholesterol elevations. Am J Cardiol. 1997;80:278–286.

22. Nissen SE, Tuzcu EM, Schoenhagen P, et al. Effect of intensive compared with moderate lipid-lowering therapy on progression of coronary atherosclerosis. JAMA. 2004;291:1071–1080.

23. Downs JR, Clearfield M, Weis S, et al. Primary prevention of acute coronary events with lovastatin in men and women with average cholesterol levels. JAMA. 1998;279:1615–1622.

24. Shepherd J, Cobbe SM, Ford I, et al. Prevention of coronary heart disease with pravastatin in men with hypercholesterolemia. N Engl J Med. 1995;333:1301–1307.

25. Collins R, Armitage J, Parish S, et al. MRC/BHF heart protection study of cholesterol lowering with simvastatin in 20536 high-risk individuals: a randomized placebo-controlled trial. Lancet. 2002;360:7–22.

26. Serruys P, de Feyter P, Macaya C, et al. Fluvastatin for prevention of cardiac events following successful first percutaneous coronary intervention: a randomized controlled trial. JAMA. 2002;287:3215–3222.

27. Sever PS, Dahlöf B, Poulter NR, et al. Prevention of coronary and stroke events with atorvastatin in hypertensive patients who have average or lower-than-average cholesterol concentrations, in the Anglo-Scandinavian Cardiac Outcomes Trial—Lipid Lowering Arm (ASCOT-LLA): a multicentre randomized controlled trial. Lancet. 2003;361:1149–1158.

28. Waters D. The AVERT trial. Eur Heart J. 2000;21:1030–1031.

29. The ALLHAT Officers and Coordinators for the ALLHAT Collaborative Research Group. The Antihypertensive and Lipid-Lowerint Treatment to Prevent Heart Attack Trial (ALLHAT-LLA). JAMA. 2002;288:2998–3007.

30. Baigenet C, Keech A, Kearney, et al. Efficacy and safety of cholesterol-lowering treatment: prospective meta-analysis of data from 90056 participants in 14 randomised trials of statins. Lancet. 2005;366:1267–1277.

31. Pignone M, Phillips C, Mulrow C. Use of lipid lowering drugs for primary prevention of coronary heart disease: meta-analysis of randomized trials. BMJ. 2000;321:983–986.

32. Studer M, Briel M, Leimenstoll B, et al. Effect of different antilipidemic agents and diets on mortality. Arch Intern Med. 2005;165:725–730.

33. Xydakis AM, Jones PH. Toxicity of antilipidemic agents: facts and fictions. Curr Atheroscler Rep. 2003;5:403–410.

34. Gotto AM Jr. Safety and statin therapy. Arch Intern Med. 2003;163:657–659.

35. Pravastatin Multicenter Study Group II. Comparative efficacy and safety of pravastatin and cholestyramine alone and combined in persons with hypercholesterolemia. Arch Intern Med. 1993;153:1321–1329.

36. Heinonen TM, Schrott H, McKenney, JM, et al. Atorvastatin, a new HMG-CoA reductase inhibitor as monotherapy and combinded with colestipol. J Cardiovasc Pharmacol Therapeut. 1996;1:117–122.

37. Lovastatin Study Group III. A multicenter comparison of lovastatin and cholestyramine therapy for severe primary hypercholesterolemia. JAMA. 1988;260:359–366.

38. Lipid Research Clinics Program. The Lipid Research Clinics Coronary Primary Prevention Trial results. I: Reduction in the incidence of coronary heart disease. JAMA. 1984;251:351–364.

39. Lipid Research Clinics Program. The Lipid Research Clinics coronary Primary Prevention Trial results. II: The relationship of reduction in incidence of coronary heart disease to cholesterol lowering. JAMA. 1984;251:365–374.

40. Blankenhorn DH, Nessim SA, Johnson RL, et al. Beneficial effects of combined colestipol-niacin therapy on coronary atherosclerosis and coronary venous bypass grafts. JAMA. 1987;257:3233–3240.

41. Brown G, Albers JJ, Fisher LD, et al. Regression of coronary artery disease as a result of intensive lipid-lowering therapy in med with high levels fo apolipoprotein B. N Engl J Med. 1990;323:1289–1298.

42. Konzem SL, Gray DR, Kashyap ML. Effect of pharmaceutical care on optimum colestipol treatment in elderly hypercholesterolemic veterans. Pharmacotherapy. 1997;17:576–583.

43. Insull W Jr, McGovern ME, Schrott H, et al. Efficacy of extended-release niacin with lovastatin for hypercholesterolemia: assessing all reasonable doses with innovative surface graph analysis. Arch Intern Med. 2004;164:1121–1127.

44. Bayes HE, Dujovne CA, McGovern ME, et al. Comparison of once-daily, niacin extended-release/lovastatin with standard doses of atorvastatin and simvastatin (the ADvicor Versus Other Cholesterol-Modulating Agents Trial Evaluation [ADVOCATE]). Am J Cardiol. 2003;91:667–672.

45. Taylor AJ, Sullenberger LE, Lee HJ, et al. Arterial biology for the investigation of treatment effects of reducing cholesterol (ARBITER) 2: a double-blind, placebo-controlled study of extended-release niacin on atherosclerosis progression in secondary prevention patients treated with statins. Circulation. 2004;110:3512–3517.

46. Brown BG, Zhao XQ, Fisher CA. Simvastatin and niacin, antioxidant vitamins, or the combination for the prevention of coronary disease. N Engl J Med. 2001;345:1583–1592.

47. Whitney EJ, Krasuski RA, Personius BE, et al. A randomized trial fo a strategy for increasing high-density lipoprotein cholesterol levels: effects on progression of coronary heart disease and clinical events. Ann Intern Med. 2005;142:95–104.

48. Grundy SM, Vega GL, McGovern ME, et al. Efficacy, safety, and tolerability of once-daily niacin for the treatment of dyslipidemia associated with type 2 diabetes: results of the assessment of diabetes control and evaluation of the efficacy of niaspan trial. Arch Intern Med. 2002;162:1568–1576.

49. Frick MH, Elo MO, Haapa K, et al. Helsinki heart study:

primary-prevention trial with gemfibrozil in middle-aged men with dyslipidemia: safety of treatment, changes in risk factors, and incidence of coronary heart disease. N Engl J Med. 1987;317:1237–1245.

50. Committee of Principal Investigators. A co-operative trial in the primary prevention of ischemic heart disease using clofibrate: report from the committee of principal investigators. Br Heart J. 1978;40:1069–1118.

51. Rubins HB, Robins SJ, Collins D, et al. Gemfibrozil for the secondary prevention of coronary heart disease in men with low levels of high-density lipoprotein cholesterol. N Engl J Med. 1999;341:410–418.

52. Maki KC, Galant R, Davidson MH. Non-high density lipoprotein cholesterol: the forgotten therapeutic target. Am J Cardiol. 2005;96[Suppl 1]:59K–64K.

53. Coronary drug project. Clofibrate and niacin in coronary heart disease. JAMA. 1975;231:360–381.

54. Ezzet F, Wexler D, Statkevich P, et al. The plasma concentration and LDL-C relationship in patients receiving ezetimibe. J Clin Pharmacol. 2001;41:943–949.

55. Feldman T, Koren M, Insull W, et al. Treatment of high-risk patients with ezetimibe plus simvastatin co-adminsstration versus simvastatin alone to attain National Cholesterol Education Program Adult Treatment Panel III low-density lipoprotein cholesterol goals. Am J Cardiol. 2004;93:1481–1486.

56. Ballantyne CM, Blazing M, King TR, et al. Efficacy and safety of ezetimibe co-administered with simvastatin compared with atorvastatin in adults with hypercholesterolemia. Am J Cardiol. 2004;93:1487–1494.

57. Goldberg AC, Sapre A, Liu J, et al. Efficacy and safety of ezetimibe coadministered with simvastatin in patients with primary hypercholesterolemia: a randomized, double-blind, placebo-controlled trial. Mayo Clin Proc. 2004;79:620–629.

58. Carroll DN, Roth MT. Evidence for the cardioprotective effects of omega-3 fatty acids. Ann Pharmacother. 2002;36:1950–1956.

59. Dietary supplementation with n-3polyunsaturated fatty acids and vitamin E after myocardial infarction: results of the GISSI-Prevenzione trial. Gruppo Italiano per lo Studio della Sopravvivenza nell'Infarto miocardico. Lancet. 1999;354:447–455.

60. Hooper L, Thompson RL, Harrison RA, et al. Omega 3 fatty acids for prevention and treatment of cardiovascular disease. Cochrane Database of Systematic Reviews. 4, 2005.

61. Palinkas LA, Kabongo ML. The use of complementary and alternative medicine by primary care patients. A SURF*NET study. J Fam Pract. 2000;49:1121–1130.

62. Stevinson C, Ptiiler MH, Ernst E. Garlic for treating hypercholesterolemia. A meta-analysis of randomized clinical trials. Ann Intern Med. 2000;133:420–429.

63. Coon JST, Ernst E. Herbs for serum cholesterol reduction: a systematic review. J Fam Pract. 2003;52:468–478.

64. Szaparay PO, Wolfe ML, Bloedon LT, et al. Guggulipid for the treatment of hypercholesterolemia. A randomized controlled trial. JAMA. 2003;290:765–772.

CHAPTER 17

Thyroid Disease

Jeri R. Reid

Thyroid problems are commonly encountered in family medicine and can lead to significant clinical consequences if undiagnosed. The initial presentation is often subtle, making clinical diagnosis challenging. Fortunately, when diagnosed, most thyroid disorders can be satisfactorily treated but will require long-term monitoring. In this chapter, the current evidence and consensus recommendations on the evaluation and management of the most common thyroid disorders will be reviewed.

HYPOTHYROIDISM

CASE

A 39-year-old woman presents to her family physician with the complaints of fatigue, constipation, and cold intolerance. On physical exam she has a diffusely enlarged, nontender thyroid gland and facial puffiness. She has no significant past medical history and takes no regular medications. However, her mother has been previously treated for an unknown type of thyroid disease. Laboratory studies reveal an elevated thyroid-stimulating hormone (TSH) and a decreased free thyroxine (FT4) level. Anti-thyroperoxidase antibodies are present in high titers.

CLINICAL QUESTIONS

1. What are the most common causes of hypothyroidism?
2. What is the role of thyroid autoantibodies in the diagnosis of hypothyroidism?
3. What are the treatment goals, and should they differ in different populations?

Hypothyroidism is defined as undersecretion of thyroid hormone and is identified biochemically by an elevated thyroid-stimulating hormone (TSH). This syndrome can be classified as congenital or acquired based on the time of onset. Congenital hypothyroidism is most commonly caused by endemic iodine deficiency. In countries with sufficient iodine this disorder is usually caused by thyroid gland dysgenesis or defective hormone synthesis. Acquired hypothyroidism occurs later in life and is usually the result of autoimmune thyroiditis (Hashimotos). Other causes include surgical removal of thyroid tissue or destruction of the thyroid by radioactive iodine, other external radiation, or toxin exposure. Certain drugs such as amiodorone and lithium interfere with glandular hormone release

and can also cause hypothyroidism. A transient hypothyroidism can also be caused by subacute or lymphocytic thyroiditis (postpartum thyroiditis) with most patients returning to a euthyroid state after 2–8 months (1). Table 17.1 lists the differential diagnosis of hypothyroidism.

Hypothyroidism can be further classified as primary and secondary. Primary hypothyroidism relates to disease that directly affects the thyroid gland. Secondary hypothyroidism refers to a central cause, such as an adenoma impinging on the hypothalamus or pituitary. Central causes are very rare and for purposes of the present discussion, hypothyroidism mentioned subsequently will refer to primary hypothyroidism.

The last classification scheme for hypothyroidism is based on severity. Clinical (overt) is distinguished from subclinical (mild) on the basis of the serum free thyroxine (FT4) level in a patient with an elevated TSH (1). Clinical hypothyroidism will be reviewed in this section, and subclinical disease will be reserved for later discussion.

The prevalence of clinical hypothyroidism in the United States is between 0.3% and 2.0%. It is approximately three times more common in African-Americans than whites, five times more common in persons aged 65 and older than in younger populations, and 10 times as frequent in women as in men (2, 3). Other risk factors include a personal or family history of thyroid or autoimmune disease, Turner's syndrome, Down syndrome, multiple sclerosis, and primary pulmonary hypertension (1).

Initial Evaluation

The most common signs and symptoms of hypothyroidism are listed in Table 17.2. Other symptoms include weight gain, hoarseness, hair loss, muscle cramping and weakness, menstrual irregularity (usually menorrhagia), and infertility. However, the clinical manifestations of hypothyroidism can be subtle, especially in the elderly. The detection of hypothyroidism is complicated by its insidious onset and the fact that the symptoms overlap with those of many other health problems (1). A recent study set out to determine a correlation between symptoms and biochemical hypothyroidism. They found that no individual symptom had a positive predictive value above 12%. However, there was a positive correlation between the number of symptoms reported and the serum TSH concentration, with the strongest association among persons who reported a change in seven symptoms over the preceding year. These individuals were nine times more likely to be hypothyroid than euthyroid (4). Occasionally, usually in very advanced disease, the presentation is dominated by hypothermia, congestive heart failure, pleural effusion, intestinal ileus, coa-

TABLE 17.1 Causes of Hypothyroidism*

Primary—due to underfunction of the thyroid gland (95% of cases)

Idiopathic (most commonly "burned out" Hashimoto's thyroiditis)

Hashimoto's thyroiditis

Irradiation of the thyroid to treat Graves' disease

Surgical removal of the thyroid

End-stage invasive fibrous thyroiditis

Severe iodine deficiency

Drug therapy (e.g., lithium, interferon)

Infiltrative systemic disease:
   sarcoidosis
   amyloidosis
   scleroderma
   hemochromatosis

Secondary—due to undersecretion of TSH (5% of cases)

Neoplasms of the pituitary gland or hypothalamus

Congenital hypopituitarism

Pituitary necrosis (Sheehan's syndrome)

* Excludes congenital hypothyroidism.

TABLE 17.2 Common Signs and Symptoms of Hypothyroidism

Symptom	Percent of Patients Affected*
Weakness	99
Lethargy	91
Cold intolerance	89
Decreased sweating	89
Forgetfulness	66
Constipation	61
Physical Findings	
Coarse or dry skin	97
Slow speech	91
Eyelid edema	90
Skin cold to touch	83
Thick tongue	82
Facial edema	79
Coarse hair	76
Skin pallor	67

*These statistics are adapted from a textbook of endocrinology. Findings may be more subtle in the primary care setting. (Adapted from Wilson JD, et al, eds. Williams Textbook of Endocrinology, 9th ed. Philadelphia, PA: Saunders, 1998. [In Hueston WJ. Treatment of hypothyroidism. Am Fam Physician. 2001;64:1717–1724.] Used with permission from Elsevier.)

gulopathy, ataxia, seizures, psychosis, severe depression, dementia, and/or coma (1).

The physical exam may reveal a diffuse or nodular goiter, sluggish movements, bradycardia, pretibial edema, facial puffiness, coarse skin, and prolongation of ankle reflex. A recent cross-sectional, double-blind study looked at the diagnostic accuracy of the physical exam in diagnosing hypothyroidism and found that no one physical sign could discriminate a euthyroid patient from a hypothyroid patient. The combination of coarse skin, bradycardia, and delayed ankle reflex had a moderate predictive value but was not considered accurate enough to guide clinical decision making (5).

Congenital hypothyroidism may present with hypothermia, poor feeding, bradycardia, jaundice, enlarged posterior fontanelle, and umbilical hernia. Most infants are asymptomatic, warranting the routine screening of all newborns (1).

LABORATORY TESTING

Making the definitive diagnosis begins with the measurement of highly sensitive TSH in a reliable laboratory. An elevated level suggests hypothyroidism and should be followed by a FT4 level. If this value is below the normal range, the diagnosis of hypothyroidism is confirmed.

A normal TSH level does not rule out secondary (central) hypothyroidism. This should be suspected in a patient with a normal TSH who exhibits clinical features of hypothyroidism and should prompt further testing with FT4. A normal TSH and T4 usually do not require further evaluation; however, severe nonthyroid illness and some drugs (e.g., glucocorticoids, dopamine, and dobutamine) can falsely lower the TSH level and mask mild hypothyroidism (1). If the T4 level is low, clinical findings suggesting pituitary dysfunction or an intracranial mass should be sought, especially in patients with sarcoidosis, cranial injury, radiotherapy, or cancers known to metastasize to the pituitary (1). These causes are rare, but many practitioners routinely order both TSH and FT4 in all hypothyroid patients to rule out this possibility. Imaging of the pituitary gland and hypothalamus would be indicated in these patients.

The measurement of thyroid autoantibodies (specifically antithyroperoxidase antibodies) confirms autoimmune thyroiditis as the cause of sustained primary hypothyroidism, since they are present in high titers in 95% of these patients (6). This diagnosis should already be clinically suspected in patients who do not have other risk factors for hypothyroidism (1). The presence of antibodies should also alert the clinician to the possibility of other autoimmune diseases in the patient or their family (7). Thyroid ultrasound or radionucleide scanning are only necessary if structural abnormalities are suspected.

Management

The treatment for hypothyroidism is hormone supplementation with levo-thyroxine (L-thyroxine). When used properly, this medication is highly effective with few side effects.

The L-thyroxine dose needs to be individualized, and controversy exists regarding the starting dose, the titration method, and the final goal of treatment. The generally accepted replacement dose is 1.6 to 1.8 mcg/kg (1, 6). Gradual titration is often used; however, a prospective, randomized, double-blind trial found no difference in adverse events between a full starting dose of 1.6 mcg per kg and a regimen that started with 25 mcg and titrated upward every 4 weeks (8). Their study excluded patients with a history of cardiac disease or those taking cardiac medications—a known risk factor for complications with rapid dosing (9); and the authors concluded that a full starting dose is safe, more convenient, more cost-effective, and should be used in all patients without cardiac disease. One critic of this study pointed out, however, that all major textbooks and consensus guidelines still recommend a more careful titration in all elderly patients and that one modestly powered study is not sufficient to change this well-accepted, more conservative approach (10). Therefore, dosages of 12.5 to 25 mcg (or 25% of the calculated replacement dose) are recommended for patients aged 65 and older or with heart disease (1, 6, 7, 9). These precautions are taken because of the concern that an abrupt increase in metabolic rate could precipitate angina, myocardial infarction, congestive heart failure, or arrhythmia in such patients (9). Dosages are titrated by 25 to 50 mcg every 6 weeks until a euthyroid state is achieved. Smaller titration doses of 12.5 mcg are sometimes advocated in persons with severe ischemic heart disease. (1)

The goal of therapy is to normalize the TSH level. Most authorities recommend that the TSH be maintained in the lower half of the normal range (0.5–2.0 mcU/ml) for young patients and in the mid-range (1.0–4.0 mcU/ml) for the elderly (7). There has been some dispute about these goals, since some studies have found that the lower range has more beneficial results in all age groups in terms of cholesterol level and cardiac function (7, 11).

L-thyroxine has a narrow therapeutic range, as well as potential interactions with several common medications. Malabsorptive states and medications such as cholestyramine, ferrous sulfate, sucralfate, calcium, and aluminum hydroxide can interfere with L-thyroxine absorption. Rifampin and sertraline accelerate L-thyroxine metabolism. Nephrotic syndrome and the anticonvulsant medications phenobarbital, phenytoin, and carbamazepine can decrease thyroid hormone binding. Warfarin doses need to be monitored closely during titration since the metabolism of clotting factors increases as thyroid function improves. Pregnancy increases thyroid hormone requirements by as much as 75% (1).

Choosing which L-thyroxine product to use is also a subject of debate. Most thyroidologists including the AACE still recommend the use of brand-name LT4 (6, 7) despite a recent study suggesting that generic products are bioequivalent (12). The preparation chosen should remain the same throughout treatment. The use of triiodothyronine in combination with LT4 for patients who remain symptomatic on LT4 alone is not currently recommended. One study found improvement in symptomatology in patients receiving T3 along with T4 (13) but these results could not be confirmed on further study (14, 15). Table 17.3 summarizes treatment recommendations for thyroid disease.

Long-term Monitoring

Because the half-life of thyroid hormone is nearly a week, it takes 3–6 weeks after initiating a dosage change for a steady state to be achieved. For this reason, the patient should be monitored, every 6 weeks during the titration process. At that time, serum TSH should be measured and the patient questioned about thyroid symptoms and medication side effects. When the TSH becomes normal, follow-up visits should be scheduled at 6 months and 1 year. If the TSH and LT4 dosage remain stable, annual visits should continue indefinitely (6). Any changes in dosage should be followed by a repeat TSH level in 6 weeks. The importance of compliance should be emphasized at each visit, because as many as 40% of patients on L-thyroxine do not receive enough medication to achieve a TSH in the normal range (16). This can have significant health consequences, because under-treated hypothyroidism can lead to cardiac dysfunction, depression, elevated cholesterol levels, and persistent symptoms. Over-treatment can lead to hyperthyroid symptoms and complications, as will be discussed in the next section (7).

CASE DISCUSSION

The case illustrates a typical presentation for hypothyroidism. Goiter is a frequent physical finding and can be diffuse or multinodular. The patient is at higher risk for developing thyroid disease based on her positive family history. The elevated autoantibodies confirm the diagnosis of Hashimoto's thyroiditis and provide important clinical information for her and her family, because they will be at an increased risk of developing other autoimmune diseases.

This patient was started on 100 mcg of L-thyroxine (1.6 mcg per kg), because she is less than 65 years old and has no history of cardiac disease. Six weeks later, her TSH was in the normal range, and she was feeling better and experiencing no side effects from the treatment. She was instructed to return for repeat testing in 6 months and to continue yearly check-ups indefinitely.

HYPERTHYROIDISM

CASE

A 23-year-old woman presents to her family physician complaining of decreased menstrual flow and fatigue, and wondering if she could be pregnant, though a home test was negative. On physical exam she is found to have lost 10 pounds from her previous visit several months ago. She has tachycardia, a fine resting tremor, and hyperreflexia. The patient recalls a recent viral illness that included soreness of her anterior neck. Her pregnancy test is negative. Several laboratory tests are ordered. The serum TSH is below the lower limit of normal; FT4 is elevated; but free triodothyronine (FT3) is normal. Radionucleide scanning shows diffusely decreased uptake.

CLINICAL QUESTIONS

1. What are the most common causes of hyperthyroidism?
2. What is the most efficient diagnostic approach?
3. Which treatment is most effective, with the fewest side effects?

TABLE 17.3 Summary of Treatment Recommendations for Thyroid Disease

Problem and Intervention	Strength of Recommendation*	Comment
Hypothyroidism		
Thyroid hormone replacement at full starting dose	B	As effective as other regimens in patients under age 65 without cardiac disease
Thyroid hormone replacement with gradual titration to replacement dose	C	This is recommended by most experts with lower starting doses and more careful titration in elderly or cardiac patients
Titration to TSH goal of 0.5–2.0	C	
Titration to TSH goal of 1.0 to 4.0	C	
Thyroid hormone replacement with generic L-thyroxine	B	Combining triiodothyronine with L-thyroxine is not supported by scientific evidence
Hyperthyroidism		
Antithyroid drugs	A	Effective in 40%–50% of patients. Less effective in smokers and larger goiters
Radioactive iodine therapy	A	Effective in 80% of cases; can be re-dosed. Treatment of choice for Graves' disease in the United States
Total thyroidectomy	A	100% effective, but carries 100% risk of permanent hypothyroidism
Subtotal thyroidectomy	A	92% effective; 25% risk of permanent hypothyroidism
Thyroid Enlargement		
Observation without treatment	C	Treatment of choice with no compressive symptoms or thyroid dysfunction. Hormone suppression to reduce goiter size has been demonstrated to be ineffective and is not recommended.
Surgery to reduce size of goiter	C	100% success with total thyroidectomy; 40% success with subtotal thyroidectomy. Postoperative L-thyroxine does not prevent recurrences.
RAI for toxic goiter	A	80% effective
RAI for nontoxic goiter	A	Typically decreases goiter size by 40%–90%
Thyroid Nodules		
Observation if nontoxic nodules and <1 cm in diameter	C	
Near-total thyroidectomy for cancers other than medullary	C	
Total thyroidectomy with lymph node resection for medullary cancer	C	
Lobectomy for indeterminate or suspicious nodules	C	
Subclinical Thyroid Disease		
L-thyroxine therapy -Symptomatic patient with TSH <10	C	Risks outweigh benefits in asymptomatic patients with TSH <10
-Asymptomatic patient with TSH >10	C	
Treatment of subclinical hyperthyroidism whenTSH <0.1	C	Risks outweigh benefits in patients with TSH above 0.1

*A = consistent, good-quality patient-oriented evidence; B = inconsistent or limited-quality patient-oriented evidence; C = consensus, disease-oriented evidence, usual practice, expert opinion, or case series. For information about the SORT evidence rating system, see *http://www.aafp.org/afpsort.xml*.

Clinical hyperthyroidism (also known as thyrotoxicosis) is caused by the direct effects of excess thyroid hormone and the indirect effects of increased beta-adrenergic activity. It occurs in 2% of women and 0.2% of men.

The most common causes, in approximate order of frequency are:

- Graves' disease. An autoimmune disease that leads to increased thyroid hormone secretion. Graves' disease accounts for 60%–80% of all cases with 15% of these cases occurring in patients over 60 years old.
- Toxic nodular goiter and solitary hyperfunctioning nodules. Toxic nodular goiter causes 5% of cases in the United States but may be more common in iodine deficient areas. This condition typically occurs in patients older than 40 with longstanding multinodular goiter. Autonomously functioning solitary nodules are found in younger patients and are associated with iodine deficiency. Both cause symptoms due to autonomous thyroid hormone production.
- Thyroiditis. A series of diseases that cause transient leakage of thyroid hormone from a damaged gland. They include subacute thyroiditis following a viral illness and lymphocytic and postpartum thyroiditis.
- Excess iodine ingestion, either from diet, radiographic contrast, or medication. Amiodorone can produce hyperthyroidism either as a result of its high iodine content or by inducing thyroiditis.
- Factitious hyperthyroidism. This occurs from intentional or accidental ingestion of excess thyroid hormone.
- Rare causes include metastatic thyroid cancer, ovarian tumors that produce thyroid hormone (struma ovarii), trophoblastic tumors, or TSH-secreting pituitary tumors (17).

Initial Evaluation

The common signs and symptoms of hyperthyroidism are listed in Table 17.4. The clinical manifestations vary depending on the duration of the illness, the age of the patient, and comorbid conditions. Elderly patients often present with decreased appetite or atrial fibrillation; however, they occasionally present with only fatigue and lethargy (apathetic hyperthyroidism). Thyroid storm is a rare complication of hyperthyroidism, usually resulting from a stressful illness in a patient with inadequately treated hyperthyroidism. It presents with fever, delirium, vomiting, diarrhea, and dehydration (18).

The physical examination may demonstrate weight loss, elevated systolic pressure, tachycardia, pretibial edema, tremor, and/or proximal muscle weakness. A tender diffuse goiter suggests subacute thyroiditis. Painless goiter is present in other forms of thyroiditis and in Graves' disease. Single or multiple nodules may be present with or without tenderness. In 50% of patients with Graves' disease, there are distinctive eye findings that include proptosis, lid retraction, extraocular muscle dysfunction, and keratitis (18, 19).

LABORATORY TESTING

The diagnosis of hyperthyroidism is outlined in Figure 17.1. The initial laboratory study that should be ordered is the TSH. If this is low or undetectable, a FT4 should be obtained. If this result is elevated, the diagnosis of hyperthyroidism is confirmed. If FT4 is normal, a free T3 should be ordered to rule out T3 toxicosis. Normal T4 and T3 indicate subclinical hyperthyroidism, which will be discussed later (17).

In determining the treatment plan, it is important to identify the cause of the hyperthyroidism. This is best accomplished by ordering a radionucleide uptake and scan. In-

---

TABLE 17.4 Common Signs and Symptoms of Hyperthyroidism

Signs and Symptoms	Patients Older than 70 Years (%)	Patients Younger than 50 Years (%)
Tachycardia	71	96
Fatigue	56	84
Weight loss	50	51
Goiter	50	94
Tremor	44	84
Apathy	41	25
Atrial fibrillation	35	2
Anorexia	32	4
Nervousness	31	84
Hyperactive reflexes	28	96
Depression	24	22
Increased sweating	24	95
Polydipsia	21	67
Heat intolerance	15	92
Increased appetite	0	57

(Adapted from Trivalle C, Doucet J, Chassagne P, et al. Differences in signs and symptoms of hyperthyroidism in older and younger patients. J Am Geriatr Soc. 1996;44:51. Used with permission.)

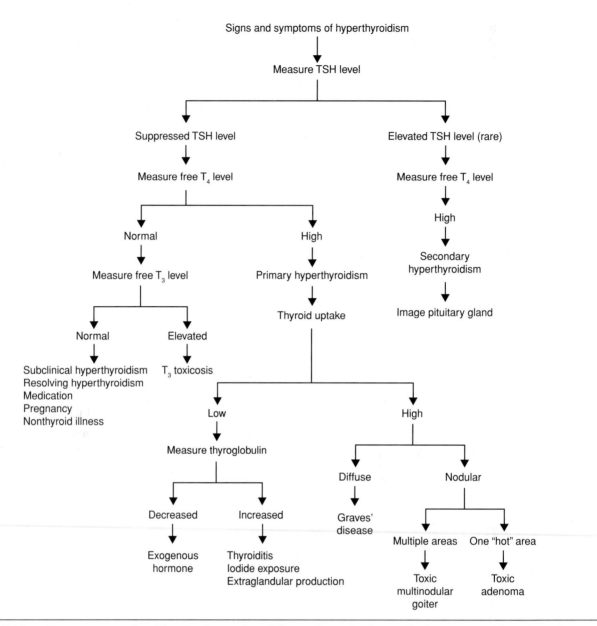

Figure 17.1 • Management algorithm for hyperthyroidism. (From Reid JR, Wheeler SF. Hyperthyroidism: diagnosis and treatment. Am Fam Physician. 2005;72:623–630. Used with permission.)

creased uptake occurs in Graves', toxic multinodular goiter and solitary hyperfunctioning nodules. However Graves' disease is easily distinguished from the nodular causes because there will be a diffuse uptake in the gland instead of a nodular or focal pattern. Thyroiditis is also easy to distinguish from Graves' because there will be a decreased uptake on the scan with thyroiditis rather than an increase (17).

Thyroid autoantibody measurement is not recommended, since it offers little assistance in differentiating between Graves' disease and thyroiditis. Antithyrotropin antibodies can help predict the success of certain treatment regimens that will be discussed below (18).

Management

The management goal is to correct the hypermetabolic state with the fewest complications. Beta-blockers can resolve many

of the adrenergic symptoms, such as tremor, tachycardia, heat intolerance, and nervousness. Propranolol titrated to doses between 80 and 320 mg per day are most commonly used. Calcium channel blockers can resolve some of the symptoms if beta-blockers cannot be tolerated. These drugs are usually the only treatment needed for thyroiditis-induced hyperthyroidism, because it is usually self-limited. Beta-blockers are safe for short-term use in pregnancy (17). Persistent hyperthyroidism is treated with antithyroid drugs, radioactive iodine, or surgery. Each of these has been shown to be effective and well tolerated if used as recommended (19).

PHARMACOTHERAPY

Antithyroid drugs (ATDs) interfere with the organification of iodine and are the preferred treatment for Graves' disease in many parts of the world outside the United States. In this country, ATDs are generally reserved for pregnant patients, children, and those who refuse radioactive iodine (RAI) therapy. They can also be used in cardiac and elderly patients to normalize thyroid function before surgery or RAI, because thyrotoxicosis can be temporarily exacerbated by these treatments (20).

Methimazole is the agent used most often in nonpregnant patients, because it can be given less frequently at maintenance doses and has a lower incidence of side effects. The starting dose is 15 to 30 mg per day divided every 8 hours. Beta-blockers can be given in conjunction with ATDs and tapered as the patient becomes euthyroid. After 4 to 12 weeks, the patient is usually euthyroid, as evidence by symptoms and T4 levels. The methimazole dose can usually be tapered to a maintenance dose of 5 to 10 mg as a single daily dose and should be continued for 12 to 18 months (20). Symptoms, rather than TSH levels, should be used to monitor early response to treatment, because TSH levels can take months to normalize.

Propothiouracil (PTU) is the alternative medication. However, it has to be dosed more frequently, has more side effects, and has been shown to reduce the effectiveness of RAI (21). Its main use is in pregnancy, because methimazole has been linked to a rare fetal scalp abnormality. Both drugs are compatible with breastfeeding.

Remission rates are estimated at 40%–50% and do not seem to be affected by the dosage or the duration of therapy beyond 18 months (21). Treatment success decreases as the severity of the hyperthyroidism and the size of the goiter increase. Smokers and those with elevated antithyrotropin-receptor antibody titers have lower remission rates. Relapse usually occurs in the first 3 to 6 months after ATDs are discontinued (22). There is no current evidence to support using T4 in combination with ATDs to improve remission rates (21).

Major side effects of ATDs include polyarthritis (1%–2%) and agranulocytosis (0.1%–0.5%). Agranulocytosis usually occurs within 3 months of starting therapy. PTU has a higher dose-related risk of this reaction, and it is very rare with methimazole doses less than 30 mg. Patients should be warned to discontinue the drug if they experience a sudden fever or sore throat. Routine monitoring of white cell counts is controversial (20) but may be beneficial in the early detection of agranulocytosis (23). PTU causes elevated liver function tests in 30% of patients, and an immunoallergic hepatitis in 0.1%–0.2%. Methimazole can cause cholestasis, but this is rare. Minor side effects occur in less than 5% of patients and include rash, fever, gastrointestinal symptoms, and arthralgias. Most of the minor side effects do not require cessation of therapy except for arthralgias, because they could be the first sign of a more serious polyarthritis syndrome (20).

Iodides block the conversion of T4 to T3 and inhibit hormone release from the gland. They can cause paradoxical hormone release and interfere with radioactive iodine or antithyroid drug treatment, so they are not routinely used. They can, however, be used preoperatively with beta-blockers for rapid control of symptoms before emergency nonthyroid surgery or to reduce the vascularity of the gland before Graves' disease surgery (24, 25).

RADIOACTIVE IODINE

Radioactive iodine (RAI) concentrates in the thyroid gland and destroys thyroid tissue. It is the treatment of choice for Graves' disease in the United States and the preferred treatment for multinodular goiter and toxic nodules in patients older than 40. When relapse occurs after ATD therapy, RAI is generally recommended. The cure rate with single-dose treatment is 80%, with thyroid function returning to normal within 2–6 months (18). The treatment is safe and cost-effective but causes permanent hypothyroidism in 82% of patients at 25 years. There is a lower incidence of hypothyroidism in patients with toxic nodules or toxic multinodular goiter, because the rest of the gland may start to function normally when the hyperthyroidism is treated (26).

RAI treatment is contraindicated in pregnancy, and conception should be delayed for 6–12 months after treatment. If these guidelines are followed, RAI poses no increased risk of future birth defects or infertility in women of childbearing age (6). RAI is also being used more often in patients younger than 20 years old but is still controversial (27). Women who are breast-feeding children should avoid RAI because it appears in breast milk.

Achieving remission and earlier onset of the hypothyroidism allows for better long-term outcome for the patient (26). If relapse does occur, RAI can be repeated as soon as 3 months (28).

Potential complications of RAI include:

- Radiation thyroiditis (1% of patients). This is reversible but can cause a transient thyrotoxicosis. Pretreatment with ATDs, preferably methimazole, can be used for cardiac and elderly patients to prevent this possibility. The drug needs to be stopped several days before RAI and can be restarted a few days after the treatment (17).
- Exacerbation of Graves' ophthalmopathy (15% of patients, especially smokers). This complication can be prevented by starting prednisone prior to RAI and continuing it for 2–3 months. Consultation with an experienced ophthalmologist is recommended. Because of this complication, many endocrinologists prefer not to treat patients with severe Graves' ophthalmolopathy with RAI (29).
- Transient neck soreness, facial flushing, and decreased taste.

Patients should avoid children and pregnant women for 24–72 hours after RAI and use frequent hand washing and flushing to minimize the exposure of others to contaminated urine, saliva, and feces during this time (17).

SURGERY

Subtotal thyroidectomy is a treatment option for pregnant women or children who cannot tolerate ATDs or in patients who are experiencing compressive symptoms from their goiters. Toxic nodules in healthy patients younger than 40 are usually removed surgically. Surgery could also be considered in a noncompliant patient, a patient who has failed ATDs but does not want RAI, or a patient with such severe disease that a recurrence would not be tolerated (17). Total thyroidectomy is curative and is indicated for patients with severe disease or large goiters.

A recent meta-analysis of thyroidectomy revealed a low morbidity rate (3%) and no mortalities. The risk of hypothyroidism with subtotal thyroidectomy was 25% and the risk of relapse was 8%. Complications include hypoparathyroidism and/or recurrent laryngeal nerve damage (In 1%–2% of patients regardless of the type of surgery performed). Patients should be rendered euthyroid with antithyroid drugs preoperatively. Iodinated contrast agents, beta-blockers, and corticosteroids may also be needed if surgery needs to be done urgently (30).

Long-term Monitoring

Patients should be monitored closely after any treatment for hyperthyroidism. After ATD treatment the patient should be monitored every 4–12 weeks until the thyroid status stabilizes; then every 3 to 4 months for the 12- to 18-month duration of therapy. When the medication is withdrawn, visits should continue at 3- to 4-month intervals for the first year, when relapse is more likely to occur.

Recommended follow-up after RAI includes frequent visits every 4–6 weeks for the first 3 months as the thyroid status normalizes and, in most cases, hypothyroidism develops. After the patient's condition has stabilized, 3-month and 6-month follow-up visits should be planned. Regardless of the treatment, annual visits should continue indefinitely because relapse can occur years later and because thyroid replacement may need to be adjusted (18).

Despite appropriate treatment, some patients with hyperthyroidism continue to experience ocular, cardiac, and psychological complications of the disease. There seems to be no significant increase in the risk of cancer mortality in these patients (31), but there may be an increased risk of mortality related to cerebrovascular, cardiac disease, and hip fractures in those treated with RAI (32). Interestingly, a recent study on bone mineral density in hyperthyroid patients showed a return to baseline bone density in women 3 years after treatment (33). It seems prudent, however, to monitor hyperthyroid patients carefully for osteoporosis and atherosclerotic risk factors.

CASE DISCUSSION

The case illustrates subacute thyroiditis, which should be included in the differential diagnosis of a patient with recent onset of symptoms of hyperthyroidism. It is caused by a viral infection and can lead to transient hyperthyroidism (sometimes followed by transient hypothyroidism) that resolves spontaneously over a 2- to 8-month period. Symptomatic treatment with β-blockers and close follow-up is indicated.

The low uptake on RAI scanning distinguishes thyroiditis from Graves' disease. However, it should be noted that most experts recommend making the diagnosis clinically and not ordering an RAI scan unless the condition persists past the expected 8 months. Antithyroid antibody testing would not have provided any helpful information unless this patient developed persistent hypothyroidism and the diagnosis of Hashimoto's thyroiditis was being considered. Interestingly, the hypomenorrhea that this patient experienced would seem contradictory to the hypermetabolic state of hyperthyroidism, but is a commonly associated symptom.

THYROID ENLARGEMENT

CASE

At a new patient appointment, a 66-year-old woman informs her family physician that she has been taking L-thyroxine therapy for several years for an enlarged thyroid gland. She was told that this medication would shrink her thyroid gland and allow her to avoid surgery. She has never experienced symptoms of thyroid disease and reports no side effects from the medication. She thinks that her thyroid gland may have gotten smaller but is not sure. She has been menopausal for 16 years, is not on hormone replacement therapy, and has never had bone density testing. She had a heart attack 10 years ago and takes medication for hypertension and elevated cholesterol. On physical examination she is found to have a firm, enlarged thyroid that contains many nodules. Her TSH level is slightly below the normal range.

CLINICAL QUESTIONS
1. What are the causes of an enlarged thyroid gland?
2. Will an enlarged thyroid gland lead to more serious thyroid disease?
3. What is the long-term management of thyroid enlargement?

Thyroid enlargement, or goiter, is the most common thyroid disorder in clinical practice. The prevalence in the United States is variable depending on the regional iodine intake but is estimated at 4%–7% (34). Goiter is 5–10 times more common in women (35). The development of goiter is influenced by autoimmune, genetic, and extrinsic factors (36). There are three general ways of describing goiter:

- Endemic versus sporadic. Goiter is termed endemic if it occurs in 10% or more of the population; otherwise it is sporadic. Endemic goiter is the result of iodine deficiency and is very rare in the United States.
- Simple or multinodular. Goiter is described as simple when the gland is diffusely enlarged. Multinodular goiters have multiple nodules within the gland.
- Nontoxic or toxic. Nontoxic goiter exhibits normal thyroid function, whereas toxic goiter refers to an enlarged gland associated with either hypo- or hyperthyroidism (35).

Certain drugs (including lithium, iodides, and amiodorone) and certain foods (including rutabagas, cabbage, turnips, soybeans, and kelp) can act as goitrogens by disrupting normal thyroid hormone synthesis and release. Cigarette smoking is also associated with goiter; this occurs because thiocyanate, a degradation product of cyanide in tobacco smoke, competes with iodine for uptake in the thyroid gland. Pregnancy can induce goiter by exacerbating an existing iodine deficiency (37).

Goiter occurs in 50% of patients with Hashimoto's thyroiditis (38) as a result of defective hormone synthesis, lymphocytic infiltration, and increased growth factor secretion. Typically there is a goiter present with Graves' disease that is caused by the effects of thyroid stimulating immunoglobulin

(39). Multinodular goiter results from the disordered growth of thyroid cells and the gradual replacement of the gland by fibrosis. A painful goiter is usually (in 90% of cases) caused by subacute thyroiditis or acute hemorrhage into a thyroid cyst or adenoma. Rare causes are acute suppurative thyroiditis or a rapidly enlarging carcinoma (38).

Initial Evaluation

Most patients with goiter are asymptomatic. History should be directed toward eliciting symptoms of hypo- or hyperthyroidism (discussed previously) and determining the presence of risk factors for thyroid disease or malignancy. The patient should be questioned about the ingestion of goitrogens, pregnancy, and smoking. Risk factors for malignancy include a family history of thyroid pathology, personal history of neck radiation therapy, previous thyroid surgery, and cervical adenopathy (40). Rarely, there could be worrisome symptoms of mechanical pressure if the goiter is very large or extends into the thorax. These could include dyspnea, dysphagia, hoarseness, cough, or symptoms of thoracic outlet syndrome (41).

Physical exam should include a thorough palpation of the thyroid gland to determine the size, tenderness, and presence of nodules. The patient should be examined for the previously described signs of hypo- or hyperthyroidism. Pemberton's sign was first described in 1946; it is used to identify intrathoracic extension of the thyroid gland. After elevating the arms above the head for 1 minute, a patient with a positive Pemberton's sign will exhibit facial plethora, dilated neck veins, cyanosis, and discomfort (42).

LABORATORY TESTING

Laboratory investigation should begin with TSH testing. If abnormal, the appropriate work-up for hypo- or hyperthyroidism should follow. Elevated levels of antithyroid antibodies occur in 15%–20% of patients with multinodular goiter and help predict the development of Graves' thyrotoxicosis and Hashimotos-induced hypothyroidism (41). Basal serum calcitonin has been associated with thyroid cancer; it has been recommended in evaluating goiter in persons with a family history of thyroid cancer or multiple endocrine neoplasia. Because of a high incidence of false positives and a lack of standardization of measured values, routine calcitonin measurement is not recommended (43).

Thyroid ultrasound should be considered in multinodular goiter to rule out the presence of a dominant nodule that would need further work-up. Some authors recommend ultrasound for all patients with goiter, because it has been estimated that up to 50% of nodules are not palpable on physical exam (36). A dominant nodule is investigated in the same way as a solitary nodule, with fine-needle biopsy (FNB).

Pulmonary function testing or a barium swallow may be needed if compressive symptoms are present. Screening for suspected tracheal compression or intrathoracic extension of goiter is indicated in all patients with large mulinodular goiters having compressive symptoms or in whom the lower margin of the goiter cannot be palpated. Chest radiographs may sometimes reveal these goiters, but CT scanning or MRI are much more sensitive tests for this purpose. Because CT scanning involves the use of iodinated contrast agents, pretreatment with ATDs may need to be considered to prevent iodine-induced thyrotoxicosis (41).

Management

The management of goiter includes monitoring without treatment, thyroidectomy, L-thyroxine suppression, or RAI. The choice of treatment is dependent on the whether the goiter is toxic or nontoxic, simple or multinodular, or associated with compressive symptomatology.

Monitoring without treatment can be considered in patients with nontoxic goiter who have no compressive symptoms. These patients should be followed with clinical exam, thyroid laboratory testing, and, possibly, ultrasound to detect growth of the thyroid, thyroid dysfunction, or the presence of dominant nodules (36).

Surgery is the treatment of choice for patients with large symptomatic goiters or those with risk factors for thyroid cancer (44, 45). Total thyroidectomy is becoming preferred over subtotal thyroidectomy because it results in no risk of recurrence and, in the hands of an experienced surgeon, carries the same rate of complications. Permanent hypoparathyroidism or damage to the recurrent laryngeal nerve occurs in 1% of patients. These complications become 3 to 10 times more likely in recurrent goiter operations. The postoperative use L-thyroxine to prevent goiter recurrence in patients undergoing partial thyroidectomy is used by many clinicians but is not supported by the current evidence (44).

Long-term suppression of TSH with the use of L-thyroxine has been extensively studied as a treatment for nontoxic goiter. In general, this therapy is not recommended because there is not a significant reduction in the size of the goiter with therapy and long-term treatment could result in subclinical hyperthyroidism (see below) (36, 44).

In the treatment of toxic goiter associated with hyperthyroidism, RAI is considered the treatment of choice. In nontoxic goiter, treatment with RAI can result in a decrease in goiter volume by more than 40% and a reduction in compressive symptoms with a low incidence of complications (41). The use of recombinant human TSH has been found to increase the uptake of RAI in multinodular goiter, allowing for lower dosages to be used (46). The incidence of hypothyroidism is 20%–45% within the first year and there is a rare chance of radiation thyroiditis or induction of Graves' disease (45). There is still reluctance among clinicians to use RAI treatment in patients without hyperthyroidism despite studies supporting its safety. Perhaps this results from the lack of evidence regarding the long-term risk of thyroid and nonthyroid cancers after treatment of these patients. When used, it tends to be restricted to patients older than 40 years of age and those with contraindications for surgery (44).

Long-term Monitoring

The natural history of nontoxic goiter is characterized by gradual growth (averaging 4.5% per year), nodule formation, and development of functional autonomy. For this reason, patients with goiter need to be followed longitudinally. Here are a few key issues to consider in following patients with goiter:

- Progression to clinical hyperthyroidism occurred in 9%–10% of patients with goiter within a 7- to 12-year follow-up period (44). Therefore, patients with goiter who do not receive treatment need to be educated about these complications and followed clinically at least annually.

- Patients who have been treated for goiter require the same diligent follow-up. Those treated with subtotal thyroidectomy need to be monitored for goiter recurrence (15%–40% of patients) and hypothyroidism (10%–20%). Of course, patients undergoing total thyroidectomy need life-long monitoring of their iatrogenic hypothyroidism. Eight percent of patients who have received RAI will experience recurrent goiter; Graves' disease associated with ophthalmopathy can occur in up to 5% of these patients (44).
- Even though L-thyroxine suppression is no longer recommended in most cases of goiter, a clinician may still encounter patients treated in this manner. It is important to monitor these patients for the development of subclinical and overt hyperthyroidism, which becomes more likely the longer the therapy is continued (44). It might be beneficial to counsel these patients about these risks so they can consider other treatment options.
- Regardless of the treatment, monitoring for the development of thyroid cancer must always be one of the goals of follow-up. Although simple goiter is not a risk factor for thyroid cancer, the tendency to form nodules over time increases the risk. The incidence of malignancy in both solitary nodules and multinodular goiter is approximately 5% (45).

CASE DISCUSSION

L-thyroxine suppression of nontoxic goiter is still commonly encountered in clinical practice, despite evidence that does not support its use. This patient does not have any compressive symptoms related to her goiter; so surgery is not indicated. L-thyroxine, especially at levels that reduce TSH below the normal range, may put this patient at risk of an exacerbation of her cardiac disease and/or the development of osteoporosis. A thorough history needs to be taken to assess her risk of thyroid cancer, and thyroid ultrasound should be considered to evaluate for dominant nodules that may need evaluation. She needs to be educated about the natural history of her disease and the risks and benefits of the treatment options. Her L-thyroxine should be reduced (and possibly discontinued) and her thyroid status monitored at least on an annual basis.

SOLITARY THYROID NODULE

CASE

A 30-year-old man presents to his family physician with symptoms of an upper respiratory infection. On physical exam of his neck, a nodule is palpated in the left lobe of his thyroid gland. It is soft, nontender, and approximately 1 cm in diameter but has a slightly irregular shape. The patient has no personal or family history of thyroid disease. His TSH is normal. He is referred for an ultrasound-guided FNB, which reveals an adequate specimen of benign follicular cells. The ultrasound shows that he has several nodules, each less than 1 cm in diameter. He is asked to follow up in 6 months.

CLINICAL QUESTIONS

1. What is the work-up for a solitary thyroid nodule?
2. What is the likelihood that a nodule will be malignant?
3. What is the management based on biopsy cytology?

Solitary thyroid nodules are frequently found incidentally during a physical examination or on nonthyroid neck imaging. Their prevalence increases with age, so that as many as half of patients older than age 60 will have a thyroid nodule (47). Many are quite small, but palpable nodules are present in 4%–7% of the adult population. Thyroid nodules are 4 to 5 times more likely in women than men (43).

As in the development of goiter, the formation of a solitary nodule depends on environmental, genetic, and autoimmune factors. Exposure to ionizing radiation or external beam radiation especially after the age of 20 increases the risk of nodules (47). Thyroid nodules are also more likely to occur in areas of low iodine intake (48). Twenty-five percent of patients with Graves' disease have nodules and as many as 15% of these may be malignant (49). Genetic mutations have also been linked to the formation of autonomously functioning nodules.

The most common type of nodule is a colloid nodule, which has no malignant potential. Cysts and thyroiditis are also common and, with colloid nodules, account for 80% of all nodules. Of the remainder, 10%–15% are benign follicular adenomas, and about 5% are cancerous (48). Papillary carcinoma is the most common malignancy (75% of cases). Other types of thyroid malignancy are follicular (10%), medullary (5%–10%), anaplastic (5%), and lymphoma (5%) (47).

Initial Evaluation

In a euthyroid patient, history and physical should be directed toward identifying risk factors for malignancy. Table 17.5 lists the clinical findings that may suggest thyroid carcinoma according to the degree of suspicion. Additionally, papillary carcinoma occurs in 4%–8% of patients with a family history of the same tumor. Patients with familial adenomatous polyposis and multiple hamartoma syndrome also have an increased risk of thyroid carcinoma (43).

The physical examination should include a thorough examination of the thyroid and surrounding lymph node beds, noting the size, tederness, and consistency of any nodule or lymph node.

LABORATORY TESTING

TSH and, if indicated, FT4 should be obtained in all patients; however, only 1% of solitary nodules cause hyper- or hypothyroidism (50). The presence of hyperthyroidism or hypothyroidism lowers the suspicion of cancer but does not exclude it. Serum calcitonin levels should be measured in patients with family history of medullary carcinoma or multiple endocrine neoplasia II, as described earlier under thyroid enlargement.

Imaging studies are not usually indicated with an easily palpable nodule in a euthyroid patient. Ultrasonography can be useful to identify additional nodules, to help distinguish solid from cystic nodules, and to guide fine needle biopsy (FNB) of small nodules. Some authors advocate ultrasonography in the diagnostic evaluation of all solitary nodules (51, 52)

TABLE 17.5 Red Flags Raising Concern for Thyroid Cancer in a Patient with a Thyroid Nodule

Data Source	Factors Raising Strong Concern	Factors Raising Moderate Concern
Clinical history	• Family history of medullary thyroid cancer or multiple endocrine neoplasia • Rapid growth of nodule	• Male sex • Patient age younger than 20 or older than 65 years • Previous radiation to the head or neck
Physical examination	• Firm or hard nodule • Nodule fixed to adjacent structures • Paralysis of vocal cords • Regional lymphadenopathy	• Nodule greater than 4 cm or partially cystic • Symptoms suggesting compression (dysphagia, hoarseness, dyspnea)

(Adapted from Hegedus L, Bonnema SJ, Bonneddback FN. Management of simple nodular goiter: current status and future perspectives. Endocr Rev. 2003;24:102–132.)

because up to 50% of nodules are not palpable (48). Ultrasound and color-flow Doppler criteria that may indicate an increased risk of malignancy include irregular margins, intranodular vascular spots, and microcalcifications (52). Computed tomography, magnetic resonance imaging, and positron emission tomography have no established role in the evaluation of thyroid nodules. Radionuclide scanning is indicated only if hyperthyroidism is diagnosed by laboratory testing. The toxic nodule is easily identified on the scan and the uptake in the rest of the gland will be reduced. The cancer risk in a toxic nodule is less than 1% (43).

FNB of a thyroid nodule is the most accurate and cost-effective way to differentiate benign from malignant nodules. The sensitivity is estimated at 93% and the specificity at 96%. The use of FNB has reduced the number of nodules for which surgery is recommended from nearly 50% to less than 20% (53). Ultrasound-guided FNB decreases the rate of unsatisfactory specimens from 15% to 3% and is especially helpful in nodules less than 1.5 cm and in all nonpalpable nodules (54).

Management

The algorithm in Figure 17.2 depicts the current recommendations for the evaluation and treatment of a clinically detected solitary thyroid nodule. Patients with no risk factors for malignancy and a nodule less than 1 cm have a very low risk of malignancy and need no further follow-up, according to American Association of Clinical Endocrinologists (AACE) guidelines (55). However, the American Thyroid Association (ATA) suggests that these patients may be followed by periodic ultrasonography (56). All nodules 1 cm or greater should be biopsied by an experienced clinician. If the specimen is found to be adequate and reveals benign follicular cells, no further treatment is needed. Because false negative results occur in 2%–3% of biopsies, the patient should be re-evaluated at 6 and 12 months and have a repeat biopsy if the nodule enlarges. The presence of malignant cells is always an indication for surgery; this is usually a near-total thyroidectomy, except in the case of medullary carcinoma, which requires total thyroidectomy and bilateral regional lymph node resection (43).

Approximately 10% of biopsy specimens will be read as "suspicious follicular lesions" or "indeterminate." Surgical ex-

cision is recommended for this diagnostic dilemma (54). The surgery performed is usually a lobectomy since this will include the margins of the nodule in 85% of cases. Frozen section at the time of surgery is not reliable (43).

The use of L-thyroxine in the suppression of benign solitary nodules is controversial. It is recommended by many clinicians as an alternative to surgery or to prevent recurrence postoperatively (58). However, the results of numerous studies on this issue have failed to provide conclusive evidence that the benefit of L-thyroxine for solitary nodules outweighs the risks of this therapy (54–56), and observation without L-thyroxine treatment is the current evidence-based choice (43, 48). Percutaneous ethanol injection and laser photocoagulation are new techniques being investigated in the treatment of solitary nodules. The safety and long-term efficacy of either technique has yet to be established through controlled clinical trials (48).

RAI treatment of thyroid nodules is restricted to hyperfunctioning nodules (17) and those with locally invasive or metastatic thyroid cancer (56).

Long-term Monitoring

The natural history of benign thyroid nodules is to grow slowly over time (59). The patient should be followed at least annually with palpation and interval history especially regarding the development of risk factors for cancer. Serum TSH should be monitored during these visits, because autonomous functioning may occur within the nodule. Although nodule size alone does not predict malignancy, all benign nodules that increase in size at annual follow-up should be rebiopsied. Many endocrinologists rebiopsy all benign nodules after 6–24 months (55), although this practice is not routinely recommended (56). The use of ultrasonography to follow nodules that are not easily palpable should be considered (52).

The primary care physician may encounter patients taking long-term L-thyroxine therapy for thyroid nodule suppression and should monitor them for thyrotoxic side effects as well as discuss the risks and benefits of continuing this therapy.

CASE DISCUSSION

The patient in the above case was appropriately referred for an ultrasound, because the nodule was irregular in size and

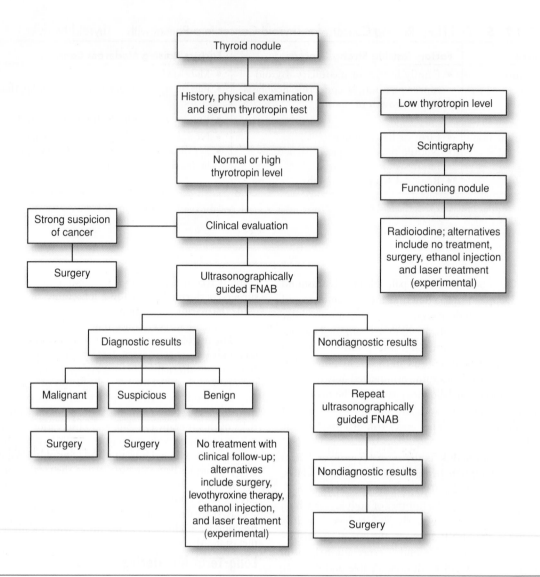

Figure 17.2 • Management algorithm for thyroid nodule. (From Hegedus L. The thyroid nodule. N Engl J Med. 2004; 351:1764–1771. Copyright 2007 Massachusetts Medical Society. All rights reserved. Used with permission.)

the presence of multiple nodules could not be ruled out. Considering that all of the nodules were less than 1 cm, this patient may not have needed to undergo FNB and could have been followed with serial physical exams and/or ultrasound. However, because his male sex is a known risk factor for malignancy, there are many who would argue that the biopsy was indicated. The results of the biopsy are reassuring but do not eliminate the need for follow-up and rebiopsy if the nodules enlarge.

SUBCLINICAL THYROID DISEASE

CASE

A 28-year-old woman is found to have an elevated TSH, at 7.9 mIU/L, during a routine exam. She is generally healthy and asymptomatic. She takes oral contraceptives

and has a positive family history of thyroid disease. On physical examination, she has no thyroid enlargement or nodules. No treatment is recommended and she is asked to return within 3 months for repeat testing. When she returns, she has another TSH level done, plus an FT4 and an antithyroid peroxidase antibody level. The TSH is again elevated at 6.8 mIU/L, but the FT4 and antibody testing are normal. She is informed about the risks and benefits of treatment for subclinical hypothyroidism and chooses to be followed without treatment.

CLINICAL QUESTIONS

1. What is the definition of subclinical thyroid disease?
2. Should you routinely screen for subclinical thyroid disease?
3. Should you treat patients with subclinical thyroid disease?

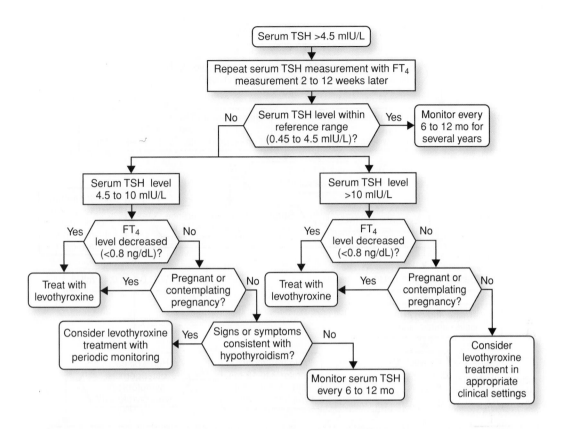

Figure 17.3 • Management algorithm for subclinical hypothyroidism. (From Col NF, Surks MI, Daniels GH. Subclinical thyroid disease: clinical applications. JAMA. 2004;291:239–243. Used with permission.)

Subclinical thyroid disease is a subject of considerable concern and debate among professional societies. Untreated subclinical thyroid disease may have significant clinical consequences. Subclinical thyroid disease is a laboratory diagnosis made when the TSH level is outside the reference range, and the freeT4 (and T3, if measured) are normal. There is some debate over the reference range used for TSH, but a recent consensus panel, with representatives from the ATA, the AACE, and the Endocrine Society concluded that the range of normal TSH is between 0.45 and 4.5 mIU/L (60).

Subclinical hypothyroidism is estimated to be present in 4%–8% of the general population and in as many as 20% of women age 60 or older (2, 3). It has been linked to adverse cardiac events, elevations in cholesterol and low-density lipoprotein (LDL) levels, and the development of systemic and neuropsychiatric symptoms. However, the consensus panel found no or insufficient evidence that it caused any of these effects, except for significantly elevated cholesterol and LDL levels in patients with TSH greater than 10 mIU/L.

Subclinical hyperthyroidism occurs in about 2% of the population. It has been associated with atrial fibrillation and other cardiac events, and with increased cardiac mortality in patients aged 60 and older. There is about a threefold increase in the incidence of atrial fibrillation, but only in patients with TSH levels below 0.1 mIU/L. Bone mineral density decreases in prolonged subclinical hyperthyroidism if TSH is below 0.1 mIU/L but there is insufficient evidence to link fractures to this condition.

Important subsets of patients to consider in subclinical thyroid disease are those who have known thyroid disease and are being treated with L-thyroxine medication. It is estimated that 20% of these patients have subclinical hypothyroidism due to inadequate thyroid replacement and 14%–20% have subclinical hyperthyroidism from overtreatment with L-thyroxine (60).

Initial Evaluation

There has been considerable debate and disagreement over who should be screened for thyroid disease. The consensus panel, based on United States Preventative Services Task Force (USPSTF) criteria, found insufficient evidence to recommend for or against routine screening for thyroid dysfunction in the general population. The panel recommended routine testing of women aged 60 and older, and all persons with previous thyroid radiation, surgery or dysfunction, type 1 diabetes or other autoimmune disease, atrial fibrillation, or a family history of thyroid disease. They also recommend screening of patients with any signs or symptoms of thyroid dysfunction including any thyroid enlargement or nodule (60).

Subclinical hypothyroidism is diagnosed when the TSH is above the normal range and the free T4 is normal. It is important to exclude other causes of elevated TSH, such as undertreated clinical hypothyroidism, early pituitary or hypothalamic disorders, and recovery from severe illness or thyroiditis. Before treatment decisions are made, the TSH should be repeated along with the free T4 measurement within 2 to

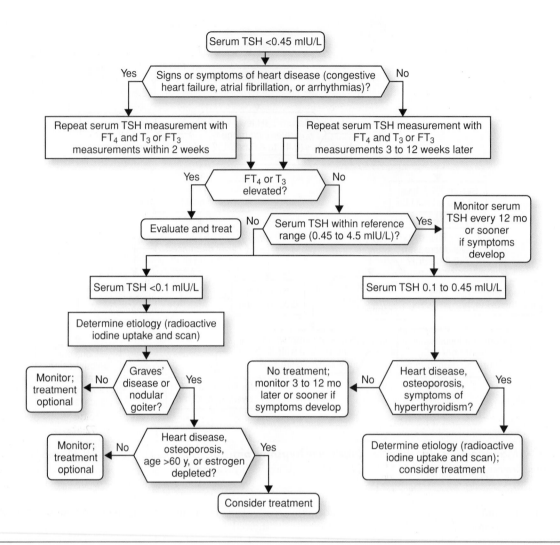

Figure 17.4 • Management algorithm for subclinical hyperthyroidism. (From Col NF, Surks MI, Daniels GH. Subclinical thyroid disease: clinical applications. JAMA. 2004;291:239–243. Used with permission.)

12 weeks, and the patient should be evaluated for signs and symptoms of hypothyroidism. Lipid profiles should be considered. Measurement of anti-thyroid antibodies are not needed to diagnose subclinical hypothyroidism, but their presence predicts about twice the likelihood of developing clinical hypothyroidism (60).

Subclinical hyperthyroidism is diagnosed when the TSH is below the normal range and the free T4 and free T3 are normal. Other causes that need to be excluded include overtreatment or inappropriate treatment with L-thyroxine, delayed recovery from treatment for hyperthyroidism, pregnancy, euthyroid sick syndrome, or treatment with certain medications (e.g., dopamine and glucocorticoids). An asymptomatic patient with a low TSH should have repeat testing with free T4 and T3 in 3 to 12 weeks. Patients with atrial fibrillation or any cardiac signs or symptoms need follow-up within 2 weeks. A radioiodine scan is useful to determine the etiology of the subclinical hyperthyroidism, as described in the hyperthyroidism section. This test is recommended in the workup of a patient with subclinical hyperthyroidism whose TSH is <0.1 mIU/L, or in patients with heart disease, osteo-

porosis, or hyperthyroid symptoms. Bone mineral density testing may also be considered (61).

Management

The decision to treat subclinical hypothyroidism with L-thyroxine must be an individual one, since the benefits of treatment based on the current literature are limited to a possible improvement in symptoms and a lowering of LDL cholesterol. The recent consensus panel did not recommend treatment of TSH levels less than 10 mIU/L. However, if there are significant hypothyroid symptoms present, a trial of L-thyroxine therapy could be considered. In patients with TSH above 10 mIU/L, L-thyroxine therapy is considered reasonable (60). These recommendations are depicted in Figure 17.3.

Figure 17.4 outlines a detailed approach to the evaluation and management of patients with subclinical hyperthyroidism. If the cause is subacute thyroiditis, symptomatic treatment may be all that is needed, because this condition resolves spontaneously. Treatments for subclinical hyperthyroidism due to Graves' disease or nodular thyroid disease are described in detail in the hyperthyroid section.

Long-term Monitoring

Close clinical follow-up is recommended for all patients with subclinical thyroid disease.

Subclinical hypothyroidism progresses to clinical disease at a rate of about 2%–5% per year (60). For subclinical hyperthyroidism the progression rate is not as well established, but in one study of 90 patients with multinodular goiter and subclinical hyperthyroidism, 8% developed overt hyperthyroidism over a period of 7 years (62).

Patients who are treated for their subclinical disease have the same long-term risks as patients with overt disease. They should be routinely monitored for therapeutic response and for adverse effects of treatment, and their medication should be adjusted as needed.

CASE DISCUSSION

This case was published by the consensus panel to illustrate one of the commonly encountered scenarios related to the screening and treatment of subclinical thyroid disease. This patient was appropriately screened for thyroid dysfunction considering her positive family history of thyroid disease. Because she was asymptomatic, there was no urgency for her to return for repeat testing any sooner than 12 weeks, and the FT4 did not need to be included until the repeated test. The inclusion of the antibody testing is controversial, but a negative test does predict a lower risk of becoming hypothyroid in the future. The only reason to recommend treatment in this asymptomatic patient would be if she were contemplating pregnancy, because there is limited evidence that untreated subclinical hypothyroidism increases the risk of fetal loss or neurologic complications in the newborn. She should be instructed to report symptoms of hypothyroidism and have repeated TSH testing annually (61).

REFERENCES

1. Roberts CR, Ladeson PW. Hypothyroidism. Lancet. 2004; 363:793–803.
2. Hollowell JG, Staehling NW, Flanders WD, et al. J Clin Endocrinol Metab. 2002;87:489–499.
3. Vanderpump MP, Tunbridge WM. Epidemiology and prevention of clinical and subclinical hypothyroidism. Thyroid. 2002;12(10):839–847.
4. Canaris GJ, Steiner JF, Ridgeway EC. Do traditional symptoms of hypothyroidism correlate with biochemical disease? J Gen Intern Med. 1997;12(9):544–550.
5. Indra R, Patil SS, Joshi R, et al. Accuracy of physical examination in the diagnosis of hypothyroidism: a cross-sectional, double-blind study. J Postgrad Med. 2004;50(1):7–11.
6. American Association of Clinical Endocrinologists. Medical guidelines for clinical practice for the evaluation and treatment of hyperthyroidism and hypothyroidism. Endocr Pract. 2002;8(6):457–466.
7. McDermott MT, Haugen BR, Lezotte DC, et al. Management practices among primary care physicians and thyroid specialists in the care of hypothyroid patients. Thyroid. 2001; 11(8):757–764.
8. Roos A, Linn-Rasker SP, van Domberg RT. The starting dose of levothyroxine in primary hypothyroidism treatment. Arch Int Med. 2005;165:1714–1720.
9. Klein I, Ojamaa K. Mechanisms of disease: thyroid hormone and the cardiovascular system. N Engl J Med. 2001;344(7): 501–509.
10. Wartofsky L. Levothyroxine therapy for hypothyroidism. Arch Int Med. 2005;165:1683–1684.
11. Danese MD, Ladeson PW, Meinert CL, et al. Effects of thyroxine therapy on serum lipoproteins in patients with mild thyroid failure: a quantitative review of the literature. J Clin Endocrinol Metab. 2000;85(9):2993–3001.
12. Dong BJ, Hauck WW, Gambertoglio JG, et al. Bioequivalence of generic and brand-name levothyroxine products in the treatment of hypothyroidism. JAMA. 1997;277(15): 1205–1213.
13. Bunevicius R, Kasanavicius G, Zalinvicius R, et al. Effects of thyroxine as compared with thyroxine plus triiodothyronine in patients with hypothyroidism. N Engl J Med. 1999; 340(6):424–429.
14. Sawka AM, Gerstein MJ, Marriott GM, et al. Does a combination of thyroxine and 3,5,3- triiodothyonine improve depressive symptoms better than T4 alone in patients with hypothyroidism? Results of a double-blind, randomized, controlled trial. J Clin Endocrinol Metab. 2003;88:4551–4555.
15. Walsh JP, Shiels L, Kim EM, et al. Combined thyroxine/liothyronine treatment does not improve well-being, quality of life, or cognitive function compared with thyroxine alone: a randomized controlled trial in patients with primary hypothyroidism. J Clin Endocrinol Metab. 2003;66:4543–4550.
16. Canaris GJ, Manowitz NR, Mayor G, Ridgeway EC. The Colorado thyroid disease prevalence study. Arch Int Med. 2000;160(4):526–534.
17. Reid JR, Wheeler SF. Hyperthyroidism: diagnosis and treatment. Am Fam Physician. 2005;72:623–630.
18. Cooper DS. Hyperthyroidism. Lancet. 2003;362:459–468.
19. Torring O, Tallstedt L, Wallin G, et al. Graves' hyperthyroidism: treatment with antithyroid drugs, surgery, or radioiodine—a prospective, randomized study. J Clin Endocrinol Metab. 1996;81:2986–2993.
20. Cooper DS. Drug therapy: antithyroid drugs. N Engl J Med. 2005;352(9):905–917.
21. Cooper DS. Antithyroid drugs in the management of patients with Graves' disease: an evidence-based approach to therapeutic controversies. J Clin Endocrinol Metab. 2003;88(8): 3474–3481.
22. Nedebro BG, Holm PI, Uhlving S, et al. Predictors of outcome and comparison of different drug regimens for the prevention of relapse in patients with Graves' disease. Eur J Endocrinol. 2002;147:583–589.
23. Tajiri J, Naguchi S, Marakami T, Marakami N. Anti-thyroid drug-induced agranulocytosis. Arch Intern Med. 1990;15: 621–624.
24. Woeber KA. Update on the management of hyperthyroidism and hypothyroidism. Arch Intern Med. 2000;160:1067–1071.
25. Fontanilla JC, Schneider AB, Sarne DH. The use of oral radiographic contrast agents in the management of hyperthyroidism. Thyroid. 2001;11(6):561–567.
26. Metso S, Jaatinen P, Huhtala H. Long-term follow-up study of radioiodine treatment of hyperthyroidism. Clin Endocrinol. 2004;51:641–648.
27. Rivkees SA. The use of radioactive iodine in the management of hyperthyroidism in children. Curr Drug Targets Immune Endocr Metabol Disord. 2001;1:255–264.
28. Gayed I, Wendt J, Haynie T, et al. Timing for repeated treatment of hyperthyroid disease with radioactive iodine after initial treatment failure. Clin Nucl Med. 2001;26(1):1–5.
29. Weetman AP. Controversy in thyroid disease. J R Coll Physicians Lond. 2000;34(4):374–380.
30. Palit TK, Miller CC, Miltenburg DM. The efficacy of thy-

roidectomy for Graves' disease: a metanalysis. J Surg Res. 2000;90:161–165.

31. Ron E, Doody MM, Becker DV, et al. Cancer mortality following treatment for adult hyperthyroidism. JAMA. 1998; 280(4):347–355.

32. Franklyn JA, Maisonneuve P, Sheppard MC, et al. Mortality after the treatment of hyperthyroidism with radioactive iodine. N Engl J Med. 1998;338:712–718.

33. Karga H, Papapetrou PD, Korakovouni A, et al. Bone density in hyperthyroidism. Clin Endocrinol. 2004;61:466–472.

34. Day TA, Chu A, Hoang KG. Multinodular goiter. Otolaryngol Clin North Am. 2003;36:35–54.

35. Hermus AD, Huysmans DA. Pathogenesis of nontoxic diffuse and nodular goiter. In: Braverman LE, Utiger RD, eds. Werner & Ingbar's The Thyroid: A Fundamental Clinical Text, 9th ed. Philadelphia, PA: Lippincott Williams & Wilkins, 2005.

36. Samuels MH. Evaluation and treatment of sporadic nontoxic goiter: some answers and more questions (editorial). J Clin Endocrinol Metab. 2001;86(3):994–997.

37. Knudsen N, Laurberg P, Perrild H, et al. Risk factors for goiter and thyroid nodules. Thyroid. 2002;12(10):879–888.

38. Slotosky J, Shipton B, Wahba H. Thyroiditis: differential diagnosis and management. Am Fam Physician. 2000;61: 1047–1052.

39. Jameson JL, Weetman AP. Disorders of the thyroid gland: Goiter and nodular thyroid disease. In Kasper DL, Braunwald E, Fauci AS, et al., eds. Harrison's Principles of Internal Medicine, 16th ed. New York: McGraw-Hill, 2005.

40. Rios A, Rodriguez JM, Canteras M, et al. Risk factors for malignancy in multinodular goiters. Eur J Surg Oncol. 2004; 30:58–62.

41. Hermus AD, Huysmans DA. Clinical manifestations and treatment of nontoxic diffuse and nodular goiter. In Braverman LE, Utiger RD, eds. Werner & Ingbar's The Thyroid: A Fundamental Clinical Text, 9th ed. Philadelphia, PA: Lippincott Williams & Wilkins, 2005.

42. O'Brien KE, Gopal V, Mazzaferri. Pemberton's sign associated with a large multinodular goiter. Thyroid. 2003;13(4): 407–408.

43. Kaplan MM. Clinical evaluation and management of solitary throid nodules. In Braverman LE, Utiger RD, eds. Werner & Ingbar's The Thyroid: A Fundamental Clinical Text, 9th ed. Philadelphia, PA: Lippincott Williams & Wilkins, 2005.

44. Hegedus L, Bonnema SJ, Benneddbaek FN. Management of simple nodular goiter: current status and future perspectives. Endocr Rev. 2003;24:102–132.

45. Bonnema SJ, Bennedbaek FN, Landenson PW, Hegedus L.

46. Albino CC, Mesa Junior CO, Olandoski M, et al. Recombinant human thyrotropin as adjuvant in the treatment of multinodular goiters with radioiodine. J Clin Endocrinol Metab. 2005;90:2775–2780.

47. Mazzaferri EL. Current concepts: Management of a solitary nodule. N Engl J Med. 1993;328(8):553–559.

48. Hegedus L. The thyroid nodule. N Engl J Med. 2004;351(17): 1764–1771.

49. Weiss RE, Lado-Abeal J. Thyroid nodules: diagnosis and therapy. Curr Opin Oncol. 2002;14:46–52.

50. Welker MJ, Orlov D. Thyroid nodules. Am Fam Physician. 2003;67:559–566.

51. Marqusee E, Benson CB, Frates MC, et al. Usefulness of ultrasonography in the management of nodular thyrid disease. Ann Intern Med. 2000;133(9):696–700.

52. Papini E, Guglielmi R, Biachini A, et al. Risk of malignancy in nonpalpable thyroid nodules: predictive value of ultrasound and color-doppler features. J Clin Endocrinol Metab. 2002;87(5):1941–1946.

53. Sriram U, Patacsil LM. Thyroid nodule. Dis Mon. 2004;50: 486–526.

54. Castro MR, Gharib H. Continuing controversies in the management of thyroid nodules. Ann Inter Med. 2005;142: 926–931.

55. American Association of Clinical Endocrinologists and the American College of Endocrinology. AACE clinical practice guidelines for the diagnosis and management of thyroid nodules. Endocr Pract. 1996;2(1):80–84.

56. Singer PA, Cooper DS, Daniels GH, et al. Treatment guidelines for patients with thyroid nodules and well-differentiated thyroid cancer. Arch Intern Med. 1996;156(19):2165–2172.

57. Pacini F, Burroni L, Ciuoli C, et al. Management of thyroid nodules: a clinicopathological, evidence-based approach. Eur J Nucl Med Mol Imaging. 2004;31:1443–1449.

58. Bennedbaek FN, Hegedus L. Management of the solitary thyroid nodule. J Clin Endocrinol Metab. 2000;85(7): 2493–2498.

59. Alexander EK, Hurwitz S, Heering JP, et al. Natural history of benign solid and cystic thyroid nodules. Ann Intern Med. 2003;138:315–318.

60. Surks ML, Ortiz E, Daniels GH. Subclinical thyroid disease: scientific reiview and guidelines for diagnosis and management. JAMA. 2004;291:228–238.

61. Col NF, Surks MI, Daniels GH. Subclinical thyroid disease: clinical applications. JAMA. 2004;291:239–243.

62. Hoogendoorn EH, den Heijer M, van Dijk APJ, Hermus AR. Subclinical hyperthyroidism: to treat or not to treat? Postgrad Med J. 2004;80:394–398.

CHAPTER 18

Nutrition and Weight Management

Margaret E. Thompson and Mary Barth Noel

CASE

J. is a 74-year-old man who has always enjoyed good health, swimming 3 miles per week and taking frequent walks with his wife. His height is 70 inches and 6 months ago he weighed 170 pounds (body mass index [BMI] 24.4). Since then, he has noted increasing right hip pain, which limits his ability to walk and to swim. His family physician evaluated his hip pain, diagnosed severe osteoarthritis of the right hip, and referred him to an orthopedic surgeon for joint replacement, which was scheduled for a month later.

By the time the date of his surgery approaches, J. is only able to ambulate using crutches. When he presents to the hospital on the day of his surgery, his weight is 155 pounds (BMI 22.2). He cannot recall any changes in his diet or food consumption over the past 6 months, and notes that his activity level has decreased.

Meanwhile, J.'s 40-year-old daughter A. presents to the same family physician complaining of increasing knee pain, especially while climbing stairs. She notes that she must have arthritis, since that is what her father has. She complains that despite the fact that she has been doing errands for her father and helping out around the house, she continues to be overweight. She is 67 inches tall and weighs 192 pounds (BMI 30.1).

CLINICAL QUESTIONS

1. How is obesity defined and measured?
2. What factors influence the nutritional status of people throughout the life cycle?
3. How does one assess the nutritional status of patients such as J. and A.?
4. What are the best treatments for undernutrition and obesity?

With the increasing interest in nutrition and obesity in the medical and lay communities, helping portray diet as neither villain nor saint is important. Diet is fundamental to health, since life must be supported by food and water. However, diet needs to be considered according to a person's genetic makeup, family, culture, and environment. There is wide variation in what, how, when, and where nutritional components are consumed. Frequently, however, the nutrition community lacks understanding of how and why these differences exist.

In trying to educate patients about nutrition, it is useful to think of diet, genetics, and environment (see Figure 18.1). It is important to consider the role of each component in relation to the other elements. It is also important to consider potential disease states and their influence on nutritional needs.

The interplay of diet, genetics, and environment in hypertension is an excellent example of this conceptual framework. Many individuals develop hypertension, but the different components play different roles in each patient. For example:

- About a third of the US population appears to have a genetic predisposition to elevated blood pressure related to sodium consumption (1).
- Many individuals may improve blood pressures from mildly abnormal to within normal by changing their diet to include more fruits, vegetables, and sources of calcium. Either genetics or diet could contribute to this result.
- Exercise is an environmental change that has a positive effect on the physiology of the arteries and blood pressure.

The Recommended Dietary Allowances and the newer Adequate Intakes acknowledge the human variation in dietary requirements. These guidelines set ranges of 2 standard deviations around the mean requirement, thus taking into account genetic, age, and health status differences. Models such as the US Department of Agriculture (USDA) food pyramid are practical illustrations of the nutrient needs for the US population based on the current medical evidence and cultural trends regarding issues such as obesity, diabetes, cancer, and heart disease. Models such as the food pyramid may be helpful for some, but the recommendations need to vary with age, health status, and genetic makeup. The 2005 iteration of the food pyramid allows customization depending on these factors (see *www.mypyramid.gov*).

A good source of evidence-based advice is the *2005 USA Nutrition and Your Health: Dietary Guidelines for Americans (2)*. Its key recommendations for healthy people over age 2 include:

- Consume a variety of nutrient-rich foods and beverages from among the various food groups.
- Limit the intake of saturated and trans fats, cholesterol, added sugars, salt, and alcohol.
- Obtain recommended intakes within caloric needs by adopting a balanced eating pattern, such as the USDA Food Guide or the Dietary Approaches to Stop Hypertension (DASH) eating plan.

The Web site incorporating these guidelines, *www.healthierus.gov/dietaryguidelines*, also makes recommen-

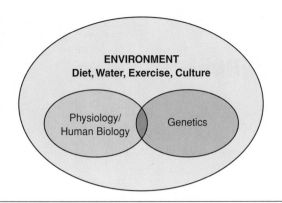

ENVIRONMENT
Diet, Water, Exercise, Culture

Physiology/
Human Biology

Genetics

Figure 18.1 • Interplay of diet, genetics, and environment.

dations for specific population groups, such as women of childbearing age and the elderly.

INITIAL EVALUATION

A nutritional assessment is the process of determining whether an individual is consuming and using appropriate amounts of the nutrients that are required for vital life processes. Almost all patients, and certainly the two in the cases presented here, deserve some level of nutritional assessment. In a relatively healthy person, the assessment may take the form of a simple screen, while a patient with risk factors for malnutrition requires a more thorough evaluation. The latter category includes patients who are over or underweight, have chronic or severe acute illness, are children, live in poverty, or have other factors that may make access to nutrients difficult.

History

All patients should receive a brief screening history that inquires about changes in weight and appetite, eating habits (e.g., the number of meals per day and the variety of foods consumed), and symptoms of chronic disease (e.g., fever, chronic pain, or fatigue). Information about the ability to perform normal activities is helpful in uncovering underlying illness.

In patients with known or newly identified chronic illness, a more thorough history is appropriate. In addition to a complete review of gastrointestinal symptoms, the physician should ask about supplemental vitamins and other products, alcohol and illicit drug use, appetite suppressants or stimulants, glucocorticoids, and laxatives. Chronic disease frequently increases nutritional requirements. For example, inflammation causes an increase in basal metabolic rate, which raises the daily caloric requirement.

In considering which patients might be at risk for poor nutrition, physicians should consider the various steps involved in nutritional intake, from acquiring food to absorbing nutrients (see Table 18.1). Poverty and other access issues impair the ability to acquire food. Age or disability may preclude preparation of proper foods. Problems with dentition or coordination may impair ingestion of nutrients. Various gastrointestinal diseases, enzyme deficiencies, and/or medications may interfere with the digestion, absorption, or metabolism of nutrients. Table 18.2 lists "red flags" that suggest the need to look especially hard for nutritional disease.

Dietary History

The dietary history should relate to both usual and recent food intake patterns. Reasonable questions include number of

TABLE 18.1	Areas to Consider in Identifying Patients at Risk for Poor Nutrition
Aspect of Nutrition	**Examples**
Acquiring food	• Poverty • Transportation needs • Infirmity • Language barriers • Inability to prepare food • Substance abuse • Depression
Ingestion of nutrients	• Poor dentition • Pain with chewing or swallowing • Lack of taste • Depression • Anxiety • Dementia • Medications • Substance abuse
Digestion	• Complete or partial gastrectomy • Pancreatic disease
Absorption	• Lack of absorptive surface due to surgery, Crohn's disease
Metabolism and excretion	• Inborn errors of metabolism • Nonabsorbable fat substitutes, leading to steatorrhea

TABLE 18.2 Red Flags Suggesting High Risk of Serious Nutritional Problems

- Weight loss of >5% in 1 month, 7.5% in 3 months, or 10% in 6 months
- Weight loss or gain associated with other systemic symptoms
- History of upper gastrointestinal surgery or disease

meals per day and examples of what is consumed at each meal. A more thorough investigation includes cultural practices, personal preferences, and the use of a food pyramid to help patients identify the numbers of servings in each food group that they consume. Clinicians may use either retrospective methods (i.e., recall) or prospective food diaries to evaluate nutrient intake. The retrospective analysis has less validity than a prospective food diary, in which the patient is assigned the task of tracking all intake over the course of 1–2 days (3).

Physical Examination

A systematic physical examination is important in evaluating nutritional status. General inspection may readily reveal overweight or underweight status. Temporal wasting, decreased muscle mass, proximal muscle weakness, scaling skin, poor wound healing, and excessive bruising are signs suggesting malnutrition. Dietitians often use anthropometric measurements, including height, weight, skin fold thickness, head circumference (especially in infants and children), and waist and hip circumferences. Clinicians tend to use the body mass index (BMI), a standardized and reliable measurement of body fat in adults (4, 5), that is calculated as follows:

$$BMI = (weight\ in\ kg)/(height\ in\ meters)^2$$

BMI tables and a downloadable tool for calculating BMI with personal digital assistants are readily available at *http:// www.nhlbi.nih.gov*. When using BMI, be aware that it may overestimate body fat in trained athletes and underestimate body fat in older patients and others who have low lean body mass, including some obese individuals.

Circumference measurements are also useful in determining nutritional status. The waist circumference assesses abdominal fat content. Increased waist circumference has been associated with cardiovascular disease (CVD) risk (6). Waist measurements of greater than 40 inches in men and 35 inches in women are independent risk factors for disease (7).

A significant weight loss is defined as a 5% weight loss in 1 month, 7.5% in 3 months, or a 10% loss in 6 months. A severe weight loss is defined as anything greater than those parameters. It is important to note, however, that acute weight loss or weight gain (over a day or two) is usually because of a change in fluid status rather than an indication of nutritional change.

Laboratory Evaluation

No single laboratory test can diagnose malnutrition. Protein status is one of the oldest and most important measures of nutritional health. Commonly used measures include serum albumin, serum transferrin, and other serum proteins, such as transthyretin (also known as prealbumin). It is important

to remember that the serum albumin level lags behind actual protein nutrition, because serum albumin has a half-life of 2 to 3 weeks. Serum proteins such as albumin and transferrin also are acute phase reactants and may actually increase under conditions of inflammation. Transferrin has a serum half-life of 8 days, and thus may be a more accurate parameter than albumin for measuring recent nutritional changes. However, the transferrin concentration is related to the overall iron status of the patient.

Assessment of micronutrients may be done directly via vitamin and mineral assays, or indirectly using tests such as the complete blood count and peripheral blood smear. Common patterns of vitamin and mineral deficiency include:

- Low levels of vitamin A, zinc, and magnesium in protein-calorie malnutrition;
- Deficiencies of fat-soluble vitamins (A, D, K, and E) in syndromes involving fat malabsorption; and
- Folic acid and iron deficiency in celiac disease

Changes in red blood cell production may result from insufficient levels of iron, vitamin B_{12}, folic acid, and other vitamins.

Patients with poor nutritional status may also demonstrate weak immune status in the form of poor T-lymphocyte responses. Evaluating the total lymphocyte count can be helpful in assessing T-cells. Using a skin test for anergy is another way of assessing T-cell function.

OBESITY

Definitions

In 1999, a National Institutes of Health consensus panel lowered the threshold for overweight from a BMI of 27 to a BMI of 25. Likewise, the cut-off for obesity has been lowered from a BMI of 32 to a BMI of 30 (8); these are presented in Table 18.3. This new classification has nearly doubled the number of people who qualify as overweight. These definitions are not without controversy, primarily because we do not know whether the risk comes from the excess weight, the genetic makeup, or the lifestyle and behaviors of the overweight population (9, 10). The weight guidelines also do not take into consideration the location of the fat and health risk. Weight carried in the abdominal region of the body, for example, seems to confer greater risk for heart disease and diabetes. Additionally, there may be differences between racial groups; for example, the increased risk associated with obesity may occur at higher BMIs for populations of African-American descent than for Asian populations.

Epidemiology

Age-adjusted figures for obesity show that in the United States, the prevalence of obesity has increased from 12.8% (including male and female subjects) in 1960–1962 to 22.6% in 1988–1994. Furthermore, Americans are not the only ones getting heavier; so is the rest of the world. The obesity epidemic also is spreading from the industrialized nations into developing countries; there are currently more than 1 billion overweight adults in the world (11).

Although obesity is common in all races, ages, and both

TABLE 18.3 Classification of Overweight and Obesity by Body Mass Index (BMI), Waist Circumference, and Associated Disease Risks

Category	Definition Based on BMI	Obesity Class	Disease Risk* Relative to Normal Weight and Waist Circumference	
			Normal	Increased Men >102 cm, Women >88 cm
Waist circumference				
Underweight	<18.5		—	—
Normal	18.5–24.9		—	—
Overweight	25.0–29.9		Increased	High
Obesity	30.0–34.9	I	High	Very high
Obesity	35.0–39.9	II	Very high	Very high
Extreme obesity	≥40	III	Extremely high	Extremely high

*Risk of developing type 2 diabetes, hypertension, and/or cardiovascular disease.
(From National Heart, Lung, and Blood Institute. Clinical guidelines on the identification, evaluation, and treatment of overweight and obesity in adults. Executive summary. Bethesda, MD: National Institutes of Health; 1998.)

genders, African-American women tend to be heavier than white and Mexican-American women (12); Mexican-American men are heavier than white men; and white men are heavier than African-American men. Men, as a group, are more overweight than women in every age group but two; the 55- to 64-year-old and the 65- to 70-year-old groups. More women, however, meet the definition of obesity than men (13). The question of whether these weight differences are attributable to gender, cultural, genetic, or racial differences is still under consideration, as is the health risk associated with these differences.

The average weight gain for most Americans during youth and middle age is about 5 pounds per year, which amounts to an excess of about 50 kilocalories (kcal) per day (/d) over the energy requirement. This weight gain usually occurs during the winter and especially the winter holidays. In effect, this means that increasing energy expenditure by an average of 50 kcal/d (the amount expended walking 2 mph for 15 minutes!) may offset this gradual weight gain.

Prejudices against overweight individuals in employment, schools, the media, and daily living have a greater effect than the health risks of obesity in creating a desire for thinness among many individuals. The prevalence of dieting is increasing, and the age at which people start dieting seems to be getting younger. Weight management programs abound, with new ones entering the market every day; sadly, nearly all of these programs have failures and disheartened participants. As a country we are spending more than $33 billion on dieting and related products (14).

Obesity as a Health Risk

Scientific knowledge and advice vary about the health implications of increased weight. Some studies indicate that a 10-lb weight gain for a woman over her lifetime significantly increases her risk of cancer (15). One study found that for people whose BMI was greater than 40, the death rate for cancer was 52% higher for men and 62% higher for women than in people of normal weight (16). Some advocate treatment of overweight individuals only if they have risk factors

for weight-related chronic diseases such as diabetes, hypertension, hyperlipidemia, atherosclerotic CVD, and sleep apnea. Others advise treatment for an increased abdominal circumference in the absence of other disease risk factors. Table 18.4 summarizes the current consensus on the health implications of overweight and obesity (13).

Diagnostic Evaluation

Overweight patients generally present to the family physician's office with a concern other than that of losing weight. Common presenting problems include type 2 diabetes mellitus, hypertension, musculoskeletal complaints (particularly knee, hip, or foot pain), and breathing difficulties. It is important to identify the excess weight or obesity as a problem, even if that is not the presenting complaint.

At some point, you will need to take a complete history of the weight problem. You should also determine the patient's risk status. Patients with established coronary heart disease, other atherosclerotic diseases, type 2 diabetes, and sleep apnea are classified as being at very high risk for disease complications and mortality (17). Also assess for the presence of other obesity-associated conditions, including polycystic ovarian disease, osteoarthritis, gallstones, and stress urinary incontinence. Table 18.5 outlines the assessment of the overweight or obese patient.

It is important to determine the patient's readiness to lose weight. Gather information on previous attempts at losing weight, and whether those were successful. Ascertain the number of meals consumed each day, and how the patient's family life may affect the eating pattern. Many overweight patients admit to skipping meals in an attempt to lose weight. This practice should be discouraged because it may actually result in lowered basal metabolic rate (BMR) as well as an increase in caloric intake during the less frequent meals, both of which retard weight loss. Some overweight patients may give a history of using medications such as laxatives and diuretics in an attempt to lose weight.

It is also important to determine a patient's activity during the day; many patients think that they are very active during

TABLE 18.4 Risks of Overweight and Obesity

Overweight and obesity are known risk factors for:	Obesity is associated with:
• Diabetes	• High blood cholesterol
• Heart disease	• Complications of pregnancy
• Stroke	• Menstrual irregularities
• Hypertension	• Hirsutism
• Gallbladder disease	• Stress incontinence
• Osteoarthritis	• Depression
• Sleep apnea	• Increased surgical risk
• Uterine, breast, colorectal, kidney, and gallbladder cancer	

Source: National Institute on Diabetes and Digestive and Kidney Disease. Statistics related to overweight and obesity. Bethesda, MD: National Institutes of Health; 2000.

TABLE 18.5 Evaluation of the Overweight or Obese Patient

History	Duration
	Dietary history
	Activity history
	Presence of heart disease; hypertension; diabetes; sleep apnea; polycystic ovaries; hypothyroidism; osteoarthritis; gallbladder disease; gout
	Medications or nutritional supplements
	Number of previous pregnancies
	Family history of overweight
	Social and emotional histories
	Employment history
Physical examination	Blood pressure
	Calculated body mass index
	Waist circumference
	Thyroid examination
	Striae, centripetal fat distribution (Cushing's syndrome)
	Leg edema
	Cellulitis
	Acanthosis nigricans (coarse hyperpigmentation seen with hyperinsulinemia)
	Intertriginous rashes
Laboratory evaluation	Electrolytes
	Liver function tests
	Complete blood counts
	Lipid profile
	Thyroid-stimulating hormone
	Fasting or random serum glucose

their jobs, and that exercise is therefore unnecessary for them. Social and emotional histories may reveal obstacles to losing weight, or even a history of emotional or physical abuse.

PHYSICAL EXAMINATION

Obese patients deserve a complete physical examination to rule out signs of secondary causes of obesity, such as Cushing's syndrome, hypothyroidism, or other pituitary abnormalities. Measurement of the waist circumference is also important.

LABORATORY EVALUATION

Obesity is a known risk factor for CVD and diabetes mellitus; therefore, other risk factors should be evaluated. Patients should undergo serum testing for hyperlipidemia and hyperglycemia.

THE UNDERWEIGHT PATIENT

The underweight patient presents unique considerations in a culture that is not sympathetic to this problem. As with the overweight person, careful assessment is needed because there are multiple causes of being underweight. A person is defined as underweight if the BMI is below 18.5. One problem of being underweight is that there is little caloric reserve as a margin of safety if there are major health problems. Another concern is that people with restricted diets frequently have inadequate intake of vitamins and trace minerals. Additionally, the insulating function of body fat is not present, and the person may feel cold and is, therefore, at risk for hypothermia.

Causes of underweight status include dieting and eating disorders, genetically low normal body weight, wasting diseases, and high activity levels. Also, movement disorders (e.g., Parkinson disease) can cause extra energy expenditure, leading to decreased weight.

Assessment of the underweight individual should consist of a good nutritional assessment, as outlined earlier in the chapter.

MANAGEMENT OF WEIGHT PROBLEMS

Many treatment modalities are available to foster weight loss. In prescribing a weight loss regimen, it is crucial to remember to set goals with the patient, to negotiate a customized plan for weight loss, and to let the patient know that you will be there with him or her over the long haul, regardless of weight loss success. Assistance from experts such as nutritionists is often helpful. The best practice is to prevent overweight and obesity from occurring by instilling in patients the healthy habits of good nutrition and avoiding a sedentary lifestyle.

As discussed above, physicians most commonly interface with overweight patients because of a visit for another complaint, such as joint pain. Although often the patient's anatomic excess may be the obvious culprit, the physician must remain sensitive to addressing the patient's primary complaint.

Once the problem is identified as weight, it is important to set appropriate goals with the patient. The National Heart, Lung, and Blood Institute (NHLBI) practice guideline suggests an initial weight loss of 10% of body weight; however,

this may not always be practical or achievable (17). In fact, even a 10-lb weight loss may ameliorate related conditions, such as hypertension and elevated blood glucose. A general time line for a 10-lb weight loss is 6 months. Additional goals should include the maintenance of weight loss over time, and prevention of further weight gain. Modification of other cardiovascular risk factors, such as smoking, hypertension, elevated cholesterol, and physical inactivity, and recognition and treatment of diabetes deserve equal emphasis in the management of overweight or obese patients.

Table 18.6 outlines the evidence regarding recognition and management of obesity. It is important to ascertain the patient's understanding of the risks of obesity. The physician should also establish the patient's willingness and ability to participate in physical activity. Table 18.7 shows expected outcomes for the various treatments of obesity (18).

Diet — The "Input" Side of the Equation

Modification of the diet affects the "energy input" side of the weight loss equation. Research continues in determining appropriate diets for weight loss. Any macronutrient—carbohydrate, protein, or fat—causes weight gain when over consumed. Conversely, diets that decrease calories, whether as carbohydrate, protein, or fat, will be effective in helping adults lose weight, and reduce cardiovascular risk (19).

Current evidence supports the use of calorie restriction for weight loss. Table 18.8 outlines a reasonable, first-step low-calorie diet. In an individual with a BMI ≥35, reducing the kcal consumed by 500 to 1,000 kcal/d would result in weight loss of 1 to 2 lb per week, and thus a 10% weight loss in 6 months. A combination of reducing calories and increasing physical activity could be used to get the 500-kcal deficit. For individuals with a BMI of 27 to 35, reducing caloric intake by 300 to 500 kcal/d will result in a weight loss of 0.5 to 1 lb/wk, and again, 10% over 6 months. Reducing the amount of fat in the diet is helpful as long as the excess calories are not added back through increased consumption of carbohydrates.

Individual goals need to be just that—individual. The balance between increased activity and decreased caloric consumption should be determined jointly by the patient and the physician. For example, the overall goal of 1 or 2 pounds per week (with a 500 to 1,000 kcal/d difference between intake and output) may be more of a change than many individuals can manage. More moderate goals (such as 1 lb/mo or developing/improving health habits), with moderate changes (the difference of about 100 kcal/d), might be more realistic.

In developing the plan for weight loss, the physician needs to investigate what the individual has done in the past that has been successful or unsuccessful. This can provide strategies to help the person now. The individual who determines how she or he will change is far more likely to implement that change. For example, a patient who is reluctant to change his or her diet may be counseled to increase activity by an amount equivalent to the required caloric deficit. A weight loss prescription should be written with specific numbers, such as number of calories and number of minutes of specific exercises. Figure 18.2 contains helpful tips to discuss with your patients.

The public needs to readjust its understanding of weight to include the idea of energy balance—calories do count. The constant and perpetual food availability in this country will

TABLE 18.6 A Summary of Evidence-Based Clinical Guidelines on the Identification, Evaluation, and Treatment of Overweight and Obesity in Adults

Recommendation	Strength of Recommendation*
Advantages of weight loss	
Lower elevated blood pressure	A
Improve hyperlipidemia	A
Lower blood glucose in obese patients with type 2 diabetes mellitus	A
Measurement of degree of overweight and obesity	
Body mass index to assess obesity and estimate relative risk	C
Waist circumference	C
Waist circumference cut-offs for patients with body mass index of 25–34.9 kg/m^2	C
Goals of weight loss	
Initial goal = 10% from baseline	A
Loss of 1–2 lb/wk for 6 mo	B
Methods of weight loss	
Dietary therapy	
Low-calorie diet	A
Reduced fat as part of a low-calorie diet	A
Diet with deficit of 500–1,000 kcal/d (will achieve weight loss of 1–2 lb/wk)	A
Physical activity	
Weight loss	A
Decreased abdominal fat	B
Increased cardiorespiratory fitness	A
Maintenance of weight loss	C
30 minutes or more of moderate-intensity physical activity on most and preferably all days of the week as an integral part of weight loss therapy and weight maintenance	B
Behavior therapy	
As adjunct to diet in promoting weight loss and weight maintenance	B
Assessment of patient's motivation and readiness to implement a plan	C
Combined low-calorie diet, increased physical activity, and behavior therapy	A
Pharmacotherapy with lifestyle modification	B
Weight loss surgery—see text for indications	B
Maintenance	
After successful weight loss, maintenance program consisting of low calorie diet, physical activity, and behavior therapy, which should be continued indefinitely	B

*A, consistent, good-quality patient-oriented evidence; B, inconsistent or limited-quality patient-oriented evidence; C, consensus, disease-oriented evidence, usual practice, expert opinion, or case series. For information about the SORT (Strength of Recommendation Taxonomy) evidence rating system, see *http://www.aafp.org/afpsort.xml*

make any countrywide attempts at managing weight extremely difficult.

Physical Activity — The "Output" Side of the Equation

When counseling a patient in techniques for losing weight, an exercise prescription is essential, unless there is a medical contraindication to exercise. Promoting an increase in "physical activity" might be a more acceptable term to patients who think that exercise is too difficult for them. You and your patient should discuss various forms of physical activity, and agree on types that are suitable, affordable, and desirable for the patient. Table 18.9 lists types of activities and the time needed to consume a given number of calories. Exercise is especially important in maintaining weight loss, and has the added benefits of decreasing insulin resistance and reducing cardiovascular risk. Exercise may also convey an increased sense of well-being.

Giving a written prescription may help the patient consider your recommendation more seriously. Some experts sug-

TABLE 18.7 Comparison of Obesity Treatment Methods*

	Average Weight Loss (%)	Time†
Low-calorie diet	8	1 y
Exercise	2.4	>1 y
Combined behavioral therapy	2–12	6 mo–5 y
Obesity drugs		
Phentermine	13	36 wk
Sibutramine hydrochloride	6–8	1 y
Orlistat	8–10	1–2 y
Obesity surgery		
Gastric bypass	25–40	3–5 y
Vertical banded gastroplasty	17–25	3–5 y

*Percentage of average weight loss refers to percentage loss of total body weight.
†Time is from initiation of treatment.
(From Atkinson RL. A 33-year-old woman with morbid obesity. JAMA. 2000;283(4):3236–3243. Used with permission.)

gest that 1 hour per day of physical activity is necessary to lose weight. This does not have to be over a continuous period of time, in contrast to the 20–30 minutes, 3 times per week needed to reduce CVD risk. Another difference between exercises for CVD and physical activity for weight loss is that physical activity for weight loss does not require a specific heart rate elevation. The goal of increased physical activity is that when combined with dietary changes, it should result in a caloric deficit of 250 to 500 kcal/d.

Behavioral Therapy

Self-monitoring of eating habits may help patients lose weight. Food diaries are a simple form of this monitoring. The risk is that some patients may become obsessed with excessive dieting behaviors; therefore, this type of monitoring is best used to gain a short-term understanding of problem areas in eating. Patients may also benefit by recognizing and avoiding food triggers and enlisting the social support of friends, relatives,

or others attempting to lose weight. Table 18.10 lists Web-based resources for both patients and clinicians.

Medications

Patients desiring weight loss should complete a trial of diet, exercise, and behavioral modification before pharmacotherapy is considered. According to the NHLBI and the US Food and Drug Administration (FDA), medications are indicated in patients who have a BMI greater than 30 kg/m^2 with no cardiac risk factors, or a BMI greater than or equal to 27 kg/m^2 with two or more risk factors (e.g., hypertension, dyslipidemia, CVD, type 2 diabetes mellitus, or sleep apnea). Medications should not be used in isolation; diet, exercise, and behavior modification are also necessary. A randomized controlled trial demonstrated that the combination of lifestyle changes (diet and exercise) with sibutramine is more effective than either of those interventions alone in losing weight and maintaining weight loss after 1 year (20).

TABLE 18.8 Guidelines for the Low-Calorie, Step 1, Weight Loss Diet

Nutrient	Recommended Intake
Calories	Approximately 500 kcal/d reduction from usual intake
Total fat	30% or less of total calories
Cholesterol	<300 mg/d
Protein	Approximately 15% of total calories
Carbohydrate	55% or more of total calories
Sodium chloride	No more than approximately 2.5 g of sodium or approximately 6 g of sodium chloride [i.e., no added salt]
Calcium	1,000 to 1,500 mg/d
Fiber	20 to 30 g/d

Modified from National Heart, Lung, and Blood Institute Practical Guide. Identification, evaluation, and treatment of overweight and obesity, 2000. Bethesda, MD: National Institutes of Health; 2000.

<u>**Cookbooks**</u>

Here are some good reliable sources of advice and recipes
• The *Cooking Light* magazine or series for each year
• The *American Heart Association Cookbook*.
• The *Better Homes and Gardens Cookbooks* are a few examples of reliable sources of advice and recipes.

<u>**Eating Out**</u>

Many Americans eat out frequently. Here are some tips that may be helpful:
• It is usually easier to control what you eat if you eat at home.
• However, if you plan ahead you can choose lower calorie options, such as baked or broiled foods; no added butter/margarine/sour cream/cream sauces to the foods
• Beware that American restaurants generally serve very large portions; share the meal, take part home, or leave part of the meal to make the portions represent portion sizes that should be consumed by most people; children's meals are actually the portion size that most children need – don't buy an extra meal for a child; adults consume more than a child needs so we often don't understand the smaller portions that the child needs and then encourage over-consumption of food with children
• Never super-size any meal or beverage; super-sizing adds more than 600 kilocalories and sometimes as much as 1000 kilocalories to the meal/beverage
• Be aware that many chain restaurants publish lists of nutritional information for each of their selections, usually at the location where the food is paid for.
• Here are two web sites you can use in planning healthy meals out:
> www.restaurant.org/nutrition/index.cfm
> www.healthy-dining.com

<u>**How to Feel Full While Eating Less**</u>

• Drink water instead of caloric drinks to quench thirst. If you have to have a flavor to the water, use lemons or limes as flavoring. Also, remember that you can sometimes feel hungry when you are thirsty instead.
• Small snacks can add up to big calories. Small candies range from 20 to 60 kilocalories apiece. If you eat 10 pieces, that could be as much as 600 kilocalories.
• Changing from one food item (such as a small candy that is 20 kilocalorie to one that is 60 kilocalories, or 1 glass of wine to 1 bottle of a wine cooler) can add significant kilocalories without any change in what is consumed noted by the body (fuller feeling or longer eating). Example of the 10 – 20 kilocalorie candy (200 kilocalories) to 10 – 60 kilocalorie candy (600 kilocalories) is an added consumption of 400 kilocalories or 1 pound weight gain in less than 10 days!

<u>**Make Changes That You Can Stick With, and Then Be Patient**</u>

• Most overweight individuals have become that way by eating only about 50 calories too many a day. So most people don't have to make big changes to start losing weight-- they just have to make and keep the changes, and then be patient.
• A combination of healthy eating with moderate diet and exercise changes is the best way to lose weight, or at the very least, improve one's health.
• Changes for weight loss in a person's diet and exercise need to be individualized. Everyone does not gain weight in the same way nor are they going to be able to lose weight and not regain it in the same way. The above suggestions are some areas that research has shown to be problematic, but these suggestions need to be tailored to each person's problematic areas of eating and physical activity.

Figure 18.2 • Tips for patients on losing weight.

There are currently four FDA-approved medications for weight loss. Sibutramine acts to inhibit reuptake of norepinephrine, dopamine, and serotonin, and works by suppressing the appetite. Phentermine and diethylpropion are also appetite suppressants. Orlistat inhibits absorption of fat, and in early 2007, was approved for sale without a prescription. Other medications that have been approved for other uses, such as anticonvulsants and antidepressants, have been associated with weight loss, but are not approved by the FDA for treating obesity. Table 18.11 lists and discusses medications for weight loss.

Both ephedrine and ephedra have been used by patients for weight loss. There is evidence that these drugs promote only a small amount of weight loss (2.5 to 10.5 pounds in six months), with the tradeoff of a relatively large risk (1/1000) of a serious adverse event (21). Hence, these drugs are not recommended for use in helping patients lose weight.

Medications achieve varying degrees of success, with the most generous additional weight loss being a few kilograms beyond that of the traditional diet and exercise programs (22, 23). These medications may be taken for weight loss and for maintenance, but they do not work for everyone. A general guideline is that if a patient taking either medication has not lost at least 2 kg after 4 weeks, the medication should be discontinued.

A large meta-analysis of data has found little evidence that herbal supplements or other alternative products result in a sustained, significant weight loss (Level of Evidence 1A) (24). Some of the substances which have been studied include chromium picolinate, chitosan, and glucomannan, none of which was shown to cause weight loss. Garcinia cambogia, a source of hydroxycitric acid, showed mixed results in helping with weight loss. There have also been studies of fiber compounds, such as psyllium, which do not appear to lead to

TABLE 18.9 Examples of Moderate Activities

Moderate physical activity uses approximately 150 calories of energy per day, or 1,000 calories/wk. Everyday chores and sports are moderate activities. Examples are listed below.

Common Chores	Sporting Activities
Washing and waxing a car for 45–60 min	Playing volleyball for 45–60 min
Washing windows or floors for 45–60 min	Walking 1.75 miles in 35 min (20 min/mile)
Gardening for 30–45 min	Basketball (shooting baskets) for 30 min
Wheeling self in wheelchair for 30–40 min	Bicycling 5 miles in 30 min
Pushing a stroller 1.5 miles in 30 min	Dancing fast (social) for 30 min
Raking leaves for 30 min	Water aerobics for 30 min
Walking 2 miles in 30 min (15 min/mile)	Swimming laps for 20 min
Stair-walking for 15 min	Basketball (playing a game) for 15–20 min
	Jumping rope for 15 min

More vigorous activities, such as running, bicycle racing, and stair climbing take less time to consume the same number of calories.

sustained weight loss, though increasing fiber in the diet may help contribute to a sense of fullness and thus less intake over time. Hydroxy-methylbutyrate and pyruvate are substances used by body builders, and they may increase lean body mass. The same large meta-analysis found that compounds related to caffeine do not cause sustained weight loss.

Surgery

Surgical procedures for weight loss should be reserved for patients in whom medical weight loss treatment has failed, and who are suffering from complications of extreme obesity. Bariatric surgery can be considered an option for patients with a BMI greater than or equal to 40 kg/m², or greater than or equal to 35 kg/m², if cardiovascular risk factors are present

(Strength of Recommendation C). Available procedures include placing a restrictive band around the stomach to reduce the capacity (gastric banding), ligating off part of the stomach (gastroplasty), or bypassing the stomach altogether (gastric bypass). Figures 18.3 and 18.4 illustrate two of these techniques.

Gastric bypass has been shown to be more effective than gastric banding for weight loss and requires fewer surgeries for revision, but has more side effects (SOR: A, systematic review). Some evidence suggests that gastric bypass produces more weight loss than gastric banding (SOR:B) (25). Improvements related to bariatric surgery are outlined in Table 18.12. It should be noted that bariatric surgery has a significant complication rate, depending on the surgeon who performs the operation (26).

TABLE 18.10 Web-Based Resources for Nutrition and Weight Management

Organization and/or Web Site	Web Address
The American Dietetic Association	http://eatright.org
The National Association of Anorexia Nervosa and Associated Disorders	http://www.anad.org
The National Academy of Sciences	http://www.nas.edu
Overeaters Anonymous	http://www.overeatersanonymous.org
National Heart, Lung, and Blood Institute	http://www.nhlbi.gov/guidelines/obesity
US Food and Drug Administration	http://www.fda.gov
National Health Information Council (a part of the Public Health Service—Office of Disease Prevention and Health Promotion)	http://nhic-nt.health.org
The National Institutes of Health information clearinghouse for diabetes, digestive diseases, and related areas such as obesity	http://www.niddk.nih.gov
US Department of Agriculture—Food and Nutrition Consumer Service (food pyramid and related materials)	http://www.mypyramid.gov
Nutrition site for all government information	http://www.nutrition.gov
Disease-specific nutrition information (Medline Plus)	http://www.medlineplus.gov

TABLE 18.11   Drugs Commonly Used for Weight Loss

Drug	Dose	FDA Approval	Action	Adverse Effects	Cost
Sibutramine (Meridia)	5, 10, 15 mg 10 mg orally daily to start, may be increased to 15 mg or decreased to 5 mg	Long-term use (controlled substance C-IV)	Norepinephrine, dopamine, and serotonin reuptake inhibitor	Increase in heart rate and blood pressure; drug interactions with CNS active drugs, including MAOIs and seratonergic medications	$$$
Orlistat (Xenical)	120 mg 120 mg orally three times daily before fat-containing meals	Long-term use	Inhibits pancreatic lipase, decreases fat absorption	Decrease in absorption of fat-soluble vitamins; soft stools and anal leakage	$$$
Phentermine (Adipex-P, Fastin, Oby-trim, Pro-fast, Zantryl)	8, 15, 18.75, 30, 37.5 mg 8 mg three times daily 30 minutes before meals, or 15–37.5 mg daily before breakfast	Short-term use (controlled substance C-IV)	Appetite suppressant	Abuse, hypertension, tachycardia, restlessness, insomnia	$
Dietylpropion (Tenuate, Tenuate Dospan, generic available)	25 mg, 75 mg SR 25 mg three times daily, 1 hour before meals, or 75 mg SR once daily in the midmorning	Short-term use (controlled substance C-IV)	Appetite suppressant	Pulmonary hypertension, arrhythmias, psychosis, dry mouth, restlessness	$

CNS, central nervous system; FDA, US Food and Drug Administration; MAOIs, monoamine oxidase inhibitors.

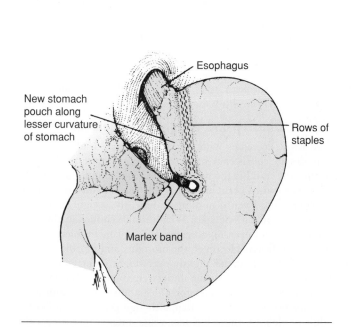

Figure 18.3 • Vertical banded gastroplasty.   (From Nettina SM. The Lippincott Manual of Nursing Practice. 7th ed. Baltimore, MD: Lippincott Williams & Wilkins; 2001.)

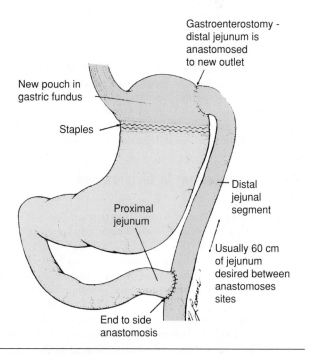

Figure 18.4 • Roux-en-Y gastric bypass.   (From Nettina SM. The Lippincott Manual of Nursing Practice. 7th ed. Baltimore, MD: Lippincott Williams & Wilkins; 2001.)

TABLE 18.12 Benefits of Bariatric Surgery

Improvement	Strength of Recommendation*
Diabetes	B
Abnormal lipid profiles	B
Decreased incidence of hypertension	B
Obstructive sleep apnea	C
Obesity hypoventilation syndrome	C
Menstrual irregularity	C
Female urinary stress incontinence	C

*A, consistent, good-quality patient-oriented evidence; B, inconsistent or limited-quality patient-oriented evidence; C, consensus, disease-oriented evidence, usual practice, expert opinion, or case series. For information about the SORT evidence rating system, see *http://www.aafp.org/afpsort.xml*.

Management of the Underweight Patient

The underweight person works with the same energy balance principles as the overweight person (kcal eaten vs. energy expended). Food, exercise, and weight goals need to take these factors into consideration. Practical food considerations include the following:

- High-fat foods do not necessarily help an underweight person gain weight because they cause the person to feel full for long periods of time and therefore can act as an appetite suppressant.
- Snacks or small frequent meals may help, if the person does not use them to replace regular meals.
- Increasing the calories in readily consumed forms (e.g., beverages), or as additives, is often helpful. An example is adding a protein-carbohydrate mix to milk each day.

A physician who is concerned with an underweight patient should investigate the problem with the same clinical tools as are used for the overweight patient. It is important to have sympathy for this weight concern; the underweight patient may be struggling as much as the overweight person. Treatment should consist of measures appropriate to the diagnosis; for example, increased calories for increased energy expenditure or mental health treatment for eating disorders.

Weight Management in Children and Adolescents

Weight prior to the last adolescent growth spurt does not seem to influence adult weight (27–30). This is good news because American children, similar to adults, also are gaining weight. For the obese child, dieting seems to be even less effective than it is in adults, and involves more risk (31). Instead, activity seems more amenable to intervention and should be a cornerstone of any weight loss efforts for children. The risks of dieting in children seem to include the increased possibility of disordered eating, psychological deprivation, rebound weight gain, and possible detrimental influences on growth.

Television watching is strongly correlated with increased weight; the more television watched, the heavier the child (32); this is independent of the number of kilocalories consumed. To date, there is only one study that evaluated eliminating television viewing, and the effects on weight of children; it showed a significant decrease in weight when time spent watching television was reduced (33).

A children's food pyramid is available at *www.mypyramid.gov*. Remember, however, that it is a suggested food pattern, and there is probably wide variation in what individual children need. For example, some children, because of high caloric need, will suffer from too few calories if the lower portion of the food pyramid is stressed too vigorously. Food choices should be from a range of healthy foods, with children determining the amounts based on their bodies' caloric demands.

Dramatic obesity is rare in children, and children's treatment programs for weight loss have not met with success in long-term weight normalization as the child grows into adulthood. Therefore, the wisest advice for children is to:

- Eat a healthy diet
- Eat to appetite (appetite will vary from day to day)
- Be active
- Avoid excess television viewing

This is the least risky approach, and may promote the best long-term health habits.

Elderly Obesity and Weight Management

The BMR decreases with age, and this may lead to weight gain despite consistency in diet and exercise patterns. In spite of this, the trend is for weight to decrease in older age. Peak weights for men occur on average at age 55, and for women at 65 (34, 35). Even if nothing is done, the weight will tend to decrease after these ages. Weight interventions in this age group have not been investigated for any conclusions regarding their efficacy. However, the mortality and morbidity data seem to show that the slightly overweight older adult fares better in longevity than the underweight older adult (36).

Nutritional guidelines for older adults can be found at *www.mypyramid.gov*. Note that, although generally similar to adult guidelines, these include: water intake, increased calcium, and selected vitamin supplements. The DASH study found that consuming increased fruits, vegetables, and calcium-containing foods, combined with physical activity, decreased hypertension. The study also recommended weight loss, but within the context of the changes suggested, the improved dietary content and physical activity seemed as important as caloric reduction (37).

One negative consequence of weight loss in the elderly, especially in women who think that they will regain a "youthful appearance," is that eating disorders, such as self-induced anorexia and bulimia, are observed in the elderly just as in younger age groups. Also, in the elderly it is possible that weight loss is an indicator of other health problems, such as cancer or polymyalgia rheumatica.

CONCLUSION

The major elements of weight loss—dieting, surgery, and medications—have not correlated with much long-term success. The general rule of thumb is that 95% of people who lose weight with any weight loss program will gain back all of the weight within 2 years, and almost all of the people will gain back more than is lost within 5 years, regardless of the program tried!

The question, then, is what works? A four-pronged approach of diet, water consumption, increased activity, and behavioral modification offers the best chance of permanent weight loss, and will be most successful if the patient helps plan and is committed to the program.

Remember, an adult who has gained 50 pounds over 10 years averaged only 50 extra kilocalories per day above his or her requirements. Thus, a relatively small change in routine, such as switching from sugared drinks to diet drinks or water, combined with a modest increase in physical activity, will reduce this pattern. The good news is that this is probably the best advice for chronic disease prevention as well as modest weight loss; the bad news is that this will NOT achieve the "cultural underweight" norms that the public would like to have.

CASE DISCUSSION

In the initial case presentation, J. suffers from unexplained weight loss. On further evaluation, we learn that he has developed chronic pain and likely some inflammation related to his degenerating joints. Despite the fact that he is moving less, his basal metabolic rate has increased because of his chronic pain and inflammation. Additionally, a dietary history or diary demonstrates that his caloric intake is decreased, as is common in patients with chronic pain. As his primary care physician, you should consider performing laboratory evaluation of J.'s nutritional status before surgery, and if necessary, remediate any protein, vitamin, and mineral deficiencies. Surgery and the stress of healing will increase J.'s nutritional requirements, so careful monitoring of his nutritional condition during and after hospitalization is very important.

A. represents a common presentation of an obese patient. She notes that she would like to get down to her college weight of 145 pounds. She has no family history of CVD or diabetes, does not smoke, and has not had a blood lipid evaluation. Upon further questioning, you learn that she rarely eats break-

fast and views skipping a meal as a good way to cut calories. She admits to rarely using the stairs in public buildings, choosing the escalator or elevator instead.

You obtain a lipid profile, which shows a total cholesterol of 190 mg/dL, a high-density lipoprotein of 56 mg/dL, and a low-density lipoprotein of 118 mg/dL. You ask A. to keep a food diary, and learn that, although she consumes few calories at breakfast and typically eats a piece of fruit or bowl of cottage cheese for lunch, she eats frequent snacks of crackers, chips, or pretzels, accompanied by soft drinks. Her portions at supper are "super-sized," and she commonly eats a hot dog or frozen diet dinner in the evening as a snack.

Your approach to A. should be two-pronged: decreasing caloric intake and increasing activity. First, it is important to set a realistic goal; her idea of losing 45 pounds (25% of her body weight) is probably not realistic. Encourage her to set a goal of a 10% (19 lbs) weight loss, or even an initial 10-lb weight loss, at a rate of a pound per week. Advise her to spread her caloric intake out across the day, consuming a balanced breakfast and cutting down on night-time snacks. She may do well to eat four smaller, balanced meals than to consume most of her calories at the end of the day. Help her to use *www.mypyramid.gov* to obtain nutritional guidelines for someone of her age and desired weight. Finally, encourage A. to increase her daily activity. Because of her knee pain, many types of exercise may be unrealistic. Work with her to find out what she can and will do, and write a prescription for increased activity.

Although she is technically a candidate for weight loss medication (BMI >30), she has not made a reasonable attempt at weight loss with diet and activity modification. Therefore, it is wise to use these modalities first. Careful follow up and encouragement are essential.

REFERENCES

1. Preuss HG. Sodium, chloride, and potassium. In: Bowman BA, Russell RM, eds. Present Knowledge in Nutrition, 8th ed. Washington, DC. International Life Sciences Press; 2001: 302–310.
2. US Department of Health and Human Services, US Department of Agriculture. Dietary Guidelines for Americans 2005. Available at *www.healthierus.gov*. Accessed February, 10, 2006.
3. Hammond KA. Dietary and clinical assessment. In: Mahan LK, Escott-Stump S, eds. Krause's Food, Nutrition, and Diet Therapy, 11th ed. Philadelphia, PA: Saunders-Elsevier; 2004. Chapter 17.
4. Balcombe NR, Ferry PG, Saweirs WM. Nutritional status and well being. Is there a relationship between body mass index and the well-being of older people? Curr Med Res Opin. 2001;17:1–7.
5. Keys A, Fidanza F, Karvonen MJ, Kmura N, Taylor HL. Indices of relative weight and obesity. J Chronic Dis. 1972; 25:329–343.
6. Dalton N, Cameron AJ, Zimmet PZ, et al. Waist circumference, whist-hip ratio and body mass index and their correlation with cardiovascular disease risk factors in Australian adults. J Intern Med. 203;254:555–563.
7. National Heart, Lung and Blood Institute. Clinical guidelines on the identification, evaluation, and treatment of overweight and obesity in adults: the evidence report. Bethesda, MD; National Institutes of Health; 1998.
8. Health United States 2000. Washington, DC: Centers for Dis-

ease Control and Prevention, National Center for Health Statistics, Division of Health Examination; 2000.

9. Hu FB, Stampfer MJ, Colditz GA, et al. Physical activity and risk of stroke in women. JAMA. 2000;238(22):2961–2967.

10. Lew EA, Garfinkel L. Variations in mortality by weight among 750,000 men and women. J Chron Dis. 1979;32: 563–576.

11. World Health Organization. Global strategy on diet, physical activity, and health. Obesity and overweight. 2003.

12. Wagner DR, Heyward VH. Measures of body composition in African-Americans and whites: a comparative review. Am J Clin Nutr. 2000;71:1392–1402

13. National Institute of Diabetes and Digestive and Kidney Diseases. Statistics related to overweight and obesity. 2005. Available at: *http://www.medhelp.org/NIHlib/GF-367.html*. Accessed February 10, 2006.

14. Kassirer JP, Angell M. Losing weight—an ill-fated New Year's resolution. N Engl J Med. 1998;338(1):52–54.

15. Manson JE, Willett WC, Stampfer MJ, et al. Body weight and mortality among women. N Engl J Med. 1995;333:677–685.

16. Calle EE, Rodriguez C, Walker-Thurmond K, Thun M. Overweight, obesity, and mortality from cancer in a prospectively studied cohort of U.S. adults. N Engl J Med. 2003;348: 1625–1638.

17. National Heart, Lung, and Blood Institute. Executive Summary. Clinical guidelines on the identification, evaluation, and treatment of overweight and obesity in adults. Bethesda, MD: National Institutes of Health; 1998.

18. Atkinson RL. A 33 year-old woman with morbid obesity. JAMA. 2000;283:3236–3243.

19. Dansinger ML, Gleason JA, Griffith JL, Selker HP, Schaefer EJ. Comparison of the Atkins, Ornish, Weight-Watchers, and Zone diets for weight loss and heart disease reduction: a randomized trial. JAMA. 2005;293:43–53.

20. Wadden TA, Berkowitz RI, Womble LG, et al. Randomized trial of lifestyle modification and pharmacotherapy for obesity. N Engl J Med. 2005;353:2111–2130.

21. Shekelle PG, Hardy ML, Morton SC, et al. Efficacy and safety of ephedra and ephedrine for weight loss and athletic performance. A meta-analysis. JAMA. 2003;289:1537–1545.

22. Wirth A, Krause J. Long term weight loss with sibutramine: a randomized controlled trial. JAMA. 2001;286:1331–1339.

23. Davidson MH, Hauptman J, DiGirolamo M, et al. Weight control and risk factor reduction in obese subjects treated for 2 years with orlistat. A randomized controlled trial. JAMA. 1999;281:235–242.

24. Pittler MH, Ernst E. Dietary supplements for body-weight reduction: a systematic review. Am J Clin Nutr. 2004;79: 529–536.

25. Everson G, Kelsberg G, Nashelsky J. Clinical inquiries. How effective is gastric bypass for weight loss? J Fam Pract. 2004; 53:914–918.

26. Buchwald H, Avidor Y, Braunwald E, et al. Bariatric surgery. A systematic review and meta-analysis. JAMA. 2004;292: 1724–1737.

27. Goran MI. Metabolic precursors and effects of obesity in children: a decade of progress, 1990–1999. Am J Clin Nutr. 2001; 73:158–171.

28. Dietz WH. Critical periods in childhood for the development of obesity. Am J Clin Nutr. 1994;59:955–959.

29. Epstein LH, Valoski A, Wing RR, McCurley J. Ten year follow-up of behavioral family-based treatment for obese children. JAMA. 1991;264:2519–2523.

30. Whitaker RC, Wright JA, Pepe MS, Seidel KD, Dietz WH. Predicting obesity in young adulthood from childhood and parental obesity. N Engl J Med. 1997;337(13):869–873.

31. Gortmaker SL, Dietz WH, Cheung LW. Inactivity, diet and the fattening of America. J Am Diet Assoc. 1990;90: 1247–1252, 1255.

32. Gortmaker SL, Must A, Sobol AM, Peterson K, Coliditz GA, Dietz WH. Television watching as a cause of increasing obesity among children in the United States. Arch Pediatr Adolesc Med. 1996;150:356–362.

33. Robinson TN. Reducing children's television viewing to prevent obesity; a randomized controlled trial. JAMA. 1999; 282(16):1561–1567.

34. Roberts SB. Energy regulation and aging: recent findings and their implications. Nutr Rev. 2000;58(4):91–97.

35. Shils ME, Olson JA, Shike M, Ross AC. Changes in weight and height with age In: Modern Nutrition in Health and Disease, 9th ed. Philadelphia, PA: Lippincott Williams & Wilkins; 1999:Appendix A73.

36. Stevens J. Impact of age on associations between weight and mortality. Nutr Rev. 2000;58(50):129–137.

37. Conlin PR, Chow D, Miller ER III, et al. The effect of dietary patterns on blood pressure control in hypertensive patients: results from the Dietary Approaches to Stop Hypertension (DASH) trial. Am J Hypertens. 2000;13(9):949–955.

CHAPTER 19

Ear Pain

William J. Hueston and Arch G. Mainous III

CASE

P.J. is a 19-month-old brought to your office in early February with a complaint of fever that started 3 days after cold symptoms appeared. P.J. has had several ear infections before and his mother is concerned that he might have another one. When you review his chart, you see that P.J. was seen in the office the end of December with a right otitis media, in early November with a left otitis, and the middle of September with the diagnosis of bilateral otitis media.

P.J. is a bit fussy, but easily consoled and entertained. His temperature is 101.1°F. His left tympanic membrane (TM) is red and retracted and does not respond to pneumatic otoscopy. The right TM appears normal and moves well with pneumatic otoscopy. The remainder of the examination reveals a congested nose with yellowish drainage, mildly red throat, and shotty cervical nodes. The lungs are clear and abdomen is benign.

You explain to his mother that he looks like he has another ear infection and recommend starting amoxicillin. She notes that the last time he had an ear infection, amoxicillin did not work and wants to try cefixime because that worked last time. One of her neighbors also told her that P.J. should have tubes put in his ears because of all his infections.

CLINICAL QUESTIONS

1. What are the primary infectious and non-infectious causes of pain in the ear?
2. How reliable are diagnostic tests for otitis media?
3. What is the optimal management for acute suppurative otitis media?
4. What strategies are most effective for preventing recurrence of otitis media in children with frequent infections?

Ear pain, and more specifically, ear infection in younger patients, is one of the most common reasons why parents seek care for their children from primary care physicians. Otitis media was the third most common reason for visiting a physician in a study of community practices associated with the WAMI (Washington/Alaska/Montana/Idaho) Residency Network (1) and ranked 11th in reasons for visits among the more than 500,000 patient problems recorded in the large Virginia Study (2). In addition, ear wax, serous otitis media, and otitis externa also ranked in the top 50 for visits in the WAMI study (1). Although these problems are infrequently life threatening, they are very common and cause a significant amount of anxiety and suffering in primary care patients as well as posing significant costs to the health care system (3).

DIFFERENTIAL DIAGNOSIS

The ear is innervated by three different neural pathways (4). The conchae and external auditory canal receive primary sensory innervation from somatic sensory fibers of the facial nerve (7th cranial nerve). Parts of the external auditory canal also receive sensory innervation from the auricular branch of the vagus (Arnold's nerve), which contains nerve fibers from the 7th cranial nerve as well as the 9th and 10th nerves. The stimulation of Arnold's nerve in the external auditory canal sometimes produces cough through vagal stimulation. Arnold's nerve also is involved in herpes zoster infections of the external ear canal.

The middle ear receives its neural innervation through branches of the glossopharyngeal nerve, the ninth cranial nerve. Since this nerve innervates the throat and tongue, it is common for throat pain to be referred to the middle ear.

The separate innervation of the middle and external ears can be useful in differentiating the source of pain. Retraction of the conchae in the case of an external otitis or trauma to the external auditory canal will cause pain because of local inflammation of the 7th cranial nerve. However, because the middle ear receives different neural innervation, stimulation of the external ear should not produce pain with an otitis media.

The most common cause of inflammation in the middle or external ears is infection. Other causes of noninfectious inflammation include local trauma, dermatoses, or tumors penetrating into the external auditory canal. Additionally, pain may be present with impaction of the external ear with foreign bodies or with excessive cerumen. Generally, cerumen impaction or foreign body presence does not produce pain, but rather results in hearing loss. However, excessive pressure in the auditory canal can cause mucosal irritation, which could result in pain. Another possible source of pain with a foreign body is penetration of the thin skin of the auditory canal by insects such as ticks.

Infection of the external ear and auditory canal results from direct trauma to the area with invasion of skin colonizing bacteria such as *Staphylococcus* or pneumococcus or, less commonly, with *Pseudomonas* The infection is defined primarily by its location:

- Perichondritis is used to describe infection of the pinna. These infections usually produce a red, painful, swollen external ear.
- Furunculosis refers to infection of the hair follicles in the outer third of the auditory canal.
- Otitis externa refers to infection of the fibrocartilaginous inner two-thirds of the auditory canal which is devoid of hair follicles and glands and has a very friable, thin skin layer.

Patients with repetitive trauma to any of these areas are at highest risk for the development of an infection.

Decreased hearing, pain, and systemic signs of infections such as fever or malaise characterize middle ear infections. The peak onset of middle ear infections is in the first 6 years of life. About one-third of children have their first episode of otitis media in the first year of life and often have repetitive episodes throughout their childhood. Another third of children have only a small number of ear infections (<3) in their childhood. The remaining third of children do not have any ear infections.

The function and integrity of the Eustachian tube is a major factor in the likelihood of a child developing middle ear infections. The role of the Eustachian tube is to ventilate the middle ear and provide mucociliary clearance for bacteria and other materials that migrate from the nasopharynx. Ventilation is controlled by the tensor veli palatini muscle, which opens and closes the Eustachian canal to normalize pressures in the middle ear. Mucociliary clearance is performed primarily in the lower half of the Eustachian tube that is provided with many mucous glands.

Dysfunction of the Eustachian tube disrupts proper ventilation of the middle ear and can result in a negative pressure that pulls fluid into the middle ear space. Stasis of this fluid combined with colonization with nasopharyngeal organisms can result in otitis media. Conditions that are associated with poor Eustachian tube function or occlusion of the lower Eustachian tube such as allergic rhinitis or upper respiratory tract infections increase the risk of otitis media. Additionally, poor function of the tensor veli palatini muscle which is seen in some families as well as in patients with Trisomy 21 (Down's syndrome) also increase the risk of otitis media. Finally, patients with craniofacial abnormalities that may involve the Eustachian tube also have higher incidences of otitis media. Table 19.1 lists the differential diagnosis for ear pain.

CLINICAL EVALUATION

History and Physical Examination

A good history is often difficult to gather from patients with ear pain since many of them are too young to relate an accurate story of their illness. Parents often interpret a child's action as indicating a problem. However, some parental cues such as a history of pulling at the ears are not associated with ear infections.

The most useful history in ear pain is the location of the pain, type of pain, and actions that make the pain worse. Outer ear infections are sensitive to touch of the ear. Otitis externa and furunculosis occur in the auditory canal and are worsened

TABLE 19.1 Differential Diagnosis of Ear Pain

Diagnosis	Frequency in Primary Care
Otitis media	Very common
Cerumen impaction	Very common
Otitis externa	Common
Referred pain from throat or temporal bone	Common
Acoustic trauma	Less common
External ear dermatitis	Less common
Perichondritis	Less common
Foreign body in the canal	Less common
Furunculosis	Rare
Mastoiditis	Rare
Ear tumors (eosinophilic granulomas, rhabdosarcomas)	Rare

by moving the ear. Otitis media is a deeper pain that is unaffected by movement of the outer ear.

Hearing loss also can be a useful historical sign. Complete hearing loss can occur with foreign bodies or complete canal occlusion with cerumen. Severe otitis externa may totally obstruct the auditory canal as well. Middle ear infections generally cause a dulling of sound, but hearing is still present.

Finally, it is important to ask about dental problems, pain with chewing, throat pain, or other problems that are affecting the throat and jaw. Referred pain to the ear is common and other sources of the problem should be sought. Temporomandibular disorders are particularly prone to ear pain (5). In patients with temporomandibular disorders, the prevalence of otalgia without infection varied between 12% and 16% (6). Patients with suspected temporomandibular disorders should be referred to a dentist for further assessment.

The first step in evaluating ear pain is differentiating middle ear pain, external ear pain, and referred pain. Manipulation of the external ear will exacerbate most pain located in the external ear or the auditory canal. However, referred pain and middle ear pain will be unaffected by this maneuver. Inspection of the outer ear and auditory canal will confirm the presence of foreign bodies or inflammation.

If manipulation of the outer ear fails to reproduce or worsen the pain, the source is more likely to be the middle ear or referred pain. The presence of an earache along with night restlessness and a fever increase the likelihood of an otitis media (7). The next step in the evaluation is visualization of the tympanic membrane plus possible ancillary testing such as pneumatic otoscopy and tympanometry to determine if the membrane is mobile. A mobile tympanic membrane suggests that no fluid is present in the middle ear making otitis media unlikely.

When examining the tympanic membrane when acute otitis medial is suspected, the most useful positive findings for otitis media include a bulging (positive likelihood ratio [LR] of 51) or cloudy (LR of 34) tympanic membrane. These findings are much better at predicting otitis media than the traditional erythematous tympanic membrane (7). A tympanic membrane that is only slightly red (LR 1.4) is not very useful at all (8). The combination of a cloudy effusion, bulging membrane, and loss of mobility has a predictive value in the mid-90th percentile (9). Another finding to look for on direct examination of the tympanic membrane is a perforation which will allow purulent material to exude into the auditory canal.

However, a classic presentation of otitis media is rare. In a study of practicing primary care doctors, in only 58% of cases could clinicians could state with confidence that the person they diagnosed with otitis media really had an infected looking ear (10). Other investigations have shown significant disagreement between expert examiners for the presence of effusion (11). When clinical otoscopy was compared to myringotomy in a study of 226 children, the sensitivity of clinical examination was only 74% and the specificity was 60% compared to myringotomy (12). The presence of erythema without a bulging or cloudy tympanic membrane is even less helpful; the positive predictive value of erythema alone was found to be only 65% in predicting otitis media when compared to myringotomy (13).

To improve diagnostic accuracy, pneumatic otoscopy has been advocated as an adjunctive maneuver to simple visualization. In this test, air is introduced into the auditory canal while the tympanic membrane is visualized. Movement of the tympanic membrane with increased air pressure is believed to indicate a mobile tympanic membrane and no middle ear effusion. However, this test does not improve positive predictive value significantly (13). Table 19.2 lists key elements of the history, physical examination, diagnostic testing.

Red Flags Signaling Problems

Another key aspect of the evaluation of ear pain is assessment for the presence of any important complications (see Table 19.3). Most ear infections are localized to the ear canal and middle ear, but contiguous spread to adjoining structures can occur infrequently.

External ear infection (perichondritis) is generally located in the body of the auricle, but spares the non-cartilaginous lobule. Involvement of the lobule of the auricle, which does not contain cartilage, is an ominous sign that suggests a more virulent infection such as erysipelas. If the lobule is involved in infection, rapid initiation of anti-streptococcal antibiotics is

imperative to keep the infection from rapidly progressing into the surround neck tissue.

In otitis externa, invasion into adjoining tissue occurs most frequently in infections caused by *Pseudomonas aeruginosa*. Infection with this organism, termed malignant otitis externa, can cause widespread local invasion and bacteremia with sepsis and death. The hallmark warning signs of *Pseudomonas* malignant otitis include a seventh nerve palsy on the affected side. Other infections, in particular, herpes zoster of the ear, also can produce a seventh nerve palsy and must be differentiated from malignant otitis externa.

Other warning signs in the auditory canal include an ulcerated or non-healing lesion in the canal. Either of these signs can indicate erosion of an adjoining tumor into the canal. If these lesions are seen, biopsy of the ulcerated or non-healing area are indicated.

A final red flag seen in otitis media is tenderness over the mastoid process of the temporal bone. This could signal mastoiditis, a chronic osseous infection that may not resolve without surgical debridement of the mastoid.

Diagnostic Testing

Tympanometry improves the sensitivity and specificity of the diagnosis of middle ear effusion. Tympanometry testing measures the amount of a test sound that is transverses the tympanic membrane at given positive and negative auditory canal pressures. The tympanometer forms an airtight seal around the auditory canal, and a sound wave is introduced by pushing a button on the instrument. The machine monitors the amount of the sound reflected back from the tympanic membrane. This procedure is repeated as various positive and negative pressures are the results are plotted based on the amount of sound transmitted. In a series of studies evaluating this test, the sensitivity of tympanometry compared to myringotomy has ranged from 79% to 95% with a corresponding specificity of 57% to 93% (9). However, the reliability of the test is influenced by the level of cooperation by the patient. In poorly cooperative children, the predictive value drops substantially (14).

Acoustic reflectometry, another adjunctive test, measures reflected sound off the tympanic membrane is measured. The amount of sound reflected is measured in decibels. The most appropriate cut-off value for a positive test is still controversial.

TABLE 19.2 Key Elements in the History, Physical Examination, and Diagnostic Testing for Ear Pain

Diagnosis	Diagnostic Maneuvers	Reliability of Diagnostic Test
Otitis externa	Pain on manipulation of outer ear	Not tested
Otitis media	Pneumatic otoscopy	Sensitivity: 74%–93%
		Specificity: 58%–60%
	Tympanometry in cooperative children	Sensitivity: 78%–95%
		Specificity: 79%–93%
	Tympanometry in uncooperative children	Sensitivity: 71%
		Specificity: 38%
	Acoustic reflectometry	Sensitivity: 79%–90%
		Specificity: 79%–86%

TABLE 19.3 Red Flags Suggesting Progressive or Life-Threatening Disease in Patients with Ear Pain

Red Flag	Diagnosis Suggested
Ear lobule erythema	Erysipelas
Seventh cranial nerve palsy	Malignant otitis externa (*Pseudomonas* infection)
Ulceration in external ear canal	Auditory canal tumor or tumor eroding into the canal such as rhabdomyosarcoma or lymphoma
Nonhealing lesion in the auditory canal	Auditory canal tumor or tumor eroding into the canal such as rhabdomyosarcoma or lymphoma
Tenderness over the mastoid	Mastoiditis

Studies of acoustic reflectometry have used either tympanometry or clinical examination as the gold standards, which limits their interpretation. Even given these weak gold standards, positive and negative predictive values are in the 80% range (9).

Recommended Diagnostic Strategy

A combination of history, physical examination, and diagnostic testing to diagnose otitis media is recommended by the Agency for Healthcare Research and Quality (AHRQ) (15). In the 1990 AHRQ technical report on otitis media and in a 2004 American Academy of Pediatrics American Academy of Family Physicians (AAP/AAFP) guideline, it was recommended that otitis media be defined as the presence of middle ear effusion (based on either diagnostic tests or physical exami-

nation findings of opacification or a full or bulging tympanic membrane) plus a rapid onset of symptoms that include either otalgia, otorrhea, fever, or irritability in an infant or toddler. Figure 19.1 illustrates a useful approach to the evaluation and treatment of ear pain.

MANAGEMENT

Cerumen Impaction

Pain from cerumen impaction usually occurs because of pressure of the cerumen against the tympanic membrane. Management includes irrigation of the auditory canal with either water or a 50:50 water-peroxide solution to soft and dislodge

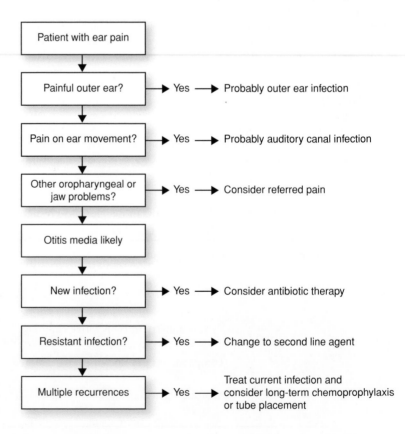

Figure 19.1 • General approach to the patient with ear pain.

cerumen. (If using water, it is important to ensure that the water temperature is tepid or as close to body temperature as possible. Use of either water that is cold or too hot can precipitate a strong vestibular nerve reaction with nystagmus and dizziness.) When this is not successful, cerumen softening agents (e.g., liquid Colace) can be used, but prolonged use may cause irritation of the canal with subsequent edema, which worsens the cerumen entrapment. As a last resort, cerumen can be removed with direct suction under direct microscopic visualization, which is usually performed by an otolaryngologist.

Perichondritis and Furunculosis

These infections of the outer ear or outer third of the auditory canal are usually caused by staphylococcal species or, occasionally, streptococcal species. Antibiotics directed against these two organisms, such as cephalosporins, are necessary. Because blood flow to the outer ear cartilage is scanty, cartilage necrosis with long-term ear deformity (cauliflower ear) can occur if treatment is delayed or inadequate.

Infection of the outer ear also is common after trauma, especially injuries such as frostbite. Close attention to tissue healing and protection against infection is an important aspect of managing outer ear frostbite or other traumas such as bites or scratches.

Otitis Externa

The most common organism cultured from the auditory canal in otitis externa is *Pseudomonas*, which can be found in association with other bacteria such as *Staphylococcus* and *Proteus* (16). Infection causes edema of the ear canal and disrupts the normal squamous cell shedding that occurs on a regular basis. This leads to the accumulation of a keratin layer in the canal along with exudate and necrotic debris. Treatment includes debridement of necrotic tissue through gentle rinsing followed by the application of a broad-spectrum antibiotic topical solution that will cover the most common organisms in what is usually a poly-microbial infection. For patients whose canal is obliterated by edema, the insertion of a gauze wick may be necessary to draw antibiotics into the infected canal.

The choice of an antibiotic for otitis externa has not been studied extensively. Neomycin/polymixin B ear drops and ofloxacin ear drops are both popular because of their ability to eradicate *Pseudomonas*. Because of ototoxicity associated with aminoglycosides, neomycin should be avoided when the tympanic membranes is ruptured or cannot be visualized well. The addition of corticosteroids is popular in some ear drops, although there is little evidence that this speeds healing or prevents recurrences.

Prevention of recurrent otitis externa includes maneuvers to reduce the intrusion of fluids or other materials into the ear. Cleaning of the ear by sticking instruments into the ear canal should be avoided. Finally, some suggest rinsing the ear with alcohol following bathing or swimming to flush out water that may pool in the canal. While probably harmless, this technique has not been evaluated to determine if it reduces recurrences.

Otitis Media

The most appropriate management of otitis media has sparked debated for many years. For example, in the United States, routine use of antibiotics for otitis media has been the tradition without evidence that this practice is superior to other strategies (16, 17). But in other countries, most notably the Netherlands, antibiotic use for otitis media is reserved for high-risk children between ages 6 months and 2 years, and for most children over the age of 2. Data from two meta-analyses showed that the routine use of amoxicillin is associated with a 12.3% (17) to 13.7% (18) lower failure rate than observation (or placebo). This translates into a number needed to treat (NNT) of 6 to prevent one case of failure in a patient not treated with antibiotics.

To help guide clinicians sort out the controversy, the AAP and the AAFP published an evidence-based guideline for treatment in 2004. For children less than 6 months of age, the AAP/AAFP guideline recommends routine antibiotic administration starting with amoxicillin at a dose of 80 to 90 mg/kg per day (19). For children over age 6 months, the AAP/AAFP recommendations for managing acute otitis media include the option to observe selected children without antibiotic treatment. This option should be based on the certainty of diagnosis, the child's age, the severity of illness, and the assurance that the patient will be able to follow-up if the symptoms do not improve in 48 to 72 hours. If the child is otherwise healthy, the diagnosis is uncertain, the illness not severe, and the child's caregiver can reliably follow-up if symptoms do not improve, then observation is a reasonable strategy. If the child returns with a more definitive examination or worsening of symptoms within 72 hours, then antibiotic therapy should be started.

When the effectiveness of multiple different antibiotics was compared in their ability to treat suppurative otitis media, there appeared to be no benefit of any one drug over any other (see Table 19.4). Antibiotics used for 5 days or less showed equal effectiveness with longer durations of therapy (20). One study has suggested, though, that 2 days of therapy with oral antibiotics is not as effective as treatment for 7 days (17). In addition to a cost benefit of shorter durations of therapy, reports have noted fewer drug-related side effects in patients taking short courses of antibiotics. One study estimated that the NNT with short-duration therapy to avoid one gastrointestinal adverse effect was eight children. In addition to short-duration therapy compared to long-duration therapy with oral antibiotics, a single intramuscular dose of ceftriaxone was just as effective as a longer duration of other antibiotics.

Because of the emergence of multiple drug resistant strains of *Streptococcus pneumoniae,* there has been some concern that standard doses of medications might not be sufficient to cover strains that are intermediately resistant. Higher-dose regimens of amoxicillin-clavulanate have been suggested to deal with this potential problem. However, two controlled studies of high-dose amoxicillin-clavulanate have shown no greater effectiveness than standard dosing regimens. It should be noted that whereas the higher doses of amoxicillin are not supported by these studies and remain theoretical, the AAP/AAFP guideline on otitis media still recommends doses of amoxicillin of 80–90 mg/kg to overcome intermediate resistance.

The treatment of recurrent otitis media after a previous resistant episode is another area of controversy. Some physicians treat recurrent infection failure with a second-line drug to avoid a treatment failure in the new episode after a previous treatment. However, recurrences several weeks after an initial

TABLE 19.4 Management of Common Causes of Ear Pain

Treatment Strategy	Strength of Recommendation*	Recommendations/Conclusions
Antibiotic for AOM Media		
Routine antibiotics use in children <6 months of age	A	Antibiotics associated with 12.3% reduction in failure rate (NNT = 6)
Observation acceptable in healthy children > 6 months of age with uncertain diagnosis, mild/moderate severity of illness, and reliable follow-up available	B	Patients have to meet all criteria for observation and those who return with continuing symptoms in 48–72 hours should receive antibiotics
Comparison of amoxicillin, penicillin, cefaclor, cefixime	A	No differences in effectiveness
Trimethoprim-sulfamethoxazole versus cefaclor	A	No difference in effectiveness
Single dose ceftriaxone versus amoxillin-clavulanate	A	No differences in effectiveness
High dose versus regular dose amoxillin-clavulanate dose	A	No differences in effectiveness
Duration of antibiotic therapy for AOM		
Multiple studies of 3–5 days of therapy versus 10 days of therapy	A	No difference in effectiveness; greater incidence of antibiotic side effects in patients treated for longer duration
Dosing frequency of amoxillin		
Twice-a-day dosing versus three-times-a-day dosing	A	No difference in effectiveness

AOM, Acute otitis media

*A, consistent, good-quality patient-oriented evidence; B, inconsistent or limited-quality patient-oriented evidence; C, consensus, disease-oriented evidence, usual practice, expert opinion, or case series. For information about the SORT evidence rating system, see *http://www.aafp.org/afpsort.xml*.

episode are usually produced by a new organism and do not necessarily have the same resistance pattern as previous infections. One non-randomized study that investigated the effectiveness of a second-line drug versus a first-line agent (amoxicillin or trimethoprim-sulfamethoxazole) showed no benefit of the broader spectrum second-line agent in a recurrent infection following a previously resistant episode (21). To reduce the development of resistance, new episodes should be treated with narrower spectrum agents.

LONG-TERM MONITORING AND PREVENTION

In children with multiple episodes of otitis media, prevention of recurrent infections may be necessary. Recurrent otitis is defined as three or more episodes in a 6-month period or 4 episodes in a year with a normal examination documented between each infection (22). The first approach in preventing recurrences is to identify conditions that predispose children to Eustachian tube dysfunction. Most commonly, this is an upper respiratory infection that cannot be prevented. However, some children have chronic allergic rhinitis that results in Eustachian tube dysfunction. Treatment of these children with antihistamines or nasal steroids may reduce their risk of a recurrent infection.

For children with no evidence of allergy, options include chronic antibiotic prophylaxis or surgical ventilation of the inner ear through the placement of tubes. Tympanostomy tubes and antibiotic prophylaxis have nearly equal effectiveness for the prevention of recurrence (22, 23), but medication use is associated with fewer side effects. Antibiotic prophylaxis can be achieved with either amoxicillin or sulfamethoxazole given as a single dose at bedtime. The usual dose is one-half of the total daily treatment dose. For children who continue to have episodes of otitis media despite antibiotic prophylaxis, the insertion of typanostomy tubes is indicated. If antibiotic prophylaxis does fail, it is most likely to fail in the first 6 months, so a short trial of antibiotic suppression is probably indicated in most patients (23). An exception to this may in children who already have language delay and recurrent infections complicated by persistent serous otitis media, for whom tympanostomy tubes are indicated as initial therapy (24). However, controlled trials showed no benefit for early insertion of tubes (25). Selected antibiotics for treatment of otitis are shown in Table 19.5.

PATIENT EDUCATION

Ear pain is very common in childhood. The symptoms experienced by children with ear disorders may create a great deal of anxiety in parents in addition to causing sleepless nights

TABLE 19.5 Drug Therapy for Otitis

Drug	Dosage	Contraindications/Cautions/Adverse Effects
Otitis externa		
Neomycin solutions	3–4 drops QID × 7 days	Rupture of tympanic membrane, potential ototoxicity with ruptured tympanic membrane
Ofloxacin solutions	Children 1–12 years: 5 drops BID × 10 days Patients ≥12 years: 10 drops BID × 10 days	Warm bottle in hands to avoid dizziness
Suppurative otitis		
Amoxicillin	40 mg/kg split BID × 5 days	Penicillin allergy, diarrhea (~2%)
Sulfamethoxazole-trimethoprim	8 mg TMP/40 mg sulfamethoxazole divided BID × 10 days	Sulfa allergy; avoid in patients with glucose-6-phosphatase deficiency; avoid in folate deficiency; light sensitivity, skin reactions (2%) with severe reactions in (<0.1%); may cause bone marrow suppression possible with chronic use
Ceftriaxone	50 mg/kg up to 1 g	Cross-reactivity with penicillin allergy; pain at injection site, diarrhea (5%–6%)
Amoxicillin-clavulanate	20–45 mg/day of amoxicillin component in 2 or 3 doses	Penicillin allergy; history of jaundice; select appropriate concentration; diarrhea (up to 40%)
Azithromycin	30 mg/kg as a single dose OR 10 mg/kg QD × 3 days OR 10 mg/kg × 1 day then 5 mg/kg on days 2 through 5	Macrolide allergy; diarrhea (~5%), nausea (~3%), abdominal pain (~3%)
Other second- or third-generation cephalosporins (e.g., cefaclor, cefuroxime, cefixime)	Varies with drug	Caution in penicillin allergy, diarrhea (3%–5%), rash
Prophylaxis for otitis		
Amoxicillin	Half daily dosage at bedtime	Penicillin allergy, diarrhea (2%)
Sulfamethoxazole-Trimethoprim	40 mg/kg sulfamethoxazol 8 mg/kg TMO QHS	Sulfa allergy, skin reactions (2%) with severe reactions in (<0.1%)

QID, four times a day; BID, twice daily; QD, once daily; TMP, trimethoprim; QHS, at bedtime.

and days off from work. When encountering the family with a young child who has ear pain, clinicians should recognize the stress that this illness places on the family as well as try to dispel myths that may have arisen regarding treatment of the problem. Some of the issues that physicians should be prepared to counsel families about include:

- Antibiotic therapy may not change outcomes in children but could cause adverse effects. Parents are accustomed to receiving antibiotics, so challenging this long-held assumption can be difficult. In addition, parents often focus on short-term successes ("Will it help me get some sleep tonight?") as opposed to long-term consequences.
- A treatment failure in one infection does not indicate that a second-line antibiotic must be used for all subsequent infections. Many parents assume that because amoxicillin did not work the last time, it is not going to work this time. This can lead to the unnecessary use of broader-spectrum, more expensive agents and speed the development of drug

resistance. When treatment failures occur, physicians should emphasize at that time that the use of a different drug should not influence the treatment if the child should get another infection in the future.
- Prevention of recurrent otitis media is indicated in few patients and non-surgical options are effective.

CASE DISCUSSION

Otitis media episodes frequently accompany upper respiratory tract infections. Occlusion of the Eustachian tube from the respiratory infection (or in cases of allergic rhinitis) results in the negative middle ear pressure that causes the effusion that characterizes otitis media. Direct visualization of the tympanic membrane is usually all that is sufficient to diagnose an acute suppurative otitis media, although pneumatic otoscopy can help detect fluid when infection is not present.

The evidence shows that for most children over the age of 6 months, otitis media symptoms usually resolve with simple observation only. Children with symptoms persisting over 48 hours benefit from antibiotic therapy. However, at least in the United States, the vast majority of otitis media patients are treated with an antibiotic. New infections should be treated with a narrow-spectrum antibiotic for 3 to 5 days. Broad-spectrum antibiotics should be reserved for persistent infections that do not respond to first-line therapy. For children with recurrent infections, prophylaxis with sulfamethoxazole-trimethoprim or amoxicillin is just as successful as the surgical placement of ventilation tubes. Both antibiotic prophylaxis and ventilation tubes seem to be equally successful at preserving speech function.

Based on evidence that new infections represent a different pathogen than the last one (and the infection being in the opposite ear, which is useful in supporting this view), you explain the rationale for using amoxicillin again. You also discuss with her the role of chronic antibiotic prophylaxis as a successful way of reducing episodes of otitis media while avoiding surgery. She seemed skeptical about the amoxicillin, but when you validated her concerns about the number of episodes and wanting to help her avoid future infections she appeared more willing to follow your recommendations.

In 2 weeks, P.J. is back. He is happy and afebrile. His ear still shows some effusion, but is no longer red or retracted. You and his mother discuss chronic antibiotic prophylaxis and start him on a nightly dose of sulfamethoxazole until the summer.

P.J.'s mother is concerned about the lingering fluid that you note behind his tympanic membrane. She remembers that when she was a child that her doctor was worried she would get "glue ear" from the fluid and suggested she have tubes put in her ears. You reassure her that serous otitis following an acute otitis media is not uncommon and is usually transient. Even in cases of persisting serous otitis, the placement of ventilation tubes is not an emergency since children's speech and hearing continues to develop normally even if insertion of tubes is delayed. You agree to recheck P.J.'s ear in 4 to 6 weeks when the fluid should be resolved.

REFERENCES

1. Kirkwood CR, Clure HR, Brodsky R, et al. The diagnostic content of family practice: 50 most common diagnoses recorded in the WAMI community practices. J Fam Pract. 1982;15:485–492.
2. Marsland DW, Wood M, Mayo F. A data bank for patient care, curriculum, and research in family practice: 526,196 patient problems. J Fam Pract. 1976;3:25–28.
3. Kaplan B, Wandstrat TL, Cunningham JR. Overall cost in the treatment of otitis media. Ped Infect Dis J. 1997;16(2 suppl):S9–S11.
4. Gulya AJ. Anatomy and embryology of the ear. In Hughes GB, Pensak ML, eds. Clinical Otology, 2nd ed. New York, NY: Thieme; 1997.
5. Luz JG, Maragno IC, Martin MC. Characteristics of chief complaints of patients with temporomandibular disorders in a Brazilian population. J Oral Rehabil. 1997;24:240–243.
6. Kuttila S, Kuttila M, Le Bell Y, Alanen P, Jouko S. Aural symptoms and signs of temporomandibular disorder in association with treatment need and visits to a physician. Laryngoscope. 1999;109:1669–1673.
7. Kontiokari T, Koivunen P, Miemela M, Pokka T, Uhari M. Symptoms of acute otitis media. Pediatr Infect Dis J 1998; 17:676–679.
8. Rothman R, Owens T, Simel DL. Does this child have acute otitis media? JAMA. 2003:290:1633–1640.
9. Stewart MH, Siff JE, Cydulka RK. Evaluation of the patient with sore throat, earache, and sinusitis: an evidence based approach. Emerg Med Clinic North Am. 1999;17:153–187.
10. Froom J, Culpepper L, Grob P, Bartelds A, et al. Diagnosis and antibiotic treatment of acute otitis media: Report from International Primary Care Network. BMJ. 1990;300: 528–586
11. Nozza RJ, Bluestone CD, Krdatzke D, Bachman R. Towards the validation of aural acoustic immittance measure for the diagnosis of middle ear effusion in children. Ear Hearing. 1992;13:442453.
12. Sassen ML, Van Aarem A, Gote JJ. Validity of tympanometry in the diagnosis of middle ear effusion. Clin Otolaryngol. 1994;19:185–189.
13. Karma PH, Penttila MA, Sipila MM, et al. Otoscopic diagnosis of middle ear effusion in acute and non-acute OM. Int J Pediatr Otolaryngol. 1989;17:37–49.
14. Koivunen P, Albo O, Ubari M, Niemala M, Luotonen J. Minitympanometry in detecting middle ear fluid. J Pediatr. 1997;131;419–422.
15. Agency for Healthcare Research and Quality. Management of acute otitis media. Evidence Report/Technology Assessment: Number 15, AHRQ publication no. 00-E009. *www.ahrq.gov/clinic/otitisum.htm.*).
16. Licameli GR. Diagnosis and management of otalia in the pediatric population. Pediatr Ann. 1999;28:364–368.
17. Institute for Clinical Systems Improvement. Postgrad Med. 2000;107:239–247.
18. Rosenfeld RM, Vertrees JE, Carr J, et al. Clinical efficacy of antimicrobial drugs for acute otitis media: metanalysis of 5400 children from thirty-three randomized trials. J Pediatr. 1994; 124:355–367.
19. Subcommittee on the Management of Acute Otitis Media. Diagnosis and management of acute otitis media. Pediatrics. 2004:113:1451–1465.
20. Koryrskyj AL, Hildes-Ripstein GE, Longstaffe SEA, et al. Treatment of acute otitis media with a shortened course of antibiotics: a meta-analysis. JAMA. 1998;279:1736–1742.
21. Hueston WJ, Ornstein S, Jenkins RG, Pan Q, Wulfman JS. Treatment of recurrent otitis media after a previous treatment failure: which antibiotics work best? J Fam Pract. 1999; 48:43–46.
22. Pizzuto MP, Volk MS, Hingston LM. Common topics in pediatric otolaryngology. Ped Clin North Am. 1998;45: 973–991.
23. Phillippe BAM, Stenstrom RJ, Feldman W, Durieux-Smith A. Randomized, controlled trial comparing long-term sufonamide therapy to ventilation tubes for otitis media with effusion. Pediatrics. 1991;88:215–222.
24. Rach GH, Zielhuis GA, van Barrle PW, can den Broek P. The effect of treatment with ventilating tubes on language development in preschool children with otitis media with effusion. Clin Otolaryngol Appl Sci. 1991;16:128–132.
25. Paradise JL, Feldman HM, Campbell TF, et al. Effect of early or delayed insertion of tympanostomy tubes for persistent otitis media on developmental outcomes at the age of three years. N Engl J Med. 2001;344:1179–1187.

CHAPTER 20

Common Eye Problems

Gary R. Gray and Rebecca Rosen

CASE 1

Mr. W. is 21 years old, and presents with a chief complaint of a red, watery and "irritated" right eye. He is concerned that he has pink eye. His symptoms started two days ago but have worsened over the past 24 hours. His vision is fine except he has to blink a lot to clear the discharge covering his eye when he awakens. He has had some "cold symptoms" consisting of a runny nose and a scratchy throat. He denies eye pain, history of trauma, irritant, or chemical exposure. He does not wear contact lenses. He has noted some very minimal itching in his eye.

He takes no medications and relates an unremarkable medical history. Examination reveals a healthy appearing male in no apparent distress. Vital signs: blood pressure 125/68; temperature 99.0; respirations 14; pulse 75. His exam is remarkable for some clear rhinorrhea. His oropharynx is normal except for some scant postnasal drip. Visual acuity is 20/30 in each eye. Ocular exam is remarkable for conjunctival injection (hyperemia) and tearing of the right eye. Pupils are equal round and reactive to light. Lids and lashes appear normal except for a slight mucoid discharge on his lower lashes. No lymphadenopathy is noted.

CLINICAL QUESTIONS

1. What are the differential diagnoses for his red eye?
2. What physical exam findings are most useful for clarifying the diagnosis?
3. What historical findings aid the physician in evaluating a patient with a red eye?
4. What key physical exam or historical findings would suggest a possible serious or vision threatening eye disorder?

CASE 2

Mrs. L. is 63 years old and presents to your office complaining of red, itchy eyes that are caked with "gunk," especially upon awakening. She states that there is a gritty feeling along the lids, and she has noticed that a lot of her eyelashes are breaking off and falling out. Her eyes are drier than they used to be, which she attributes to the dry climate. She has suffered with these symptoms for the last 2 to 3 years, but 2 weeks ago she noticed a small bump along her left lower eyelid that has been increasing in size. The bump

was initially red but now it is neither red nor painful, but she finds it unsightly and wants it removed as soon as possible. On exam, all of Mrs. L.'s observations are confirmed. Also noted are small flakes at the bases of the lashes. The left lower eyelid mass is about 1 × 0.5 cm and nontender. Her visual acuity is normal. On general exam, she is noted to have a slightly red nose and chin, fine telangiectasias on her cheeks, and some pustules over her cheeks and nose. When asked, she admits to frequent bouts of facial flushing as well.

CLINICAL QUESTIONS

1. Does Mrs. L. need to be referred to an ophthalmologist to have the bump removed?
2. Does Mrs. L. have an underlying condition that should be addressed in addition to her other complaints?
3. What are your treatment recommendations? Does she need an antibiotic?

CASE 3

Mr. D. is 55 years old and presents to your office complaining of the sudden appearance of floaters after a "shower of black dots" in his right eye this morning. These floaters move with eye movement. He also thinks that his vision in his right eye may not be as sharp as in his left eye. He wears glasses for his nearsightedness and has always had one or two floaters in the same eye. He denies any recent trauma or any "foreign body" sensation. He is anxious and worried that he might be going blind in his right eye, and he is also worried about the same thing happening in the left eye.

CLINICAL QUESTIONS

1. What further history do you want to know?
2. In addition to your bilateral fundus exam, what are the other key aspects of the physical exam?
3. What is your differential diagnosis, and what prognostic information can you tell Mr. D.?

Red eye is the most common ophthalmic disorder encountered in the family physicians' office practice (1). Although most cases represent a relatively benign self-limited process, the physician must be able to accurately assess the patient and rule out potential vision-threatening disorders. Therefore, a thorough understanding of the potential etiologies coupled with a careful history and physical exam is essential.

Infectious and inflammatory disorders of the eyelids are frequently encountered in the family physician's office practice. Many conditions may be successfully treated by the family physician, though some require surgical intervention and referral to an ophthalmologist.

Although it is not commonly encountered in their daily practices, most family physicians will be faced with a patient suffering from sudden visual loss. An accurate, quick assessment is the key to preserving vision.

There is considerable overlap in the symptomatology and differential diagnosis of ocular conditions. Patients' descriptions are often not precise, and they may focus only on the particular symptom that is most bothersome to them, overlooking other symptoms that a physician would find more alarming. A systematic approach is recommended.

DIFFERENTIAL DIAGNOSIS OF THE RED EYE

Conjunctivitis, inflammation of the conjunctiva, a thin transparent membrane covering the sclera and inner surfaces of the eyelids, is the most common cause of red eye (1, 2). The four main causes of painful red eye—corneal lesions, uveitis, acute glaucoma, and scleritis—all represent involvement of deeper eye structures (3). Subconjunctival hemorrhages are a commonly encountered cause of a painless red eye.

Historical clues and clinical findings guide the physician to the appropriate diagnosis and plan of action. Table 20.1 summarizes the differential diagnosis of red eye. Although the frequency of more serious diseases is low in the family physicians' office, they must always be considered.

Conjunctivitis

Conjunctivitis includes both infectious and noninfectious etiologies. The true incidence of conjunctivitis is not clearly defined though it is likely the number one acute ocular condition seen in primary care practices (2). Table 20.2 describes the most common etiologies of conjunctivitis. Although widely used, the actual diagnostic usefulness of specific signs and symptoms in conjunctivitis is poor. There is little evidence to either support or refute their use (4). Conjunctival hyper-

TABLE 20.1 Differential Diagnosis of the Patient with a Red Eye

Diagnosis	Frequency
Conjunctivitis	Very common
Keratitis	Uncommon
Uveitis	Uncommon
Corneal lesions/abrasions	Common
Scleritis	Uncommon
Acute glaucoma	Uncommon
Subconjunctival hemorrhage	Common

emia (redness) is a common finding in all cases of conjunctivitis. Tearing, itching, foreign body sensation, and ocular discharge are all characteristic of conjunctivitis, although these findings vary according to underlying etiology.

Infectious conjunctivitis can be caused by a variety of viruses and bacteria. The most common infectious etiologies are listed in Table 20.2. Clinical findings and history serve as primary guidance for diagnosis. For example, a purulent ocular discharge is more likely to be associated with a bacterial etiology, whereas a serous discharge is more likely associated with a viral cause.

Allergic conjunctivitis is often seasonal and found in persons with an individual history of allergic rhinitis, asthma, or atopic dermatitis. Clinical clues include bilateral involvement, ocular itching, and watery or mucoid discharge.

Mechanical or irritative conjunctivitis may be associated with contact lens use, chemical exposure, and dry eyes (keratoconjunctivitis sicca). A detailed history is crucial. Patients should be asked specifically about contact lens wear, including the use of sterilizing and wetting solutions. Thimerosal, a mercury-based preservative in contact lens solutions, has been associated with irritation. Potential workplace irritants include ultraviolet light, dust, chemicals, and tobacco smoke. Patients who use topical capsaicin for musculoskeletal pain may complain of irritation if they touch their eyes while their fingers are contaminated with the medication.

Acute Narrow Angle Glaucoma

Acute narrow angle closure glaucoma is an ophthalmologic emergency. Its pathophysiology involves blockage of the aqueous humor flow through the canal of Schlemm, resulting in an increased intraocular pressure. Most patients with acute narrow angle glaucoma have preexisting shallow anterior chamber angles (between the iris and the cornea). Acute angle closure may be precipitated by pupillary dilation from medications with anticholinergic and sympathomimetic effects. The following are associated with an increased risk for acute angle closure (5):

- Hyperopia
- Family history of angle closure glaucoma
- Advancing age
- Female
- Asian or Inuit descent

Patients with acute angle closure glaucoma have a dramatic presentation of pain and blurred vision. Patients may see halos around lights. Characteristic physical findings include conjunctival hyperemia, corneal cloudiness, and papillary dilation, with a sluggish or absent response to light.

Subconjunctival Hemorrhage

A subconjunctival hemorrhage is an easily recognized condition in which blood accumulates between the conjunctiva and sclera. Usually a benign process, it may be caused by minor trauma, excessive coughing, pushing in labor and delivery, vomiting, or other conditions associated with a significant Valsalva maneuver (6.) Patients with hypertension and diabetes are more susceptible, as well as those taking anticoagulant medications.

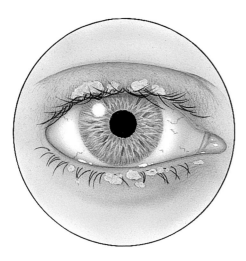

Figure 20.2 • Red-rimmed eyelids with scaling and debris at the eyelash base and broken lashes in blepharitis. (Asset provided by Anatomical Chart Company.)

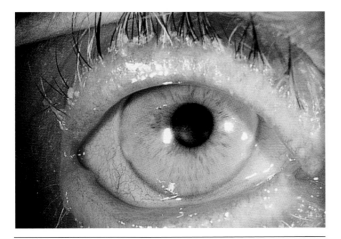

Figure 20.3 • Blepharitis. (From Weber J, Kelly J. Health Assessment in Nursing, 2nd ed. Philadelphia: Lippincott Williams & Wilkins; 2003.)

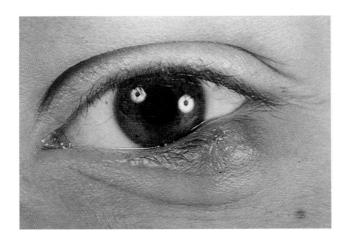

Figure 20.4 • Hordeolum: note the localized swelling and erythema with eyelash follicle involvement. (From Goodheart HP. Goodheart's Photoguide of Common Skin Disorders, 2nd ed. Philadelphia: Lippincott Williams & Wilkins; 2003.)

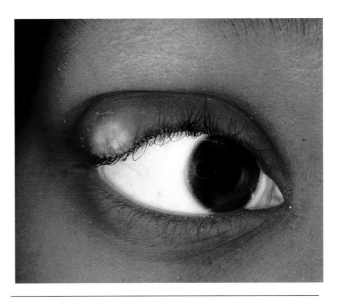

Figure 20.5 • Internal hordeolum. A 9-year-old female presented with a 3-day history of a painful, fast growing lesion on her right upper eyelid. (From Fleisher GR, Ludwig W, Baskin MN. Atlas of Pediatric Emergency Medicine. Philadelphia: Lippincott Williams & Wilkins; 2004.)

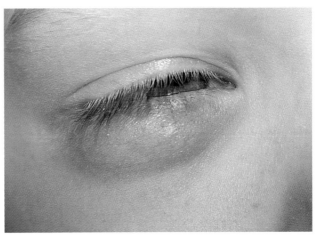

Figure 20.6 • Chalazion. A 7-year-old male presented with a large, slow growing, painless mass that developed on his lower lid over 4 months. (From Tasman W, Jaeger E. The Wills Eye Hospital Atlas of Clinical Ophthalmology, 2nd ed. Baltimore: Lippincott Williams & Wilkins; 2001.)

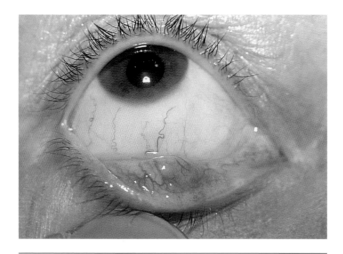

Figure 20.7 • Chalazion. Note the conjunctival component with the lower eyelid everted. (From Tasman W, Jaeger E. The Wills Eye Hospital Atlas of Clinical Ophthalmology. 2nd ed. Baltimore: Lippincott Williams & Wilkins; 2001.)

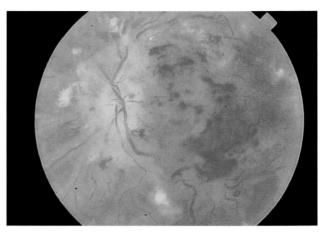

Figure 20.9 • Retinal hemorrhages. Abnormal retinal vessels and background. Note the ``flame-shaped'' hemorrhages—the linear red streaks on the retina. (From Weber J, Kelly J. Health Assessment in Nursing. 2nd ed. Philadelphia: Lippincott Williams & Wilkins; 2003.)

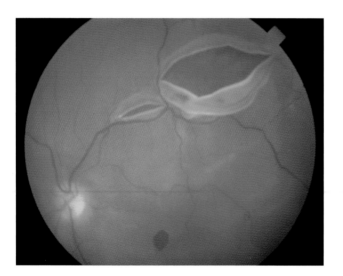

Figure 20.8 • Two retinal tears due to trauma. Note the macular tear inferiorly. (From Tasman W, Jaeger E. The Wills Eye Hospital Atlas of Clinical Ophthalmology. 2nd ed. Baltimore: Lippincott Williams & Wilkins; 2001.)

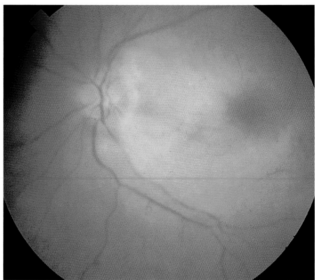

Figure 20.10 • Retinal artery occlusion resulting in retinal edema and a ``cherry red'' macula. (From Gold DH, Weingeist TA. Color Atlas of the Eye in Systemic Disease. Baltimore: Lippincott Williams & Wilkins; 2001.)

TABLE 20.2 Common Causes of Conjunctivitis and Associated Symptoms and Clinical Findings

Etiology	Symptoms and Clinical Findings
Infectious Conjunctivitis	
1. Viral Conjunctivitis:	**Viral Conjunctivitis:**
Adenovirus: Pharyngoconjunctival fever types 3 and 7, epidemic keratoconjunctivitis types 8 and 19	Unilateral involvement. Minimal itching marked tearing, minimal exudative discharge.
Enterovirus: Hemorrhagic conjunctivitis	
Herpes simplex	May be associated with URI symptoms (adenovirus).
Varicella zoster	Preauricular adenopathy common
2. Bacterial Conjunctivitis:	**Bacterial Conjunctivitis:**
Pneumococcus	Unilateral involvement.
Haemophilus influenzae	Minimal itching, moderate tearing.
Staphylococcus aureus	Profuse exudative (purulent) discharge.
Neisseria gonorrhoeae Chlamydia	Preauricular adenopathy uncommon.
Allergic Conjunctivitis	Bilateral involvement. Marked ocular itching, moderate tearing. Watery or mucoid discharge.

Corneal Abrasions

Corneal abrasions represent mechanical damage to the corneal epithelium. Symptoms include pain, photophobia, and a foreign body feeling associated with excess tearing (7). The history is often notable for a distinct precipitating event.

Scleritis, Uveitis, Keratitis

These inflammatory conditions of the deeper eye structures are significantly less common causes of red eye than conjunctivitis (8). The hallmark clinical finding in these conditions is ocular pain. Reduced visual acuity is common in both uveitis and keratitis and may accompany scleritis as well. Keratitis represents the clinical manifestation of inflammation involving the corneal epithelium. Underlying causes include (8):

- Dry eyes
- Severe viral conjunctivitis
- Ultraviolet light exposure (sunburn)
- Contact lens use

Uveitis represents inflammation of the iris and ciliary body. This condition is also commonly termed iritis or iridocyclitis and is associated with several common autoimmune diseases including (8):

- Juvenile rheumatoid arthritis
- Ankylosing spondylitis
- Systemic lupus erythematosus (SLE)
- Sarcoidosis

Scleritis refers to inflammatory conditions involving the sclera and has been associated with SLE, rheumatoid arthritis, and polyarteritis nodosa (8).

DIFFERENTIAL DIAGNOSIS OF EYELID DISORDERS

Blepharitis

Blepharitis, one of the most common ocular disorders (9), is a chronic bilateral inflammatory process affecting the eyelid margins. There are two types of blepharitis, defined by their anatomic location—anterior or posterior. The two main causes of anterior blepharitis are seborrheic dermatitis and staphylococcal infection, or a combination of the two (10, 11). Posterior blepharitis is caused by Meibomian gland dysfunction in which the openings of the Meibomian glands become clogged, resulting in thickening of the eyelids, chalazion, and eventual atrophy of the Meibomian glands (9). The Meibomian glands are important because they secrete oils that prevent the tear layer from evaporating too quickly and thus play an important role in keeping the surface of the eye moist and hydrated. If the glands atrophy and the oils dry up, the tear layer will evaporate rapidly, resulting in dry eye and possible subsequent conjunctivitis and keratitis. Anterior and posterior blepharitis may exist simultaneously. Blepharitis can begin in childhood but occurs more commonly in the 6th and 7th decades (10, 11) and in people who suffer from acne rosacea or seborrheic dermatitis of the face and scalp. Other more acute causes include contact dermatitis, head lice (pediculosis), and association with the use of isotretinoin (Accutane) (9).

Hordeolum and Chalazion

A hordeolum or sty is an acute suppurative infection of either the Meibomian gland (internal hordeolum) or of the eyelash follicle or tear gland (external hordeolum). The main causative organism is usually *Staphylococcus aureus*.

A chalazion is a chronic, sterile, granulomatous lesion of the Meibomian glands (deep chalazion) or of the Zeis glands (superficial), which results from gland obstruction. An acute chalazion may appear and present similarly to a hordeolum, or may result from a persistent hordeolum. Chalazia, as discussed above, are often associated with chronic blepharitis, acne rosacea, seborrhea, conjunctivitis, and hordeolum.

DIFFERENTIAL DIAGNOSIS OF VISUAL LOSS

Causes of painless loss of vision, with and without floaters, that the family physician may encounter, include retinal detachment, vitreous hemorrhage, central or branch retinal vein occlusion, and central retinal artery occlusion.

Retinal Detachment

To understand retinal detachment, it is important to understand the physiology of the vitreous and retina. The vitreous is composed of a gel-like substance that makes up 80% of the ocular globe volume (12). Mostly water interwoven by collagen fibrils, this gel also contains salts, soluble proteins, glycoproteins, and glycosaminoglycans. Over time, the vitreous undergoes liquefaction; this liquefaction, or synersis, is more common in the elderly population, and in people with high myopia (12). Retinal detachment occurs when the pigmented retina separates from the inner sensory retina, allowing the liquid vitreous to seep between the two layers. The pigmented layer and its underlying choroid perfuse the neurosensory retina; if this continuity is disrupted, the neurosensory retina becomes ischemic, and the photoreceptors degenerate resulting in vision loss.

There are several different etiologies of retinal detachment. They are divided into two categories: rhegmatogenous (from *rhegma*, the Greek word for tear) and nonrhegmatogenous retinal detachment. The causes of rhegmatogenous tears (RDD) are atrophic retinal holes caused by lattice degeneration (an atrophic process that leads to focal thinning of the retina), posterior vitreous detachment, and traumatic (blunt or penetrating ocular injury). Nonrhegmatogenous retinal detachment occurs primarily from vitreous traction on the retina. In patients who have neovascularization and diabetic proliferative retinopathy, there are areas of adhesion created between the vitreous and the retina (as a result of fibrosis and neovascularization). If there is shrinking or contraction of the vitreous, the neurosensory retina, at the point of adhesion, is pulled away from the pigmented retina resulting in detachment without a retinal tear. The presenting symptoms are usually flashes of light or photopsia, which result from the retinal traction and not from direct retinal stimulation, and a sudden shower of black dots, which are red blood cells in the vitreous after rupture of a retinal vessel.

The incidence of RDD is approximately 10 to 15 per 100,000 persons per year (13) or one in 10,000 per year (14). It occurs more commonly in men, in the elderly, and in people with degenerative myopia (15). Risk factors include myopia, lattice degeneration, cataract surgery, trauma, history of RDD in the other eye (13), and, to a lesser extent, family history of rhegmatogenous retinal detachment (RRD) (14). A combination of any of these risk factors increases the risk. People with nontraumatic RDD have a 10% increased risk of RRD in the opposite eye. Early diagnosis and referral to an ophthalmologist for timely treatment are critical to preserve vision.

Vitreous or Retinal Hemorrhage

Vitreous hemorrhage, caused by rupture of the retinal vessels, has multiple etiologies. The rupture of the blood vessel releases red blood cells into the avascular vitreous, which are interpreted by the patient as floaters or dark lines. If there is significant hemorrhage, there can be a sudden, painless loss of vision resulting in only light perception due to obscuring by the blood. Among the most common etiologies are: 1) tears in the abnormal vessels of neovascularization as seen in diabetic retinopathy (most common etiology) or in the retinopathy that accompanies sickle cell disease; 2) retinal detachment; 3) posterior vitreous detachment; 4) central or branch retinal vein occlusion; and 5) trauma.

Central or Branch Retinal Vein Occlusion and Central Retinal Artery Occlusion

Central or branch retinal vein occlusion represents a blockage of retinal venous flow. The two conditions share a similar pathophysiology, with branch retinal vein occlusion being more common. Risk factors for these conditions are similar to those associated with other thrombotic conditions such as stroke and myocardial infarction. Risk factors include:

- Hypertension
- Smoking
- Diabetes
- Advancing age

Central retinal artery occlusion (CRAO) is an ocular emergency as permanent blindness can result caused by infarction of the retina. In CRAO, an embolic or thrombotic event results in sudden, painless vision loss (16). Embolic etiologies include cardiogenic or carotid emboli. Thrombosis may result from arteriosclerosis, which is the most common underlying systemic etiology (17), giant cell arteritis, collagen vascular diseases, or hypercoagulable states (16).

CLINICAL EVALUATION

History and Physical Examination

Important general elements of the history and physical examination are summarized below, and in Tables 20.3 and 20.4. The history should focus on the duration of symptoms, unilateral versus bilateral involvement, and presence and characterization of any discharge. Inquire about sys-temic illnesses (e.g., connective tissue diseases, Marfan's syndrome) that may have ocular manifestations. A medication history is useful to identify systemic and topical agents that may cause ocular symptoms, such as dryness or blurred vision. A sexual history may identify those patients at risk for *Chlamydia trachomatis* and *Neisseria gonorrhoeae* eye infection. Penetrating trauma is an ophthalmic emergency requiring immediate ophthalmic attention. One should always inquire regarding decreased visual acuity, photophobia, and globe pain, which signify involvement of the deeper structures of the eye, necessitating referral to an ophthalmologist (see Table 20.5).

Ask follow-up questions to uncover exactly what the pa-

TABLE 20.3	Key Historical Elements

1. Symptoms and signs: itching, discharge, irritation, pain, photophobia
2. Duration of symptoms
3. Unilateral or bilateral disease
4. Type of discharge: mucoid, watery, purulent
5. Exposure to infection
6. History of trauma
7. Contact lens wear
8. Use of eye cosmetics
9. Signs of systemic disease: urethritis, cervicitis, skin lesions
10. History of atopy
11. Decreased vision

TABLE 20.5	Red Flags for Patients Presenting With a Red Eye

Globe pain
Decreased visual acuity
Sluggish papillary reflex
Dendritic corneal lesions suggesting herpes simplex infection
Vesicular lesions suggesting herpes zoster

Prompt ophthalmologic consultation indicated

tient is experiencing. Blurred vision is a very nonspecific term, and may be used by patients to describe a variety of disparate complaints, including glare, diplopia, refractive errors, impaired accommodation, photophobia, and others. Accurate identification of the patient's true complaint is essential for the formulation of the differential diagnosis. This will help to focus the physical examination on the relevant findings.

The physical examination of the eye should begin with a visual acuity exam. If the patient wears eyeglasses, test acuity with and without glasses. Regional lymphadenopathy, especially preauricular adenopathy, suggests adenoviral conjunctivitis. The presence of vesicular skin lesions associated with ocular complaints suggests herpes simplex or varicella zoster. If available, fluorescein staining and a slit-lamp exam should be performed and an evaluation for foreign bodies, corneal ulcerations, abrasions, or other lesions. Pupillary abnormalities suggest a serious process, such as acute glaucoma, uveitis, scleritis or keratitis. Check for eyelid eversion (ectropion) or entropion, which may cause irritation. Assess the function of extraocular muscles and check for foreign bodies. Eversion of the

upper eyelid, gently folding it over a soft swab stick, allows inspection of the inner surface for lesions or embedded foreign bodies. An algorithm for evaluation of the red eye is provided in Figure 20.1.

Diagnostic Testing

Cultures and other laboratory evaluations are generally not useful or required. Specific instances where culture is indicated include: neonatal conjunctivitis, recurrent or severe purulent conjunctivitis, and suspected *N. gonorrhoeae* or *Chlamydia* infections. Radiologic imaging is not helpful unless a foreign body is suspected. Magnetic resonance imaging (MRI) may be contraindicated, if it causes movement of a metallic object.

Special Considerations
BLEPHARITIS

Patients with blepharitis complain of a burning or gritty sensation in their eyes as well as itching, irritation, and redness of the eyelid margins. They also complain of their eyelids sticking together, especially upon awakening. The history should include questions directed at systemic symptoms, exacerbating factors, duration, allergies, infected contacts, and previous and current medications (9). The physical exam should be performed in a well-lit room. The patient's skin and scalp should be inspected for signs of seborrheic dermatitis, rosacea, atopic dermatitis, or head lice. On physical exam, the lid margins are erythematous and swollen, and there are fine flakes or debris and scales or collarettes (a crust that encircles the base of an eyelash) clinging to the base of the lashes, which are themselves often small, thin, broken, or sometimes white (9, 10). There may also be vesicles or ulcers along the eyelid margin, and a hordeolum or chalazion may also be present (see Color Plate Figures 20.2 and 20.3).

HORDEOLUM

The patient presents with the complaint of a swollen, painful, and often red mass along the lid margin. This mass may be indurated and may rupture (see Color Plate Figures 20.4 and 20.5). On exam, in addition to the above findings, there may also be preauricular lymphadenopathy (18).

TABLE 20.4	Physical Examination

1. Visual acuity
2. Slit-lamp examination (if available)
3. Fluorescein testing
4. External examination:
   a. Regional lymphadenopathy
   b. Conjunctiva: injection, hemorrhage, discharge
   c. Cornea exam facilitated by dye staining: abrasions, erosions, ulcerations, presence of dendritic lesions
   d. Eye lashes and lids: swelling, lesions, crusting
   e. Pupillary reflex

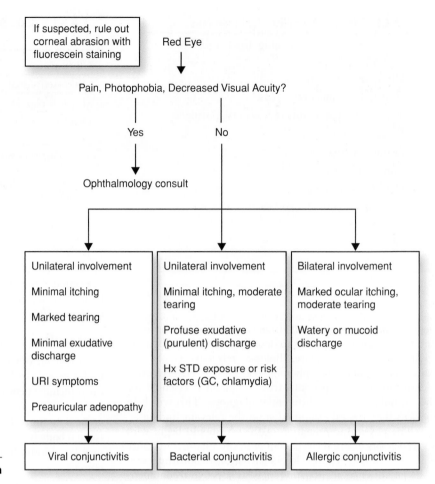

If suspected, rule out corneal abrasion with fluorescein staining	Red Eye

Pain, Photophobia, Decreased Visual Acuity?

Yes   No

Ophthalmology consult

Unilateral involvement	Unilateral involvement	Bilateral involvement
Minimal itching	Minimal itching, moderate tearing	Marked ocular itching, moderate tearing
Marked tearing	Profuse exudative (purulent) discharge	Watery or mucoid discharge
Minimal exudative discharge	Hx STD exposure or risk factors (GC, chlamydia)	
URI symptoms		
Preauricular adenopathy		
Viral conjunctivitis	Bacterial conjunctivitis	Allergic conjunctivitis

Figure 20.1 • Diagnostic approach to red eye.

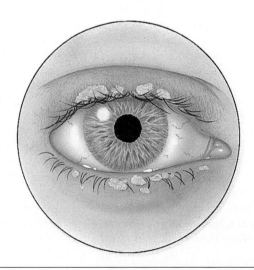

Figure 20.2 • Red-rimmed eyelids with scaling and debris at the eyelash base and broken lashes in blepharitis. (Asset provided by Anatomical Chart Company.)

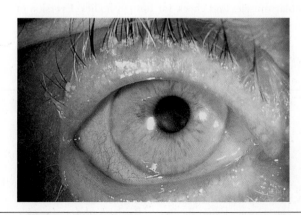

Figure 20.3 • Blepharitis. (From Weber J, Kelly J. Health Assessment in Nursing, 2nd ed. Philadelphia: Lippincott Williams & Wilkins; 2003.)

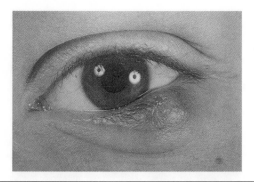

Figure 20.4 • Hordeolum: note the localized swelling and erythema with eyelash follicle involvement. (From Goodheart HP. Goodheart's Photoguide of Common Skin Disorders, 2nd ed. Philadelphia: Lippincott Williams & Wilkins; 2003.)

CHALAZION

Although the initial presentation may involve a tender, erythematous swelling or nodule, a chalazion is usually a painless lump on the eyelid. If large enough, chalazia may cause discomfort and even compress the cornea causing astigmatism. Patients may complain of nothing else, but the fact that chalazia can be cosmetically disfiguring (see Color Plate Figures 20.6 and 20.7).

RETINAL DETACHMENT

The evaluation of a patient with suspected retinal detachment includes a fundus exam with the ophthalmoscope. The key points in the patient's history should include:

- Symptoms like flashing lights or increased floaters
- Family history
- Prior eye trauma/surgery

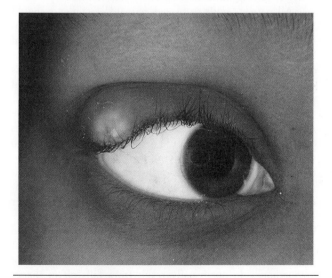

Figure 20.5 • Internal hordeolum. A 9-year-old female presented with a 3-day history of a painful, fast growing lesion on her right upper eyelid. (From Fleisher GR, Ludwig W, Baskin MN. Atlas of Pediatric Emergency Medicine. Philadelphia: Lippincott Williams & Wilkins; 2004.)

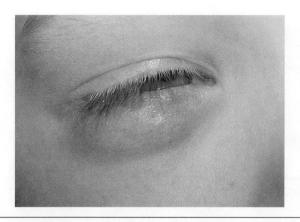

Figure 20.6 • Chalazion. A 7-year-old male presented with a large, slow growing, painless mass that developed on his lower lid over 4 months. (From Tasman W, Jaeger E. The Wills Eye Hospital Atlas of Clinical Ophthalmology, 2nd ed. Baltimore: Lippincott Williams & Wilkins; 2001.)

- Myopia
- History of cataract surgery (13)

In patients with a retinal detachment, the fundus appears gray and thin. A horseshoe-shaped tear may be visible (see Color Plate Figure 20.8).

Physical exam findings in patients with vitreous or retinal hemorrhage include a blood meniscus or collection of blood, which can be seen in the vitreous, or pre-retinal space. In the case of a retinal hemorrhage, areas of red or yellow punctuations, or streaks, or "flame-like" lesions can be appreciated on the retinal surface (see Color Plate Figure 20.9).

Patients with central or branch retinal vein occlusion will present with painless unilateral vision loss or diminished visual acuity; they may also complain of floaters. These patients may present to urgent care or to the emergency department instead of seeking immediate care from an ophthalmologist. It is very important to obtain a thorough medical history as hypertension, diabetes mellitus, atherosclerosis, glaucoma, co-

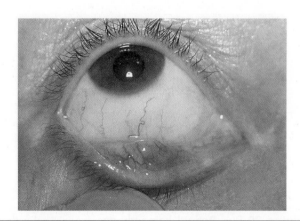

Figure 20.7 • Chalazion. Note the conjunctival component with the lower eyelid everted. (From Tasman W, Jaeger E. The Wills Eye Hospital Atlas of Clinical Ophthalmology. 2nd ed. Baltimore: Lippincott Williams & Wilkins; 2001.)

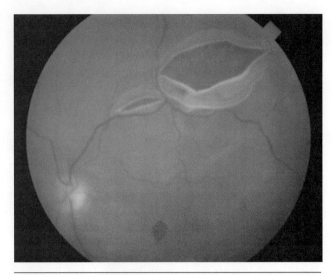

Figure 20.8 • Two retinal tears due to trauma. Note the macular tear inferiorly. (From Tasman W, Jaeger E. The Wills Eye Hospital Atlas of Clinical Ophthalmology. 2nd ed. Baltimore: Lippincott Williams & Wilkins; 2001.)

agulation disorders, hyperlipidemia, anticardiolipin antibodies, and vasculitis are among some of the common risk factors (19). Central retinal vein occlusion (CRVO) affects mainly older patients, usually 50 years or older (19). Visual acuity may be 20/15 or decrease to 20/100–20/200, or be reduced to just light perception (19). The patient may also have visual field defects, especially if the occlusion is in a branch of the central retinal vein. On exam, it is common to see retinal hemorrhages, cotton wool spots (retinal ischemia), a swollen optic disc (RVO inhibits venous return from the retina leading to increased ocular pressure), and dilated and tortuous veins along the retinal surface (see Color Plate Figure 20.10).

The funduscopic exam in cases of CRAO may show diffuse whitening of the fundus because of ischemia as well as a pathognomonic cherry-red spot, which is the choroid showing

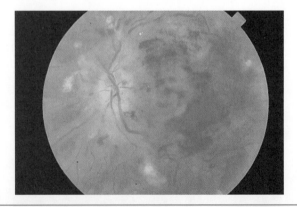

Figure 20.9 • Retinal hemorrhages. Abnormal retinal vessels and background. Note the "flame-shaped" hemorrhages—the linear red streaks on the retina. (From Weber J, Kelly J. Health Assessment in Nursing. 2nd ed. Philadelphia: Lippincott Williams & Wilkins; 2003.)

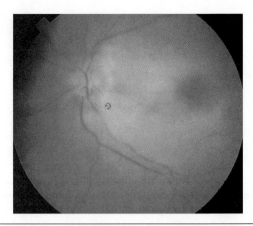

Figure 20.10 • Retinal artery occlusion resulting in retinal edema and a "cherry red" macula. (From Gold DH, Weingeist TA. Color Atlas of the Eye in Systemic Disease. Baltimore: Lippincott Williams & Wilkins; 2001.)

through the ischemic macula. There may also be "box car" segmentation of the venous vessels, which represents occlusion of the circulation, and sometimes emboli can be visualized. The physical exam should include auscultation of the heart and carotids and, once the immediacy of the situation has passed, imaging of the heart and the carotids should be performed as well.

MANAGEMENT

Patients with scleritis, uveitis, and keratitis should generally not be managed by primary care physicians, as they all have a potential to cause permanent visual impairment. Acute narrow-angle glaucoma is an absolute ophthalmologic emergency requiring immediate specialty consultation.

All patients with suspected retinal detachments should be immediately referred to an ophthalmologist. If the symptoms are consistent with retinal detachment, and both visual acuity and funds exam appear normal, the patient still requires evaluation by an ophthalmologist. The treatment for RDD is surgical, re-approximating the sensory retina to the retinal pigmented epithelium; 95% can be repaired (13, 15).

Patients with vitreous or retinal hemorrhages should be referred for evaluation by an ophthalmologist. However, it is the family doctor who should work with their patients to treat and control the underlying diabetes, hypertension, and hyperlipidemia that are among the risk factors for retinal and vitreous hemorrhage. Vitreous or retinal hemorrhages in infants and children less than 3 years old (20), especially after 1 month of age when most birth trauma retinal hemorrhages have resolved (21), are considered pathognomonic for child abuse, i.e., the shaken baby syndrome, and these cases must be addressed and investigated immediately. These types of hemorrhages do not usually result from falls off of diaper tables or beds (20).

Referral to an ophthalmologist is imperative for diagnosis of branch and CRVOs. The contralateral eye may be affected in 12% of patients within 4 years (22). There is no established treatment except to prevent further damage through treatment of the underlying disorders. Blood pressure control, treatment of glaucoma, treatment of hyperlipidemia, and addressing other atherosclerotic risk factors, such as smoking and diabetes, are essential.

Treatment of CRAO involves lowering of intraocular pressure and/or vasodilation to dislodge or move the thrombus distally into more peripheral arterioles, thereby reducing the area of infarct (17). Vasodilation can be attempted through compression and rapid decompression of the eye by putting pressure on the globe and then letting go suddenly for several attempts, with intermittent fundal exams to assess blood flow (17). Other treatment modalities include topical beta blockers, oral nitrates, paracentesis of aqueous humor, retrobulbar anesthetic block, hyperbaric oxygen, inhalation of carbogen (a mixture of 95% oxygen and 5% carbon dioxide), and direct infusion of thrombolytics into the ophthalmic artery (17, 23). Despite these varied modalities, prognosis for vision recovery is poor. However, prompt diagnosis and initiation of treatment correlates with better prognosis (23). A transient, painless monocular loss, blurring of vision, or amaurosis fugax is a symptom usually associated with strokes. However, it may also precede CRAO. Any patient presenting with amaurosis fugax requires prompt attention and work-up to assess and then treat, if possible, the underlying disease processes that could lead to further morbidity and mortality.

Conjunctivitis

Most cases of conjunctivitis can be managed by the primary care physician. Herpes simplex and varicella zoster infections are indications for ophthalmologic evaluation, and require treatment with oral antiviral mediations. Patients with suspected glaucoma and inflammatory disorders of the deeper eye structures should also be urgently referred for specialty care.

The management of conjunctivitis is specific to the underlying etiology. Viral conjunctivitis (excluding herpesviruses) is a self-limited process. Adenoviral conjunctivitis can be treated with local measures, such as cool compresses, artificial tears, and topical vasoconstrictor drops. Although commonly prescribed, antibiotics are of no value, and the incidence of secondary bacterial infection is low (1). Topical corticosteroids have been demonstrated to reduce scarring in cases of severe conjunctivitis, but their use should be guided by ophthalmic consultation because of the risk of adverse events, including herpesvirus infection. Herpes simplex and varicella infections are treated with oral antiviral therapy; ocular steroid preparations should be avoided. Patients with suspected adenoviral conjunctivitis should be reminded that they will remain contagious for up to 7 to 10 days and should pay particular attention to hand washing and avoiding contact with others.

The treatment of bacterial conjunctivitis usually involves prescribing topical ophthalmic antibiotic drops or ointment. Nonsexually transmitted bacterial infections may be self limiting, although expert consensus generally supports treatment to reduce illness duration, decrease disease communicability, and reduce complication rate. Systemic antibiotics are indicated in gonococcal and chlamydial infections, and necessitate a referral to an ophthalmologist. Commonly used ophthalmic antibiotics are listed in Table 20.6. It is generally advisable to use ointments in young children, as applying drops can be difficult. Specific antibiotic selection is not critical, although generally quinolones are unnecessary in cases of simple bacterial conjunctivitis. Erythromycin, bacitracin-polymyxin B, sul-

TABLE 20.6 Common Ophthalmic Antibiotics

Drug	Cautions	Dosage	Relative Cost*
Bacitracin-polymyxin B (ointment)	History of allergy	Small ribbon of ointment to eye every 3–4 hours	$
Gramicidin-neomycin-polymyxin B (solution)	History of allergy	1–2 drops every 4 hours	$$
Erythromycin (ointment)	History of allergy	Small ribbon of ointment to eye every 4 hours	$
Sulfacetamide (10% solution) (10% ointment)	History of allergy Contact lenses Age <2 months	1–2 drops every 4 hours, small ribbon of ointment to eye every 3–4 hours	$
Gentamycin (solution and ointment)	History of allergy	1–2 drops every 4–6 hours, small ribbon of ointment to eye every 8 hours	$
Tobramycin (solution and ointment)	History of allergy	1–2 drops every 4–6 hours, small ribbon of ointment to eye every 8 hours	$$
Ciprofloxacin (solution and ointment)	History of allergy Age <1 year	1–2 drops every 4 hours, small ribbon of ointment to eye every 8 hours × 2 days then BID	$$
Ofloxacin (solution)	History of allergy Age <1 year	1–2 drops every 4 hours	$$$

Relative cost: $, <$33.00; $$, $34.00–$66.00; $$$, >$67.00

facetamide, and aminoglycosides all remain reasonable first-line choices. Topical antibiotics should generally be continued until resolution is noted. Aminoglycosides such as neomycin and gentamycin have been associated with ocular allergic reactions, a consideration if the patient notes worsening symptoms with the use of these agents. Many providers recommend that antibiotics be stopped 24 hours after the initial resolution of redness and other symptoms. Follow-up is generally unnecessary, although patients should be told to return if their symptoms fail to improve over several days, or worsen.

Allergic conjunctivitis is treated symptomatically with topical antihistamine drops, either alone or in combination with a vasoconstrictor. Persistent symptoms may be treated with topical mast cell stabilizers. Ketorolac, a topical nonsteroidal anti-inflammatory drug (NSAID), may help with allergic conjunctivitis, and oral antihistamines may provide symptomatic relief. Ophthalmic corticosteroids, while beneficial, should be used only with the recommendation of an ophthalmologist. Commonly used ophthalmic allergy preparations are listed in Table 20.7.

Corneal Abrasion

The recommended management of corneal abrasions has changed over the past decade. Historically, eye patching was commonly used in patients with corneal abrasions. This habit has proven hard to break despite evidence that it may increase pain and slow the healing process (7). Appropriate management of corneal abrasions should include (7):

- Analgesics, oral or topical NSAIDs
- Topical antibiotics (ointments are more lubricating)
  a. Erythromycins and bacitracin are reasonable first choices.
  b. Antipseudomonal coverage with gentamycin or quinolones is indicated in contact lens wearers

- No contact lens worn in the affected eye until the abrasion has healed
- Follow-up within 24 hours
- Instructions regarding primary prevention of eye injuries with eye shields and safety glasses

Common pitfalls in management include the continued use of ophthalmic anesthetics, which may mask worsening symptoms.

Subconjunctival Hemorrhage

Subconjunctival hemorrhages require no specific treatment. Patients should be reassured that resolution should occur within approximately 2 weeks. Failure to resolve warrants a referral to an ophthalmologist to evaluate for less common causes, such as Kaposi's sarcoma (6).

Blepharitis

Although there is treatment for blepharitis, this condition is chronic, with frequent relapses. It is important to treat any underlying conditions, to maintain lid hygiene, and to avoid any exacerbating triggers (eye makeup, medications). The treatment includes warm compresses, for about 3–5 minutes once or twice daily, to loosen and then remove the matted material and debris from the lids. The compresses can also be used to perform gentle massage of the Meibomian glands to express secretions and unclog the gland openings. It is important to avoid over manipulation of the eyelids, as this can cause mechanical irritation. The compresses can be followed by cleansing of the lid margins with a cotton tip applicator soaked in a solution of diluted baby shampoo (3 oz. of water plus 3 drops of baby shampoo) (11) or with over-the-counter solutions (EyeScrub or OcuClenz), used daily 2 to 3 times a week, as needed (9). Patients should be advised to discard their current eye makeup (in case of staph infection), to never share eye makeup, to choose eyeliner and mascara that wash

TABLE 20.7 Common Ophthalmic Allergy Drugs

Drug	Cautions	Dosage	Relative Cost
Mast cell stabilizers			
Lodoxamide	Age <2 years	1–2 drops QID	$$$
Cromolyn	Age <4 years	1–2 drops QID	$$
Nedocromil	Age <3 years	1–2 drops BID	$$$
NSAID			
Ketorolac	Aspirin or NSAID induced asthma or allergy Age <3 years	1 drop QID	$$$
Antihistamines			
Levocabastine	Age <12 years	1 drop QID	$$$
Olopatadine	Age <3 years	1 drop BID	$$$
Antihistamine/vasoconstrictor Naphazoline/pheniramine	Age <6 years Narrow angle glaucoma MAO use	1–2 drops QD-QID as needed	$ OTC

BID, twice a day; OTC, over the counter; QID, four times a day.

off easily (avoid waterproof), and to replace eye makeup every 6 months.

In more recalcitrant cases, topical antibiotic ointments like bacitracin, erythromycin, and sulfacetamide can be applied once to twice daily with a cotton swab (11); bedtime is usually more convenient, as the ointment may lead to blurry vision and make daily activities more difficult. If eyelid hygiene and topical antibiotics do not relieve symptoms in patients with Meibomian gland dysfunction, a course of oral antibiotics may be warranted, either doxycycline 50 mg twice daily or tetracycline 250 mg four times daily, may be required for up to 6 to 9 months of treatment; the antibiotics can then be tapered as symptoms regress. In patients who have rosacea or severe inflammation, systemic tetracycline can be added (erythromycin in children and pregnant women) (11). In some cases, topical corticosteroids applied sparingly may also help. Patients should be made aware that this is a chronic condition, and that lid hygiene may need to be continued indefinitely. They should avoid allergens and other exacerbating factors, and they should work with their doctor to treat underlying systemic diseases. The physician should also review with the patient "return to office precautions" if the condition is worsening or not improving with the given measures.

Patients should be referred to an ophthalmologist if there is vision loss, moderate to severe pain, corneal involvement, recurrence, lack of response to therapy, or suspicion of cancer (unilateral involvement) (9).

Differential Diagnosis of Blepharitis:

- Atopic dermatitis
- Contact dermatitis
- Mechanical irritation (allergic conjunctivitis → increased rubbing)
- Sebaceous cell CA (asymmetric eyelash loss)
- Ocular rosacea
- Contact lens complications
- Conjunctivitis
- Dry eye syndrome
- Herpetic eye disease

Hordeolum

Treatment includes warm compresses for 10 to 15 minutes three to five times a day (with a clean washcloth). Compresses alone are often sufficient intervention. However, because this is a bacterial infection and may spread to other glands or follicles, the use of topical antibiotics is recommended as well. Culture is seldom required unless initial treatments are unsuccessful, and an organism needs to be identified (10).

An erythromycin or sulfacetamide ophthalmic ointment applied four times a day for 7 days hastens recovery. If the patient also suffers from blepharitis, which may have been the inciting factor, the underlying blepharitis should be treated as well. If the lesion does not show improvement in 48 hours, referral to an ophthalmologist for incision and drainage is necessary.

Chalazion

Chalazion is one of the most common eye diseases managed by non-ophthalmologists (24), and approximately 25% resolve spontaneously. The treatment for chalazion is similar to that of hordeolum. Warm compresses are applied three to four times a day. This conservative treatment is often sufficient and, as this is a lipogranuloma and not an infection, antibiotics are not indicated, unless infection is suspected. If the chalazion persists or is causing visual changes, referral to an ophthalmologist is appropriate. The chalazion can be excised or injected with steroids, although steroid injections are not always successful (18, 25). Treatment of any associated underlying condition is necessary.

CASE 1 DISCUSSION

Mr. W. has unilateral eye involvement, tearing with only minimal itching, and a nonexudative discharge. His vision is normal, and he denies photophobia or globe pain. These clinical findings associated with his upper respiratory infection support the diagnosis of viral conjunctivitis. You prescribe symptomatic treatment with artificial tears and cool compresses, and tell him that he should note improvement over the next 7 to 10 days. He is instructed to follow-up if his symptoms persist or worsen. He is specifically instructed to seek care if he develops eye pain or notes decreased vision.

CASE 2 DISCUSSION

Mrs. L.'s signs and symptoms are consistent with blepharitis. She probably suffers from posterior blepharitis as she complains of dry eye symptoms, which may mean that the Meibomian glands are becoming atrophied. The left lower eyelid bump is a chalazion and not a hordeolum (it is neither painful nor erythematous). The chalazion also points toward Meibomian gland involvement as it is the result of a clogged Meibomian gland.

You explain that the bump is a clogged oil gland in the eyelid, and that most of these lesions will resolve with warm compresses, massage, and sometimes with expressing the gland's contents. If these measures do not work after a one to two week trial, you will refer her to an ophthalmologist for removal or for steroid injection.

The reddened nose and chin with pustules and telangiectasia are features of acne rosacea, which predispose Mrs. L. to blepharitis. Treating the rosacea, usually with oral tetracycline, may help alleviate the blepharitis. It is important that Mrs. L. understand that blepharitis is a chronic condition, and that she will have to "keep on top of the treatment" to avoid recurrence of her symptoms. The treatment, as discussed above, includes twice daily warm compresses to loosen the debris on the lashes, followed by eyelid scrubs using a cotton tipped applicator dipped in either a homemade baby shampoo solution or an over-the-counter lid cleanser. You will follow up in 2 weeks to assess her progress. Tetracycline would help treat her rosacea and may also help in the amelioration of her blepharitis as well. However, at this point, there is no evidence of anterior blepharitis, superinfection, or hordeolum and therefore no current need for topical antibiotics. If in 2 weeks the symptoms do not abate, topical antibiotics might help. Mrs. L. also may benefit from artificial tears to help with the dry eye feeling. In addition you should advise Mrs. L. to avoid eye makeup until the symptoms resolve, and possibly refrain from using it at all.

CASE 3 DISCUSSION

The important historical elements to elicit from Mr. D. include the history of similar symptoms; a family history of eye problems; and a personal history of diabetes, hypertension, hyperlipidemia, glaucoma, tobacco use, or previous eye surgery. This presentation is most consistent with retinal tear/detachment. However, it is very important to rule out the more serious and potentially more vision threatening retinal vein and retinal artery occlusions. The exam should include evaluation of blood pressure, examination of the carotids and the heart, as well as a visual acuity assessment and a thorough ophthalmoscopic exam.

Mr. D. should be referred to an ophthalmologist within 48 hours, sooner if symptoms are worsening. Further testing for diabetes, hyperlipidemia, and hypercoagulable states can be done at follow-up once the patient has seen an ophthalmologist. As you suspect retinal detachment and think that you can see evidence of a small retinal tear on funduscopic exam, you should try to reassure Mr. D. by letting him know that if the ophthalmologist confirms retinal detachment, the success rate for repair is 95%. The fact that Mr. D. presented so promptly is also promising, as interventions may be performed before the tear enlarges. You also let him know that he is at greater risk for developing retinal detachment in the contralateral eye, but that he will be followed closely by the ophthalmologist. If there is evidence that he is developing a retinal tear in the left eye, early intervention will be possible.

REFERENCES

1. Morrow GL, Abbott RL. Conjunctivitis. Am Fam Physician. 1998;57(4):735–746.
2. Matoba AY, Harris DJ, Meisler DM, et al. Preferred practice pattern conjunctivitis. American Academy of Ophthalmology. 2003. Available at: *http://www.aao.org/education/library/ppp/index.cfm*. Accessed May 1, 2006.
3. Vafidis G. When is red eye not just conjunctivitis? Practitioner. 2002;246:469–481.
4. Rietveld RP, van Weert HCPM, ter Riet G, Bindels PJE. Diagnostic impact of signs and symptoms in acute infectious conjunctivitis: systematic literature search. BMJ. 2003;327:789.
5. Gaasterland DE, Allingham RR, Gross EL, et al. Preferred practice pattern primary angle closure. American Academy of Ophthalmology. 2003. Available at: *http://www.aao.org/education/library/ppp/index.cfm*. Accessed May 1, 2006.
6. Leibowitz H. M. The red eye. N Engl J Med. 2000;343:345–351.
7. Wilson SA, Last A. Management of corneal abrasions. Am Fam Physician. 2004;70(1):123–128.
8. Patel SJ, Lundy DC. Ocular manifestations of autoimmune disease. Am Fam Physician. 2002;66(6):991–998.
9. Matoba AY, Harris DJ, Meisler DM, et al. Prescribed practice patterns blepharitis. American Academy of Ophthalmology. 2003. Available at: *http://www.aao.org/education/library/ppp/index.cfm*. Accessed May 1, 2006.
10. Sullivan JH, Shetlar DJ, Whitcher JP. Lids, Lacrimal apparatus, and tears. In: Vaughan D, Asbury T, Riordan-Eva P, eds. General Ophthalmology. 16th ed. New York: Appleton & Lange/McGraw-Hill; 2004:80–82.
11. Shields SR. Managing eye disease in primary care: how to recognize and treat common eye problems. Postgrad Med. 2000;108(5):83–95.
12. Margo CE, Harmon LE. Posterior vitreous detachment. 2005; 117(3):37–42.
13. Chew EY, Benson WE, Boldt HC, et al. Prescribed practice patterns posterior vitreous detachment, retinal breaks, and lattice degeneration. American Academy of Ophthalmology. 2003. Available at: *http://www.aao.org/education/library/ppp/index.cfm*. Accessed May 1, 2006.
14. Gariano RF, Kim CH. Evaluation and management of suspected retinal detachment. Am Fam Physician. 2004;9(7):1691–1698.
15. Newell FW. Diseases and injuries of the eye. In: Ophthalmology Principles and Concepts, 8th ed. St. Louis: Mosby; 1996:204–207.
16. Appen RE, Wray SH, Cogan DG. Central retinal artery occlusion. Am J Ophthalmol. 1975;79(3):374–381.
17. Shields SR. Managing eye disease in primary care: when to refer for ophthalmologic care. Postgrad Med. 2000;108(5):99–106.
18. Newell FW. Diseases and injuries of the eye. In: Ophthalmology Principles and Concepts, 8th ed. St. Louis: Mosby; 1996:322–324.
19. Bhagat N, Goldberg MF, Gascon P, et al. Central retinal vein occlusion: review of management. Eur J Ophthalmol. 1999;9(3):165–180.
20. Buys YM, Levin AV, Enzenauer RW. Retinal findings after head trauma in infants and young children. Ophthalmology. 1992;99(11):1718–1723.
21. Emerson MV, Pieramici, DJ, Stoessel KM, et al. Incidence and rate of disappearance of retinal hemorrhage in newborns. Ophthalmology. 2001;108(1):36–39.
22. Paulman A, Paulman P. Sudden loss of vision. J Fam Pract. 2004;53(4):269–273.
23. Hardy RA, Shetlar DJ. Retina. In: Vaughan D, Asbury T, Riordan-Eva, P, eds. Vaughan and Asbury's General Ophthalmology, 16th ed. New York: Appleton & Lange/McGraw-Hill; 2004:206–207.
24. Carter SR. Eyelid disorders: diagnosis and management. Am Fam Physician. 1998;57(11):2695–2702.
25. Ho S, Lai J. Subcutaneous steroid injection as treatment for chalazion: prospective case series. Hong Kong Med J. 2002; 8(1):18–20.

CHAPTER 21

Sore Throat

Mark H. Ebell

CASE

A 12-year-old boy and his mother present to your family practice office with a complaint of 2 days of fever, sore throat, and headache. He denies a cough. On examination he has tonsillar exudates and significant anterior cervical lymphadenopathy. His mother wonders whether he might have "mono" because his best friend has this disease, and she demands a blood test for infectious mononucleosis.

CLINICAL QUESTIONS

1. Does this patient have an infectious or noninfectious cause of sore throat?
2. If infectious, is it streptococcal pharyngitis or infectious mononucleosis?
3. Which treatments will help the patient feel better sooner and prevent complications?

Sore throat is one of the most common symptoms evaluated in primary care and has been well studied as a model for clinical decision-making. Approximately 4.6% of patients seeing a family physician report "sore throat" as the primary reason for the visit, making it the second-most common reason for an office visit (1). Patients often present to the physician with the preconceived notion that they have a "strep throat" and expect antibiotic therapy. However, streptococcal pharyngitis is responsible for only a minority of cases of sore throat, and you should thoroughly consider all possible infectious and noninfectious causes of the symptom.

Antibiotic therapy for streptococcal pharyngitis reduces the duration of symptoms by about 1 day, the incidence of complications such as abscess formation, the risk of spread to others, and the incidence of rheumatic fever (2–4). However, the incidence of rheumatic fever in particular has declined substantially over the past 40 years (since the widespread introduction of penicillin) from approximately 20 cases per million to 1.5 cases per million (5). Because complications are rare in the modern era and overtreatment increases the development of resistant strains of bacteria, an accurate diagnosis is important. This chapter presents an approach to therapy that builds on our knowledge of the differential diagnosis for different ages, a rational approach to the history and physical examination, and judicious use of the laboratory.

DIFFERENTIAL DIAGNOSIS

Sore throat can be caused by bacterial, viral, or fungal infection of the posterior pharynx and tonsillar tissue. Infection by group A β-hemolytic streptococcal (GABHS) bacteria is the most important cause of bacterial infection because of rare but serious possible complications such as peritonsillar abscess, rheumatic fever, and acute glomerulonephritis. Other serotypes (notably group B and group C) are relatively common in the posterior pharynx but are not thought to cause sore throat. An exception may be large colony count group C strep, although there is no evidence that antibiotics reduce symptoms in these patients (6).

The role of other bacterial pathogens such as *Chlamydia pneumoniae*, *Branhamella* species, *Haemophilus* species, and *Mycoplasma pneumoniae* remains controversial. These diagnoses should be considered in patients with lingering infections who do not have evidence of GABHS pharyngitis. *M. pneumoniae* in particular is more common in patients who are older, are less ill, and have less evidence of pharyngeal inflammation (7). Although uncommon in most settings, gonococcal pharyngitis should be considered in patients who are otherwise at higher risk for sexually transmitted infection.

Most episodes of pharyngitis are caused by viruses, including adenoviruses, influenza viruses, parainfluenza virus, and respiratory syncytial virus (8). However, it is not usually necessary or important to determine the specific virus responsible for an episode of viral pharyngitis. An exception is pharyngitis caused by Epstein-Barr virus (EBV) infection, also known as infectious mononucleosis (IM), because of the protracted course and rare but potentially serious complications of this illness (such as splenic rupture and respiratory compromise due to severe tonsillar hypertrophy and cervical adenopathy) (9).

Acute cytomegalovirus infection is a rare cause of pharyngitis, and although it resembles infectious mononucleosis in some respects, it is associated with a greater degree of hepatic involvement. Candidiasis is a rare cause of sore throat. It should be considered in immunosuppressed patients, especially those with AIDS, and in patients using nasal or inhaled steroid preparations.

Gastroesophageal reflux disease (GERD) causes pain by direct irritation of the pharyngeal tissue by stomach acid. Allergic rhinitis or sinusitis, with chronic posterior drainage from the nasopharynx, can cause pharyngeal irritation through a combination of chemical irritation and repeated drying. Persistent coughing can cause sore throat without any direct infection of the pharynx. Acute thyroiditis causes anterior neck pain that may be mistaken for pharyngitis but is typically associated with more local tenderness to palpation. Other causes of throat pain include trauma (either external or internal, such as from a fish bone) and referred dental pain.

TABLE 21.1 Differential Diagnosis of Sore Throat*

Cause		Probability (%)
Infectious causes		
Viral		50–80
Streptococcal (group A)		
	Adult	5–10
	Child	20–35
Epstein-Barr virus		1–10
Chlamydia pneumoniae		2–5
Mycoplasma pneumoniae		2–5
Neisseria gonorrhoeae		1–2
Haemophilus influenzae type B		1–2
Candidiasis		<1
Noninfectious causes		
Gastroesophageal reflux disease		NA
Postnasal drainage due to allergic rhinitis and other upper respiratory conditions		NA
Acute thyroiditis		NA
Persistent cough		NA

*Data are from Komaroff AL, Pass TM, Aronson MD, et al. The prediction of streptococcal pharyngitis in adults. J Gen Intern Med. 1986;1:1–7; Hoffman S. An algorithm for a selective use of throat swabs in the diagnosis of group A streptococcal pharyngo-tonsillitis in general practice. Scand J Prim Health Care. 1992;10:295–300; Komaroff A, Aronson MD, Pass TM, Ervin CT, Branch WT. Serologic evidence of chlamydial and mycoplasmal pharyngitis in adults. Science. 1983;222:927–928.

The differential diagnosis of sore throat in the primary care setting is summarized in Table 21.1. No reliable estimates are available for the likelihood of noninfectious causes of sore throat. Depending on the age of the patient and the setting in which they present, the prevalence of GABHS pharyngitis varies from 5% to 36%; estimates of the likelihood of streptococcal pharyngitis by age are shown in Table 21.2. GABHS pharyngitis is more common in children, in emergency departments, and in the fall and winter (10–13).

The incidence of infectious mononucleosis peaks between the ages of 10 and 29 years and is rare in patients over age 40 or under age 10. Although the infection is thought to occur relatively often in younger children, it generally results in a mild or subclinical infection, so blood tests for infectious mononucleosis are only rarely ordered. Few data are available on the precise likelihood of mononucleosis in patients presenting to a family physician with a complaint of sore throat; estimates by age and setting are shown in Table 21.2 (14–17). These estimates were derived by combining incidence data (in cases/100,000 population) with reports of the likelihood of infectious mononucleosis among specific age groups.

CLINICAL EVALUATION

In most cases, the history will help you determine whether the sore throat is due to an infectious or noninfectious cause. Noninfectious causes should be suspected in patients who are afebrile or who have no other signs of upper respiratory infection, have had symptoms longer than 1 to 2 weeks, and have associated symptoms such as heartburn, postnasal drip, or itchy eyes. Current use of anti-acid medications or a history of peptic ulcer disease should alert you to the possibility of gastroesophageal reflux disease (GERD). Symptoms are typically worse late at night or early in the morning, and patients will often report a bitter or unpleasant taste in the back of the throat upon awakening.

When evaluating a patient with sore throat, be alert for red flags (summarized in Table 21.3). These patients need more rapid assessment and may require urgent referral. Otherwise, the key clinical questions for the patient with infectious sore throat are whether it is caused by GABHS pharyngitis or infectious mononucleosis. The remainder of this section focuses on the history, physical examination, and laboratory testing for these diagnoses.

History and Physical Examination
GABHS PHARYNGITIS

The signs and symptoms most strongly associated with GABHS pharyngitis are a measured or reported (subjective) fever, absence of cough, tonsillar or pharyngeal exudate, cervical adenopathy, and tonsillar enlargement. Myalgias, recent strep exposure, a brief duration of illness prior to presentation, and headache also increase the likelihood of GABHS pharyngitis somewhat. Pharyngeal injection is commonly noted, but the sensitivity and specificity vary greatly, probably because

TABLE 21.2 Likelihood of Group A β-Hemolytic Streptococcal (GABHS) Pharyngitis and Infectious Mononucleosis in the Primary Care Setting by Age*

Infection	Age (Years)	%
GABHS pharyngitis	0–4	15
	5–9	30
	10–19	15
	Adult	5–10
Infectious mononucleosis	0–4	<1
	5–14	1–2
	15–24	5–10
	25–34	1–2
	>34	<1

*Data are from Ehrlich TP, Schwartz RH, Wientzen R, Thorne MM. Comparison of an immunochromatographic method for rapid identification of group A streptococcal antigen with culture method. Arch Fam Med 1993;2:866–869; Holmberg SD, Faich GA. Streptococcal pharyngitis and acute rheumatic fever in Rhode Island. JAMA. 1983;250:2307–2312; Wigton RS, Connor JL, Centor RM. Transportability of a decision rule for the diagnosis of streptococcal pharyngitis. Arch Intern Med. 1986;146:81–83; Komaroff AL, Pass TM, Aronson MD, et al. The prediction of streptococcal pharyngitis in adults. J Gen Intern Med. 1986;1:1–7; Hoffman S. An algorithm for a selective use of throat swabs in the diagnosis of group A streptococcal pharyngotonsillitis in general practice. Scand J Prim Health Care. 1992;10:295–300; Fry J. Infectious mononucleosis: some new observations from a 15-year study. J Fam Pract. 1980;10: 1087–1089; Everett MT. The cause of tonsillitis. The Practitioner. 1979;223:253–259; Hanson CJ, Higbee JW, Lednar WM, Garrison MJ. The epidemiology of acute pharyngitis among soldiers at Ford Lewis, Washington. Mil Med. 1986;7:389–394.

physicians define it differently. The typical scarlatina rash (a fine sandpapery eruption) only occurs in about 4% of patients with GABHS pharyngitis, but is highly specific and when present, is strong evidence in favor of the disease. Coryza and itchy eyes are less common in patients with streptococcal pharyngitis than in other causes of sore throat (18). The test characteristics for symptoms associated with streptococcal pharyngitis are shown in Table 21.4. No single symptom will rule in or rule out the diagnosis of streptococcal pharyngitis, but combinations of symptoms and signs have been used successfully in clinical prediction rules (see Table 21.5 and discussion in the Management section of this chapter).

Patients with a more toxic appearance, and those who have a muffled or "hot potato" voice, should be carefully examined for peritonsillar abscess. This condition is usually unilateral; the tonsil on the affected side is often pushed out to the midline, giving the uvula, tonsil, and surrounding structures an asymmetric appearance. Patients with peritonsillar abscess have fluctuance over the abscess and are extremely sensitive to direct palpation of the tonsillar tissue by a gloved hand.

INFECTIOUS MONONUCLEOSIS

Sore throat caused by infection with Epstein-Barr virus (infectious mononucleosis) typically follows a 30- to 50-day incubation period and a 3- to 5-day prodrome characterized by fever, malaise, myalgias, and headache. In a series of 500 patients with confirmed infectious mononucleosis, at least 98% had sore throat, lymph node enlargement, fever, and tonsillar enlargement. Other common physical signs included pharyngeal inflammation (85%) and transient palatal petechiae (50%). This presentation is typical in adolescents. Older adults are less likely to have sore throat and adenopathy but more likely to have hepatomegaly and jaundice (9, 14).

Although symptoms in general may be similar to those of streptococcal pharyngitis (sore throat, fever, chills, malaise, and headache) and the two coexist in 5% to 30% of patients, fatigue is a much more-prominent symptom in infectious mononucleosis, and often interferes significantly with the patient's ability to function (9). Approximately 4% of patients have mild abdominal pain in the left upper quadrant; if this pain is severe, splenic rupture should be suspected and a surgical consultation obtained.

TABLE 21.3 Red Flags Suggesting Progressive or Life-Threatening Disease in Patients with Sore Throat

Finding	Condition
Hot-potato voice, toxic appearance, altered mental status	Peritonsillar abscess
Splenic enlargement	Infectious mononucleosis with increased risk for splenic rupture
Increased respiratory rate, extremely enlarged tonsils, and significant cervical adenopathy	Respiratory compromise due to upper airway obstruction, rarely associated with GABHS pharyngitis and infectious mononucleosis

TABLE 21.4 Key Elements of the History and Physical Examination for Sore Throat and Their Test Characteristics for the Detection of GABHS Pharyngitis*

Symptoms and Signs	Sensitivity	Specificity	LR+	LR−
Tonsillar or pharyngeal exudates	21%–58%	69%–92%	1.5–2.6	0.7–0.9
Fever (subjective)	30%–92%	23%–90%	1.0–2.6	0.3–1.0
Fever (measured temp >37.8°C or 101°F)	11%–84%	43%–96%	1.1–3.0	0.3–0.9
Cervical adenopathy	55%–82%	34%–73%	0.5–2.9	0.6–0.9
Enlarged tonsils	56%–86%	56%–86%	1.4–3.1	0.6
No cough	51%–79%	36%–68%	1.1–1.7	0.5–0.9
No coryza	42%–84%	20%–70%	0.9–1.6	0.5–1.4
Myalgias	49%	52%–69%	1.4	0.9
Headache	48%	50%–80%	0.8–2.6	0.5–1.1
Pharynx injected	43%–99%	3%–62%	0.7–1.6	0.2–6.4
Duration <3 days	26%–93%	59%	0.7–3.5	0.2–2.2
Palatine petechiae	7%	95%	1.4	1.0
Strep exposure previous 2 wks	19%	87%–94%	1.9	0.9
Scarlatina rash	4%	79%–99%	0.1–0.3	0.9–1.1

Note: These data are from a meta-analysis[†] of high quality diagnostic studies. Signs and symptoms are organized from greatest accuracy (as measured by area under the receiver-operating characteristic curve) to least accuracy. A range is provided when the studies were heterogeneous, and a point estimate when they were homogeneous.
*Ebell MH, Smith MA, Barry HC, Ives K, Carey M. Does this patient have strep throat? JAMA. 2000;284:2912–2918.
[†]Ho-Yen DO, Martin KW. The relationship between atypical lymphocytosis and serological tests in infectious mononucleosis. J Infect. 1981;3:324–331.

TABLE 21.5 Clinical Prediction Rule for the Diagnosis of Group A β-Hemolytic Streptococcal (GABHS) Pharyngitis*

1. Add up the points for your patient

Symptom or Sign	Points
History of fever or measured temperature >38°C	1
Absence of cough	1
Tender anterior cervical adenopathy	1
Tonsillar swelling or exudates	1
Age <15 years	1
Age ≥45 years	-1
Total:	

2. Find their risk of strep below

Points	Likelihood Ratio	Percentage with Strep (Patients with Strep/Total)
-1 or 0	0.05	1% (2/179)
1	0.52	10% (13/134)
2	0.95	17% (18/109)
3	2.5	35% (28/81)
4 or 5	4.9	51% (39/77)

Note: Baseline risk of strep = 17% in this population. This rule was validated in a group of 167 children over the age of 3 and 453 adults in Ontario, Canada.
*Data are from McIsaac WJ, Goel V, To T, Low DE. The validity of a sore throat score in family practice. CMAJ. 2000; 163:811–815.

Cervical adenopathy and fever are present in over 99% of patients with infectious mononucleosis (9). In fact, if a patient does not have cervical adenopathy (either anterior or posterior) and fever (either by history or measured in the office), you can effectively rule out infectious mononucleosis. Because 90% of patients with mononucleosis have posterior cervical adenopathy, patients without this finding also have a very low probability of disease (5) unless they have other history or physical findings pointing strongly toward mononucleosis (e.g., recent exposure to someone with the disease, a protracted course, severe fatigue, or splenomegaly). Other signs found in patients with infectious mononucleosis include splenomegaly (present in 50%) (5), palatal petechiae (50%), jaundice (10%), and rash (3%) (9).

Diagnostic Testing
GABHS

A variety of rapid antigen tests and cultures are available to test for the presence of GABHS bacteria in the pharynx. Rapid antigen tests include enzyme immunoassays, latex agglutination tests, liposomal assays, and immunochromatographic assays. Their test characteristics vary considerably and are summarized in Table 21.6. You should know the type of test used in your office and its test characteristics in real clinical use. Relying on rapid antigen tests, even when strep is relatively common, will miss less than 5% of cases of strep throat (19).

Although the throat culture test is often considered a gold standard, a second throat culture taken simultaneously from a patient with an initial positive throat culture is only positive 90% of the time. Also, a small but significant percentage of sore throat patients with a positive throat culture for GABHS bacteria are actually carriers, in which a pathogen or mechanism other than GABHS bacteria is responsible for the sore throat.

INFECTIOUS MONONUCLEOSIS

Two types of laboratory tests are useful for confirming the diagnosis of infectious mononucleosis: the complete blood count (CBC) with differential, and a variety of serologic tests. Most patients with infectious mononucleosis develop a lymphocytosis, which usually peaks 2 weeks after the onset of symptoms. Approximately 95% of patients have more than 60% lymphocytes; having less than that at 10 to 14 days after the onset of symptoms largely rules out the diagnosis. The total white blood cell (WBC) count peaks above 10,000 cells/mm^3 in 77% of patients (9). Atypical lymphocytes are also common in patients with infectious mononucleosis. In fact, in one study all patients with more than 40% atypical lymphocytes and clinically suspected infectious mononucleosis had serologic evidence of acute Epstein-Barr virus infection. In the same study, 69% of patients with 20% to 40% atypical lymphocytes had evidence of EBV infection (20, 21). The likelihood ratios for different levels of atypical lymphocytosis are shown in Table 21.6. If the patient has more than 20% atypical lymphocytes, or more than 50% lymphocytes with 10% or more atypical lymphocytes, infectious mononucleosis is quite likely, and further confirmation of the diagnosis is not needed.

Serologic tests are often negative in the first week of infection because they rely on the body's immune response. The traditional test is based on the fact that heterophil antibodies produced in patients with infectious mononucleosis agglutinate sheep erythrocytes; the "Monospot" test that is still widely used is a rapid latex agglutination test based on the same principle. However, up to 20% of patients may not produce this antibody. Viral capsid antigen (VCA) IgM antibodies are produced relatively early in infection and do not persist once the acute infection is over. This test is quite sensitive and specific, although like the Monospot test, the sensitivity improves during the second week of the illness. Other laboratory tests that are sometimes abnormal in patients with infectious mononucleosis include aspartate aminotransferase (>40 μ/L in 76% of patients) and alkaline phosphatase (elevated in 71% of patients) (14). Characteristics of serologic tests are summarized in Table 21.6.

Recommended Diagnostic Strategy

The recommended approach to management of sore throat is summarized in Figure 21.1. If an infectious cause of sore throat seems likely, the physician should consider whether infectious mononucleosis is a possibility. If unlikely, the validated McIsaac clinical decision rule shown in Table 21.5 should be used to estimate the probability of strep (22). This score assigns one point for each of the following four signs or symptoms: tonsillar swelling or exudate, tender anterior cervical adenopathy, absence of a cough, and a history of fever or a measured temperature >38°C (100.4°F). An additional point is given for age under 15 years, and a point is subtracted for age over 45 years. When prospectively validated in a group of 167 children and 453 adults, the probability of GABHS pharyngitis in patients with −1 or 0 points was 1%, in those with 1 or 2 points was 13%, in those with 3 points was 35%, and in those with 4 or 5 points was 51%.

The decision to order further testing, such as a rapid strep test, depends on this probability estimate. Using this kind of a patient-centered, individualized, and evidence-based approach has even been shown to reduce cost and increase the quality of care (21).

MANAGEMENT

Viral pharyngitis is a self-limited condition, and only symptomatic treatment is indicated. Strategies for symptomatic treatment include nonsteroidal anti-inflammatory drugs (NSAIDs; e.g., ibuprofen, naproxen sodium) or acetaminophen for fever and throat pain, gargling with 2% viscous lidocaine for patients with severe throat pain, and over-the-counter (OTC) topical sprays (e.g., Chloraseptic spray). Gargling with salt water is soothing and may reduce inflammation. Although none of these strategies have been evaluated in controlled clinical trials, they are safe and seem to be effective. Herbal tea has been shown in a randomized trial to be more effective than placebo for short-term relief of pain (23).

Treatment of other bacterial causes of pharyngitis (i.e., *Chlamydia, M. pneumoniae*) is less important than treatment of streptococcal pharyngitis because of the absence of risk of rheumatic fever. There is also no evidence that treatment of these infections reduces the duration of symptoms or decreases the likelihood that the disease will be spread to others. Gonococcal pharyngitis is generally only minimally symptomatic, but should be treated if detected to prevent spread to others. Recommended treatment for gonococcal pharyngitis is ceftri-

TABLE 21.6 Characteristics of Tests Used to Detect Group A β-Hemolytic Streptococcal (GABHS)
Pharyngitis and Infectious Mononucleosis

Test	Sensitivity	Specificity	LR+	LR−
GABHS pharyngitis				
Enzyme immunoassay[a–d]	60%	89%	5.5	0.45
Latex agglutination[e–g]	81%	91%	9.0	0.21
Liposomal method[h,i]	79%	84%	4.9	0.25
Immunochromatographic[j]	97%	97%	32.3	0.03
Office culture[k]	89%	95%	17.8	0.11
Laboratory culture[k]	90%	99%	90.0	0.10
Infectious mononucleosis				
> 40% atypical lymphocytes[l]				39
36–40% atypical lymphocytes[l]				3.1
31–35% atypical lymphocytes[l]				1.2
20–30% atypical lymphocytes[l]				0.44
50% lymphocytes and > 10% atypical cells[m]	39%	99%	39	0.61
Rapid slide agglutination				
(Monospot)[m]	86%	99%	86	0.14
1st week	69%	88%	5.7	0.35
2nd week	81%	88%	6.7	0.21
VCA-IgM[n]				
1st week	0.80	0.99	80	0.20
2nd week	0.85	0.99	85	0.15
3rd week	0.97	0.99	97	0.03
Anti-EBV ELISA (Biotest anti-EBV recombinant)[o]	0.99	0.99	99	0.01

[a]Egger P, Siegrist CA, Strautmann G, Belli D, Auckenthaler R. Evaluation of two ELISA tests for the rapid detection of group A streptococci. Eur J Pediatr. 1990;149:256–258.

[b]Macknin ML, Indich N, Easley KA, Imrie R. Comparison of two rapid diagnostic tests for group A streptococcus. Pediatr Infect Dis J. 1988;7:735–736.

[c]Carey RD, Tilyard MW, Morris RW. Evaluation of a rapid diagnostic test for group A b-hemolytic streptococcus in general practice. N Z Med J. 1991; 104:401–403.

[d]Wagner DL, Witte DL, Schrantz RD. Insensitivity of rapid antigen detection methods and single blood agar plate culture for diagnosing streptococcal pharyngitis. JAMA. 1992;267:695–697.

[e]Gerber MA, Spadaccini LJ, Wright LL, Deutsch L. Latex agglutination tests for rapid identification of group A streptococci directly from throat swabs. J Pediatr 1984;105:702–705.

[f]Taubman B, Barroway RP, McGowan KL. The diagnosis of group A, β-hemolytic streptococcal pharyngitis in the office setting. Am J Dis Child. 1989; 143:102–104.

[g]Reed BD, Huck W, French T. Diagnosis of group A β-hemolytic streptococcus using clinical scoring criteria, Directigen 1-2-3 group A streptococcal test, and culture. Arch Intern Med. 1990;150:1727–1732.

[h]Hoffman S. An algorithm for a selective use of throat swabs in the diagnosis of group A streptococcal pharyngo-tonsillitis in general practice. Scand J Prim Health Care. 1992;10:295–300.

[i]Gerber MA, Randolph MF, DeMeo KK. Liposome immunoassay for rapid identification of group A Streptococci directly from throat swabs. J Clin Microbiol. 1990;28:1463–1464.

[j]Ehrlich TP, Schwartz RH, Wientzen R, Thorne MM. Comparison of an immunochromatographic method for rapid identification of group A streptococcal antigen with culture method. Arch Fam Med. 1993;2:866–869.

[k]Centor RM, Meier FA, Dalton HP. Throat cultures and rapid tests for diagnosis of group A streptococcal pharyngitis. Ann Intern Med. 1986;105: 892–899.

[l]Ho-Yen DO, Martin KW. The relationship between atypical lymphocytosis and serological tests in infectious mononucleosis. J Infect. 1981;3:324–331.

[m]Fleischer GR, Collins M, Fager S. Limitations of available tests for diagnosis of infectious mononucleosis. J Clin Microbiol. 1983;17:619–624.

[n]Evans AS, Niederman JC, Cenabre LC, et al. A prospective evaluation of heterophile and Epstein-Barr virus-specific IgM antibody tests in clinical and subclinical infectious mononucleosis: specificity and sensitivity of the tests and persistence of the antibody. J Infect Dis. 1975;132:546–554.

[o]Farber I, Wutzler P, Wohlrabe P, et al. Serological diagnosis of infectious mononucleosis using three anti-Epstein Barr virus-recombinant ELISAs. J Virol Methods. 1993;42:301–308.

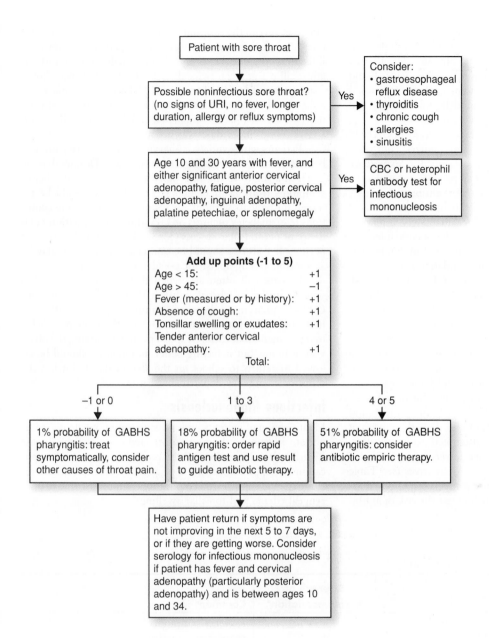

Figure 21.1 • General approach to the patient with sore throat.

axone 125 mg intramuscularly in a single dose or ciprofloxacin 500 mg orally in a single dose; azithromycin 1 g orally in a single dose (or doxycycline 100 mg orally twice daily for 7 days) should also be given if chlamydial infection is not ruled out (24).

GABHS Pharyngitis

Patients at very low risk for GABHS pharyngitis based on their demographics, history, and physical examination should be reassured that they do not seem to have a bacterial cause for their sore throat. Most patients with 0 or −1 points in the clinical prediction rule in Table 21.5 fall into this category. Although many patients have come to expect an antibiotic, a simple explanation of why they are very unlikely to have GABHS pharyngitis and why that is the only type of sore throat to benefit from antibiotics is usually satisfying to the patient.

Studies have shown that although many patients expect antibiotics, physicians are not good at guessing which patients want an antibiotic, and the patient's ultimate satisfaction with the encounter depends on the quality of the explanation and the length of time spent with the physician, rather than whether they got an antibiotic prescription (25). Also, giving antibiotics for a self-limited viral illness "medicalizes" it in the patient's mind, and may make the patient more likely to seek medical attention and antibiotics with their next illness (26).

Patients with a very high probability of GABHS pharyngitis, based on the history and physical examination, can be considered for empiric treatment without further laboratory testing, because the likelihood of disease even in the presence of a negative rapid antigen test remains more than 5% due to the number of false-negative results. Another (although more expensive) strategy is to use a rapid antigen test in these patients, and order a throat culture if the rapid test is negative. Patients with an intermediate probability of GABHS pharyngitis should be evaluated using a rapid antigen test and only receive an antibiotic if that test is positive. All patients should have adequate follow-up to ensure that they are responding to therapy; at a minimum they should be told to return if their symptoms are worsening or changing.

The symptomatic benefit of antibiotic therapy in GABHS pharyngitis is actually quite modest. Randomized controlled trials have shown that patients given penicillin experience about one fewer day of sore throat than patients given placebo (approximately 4 days of symptoms with antibiotic versus 5 days without). They also have a 20% rate of antibiotic-related adverse effects compared with 5% for patients given placebo (27). The levels of evidence for pharmacotherapeutic interventions in GABHS pharyngitis are summarized in Table 21.7.

The traditional antibiotic recommendation is for penicillin V, 250 mg given four times a day for 10 days. The risk of a serious allergic reaction is small when the drug is given orally, approximately 0.025% compared with a risk of 0.64% when given intramuscularly (27). A recent meta-analysis combined data from 35 studies of GABHS pharyngitis treatment, and found a higher clinical cure rate with cephalosporins than with penicillin (93.6% vs. 85.8%; number needed to treat = 13). The only exceptions were cefaclor and loracarbef (29).

Compliance is important because the treatment failure rate has been shown to be only 12% in compliant patients and 34% in those who are noncompliant (30). It is therefore not surprising that several studies have attempted to identify alternate antibiotic regimens that involve fewer doses per day, a shorter course of treatment, or both. Alternatives (see Table 21.8) are associated with more adverse effects (especially diarrhea), are more expensive, and may increase the risk of antibi-otic resistance in the community more than use of older antibiotics. An effective regimen (as long as patients do not have infectious mononucleosis in whom it will cause a rash) is amoxicillin 1 g, given twice daily for 6 days. This was shown to be just as effective as penicillin V 500 mg, given three times a day for 10 days in a randomized controlled trial, and is no more expensive (31). A comparison of 3 days of penicillin with 7 days found that 3 days was not as effective (6).

Patients with exudative pharyngitis and severe pain may benefit from intramuscular corticosteroids. Dexamethasone given in a single 10 mg injection halved the time to relief of symptoms from 33 to 15 hours. This therapy should be reserved for patients without any immunocompromising conditions (e.g., diabetes mellitus or HIV disease) and with no evidence of peritonsillar abscess (32, 33). Patients with suspected peritonsillar abscess should be evaluated on the same day by an otorhinolaryngologist for possible incision and drainage.

Parents will often ask when their child can return to school. Studies of throat cultures show that patients with GABHS pharyngitis become "culture-negative" within 24 hours of initiating antibiotic therapy. It is therefore reasonable to recommend that children spend the day following the office visit at home, but if feeling better and afebrile should be allowed to return to school on the second day following the office or emergency department visit (34).

Infectious Mononucleosis

Identification of patients with infectious mononucleosis is important because of the more protracted course of the disease (typically 1 to 2 months) and the possibility of serious complications in approximately 1% of patients. Complications include splenic rupture and respiratory compromise due to pharyngeal edema and tonsillar swelling.

TABLE 21.7 Treatment of Sore Throat

Treatment	Strength of Recommendation*	Comment
Antibiotics (cephalosporin for 7 to 10 days, penicillin VK 250 mg PO QID for 10 days, or amoxicillin 1 g PO BID for 6 days) for GABHS pharyngitis[b]	A	Reduces symptoms by about 1 day and reduces risk of rheumatic and suppurative complications
Dexamethasone 10 mg IM injection for severe pain and tonsillar enlargement[c]	B	Not in immunocompromised patients or those with peritonsillar abscess
2% viscous lidocaine gargle, salt water gargle, or throat lozenges	C	For relief of pharyngeal pain
Nonsteroidal anti-inflammatory drugs or acetaminophen	C	For relief of pain, fever, myalgias, headache. May also reduce pharyngeal pain.
Activity restriction for infectious mononucleosis	C	
Herbal tea	B	To relieve pain of sore throat

*A, consistent, good-quality patient-oriented evidence; B, inconsistent or limited-quality patient-oriented evidence; C, consensus, disease-oriented evidence, usual practice, expert opinion, or case series. For information about the SORT evidence rating system, see *http://www.aafp.org/afpsort.xml*.
[b]Peyramond D, Portier H, Geslin P, Cohen R. 6-day amoxicillin vs. 10-day penicillin V for group A β-hemolytic streptococcal acute tonsillitis in adults: a French Multicentre, open-label randomized study. Scand J Infect Dis. 1996;28:497–501.
[c]O'Brien JF, Meade JI, Falk JL. Dexamethasone as adjuvant therapy for severe acute pharyngitis. Ann Emerg Med. 1993;22:212–215.

TABLE 21.8 Pharmacotherapy Recommended for the Treatment of Group A β-Hemolytic Streptococcal (GABHS) Pharyngitis

Drug	Dosing Range	Adverse Effects	Comment
First-line drugs			
Penicillin VK	Children <12 yo: 25–50 mg/kg/day divided, Q 6–8 hours (max 3 g/day) Adults/children >12 yo: 250 mg PO QID for 7 to 10 days or 500 mg PO TID for 7 to 10 days	Mild diarrhea, vomiting, nausea	Compliance a problem, especially with QID dosing. Adjust dose for renal insufficiency. Available in suspension.
Amoxicillin*	Adults/children >12 yo: 500 mg PO TID for 7 to 10 days or 1 g PO BID for 6 days. Children <12 yo: 25–100 mg/kg/day divided Q 8 hours (max 2–3 g/day)	Rash in patients with infectious mononucleosis	Available as tablet, capsule, chewable tablet and oral suspension.
Erythromycin ethyl succinate	400 mg PO TID for 7 to 10 days Children <2 yo: 40 mg/kg/day in 2 divided doses (max 1600 mg/day)	Nausea or vomiting, abdominal pain	For penicillin- and amoxicillin-allergic patients. May cause drug to drug interactions. Available as tablet or oral suspension.
Alternate (second-line) drugs			
Azithromycin	Adults: 500 mg PO QD on day 1, 250 mg PO QD on days 2–5 Children >2 yo: 12 mg/kg (days 1–5)		Available as tablet or oral suspension.
Cefixime	8 mg/kg (children) PO QD for 10 days. Children >50 kg or >12 yo and Adults: 400 mg/day divided Q 12–24 hours		
Dexamethasone†	10 mg IM injection once for ages 12 and older		For severe sore throat only or pharyngeal edema

*Peyramond D, Portier H, Geslin P, Cohen R. 6-day amoxicillin vs. 10-day penicillin V for group A b-hemolytic streptococcal acute tonsillitis in adults: a French Multicentre, open-label randomized study. Scand J Infect Dis. 1996;28:497–501.

†O'Brien JF, Meade JI, Falk JL. Dexamethasone as adjuvant therapy for severe acute pharyngitis. Ann Emerg Med. 1993;22:212–215.

You should have a high index of suspicion for infectious mononucleosis in younger patients, particularly those aged 15 to 24 years, and in patients with posterior cervical adenopathy. Patients without anterior or posterior cervical adenopathy and fever are extremely unlikely to have the diagnosis, as are those over age 35, which will help rule it out in many patients. Diagnostic tests are relatively insensitive during the first week of illness when many patients present.

Patients with infectious mononucleosis should be treated symptomatically with rest, oral fluids, and NSAIDs or acetaminophen for fever and myalgias. Aspirin should be avoided because Reye's syndrome has been reported in association with infectious mononucleosis. Based on clinical experience and case reports, corticosteroids are recommended in patients with significant pharyngeal edema that causes or threatens respiratory compromise (35, 36).

Participation in contact sports (e.g., cheerleading, basketball, hockey, football, soccer) should be restricted during the acute phase of the illness and continue to be restricted for at least four weeks and as long as the spleen is palpable. One study followed 150 patients with newly diagnosed infectious mononucleosis for 6 months. The researchers found that sore throat, fever, headache, rash, cough, and nausea had largely resolved 1 month after the onset of symptoms. Fatigue resolved more slowly (77% initially, 28% at 1 month, 21% at 2 months, and 13% at 6 months), as did sleeping too much (45% initially, 18% at 1 month, 14% at 2 months, and 9% at 6 months) and sore joints (23% initially, 15% at 1 month, 6% at 2 months, and 9% at 6 months). Patients required about 2 months to achieve a stable level of recovery as measured by their functional status (37).

Patients with coexisting streptococcal pharyngitis or those at high risk for streptococcal pharyngitis based on their signs and symptoms (see Table 21.5) should be started on an antibiotic. Use an antibiotic other than amoxicillin, because it causes a rash in approximately 80% of patients with infectious mononucleosis. The mechanism of this reaction is not well understood. The level of evidence for treatment recommendations in infectious mononucleosis is shown in Table 21.7.

PATIENT EDUCATION

Education of the patient with sore throat has several goals. First, patients should understand that only a minority of sore throats are caused by streptococcal pharyngitis or other bacteria, and that symptomatic treatment is usually sufficient. They should also be told how to relieve the symptoms of sore throat, using salt water gargles, NSAIDs, OTC throat sprays, and OTC lozenges (e.g., Chloraseptic). Finally, patients should know the symptoms of bacterial or complicated sore throat, such as fever, chills, sweats, swollen glands, and respiratory impairment, that require physician evaluation.

CASE DISCUSSION

Based on his symptoms and age, you refer to Table 21.5 and find that his pretest probability of GABHS pharyngitis is 53%. You decide to treat empirically with a cephalosporin, because even if one of the confirmatory tests was negative, he would still have an unacceptably high chance of disease. You avoid amoxicillin because of the recent exposure to infectious mononucleosis.

Regarding the blood test for infectious mononucleosis, you should explain to the patient's mother that you will certainly order the blood test if he is still experiencing symptoms next week, but that the test is not very accurate this early in the course of the illness. In addition, a positive test would not change your management of the patient during the next week. You arrange a follow-up visit for the boy to assure that he is improving, and will check a CBC, Monospot, and/or VCA-IgM if he is still symptomatic.

REFERENCES

1. National Ambulatory Medical Care Survey. Hyattsville, MD: National Center for Health Statistics, 1993.
2. Randolph MF, Gerber MA, DeMeo KK, Wright L. Effect of antibiotic therapy on the clinical course of streptococcal pharyngitis. J Pediatr. 1985;106:870–875.
3. Bennike T, Brochner-Mortensen K, Kjaer E, Skadhange K, Trolle E. Penicillin therapy in acute tonsillitis, phlegmonous tonsillitis, and ulcerative tonsillitis. Acta Med Scand. 1951; 139:253–274.
4. Poskanzer DC, Feldman HA, Beadenkopf WG, Kuroda K, Drislane A, Diamond EL. Epidemiology of civilian streptococcal outbreaks before and after penicillin prophylaxis. Am J Public Health. 1956;46:1513–1524.
5. McWhinney I. A Textbook of Family Medicine, 2nd ed. Oxford, England: Oxford University Press, 1997:261.
6. Zwart S, Sachs AP, Ruijs GJ, Gubbels JW, Hoes AW, de Melker RA. Penicillin for acute sore throat: randomised double blind trial of seven days versus three days treatment or placebo in adults. BMJ. 2000;320(7228):150–154.
7. Williams WC, Williamson HA Jr, LeFevre ML. The prevalence of *Mycoplasma pneumoniae* in ambulatory patients with nonstreptococcal sore throat. Fam Med. 1991;23:117–121.
8. Del Mar C. Managing sore throat: a literature review. I. Making the diagnosis. Med J Aust. 1992;156:572–575.
9. Hoagland RJ. Infectious mononucleosis. Primary Care. 1975; 2:295–307.
10. Holmberg SD, Faich GA. Streptococcal pharyngitis and acute rheumatic fever in Rhode Island. JAMA. 1983;250: 2307–2312.
11. Wigton RS, Connor JL, Centor RM. Transportability of a decision rule for the diagnosis of streptococcal pharyngitis. Arch Intern Med. 1986;146:81–83.
12. Komaroff AL, Pass TM, Aronson MD, et al. The prediction of streptococcal pharyngitis in adults. J Gen Intern Med. 1986; 1:1–7.
13. Hoffman S. An algorithm for a selective use of throat swabs in the diagnosis of group A streptococcal pharyngo-tonsillitis in general practice. Scand J Prim Health Care. 1992;10: 295–300.
14. Axelrod P, Finestone AJ. Infectious mononucleosis in older adults. Am Fam Physician. 1990;42:1599–1606.
15. Fry J. Infectious mononucleosis: some new observations from a 15-year study. J Fam Pract. 1980;10:1087–1089.
16. Everett MT. The cause of tonsillitis. Practitioner. 1979;223: 253–259.
17. Hanson CJ, Higbee JW, Lednar WM, Garrison MJ. The epidemiology of acute pharyngitis among soldiers at Ford Lewis, Washington. Mil Med. 1986;7:389–394.
18. Ebell MH, Smith MA, Barry HC, Ives K, Carey M. Does this patient have strep throat? JAMA. 2000;284:2912–2918.
19. Gieseker KE, Roe MH, MacKenzie T, Todd JK. Evaluating the AAP diagnostic standard for Streptococcus pyogenes pharyngitis: backup culture versus repeat rapid antigen testing. Pediatrics. 2003;111:e666–e670
20. Ho-Yen DO, Martin KW. The relationship between atypical lymphocytosis and serological tests in infectious mononucleosis. J Infect. 1981;3:324–331.
21. Centor RM, Meier FA, Dalton HP. Throat cultures and rapid tests for diagnosis of group A streptococcal pharyngitis. Ann Intern Med. 1986;105:892–899.
22. McIsaac WJ, Goel V, To T, Low DE. The validity of a sore throat score in family practice. CMAJ. 2000;163:811–815.
23. Brinckmann J, Sigwart H, van Houten Taylor L. Safety and efficacy of a traditional herbal medicine (Throat Coat) in symptomatic temporary relief of pain in patients with acute pharyngitis: a multicenter, prospective, randomized, double-blinded, placebo-controlled study. J Altern Complement Med. 2003;9:285–298.
24. Centers for Disease Control and Prevention. Sexually transmitted diseases treatment guidelines 2002. MMWR. 2002: 51(No. RR-6).
25. Hamm RM, Hicks RJ, Bemben DA. Antibiotics and respiratory infections: are patients more satisfied when expectations are met? J Fam Pract. 1996;43:56–62.
26. Little P, Gould C, Williamson I, Warner G, Gantley M, Kinmonth AL. Reattendance and complications in a randomised trial of prescribing strategies for sore throat: the medicalising effect of prescribing antibiotics. BMJ. 1997; 315(7104):350–352.
27. DeMeyere M, Mervielde Y, Verschraegen G, Bogaert M. Effect of penicillin on the clinical course of streptococcal pharyngitis in general practice. Eur J Clin Pharmacol. 1992;43: 581–585.
28. Tompkins RK, Burnes DC, Cable WE. An analysis of the cost-effectiveness of pharyngitis management and acute rheumatic fever preventions. Ann Intern Med. 1977;86:481–489.
29. Casey JR, Pichichero ME. Meta-analysis of cephalosporin versus penicillin treatment of group A streptococcal tonsillopharyngitis in children. Pediatrics. 2004;113:866–882.
30. Shulman ST, Gerber MA, Tanz RR, Markowitz M. Streptococcal pharyngitis: the case for penicillin therapy. Pediatr Infect Dis J. 1994;13:1–7.
31. Peyramond D, Portier H, Geslin P, Cohen R. 6-day amoxicillin vs. 10-day penicillin V for group A b-hemolytic streptococcal acute tonsillitis in adults: a French Multicentre, open-label randomized study. Scand J Infect Dis. 1996;28:497–501.
32. O'Brien JF, Meade JI, Falk JL. Dexamethasone as adjuvant therapy for severe acute pharyngitis. Ann Emerg Med. 1993; 22:212–215.

33. Olympia RP, Khine H, Avner JR. Effectiveness of oral dexamethasone in the treatment of moderate to severe pharyngitis in children. Arch Pediatr Adolesc Med. 2005;159:278–282.

34. Snellman LW, Stang HJ, Stang JM, et al. Duration of positive throat culture for group A streptococci after initiation of antibiotic therapy. Pediatrics. 1993;91:1166–1170.

35. Roy M, Bailey B, Amre DK, Girodias JB, Bussieres JF, Gaudreault P. Dexamethasone for the treatment of sore throat in children with suspected infectious mononucleosis: a randomized, double-blind, placebo-controlled, clinical trial. Arch Pediatr Adolesc Med. 2004;158:250–254.

36. Centers for Disease Control: Epstein-Barr virus and infectious mononucleosis. Available at *http://www.cdc.gov/ncidod/diseases/ebv.htm*. Accessed August 16, 2004.

37. Rea TD, Russo JE, Katon W, Ashley RL, Buckwald DS. Prospective study of the natural history of infectious mononucleosis caused by Epstein-Barr virus. J Am Board Fam Pract. 2001;14:234–242.

CHAPTER 22

Abdominal Pain

John Smucny, John Epling, and Joseph Thompson

CASE 1

A previously healthy 35-year-old woman has severe right lower quadrant abdominal pain that began yesterday and became worse today. She reports a low-grade fever and some nausea, but denies diarrhea, vomiting, urinary complaints, respiratory or systemic symptoms, or use of any medications or illicit drugs. She has no history of prior abdominal or pelvic symptoms. Her last menses were 5 weeks ago. On examination, she appears mildly uncomfortable. Vital signs are normal. She has right lower quadrant tenderness, but no guarding or mass.

CASE 2

A 30-year-old woman complains of recurrent lower abdominal pain for 2 months, often associated with frequent, loose stools. The pain is relieved with defecation. She also notes intermittent lower abdominal bloating. She denies any weight loss, blood in the stools, nocturnal symptoms, or other red flags for serious diseases. Medical history and review of systems are unremarkable. She has been under some increased stress recently at work. Her physical examination results are normal.

KEY CLINICAL QUESTIONS

1. Which patients with abdominal pain need urgent evaluation and treatment?
2. Are diagnostic tests or specialty consultation necessary?
3. What is the best approach to initial management?

Although only a minority of adults with abdominal pain seek medical attention, it is still one of the most common presenting symptoms in primary care (1). Abdominal pain was the seventh most common principal reason for patient visits to ambulatory care settings in the United States in 1997, accounting for 2% of all visits (2). Data from the 2000 United States National Center for Health Statistics (USNCHS) reveal an incidence of abdominal pain of 63 in 1000 emergency department (ED) visits with admission rates for abdominal pain varying from 18% to 42% (the rate increases as patients get older). Although diagnostic technologies have advanced, a thorough and appropriately focused history and physical ex-

amination remain the key to effective diagnosis and management of abdominal pain.

DIFFERENTIAL DIAGNOSIS AND PATHOPHYSIOLOGY

Pathophysiology

Conditions that cause abdominal pain range in severity from the life-threatening to the benign and self-limited, and may result from either intra- or extra-abdominal pathology (Figure 22.1). Intra-abdominal conditions cause visceral and parietal pain. Visceral pain is caused by spasm or stretching of the muscle wall of a hollow viscus, distention of the capsule of a solid organ, or ischemia or inflammation of a visceral structure. The pain is typically deep, dull, and diffusely located in the midline. Epigastric visceral pain is caused by pathology in either thoracic or upper abdominal organs; periumbilical pain from the small intestine, cecum, or appendix; and hypogastric pain from the colon, rectum, or pelvis.

Parietal pain is caused by irritation of the parietal peritoneum from a contiguous, diseased intra-abdominal organ. This type of pain is sharper and more localized than visceral pain and worsens with movement. It is usually located in one of the four quadrants directly over the anatomic location of the diseased organ. Diffuse parietal pain can be caused by generalized peritonitis that occurs with perforation or rupture of an organ.

A few conditions characteristically progress from visceral to parietal pain (e.g., appendicitis progresses from periumbilical visceral pain to right lower quadrant parietal pain; diverticulitis, from the hypogastrium to the left lower quadrant; acute cholecystitis, from the epigastrium to the right upper quadrant). Pain can also radiate from one location to another. Pancreatic pain can radiate from the epigastrium to the middle of the back, and pain in cholecystitis can radiate to the right subscapular area. Finally, some diseases refer pain to extra-abdominal locations, such as subphrenic abscesses, which can cause ipsilateral shoulder pain.

Pain from extra-abdominal disease can radiate or be referred to the abdomen. Myocardial infarction can present with epigastric pain, lower lobe pneumonia with ipsilateral upper quadrant pain, and testicular torsion with ipsilateral lower quadrant pain. Pain can radiate to the abdomen from the back as a result of any condition that causes spinal nerve root irritation. Abdominal wall conditions, such as muscle strains and rectus sheath hematomas, cause pain from inflammation of the associated tissues. This pain is usually constant and

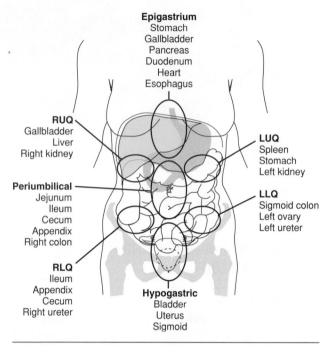

Epigastrium
Stomach
Gallbladder
Pancreas
Duodenum
Heart
Esophagus

RUQ
Gallbladder
Liver
Right kidney

LUQ
Spleen
Stomach
Left kidney

Periumbilical
Jejunum
Ileum
Cecum
Appendix
Right colon

LLQ
Sigmoid colon
Left ovary
Left ureter

RLQ
Ileum
Appendix
Cecum
Right ureter

Hypogastric
Bladder
Uterus
Sigmoid

Figure 22.1 • Structures that commonly cause abdominal pain, grouped by type and site of pain. LLQ, left lower quadrant; LUQ, left upper quadrant; RLQ, right lower quadrant; RUQ, right upper quadrant. (Redrawn and printed with permission from Currie DJ. Abdominal Pain. Washington, DC: Hemisphere Publishing; 1979.)

TABLE 22.1	Causes of Abdominal Pain in Adults in Family Practice
Diagnosis	**% of All Patients Who Presented with Abdominal Pain (n = 556)**
Nonspecific abdominal pain	50.4
Acute gastroenteritis	9.2
Urinary tract infection	6.7
Irritable bowel syndrome	5.8
Pelvic inflammatory disease	3.8
Hiatal hernia or reflux	2.3
Diverticulosis	2.2
Diarrhea	<2
Cholelithiasis/cholecystitis	<2
Benign tumor	<2
Duodenal ulcer	<2
Urolithiasis	<2
Appendicitis	<2
Ulcerative colitis	<2
Muscle strain	<2
Other*	9.5
Percent admitted	9.2
Percent undergoing surgery	4.7

*Other includes endometriosis, malignant tumor, esophagitis, gastritis, gastric ulcer, hepatitis, spontaneous abortion, anxiety, and depression. (Adapted and reprinted with permission from Adelman A. Abdominal pain in the primary care setting. J Fam Pract. 1987;25:27–32.)

aching, and increases with voluntary tightening of the abdominal wall.

Many systemic and toxic conditions can cause abdominal pain. Common causes are sickle cell disease, diabetes mellitus, and uremia; rare causes include porphyria, lead poisoning, and black widow spider bites. Psychological conditions can also lead patients to complain of abdominal pain. Patients with underlying stress, psychological illness, or a history of abuse are more likely to present with functional gastrointestinal disorders and chronic pelvic pain.

Differential Diagnosis

A relatively limited number of conditions cause the great majority of episodes of abdominal pain in family medicine (see Table 22.1). Nonspecific abdominal pain (NSAP) is the most common diagnosis coded by family physicians for patients who present with abdominal pain (3). A variety of conditions cause NSAP, and patients generally have a good prognosis. Comparison of the diagnostic coding with the medical records for patients in a family medicine office showed that 60% coded as having NSAP actually had more specific diagnoses listed in the physicians' notes (4). The most common diagnoses were irritable bowel syndrome, infectious diarrhea, gastritis, muscle strains, ovarian cysts, and peptic ulcer disease. Most patients with NSAP have improvement or resolution of pain within days to months of presentation.

There is a bimodal distribution, with patients over age 50 years more likely to have serious disease and less likely to be diagnosed with NSAP. In a series of 360 older patients presenting to the ED with abdominal pain, 58% were admitted, 18% required surgery, and 5% died; only 15% were diagnosed with NSAP. The most common specific diagnoses in this series of patients were urinary tract infection, bowel obstruction, diverticulitis, and gastroenteritis (5).

CLINICAL EVALUATION

Evaluation of patients with abdominal pain should begin with an assessment of whether there is a condition that requires urgent treatment and/or surgery. Red flags (see Table 22.2) for such conditions can be detected rapidly. For patients without red flags, you can develop a reasonable differential diagnosis from a careful history and physical examination. See Figure 22.2 for an algorithmic approach to the diagnosis of abdominal pain and Table 22.3 for information on the accuracy of key elements of the history and physical examination.

History

The location, quality, timing, and severity of pain are the most important elements of the history. The location and quality of the pain can help you determine whether the pain is due

TABLE 22.2 Red Flags Suggesting Life-Threatening Disease in Patients with Abdominal or Pelvic Pain

	Diagnoses Suggested
History	
Abrupt onset of pain	Perforation or rupture (ulcer, appendix, gallbladder, colon, ectopic pregnancy, spleen, abdominal aortic aneurysm) Acute vascular event (mesenteric infarction, aortic dissection, myocardial infarction, pulmonary embolus) Volvulus, strangulated hernia, ovarian torsion, pancreatitis
Examination	
Shock	Perforation or rupture (see above) with intra-abdominal hemorrhage or peritonitis Severe pancreatitis, acute vascular event (see above), gastrointestinal hemorrhage
Distention	Bowel obstruction, ileus, volvulus, toxic megacolon, bowel ischemia, intra-abdominal hemorrhage, abdominal aortic aneurysm, ascites
Diffuse peritoneal signs	Perforation or rupture (see above), severe pancreatitis, mesenteric infarction
Focal peritoneal signs	Appendicitis, diverticulitis, cholecystitis, cholangitis, abscess, pelvic inflammatory disease, pancreatitis

to a visceral, parietal, or extra-abdominal source. Timing and severity are important because the abrupt onset of severe pain often signifies a life-threatening condition (see Table 22.2). Gradual onset of pain over a few hours to a few days is more likely to represent an inflammatory process or intestinal obstruction. The abrupt worsening of such pain may signal the perforation of the inflamed or obstructed organ.

The temporal progression of pain is also helpful. Progression from visceral to parietal pain is characteristic of certain conditions as noted above (e.g., appendicitis, diverticulitis, and acute cholecystitis). Colicky pain that comes and goes often represents gastroenteritis, a partial bowel obstruction, obstructing renal calculus, or irritable bowel syndrome. Additional items of possible importance in the history are associated symptoms; precipitating and/or alleviating factors; underlying medical conditions; psychosocial factors; and potentially toxic, infectious, or drug exposures. A menstrual history should be taken in all women of child-bearing age.

Physical Examination

The physical examination should first be directed toward determining whether the patient needs urgent referral. Urgent conditions are usually accompanied by shock, abdominal distention, or peritonitis (see Table 22.2). A clinical maneuver that can help diagnose peritonitis from any cause is the cough test (worsening of pain when the patient coughs in response to your request to do so; LR+ = 3.0). Worsening pain with inspiration or expiration also suggests peritonitis, and the presence of all three strongly predicts peritonitis (16).

The examination of patients with abdominal pain should include examination of the abdomen, back, and thorax; palpation of all hernia orifices; a pelvic examination for women; a genital examination for men; and a rectal examination. Patients with severe disease may present with more subtle findings from the history and physical examination than described above. This is particularly true in the elderly and the immunocompromised, and you should have a lower threshold for more aggressive evaluation and referral of these patients.

Diagnostic Tests

Traditionally, because of the large number of conditions that can lead to abdominal pain, there are no specific diagnostic tests recommended for all patients. You should base your diagnostic strategy on an assessment of the most likely diagnoses and the serious conditions that must be excluded (e.g., a pregnancy test should be performed in women of child-bearing age to help exclude ectopic pregnancy). Some patients, such as those with mild symptoms and normal examination results, may require no diagnostic testing at all. In these cases, watchful waiting alone is a useful and appropriate diagnostic tool. Nonetheless, computed tomography (CT) scanning has become an invaluable tool in the rapid and accurate evaluation of abdominal pain. In the past decade, CT scanning has proved useful in diagnosing and differentiating between various causes of acute abdominal pain like appendicitis, diverticulitis, pancreatitis, and renal calculi. A prospective study in patients presenting to the ED with abdominal pain found that nonenhanced helical CT was the single most useful test (17). Table 22.4 summarizes the accuracy of diagnostic tests for common conditions.

SPECIFIC CONDITIONS

The remainder of this chapter discusses the approach to common important conditions that present primarily as abdominal pain in adults. Abdominal pain in children, with trauma, and occurring beyond the first trimester of pregnancy is beyond the scope of this chapter. Diseases that may include abdominal pain as part of the symptom complex but that generally have other more distinguishing characteristics are also excluded. Examples of the latter (with their typical presentations) include gastroesophageal reflux (heartburn, Chapter 24), hepatitis (jaundice), gastroenteritis (vomiting and/or diarrhea), inflammatory bowel disease (diarrhea), pyelonephritis (flank pain; Chapter 28), renal calculi (flank pain radiating to the groin), cystitis (dysuria; Chapter 28), and hernias (symptomatic

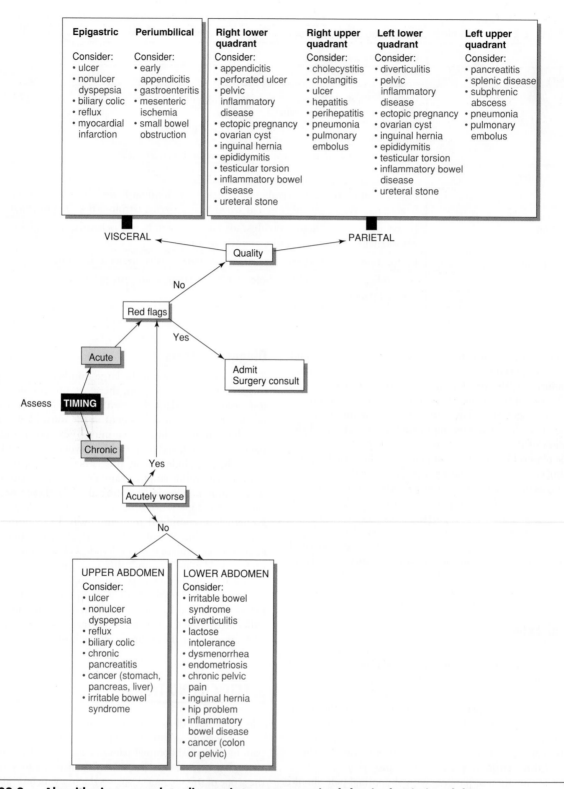

Figure 22.2 • Algorithmic approach to diagnosing nontraumatic abdominal pain in adults.

TABLE 22.3 Key Elements of the History and Physical Exam for Adults with Abdominal or Pelvic Pain

Diagnosis/Element	Sensitivity	Specificity	LR +	LR −
Acute cholecystitis (in emergency department patients with acute upper abdominal pain)				
h/o fever (6)	0.15	0.99	15.0	0.9
h/o chills (6)	0.13	0.95	2.6	0.9
h/o or presence of jaundice (6)	0.02	0.99	2.0	1.0
Palpable gallbladder (6)	0.02	0.99	2.0	1.0
Rebound/guarding (6)	0.02	0.85	0.1	1.1
Murphy's sign (adults) (6)	0.97	0.48	1.9	0.1
Murphy's sign (in elderly patients) (7)	0.48	0.79	2.3	0.7
Bowel obstruction (in patients with abdominal pain)				
Previous abdominal surgery (8)	0.69	0.74	2.7	0.4
Age over 50 (8)	0.60	0.73	2.2	0.5
Constipation (8)	0.44	0.95	8.8	0.6
Vomiting (8)	0.75	0.65	2.1	0.4
Abdominal distention (8)	0.63	0.89	5.7	0.4
Increased bowel sounds (8)	0.40	0.89	3.6	0.7
Appendicitis (in hospitalized or emergency department patients with abdominal pain)				
RLQ pain (9)	0.81	0.53	1.7	0.4
Migration (9)	0.64	0.82	3.6	0.4
Pain precedes vomiting (9)	0.99	0.64	2.8	0.01
Fever (9)	0.67	0.79	3.2	0.4
Rebound tenderness (9)	0.63	0.69	2.0	0.5
Rigidity (9)	0.27	0.83	1.6	0.9
Psoas sign (9)	0.16	0.95	3.2	0.9
Surgeon's clinical impression (10)	0.63	0.82	3.5	0.4
Irritable bowel syndrome (vs. organic disease in patients with abdominal pain, constipation, or diarrhea)				
# of Manning's criteria present				
4 or more (11)	0.5	0.88	4.2	0.6
3 or more (11)	0.84	0.76	3.5	0.2
2 or more (11)	0.93	0.55	2.1	0.1
Ectopic pregnancy (in pregnant patients with abdominal pain or bleeding presenting to an emergency department)				
Vaginal bleeding and pain (for ectopic *or* abnormal pregnancy requiring surgical therapy) (12)	0.72	0.57	1.7	0.5
Overall clinical examination for predicting ectopic pregnancy (13)	0.19	0.99	19.0	0.8
Two-stage prediction model for predicting ectopic pregnancy				
1. High risk criteria (signs of peritoneal irritation or definite cervical motion tenderness) (14)	0.32	0.95	6.1	0.7
2. Intermediate risk criteria (no fetal heart tones by Doppler, no tissue at cervical os, or any pelvic pain or tenderness, and no high-risk criteria) (14)	0.99	0.28	1.4	0.03
Endometriosis (in infertile women)				
Uterosacral nodularity (15)	0.06	0.99	6.0	0.9
Uterosacral pain (15)	0.08	0.98	4.0	0.9
Obstructed pouch of Douglas (15)	0.06	0.98	3.0	1.0

Abbreviations: h/o, history of; LR +, positive likelihood ratio; LR −, negative likelihood ratio.

TABLE 22.4 Characteristics of Diagnostic Tests Useful for Adults with Abdominal or Pelvic Pain

Diagnosis/Test	Sensitivity	Specificity	LR+	LR–
Cholelithiasis				
Transabdominal ultrasound (18)	0.89	0.97	30.0	0.1
CT scan (18)	0.79	0.99	79.0	0.2
Oral cholecystogram (18)	0.75	0.96	19.0	0.3
Acute calculous cholecystitis				
Cholescintigram (18)	0.97	0.90	9.7	0.03
Transabdominal ultrasound (18, 19)	0.60–0.91	0.79	3.0–4.3	0.1–0.5
Choledocholithiasis				
MRCP (20)	0.92	0.97	30.0	0.08
ERCP (18)	0.90	0.99	90.0	0.1
Endoscopic ultrasound (18)	0.93	0.97	31.0	0.1
Helical CT scan (18)	0.88	0.97	29.0	0.1
Transabdominal ultrasound (18)	0.25	0.95	5.0	0.8
Acute pancreatitis				
Contrast CT scan (21)	0.92	0.99	92.0	0.1
Transabdominal ultrasound (21)	0.62–0.95	0.97	21–32	0.1–0.4
Serum lipase (22)	0.94	0.96	24.0	0.06
Serum amylase (22)	0.82	0.91	9.1	0.2
Chronic pancreatitis				
ERCP (23)	0.9	0.99	90.0	0.1
Plain abdominal radiograph (23)	0.3	0.98	15.0	0.7
CT scan (22)	0.8	0.85	5.3	0.2
ECHO-enhanced power Doppler sonogram (24)	0.85	0.99	85	0.15
Transabdominal ultrasound (22)	0.65	0.85	4.3	0.4
Pancreatic cancer				
ERCP (25)	0.95	0.97	32.0	0.05
CT scan (25)	0.85	0.9	8.5	0.2
ECHO-enhanced power Doppler sonogram (24)	0.87	0.94	15	0.14
Transabdominal ultrasound (25)	0.7	0.85	4.7	0.3
Bowel obstruction				
Plain abdominal radiograph (26)	0.77	0.50	1.5	0.5
Transabdominal ultrasound (26)	0.83	0.99	83.0	0.2
CT scan (26)	0.93	0.99	93.0	0.1

(continued)

TABLE 22.4   Characteristics of Diagnostic Tests Useful for Adults with Abdominal or Pelvic Pain (*continued*)

Diagnosis/Test	Sensitivity	Specificity	LR +	LR −
Appendicitis				
Elevated WBC (27)	0.53	0.65	1.5	0.7
Elevated CRP (28)	0.70	0.62	3.0	0.5
Transabdominal ultrasound (29)	0.85	0.9	8.5	0.2
Transabdominal ultrasound with inconclusive clinical picture (30)	0.95	0.9	9.5	0.06
CT scan with rectal contrast (for "definitely" or "probably" appendicitis) (31)	0.98	0.98	49	0.02
Transabdominal ultrasound followed by CT scan with rectal contrast (if needed) in children (32)	0.94	0.94	15.7	0.06
Diverticulitis				
Water-soluble contrast enema (9)	0.94	N/A	N/A	N/A
Transabdominal ultrasound (33)	0.85	0.84	5.3	0.2
CT scan (traditional) (33)	0.91	0.77	4.0	0.1
Helical CT scan (rectal contrast only) (34)	0.97	1.00	97	0.03
Ectopic pregnancy				
Endometrial pipelle (35)	0.30	0.99	30	0.3
Transvaginal ultrasound shows noncystic adnexal mass (14)	0.84	0.99	84.0	0.2

Abbreviations: CRP, C-reactive protein; CT, computed tomography; ERCP, endoscopic retrograde cholangiopancreatography; LR +, positive likelihood ratio; LR −, negative likelihood ratio; MRI, magnetic resonance imaging; N/A, not available.

bulge). Dyspepsia is the prime subject matter in Chapter 24, and Chapter 33 covers additional causes of pelvic pain.

Gallbladder Disease

By age 75, 35% of women and 20% of men have developed gallstones; fortunately, most are asymptomatic (36). Complications from gallstones include biliary pain (biliary colic), acute cholecystitis, choledocholithiasis (common bile duct stones), cholangitis, pancreatitis, gallstone ileus, and gallbladder cancer.

Biliary pain is characterized by recurrent episodes of steady, severe pain in the epigastrium or right upper quadrant (RUQ) that lasts for more than 15 minutes (37). The pain often awakens the patient, can radiate to the back or right scapular area, and is often precipitated by meals or associated with nausea and emesis (37). Acholic stools (tan or yellow and steatorrheous) are sometimes reported. The physical examination between episodes is usually unremarkable. The best initial imaging study for detecting gallstones is ultrasonography (Table 22.3). CT scans and oral cholecystograms are less sensitive, but may be used when ultrasound is technically inadequate (18).

Acute calculous cholecystitis (inflammation of the gall-bladder secondary to persistent obstruction of the cystic duct) occurs in fewer than 2% of individuals with gallstones per year (38). This condition usually begins as typical biliary pain, but the pain persists. On physical examination, most patients have RUQ tenderness, and Murphy sign (cessation of inspiration caused by pain with palpation of the RUQ; Table 22.4). Although symptoms and signs like fever, chills, jaundice, a palpable gallbladder, RUQ tenderness and Murphy sign may be useful for ruling in acute cholecystitis, none have been especially reliable (39). These signs are less helpful in the elderly, who often present with mental status changes, no Murphy sign, and less fever (7). Laboratory tests may show leukocytosis and mild elevations of liver function test results and enzymes (38). Cholescintigrams are the most accurate tests for detecting acute cholecystitis (Table 22.3), but ultrasounds are often preferred initially because of convenience and because they can detect other conditions that may be causing a patient's symptoms (38).

About 10% of patients with cholelithiasis have common bile duct stones (11). Although most of these pass asymptomatically into the duodenum, obstruction of the common bile duct may occur, which can lead to acute cholangitis. Cholangitis is potentially lethal, particularly if not treated urgently. The classic presentation of acute cholangitis (Charcot's triad of pain, fever, and jaundice) occurs in 50% to 60% of patients; RUQ tenderness with peritoneal signs is present in 67% (40).

Laboratory studies commonly show leukocytosis and elevations of transaminases, alkaline phosphatase, and bilirubin; amylase is also elevated in 33%. Ultrasonography is not sensitive for detecting common bile duct stones. Endoscopic retrograde cholangiopancreatography (ERCP) is recommended for acutely ill patients because it is the most accurate test and offers the additional benefit of stone removal. However, because ERCP can cause pancreatitis, cholangitis, or aspiration pneumonia, magnetic resonance cholangiopancreatography (MRCP), helical CT, and endoscopic ultrasonography (Table 22.4) (38) are becoming more widely used (20).

Some patients have typical biliary pain but no detectable gallstones. Their symptoms may be attributable to sludge, microlithiasis, or gallbladder dysfunction (41). Endoscopic ultrasound is more sensitive than transabdominal ultrasonography in detecting sludge and microlithiasis. Gallbladder dysfunction (also called biliary dyskinesia) may be diagnosed by a gallbladder ejection fraction <40% on cholecystokinin-stimulated cholescintigraphy. However, a positive cholesystokinin provocation test is not highly predictive of patients who might benefit from an operation (42).

Pancreatic Disease

Acute pancreatitis is an acute inflammatory process of variable severity. Most cases are caused by excessive alcohol use (50%) or gallstones (30%) (22). The remainder are caused by hypertriglyceridemia, trauma, a variety of drugs or infections, and a host of uncommon causes; about 10% are idiopathic. Approximately 25% of patients develop severe complications; the overall mortality rate is as high as 10% to 15% in some series (43).

Typical symptoms of acute pancreatitis include upper abdominal pain (90%) that often radiates to the back, anorexia (85%), nausea and vomiting (75%), and fever (60%). The pain is usually sudden in onset and increases in severity over several hours. Common signs include decreased bowel sounds (60%) and abdominal rigidity (50%). Less common presentations include shock (15%), jaundice (15%), and hematemesis (10%) (43).

Serum lipase is the most accurate blood test for diagnosing acute pancreatitis (Table 22.4). Elevated serum aminotransaminases and/or bilirubin suggest gallstones as the etiology (44). Somewhat useful is an aspartate aminotransferase level >60 IU/L on admission; this has an LR+ of 5.8 and LR− of 0.2 for gallstone pancreatitis among patients with pancreatitis (44).

Abdominal and chest radiographs may show suggestive findings (such as hemidiaphragmatic elevation, pleural effusion, sentinel loops of small bowel, or a colon cutoff sign) or pancreatic calcifications (which are diagnostic of chronic pancreatitis). Plain films can also detect free air in the abdomen as a result of a perforated viscus as the cause of the patient's symptoms. Ultrasonography has poor sensitivity because it is often technically inadequate in patients with suspected pancreatitis (see Table 22.4). Nonetheless, it is recommended as the initial imaging study because it is diagnostic when positive and can also detect cholelithiasis as a presumptive cause. Abdominal CT scans are more accurate at diagnos-

ing pancreatitis, can more accurately show complications such as necrosis and pseudocysts, and can provide prognostic information. A CT scan is therefore recommended for patients with clinically severe disease, when the diagnosis is in question, or when patients do not improve within 48–72 hours (44). Additionally, urine trypsinogen may predict severity (45) but otherwise offers no advantage over lipase or amylase.

Chronic pancreatitis is usually caused by chronic, excessive alcohol consumption. Most patients present with recurrent upper abdominal pain and tenderness (45). Symptoms or signs of exocrine or endocrine insufficiency (such as steatorrhea, weight loss, or diabetes) may also be present after 90% of the gland is affected. Serum amylase and lipase levels are often normal or only slightly elevated. Abdominal plain films are diagnostic if they show calcifications (LR+, 15.0), but cannot rule out disease if negative (LR−, 0.7). CT scanning is more accurate than ultrasonography, but not as accurate as ERCP (see Table 22.3). However, because ERCP is invasive, expensive, and may cause complications, it is usually performed only if the other test results are nondiagnostic. Tests of exocrine function are used for patients with persistent pain and normal imaging study results (46).

The incidence of pancreatic cancer is 11 in 100,000 and increasing. It is responsible for 5% of all cancer deaths and has the worst prognosis of all malignancies, with a 5-year survival rate of <5% (46). Risk factors for pancreatic cancer include chronic pancreatitis, diabetes mellitus, and smoking. Most patients are 60 to 80 years old and present with weight loss (95%), abdominal pain (80%), and/or jaundice (50%). The visceral, epigastric pain radiates to the back in 50% of cases. Cancers in the head of the pancreas may cause jaundice, hepatomegaly, and a palpable gallbladder (Courvoisier sign). ERCP is the most accurate diagnostic procedure, but is invasive. Among noninvasive imaging tests, CT scans are more accurate than transabdominal ultrasounds although echo-enhanced power Doppler sonography is quite accurate (see Table 22.4) (25, 47). Endoscopic ultrasonography and positron-emission tomography are promising new diagnostic modalities.

Bowel Obstruction

The most common cause of bowel obstruction is adhesions from prior surgery (up to 70%) (48). Other causes are neoplasms, gallstones, congenital bowel abnormalities, and ingested materials. The pain is usually intermittent and generalized; it may be relieved by vomiting and worsened by eating. Strangulation (vascular compromise by the obstruction) occurs early in patients with an obstructed hernia or volvulus, and in up to 38% of patients with complete small bowel obstruction (49). Strangulation becomes more likely as time passes, and requires immediate surgical intervention. Patients with strangulation may have more marked tenderness and signs of peritonitis. A tender, nonreducible inguinal mass is present if the strangulation is caused by an inguinal hernia.

Bowel obstruction should be suspected and further tests ordered if two or more of the following findings are present: distended abdomen, increased bowel sounds, history of constipation, previous abdominal surgery, age over 50 years, and/or vomiting. It is unlikely if none or only one of those findings is present (8) (see Table 22.3). Plain abdominal radiographs are the initial imaging study obtained because of their low cost and convenience. They may reveal air-fluid levels or bowel distention, but if clinical suspicion remains high after negative plain films, ultrasound or CT should be performed (see Table 22.4). CT has the additional benefit of localizing the cause of the obstruction 87% of the time (26).

Appendicitis

Acute appendicitis is the most common condition leading to surgery among patients with abdominal pain. A balance between underdiagnosis and overdiagnosis is crucial. Older studies have reported a normal appendix in 15% to 35% of patients undergoing appendectomy. However, a more recent series noted that the negative appendectomy rate has fallen from 20% to 3% between 1996 and 2003 (50). This appears to be a result of the advent of the spiral CT scanning protocol about five to ten years ago. That the drop in the negative appendectomy rate has been gradual over the past decade is likely because of the learning curve experienced by radiographic operators in reading helical computed tomograms as well as improved technology. Mortality and significant morbidity are more likely if surgery is delayed until appendiceal perforation (9). Delay of the diagnosis past 48 hours is associated with a higher risk of perforation than earlier diagnosis (71% versus 24%) (51).

Distention of the appendix initially leads to poorly localized epigastric or periumbilical visceral pain, which may be accompanied by anorexia, nausea, or vomiting. In fact, pain almost always precedes vomiting in appendicitis; if vomiting precedes pain, appendicitis is very unlikely (LR−, 0.01) (51). Physical examination at this stage reveals no specific findings. With peritoneal involvement, the pain becomes localized to the right lower quadrant, often at McBurney point (5 cm from the anterior superior iliac spine on a line running to the umbilicus). Physical examination at this point will frequently reveal guarding, rigidity, rebound tenderness, a positive cough test result, Rovsing sign (referred rebound tenderness on the right lower quadrant from palpation of the left lower quadrant), or a psoas sign (pain with resisted thigh flexion). See Table 22.3 for the accuracy of some of these maneuvers.

With rupture of the appendix, the pain may decrease for a brief time, then becomes much more intense. The temperature then increases, the patient shows increasing signs of toxicity, and the abdomen may develop a board-like rigidity. Not all patients experience this classic sequence. The pain may localize at different times and locations for each patient. For these patients, a rectal or pelvic examination may be diagnostically useful. Diagnosing appendicitis is more difficult in the elderly, but overall, right lower quadrant pain, right lower quadrant tenderness, and abdominal wall rigidity are the most helpful signs (52). Young women have a broader differential diagnosis for lower abdominal pain including ovarian cysts, mittelschmerz, pelvic inflammatory disease, ectopic pregnancy, endometriosis, and other gynecologic conditions.

An elevated white blood cell count or C-reactive protein (CRP) level increases the risk of appendicitis slightly if the results are positive, but does not rule it out if normal (see Table 22.4) (28). Abdominal ultrasound when used in conjunction with a clinical scoring system is useful for patients who have an intermediate probability of appendicitis, but should not be used to change a strong initial clinical impression for or against appendicitis (30). Helical CT with 3% diatrizoate rectal contrast is very accurate in diagnosing appendicitis, and can assist in avoiding unnecessary hospitalization and surgery. Although addition of rectal contrast to helical CT scanning in adults confers higher predictive values, the sensitivity, specificity, and likelihood ratios are compelling enough to make the diagnosis without need for contrast (see Table 22.4). This does not hold true for children where rectal contrast confers significant advantage in the diagnosis of appendicitis. In children suspected of having appendicitis, the protocol of ultrasound followed by limited CT with rectal contrast (if the ultrasound result was negative or indeterminate) can also rule out appendicitis (32).

Diverticulitis

The prevalence of diverticulosis (diverticula in the colon) increases with age. It is present in fewer than 10% of people under 40 years of age, compared with up to 66% of those over age 80. Acute inflammation leading to symptoms of diverticulitis affects only 10% to 25% of patients with diverticula over their lifetime (53). The mortality rate may be as high as 18% in hospitalized patients. More than 90% of inflamed diverticula are located in the sigmoid colon and lead to left lower abdominal pain. Typical symptoms of diverticulitis include gradual onset and continuous left lower quadrant pain. Fever, change in bowel habits, and vomiting may be associated symptoms. Urinary frequency or urgency may be present if the inflamed bowel lies adjacent to the bladder (54).

In acute diverticulitis, an elevated white blood cell count has a sensitivity of only 53% (55), and plain radiographs are abnormal in only one third of patients (55). A contrast enema with a water-soluble agent, an ultrasound, or a CT scan can all be used to accurately diagnose acute diverticulitis (see Table 22.4). In patients with an atypical or severe presentation, CT should be used to rule out other pathology or an acute surgical problem. Helical CT with rectal contrast is very accurate and avoids oral or intravenous contrast administration.

Irritable Bowel Syndrome

Irritable bowel syndrome (IBS) is a common functional disorder characterized by chronic abdominal pain that is associated with defecation or a change in the frequency or appearance of stool (56). Symptoms consistent with IBS are found in approximately 15% of the population (57). Possible etiologies for IBS include altered gastrointestinal motility, visceral hypersensitivity, and luminal irritation. Risk factors for developing IBS include a recent episode of bacterial gastroenteritis (58), female sex, and lower household income. Psychiatric conditions are more common in patients who choose to seek medical help for IBS than in controls, but are not more common in individuals who report IBS-compatible symptoms in population-based surveys. Other functional conditions such as non-ulcer dyspepsia (some are patients with a confusing picture of non-urgent, non-specific upper and lower GI complaints), fatigue, and urogenital dysfunction may coexist with IBS.

The diagnosis of IBS is made by obtaining a history of symptoms compatible with IBS and by excluding other conditions. The pain of IBS varies but is usually located in the lower abdomen and is cramp-like or aching. Patients may have alternating diarrhea and constipation, or predominantly one or the other. The Manning criteria (59) are useful historical clues to the diagnosis, particularly in women and the nonelderly (see Table 22.4). These are:

1. Pain relief with bowel action
2. More frequent stools with the onset of pain
3. Looser stools with the onset of pain
4. Passage of mucus
5. Sensation of incomplete evacuation
6. Abdominal distention as evidenced by tight clothing or visible appearance

The presence of fewer than two of these criteria is strong evidence to rule out IBS. Clues in the history to other diagnoses include abdominal pain that is severe, localizing, or awakens the patient; weight loss; fever; diarrhea that awakens the patient; or stools suggestive of malabsorptive or secretory diarrhea or bleeding. The physical examination in patients with IBS is generally unremarkable. When present, abdominal tenderness is unimpressive.

A recommended routine evaluation based on expert opinion to help exclude other causes includes checking the complete blood count; sedimentation rate; chemistries; and stool for pathogens, white blood cells, and blood (59). Colonoscopy or flexible sigmoidoscopy and/ or barium enema should be offered to patients older than 45 years or those over age 40 with a family history of colon cancer.

Ectopic Pregnancy

Ectopic pregnancy should be considered in the differential diagnosis of every woman of childbearing age who presents with lower abdominal or pelvic pain. Major risk factors are a history of prior ectopic pregnancy, tubal surgery, tubal pathology, or diethylstilbesterol (DES) exposure in utero. Minor risk factors are a history of genital infections, past intrauterine device use, and more than one lifetime sexual partner (60). Classic findings include pain in the lower abdomen, back, or pelvis; vaginal spotting or bleeding; and a missed menstrual period. The diagnosis is initially missed in up to 40% of women (61) because these symptoms are common with spontaneous abortion or normal pregnancy. Vaginal bleeding may be absent, and up to 15% of women with ectopic pregnancies will not have missed a period. If the patient is examined before rupture of the ectopic pregnancy, there may be lower abdominal tenderness and rebound. Pelvic examination often reveals adnexal tenderness, a tender adnexal mass, or pain on movement of the cervix (see Table 22.3). After rupture, patients have increased tenderness, rigidity, and other signs of generalized peritoneal irritation, or shock.

Although no single element of the examination is very useful, the overall impression of a skilled clinician is very accurate when positive (LR +, 19) but not useful when negative (LR −, 0.8) (12).

Serum human chorionic gonadotropin (HCG) and transabdominal or transvaginal ultrasound are the most helpful investigations (62). A serum HCG that is negative or >50,000 mIU/mL rules out an ectopic pregnancy. If the quantitative serum HCG is >6500 mIU/mL, a transabdominal ultrasound should be able to detect an intrauterine pregnancy if one is present. With transvaginal ultrasonography (TVUS), this threshold decreases to a level of 1500 to 2000 mIU/mL. At this level, TVUS that shows a noncystic adnexal mass in the absence of an intrauterine pregnancy diagnoses ectopic pregnancy. If nothing is seen in the adnexae, then either careful observation or diagnostic laparoscopy is warranted (14).

Endometriosis

Endometriosis is characterized by the presence of endometrial glands and stroma outside the uterine cavity in a variety of locations, including the pelvic peritoneum, ovaries, and uterine ligaments. The pathologic findings of endometriosis can be found in up to 20% of asymptomatic women, 30% of subfertile women, and 60% of women with dysmenorrhea.

Endometriosis causes cyclic or noncyclic pelvic pain, dyspareunia, and/or infertility. Dysmenorrhea may also be present but is not predictive of endometriosis (15). The dyspareunia is described as deep pain and may continue for several hours postcoitus. Women may also have abnormal menses or premenstrual spotting, pain on defecation or urination, urinary frequency, hematuria, constipation, or diarrhea (63). Abnormal physical findings are most likely to be present during menses. Painful nodules along the uterosacral ligaments, uterosacral pain, or an obstructed pouch of Douglas are useful when present (LR +, 3.0 to 6.0), but failure to detect them does not rule out endometriosis (see Table 22.3). Although MRI is very predictive of endometrial cysts (LR + 45, and LR − 0.1), laparoscopy remains the gold standard for diagnosis of endometriosis (64).

Chronic Pelvic Pain

Chronic pelvic pain is a common disorder in women of reproductive age. It is defined as pelvic pain in the absence of a known cause (such as endometriosis, chronic pelvic inflammatory disease, or primary dysmenorrhea). Most patients do not have a clear diagnosis based on anatomic pathology, and the disorder can be frustrating for both patient and physician. An irritable bowel–like syndrome, pelvic vascular congestion, and altered pelvic neural sensation are proposed theories of etiology. There is an association between chronic pelvic pain and physical or sexual abuse. Symptoms can include noncyclic pain, dysmenorrhea, and dyspareunia. Patients often have a reduced quality of life and sense of well-being (65).

MANAGEMENT

Treatment of abdominal pain can be either directed specifically at the established diagnosis or used empirically if an exact diagnosis is not essential. In some cases, such as patients with nonspecific abdominal pain, symptomatic treatment or reassurance may be the only treatment needed. Regardless of the initial treatment, good follow-up is important; the timing depends on the seriousness of the problem. Of course, patients with peritoneal signs or other red flags for life-threatening conditions require immediate consultation with a surgeon. In this section, the focus is primarily on conditions treated by family physicians.

Gallbladder Disease

Asymptomatic gallstones usually do not require treatment. The treatment of choice for symptomatic cholelithiasis is cholecystectomy, usually performed laparoscopically. This operation successfully eliminates symptoms in more than 90% of patients (66). Nonetheless, some patients with uncomplicated gallstones may benefit from diet modification and choose watchful waiting over immediate surgery, although most will eventually require surgery (67). Before surgery, parenteral nonsteroidal anti-inflammatory drugs (NSAIDs), opioids, and/or antispasmodics can be used to treat episodes of biliary pain. Treatment options for patients who are too ill or unwilling to undergo surgery include dissolution therapy or lithotripsy. However, fewer than one-third of patients are appropriate candidates for these treatments and stones often recur. Cholecystectomy may also be a useful treatment for biliary dyskinesia.

Initial treatment of acute cholecystitis consists of bowel rest, intravenous hydration, broad-spectrum antibiotics, analgesics, and nasogastric suction (if an ileus is present). Cholecystectomy is usually performed within a few days of admission. The traditional approach is to allow a "hot" gallbladder to "cool off" before operating. However, a meta-analysis of randomized trials (68) suggests that early cholecystectomy (open or laparotomy) actually reduces mortality and morbidity, and results in shorter hospital stays and lower costs. Concomitant common bile duct stones are removed either preoperatively via ERCP or at the time of surgery. Acute cholangitis is treated similarly, although urgent endoscopic or percutaneous decompression is advocated for severe illness or when patients do not rapidly improve (41).

Pancreatic Disease

Management of acute pancreatitis begins by determining the severity of the episode because patients with severe disease require more aggressive and intensive care. Clinical scoring systems such as the Ranson criteria and/or CRP levels are useful for initial stratification of risk (43, 44). (See Table 22.5 for Ranson criteria and their interpretation.) A CRP level >150 mg/L drawn 48 hours after admission has an LR+ of 2.2 and an LR- of 0.2 for predicting a complicated case (71). It is therefore better at ruling out complications than at ruling them in. Treatment is aimed at correcting any underlying predisposing factors and inflammation (like obstructing gallstones, hypercalcemia, precipitating drugs, poorly controlled diabetes with elevated triglycerides). Mild cases of acute pancreatitis respond to aggressive hydration, pancreatic rest, analgesics, and nasogastric suctioning (if vomiting is present) (43). In severe cases, useful therapies include broad-spectrum antibiotics, peritoneal lavage, somatostatin, octreotide, and gabexate mesilate (not available in the United States) (72). Patients who have biliary pancreatitis may benefit from early endoscopic retrograde cholangiography with sphincterotomy (73, 74). They should then undergo cholecystectomy as soon as they are well enough to tolerate the surgery.

TABLE 22.5 Ranson Criteria for Prognosis in Acute Pancreatitis*

1. Add up the number of risk factors for your patient:

Risk Factor	Points
At admission or diagnosis	
Age over 55 years	1
White blood cell count >16,000/mm^3	1
Blood glucose >200 mg/dL	1
Serum LDH >350 IU/L	1
Serum AST (AST) >250 IU/L	1
During the initial 48 hours	
Hematocrit decrease >10 percentage points	1
Blood urea nitrogen increase >5 mg/dL	1
Serum calcium <8.0 mg/dL	1
Room air Pao$_2$ <60 mm Hg	1
Base deficit >4 mEq/L	1
Fluid sequestration >6 L	1
Total:	

2. The risk of severe disease and death is shown below:

Score	Number in Group	% with Severe Disease	% Who Died
0	20	15	5
1	28	25	14
2	23	39	22
3	14	57	43
≥4	6	50	50

Data from Refs. 89 and 90.
Abbreviations: AST, aspartate aminotransferase; LDH, lactic dehydrogenase

Treatment of chronic pancreatitis is directed at avoiding or controlling pain. Avoidance of alcohol, a low-fat diet, and nonopiate analgesics are first-line therapy (75). Opiate analgesics, nerve blocks or ablation, endoscopic therapies, and surgical decompression or pancreatic resection are options for patients with persistent pain (76). Lithotripsy is also used, although it has not been shown to be clearly beneficial (77). The exocrine insufficiency from chronic pancreatitis can be treated with low-fat diets, medium-chain triglycerides, and pancreatic enzyme replacements.

The only definitive treatment for pancreatic cancer is surgery. Unfortunately, fewer than one-third of tumors are resectable once diagnosed, and only one-third of those are curable. Pain control may be provided with sufficient doses of opiate analgesics and celiac plexus nerve blocks.

Bowel Obstruction

Patients whose obstruction is accompanied by strangulation require immediate surgery. Often, patients with a non-strangulating bowel obstruction will respond to fluid replacement and bowel decompression, but surgery is indicated when the obstruction does not promptly resolve (43). In patients with terminal abdominal or pelvic carcinoma for whom palliative care is appropriate, fluid replacement and decompression are not indicated. Corticosteroids show a trend toward relieving obstruction in these patients (78).

Appendicitis

Once appendicitis is diagnosed, early surgery provides the best opportunity to avoid the complications associated with appendiceal rupture. When the diagnosis is unclear, a period of close observation with repeated examination by a skilled clinician can be helpful. Appendectomy is a relatively simple procedure and leads to few complications. Laparoscopic appendectomy is more expensive than an open procedure and requires longer operating times, but it leads to fewer wound infections, shorter hospital stays, and a quicker return to work or usual activities (79). It is noteworthy that CT scanning technology has led to a significant reduction in the negative appendectomy rate in the past decade (50).

Diverticulitis

If good oral intake is maintained and there is help at home, many patients with diverticulitis canbe managed as outpatients with oral antibiotics directed against gram-negative and anaerobic organisms (for example, a quinolone or trimethoprim/sulfamethoxazole combined with metronidazole). More severely ill patients require intravenous fluids, antibiotics, and bowel rest in the hospital. Up to 30% of patients with diverticulitis and evidence of gross perforation require immediate surgery (50). Surgical consultation should also be obtained for failure of conservative management or if complications (abscess or perforation) are suspected. A cost-effectiveness analysis found that surgery should be considered after at least three episodes of recurrent, uncomplicated diverticulitis leading to hospitalization (80). After recovery, a colon evaluation, usually with colonoscopy, is recommended to confirm the diagnosis and rule out other pathology. Although a low-fiber diet, clear liquids, or no feeding at all is usually advocated during episodes, a high-fiber diet may help prevent recurrences between episodes (81). It has also been traditional to counsel patients with diverticula to avoid seeds, nuts, and other foods that are presumed to occlude the diverticular orifices.

Irritable Bowel Syndrome

On average, IBS spontaneously resolves within 5 years in more than 50% of patients. Favorable prognostic factors include a good patient–physician relationship, a shorter duration of symptoms at the time of diagnosis, and no associated psychiatric problems (82). Initial treatment should include interventions that are safe, such as education, reassurance, and a trial of additional fiber and/or lactose restriction. For patients with persistent symptoms, drugs that are most likely to be effective are smooth-muscle relaxants (e.g., dicyclomine) and loperamide (see Table 22.6) (83). The 5-HT receptor antagonist alosetron is effective for some women with severe diarrhea-predominant IBS, but was initially withdrawn from the market in 2000 because it led to ischemic colitis, severe constipation, and even death in some patients. It has since been reintroduced with restricted access for women who meet strict criteria. The 5-HT receptor partial agonist, tegaserod, has been shown to be effective but only for women with constipation-predominant IBS (84). Peppermint oil, Chinese herbal medicine, antidepressants, and behavioral therapy may also be helpful, but these approaches are not as well supported by the available data (89).

Ectopic Pregnancy

Laparoscopic surgery is the treatment of choice for management of tubal ectopic pregnancy. Systemic methotrexate therapy is an alternative but has a high rate of adverse drug effects. This method requires a hemodynamically stable patient with low HCG levels (<3000 IU/L) and no signs of bleeding. The patient should then be followed with weekly HCG determinations until no level is detectable (90).

Endometriosis

The management of endometriosis depends on the severity of the symptoms and the woman's desires concerning future pregnancies. NSAIDs, oral contraceptives, danazol, progesterones, and gonadotropin-releasing hormone (GnRH) antagonists like leuprolide (91) may all control mild to moderate pain but do not improve fertility (see Table 22.6). Although laparoscopic procedures that ablate the uterine nerve or endometrial deposits may improve symptoms and fertility, there is insufficient evidence to recommend its routine use (92). Women with severe pain may require total abdominal hysterectomy with bilateral salpingo-oophorectomy.

Chronic Pelvic Pain

As the pathophysiology of chronic pelvic pain is poorly understood, treatment is directed toward symptom relief. A multifaceted approach begins with the development of a clear sense of goals and boundaries in the therapeutic relationship. Supportive counseling, ultrasound examination or laparoscopy to rule out pathology, and progestagen therapy are effective treatment options (93). Surgery (hysterectomy and/or neural interruption) is a final option.

TABLE 22.6 Outpatient Pharmacologic Management of Common Causes of Chronic Abdominal and Pelvic Pain

Condition	Drug	Regimen	Strength of Recommendation*	Comments
IBS (83,84)	Loperamide	2 mg 2 times/d	A	For diarrhea-predominant IBS
	Dicyclomine	10–20 mg 3 times/d	B	For pain-predominant IBS
	Amitriptyline	10–25 mg at night	B	For pain-predominant IBS
	Tegaserod	6 mg 2 times/d	A	For constipation-predominant IBS
	Alosetron	0.5–1 mg 2 times/d	A	For diarrhea-predominant IBS
Endometriosis (85–88)	Oral contraceptives	Many brands	A	First-line recommendation
	Danazol	400–800 mg/day divided 2 times/d	A	Androgenic side effects, rare pseudotumor cevebii and intracranial hypertension, cases of thromboembolism reported
	Progestagens/antiprogestagens	Several types	A	Use throughout cycle
	GnRH analogues	Several types	A	No advantage over other therapies

Abbreviations: GnRH, gonadotropin-releasing hormone; IBS, irritable bowel syndrome.
*A = consistent, good-quality patient-oriented evidence; B = inconsistent or limited-quality patient-oriented evidence; C = consensus, disease-oriented evidence, usual practice, expert opinion, or case series. For information about the SORT evidence rating system, see *http://www.aafp.org/afpsort.xml*.

CASE 1 DISCUSSION

Acute appendicitis, pelvic inflammatory disease, and ectopic pregnancy are potentially serious diagnoses that must be considered. Diverticulitis is less likely because of the patient's age and the right-sided location of the pain. Ovarian cyst and nonspecific abdominal pain are also in the differential diagnosis, but are less likely because of the severity of the pain. Urinary tract infection is also a possibility, but is less likely because of the absence of urinary symptoms such as frequency or dysuria.

A serum HCG, urinalysis, and a pelvic examination should be performed. A negative HCG result would rule out ectopic pregnancy. Cervical motion tenderness and bilateral adnexal tenderness would suggest pelvic inflammatory disease (see Chapter 33). Right adnexal tenderness or mass would be consistent with ectopic pregnancy, appendicitis, or pelvic inflammatory disease with a tubo-ovarian abscess. If a mass is present, a sonogram may be helpful in differentiating between these conditions. An elevated white blood cell count or CRP would suggest an acute infective process such as appendicitis or pelvic inflammatory disease, but a normal white blood cell count would not rule out these diagnoses.

CASE 2 DISCUSSION

The patient probably has irritable bowel syndrome, with predominantly pain and diarrhea. She has four Manning criteria, and no evidence of other disease from the history and physical examination. You should consider doing a basic laboratory evaluation (complete blood count [CBC], erythrocyte sedimentation rate, and stool tests for blood, white blood cells, and pathogens). If these test results are negative, then reassurance, increased dietary fiber, a trial of lactose reduction, stress reduction, and follow-up would be an appropriate initial plan. If the symptoms persist, you could prescribe loperamide.

Acknowledgment

This chapter was originally authored by Drs. Smucny and Epling and then revised by Dr. Thompson. Dr. Thompson would like to acknowledge the assistance of Drs. Paul Lazar and Kenny Luong with the revision.

REFERENCES

1. Adelman A, Revicki D, Magaziner J, Hebel R. Abdominal pain in an HMO. Fam Med. 1995;27:321–325.
2. Schappert SM. Ambulatory care visits to physician offices, hospital outpatient departments, and emergency departments: United States, 1997. National Center for Health Statistics. Vital Health Stat 13. 1999;13(143):1–39.
3. Adelman A. Abdominal pain in the primary care setting. J Fam Pract. 1987;25:27–32.
4. Klinkman MS. Episodes of care for abdominal pain in a primary care practice. Arch Fam Med. 1996;5:279–285.
5. Lewis LM, Banet GA, Blanda M, et al. Etiology and clinical course of abdominal pain in senior patients: a prospective, multicenter study. J Gerentol A Biol Sci Med Sci. 2005;60(8):1071–1076.
6. Singer A, McCracken G, Henry M, Those HJ, Cabajug C. Correlation among clinical, laboratory, and hepatobiliary scanning findings in patients with suspected acute cholecystitis. Ann Emerg Med. 1996;28:267–272.

7. Adedeji OA, McAdam WA. Murphy's sign, acute cholecystitis, and elderly people. J R Coll Surg Edinb. 1996;41:88–89.

8. Bohner H, Yang Q, Frank C, Verreet PR, Ohmann C, and the Study Group Acute Abdominal Pain. Simple data from history and physical examination help to exclude bowel obstruction and avoid radiographic studies in patients with acute abdominal pain. Eur J Surg. 1998;164:777–784.

9. Wagner JM, McKinney WP, Carpenter JL. Does this patient have appendicitis? JAMA. 1996;276:1589–1594.

10. Wade DS, Marrow SE, Balsara ZN, Burkhard TK, Goff WB. Accuracy of ultrasound in the diagnosis of acute appendicitis compared with the surgeon's clinical impression. Arch Surg. 1993;128:1039–1044; discussion 1044–1046.

11. Manning AP, Thompson WG, Heaton KW, Morris AF. Towards a positive diagnosis of the irritable bowel. BMJ. 1978; 2:653–654.

12. Barnhart K, Mennuti MT, Benjamin I, Jacobson S, Goodman D, Coutifaris C. Prompt diagnosis of ectopic pregnancy in an emergency department setting. Obstet Gynecol. 1994;84: 1010–1015.

13. Buckley RG, King KJ, Disney JD, et al. History and physical examination to estimate the risk of ectopic pregnancy: validation of a clinical prediction model. Ann Emerg Med. 1999; 34:589–594.

14. Brown DL, Doubilet PM. Transvaginal sonography for diagnosing ectopic pregnancy: Positivity criteria and performance characteristics. J Ultrasound Med. 1994;13:259–266.

15. Matorras R, Rodriguez F, Pijoan JI, Soto E, Perez C, Ramon O, et al. Are there any clinical signs and symptoms that are related to endometriosis in infertile women? Am J Obstet Gynecol. 1996;174:620–623.

16. Taylor S, Watt M. Emergency department assessment of abdominal pain: Clinical indicator tests for detecting peritonism. Eur J Emerg Med. 2005;12:275–277.

17. Gerhardt RT, Nelson BK, Keenan S, et al. Derivation of a clinical guideline for the assessment of non-specific abdominal pain: the guideline for abdominal pain in the ED Setting (GAPEDS) Phase 1 Study. Am J Emerg Med. 2005;23: 709–717.

18. Richard EA, Greene RA. Cholelithiasis and acute cholecystitis. In: Black ER, Bordley DR, Tape TG, Panzer RJ, eds. Diagnostic Strategies for Common Medical Problems, 2nd ed. Philadelphia: ACP-ASIM; 1999:158–169.

19. Bingener J, Schwesinger WH, Chopra S, Richards ML, Sirinek KR. Does the correlation of acute cholecystitis on ultrasound and at surgery reflect on mirror image? Am J Surg. 2004 Dec; 188(6):703–707.

20. Romagnuolo J, Bardou M, Rahme E, Joseph L, Reinhold C, Barkun AN. Magnetic Resonance Cholangiopancreatography: a meta-analysis of test performance in suspected billiary disease. Ann Intern Med. 2003 Oct 7;139(7):547–557.

21. Agarwal N, Pitchumoni CS, Sivaprasad AV. Evaluating tests for acute pancreatitis. Am J Gastroenterol. 1990;85:356–366.

22. Corsetti JP, Arvan DA. Acute pancreatitis. In: Black ER, Bordley DR, Tape TG, Panzer RJ, eds. Diagnostic Strategies for Common Medical Problems, 2nd ed. Philadelphia: ACP-ASIM; 1999:204–212.

23. Owyang C, Levitt MD. Chronic pancreatitis. In: Yamada T, Alpers DH, eds. Textbook of Gastroenterology, 2nd ed. Philadelphia: JB Lippincott; 1995:2091–2112.

24. Rickes S, Unkrodt K, Neye H, Ocran KW, Wermke W. Differentiation of pancreatic tumours by conventional ultrasound, unenhanced and echo-enhanced power Doppler sonography. Scand J Gastroenterol. 2002 Nov;37(11): 1313–1320.

25. Panzer RJ. Pancreatic masses. In Black ER, Bordley DR, Tape TG, Panzer RJ, eds. Diagnostic Strategies for Common

26. Suri S, Gupta S, Sudhakar PJ, Venkataramu NK, Sood B, Wig JD. Comparative evaluation of plain films, ultrasound and CT in the diagnosis of intestinal obstruction. Acta Radiologica. 1999;40:422–428.

27. Chi CH, Shiesh SC, Chen KW, Wu MH, Lin XZ. C-reactive protein for the evaluation of acute abdominal pain. Am J Emerg Med. 1996;14:254–256.

28. Hallan S, Asberg A. The accuracy of C-reactive protein in diagnosing acute appendicitis—a meta-analysis. Scand J Clin Lab Invest. 1997;57:373–380.

29. Orr RK, Porter D, Hartman D. Ultrasonography to evaluate adults for appendicitis: decision-making based on meta-analysis and probabilistic reasoning. Acad Emerg Med. 1995;2: 644–650.

30. Douglas CD, Macpherson NE, Davidson PM, Gani JS. Randomised controlled trial of ultrasonography in diagnosis of acute appendicitis, incorporating the Alvarado score. BMJ. 2000;321:1–6.

31. Rao PM, Rhea JT, Novelline RA, Mostafavi AA, McCabe CJ. Effect of computed tomography of the appendix on treatment of patients and use of hospital resources. N Engl J Med. 1998;338:141–146.

32. Garcia Pena BM, Mandl KD, Kraus SJ, et al. Ultrasonography and limited computed tomography in the diagnosis and management of appendicitis in children. JAMA. 1999;282: 1041–1046.

33. Pradel JA, Adell J, Taourel P, Djafari M, Monnin-Delhom E, Bruel J. Acute colonic diverticulitis: Prospective comparative evaluation with US and CT. Radiology. 1997;205:503–512.

34. Rao PM, Rhea JT, Novelline RA, Dobbins JM, Lawrason JN, Sacknoff R, Stuk JL. Helical CT with only colonic contrast material for diagnosing diverticulitis: prospective evaluation of 150 patients. Am J Roentgenol. 1998;170:1445–1449.

35. Nyhlin H, Elsborg L, Silvennoinen J, Holme I, Ruegg P, Jones J, Wagner A. A double-blind placebo-controlled randomized study to evaluate the efficacy, safety, tolerability of tegaserod in patients with IBS. Scand J Gastroenterol. 2004 Feb;39(2):119–126.

36. Anonymous. Guidelines for the treatment of gallstones. Ann Intern Med. 1993;119:620–622.

37. Kraag N, Thijs C, Knipschild P. Dyspepsia—how noisy are gallstones? Scand J Gastroenterol. 1995;30:411–421.

38. Friedman G. Natural history of asymptomatic and symptomatic gallstones. Am J Surg. 1993;165:399–404.

39. Trowbridge RL, Rutkowski NK, Shojania KG. Does this patient have acute cholecystitis? JAMA. 2003 Jan 1;289(1): 80–86.

40. Kadakia SC. Biliary tract emergencies—acute cholecystitis, acute cholangitis, and acute pancreatitis. Med Clin North Am. 1993;77:1015–1036.

41. Corazziari E, Shaffer EA, Hogan WJ, Sherman S, Toouli J. Functional disorders of the biliary tract and pancreas. Gut. 1999;45(suppl II):II48–II54.

42. Smythe A., Majeed AW, Fitzhenry M, Johnson AG. A requiem for cholecystokinin provacation test? Gut. 1998 Oct; 43(4):571–574

43. Anonymous. United Kingdom guidelines for the management of acute pancreatitis. Gut. 1998;42(suppl 2):1S–13S.

44. Mayer AD, McMahon MJ. Biochemical identification of patients with gallstones associated with acute pancreatitis on the day of admission to hospital. Ann Surg. 1985;201:68–75.

45. Steer M, Waxman I, Freedman ST. Chronic pancreatitis. N Engl J Med. 1995;332:1482–1490.

46. DiMagno E. Pancreatic adenocarcinoma. In Yamada T, Alp-

ers D, eds. Textbook of Gastroenterology, 2nd ed. Philadelphia: JB Lippincott; 1995:2113–2130.

47. Rickes S, Unkrodt K, Neye H, et al. Differentiation of pancreatic tumors by conventional ultrasound, unenhanced, and echo-enhanced power Doppler sonography. Scand J Gastroenterol. 2002;37:1313–1320.

48. Wilson MS, Ellis H, Menzies D, Moran BJ, Parker MC, Thompson JN. A review of the management of small bowel obstruction. Ann R Coll Surg Engl. 1999;81:320–328.

49. Frager D, Medwid SW, Baer JW, Mollinelli B, Friedman M. CT of small-bowel obstruction: value in establishing the diagnosis and determining the degree and cause [see comments]. AJR Am J Roentgenol. 1994;162:37–41. Comment in: AJR Am J Roentgenol. 1996 May;166(5):1227.

50. Rhea JT, Halpern EF, Ptak T, Lawrason JN, Sacknoff R, Novelline RA. The status of appendiceal CT in an urban medical center 5 years after its introduction: experience with 753 patients. Am J Roentgenol. 2005;184(6):1802–1808

51. Cappendijk VC, Hazebrook FWJ. The impact of diagnostic delay on the course of acute appendicitis. Arch Dis Child. 2000;83:64–66.

52. Eskelinen M, Ikonen J, Lipponen P. The value of history-taking, physical examination and computer assistance in the diagnosis of acute appendicitis in patients more than 50 years old. Scand J Gastroenterol. 1995;30:349–355.

53. The Standards Task Force of the American Society of Colon and Rectal Surgeons. Practice parameters for the treatment of sigmoid diverticulitis. Dis Colon Rectum. 2000;43:289–297.

54. Ambrosetti P, Robert JH, Witsig J, Mirescu D, Mathey P, Borst F, Rohner A. Acute left colonic diverticulitis: A prospective analysis of 226 consecutive cases. Surgery. 1994;115:546–550.

55. Morris J, Stellato TA, Haaga JR, Lieberman J. The utility of computed tomography in colonic diverticulitis. Ann Surg. 1986;204:128–132.

56. Thompson WG, Longstreth GF, Drossman DA, Heaton KW, Irvine EJ, Muller-Lissner SA. Functional bowel disorders and functional abdominal pain. Gut. 1999;45(suppl II):II43–II47.

57. Taub E, Cuevas JL, Cook EW III, Crowell M, Whitehead WE. Irritable bowel syndrome defined by factor analysis. Gender and race comparisms. Dig Dis Sci. 1995; 40(12):2647–2655.

58. Rodriguez LAG, Ruigomez A. Increased risk of irritable bowel syndrome after bacterial gastroenteritis: cohort study. BMJ. 1999;318:565–566.

59. Anonymous. American Gastroenterological Association medical position statement: irritable bowel syndrome. Gastroenterology. 1997;112:2118–2119.

60. Ankum WM, Mol BWJ, Van der Veen F, Bossuyt PMM. Risk factors for ectopic pregnancy: a meta-analysis. Fertil Steril. 1996;65:1093–1099.

61. Kaplan BC, Dart RG, Moskos M, Kuligowska E, Chun B, Adel HM, et al. Ectopic pregnancy: prospective study with improved diagnostic accuracy. Ann Emerg Med. 1996;28:10–17.

62. Gracia CR, Barnhart RT. Diagnosing ectopic pregnancy: decision analysis comparing six strategies. Obstet Gynecol. 2001 Mar;97(3):464–470.

63. Damewood MD. Pathophysiology and management of endometriosis [see comments]. J Fam Pract. 1993;37:68–75.

64. Togashi K, Nishimura K, Kimura I, Tsuda Y, Yamashita K, Shibata T, et al. Endometrial Cysts: diagnosis with MR imaging Radiology. 1991 Jul;180(1):73–78.

65. Zondervan KT, Yudkin PL, Vessey MP, Dawes MG, Barlow DH, Kennedy SH. The prevalence of chronic pelvic pain in women in the United Kingdom: a systematic review. Br J Obstet Gynecol. 1998;105:93–99.

66. NIH Planning Committee. National Institutes of Health Consensus Development Conference Statement on Gallstones and Laparoscopic Cholecystectomy. Am J Surg. 1993;165:390–398.

67. Vetrhus M, Soreide O, Solhang JH, Nesrik I, Soridenaa K. Symptomatic, non-complicated gallbladder stone disease. Operation or observation? A randomized clinical study. Scand J Gastroenterol. 2002 Jul;37(7):834–839.

68. Papi C, Cartarci M, D'Ambrosio L, et al. Timing of Cholecystectomy for acute calculous cholecystitis: a meta-analysis. Am J Gastroentorol 2004 Jan;99(1):147–155.

69. de Bernardinis M, Violi V, Roncoroni L, Montanari M, Peracchia A. Automated selection of high-risk patients with acute pancreatitis. Crit Care Med. 1989;17:318–322.

70. Ranson JHC, Rifkind KM, Turner JW. Prognostic signs and nonoperative peritoneal lavage in acute pancreatitis. Surg Gynecol Obstet. 1976;143:209–219.

71. Neoptolemos JP, Kemppainen EA, Mayer JM, Fitzpatrick JM, Raraty MGT, Slavin J, et al. Early prediction of severity in acute pancreatitis by urinary trypsinogen activation peptide: a multicentre study. Lancet. 2000;355:1955–1960.

72. Andriulli A, Leandro G, Clemente R, Festa V, Caruso N, Annese V, et al. Meta-analysis of somatostatin, octreotide and gabexate mesilate in the therapy of acute pancreatitis. Aliment Pharmacol Ther. 1998;12:237–245.

73. Sharma VK, Howden CW. Metaanalysis of randomized controlled trials of endoscopic retrograde cholangiography and endoscopic sphincterotomy for the treatment of acute biliary pancreatitis. Am J Gastroenterol. 1999;94:3211–3214.

74. Evidence Report/Technology assessment no.50, Endoscopic Retrograde Cholangiopancreatography. AHRQ publication no. 02-E017.

75. Anonymous. American Gastroenterological Association medical position statement: treatment of pain in chronic pancreatitis. Gastroenterology. 1998;115:763–764.

76. Anonymous. Surgical treatment of chronic pancreatitis. J Gastrointest Surg. 1998;2:489–490.

77. Adamek HE, Jakobs R, Buttmann A, Adamek MU, Schneider ARJ, Riemann JF. Long term follow up of patients with chronic pancreatitis and pancreatic stones treated with extracorporeal shock wave lithotripsy. Gut. 1999;45:402–405.

78. Feuer DJ, Broadley KE. Corticosteroids for the resolution of malignant bowel obstruction in advanced gynaecological and gastrointestinal cancer (Cochrane Review). In: The Cochrane Library. Oxford, England: Update Software; 2000:Issue 3.

79. McCall JL, Sharples K, Jadallah F. Systematic review of randomized controlled trials comparing laparoscopic with open appendectomy. Br J Surg. 1997;84:1045–1050.

80. Richarts RJ, Hammitt JR. Timing of prophytactic surgery in the prevention of diverticulitis recurrence: a cost-effective analysis. Dig Dis Sci. 2002 Sept;47(9):1903–1908.

81. Leahy AL, Ellis RM, Quill DS, Peel AL. High fibre diet in symptomatic diverticular disease of the colon. Ann R Coll Surg Engl. 1985;67:173–174.

82. Janssen HAM, Muris JWM, Knotterus JA. The clinical course and prognostic determinants of the irritable bowel syndrome: a literature review. Scand J Gastroenterol. 1998;33:561–567.

83. Jailwala J, Imperiale TF, Kroenke K. Pharmacologic treatment of the irritable bowel syndrome: a systematic review of randomized, controlled trials. Ann Intern Med. 2000;133:136–147.

84. American College of Gastroenterology Functional Gastrointestinal Disorders Task Force. Evidence-based position paper

on the management of irritable bowel syndrome in North America. Am J Gastroenterol. 2002;97:S1–S5.

84. Moore J, Kennedy S, Prentice A. Modern combined oral contraceptives for pain associated with endometriosis (Cochrane Review). In: The Cochrane Library. Oxford, England: Update Software; 2000:Issue 3.

85. Selak V, Farquhar C, Prentice A, Singla A. Danazol for pelvic pain associated with endometriosis (Cochrane Review). In: The Cochrane Library. Oxford, England: Update Software; 2000:Issue 3.

86. Prentice A, Deary AJ, Bland, E. Progestagens and antiprogestagens for pain associated with endometriosis (Cochrane Review). In: The Cochrane Library. Oxford, England: Update Software; 2000:Issue 3.

87. Prentice A, Deary AJ, Goldbeck-Wood S, Farquhar C, Smith SK. Gonadotrophin-releasing hormone analogues for pain associated with endometriosis (Cochrane Review). In: The Cochrane Library. Oxford, England: Update Software; 2000: Issue 3.

89. Drossman DA, Toner BB, Whitehead WE, et al. Cognitive-behavioral therapy versus education and desipramine versus placebo for moderate to severe functional bowel disorders. Gastroenterology. 2003 Jul;125(1):19–31.

90. Hajenuis PJ, Mol BW, Bossuyt PM, Ankrum WM, Van Der Veen F. Interventions for tubal ectopic pregnancy (Cochrane Review). In: The Cochrane Library. Oxford, England: Update Software; 200:Issue 2.

91. Ling F. Randomized control trial of depot leuprolide in patients with chronic pelvic pain and clinically suspected endometriosis. Pelvic Pain Study Group. Obstet Gynecol. 1999 Jan;93(1): 51–58.

92. Proctor ML, Latthe PM, Farquhar CM, Khan KS, Johnson NP. Surgical interruption of pelvic nerve pathways for primary and secondary dysmenorrhea. Cochrane Database Syst Rev. 2005 Oct 19;4:CD001896. Chichester, U.K.: John Wiley and Sons, Ltd.

93. Stones W, Cheong YC, Howard FM. Interventions for treating chronic pelvic pain in women. In Cochrane Review, Issue 4, 2005. Chichester, U.K.: John Wiley and Sons, Ltd.

CHAPTER 23

Chronic Liver Disease

Kenneth W. Lin

CASE 1

B.J. is a 48-year-old man whose medical problems include obesity, hypertension, type 2 diabetes, and hyperlipidemia. Because exercise and dietary modification have not lowered his cholesterol to target levels, his physician decides to start him on a statin and obtains baseline liver function tests before starting the medication. Testing reveals an elevated alanine transaminase of 87 and aspartate transaminase of 98. What further history, physical examination, and diagnostic testing should be undertaken at this point?

CASE 2

D.M. is a 36-year-old male patient who presents for a routine physical examination. His medical and social history are significant for a history of injection drug use and unprotected sex with multiple female partners 10 years ago. He has no history of significant alcohol use, and he denies symptoms of abdominal pain or jaundice. He has never received the hepatitis B vaccine. Why is D.M. at risk for chronic liver disease (CLD)?

CLINICAL QUESTIONS

1. What are common causes of CLD, and who is at increased risk?
2. How is CLD treated?
3. What primary and secondary preventive strategies are available for CLD?

Chronic liver disease (CLD) is estimated to affect at least 20 million Americans and is the 10th leading cause of death in U.S. adults (1). In many patients, CLD is diagnosed during routine laboratory testing for other conditions, but certain demographic risk factors and exposures may suggest the need for disease-specific testing. Because CLD has many distinct etiologies, establishing the diagnosis in asymptomatic patients can be challenging. This chapter will discuss causes of CLD in patients who present to family physicians. The most common noninfectious and infectious causes of CLD include: alcoholic hepatitis, nonalcoholic fatty liver disease, and viral hepatitis. All of these conditions may lead to cirrhosis and end-stage liver disease. Prevention and treatment of secondary complications of CLD are important because they reduce morbidity and mortality.

COMMON CAUSES OF ABNORMAL LIVER TRANSAMINASES

Although they are often called markers of liver "function," elevated alanine transaminase (ALT) and aspartate transaminase (AST) levels more accurately reflect hepatocellular injury. The destruction of hepatocytes causes these enzymes to be released into the bloodstream. Although levels may sometimes be normal in CLD, unexplained elevations in transaminases should increase suspicion of its presence.

To rule out iatrogenic causes and identify risk factors for CLD, a patient with an unexplained elevation in ALT or AST should be questioned about medication use (including herbal and "alternative" medications and dietary supplements), alcohol and injection drug use, and sexual history. If possible, potentially hepatotoxic medications should be discontinued. Although a history of injection drug use or multiple sexual partners increases the risk for viral hepatitis, all patients with elevated transaminases should undergo testing for hepatitis A, B, and C. Hemochromatosis is an inherited, treatable cause of abnormal transaminases. The best single test to detect hemochromatosis is the transferrin saturation, although ferritin may also be elevated (2–4).

Most asymptomatic patients presenting to a family physician with isolated elevated transaminases and normal viral hepatitis serologies and iron studies will ultimately be diagnosed with either alcoholic hepatitis or nonalcoholic fatty liver disease (NAFLD). NAFLD often has a benign course, with a relatively small percentage of affected patients developing nonalcoholic steatohepatitis (NASH) and clinically significant liver dysfunction. Continued alcohol use in the presence of alcoholic hepatitis is more likely to lead to cirrhosis, liver failure, and hepatocellular cancer (HCC).

Although there is no evidence from randomized controlled trials to guide the most efficient work-up of elevated liver transaminases, the American Gastroenterological Association recommends an algorithmic approach (see Figure 23.1). When viral hepatitis serologies and iron studies are normal in a patient without acute hepatic decompensation, a diagnosis of NAFLD is presumed and 6 months of lifestyle modification should be initiated to reduce weight and improve control of diabetes, if present (5). The persistence of ALT or AST abnormalities beyond this period should cause the clinician to consider additional testing for rare causes.

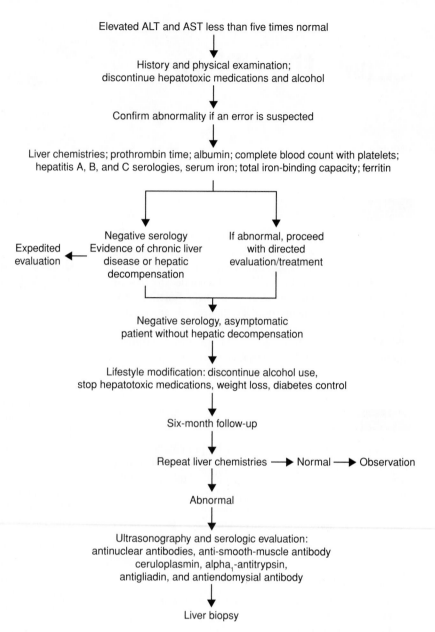

Figure 23.1 • Management of ALT and AST abnormalities (less than 5 times upper limit of normal). Algorithm reproduced from Giboney PT. Mildly elevated liver transaminase levels in the asymptomatic patient. Am Fam Physician. 2005;71:1105–1110. Available at *http://www.aafp.org/afp/20050315/1105.html.*

This algorithm should not be used if other liver function tests, such as alkaline phosphatase, bilirubin, prothrombin time, or albumin are also significantly abnormal, or if the AST or ALT are elevated more than 5 times the upper limit of normal. This may indicate more serious disease or disease originating outside of the liver. The clinician should also keep in mind "red flags" that make serious disease more likely, and expeditious diagnosis imperative (see Table 23.1).

Both alcoholic hepatitis and NAFLD can be definitively diagnosed only on biopsy. Because of the risks of biopsy and the uncertain benefits of treatment, it is controversial which patients with unexplained LFT elevations should undergo biopsy. A prospective study of 36 adult patients with LFT elevations for greater than 6 months found that liver biopsy changed the presumptive diagnosis in only 14% of cases and did not significantly alter treatment recommendations (6).

TABLE 23.1 Red Flags for Patients with Elevated Transaminases Indicating More Serious Disease

Red Flags
Abdominal pain
Elevations of other markers of liver function Hematemesis Rectal bleeding
Signs of advanced liver failure: - spider angiomas - lower extremity edema - congestive heart failure - hepatojugular reflex

TABLE 23.2 Risk Factors for NAFLD/NASH

Risk Factors
Age >45
Diabetes
Family history of cryptogenic cirrhosis
Hyperlipidemia
Hypertension
Obesity

Information from References 8, 12, 13.

Alcoholic Hepatitis

Although the minimum level of alcohol consumption that causes hepatitis is not known, a history of >40 g of alcohol, or three drinks per day, is a generally accepted threshold for increased risk. In the absence of a suggestive history, the AST to ALT ratio is useful in distinguishing alcoholic hepatitis from NASH. A retrospective case-control study found that an AST to ALT ratio of >2 was strongly associated with alcoholic liver disease, whereas a ratio of <1 suggested NASH. The ratio was less reliable in the presence of cirrhosis (7). Because histologic findings are virtually identical, a liver biopsy is not useful in distinguishing alcoholic hepatitis from NASH (8).

Discontinuation of alcohol use is the only effective treatment for alcoholic hepatitis. A systematic review and meta-analysis concluded that brief (5–10 minute) office counseling delivered by primary care providers is effective in reducing alcohol consumption at 6 and 12 months (9). A variety of behavioral approaches and medications have been shown to be effective in achieving and maintaining abstinence from alcohol (10, 11).

Nonalcoholic Fatty Liver Disease

Although it is the most common cause of liver test abnormalities in asymptomatic patients, NAFLD is largely a diagnosis of exclusion. NAFLD exists along a pathologic spectrum of four types of fatty infiltration of the liver, the more severe of which are associated with the development of liver fibrosis

and poor clinical outcomes (8). Certain conditions and risk factors increase the risk of NAFLD and NASH in the general population (see Table 23.2).

Although abdominal ultrasound, computed tomography, and magnetic resonance imaging are all useful in identifying fatty infiltration of the liver, a prospective study of patients with biopsy-proven NAFLD found that none of these imaging modalities was able to accurately distinguish fatty liver from NASH (14). Although biopsy remains the "gold standard" for diagnosing NASH and providing prognostic information, some experts have argued that it is not necessary, especially in primary care settings where the disease is common, to routinely perform a biopsy to confirm the diagnosis (6, 8).

Although there is no controlled trial evidence of improved patient-oriented outcomes with any therapy for NAFLD, the mainstay of treatment at all stages of disease is weight loss, exercise, and optimal control of co-existing diabetes and hyperlipidemia (8, 13). Patients with NAFLD should also be counseled to avoid consumption of alcohol and potentially hepatotoxic medications (including nonsteroidal anti-inflammatory drugs) and dietary supplements (15).

CHRONIC VIRAL HEPATITIS

Epidemiology

Hepatitis B and hepatitis C are viruses that infect hepatocytes; both are common and preventable causes of CLD. An estimated 1.25 million persons in the United States are infected with hepatitis B (16), and 3.2 million persons with hepatitis C (17). Although hepatitis B and C have many characteristics in common, they also have notable differences (see Table 23.3).

The incidence of hepatitis B in the United States has declined dramatically since the institution of large-scale vaccination programs. Although a hepatitis B vaccine was developed in 1982, it was initially administered only to individuals thought to be at high risk for infection and thus was only moderately effective at reducing the overall disease burden. An estimated 16,000 children younger than 10 years were acutely infected with hepatitis B in 1991, the year that universal infant vaccination was instituted (18). The current recommendations for a first birth dose and catch-up vaccination of all children under the age of 18 have accelerated the disease's

TABLE 23.3 Comparing Hepatitis B and C

	Hepatitis B	Hepatitis C
Rate of progression from acute to chronic infection	15%–20%	80%–85%
Vaccine exists	Yes	No
Predominant mode of transmission	Sexual intercourse	Intravenous drug use
Perinatal infection	Yes	Yes
Increased risk of HCC	Yes	Yes

HCC, hepatocellular cancer
Original table.

decline. In contrast, the prevalence of hepatitis C has remained roughly stable over the past 10–15 years (17). No vaccine exists, and available treatments have limited effectiveness in a minority of patients.

Natural History

Both hepatitis B and C cause acute and chronic infections. A chronic infection results when the immune system fails to completely eliminate the virus following an acute infection. Whereas only 15%–20% of patients acutely infected with hepatitis B develop a chronic infection, 80%–85% of those infected with acute hepatitis C develop a chronic infection. The risk of chronic infection is higher in infants and persons with impaired immunity (e.g., due to HIV infection).

Even after a chronic infection is established, the immune system continues to identify and destroy infected hepatocytes. Over time, repeated cycles of destruction of hepatocytes may lead to cirrhosis, liver decompensation, and hepatocellular cancer. An estimated 12% of patients with chronic hepatitis B infection develop cirrhosis annually. However, large numbers of patients with chronic hepatitis C do not develop clinical liver disease for many years. A community-based cohort of 1,667 patients who had acquired hepatitis C from injection drug use demonstrated persistent viremia in most; however, only 40 developed end-stage liver disease (ESLD) over a median follow-up period of 8.8 years. The risk of ESLD increased with age and amount of reported alcohol consumption (19).

Initial Evaluation: Confirming Chronic Infection

The presence of circulating antibodies to hepatitis B or C does not necessarily mean that the patient is chronically infected. Hepatitis B has several laboratory markers that may be interpreted to represent a number of infectious states (see Table 23.4).

The majority of patients with a positive hepatitis C antibody titer will also have chronic infection, indicated by the presence of hepatitis C RNA. Elevated liver enzyme levels correlate poorly with severity of infection in either hepatitis B or C but are an important consideration in the decision to begin antiviral therapy.

Treatment of Hepatitis B and C

Existing treatments for hepatitis B and hepatitis C are often not curative and can have significant adverse effects. As a rule, treatment should be instituted only in patients who are most likely to benefit in terms of reduced mortality or future complications (20–22). Although precise criteria for treatment are constantly evolving, the general principle of antiviral therapy for hepatitis is to suppress viral replication in patients at highest risk of immune-mediated liver damage. For some patients with hepatitis C, viral eradication within a finite treatment period is an achievable goal. On the other hand, responses to hepatitis B treatment are usually transient, and optimal duration of treatment is uncertain.

HEPATITIS B

The options for treatment of hepatitis B are rapidly changing. Until 1999, the only U.S. Food and Drug Administration–approved medication was interferon alpha-2b, which assists the immune system in suppressing viral replication by upregulating cytokines involved in the response to viral infection. Interferon is limited by significant side effects and incomplete effectiveness. Three other drugs are now available that slow disease by directly inhibiting viral replication (see Table 23.5). Although these drugs are better tolerated than interferon, they often need to be continued indefinitely and over time lead to high rates of viral resistance.

HEPATITIS C

Unlike treatment for hepatitis B, there is expert consensus on a single most effective medication regimen for hepatitis C in eligible patients: pegylated interferon alfa and ribavirin (see Table 23.6). The sustained viral response rate to this combination of treatments varies by hepatitis C viral genoype. Al-

---

TABLE 23.4 Laboratory Markers for HBV Infection

Hepatitis B surface antigen (HBsAg): present in acute or chronic infection

Hepatitis B surface antibody (anti-HBs): marker of immunity acquired through natural HBV infection, vaccination, or passive antibody (immune globulin)

Hepatitis B core antibody (anti-HBc):

IgM—indicative of infection in the previous 6 months

IgG—indicative of more distant HBV infection that may have been cleared by the immune system or that may persist; positive HBsAg and anti-HBc IgG—indicative of persistent chronic HBV infection

Hepatitis B e antigen (HBeAg)*: correlates with a high level of viral replication; often called a "marker of infectivity"

Hepatitis B e antibody (anti-HBe): correlates with low rates of viral replication

HBV DNA: correlates with active replication; useful in monitoring response to treatment of HBV infection, especially in HBeAg-negative mutants

HBV, hepatitis B virus.
*A small but significant number of persons infected with a mutant strain of HBV cannot synthesize HBeAg; nevertheless, HBeAg is associated with a high rate of viral replication and infectivity.
Reproduced from Reference 16.

TABLE 23.5 Treatments for Hepatitis B

Drug	Contraindications/Cautions/Adverse Effects	Dosage	Relative Cost*
Interferon alpha-2b	May cause or aggravate fatal or life-threatening neuropsychiatric, autoimmune, ischemic, or infectious disorders.	Adults—5 million IU SC per day, or 10 million IU SC three times per week; children—3 million IU per m^2 SC three times in the first week, 6 million IU per m^2 SC three times per week after	$$$
Lamivudine	Lactic acidosis and severe, possibly fatal, hepatomegaly have been reported.	Adults—100 mg orally per day; children—3 mg per kg orally per day (maximum: 100 mg per day) <u>Note:</u> medication must be renally dosed	$$$
Adefovir	Nephrotoxicity in patients at high risk for underlying renal dysfunction. Lactic acidosis and hepatic steatosis	10 mg orally per day <u>Note:</u> medication must be renally dosed	$$$
Entecavir	Lactic acidosis and steatosis	0.5 mg orally per day; If lamivudine-resistant, 1 mg orally per day	$$$

* $, inexpensive, $$, moderate, $$$, expensive.
Portions adapted from Table 7 of Reference 16 (*http://www.aafp.org/afp/20040101/75.html*)

though genotypes 2 and 3 have an 80% response rate, genotype 1 has only a 45% response rate (23). Patients who have undetectable viral RNA levels 24 weeks after completing treatment have a 95% chance of remaining virus-free 5 years later (24). Although there are no long-term randomized trial data showing mortality benefits from treatment, a prospective cohort study of patients with chronic hepatitis C who either accepted or declined interferon therapy showed lower rates of hepatocellular cancer and improved survival in the interferon group (25).

Screening and Prevention

Screening for viral hepatitis remains controversial. Chronic hepatitis B and C have an indolent clinical course in many patients, and it is uncertain whether the benefits outweigh the harms of treatment in patients identified by screening. Citing the lack of good quality evidence that identifying and treating asymptomatic patients reduces long-term mortality, the United States Preventive Services Task Force (USPSTF) gives screening for hepatitis C in high-risk persons an "I" recommendation (26). Other organizations such as the Centers for Disease Control and Prevention (CDC) have contended that routinely offering testing to persons at high risk has the potential to reduce the future disease burden of cirrhosis and liver failure (27).

Because universal prenatal screening reduces transmission of hepatitis B virus (HBV) from mother to infant, the USPSTF strongly recommends screening all pregnant women for hepatitis B at their first prenatal visit. The USPSTF recommends against screening the general population for hepatitis B because of the low prevalence of chronic infection in adults but does not take a position on high-risk groups (intravenous drug users, persons with a history of a sexually transmitted disease, men who have sex with men, immigrants and

TABLE 23.6 Treatments for Hepatitis C

Drug	Contraindications/Cautions/Adverse Effects	Dosage	Relative Cost*
Pegylated interferon alfa	Neutropenia, anemia, thrombocytopenia, depression	180 mcg subcutaneously once weekly	$$$
Ribavirin	Hemolytic anemia, cardiac disease, birth defects	800–1200 mg orally per day in two divided doses depending on baseline disease (e.g., genotype), response to therapy, and tolerability of regimen	$$$

* $, inexpensive, $$, moderate, $$$, expensive.
Information from Reference 24.

children of immigrants from areas with a high prevalence of HBV infection) (28).

Unlike hepatitis C, hepatitis B has been preventable since the first vaccine was licensed in 1982. The current vaccine requires a 3-dose series, the second and third doses being given at 1 and 6 months after the first dose, respectively. Routine infant hepatitis B vaccination became the norm in the United States in 1991, the first dose being administered in the newborn period or at 1 to 2 months of age. Concerns about the risk of neonatal infection and evidence showing decreased vaccine series completion rates among children who did not receive their first hepatitis B vaccine in the hospital caused the CDC's Advisory Committee on Immunization Practices (ACIP) in 2005 to strongly recommend administering the first dose at birth except in rare circumstances (29).

There has been a marked decline in hepatitis B infections due to routine infant, childhood, and adolescent vaccination. An analysis of CDC surveillance data from 1990–2002 showed an 89% decrease in the rate of acute hepatitis B in children under 18 years of age, even though routine vaccination of this age group was not completely instituted until 1999 (30). Vaccinating at-risk adults has been more challenging. From 1999 to 2002, the incidence of acute hepatitis B actually increased in men and women over 40 years, and men aged 20–39 (31). Although most of these infections do not lead to CLD, they permit the virus to persist in the community. At current adult vaccination rates, elimination of the disease will not be possible for decades (32). Consequently, in 2006 the ACIP released an updated adult immunization strategy that recommends universal hepatitis B vaccination in high-risk care settings and the implementation of standing orders in primary care and specialty medical settings to identify and vaccinate adults with one or more risk factors for HBV infection (34).

CIRRHOSIS

Unfortunately, most CLD is incurable. However, only a minority of patients with CLD will develop cirrhosis or hepatocellular cancer. Cirrhosis occurs when changes from CLD have become irreversible. Decision rules have been developed to predict the probability of cirrhosis in patients with hepatitis C, based on noninvasive laboratory markers (33). Because these rules were developed and validated at large specialty referral centers, they may overestimate the likelihood of cirrhosis when applied to primary care populations (35).

Prevention of Complications

Secondary preventive strategies in CLD include abstinence from alcohol, vaccinations against hepatitis A and B in susceptible patients, avoidance of hepatotoxic medications and dietary supplements (see Table 23.7), and weight loss if obesity is present (36). Although hepatitis A and B vaccinations are less effective in advanced liver disease, it is safe to administer them at any stage of liver disease, and they are recommended to avoid the high mortality associated with co-infections with hepatitis C (37). Patients with cirrhosis should also receive pneumococcal and annual influenza vaccines.

Prognosis

Once cirrhosis has developed, the only cure is liver transplantation. To prioritize transplant resources, two major scoring systems have been developed to estimate prognosis. The modified Child-Pugh score divides patients into three classifications (A, B, and C) based on serum bilirubin and albumin levels, international normalized ratio for prothrombin time, and presence and severity of ascites and encephalopathy (see Table 23.8). Class C patients have the worst prognosis, with a mean survival of 1–3 years (35). The Model for End-Stage Liver Disease (MELD) score substitutes serum creatinine for albumin and does not include subjective clinical parameters (38). The MELD score estimates a patient's risk of dying from liver disease within three years. Although the MELD score (available online at *http://www.unos.org/resources/MeldPeldCalculator.asp?index = 98*) is currently used in the United States to determine transplantation priority, the modified Child-Pugh score's simplicity and clearly defined cut-off values may be easier to apply to individuals (39).

TABLE 23.7 Selected Potentially Hepatotoxic Medications

All nonsteroidal anti-inflammatory drugs Lipid-lowering agents: statins, nicotinic acid (niacin; Nicolar)

Antidiabetic agents: acarbose (Precose), pioglitazone (Actos), sulfonylureas

Antibiotics: amoxicillin clavulanate potassium (Augmentin), erythromycin, isoniazid (INH), nitrofurantoin (Furadantin), tetracycline

Antifungal agents: fluconazole (Diflucan), itraconazole (Sporanox), ketoconazole (Nizoral)

Retinoids: etretinate (Tegison)

Anticonvulsant agents: phenytoin (Dilantin), valproic acid (Depakene)

Psychotropic agents: bupropion (Wellbutrin), chlorpromazine (Thorazine), tricyclic antidepressants

Hormones: tamoxifen (Nolvadex), testosterone

Others: halothane (Fluothane), methotrexate (Rheumatrex)

Reproduced from Reference 15. Available at: *http://www.aafp.org/afp/20011101/1555.html.*

TABLE 23.8 Estimating Prognosis in Cirrhosis: The Modified Child-Pugh Score

Points Assigned to Laboratory Values and Signs*

Parameters	1	2	3
Laboratory value			
Total serum bilirubin level	<2 mg per dL (34 μmol per L)	2 to 3 mg per dL (34 to 51 μmol per L)	>3 mg per dL
Serum albumin level	>3.5 g per dL (35 g per L)	2.8 to 3.5 g per dL (28 to 35 g per L)	<2.8 g per dL
International Normalized Ratio	<1.70	1.71 to 2.20	>2.20
Signs			
Ascites	None	Controlled medically	Poorly controlled
Encephalopathy	None	Controlled medically	Poorly controlled

*—Based on total points, a patient with cirrhosis is assigned to one of three classes: Child class A = 5 to 6 points; Child class B = 7 to 9 points; Child class C = 10 to 15 points.
Reproduced from Reference 35. Available at: *http://www.aafp.org/afp/20011115/1735.html.*

Management of Complications
VARICES

Gastroesophageal varices are dilated blood vessels that result from the increased portal-to-systemic venous pressure in cirrhosis. Bleeding from varices may be life-threatening. All patients with cirrhosis should undergo a screening endoscopy that should be repeated every 2 years if gastroesophageal varices are absent on initial screening. If medium or large gastroesophageal varices are present, primary prophylaxis against bleeding should be initiated with the nonselective beta-blockers propranolol or nadolol, titrated to a resting heart rate between 50 and 60 beats/minute. Patients who are unable to tolerate these medications should be offered endoscopic variceal band ligation, which has been shown to be similarly effective in reducing the risk of bleeding by up to 50% (40). It is unclear whether combining these two preventive therapies results in any additional benefit compared to using either alone (41).

ASCITES AND SPONTANEOUS BACTERIAL PERITONITIS

Ascites are collections of fluid that form in the abdomen from changes in intestinal capillary pressure and permeability resulting from increased portal resistance. The presence of ascites in cirrhosis is a poor prognostic sign and an indicator for transplantation. A low-sodium diet is recommended to control clinically undetectable ascites that are only seen on abdominal ultrasound. For ascites that can be palpated on examination, diuretics (aldactone or amiloride) and therapeutic paracentesis are both used. Patients who do not respond adequately to these treatments may undergo a transjugular intrahepatic portosystemic shunt (TIPS) procedure, connecting the hepatic to the portal vein, and bypassing the increased resistance of the liver. However, TIPS has not been shown to offer any improvement in survival over repeated large-volume paracentesis (42).

In 10% to 30% of patients, ascites may be infected by intestinal bacteria, causing spontaneous bacterial peritonitis (SBP). SBP should be considered when a cirrhotic patient presents with unexplained abdominal pain and fever, and a diagnostic paracentesis should be performed. Intravenous third-generation cephalosporins are the recommended treatment for SBP; SBP recurs in 70% of affected patients after 1 year. Prophylaxis with fluoroquinolone antibiotics effectively reduces subsequent episodes, but bacterial resistance is increasingly complicating the prevention and treatment of SBP (40, 42).

ENCEPHALOPATHY

Hepatic encephalopathy is a clinical syndrome of mental status changes that is thought to be secondary to the buildup of circulating nitrogenous waste products that bypass the blood-brain barrier. Standard treatment aimed at removing these waste products via the intestine includes oral lactulose and antibiotics directed against nitrogen-producing bacteria (40).

Screening for HCC

HCC is commonly associated with cirrhosis, and most organizations recommend screening for HCC in viral hepatitis with periodic ultrasonography or alpha-fetoprotein (23, 43). However, evidence that screening reduces mortality from HCC is scant. A Cochrane systematic review found only two randomized trials that suggested increased survival from HCC screening versus no screening and concluded that better designed studies are needed to establish conclusively the benefit of and optimal interval for screening (44).

CONCLUSION

A recent cohort study found that men with diabetes had twice the risk of having CLD and HCC as men without diabetes (45). Further studies are needed to determine if this association is simply the result of shared risk factors, or if diabetes actually causes CLD. While the proportion of CLD secondary to alco-

TABLE 23.9 Key Recommendations for Practice

Recommendation	Strength of Recommendation*	References
Initial management for a patient with mildly elevated AST or ALT and normal viral hepatitis serologies and iron studies should be six months of lifestyle modification.	C	5
Family physicians should offer brief office counseling for patients with alcohol problems, since it has been shown to reduce alcohol consumption and injuries at 6 and 12 months.	B	9
Patients with CLD should avoid consumption of alcohol and potentially hepatotoxic medications (including nonsteroidal anti-inflammatory drugs) and dietary supplements.	B	15
Patients with NAFLD should be encouraged to lose weight, exercise, and attain optimal control of diabetes and hyperlipidemia, if present.	C	8, 13
All patients with CLD should receive vaccinations against hepatitis A and hepatitis B if not already immune from previous infection.	B	36
Nonselective beta-blockers should be initiated in patients with cirrhosis and gastroesophageal varices to prevent variceal bleeding.	A	39

AST, aspartate transaminase; ALT, alanine transaminase; CLD, chronic liver disease; NAFLD, nonalcoholic fatty liver disease
*A = consistent, good-quality patient-oriented evidence; B = inconsistent or limited-quality patient-oriented evidence; C = consensus, disease-oriented evidence, usual practice, expert opinion, or case series. For information about the SORT evidence rating system, see *http://www.aafp.org/afpsort.xml*.

holism and hepatitis B is declining in the United States, the aging of the population infected with hepatitis C, and the rising prevalence of obesity and NAFLD, make it likely to remain a common problem encountered by family physicians. Until more effective treatments are developed, improving primary and secondary prevention will be the key to reducing morbidity and mortality from CLD. Key recommendations for practice are summarized in Table 23.9.

CASE 1 DISCUSSION

Given his medical history, B.J. most likely has nonalcoholic fatty liver disease. However, testing for viral hepatitis and iron studies should be performed to rule out other causes. If there is no clinical evidence of other gastrointestinal disorders or hepatic decompensation, B.J. should be instructed to abstain from alcohol and work with his physician to achieve better control of his weight, diabetes, and cholesterol. After 6 months, his liver chemistries should be repeated. If they are persistently abnormal, further testing should be performed, and liver biopsy may be considered.

CASE 2 DISCUSSION

D.M.'s history of injection drug use and unprotected sex puts him at risk for hepatitis B and hepatitis C. Although routine screening of individuals at high-risk has not been endorsed by the United States Preventive Services Task Force, it is reasonable to offer testing to D.M. A positive screening test (hepatitis B surface antigen/hepatitis C antibody) should be

followed by additional testing to confirm chronic infection. If D.M. does have hepatitis B or C, liver enzyme levels may be useful in guiding the decision to treat. If he is uninfected and does not have natural immunity to hepatitis B infection, he is eligible to receive the 3-dose vaccine.

REFERENCES

1. Kim WR, Brown RS Jr, Terrault NA, El-Serag H. Burden of liver disease in the United States: summary of a workshop. Hepatology. 2002;36:227–242.
2. Giboney PT. Mildly elevated liver transaminase levels in the asymptomatic patient. Am Fam Physician. 2005;71:1105–1110.
3. Pratt DS, Kaplan MM. Evaluation of abnormal liver-enzyme results in asymptomatic patients. N Engl J Med. 2000;342:1266–1271.
4. Mallory MA, Lee SW, Kowdley KV. Abnormal liver test results on routine screening. Postgrad Med. 2004;115:53–66.
5. American Gastroenterological Association medical position statement: evaluation of liver chemistry tests. Gastroenterology. 2002;123:1364–1366.
6. Sorbi D, McGill DB, Thistle JL, Therneau TM, Henry J, Lindor KD. An assessment of the role of liver biopsies in asymptomatic patients with chronic liver test abnormalities. Am J Gastroenterol. 2000;95:3206–3210.
7. Sorbi D, Boynton J, Lindor KD. The ratio of aspartate aminotransferase to alanine aminotransferase: potential value in differentiating nonalcoholic steatohepatitis from alcoholic liver disease. Am J Gasteroenterol. 1999;94:1018–1022.
8. Adams LA, Angulo P, Lindor KD. Nonalcoholic fatty liver disease. CMAJ. 2005;172:899–905.
9. Bertholet N, Daeppen JB, Wietlisbach V, Fleming M, Burnand B. Reduction of alcohol consumption by brief alcohol intervention in primary care: systematic review and meta-analysis. Arch Intern Med. 2005;165:986–995.

10. Enoch MA, Goldman D. Problem drinking and alcoholism: diagnosis and treatment. Am Fam Physician. 2002;65: 441–448.

11. Williams SH. Medications for treating alcohol dependence. Am Fam Physician. 2005;72:1775–1780.

12. McCullough AJ. The clinical features, diagnosis and natural history of nonalcoholic fatty liver disease. Clin Liver Dis. 2004;8:521–533.

13. Angulo P. Nonalcoholic fatty liver disease. N Engl J Med. 2002;346:1221–1229.

14. Saadeh S, Younossi ZM, Remer EM, et al. The utility of radiological imaging in nonalcoholic fatty liver disease. Gastroenterology. 2002;123:745–750.

15. Riley TR, Bhatti AM. Preventive strategies in chronic liver disease: part I. Alcohol, vaccines, toxic medications and supplements, diet and exercise. Am Fam Physician. 2001;64: 1555–1560.

16. Lin KW, Kirchner JT. Hepatitis B. Am Fam Physician. 2004; 69:75–82.

17. Armstrong GL, Wasley A, Simard EP, McQuillan GM, Kuhnert WL, Alter MJ. The prevalence of hepatitis C virus infection in the United States, 1999 through 2002. Ann Intern Med. 2006;144:705–714.

18. Armstrong GL, Mast EE, Wojczynski M, Margolis HS. Childhood hepatitis B virus infections in the United States before hepatitis B immunization. Pediatrics. 2001;108: 1123–1128.

19. Thomas DL, Astemborski J, Rai RM, et al. The natural history of hepatitis C virus infection. Host, viral, and environmental factors. JAMA. 2000;284:450–456.

20. Aggarwal R, Ranjan P. Preventing and treating hepatitis B infection. BMJ. 2004;329:1080–1086.

21. Wong SN, Lok AS. Treatment of hepatitis B: who, when, and how? [Editorial] Arch Intern Med. 2006;166:9–12.

22. Hoofnagle JH. Hepatitis B—preventable and now treatable. [Editorial] N Engl J Med. 2006;354:1074–1076.

23. National Institutes of Health. Consensus Statement: management of hepatitis C: 2002. NIH Consens State Sci Statements 2002;19:1–46.

24. Ward, RP, Kugelmas M. Using pegylated interferon and ribavirin to treat patients with chronic hepatitis C. Am Fam Physician. 2005;72:655–662.

25. Shiratori Y, Ito Y, Yokosuka O, et al. Antiviral therapy for cirrhotic hepatitis C: association with reduced hepatocellular carcinoma and improved survival. Ann Intern Med. 2005; 142:105–114.

26. US Preventive Services Task Force. Screening for hepatitis C virus infection in adults: recommendation statement. Ann Intern Med. 2004;140:462–464.

27. Alter MJ. Integrating risk history screening and HCV testing into clinical and public health settings. [Editorial] Am Fam Physician. 2005;72:576–579.

28. US Preventive Services Task Force. Screening for hepatitis B virus infection: recommendation statement. *http://www.ahrq.gov/clinic/uspstf/uspshepb.htm*

29. Centers for Disease Control and Prevention. A comprehensive immunization strategy to eliminate transmission of hepatitis B infection in the United States. MMWR. 2005;54(No. RR 1–16):1–39.

30. Centers for Disease Control and Prevention. Acute hepatitis B among children and adolescents—United States, 1990–2002. MMWR. 2004;53(43):1015–1018.

31. Centers for Disease Control and Prevention. Incidence of acute hepatitis B—United States, 1990–2002. MMWR. 2004; 52(51–52):1252–1254.

32. Alter MJ. Epidemiology and prevention of hepatitis B. Semin Liver Dis. 2003;23:39–46.

33. Kaul V, Friedenberg FK, Braitman LE, et al. Development and validation of a model to diagnose cirrhosis in patients with hepatitis C. Am J Gastroenterol. 2002;97:2623–2628.

34. Centers for Disease Control and Prevention. A comprehensive immunization strategy to eliminate transmission of hepatitis B virus infection in the United States. MMWR. 2006; 55(No. RR-16): 1–33.

35. Ebell MH. Probability of cirrhosis in patients with hepatitis C. Am Fam Physician. 2003;68:831–832.

36. Propst A, Propst T, Zangerl G, Ofner D, Judmaier G, Vogel W. Prognosis and life expectancy in chronic liver disease. Dig Dis Sci. 1995;40:1805–1815.

37. Keeffe EB. Acute hepatitis A and B in patients with chronic liver disease: prevention through vaccination. Am J Med. 2005;118:21S–27S.

38. Kamath PS, Wiesner RH, Malinchoc M, et al. A model to predict survival in patients with end-stage liver disease. Hepatology. 2001;33:464–470.

39. Durand F, Valla D. Assessment of the prognosis of cirrhosis: Child-Pugh versus MELD. J Hepatol. 2005;42:S100–S107.

40. Cardenas A, Gines P. Management of complications of cirrhosis in patients awaiting liver transplantation. J Hepatol. 2005;42:S124–S133.

41. Chalasani N, Boyer TD. Primary prophylaxis against variceal bleeding: beta blockers, endoscopic ligation, or both? [Editorial] Am J Gastroenterol. 2005;100:805–807.

42. Gines P, Cardenas A, Arroyo V, Rodes J. Management of cirrhosis and ascites. N Engl J Med. 2004;350:1646–1654.

43. Lok AS, McMahon BJ. Chronic hepatitis B. Hepatology. 2001;34:1225–1241.

44. Wun YT, Dickinson JA. Alpha-fetoprotein and/or liver ultrasonography for liver cancer screening in patients with chronic hepatitis B (Cochrane Review). In: The Cochrane Library. Oxford, England: Update Software; 2006:Issue 1.

45. El-Serag HB, Tran T, Everhart JE. Diabetes increases the risk of chronic liver disease and hepatocellular carcinoma. Gastroenterology 2004;126:460–468.

CHAPTER 24

Dyspepsia

William Y. Huang and Fareed M. Khan

CASE 1

A 35-year-old nonsmoking man complains of heartburn relieved by belching. These symptoms occur daily. He also complains of an occasional nighttime sour taste in the mouth followed by an episode of coughing usually after a fatty meal and/or alcohol consumption. The symptoms began a few years ago. The patient denies a loss of appetite, dysphagia, or weight loss. He attributes the symptoms to gastroesophageal reflux and excessive coffee drinking. The patient occasionally takes antacids as needed and they relieve his symptoms. He asks you about the need for an upper endoscopy to investigate his symptoms further.

CASE 2

A 44-year-old man presents with a history of frequent epigastric pain for the past month that is burning in nature. He notes it is relieved after eating a meal or drinking milk. He has no change in his bowel movements and no melena or hematochezia. A friend gave him some esomeprazole tablets which helps when used. On examination, the patient has stable vital signs and is in no distress. At the time of your exam, he has no epigastric tenderness. His rectal exam shows heme-negative stool. He asks for a prescription of esomeprazole to relieve his symptoms.

CLINICAL QUESTIONS

1. What are the most common and important causes of dyspepsia?
2. What is the best strategy for the family physician to use in diagnosing the cause of a patient's dyspepsia?
3. What are the most effective treatments for different causes of dyspepsia?

Dyspepsia is defined as "episodic or persistent symptoms that include abdominal pain or discomfort and which are referable to the upper gastrointestinal tract" (1). In addition to pain and discomfort, patients may note other symptoms including early satiety, fullness, upper abdominal bloating, and nausea (2). While the formal definition excludes patients whose only symptom is heartburn, in reality, reflux esophagitis is a common finding in patients evaluated for dyspepsia. Therefore, gastroesophageal reflux disease (GERD) should be included in the differential diagnosis of an undiagnosed patient who presents with dyspepsia and is addressed in this chapter.

In the 2002 National Ambulatory Medical Survey, "stomach pain, cramps, and spasms" was the 11th most frequent reason for patients to present to their physicians, estimated to account for more than 13.5 million visits per year (3). About 25% of persons in the United States or other western countries experience recurrent upper abdominal pain during a typical year. If one adds heartburn, then the prevalence is closer to 40% (4).

If no alarm symptoms or signs are present, the family physician can effectively manage most patients through the use of simple diagnostic tests and medication. Patients who have alarm symptoms or fail to improve with standard treatment may require referral to a gastroenterologist for further testing, including an upper endoscopy in most cases.

DIFFERENTIAL DIAGNOSIS AND PATHOPHYSIOLOGY

The most common causes of dyspepsia are functional dyspepsia (a diagnosis of exclusion), peptic ulcer disease (PUD), and gastroesophageal reflux disease (GERD). Esophageal or gastric cancer are rare causes (See Table 24.1) (4). Other rare, but identifiable causes include carbohydrate malabsorption, mucosal disorders of the small intestine (e.g., sprue), intestinal parasites, chronic pancreatitis, infiltrative diseases of the stomach (e.g., Crohn's disease), metabolic disorders (e.g., hypothyroidism, hypercalcemia) and certain medications (e.g., erythromycin) (4, 5). Cardiac (e.g., inferior myocardial ischemia) and pulmonary (e.g., lower lobe pneumonia) conditions may on occasion also present with upper abdominal discomfort.

Gastroesophageal Reflux Disease

Gastroesophageal reflux disease (GERD) is a condition in which the reflux of gastric contents into the esophagus results in symptoms such as heartburn or a bitter taste in the back of the mouth. It may also cause evidence of inflammation (esophagitis) and erosions in the esophageal mucosa (6). Our understanding of the underlying pathophysiology is evolving. One important causative factor is esophago-gastric junction (EGJ) incompetence that can occur from transient lower esophageal sphincter relaxations, lower esophageal sphincter hypotension, or anatomic deformities of the EGJ such as a hiatal hernia. After the reflux occurs, another key factor is ineffective esophageal clearance of acid and reflux material that may result from impaired esophageal emptying, esopha-

TABLE 24.1 Differential Diagnosis of the Patient with Dyspepsia Based on Endoscopic Results from 36 Studies[*]

Diagnosis	Frequency
Functional dyspepsia	60%
Peptic ulcer disease	15%–25%
Reflux esophagitis[†]	5%–15%
Gastric or esophageal cancer	<2%
Rare causes of dyspepsia	
Carbohydrate malabsorption	
Small intestinal mucosal disorders (e.g., sprue)	
Intestinal parasites	
Chronic pancreatitis	
Infiltrative diseases of the stomach (e.g., Crohn's disease)	
Metabolic disorders (e.g., hypothyroidism, hypercalcemia)	
Medications (e.g., erythromycin)	
Cardiac conditions (e.g., inferior myocardial ischemia)	
Pulmonary conditions (e.g., lower lobe pneumonia)	

[*]Compiled using data from References 4 and 5.
[†]Patients with gastroesophageal reflux disease do not always have evidence of reflux esophagitis on endoscopy

geal peristalsis dysfunction and/or decreased salivary neutralizing capacity (7). There is a poor correlation between endoscopic findings and symptoms. A recent hypothesis is that in patients with heartburn but no erosions seen on endoscopy, the heartburn results from abnormal tissue resistance and damage at the microscopic level that is not visible on endoscopy (8).

There are a number of potential risk factors for GERD including an immediate family history, increased body-mass index, history of smoking, and alcohol use (9). Certain foods such as chocolate, alcohol, peppermint, caffeine, and onions have been demonstrated to decrease lower esophageal sphincter pressure and may cause reflux symptoms (6). Reflux events occur more often in the lying position as opposed to the upright position.

Peptic Ulcer Disease (PUD)

The primary causes of PUD are *Helicobacter pylori* infection and nonsteroidal anti-inflammatory drug (NSAID) use. While either of these alone is a significant cause, these two factors can act synergistically to further increase the risk of PUD (10). Cigarette smoking is an additional risk factor that may impair the healing of an ulcer and increase the likelihood of recurrence after successful treatment (11). Zollinger-Ellison syndrome is an uncommon cause of PUD that results from tumors of the small intestine or pancreas that secrete excessive amounts of gastrin hormone which leads to an overproduction of stomach acid.

Functional Dyspepsia

In up to 60% of patients with dyspepsia, there is no identifiable cause on endoscopy. In this case, the patient is diagnosed as having functional dyspepsia. Three major potential pathophysiologic mechanisms of functional dyspepsia have been identified. The first is delayed gastric emptying that occurs in about 30% of patient with functional dyspepsia and is associated with postprandial fullness, nausea and vomiting. Another is impaired gastric accommodation that occurs in about 40% of patients with functional dyspepsia and is associated with early satiety. Finally, hypersensitivity to gastric distention is noted in approximately 37% of patients with functional dyspepsia, and is associated with postprandial pain, belching and weight loss (12).

H. pylori gastritis may be the etiology of functional dyspepsia in a few cases (13). It may also be caused by other motility disorders (small intestinal dysmotility, gall bladder/biliary tract motor dysfunction), or psychiatric disorders (5).

CLINICAL EVALUATION

Alarm Symptoms

There are certain red flags to look for which may indicate the possibility for serious disease such as a complicated peptic ulcer or malignancy (see Table 24.2). Clinicians should look for the following alarm symptoms and signs: anorexia, unexplained recent weight loss, dysphagia, odynophagia, persistent vomiting, hematemesis, longstanding gastroesophageal reflux symptoms, melena, blood in the stool, anemia, previous gastric surgery, a palpable abdominal mass, gastrointestinal perforation, or jaundice (6, 14). Although it is important to fully evaluate patients with any of these red flags, the positive predictive value of these symptoms is low (4% for cancer,

TABLE 24.2 Red Flags Suggesting Progressive or Life-Threatening Diseases in Patients with Dyspepsia*

Disease	Symptoms, Signs, or Laboratory Test
Cancer	Unexplained weight loss, anorexia, dysphagia, hematemesis, melena, anemia, heme-positive stool, long-standing reflux symptoms
Bleeding ulcer	Hematemesis, melena, hematochezia, heme-positive stool, orthostatic hypotension, shock, anemia
Obstruction	Dysphagia, odynophagia, early satiety, recurrent vomiting, weight loss
Perforated ulcer	Sudden onset of severe abdominal pain, rigid board-like abdomen or other peritoneal signs, shock

*Compiled using data from References 6, 14, 15, and 16.

13%–14% for ulcer disease or esophagitis) (15, 16). Age is another important factor; current guidelines recommend that all patients who are above 55 years of age with the new onset of dyspepsia should receive an endoscopy to evaluate for more serious disease (17, 18).

Some conditions that present with dyspepsia may cause gastrointestinal bleeding. When the gastrointestinal bleeding is severe, it may present with alarm symptoms and signs including hematemesis, melena, hematochezia, hypotension, tachycardia, anemia, syncope and shock. Other emergency presentations include an obstructed viscus or perforated ulcer. In all of these conditions, the physician must urgently stabilize the patient and identify the cause the symptoms.

History and Physical Examination

In taking a focused history, the physician should ask about the location of discomfort, duration, quality, severity, associated symptoms and both alleviating and exacerbating factors and use that information to refine the differential diagnosis of the patient's dyspepsia. Inquiring about a history of similar symptoms, use of medications, history of smoking, and the presence of any red flag symptoms also is important. In performing a focused examination, the patient's vital signs and appearance may give a clue on how urgent the patient's condition is. A careful examination of the abdomen is essential, although one must also realize that a patient with dyspepsia usually does not have any abnormal findings. A lung and cardiovascular examination may be useful in assessing whether an extraabdominal cause of the patient's symptoms is present. If there are any alarm symptoms or concern about gastrointestinal bleeding, a rectal examination with stool heme testing is indicated. A discussion of additional items to look for during the history and physical examination follows in the next section.

GASTROESOPHAGEAL REFLUX DISEASE

Patients with GERD commonly present with heartburn, which is a sensation of a burning pain in the substernal area. This is frequently accompanied by acid regurgitation and a sour taste in the mouth (waterbrash). Symptoms may be aggravated by the foods discussed earlier, or by certain body positions such as bending forward or lying down. Food or antacids may alleviate the symptoms. The physical examination is usu-

ally normal. GERD may also cause noncardiac chest pain, chronic hoarseness, asthma, or a chronic cough. Therefore, the clinician should think of GERD when seeing patients with any of these associated conditions (19).

PEPTIC ULCER DISEASE

The classic presentation of PUD is epigastric abdominal pain that is burning or gnawing in character. Duodenal ulcers typically occur on an empty stomach or at least 2 hours after eating and are relieved by eating food or taking antacids. Gastric ulcers may occur sooner after eating and are less frequently relieved by food or antacids. A variety of other symptoms, including vomiting, loss of appetite, and flatulence may also be present (20). Epigastric tenderness may or may not be present on physical examination. The patient's stool may be heme-positive if bleeding has occurred.

FUNCTIONAL DYSPEPSIA

Functional dyspepsia is defined as having at least 12 weeks (not necessarily consecutive) of the following symptoms within the previous 12 months: 1) "persistent or recurrent dyspepsia" (upper abdominal pain or discomfort); 2) "no evidence of organic disease" (on endoscopy or other tests) that probably accounts for the symptoms; 3) It is not "exclusively relieved by defecation or associated with the onset of a change in stool frequency or stool form" and therefore, unlikely to be irritable bowel syndrome (2). Again, it is likely that the physical examination will be normal. Since the absence of organic disease is part of the definition, a history and physical examination alone is not sufficient to make this diagnosis. Table 24.3 lists the accuracy of key elements of the history and physical examination of the dyspepsic patient.

Diagnostic Testing

GASTROESOPHAGEAL REFLUX DISEASE

There is no clear standard of diagnosis for GERD. Also, generalists may differ quite appropriately from specialists in their approach to GERD and the subsequent use of diagnostic testing because of differences in the frequency of serious disease between primary care and specialty settings. Generalists often make a presumptive diagnosis based on symptoms and empirically begin treatment. They aim to "minimize danger" and

TABLE 24.3 Accuracy of Key Elements of the History and Physical Examination in Patients with Dyspepsia

Diagnosis Suggested	Clinical Finding	Sens	Spec	LR+	LR−	Comments
Esophagitis (24)	Overall clinical impression by GPs	62%	71%	2.14	0.54	Gold standard = endoscopic evidence of esophagitis
	Overall clinical impression by gastroenterologists	64%	81%	3.37	0.44	
Peptic ulcer disease (24)	Overall clinical impression by GPs	61%	73%	2.26	0.53	Gold standard = endoscopic evidence of peptic ulcer disease
	Overall clinical impression by gastroenterologists	55%	84%	3.44	0.54	
Functional dyspepsia (24)	Overall clinical impression by GPs	37%	76%	1.54	0.83	Other diagnoses excluded by endoscopy
	Overall clinical impression by gastroenterologists	58%	72%	2.11	0.57	
Peptic ulcer disease (vs other condition suchas gastritis, duodenitis, malignancy or esophagitis	Male gender	61%	58%	1.45	0.67	Gold standard = confirmed peptic ulcer disease, method of diagnosis not specified
	Main symptom is pain	77%	45%	1.40	0.51	
	Duration <2 years	66%	65%	1.89	0.52	
	Episodic pain	80%	50%	1.60	0.40	
	Epigastric pain	68%	62%	1.79	0.52	
	Food reduces pain	39%	88%	3.25	0.69	
	Symptoms awaken patient at night and are relieved with food	48%	83%	2.82	0.63	
	Vomiting	33%	75%	1.32	0.89	
	Waterbrash	42%	77%	1.83	0.75	
	Heartburn	65%	45%	1.18	0.78	
	Flatulence	58%	52%	1.21	0.81	
	Loss of appetite	50%	63%	1.35	0.79	
	Family history of ulcer	47%	70%	1.57	0.76	
	Smoker	73%	50%	1.46	0.54	
	Epigastric tenderness to deep palpation	52%	27%	0.71	1.78	Gold standard = endoscopic evidence of peptic ulcer disease

identify those who may need more definitive diagnosis because of alarm symptoms or other urgent reasons. This is appropriate in a setting where serious disease is quite rare. Gastroenterologists typically see patients who have been referred to them for a failure to respond to usual therapy or because of worrisome symptoms and seek to "minimize uncertainty" by using invasive methods to establish a diagnosis (21). This is also appropriate given the referral nature of their population and the greater likelihood of serious disease. Thus, it is important to keep in mind the setting and prevalence of serious disease when deciding whether to order invasive or expensive diagnostic tests.

The response to proton pump inhibitors (PPIs) has been evaluated as a diagnostic test for gastroesophageal reflux.

Studies have investigated different dosages and drugs (mostly using higher than standard doses) and varying lengths of time of medication use, from 1 to 4 weeks (22, 23). As shown in Table 24.4, the test characteristics depend to some extent on the population studied and the reference standard used. The meta-analysis using a 24-hour pH probe or endoscopy as the reference standard found that given a 50% pretest probability of GERD, a positive response to a trial of a PPI increases the likelihood of GERD to 75%, whereas a negative test reduces it to 21% (23). The PPI test can therefore be use as an initial diagnostic approach by primary care physicians when GERD is suspected.

Endoscopy has the advantage of allowing direct visualization of the esophageal mucosa and documentation and biopsy

TABLE 24.4 Accuracy of Diagnostic Tests Useful in Patients with Dyspepsia

Test	Sensitivity	Specificity	LR+	LR−	Comment
Gastroesophageal reflux disease					
Proton pump inhibitor test* (22)	78% (meta-analysis of five studies)	54% (meta-analysis of five studies)	1.70	0.41	Gold standard = abnormal 24-hour esophageal pH
Proton pump inhibitor test* (22)	68% (meta-analysis of six studies)	46% (meta-analysis of six studies)	1.26	0.70	Gold standard = esophagitis on endoscopy
Proton pump inhibitor test in patients with non-cardiac chest pain* (23)	80% (meta-analysis of six studies)	74% (meta-analysis of six studies)	3.08	0.27	Gold standard = esophagitis on endoscopy and/or abnormal esophageal pH
Endoscopy (72)					Gold standard = abnormal esophageal pH
- Esophageal erythema	22%	74%	0.85	1.05	
- Esophageal erosions or ulcerations	48%	64%	1.33	0.81	
24 hour pH monitoring (73)					
- Clinical impression of a gastroenterologist as the gold standard	72%	60%	1.79	0.47	
- Esophagitis on endoscopy as the gold standard	79%	44%	1.41	0.48	
- Esophageal erosions as the gold standard	93%	41%	1.58	0.17	
Peptic ulcer disease					
- Endoscopy (74)	92%	100%[†]	92	0.08	Final diagnosis jointly made by radiologists and endoscopists
- Upper GI (74)	54%	91%	6	0.51	
Gastric ulcer (75)					No gold standard. Method of Hui and Walter (76) used for calculations
- Endoscopy	85%	98%	42.5	0.15	
- Upper GI	91%	99%	91	0.09	
Duodenal ulcer (75)					
- Endoscopy	99%	100%[†]	99	0.01	
- Upper GI	50%	99%	50	0.51	
H. pylori infection					
- Urea breath test (25)	95% (mean of 6 studies)	96% (mean of 6 studies)	22.02	0.06	Most studies used an endoscopic based method of confirming H. pylori as the gold standard.
- Stool antigen test (28)	92% (systematic review of 43 studies)	92% (systematic review of 43 studies)	11.41	0.08	
- Serum IgG antibody tests (27)	85% (meta-analysis of 21 studies)	79% (meta-analysis of 21 studies)	4.05	0.19	
- Whole-blood antibody tests (25)	71% (mean of 8 studies)	88% (mean of 8 studies)	5.73	0.33	

*In studies reporting the use of proton pump inhibitor tests, patients were given a PPI at a standard or high dose for a period of 1–4 weeks. Depending on the study, a positive test response was defined as a complete resolution of symptoms or a partial improvement of symptoms as measured by the use of a symptom questionnaire. All patients had an objective diagnosis of GERD confirmed by either an abnormal esophageal pH study or evidence of esophagitis or erosions on upper endoscopy.

[†]Specificities of 100% were changed to 99% to calculate positive likelihood ratios.

of lesions such as erosions, esophagitis, Barrett's esophagus and cancer. However, it is also important to understand that the endoscopic findings do not correlate with the severity of symptoms or the response to treatment. Patients without endoscopic findings may still have significant symptoms and require strong medication for control of symptoms (6).

Esophageal pH monitoring may be useful in documenting persistent acid reflux events in patients with symptoms that have not responded to usual treatment and have no endoscopic findings. This test may also be helpful in patients with atypical symptoms (such as a cough) and to followup reflux symptoms in patients after a trial of medication or surgery (6).

PEPTIC ULCER DISEASE AND MALIGNANCY

Both generalist physicians and gastroenterologists have difficulty in making the diagnosis of peptic ulcer disease based on history and physical alone (24). Therefore, other diagnostic studies for peptic ulcer disease such as upper endoscopy or an upper gastrointestinal series (UGI) are needed to confirm the diagnosis. Upper endoscopy is very sensitive and specific (see Table 24.4) and has the added advantages of direct observation of the esophageal, gastric, and duodenal mucosa and the ability to perform biopsies of any lesions of concerns for cancer or for *H. pylori* infection. Patients who are noted to have a gastric ulcer on UGI should have an upper endoscopy and biopsy of the lesion given that as many as 3% of gastric ulcers may be malignant (4). The risk of complications from an upper endoscopy is extremely low (<0.3%) (4). Although a UGI is less sensitive and specific (see Table 24.4) and results in radiation exposure for the patient, it may still have a role in the diagnosis if the patient is not able to tolerate endoscopy or if a trained endoscopist is not available in the community.

Because *H. pylori* infection is the most common cause of peptic ulcer disease, the presence or absence of an *H. pylori* infection should guide the management of a patient with dyspepsia and suspected PUD (see Management section). Available methods of diagnosing an *H. pylori* infection include ^{13}C and ^{14}C urea breath tests, serologic tests, and stool antigen tests. Breath tests are highly sensitive and specific (Table 24.4) (25). However, PPIs may increase the likelihood of false-negative results on breath tests for up to 2–4 weeks after stopping the PPI (26). Serologic tests include both serum antibody tests performed in a reference laboratory and whole blood tests performed at the point of care. The most commonly used serum antibody tests are enzyme-linked immunosorbent assays (ELISAs). There is no significant difference in the accuracy of commonly used serum antibody kits (27). Although whole blood tests used in the ambulatory setting may be more convenient for the physician and patient, they are less sensitive than serum antibody tests performed in a reference laboratory (71% vs. 85%) (25). Finally, stool antigen tests detect *H. pylori* antigen in the stool and are more accurate than whole blood or serologic tests, although somewhat less convenient (28). They can also be used to confirm eradication because they are an antigen and not an antibody test. However, concurrent use of PPIs can cause false negative stool antigen results (29).

Current guidelines recommend breath tests or stool antigen tests as the preferred initial test to detect *H. pylori* infection (30). Serologic tests at a reference laboratory are an alternative if breath tests or stool antigen tests are not available or if the patient has recently taken a PPI.

FUNCTIONAL DYSPEPSIA

In making the diagnosis of functional dyspepsia, history and physical findings alone are not sensitive or specific (24). Because this is a diagnosis of exclusion, a diagnostic evaluation, as described below, should be performed to exclude other conditions such as peptic ulcer disease, GERD and cancer. Extensive diagnostic testing is not recommended in patients with functional dyspepsia, unless the patient's symptoms and signs suggest an alternate diagnosis.

Recommended Diagnostic Strategy

The recommended strategy outlined here is based on evidence-based guidelines published in 2005 on the management of dyspepsia from the American Gastroenterological Association (AGA) (18, 31) and management of GERD from the American College of Gastroenterology (6). Figure 24.1 presents an algorithm for diagnosing and managing patients with dyspepsia. The first step is to note whether the patient is above the age of 55 with the new onset of symptoms or has any of the alarm symptoms or signs described earlier in the Clinical Evaluation section. If so, one must initially arrange an endoscopy to evaluate the patient for a more serious cause such as malignancy or complicated peptic ulcer. Patients in severe pain or with unstable vital signs, dehydration from recurrent vomiting, acute gastrointestinal bleeding, or acute abdomen require immediate, emergent stabilization, diagnosis, and management.

For patients with typical GERD symptoms of heartburn and acid regurgitation and without alarm symptoms, empirical treatment with a PPI is an option. If patients respond to the treatment, GERD is the likely diagnosis and one can continue the treatment. However, if the patient does not respond to initial treatment, further diagnostic evaluation such as an endoscopy may be considered.

Patients taking an NSAID or cyclooxygenase-2 inhibitor should discontinue the drug or add a PPI. For patients with typical dyspeptic symptoms who are 55 years of age or below and have no alarm symptoms, a "test and treat" strategy is recommended. Using this strategy, one initially tests the patient with dyspepsia for an *H. pylori* infection. Patients with a positive test result are treated with medication to eradicate *H. pylori*. Those with negative test results are given acid suppression treatment with a PPI to control their symptoms. If they still have no response to a PPI, endoscopy may be considered although the yield is generally low. Other diagnoses such as pancreatitis, gall bladder disease, irritable bowel syndrome (IBS), delayed gastric emptying, and psychological problems should be considered in these patients as well (18, 31).

In comparing the test and treat strategy with a strategy of giving all patients initial acid suppression medication, the test and treat strategy was slightly more effective in reducing dyspeptic symptoms in the subgroup of *H. pylori*–positive patients at 1 year of follow-up (32). In comparing the test and treat strategy with a strategy of immediate endoscopy for all patients, there were no significant differences between these

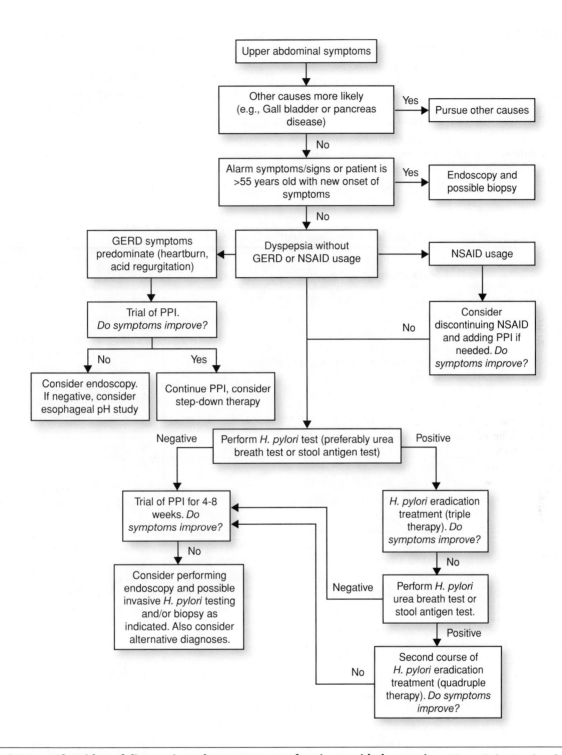

Figure 24.1 • Algorithm of diagnosis and management of patients with dyspepsia. (Compiled using data from References 6, 17, 18, 30, 31.)

two strategies in improving patients' dyspeptic symptom at 1 year of follow-up (32). After a longer follow-up (median of 6.7 years), the test and treat strategy was more cost-effective than the immediate endoscopy strategy by resulting in fewer endoscopies and less antisecretory medication (33). Despite the demonstrated improvements in symptoms using the "test and treat" strategy, one must realize that a fair number of *H.*

pylori–positive patients may continue to have symptoms of dyspepsia 1 year after the eradication treatment (34). For patients who are tested using this strategy and found to be *H. pylori* negative, there is short-term evidence that a PPI is helpful for up to 6 months, but again, some patients may continue to have symptoms on this or other acid suppression medication (35).

MANAGEMENT

Pharmacotherapy options for the treatment of dyspepsia are listed in Table 24.5. Key recommendations for practice are listed in Table 24.6.

Gastroesophageal Reflux Disease

With the demonstrated association of GERD and certain body positions and different types of foods, there are a number of lifestyle measures that may help reflux symptoms. These include elevating the head of the bed, not lying down for at least 2 hours after eating, smoking cessation, minimizing alcohol intake, losing weight, and avoiding large meals and exacerbating foods (e.g., chocolate, caffeine, onions, and peppermint). The low cost and absence of harm of these lifestyle measures makes them reasonable to consider as part of an initial treatment plan, although lifestyle changes by themselves may not control the patient's symptoms.

A number of medications have been used to treat GERD. Over-the counter medications such as antacids, alginic acid, and histamine$_2$ receptor antagonists (H$_2$RAs) alleviate reflux symptoms. Prokinetic agents have the theoretic potential to

TABLE 24.5 Medications Options for the Treatment of Dyspepsia

Drug	Contraindications/Cautions/Adverse Effects	Dosage	Relative Cost*
Gastroesophageal reflux disease, peptic ulcer disease and functional dyspepsia			
- H$_2$RA	Headache, constipation, diarrhea, nausea/vomiting, abdominal pain are rare adverse effects. Cimetidine interacts with some medications such as warfarin, theophylline and phenytoin; adjust for renal function.	Higher doses may be needed in GERD	$
- PPI	Diarrhea, abdominal pain and bloating are rare adverse effects	Standard dose Q day	$$$
***H. pylori* eradication therapy**			
- **Triple therapy:**			
— PPI	See above	Standard dose 2 times/d	$$$
— Clarithomycin	Nausea, abnormal taste, headache or exacerbation of dyspepsia; diarrhea or antibiotic-associated colitis; not recommended for pregnant women; may interact with medication metabolized by the CYP3A system such as certain statin drugs	500 mg po 2 times/d	$$
— Amoxicillin (Substitute with metronidazole if allergic to penicillin)	Rash or drug allergy, diarrhea, antibiotic-associated colitis	1,000 mg po 2 times/d for amoxicillin (500 mg po 2 times/d for metronidazole)	$
- **Quadruple therapy** (if triple therapy fails)			
— PPI	See above	Standard dose 2 times/d	$$$
— Bismuth subsalicylate/ subcitrate	Bismuth subsalicylate can not be used in aspirin-allergic patients. May cause a darkened tongue and dark stools.	120 mg po 4 times/d	$
— Metronidazole	May cause a metallic taste in the mouth. Causes a disulfiram-like reaction if the patient drinks alcohol while on this. Not recommended in the first trimester of pregnancy. Interacts with medications such as warfarin.	500 mg po 3 times/d	$
- Tetracycline	Not for use in pregnancy or children. Better absorbed on an empty stomach. Antacids may decrease its efficacy. Photosensitivity reactions are possible.	500 mg po 4 times/d	$

*Relative cost: $, <$33.00; $$, $34.00 - $66.00; $$$, >$67.00

TABLE 24.6 Key Recommendations for Practice

Recommendation	Strength of Recommendation*	References
Initial evaluation		
— If alarm symptoms or above the age of 55 years old with new symptoms, arrange endoscopy as the initial test	B	17, 18
Gastroesophageal Reflux Disease		
— If GERD is suspected, give a trial of a PPI as a diagnostic test	B	22, 23
— Recommend lifestyle measures such as elevation of the head of bed, staying upright for two hours after eating, smoking cessation, minimizing alcohol intake, weight loss, avoidance of exacerbating foods	C	6
— Use a PPI as the initial medication to relieve symptoms	A	36
— Use a PPI to maintain symptom relief and heal esophagitis	A	38
Uninvestigated Dyspepsia Without Alarm Symptoms and Age of 55 or Below		
— Test and treat for *H. pylori* infection as the initial diagnostic strategy	A	18
— If *H. pylori* positive, give a triple therapy regimen to eradicate the *H. pylori* infection	A	32
— If *H. pylori* negative, use a PPI to control symptoms	B	35
Documented Peptic Ulcer Disease		
— If *H. pylori* positive, give a triple therapy regimen to heal duodenal ulcers, prevent recurrent ulcers and ulcer-related hemorrhage	A	58, 59
— If *H. pylori* negative, but the ulcer is NSAID-related, give a PPI to heal ulcer and prevent recurrent ulcers	B	61, 62
— If *H. pylori* negative and the ulcer is not NSAID-related, give a PPI	C	63
— Perform an initial biopsy of gastric ulcers and repeat biopsy after appropriate treatment	C	64
Functional Dyspepsia (other conditions ruled out)		
— If *H. pylori* positive, give a triple therapy regimen to improve symptoms	B	66
— If *H. pylori* negative, give a PPI or H₂RA to relieve symptoms	B	68

*A = consistent, good-quality patient-oriented evidence; B = inconsistent or limited-quality patient-oriented evidence; C = consensus, disease-oriented evidence, usual practice, expert opinion, or case series. For information about the SORT evidence rating system, see *http://www.aafp.org/afpsort.xml*.

correct the disturbances in gastro-esophageal motility and improve symptoms. However, because of their poor efficacy in clinical trials and potential for adverse effects, they are not recommended for routine use in the treatment of GERD. PPIs are more effective than H_2RAs in empirically relieving symptoms of heartburn for the short term (36) and have emerged as the medication of choice for most patients. A number of PPIs are now available and one, omeprazole, is available over the counter in a standard dose of 20 mg.

Whereas most patients will have an immediate response to PPIs, intermittent use of PPIs may not maintain symptom relief in patients with esophagitis (37), suggesting that chronic, regular use of medication is needed. Standard doses of PPIs are superior to H_2RAs or placebo in maintaining symptom relief and healing of endoscopically proven esophagitis (38). However, a meta-analysis of 19 studies with more than 9,000 patients found no differences between individual PPIs at equivalent doses (39). Standard dose of PPIs also are the best agents to prevent esophageal strictures, a complication of

GERD (number needed to treat [NNT] = 8 to prevent one recurrent stricture after 1 year) (40). A double dose of a PPI may be used when patients do not completely respond to the standard dose or initially improve and then have a recurrence of symptoms on the standard dose. Patients with esophageal dysmotility may also benefit from a double dose of a PPI (6).

Once the patient's symptoms are under control, at least one-third of patients can "step down" to a lower intensity of treatment, with some patients maintaining symptom relief on H_2RAs or on a lower dose of PPIs than initially used to control symptoms (41, 42). However, most patients will need chronic, maintenance treatment for GERD symptoms and the clinician should use the medication that works best for an individual patient at an appropriate dosage that controls the symptoms.

Patients with persistent reflux symptoms for more than 10 years are predisposed to the development of Barrett's esophagus (43). Other risk factors for the development of Barrett's esophagus include the male sex, an increased body mass index (BMI), white ethnicity, and higher socioeconomic status (44,

whom colonoscopy does not diagnose the source of bleeding, other diagnostic tests may be necessary as described below.

Differential Diagnosis

Among adult patients undergoing diagnostic evaluation, the most common causes of LGI bleeding are diverticular disease, ischemic colitis, angiodysplasia, neoplasm, and benign anorectal bleeding (1) (see Table 25.1). The causes of LGI bleeding in children are different, and include disorders such as juvenile polyposis (including hereditary polyposis syndromes), inflammatory bowel disease, Meckel's diverticulum, and intussusception. The remainder of this discussion will focus on bleeding in adults.

Clinical Evaluation

The history and physical exam should serve to identify correctable or modifiable causes of LGI bleeding, and to evaluate the severity of resulting anemia or volume loss.

HISTORY AND PHYSICAL EXAMINATION

The history should identify previous episodes of GI bleeding and any associated workup; attempt to quantify the amount of blood lost and the frequency of bleeding; and identify patient symptoms such as abdominal pain, diarrhea, passage of mucus, perianal discomfort, fever, or other complaints. Patients should also be asked specifically about contributory medical conditions, including: peptic ulcer disease; liver disease or alcohol use; bleeding disorders or bruising; and use of any medications such as nonsteroidal anti-inflammatory drugs (NSAIDs), warfarin, aspirin, or other antiplatelet agents.

The role of the physical examination is primarily to assess the degree of hemodynamic compromise (blood pressure, orthostatis vital signs, overall clinical appearance, signs of anemia, or volume loss), although some clinical conditions causing LGI bleeding also have physical exam findings. Examples include stigmata of cirrhosis (spider angiomas, hepatomegaly, jaundice), bruising, and malnutrition from colorectal cancer. Perianal examination should be performed to evaluate for fissures, hemorrhoids, or fistulae. The role of hemoccult testing in patients who already complain of rectal bleeding is unclear, and a negative hemoccult test should not impede further investigation of a reliable history of rectal bleeding.

DIAGNOSTIC TESTING

Most patients with LGI bleeding should have a complete blood count (CBC) performed to evaluate for anemia or thrombocytopenia. Serum ferritin, reticulocyte count testing, and other studies as indicated should be ordered if the cause of anemia remains unclear. Routine chemistry testing (including serum albumin if poor nutritional status is suspected) and coagulation studies may provide diagnostic clues in some patients. A large number of imaging and functional tests are available to assess for LGI bleeding; the indications and use of these tests is summarized below and in Table 25.2.

RECOMMENDED DIAGNOSTIC STRATEGY

The first diagnostic step should be to attempt to exclude UGI bleeding. Approximately 2% to 15% of patients presenting with LGI bleeding will have an UGI source (1). Nasogastric lavage containing gross blood, 25% blood-tinged fluid, or

TABLE 25.1 Common Causes of Lower Intestinal Bleeding

Diagnosis	Typical Presentation	Frequency*
Diverticulosis	Painless bleeding, possibly constipation	24%
Other colitis (infectious, antibiotic-associated)	Bloody diarrhea, abdominal pain, fever	14%
Ischemic colitis	Maroon-colored stools, abdominal pain, other vascular disease	12%
Benign anorectal disease (hemorrhoids, anal fissure, fistula)	Fissures: perianal itching or tearing Internal hemorrhoids: painless bleeding, possibly external hemorrhoids or perianal itching or burning Fistula: history of inflammatory bowel disease, perianal discharge, visible fistula opening	12%
Colorectal cancer	Microscopic blood (positive hemoccult), microcytic anemia, weight loss, altered bowel habits	7%
Postpolypectomy	Bleeding following procedure	5%
Inflammatory bowel disease	Diarrhea with bleeding, abdominal pain, weight loss	3%
Arteriovenous malformation (angiodysplasia)	Painless bleeding, may be recurrent without previously identified cause	2%
Any small bowel or upper gastrointestinal cause	Chronic gastritis: alcohol use, nonsteroidal anti-inflammatory drug (NSAID) use Variceal bleeding: chronic liver disease Peptic ulcer: gnawing abdominal pain, NSAID use	7%
Unknown		12%

* This is a non-weighted average frequency from studies in Reference 1, consisting primarily of patients hospitalized for lower gastrointestinal bleeding

TABLE 25.2 Diagnostic Studies for Lower Intestinal Bleeding*

Test	Description	Clinical Diagnostic Role
Colonoscopy	Direct visualization of entire colon	Preferred test for initial and recurrent bleeding, allows biopsy and local treatment as well as diagnosis
Anoscopy	Direct visualization of distal rectum and anus	Evaluate for internal hemorrhoids especially if history of constipation or external hemorrhoids on examination
Double-contrast barium enema	Air injected into bowel to contrast with residual barium to visualize bowel mucosa	Option if colonoscopy cannot be performed
Small bowel "push" enteroscopy	Extension of upper endoscopy to visualize 15–160 cm of small bowel distal to Treitz ligament	Potentially long procedure times and patient discomfort but higher diagnostic yield than small bowel radiography
Small-bowel follow-through (SBFT)	Timed radiographic imaging following ingestion of contrast dye	May identify signs of colitis or structural lesion causing small bowel bleeding
Enteroclysis	Barium delivered via tube directly to small intestine with radiographic imaging	More uncomfortable but higher diagnostic yield and sensitivity than SBFT
Capsule endoscopy	Swallowed radiotelemetry capsule allows visualization of entire small intestine	Higher diagnostic yield than enteroscopy with improved patient comfort
Technetium-99m-tagged red blood cell scan	Nuclear medicine imaging 12–24 hours after injection of labeled RBCs, no bowel preparation required	May be helpful to localize site of bleeding exceeding 0.1–0.4 ml/min
Meckel's scan	Nuclear medicine imaging of abdomen following intravenous radioactive isotope	Helpful to identify small bowel bleeding only if positive; does not rule out small bowel bleed if negative*
Arteriography	Intravenous contrast agent with subsequent imaging of vascular supply, no bowel preparation required	Identifies bleeding into gut lumen if rate >0.5 ml/min; may identify typical vascular patterns in non-actively-bleeding angiodysplasia or neoplasia. Allows therapeutic interventions but some risk for complications
Abdominal computed tomography scan	Contrast two-dimensional imaging of abdomen	May identify larger neoplasms or non-specific inflammatory changes, but cannot identify source of bleeding

*Information drawn from References 1 through 4

strongly hemoccult positive dark fluid is highly specific for an UGI source of bleeding, but is not very sensitive (approximately 40%) and is best reserved for patients with brisk bleeding in whom EGD is not already planned (1, 5). The blood urea nitrogen to creatinine ratio has not been shown to be sufficiently accurate to guide clinical decision making. Although highly specific if greater than 36, it is insensitive at that level (approximately 10%) (6). Diagnostic approaches for different patient presentations are outlined below.

Occult Bleeding (Anemia or Positive Hemoccult)

Symptoms associated with occult bleeding do not accurately predict the diagnosis, and current guidelines do not firmly indicate an order for investigation (i.e., EGD or colonoscopy

first) (2). Approximately half of occult bleeding cases remain undiagnosed; depending on age, colon cancer is identified in 2% to 17% of cases.

EGD should be the initial diagnostic test in patients with suspected UGI bleeding or evidence of chronic, slow intestinal bleeding. In patients with suspected LGI bleeding, or in whom EGD is unrevealing, colonoscopy remains the most appropriate initial diagnostic test. This study can provide direct visualization of the entire large bowel and allows diagnostic biopsy sampling as well as therapeutic intervention. Colonoscopy has been shown to have higher positive predictive value than double-contrast barium enema in identifying all colonic lesions.

Many cases of occult bleeding will not evolve into evident or gross bleeding. Thus, patients without a diagnosis after initial upper and lower endoscopy may be followed conservatively, with monitoring for worsening anemia or grossly evident bleeding. Such patients require regular colonoscopic surveillance but might be cautiously reassured that no colorectal cancer was identified on initial testing. Fortunately, less than 1% of patients under age 40 with nonacute rectal bleeding have cancer (7).

Nonmassive Gross Bleeding (Hematochezia)

The evaluation of patients with grossly evident rectal bleeding should begin with an assessment of vitals and fluid status, physical examination for benign anorectal disease, abdominal examination, and CBC. A nontender abdominal examination actually increases the risk of severe bleeding because vascular and diverticular bleeding are typically more severe but are nonpainful and nontender to examination. Patients should undergo EGD for suspected UGI bleeding and colonoscopy if the diagnosis remains unclear, or if LGI bleeding seems most likely. Patients who are under age 40 have a very low incidence of colorectal cancer (8), but evaluation of the entire colon may still be necessary for cases of undiagnosed, severe, or recurrent LGI bleeding.

The timing of a colonoscopy can be determined by stratifying patients into high- or low-risk groups for severe bleeding after initial presentation. A validated clinical decision rule has identified key risk factors for "severe bleeding," defined as continued bleeding within 24 hours of hospital admission and/ or recurrent bleeding after 24 hours of stability (Table 25.3). Patients with three or more of these risk factors have a high (approximately 80%) risk of severe bleeding, and patients with no risk factors have a much lower risk (approximately 10%) (9). Whereas patients at high risk for severe bleeding have improved outcomes with urgent colonoscopy (within 12 hours

of admission), patients at low risk might safely be referred for less urgent evaluation.

Obscure bleeding, defined as LGI bleeding that persists or recurs after negative initial endoscopic evaluation (2), remains a diagnostic challenge, and there is not sufficient evidence to provide clear guidelines on the procedure of choice in these circumstances. An evidence-based guideline from the American Gastroenterological Association (AGA) recommends (2) repeat upper and/or lower endoscopy if there is no evidence of active bleeding, given the difficulty of detecting small bleeding lesions on endoscopy and other causes of false negative initial testing. The diagnostic yield of this "second look" endoscopy, especially for neoplasms and angiodysplasia, is sufficient to justify this approach before proceeding with other tests to evaluate the small bowel or localize bleeding. Table 25.2 summarizes the diagnostic roles for further tests to evaluate such patients for large and small bowel bleeding sources.

In cases of continued active bleeding, AGA recommendations (2) include a stepped work-up, with nuclear red blood cell scan or angiography, followed by small bowel evaluation via enteroscopy, enteroclysis, small bowel series, or capsule endoscopy. Currently, capsule endoscopy seems to have a higher diagnostic yield (55% to 70%) than push enteroscopy (25% to 30%), but retained stool, limited battery life, and poor field of vision may limit the ability to identify colonic bleeding sources (1, 4).

If bleeding persists after this degree of evaluation, physicians should discuss with patients in detail the risks versus benefits of continued diagnostic evaluation. It may be appropriate in such patients to observe, transfuse, or treat empirically with iron supplementation, managing their anemia empirically, with relative confidence that worrisome causes of bleeding have been ruled out.

Massive Lower Intestinal Bleeding

Angiodysplasia and diverticular disease are the most common causes of acute, massive LGI bleeding. Colonoscopy remains the diagnostic study of choice in these cases, with a high diagnostic yield limited only by poor visualization in cases of active, profuse bleeding. In patients who are hemodynamically stable, colonoscopy may be performed urgently (within 12 hours of admission) to identify the source of bleeding. Colonic preparation, ideally with colonoscopy within 1 hour of the colon prep, improves visualization, and allows the therapeutic and diagnostic advantages of urgent colonoscopy to be achieved. Earlier colonoscopy has been associated with a shorter hospital length of stay, due primarily to diagnostic yield rather than treatment interventions (10). Second-line investigations of massive bleeding include arteriography, tagged red blood cell scan, and helical CT scan. Emergent exploratory laparotomy may be indicated in patients with continued bleeding, hemodynamic compromise, and no identified source with the above tests.

Management

Diverticular bleeding may be controlled endoscopically (11) with epinephrine injection, bipolar probe coagulation, or metallic clips; medical therapy includes stool softeners and other measures to control constipation, and abstinence from aspirin or other anticoagulant medications. Although avoidance of

---

TABLE 25.3 Clinical Risk Factors for Severe Acute Lower Gastrointestinal Bleeding*

Heart rate ≥100 beats/minute
Systolic blood pressure ≤115
Syncope
Nontender abdominal examination
Bleeding per rectum during first 4 hours of evaluation
Aspirin use
More than 2 active comorbid conditions (heart failure, ischemic heart disease, renal failure, liver failure, cancer, etc.)

Interpretation:
- ≥3 risk factors: high (approximately 80%) risk of severe bleeding
- 1 to 3 risk factors: moderate (approximately 45%) risk of severe bleeding
- 0 risk factors: low (approximately <10%) risk of severe bleeding

*Data are from Reference 9.

small, hard seeds or nuts has traditionally been recommended for patients with diverticular disease, evidence for this recommendation is limited. Surgical resection of bowel prone to profuse bleeding may be required in patients with recurrent or massive hemorrhage.

Colonic angiodysplasia may be managed endoscopically by epinephrine injection or bipolar laser coagulation. Transcatheter embolization or vasopressin infusion are vascular interventions that may be helpful also. Medical therapy is indicated for patients with diffuse vascular lesions, lesions inaccessible to endoscopic therapy, recurrent bleeding despite local therapy or surgical resection, or an unknown diagnosis, with vascular bleeding suspected (2). Options for medical therapy in these cases include hormonal therapy, vasopressin, octreotide, and others. Octreotide has been shown effective for variceal bleeding, and has been reported to be effective in obscure lower intestinal bleeding (12, 13), but has not been evaluated in randomized trials for this purpose.

The option of blind surgical resection for obscure bleeding in patients with recurrent bleeding and continued requirements for transfusion is a complex decision. Every effort should be made to identify the source of bleeding, and the likelihood of rebleeding following resection, from multifocal mucosal angiodysplasia or other lesions, should be considered (2). Table 25.4 summarizes key recommendations regarding LGI bleeding.

ACUTE DIARRHEA

Clinical Questions

1. What findings on history, physical examination, and routine tests help distinguish *Clostridium difficile*–induced colitis from other causes of antibiotic-associated diarrhea?
2. When are stool cultures or other studies warranted to evaluate acute infectious diarrhea?
3. What clinical features of chronic diarrhea warrant further diagnostic testing?

Diarrhea can be defined as an alteration in normal bowel movements characterized by an increase in frequency, water content, or volume of stools. Recent evidence-based guidelines

---

TABLE 25.4 Key Recommendations for Practice

Recommendation	Strength of Recommendation*
Lower Gastrointestinal Bleeding (LGI)	
Urgent colonoscopy should be the initial diagnostic step for massive LGI bleeding (2, 9)	B
Colonoscopy is the initial diagnostic test for occult LGI bleeding (1, 2)	A
Repeating upper and lower endoscopy may be preferred prior to other diagnostic tests for colonic or small bowel bleeding (2, 9)	C
Clinical criteria can accurately identify patients at lower and higher risk for severe LGI bleeding (9)	C
Acute and Chronic Diarrhea	
Manage acute infectious diarrhea primarily by initiating rehydration, using the oral route when possible (14)	A
Classify chronic diarrhea as inflammatory, watery, or fatty to guide further diagnostic studies (19)	C
Diagnose irritable bowel syndrome based on clinical criteria, reserving testing for patients with "alarm symptoms" (21)	B
Constipation	
Routine laboratory testing and plain abdominal radiographs have limited evidence to support or reject their use, but may be useful to exclude secondary causes in selected patients (32)	C
Patients with rectal bleeding, iron deficiency, weight loss, or other concerning symptoms should have colonoscopy (33)	B
Constipated patients without "alarm" symptoms or signs suggesting neoplasm do not routinely need colonoscopy or other imaging studies unless indicated for routine screening purposes due to age (33)	B
Treatment of idiopathic normal-transit constipation should begin with fiber or other bulk-forming agents and inexpensive saline laxatives (32)	B

*A = consistent, good-quality patient-oriented evidence; B = inconsistent or limited-quality patient-oriented evidence; C = consensus, disease-oriented evidence, usual practice, expert opinion, or case series. For information about the SORT evidence rating system, see *http://www.aafp.org/afpsort.xml*.

from the Infectious Disease Society of America (IDSA) (14) cite infectious diarrheal diseases as the second leading cause of morbidity and mortality worldwide, and the cause of 1.8 million hospitalizations and 3,100 deaths in the United States annually. Beyond acute morbidity and risk of death, some causes of infectious diarrhea may result in long-term complications such as hemolytic-uremic syndrome or renal failure (Shiga toxin-producing *Escherichia coli*), Guillian-Barre syndrome (*Campylobacter jejuni* infection), or malnutrition with a variety of enteric infections. In the United States, an estimated $23 billion is spent annually on diarrhea, including $6 billion on foodborne illnesses, which account for 250,000 patients requiring hospitalization.

The first step in evaluating patients with diarrhea is to establish the severity of the symptoms and to classify the presentation as acute (presumably infectious) diarrhea lasting less than 14 days, or chronic intermittent diarrhea (discussed in the next section of this chapter) (15). The differential diagnosis, evaluation, and management strategies are very different for these two scenarios.

Differential Diagnosis

The differential diagnosis for acute diarrhea focuses primarily on infectious agents, although there are a number of noninfec-

tious causes that should also be considered. These include drug-induced diarrhea, first presentation of inflammatory bowel disease or other "chronic diarrhea" conditions, or toxin-induced diarrhea; these can usually be identified from the patient's history. The most common infectious disorders among adults in industrialized nations are listed in Table 25.5, along with their most common epidemiologic settings or modes of transmission. Patients with persistent diarrhea (greater than 7 days), without any identified cause, should be evaluated for noninfectious diarrhea, including irritable bowel syndrome (IBS), inflammatory bowel disease, ischemic bowel disease (especially in older patients with vascular disease), laxative abuse, partial bowel obstruction, malabsorption syndromes, or other causes.

Clinical Evaluation

Initial evaluation of the patient with acute diarrhea should include an assessment of the need for intravenous rehydration and the need for symptomatic treatment. Although detailed recommendations for oral versus intravenous rehydration are beyond the scope of this chapter, every attempt should be made to rehydrate the patient using oral rehydration solution. Symptomatic relief with bismuth subsalicylate or loperamide

TABLE 25.5 Exposures and Symptoms Suggesting Specific Infectious Diarrheal Disorders*

Finding	Infectious Organism suggested
Epidemiologic	
Consumption of undercooked poultry or employment in poultry industry	*Campylobacter*
Recent use of antibiotics	*C. difficile*
Community outbreak during winter in clusters or on cruise ships	Norovirus
Ingestion of untreated water by traveler or hiker	*Giardia, Cryptosporidium*
Travel to a developing area	*Cyclospora, Cryptosporidium, Entamoeba histolytica*
Daycare center attendance or employment	*Shigella, Giardia, Cryptosporidium*
Swimming in or drinking untreated fresh surface water from a lake or stream	*Giardia, Cryptosporidium*
Seafood	*Vibrio*
Visiting a farm or petting zoo, having contact with animals with diarrhea	*E. coli*
Community-acquired, foodborne transmission	*Salmonella, Yersinia, Campylobacter, E. coli* (including O157-H7)
Community-acquired, person-to-person transmission	*Shigella*, norwalk, rotavirus, other enteric viruses
Receptive anal intercourse or oral-anal sexual contact	*Giardia, Clostridium histolyticum*
Clinical	
Incubation period <6 hours	*Staphylococcus aureus* or *Bacillus cereus* toxin–induced
Incubation period 6–24 hours	*Clostridium perfringens* or *B. cereus* more likely
Fever, abdominal pain, bloody stools	*Salmonella, Campylobacter, Shigella*
Afebrile, abdominal pain, bloody stools	Shiga toxin-producing *E. coli*

*Data are from References 14 and 15.

for noninflammatory diarrhea should be initiated as the diagnostic work-up proceeds.

HISTORY AND PHYSICAL EXAMINATION

Most cases of acute infectious diarrhea are caused by self-limited viral gastroenteritis; the acute onset of vomiting, watery diarrhea, and mild abdominal pain in a healthy patient with no unusual exposures and no worrisome symptoms suggests such a routine viral infection. The patient history should focus on identifying features that (a) indicate a specific organism or other concerning cause of the diarrhea or (b) warrant further diagnostic evaluation. Public health measures may be required if a reportable infection is identified, and the history should include questions about possible disease outbreaks. A number of symptoms or other historical features can help to suggest specific causes of diarrhea (Table 25.5).

Fever, severe abdominal pain, bloody bowel movements, and vomiting are more likely to occur with infectious (and especially bacterial) enteritis, but the predictive value of any single finding is low (14). Shigellosis, salmonellosis, and campylobacteriosis are "inflammatory diarrheas" typically characterized by fever, abdominal pain, bloody stools, fecal leukocytes, fecal lactoferrin, or occult blood.

DIAGNOSTIC TESTING

Although many patients with acute diarrhea are asked to provide samples for stool culture, fecal leukocytes, and examination for ova and parasites in the stool, such testing may be overused. Most cases of acute infectious diarrhea are self-limited, and stool testing results are available only after the patient's illness has resolved (14). One study of stool samples tested by labs in the FoodNet foodborne diseases surveillance network (14) found only a 1%–2% positive yield of stool studies for salmonella, shigella, campylobacter, and *E. coli* O157, at a cost of more than $1,000 per positive result. In particular, the yield of diagnostic testing for routine stool cultures and ova or parasite examination is very low for patients hospitalized greater than 3 days (many of whom have *Clostridium difficile* colitis). Diagnostic testing should be limited to patients with a higher likelihood of a specific organism (e.g., over age 65, neutropenic, HIV positive), and where such testing will aid either treatment decisions or public health investigation (16).

RECOMMENDED DIAGNOSTIC STRATEGY

Diagnostic testing is not generally indicated for suspected viral, self-limited gastroenteritis, nor should broad stool testing be pursued without consideration for the specific organisms involved. IDSA guidelines (14) recommend the strategy outlined in Table 25.6.

One important challenge is distinguishing *C. difficile* colitis from other causes of antibiotic-associated diarrhea. *C. difficile* infection causes a toxin-mediated enteritis, and is most commonly associated with use of clindamycin, cephalosporins, and penicillins. However, other mechanisms and other antibiotics can cause diarrhea, and only 10% to 20% of stool specimens tested for *C. difficile* toxin are positive (17). The primary mechanisms for other antibiotic-associated, non–*C. difficile* diarrhea primarily include direct effects of antibiotics on the intestinal mucosa and the metabolic consequences of reductions in intestinal flora. Patients with antibiotic-associated, non–*C. difficile* diarrhea usually have a previous history of similar responses to antibiotics; typically have more moderate diarrhea without fever, cramps, fecal leukocytes, or rectal bleeding; and typically are not markedly ill, though they may be mildly dehydrated. Non–*C. difficile*–associated diarrhea usually readily resolves upon withdrawal of the implicated antibiotic, while *C. difficile* colitis does not.

Management

Oral rehydration and general supportive care remain the most important factors in patient management. Primary care physi-

---

TABLE 25.6 Guidelines for Diagnostic Testing in Selected Patients with Acute Diarrhea

Clinical Situation	Tests
Suspected viral gastroenteritis	None
Community-acquired or traveler's diarrhea (especially with significant fever or blood in stool)	Culture for *Salmonella*, *Shigella*, *Campylobacter*, *E. coli* O157:H7
Diarrhea is bloody, associated with tenesmus, or associated with nosocomial outbreak	Perform stool culture and test for shiga toxin
Antibiotic use or chemotherapy in recent weeks	Test for *C. difficile* toxins A and B
Nosocomial diarrhea, onset after 3 days in the hospital	Test for *C. difficile* toxins A and B
Persistent diarrhea >7 days (especially if immunocompromised)	Test for ova and parasites (*Giardia*, *Cryptosporidium*, *Cyclospora*, *Isospora belli*)
Patient is HIV positive	Test for *Microsporidia* and *M. avium* complex in addition to stool culture as above

*Data are from Reference 14.

TABLE 25.7 Selected Antibiotic Therapy for Specific Infectious Diarrheal Conditions*

Target Disorder	Intervention
Shigellosis	Levofloxacin 500mg once daily for 3 days, or trimethoprim/sulfimethoxazole 160/800 mg twice daily for 3 days if susceptible
Non-*typhi* salmonellosis	Treatment not routinely recommended†
Campylobacteriosis	Erythromycin 500 mg twice daily for 5 days
E. coli enteritis	Trimethoprim/sulfimethoxazole 160/800 mg twice daily for 3 days (fluoroquinolone regimens also effective, see detailed guidelines)
Yersinia species	Treatment not routinely recommended
Vibrio cholerae	Doxycycline 300 mg single dose (other regimens may also be effective, see detailed guidelines)
C. difficile colitis	Metronidazole 500 mg three times daily for 10 days
Giardiasis	Metronidazole 250–750 mg three times daily for 7–10 days

*Data are from Reference 15.
†Patients <6 months old, >50 years old, or with valvular heart disease or other conditions may require specific treatment—see detailed guidelines.

cians who suspect a disease outbreak should contact local public health authorities. Outbreaks might be suspected on the basis of diarrheal illness in a daycare attendee or employee, or a resident of an institutional facility (nursing home, hospital, military facility, prison), or similar presentations or diagnoses among a defined group of individuals.

The management of the full spectrum of infectious diarrheal illnesses is complex; patient immune status, age, duration of illness, and general medical conditions are all important factors in determining the need and duration of specific treatment. The selected treatment recommendations in Table 25.7 apply to immunocompetent adults; IDSA guidelines (14) or other resources should be consulted before prescribing specific treatment.

CHRONIC DIARRHEA

Diarrhea lasting more than 4 weeks may occur in up to 3% to 5% of the population (18); frequently it is not the quantity of stool that patients characterize as diarrhea, however, but the liquidity or consistency of the stools that becomes abnormal (19). The impact on patients' quality of life, in terms of the effect of symptoms, lost time from work, and the need for treatment, can be considerable. Evaluation is driven primarily by a careful history to search for clues to the underlying diagnosis, with directed testing for specific disorders or to categorize the type of diarrhea. Most of the recommendations for evaluating and managing chronic diarrhea are based on expert opinion, rather than properly designed epidemiologic studies or controlled trials (19).

Differential Diagnosis

AGA guidelines (18) classify chronic diarrhea into four categories (Table 25.8). Secretory diarrhea is the most common type according to two case series from a tertiary referral center (20).

Clinical Evaluation
HISTORY AND PHYSICAL EXAMINATION

The history should include clarifying details for the onset, timing, pattern, and duration of symptoms, as well as the quality of the stools, including whether stools are watery, bloody, or fatty. Pain, weight loss, and bloody diarrhea suggest inflammatory bowel disease. Weight loss and fatty diarrhea also suggest malabsorption. Travel or exposure to untreated water raises the possibility of chronic infectious colitis, such as that caused by *Giardia lamblia*. Medications, radiation, and cholecystectomy or colectomy can all lead to chronic diarrhea. Rarely, patients will also overuse laxatives, leading to a factitious diarrhea. The effect of stress or diet on symptoms should also be elicited. Finally, the history should include a review of systems to address symptoms of systemic illnesses, such as hyperthyroidism, diabetes, acquired immunodeficiency syndrome, or collagen vascular diseases.

The diagnosis of IBS can be made on clinical grounds—the Rome II criteria (Table 25.9) have a high positive predictive value. Patients who meet these criteria and do not have "alarm symptoms" (e.g., bleeding, fever, family history of colorectal cancer, chronic severe diarrhea, weight loss, or malnutrition) can be treated for IBS without further testing (22, 23).

The physical examination may occasionally offer clues to the diagnosis for a patient's diarrhea (e.g., thyromegaly suggesting hyperthyroidism, rash suggesting celiac sprue, perianal fistula suggesting Crohn's disease, etc.) but typically the most important finding from the physical examination is an assessment of the extent of dehydration or nutrient deficiency.

DIAGNOSTIC TESTING

Routine laboratory testing may provide additional clues to the underlying diagnosis and can help establish the severity of dehydration or nutrient-related anemia or electrolyte disor-

TABLE 25.8 Causes of Chronic Diarrhea*

Mechanism	Disorder
Secretory diarrhea	Nonosmotic laxative abuse
	Inflammatory bowel disease
	Ileal bile acid malabsorption
	Neuroendocrine tumors (carcinoid syndrome, vipoma, gastrinoma)
	Disordered motility (postvagotomy, hyperthyroidism, autonomic neuropathy, irritable bowel syndrome)
Osmostic diarrhea	Magnesium, phosphate, sulfate ingestion
	Carbohydrate malabsorption (lactose intolerance)
Fatty diarrhea	Malabsorption syndromes (short-bowel syndrome, postresection diarrhea, celiac and other mucosal disease, mesenteric ischemia)
	Maldigestion (pancreatic insufficiency, bile acid deficiency)
Inflammatory diarrhea	Inflammatory bowel disease
	Infectious disease (cytomegalovirus)
	Radiation colitis
	Neoplasia (colon cancer, lymphoma)

*Data are from Reference 18.

ders. Complete blood counts may identify leukocytosis consistent with an infection, and eosinophilia may suggest neoplasm, allergy, parasitic infection, or other causes. An elevated sedimentation rate suggests inflammatory bowel disease (IBD). Antigliadin antibodies may be considered for patients with suspected celiac disease; these patients represent about 1% of the United States population (23).

Colonoscopy or flexible sigmoidoscopy is helpful when IBD or malignancy is suspected in patients with alarm symptoms. Anti–*Saccharomyces cerevisiae* antibodies and anti-neutrophil cytoplasmic antibodies are specific but nonsensitive tests for IBD, which are helpful when positive to rule in disease. Negative tests do not rule out IBD, though (24).

RECOMMENDED DIAGNOSTIC STRATEGY

Evidence-based guidelines from the AGA (18) describe a "categorize, test, and treat" strategy, where chronic diarrhea is categorized as watery (either osmotic or secretory), fatty, or inflammatory to guide further evaluation and treatment. Gross inspection of the stool by physician or patient may often be sufficient to establish this categorization (18), although AGA guidelines recommend simple stool analysis to provide more definitive information. Although extensive tests are available to fully evaluate 48- or 72-hour stool collections, evaluation of a single, randomly collected stool specimen can often provide sufficient clues to categorize the diarrhea. The accuracy of these tests are generally unknown (19), and the use of stool evaluation should be guided by the physician's overall impression of the patient's most likely diagnosis. Table 25.10 describes some available stool sample tests and their possible diagnostic impact. AGA guidelines (19) also suggest that stool cultures be performed in many patients with chronic diarrhea despite limited diagnostic impact.

Management

Management of chronic diarrhea primarily involves treating or correcting the underlying cause, such as infection, IBD, or malabsorption syndrome. Empiric therapy is indicated for symptomatic relief pending additional testing, when testing

TABLE 25.9 Rome II Criteria for Irritable Bowel Syndrome*

At least 12 weeks (which need not be consecutive) in the preceding 12 months, of abdominal discomfort or pain that has two out of three of these features:
- relieved with defecation; and/or
- onset associated with a change in frequency of stool; and/or
- onset associated with a change in form (appearance) of stool

Symptoms that cumulatively support the diagnosis of irritable bowel syndrome
- abnormal stool frequency (for research purposes abnormal may be defined as greater than three bowel movements per day and less than three bowel movements per week)
- abnormal stool form (lumpy/hard or loose/watery stool)
- abnormal stool passage (straining, urgency, or feeling of incomplete evacuation)
- passage of mucus
- bloating or feeling of abdominal distension

*Data are from Reference 21.

TABLE 25.10 Stool Specimen Testing and Suggested Diarrhea Category*

Stool Analysis	Disorder or Diarrhea Category Suggested	Clinical or Diagnostic Role
Occult blood	Celiac sprue, inflammatory diarrhea, neoplasm	50%–70% of patients with celiac sprue are hemoccult positive, unclear role for other conditions
Wright's stain or microscopy for white blood cells	Infectious or inflammatory cause of diarrhea	Reported "few WBC" may be false positive
Latex agglutination test for neutrophil product lactoferrin	Acute infectious diarrhea including *C. difficile* colitis	Unclear role in chronic diarrhea
Sudan staining for stool fat	Malabsorption syndrome	Semiquantitative measure for stool fat content provides similar information
Fecal culture	Bacterial colitis	Identify rare bacterial causes of chronic diarrhea, especially for aeromonas or pseudomonas species in patients exposed to untreated well water
Microscopic evaluation for ova and parasites	Protozoal or parasitic infection, e.g., Giardiasis	Undefined predictive value in immunocompetent patients in developed countries; *Giardia*-specific antibody ELISA may be more sensitive and specific
Stool pH and electrolytes	Osmotic or secretory diarrhea pH <5.3 suggests carbohydrate malabsorption	Osmotic gap elevated (>125 mOsm/kg) in pure osmotic diarrhea, and low (<50 mOsm/kg) in pure secretory diarrhea
Stool laxative testing	Factitious diarrhea, laxative abuse	Patient history and/or search of hospital room for laxatives may have higher sensitivity than stool testing

*Data are from Reference 19.

has failed to reveal a diagnosis, or when no specific therapy is available (19). Opioids remain the most effective empiric medical therapy for diarrhea; loperamide or diphenoxylate are used for more mild cases of chronic diarrhea, although morphine is occasionally effective for severe, intractable cases. Cholestyramine, bismuth, or dietary fiber are also useful empiric treatments in some patients. None of these agents have been studied prospectively for this purpose, though extensive experience supports their benefit (19).

IBS is a common cause of chronic diarrhea; the management of this disorder requires careful patient education, dietary adjustments, and individualized medical treatment that is detailed elsewhere. An evidence-based guideline from the American College of Gastroenterology (23) recommends bulking agents and loperamide to improve stool frequency and tricyclic antidepressants for abdominal pain. However, neither of these treatments improves global IBS symptoms. Hypnotherapy, relaxation therapy, cognitive therapy, paroxetine, and psychotherapy may improve IBS symptoms, although the quality of studies is poor. Tegaserod, a 5-HT4 agonist, is helpful in patients with constipation-predominant IBS, whereas alosetron, a 5-HT3 antagonist, is helpful in patients with diarrhea-predominant IBS. However, the latter was withdrawn from the market after the deaths of five women were attributed to the drug. It has now been re-released, but only for women with severe diarrhea-predominant symptoms (23, 25).

A detailed discussion of treatment of IBD is beyond the scope of this chapter. In general, Crohn's disease and ulcerative colitis should be considered in patients presenting with chronic diarrhea, especially if abdominal pain or rectal bleeding are present. These conditions can be effectively managed using a combination of oral and topical aminosalicylates, corticosteroids, antibiotics, and other agents. Recent evidence-based reviews provide additional details regarding the diagnosis and management of IBD (26, 27). Table 25.4 lists key recommendations regarding acute and chronic diarrhea.

CONSTIPATION

Clinical Questions

1. What findings on history, physical examination, and routine tests help diagnose chronic constipation as a cause of patients' abdominal pain or other presenting symptom?
2. What symptoms or signs warrant more detailed diagnostic evaluation for specific conditions causing chronic constipation?
3. What are the most effective management strategies to provide short-term and long-term relief of chronic constipation?

Although many people experience transient constipation, at times it becomes a chronic condition requiring medical intervention. Patients suffering from chronic constipation can present with a wide variety of symptoms, including altered bowel habits, abdominal pain or bloating, hard or small stools, early satiety, or lower back pain. An important step in identifying chronic constipation as a diagnosis is to keep the disorder in mind and include questions about bowel habits while reviewing systems for these presenting concerns.

There is no single definition of chronic constipation, although it is often defined in research studies (28) as the inability to evacuate stool completely and spontaneously three or more times per week. Patients may describe any of the following as constipation: small or hard stools, infrequent bowel movement (fewer than three per week), the need to strain to have a bowel movement, a sense of fullness or bloating, a sense of incomplete evacuation, or an inability to have a bowel movement without excessive straining or time on the toilet.

It is useful to keep in mind the physiologic steps required to achieve normal bowel movements. These include absorption of water; segmental bowel contractions that mix stool and move feces short distances; high-amplitude contractions that move fecal waste larger distances in the colon; synchronized voluntary striated muscle contraction and involuntary smooth muscle contraction for defecation; and unimpaired passage of stool through the colon and rectum.

Risk factors for chronic constipation in adults include female sex, non-white ethnicity, older age, physical inactivity, limited education, and depression. Constipation in children has a different spectrum of disorders and may represent a neurologic disorder, a functional or emotional problem, or a manifestation of sexual abuse. The diagnosis and management of chronic constipation in children at various ages is quite different from that in adults; this section will focus on adult patients.

Differential Diagnosis

It is probably easiest for clinicians to classify causes of constipation by etiology, as shown in Table 25.11, rather than physiology. Physiologically, constipation can be divided (28) into broad categories of normal-transit constipation (most common, affecting 59% of patients), defecatory disorders, or slow-transit constipation. Up to 3% of patients have a combination of causes. Among patients with severe, intractable constipation, the most common causes are IBS, pelvic floor dysfunction, isolated slow-transit constipation, or combinations of these (29).

Normal-transit constipation ("functional" constipation) entails normal rate of stool passage through the colon and normal stool frequency, yet patients feel they are constipated. The perception of constipation may be because of difficulty with evacuation, hard stools, abdominal pain or bloating, constipation, or other symptoms. Symptoms typically respond to treatment with dietary fiber, with or without an osmotic laxative.

Defecatory disorders may be caused by dysfunction of the pelvic floor or anal sphincter, structural abnormalities (rectal intussusception, etc.), or failure to effectively coordinate the muscular functions of defecation because of a variety of conditions. Slow-transit constipation is considered an idiopathic disorder, primarily in young women with chronic constipation beginning in adolescence, due to a disorder of the myenteric plexus neurons. Symptoms of bloating and abdominal discomfort are the presenting symptoms rather than constipation.

Clinical Evaluation

Given the frequency with which chronic constipation is caused by functional or readily identifiable factors, the history alone is often sufficient to determine the underlying cause. The physical examination may provide only limited information to aid diagnosis but may be useful to identify or to rule out specific local perianal conditions or selected "alarm symptoms" of possible serious illness, e.g. hemoccult positive, weight loss, stool impaction.

HISTORY AND PHYSICAL EXAMINATION

Patients complaining of abdominal pain, back pain, rectal bleeding, nausea, early satiety, bloating, or other symptoms should be asked about constipation symptoms. If patients are directly asked, "Are you constipated?" the answer may vary depending on that patient's definition of this problem; likewise patients who complain of constipation may have many different symptoms and normal stool patterns. All patients with constipation and/or suggestive symptoms should be asked in detail about stool frequency, consistency, discomfort, straining, bleeding, and any need for medical or manual assistance to have an effective bowel movement.

Functional constipation, IBS, medications (especially opioids), neurologic or spinal cord injury, marked physical inactivity, and symptoms of thyroid disorders are readily identified in the patient history and may be sufficient to establish the diagnosis. Patients should be specifically asked about their use of over-the-counter laxatives, including which agents are used, how often, and for how long. A typical pattern of alternating diarrhea with constipation may suggest IBS (Table 25.9); recent changes in medication may suggest an adverse effect of medication. The history should also focus on specifically inquiring about "alarm" symptoms (Table 25.12) that may suggest specific secondary causes.

The physical examination does not usually provide additional information to confirm the diagnosis or the cause of chronic constipation. However, the exam may help to identify a few specific abnormalities, including: thyromegaly; marked abdominal distension suggesting obstruction; local perianal abnormalities such as hemorrhoids or fissure; altered rectal tone suggesting neurologic impairment; or obstructing masses such as tumors or rectocele.

Pelvic floor dysfunction is increasingly recognized as an important cause of chronic constipation, and it is helpful to identify this problem early because symptoms do not respond to, and may be worsened by, routine recommendations for dietary changes, stool softeners, and laxatives. The primary defect is the inability to evacuate stool from the rectum because of inappropriate contraction or relaxation of the pelvic floor muscles and external anal sphincter. Symptoms may include prolonged or excessive straining before defecation, the need for perineal or vaginal pressure to allow bowel movement, difficulty passing even liquid stools or enema liquid, or the need for manual removal of stool by the patient.

DIAGNOSTIC TESTING

The role of diagnostic tests for chronic constipation in selected patients is summarized in Table 25.13. However, evidence-based guidelines do not recommend obtaining these tests routinely for all or even most patients. Plain abdominal radiographs may help identify large amounts of stool in the colon,

TABLE 25.11 Differential Diagnosis of the Patient with Chronic Constipation*

Diagnosis	
Primary Constipation	• Hypokalemia
Functional constipation†	• Uremia
• Idiopathic functional constipation†	• Heavy metal poisoning
• Irritable bowel syndrome†	Mechanical obstruction
• Pelvic floor dysfunction (anismus)	• Colon cancer†
• Slow-transit constipation	• Compression by extra-colonic tumor
Secondary Constipation	• Stricture (diverticular, post-ischemic)
Medications*	• Large rectocele
• Iron supplements†	• Postsurgical changes
• Calcium channel blockers (verapamil)†	• Anal stenosis from anal fissure, etc.
• Diuretics	• Crohn's disease, megacolon
• Opioids†	Neuropathies
• Anticholinergics, antihistamines	• Spinal cord injury or tumor
• Anticonvulsants	• Parkinson's disease
• Antidepressants	• Cerebrovascular disease
• Antipsychotics	• Multiple sclerosis
• Laxatives (chronic abuse)	• Hirschprung's disease
• Nonsteroidal anti-inflammatories	• Others (Chagas disease, congenital anal sphincter myopathy, hyperganglionosis)
• Calcium supplements	Other conditions
• Antacids	• Depression
Metabolic/Endocrine	• Degenerative joint disease, immobility
• Hypothyroidism†	• Autonomic neuropathy
• Hypomagnesemia	• Cognitive impairment
• Hypercalcemia	• Cardiac disease

*Data are from References 29 and 30.
†Indicates common causes

confirming the presence of chronic constipation, and may show evidence of obstruction or ileus. Typically these films do not help identify the cause of constipation, however. No high-quality studies have evaluated the role of routine plain films in patients with chronic constipation (31). Although barium enema testing may provide additional anatomic information and has the potential to identify obstructing lesions or narrowed bowel segments, it adds little to information that can be obtained from plain radiographs. Compared to colonoscopy, barium enema testing may not be sufficiently accurate to exclude small polyps or other concerning lesions (31).

RECOMMENDED DIAGNOSTIC STRATEGY

Current guidelines (32) indicate that in the absence of alarm signs or symptoms (age 50 years or older), there is no evidence

to recommend the routine use of flexible sigmoidoscopy, colonoscopy, barium enema, thyroid function tests, serum calcium, or other diagnostic tests in patients presenting with constipation.

Adult patients over 50 years of age with chronic constipation should be evaluated by colonoscopy to rule out colon cancer, IBD, or other obstructing lesions. Guidelines for using colonoscopy in patients with constipation (33) report that the yield of colonoscopy in identifying neoplasm in patients with chronic constipation but no concerning symptoms is comparable to that in asymptomatic patients. Therefore, colonoscopy may not be necessary in such patients, unless age or other factors indicate a need for such testing. A systematic review (31) of diagnostic modalities for chronic constipation (34) identified a yield of 2.0% for colonoscopy in detecting colon cancer

TABLE 25.12 Alarm Signs and Symptoms for Patients with Chronic Constipation Indicating More Serious Disease

Red Flags	Suggested Cause
Progressive symptoms	Obstruction due to colon cancer or extracolonic mass
Lower intestinal bleeding	Colon cancer, Crohn's disease
Weight loss >10 pounds	Colon cancer
Anemia	Colon cancer
Family history of colon cancer or inflammatory bowel disease	Colon cancer, inflammatory bowel disease
Rectal pain, urinary stress incontinence	Defecatory disorder
Need to manually remove stool, apply perineal pressure, or strain excessively to have a bowel movement	Pelvic floor dysfunction

in a large retrospective study of patients with constipation and a yield of 1.0% for flexible sigmoidoscopy.

The guidelines (33) recommend the following:

- patients with constipation should undergo colonoscopy if they have rectal bleeding, heme-positive stool, iron deficiency anemia, weight loss, obstructive symptoms (such as excessive straining), recent onset of constipation, rectal prolapse, or change in stool caliber
- chronic constipation may be a risk factor for colorectal cancer; patients over age 50 with constipation who have not had colon cancer screening should have a colonoscopy
- flexible sigmoidoscopy may be adequate in younger patients
- colonoscopy allows dilation of benign colonic strictures in some patients

Additional testing for defecatory and pelvic floor dysfunction, or other testing suggested by suspected or likely di-

agnosis, are usually pursued in consultation with a gastroenterologist.

Management

Initial management of patients with chronic constipation should address resolving correctable factors, such as removing offending medications, treating metabolic or endocrine conditions, improved hydration, increasing physical activity or mobility, or surgically removing obstructing tumors, as much as possible.

Patients with symptoms suggesting pelvic floor dysfunction should be referred for appropriate diagnostic testing. Patients with this condition do not respond well to increasingly aggressive regimens of stool softeners and laxatives, and should be referred for intensive pelvic floor retraining or biofeedback programs.

In most patients with idiopathic, normal-transit constipa-

TABLE 25.13 Role of Diagnostic Tests for Selected Patients with Chronic Constipation

Test	Recommended Role
Routine blood counts, thyroid profile, and chemistry profile	To exclude metabolic or endocrine cause in patients with suggestive signs or symptoms
Plain abdominal x-ray	To confirm chronic constipation, but no role in determining diagnosis
Barium enema	To identify structural bowel lesions when colonoscopy cannot be performed
Colonoscopy (or flexible sigmoidoscopy)	For patients who have "alarm" signs or symptoms, or who are over 50 years of age
Colonic transit study*	For patients with symptoms suggesting slow-transit constipation
Anorectal manometry, balloon expulsion test, or defecography*	To identify pelvic floor dyssynergia or other defecatory disorder

* Used primarily in patients referred to tertiary care centers for severe chronic idiopathic constipation, unresponsive to other therapy (31)

TABLE 25.14 Treatment Options for Chronic Constipation*

Drug	Contraindications/Cautions/Adverse Effects	Dosage	Relative Cost *
Bulk-forming agents			
Dietary fiber (bran)	Bloating, flatulence, diminished iron and calcium absorption	1 cup per day	$
Psyllium (e.g., Metamucil, konsyl, perdiem with fiber)	Bloating, flatulence	1 teaspoon up to three times a day with water	$
Methylcellulose (e.g., Citrucel)	Less bloating	1 teaspoon up to tid with water	$
Calcium polycarbophil (e.g., Fibercon)	Bloating, flatulence	2–4 tablets daily	$
Stool softener			
Docusate sodium (e.g., Colace)		100 mg twice a day	$
Saline laxatives			
Magnesium (e.g., Milk of Magnesia, Haley's MO)	Dehydration, abdominal cramps, magnesium toxicity	15–30 mL once or twice daily	$
Hyperosmolar laxatives			
Lactulose (e.g., Chronulac)	Transient abdominal cramps, flatulence	15–30 mL once or twice daily	$$
Polyethylene glycol (e.g., Golytely, Colyte, Miralax)	Stool incontinence due to potency	8–32 oz daily	$$
Stimulant laxatives			
Bisacodyl (e.g., Dulcolax)	Incontinence, abdominal cramps, rectal burning with daily use	10 mg suppositories up to 3 times per week	$
Sennosides (senna) (e.g., Senokot)	Unproven degeneration of Meissner's and Auerbach's plexus, malabsorption	2 tablets daily up to 4 tablets bid	$
Serotonin receptor agonist			
Tegaserod (Zelnorm)	Increased frequency of diarrhea	6 mg twice a day before meals	$$$

Relative cost: $ = <$33.00; $$ = $34.00 - $66.00; $$$ = >$67.00
*Data are from Reference 29.

tion, management should begin with recommendations for dietary fiber and/or the routine use of stool softener agents (Table 25.14). The prescription for dietary fiber should be specific—the target dosage should be 20–25 grams of dietary fiber daily beyond usual intake, and patients should be instructed to begin with a lower, twice-daily dose and slowly increase to the target dose over 2–4 weeks. Patients should be warned that fiber supplements increase gaseousness, but symptoms may improve over several days (29).

Obtaining sufficient dietary fiber through fruits and vegetables may be difficult (typically 1 g per serving or less), and dietary changes should emphasize bran cereals (4–10 g per serving), raspberries or blackberries (4–5 g per serving), bran muffins, or beans (2–3 g per serving). Other over-the-counter bulk-forming agents may be used according to patient preference; these should be taken with water, and patients should be advised of likely side effects. For all these agents, patients should be instructed that improvement may take some weeks. Fair evidence suggests that psyllium increases stool frequency in patients with chronic constipation, but there is insufficient evidence regarding the efficacy of other bulk-forming agents. Likewise there is insufficient evidence for the efficacy of stool softeners in patients with chronic constipation (32), although all of these agents may be effective in some patients.

Patients who do not respond to these measures should next try inexpensive saline laxative agents to achieve soft, but not liquid, stools. These agents promote osmotic retention of fluid in the intestinal lumen. Patients with persistent symptoms should be prescribed either more expensive hyperosmolar laxatives, or stimulant laxatives, such as those listed in Table 25.14. Polyethylene glycol (PEG) and lactulose have been shown to be effective at improving stool frequency and consistency in patients with chronic constipation (32); there is insufficient evidence for the efficacy of saline laxatives, although their low cost may make their use more acceptable to patients. Patients may need to try multiple agents to find the most effective regimen. Dietary changes and stool softener treatment should be continued as laxatives are tried. Stimulant laxatives (including enemas or suppositories), such as those listed in Table 25.14, should be recommended only for intermittent, as-needed use of severe flare-ups of chronic constipation. There is insufficient evidence to make firm recommendations regarding their use in patients with chronic constipation, but for some patients these agents seem to be highly effective in alleviating constipation symptoms.

The safety of long-term laxative use, especially stimulant laxatives, has been questioned for many years, with concerns of possible damage to the colonic myenteric system, increased risk of cancer, and tolerance or even addiction to these laxatives. It is true that some patients with chronic constipation may depend on these agents over a long period of time for appropriate stool frequency, and some patients may abuse laxatives by using many times the recommended dose. However, available evidence suggests that there are no harmful effects on the colon and no significantly increased risk for addiction or colorectal cancer from using laxatives at recommended doses on a chronic basis to control symptoms (35).

Tegaserod is effective at improving stool frequency and consistency, and reducing straining in patients with chronic constipation, although it is expensive (32). Patients with truly intractable constipation or slow-transit constipation ("colonic inertia") represent a complex management challenge—these may include patients with inoperable obstructing tumors, scleroderma, neurologic injury, amyloidosis, or other conditions. Aggressive use of laxatives (stimulant, saline, PEG solutions, lactulose) may be effective (29), or patients may be candidates for surgical intervention, such as total colectomy with ileorectal anastomosis, continent sigmoid colon conduit, or other procedures. Key recommendations for chronic constipation are listed in Table 25.4.

CASE 1 DISCUSSION

Despite the relative absence of risk factors, given T.G.'s repeatedly negative colonoscopy, UGI endoscopy would be an appropriate next test in this patient. Transfusion and possibly active treatment for his bleeding should be sufficient to control his symptoms; if bleeding stops, repeat upper and lower endoscopy in a few months might be reasonable, if no lesion is identified. Alternatively, or if bleeding persists, angiography (possibly preferred to RBC scan because bleeding is not profuse) or small bowel evaluation by small bowel series or capsule endoscopy could help identify a source of bleeding.

CASE 2 DISCUSSION

R.G. most likely has functional constipation caused by a number of factors, including inactivity, laxative over-use, dietary factors, and possibly opioid medications if used for her arthritis. Initial testing should include routine blood counts (anemia possibly suggesting colon cancer), chemistry, and thyroid function. Fiber, fluid, stool softeners, and as-needed laxatives should be the initial treatment. Assuming that adequate colon cleansing can be achieved, a repeat colonoscopy may be warranted to evaluate for neoplasm since her last test was 6 years ago.

REFERENCES

1. Strate LL. LGI bleeding: epidemiology and diagnosis. Gastroenterol Clin North Am. 2005;34:643–664.
2. American Gastroenterologic Association. Medical position statement: evaluation and management of occult and obscure gastrointestinal bleeding. Gastroenterology. 2000;118(1):197–200.
3. Mitchell SH. A new view of occult and obscure gastrointestinal bleeding. Am Fam Physician. 2004;69:875–881.
4. Mylonaki M. Wireless capsule endoscopy: a comparison with push enteroscopy in patients with gastroscopy and colonoscopy negative gastrointestinal bleeding. Gut. 2003;52:1122–1126.
5. Witting MD. Usefulness and validity of diagnostic nasogastric aspiration in patients without hematemesis. Ann Emerg Med. 2004;43(4):525–532.
6. Chalasani N. Blood urea nitrogen to creatinine concentration in gastrointestinal bleeding: a reappraisal. Am J Gastroenterol. 1997;92(10):1796–1799.
7. Mulcahy HE. Yield of colonoscopy in patients with nonacute rectal bleeding: a multicenter database study of 1766 patients. Am J Gastroenterol. 2002;97(2):328–333.
8. Lewis JD. Endoscopy for hematochezia in patients under 50 years of age. Dig Dis Sci. 2001;46(12):2660–2665.
9. Strate LL. Validation of a clinical prediction rule for severe acute lower intestinal bleeding. Am J Gastroenterol. 2005;100:1821–1827.
10. Strate LL. Timing of colonoscopy: impact on length of hospital stay in patients with acute lower intestinal bleeding. Am J Gastroenterol. 2003;98(2):317–322.
11. Kovacs TOG, Jensen DM. Recent advances in the endoscopic diagnosis and therapy of upper gastrointestinal, small intestinal, and colonic bleeding. Med Clin North Am. 2002;86(6):1319–1356.
12. Gotzsche PC. Somatostatin analogues for acute bleeding oesophageal varices. Cochrane Database Syst Rev. 2005 Jan 25;(1):CD000193.
13. Nardone G. The efficacy of octreotide therapy in chronic bleeding due to vascular abnormalities of the gastrointestinal tract. Aliment Pharmacol Ther. 1999;13(11):1429–1436.
14. Guerrant RL, Van Gilder T, Steiner TS, et al; Infectious Diseases Society of America. Practice guidelines for the management of infectious diarrhea. Clin Infect Dis. 2001;32:331–351.
15. Thielman NM, Guerrant RL. Acute infectious diarrhea. N Engl J Med. 2004;350(1):38–47.
16. Bauer TM. Derivation and validation of guidelines for stool cultures for enteropathogenic bacteria other than *Clostridium difficile* in hospitalized adults. JAMA. 2001;285:313–319.
17. Bartlett JG. Antibiotic-associated diarrhea. N Engl J Med. 2002;346(5):334–339.
18. Schiller LR. Chronic diarrhea. Gastroenterology. 2004;127(1):287–293.
19. Fine KD, Schiller LR. AGA technical review on the evaluation and management of chronic diarrhea. Gastroenterology. 1999;116:1464–1486.
20. Kruszka PS. What is the differential diagnosis of chronic diarrhea in immunocompetent patients? J Fam Pract. 2002;51(3):212.
21. Longstreth GF. Definition and classification of irritable bowel syndrome: current consensus and controversies. Gastroenterol Clin. 2005;34(2):173–187.
22. Olden KW. Diagnosis of irritable bowel syndrome. Gastroenterology. 2002;122(6):1701–1714.

TABLE 27.2 Contraceptive Methods

Method	% Unintended Pregnancy During First Year of Use		Noncontraceptive Benefits	Common Side Effect/ Potential Complications	Cost to Patient (estimate)*
	Perfect Use	Typical Use			
No contraceptive use	85	85	N/A	N/A	N/A
Oral contraceptive	0.3	8	Protection against ovarian and endometrial cancer, benign breast tumors, ovarian cysts, dysmenorrhea and blood loss; reduces acne, suppression of endometriosis, treatment of menopause-related hot flashes	Amenorrhea, spotting and BTB, nausea, acne, breast pain/tenderness, increased vaginal discharge, melasma, decreased libido, VTE, hyperkalemia (only Yasmin®), increased risk of benign hepatic tumor, increased risk of MI and stroke	$35–$50/month (brand) $24–$30/ month (generic)
Progestin-only oral contraceptive	0.3	8	Protection against ovarian and endometrial cancer, compatible with breastfeeding; reduced risk of PID and VTE associated with estrogen-containing OC	Menstrual changes (unpredictable, frequent or absent bleeding) and amenorrhea; narrow margin of error for contraceptive efficacy (late or missed pills); some users continue to ovulate	$52/month
Patch (Ortho-Evra®)	0.3	8	Similar to OC	Local skin irritation at site of patch; other side effects are similar to OC Possible increased risk of VTE compared with OC; other complications are similar to OC	$42 for 24 patches
Vaginal ring (NuvaRing®)	0.3	8	Similar to OC	Decreased spotting and BTB compared with OC; increased risk of vaginal discomfort and discharge; other side effects and potential complications are similar to OC	$43/month
Injectable medroxy-progesterone acetate (Depo-Provera®)	0.3	3	Protection against ovarian and endometrial cancer; compatible with breastfeeding; reduced risk of PID and VTE associated with estrogen-containing OC	Menstrual changes and amenorrhea, weight gain, headaches, transient decrease in bone density, adverse effect on lipids, slow return of fertility (average 10 months)	$60 every 12 weeks
IUD Tcu380A (Paragard®) LNG-IUS (Mirena®)	0.6 0.1	0.8 0.1	Protection against endometrial cancer; decreased menstrual blood loss and pain	Menstrual cramping and increased or irregular bleeding†; rarely PID following insertion	Tcu380A: $270† LNG-IUS: $360†

(*continued*)

TABLE 27.2 Contraceptive Methods *(continued)*

Method	% Unintended Pregnancy During First Year of Use		Noncontraceptive Benefits	Common Side Effect/ Potential Complications	Cost to Patient (estimate)*
	Perfect Use	Typical Use			
Diaphragm with spermicide	6	16	Possible protection against some STI (gonorrhea, chlamydia, trichomonas); reduced risk of cervical cancer	Vaginal and urinary tract infections; increased risk for TSS, latex allergy, cervical irritation	$30–$50
	2 5	15 21	Protection against STI	Condom Male Female	$0.5–$1 each (male) $3 each (female)
Spermicide	18	29		Temporary skin or vaginal irritation due to allergy or sensitivity to the spermicide product Risk for recurrent UTI	Various‡ $9–$14
Sponge (Today® Sponge) Nulliparous woman Parous woman	9 20	16 32	Possible protection against some STI (gonorrhea, chlamydia, trichomonas)	Difficulty with removal; increased risk for vaginal and urinary tract infections; TSS	$2.50 each
Sterilization Female Male	0.5 0.10	0.5 0.15	Female: reduced risk of ovarian cancer; may protect against PID	Short-term: postsurgical pain and risk of infection	Female: $1400 male: $365–$450

BTB, breakthrough bleeding; PID, pelvic inflammatory disease; STI, sexually transmitted infections; TSS, toxic shock syndrome; UTI, urinary tract infection; VTE, venous thromboembolism.

*Cost estimates obtained at *http://www.drugstore.com*. For surgical methods and contraceptives provides at the prescriber's office, cost estimate were obtained from Planned Parenthood and a university gynecologic service in Michigan.

†Users of the Tcu390A typically have heavier menses, and irregular bleeding is common in the initial months of use. Women using the LNG-IUS typically have irregular, light bleeding or spotting during the initial months of use. After several months, about 20% of women using the LNG-IUS experience amenorrhea. Costs include insertion fee.

‡$13 per 17 g container (Delfen® Foam). $14 per 1108-g tube (Gynol II® jelly). $9 for 6 Ortho Options prefilled gel, $9 for 12 vaginal inserts (Encore®). (From Table 2 in RX Consultant – Contraceptives by Leslie A. Shimp. Volume XV, Number 4, April 2006 1-800-798-3353, Terry Baker, PharmD, editor.)

creased risk for ischemic stroke (9). It is recommend that women over age 35 who have migraine headaches (with or without auras or focal neurologic symptoms) not use OCs and women of any age with migraines with auras should not use OCs (9).

VTE is the most common cardiovascular risk associated with OCs. Among reproductive aged women, VTE occurs at a rate of 3–6 per 100,000 women (22). For users of low-dose OCs, the rate is increased three- to six-fold; comparatively, the risk of VTE during pregnancy is 48–60 per 100,000 (22, 29). Risk for VTE is highest during the first 2 years of OC use and smoking adds to this risk (15, 22) VTE risk is also greater in women, with inherited (genetic) conditions including factor V Leiden mutation, and Protein S or C synthesis disorders. The factor V Leiden mutation is present in about 5% of white women but only 2% or fewer of women of other races. Women who are heterozygous for the factor V Leiden mutation have a six to eight-fold increased risk for VTE; those who are homozygous have a ten-fold increase in VTE risk. The combination of the factor V Leiden mutation with OC use increases the risk of VTE to 120–150 per 100,000 per year (15).

The composition of the OC also alters risk for VTE (29, 30). Use of third-generation progestins (e.g., desogestrel) increases the risk of VTE (OR 1.7, 95% CI 1.4–2), but the additional risk associated with these OCs is small (1.5 per 10,000 women per year) (30).

The relationship between breast cancer and OC use is unclear. A recent well-designed case-control study found no increased risk of breast cancer with use of the OC for either current or former users (31). Even women with first-degree relatives who have been diagnosed with breast cancer do not routinely need to avoid OC use (32). In contrast, the International Agency for Research on Cancer (IARC) concluded that OCs are associated with a small increased risk of breast cancer for current and recent users and this increase was particularly noted in women <35 years of age who had begun use of oral contraceptives when < 20 years of age (33). Fortunately, the risk of cancer is quite low in young women and the excess risk for breast cancer with the typical pattern of use for the OC is likely very small. Among women at high risk for breast cancer because of BRCA1 genetic mutation, use of the OC for longer than 5 years, and use before age 30 years increased the risk of breast cancer (OR 1.33; CI 1.11–1.6 and OR 1.29; CI 1.09–1.52, respectively). Nonetheless, use of OC to prevent ovarian cancer, especially after age 30, is still widely supported (34).

Some data suggest that the OC increases risk for the development of cervical cancer (33). This risk appears to increase with increased duration of use but declines when OC use is discontinued. However, among women infected with the human papilloma virus (HPV), the main cause of cervical cancer, OC use was not associated with an increased risk of cervical cancer (33, 35).

Some women are not candidates for OC use. Contraindications to use of the OC are listed in Table 27.3 (36). Because thrombotic complications are the most common serious side effects, providers should refrain from providing OCs to women with current or past deep vein thromboses or pulmonary emboli, major surgery with immobilization, structural heart disease, diabetes mellitus with complications (presence of nephropathy, neuropathy, retinopathy) or if long-standing (>20 years), hypertension, or for women who are over 35 and heavy smokers.

Drug interactions

Drug interactions are common with OCs (Table 27.4). One controversial drug interaction is the theoretical decreased efficacy of OCs with concomitant use of common antibiotics (e.g., tetracycline, amoxicillin, erythromycin). The proposed mechanism for the interaction is antibiotic-induced reduction in enterohepatic recirculation of contraceptive hormones by alteration of intestinal bacteria. However, the reduction in serum levels of hormones is not clinically significant and levels remain within the therapeutic range for almost all women (15). In a study comparing the occurrence of pregnancy among OC users taking or not taking broad-spectrum antibiotics, there were more pregnancies among antibiotic users (1.6 pregnancies vs. 0.96 per 100 women-years) but the difference was not statistically significant and there was no greater overall failure rate of the OC (37). One well-respected clinician group believes that concurrent use of these antibiotics does not reduce the efficacy of the OCs and does not recommend use of back-up methods during antibiotic use (15). Given the small likeli-

TABLE 27.3 Contraindications to Oral Contraceptive Use

Contraindication	Potential Risk
Breastfeeding <6 weeks postpartum >6 weeks to <6 months postpartum*	Infant exposure to contraceptive steroids Decreased quantity of breast milk and shortened duration of lactation
Immediately postpartum (<21 days)	Thrombosis
Smoking plus age >35 years	CVD, especially MI
CVD (HTN†, CHD, stroke) or high-risk for CVD‡	CVD events such as MI, stroke, and peripheral arterial disease
Presence of DVT/PE or history of DVT/PE	Thrombosis
Major surgery with prolonged immobilization	Thrombosis
Thrombogenic mutations (e.g., Factor V Leiden)	Thrombosis
Migraine headache (with aura or age >35)	Stroke
Breast cancer	May worsen cancer prognosis
DM with end-stage organ involvement§, or with other vascular disease, or if >20 years' duration	CVD and thrombosis
Gall bladder disease	Worsening gall bladder disease
Liver disease (viral hepatitis, cirrhosis, tumor)	Increased adverse affects from OC, increased growth of liver tumors

CHD, coronary heart disease; CVD, cardiovascular disease; DM, diabetes mellitus; DVT, deep venous thrombosis; HTN, hypertension; MI, myocardial infarction; PE, pulmonary embolism.
*Other guidelines allow for use after 8 weeks in select circumstances.
†Women with controlled HTN are at less risk for CVD events than women with untreated HTN.
‡Multiple risk factors such as age, smoking, DM, HTN.
§Nephropathy, neuropathy, retinopathy.
(From Table 1 in–Shimp, LA. Contraceptives. RX Consultant. 2006 Apr;XV(4).

TABLE 27.4 Selected Clinically Significant Interactions with Oral Contraceptives*

These Drugs May Reduce the Efficacy of Oral Contraceptives:

Antibiotics[1] (i.e., penicillins, tetracyclines)	Aprepitant[2] Felbamate[2] Griseofulvin[2] Hydantoins (e.g., phenytoin, mephenytoin, ethofoin)[2] Modafinil[2] Nevirapine[2] Protease inhibitors[2] (nelfinavir, ritonavir, lopinavir, tipranavir) Rifamycins (e.g., rifampin)[2] St. John's wort[2]	Barbiturates[3] Carbamazepine[3] Primidone[3] Oxcarbazepine[3] Topiramate[3] Isotretinoin[4]

1. Reduced efficacy is unlikely, but contraceptive failure may be a possibility in a very small percentage of women. For women taking a 20–35 mcg OC who wish to avoid any possible increase in pregnancy risk, use of a BUM during antibiotic therapy or for 14 days (whichever is shorter) plus 7 days can be recommended.
2. Use an alternative contraceptive, or use an additional nonhormonal BUM during concurrent therapy. For aprepitant and modafinil, use a nonhormonal BUM and continue use for at least 1 month after stopping therapy.
3. Use an alternative contraceptive, or use a higher estrogen dose OC (titrate estrogen dose to avoid BTB) during concurrent therapy.
4. Use more than one method of contraception concurrently during the use of isotretinoin.

Oral contraceptives may increase the adverse effects and toxicity of these drugs:

Cyclosporine[5] Troleandomycin[5]	Alprazolam[6] (and perhaps other benzodiazepines) Prednisone[6], methylprednisolone[6] Selegriline[6] Theophylline[6] Tizanidine[6]

5. Avoid concurrent use.
6. Monitor for adverse effects and reduce the dose as needed.

Other interactions:
Lamotrigine[7]
Licorice (herbal)[8]
Red clover[9]
Caffeine[10]

7. Potential decreased effect of lamotrigine; adjust dose as needed.
8. Interaction is possible with herbal licorice (*Glycyrrhize glabra*). Potential for elevated blood pressure and fluid retention; monitor blood pressure and stop licorice use if blood pressure increases.
9. Possible loss of contraceptive efficacy or increased estrogen toxicity; avoid concurrent use.
10. May result in increased CNS stimulation; decrease caffeine intake if this occurs.

*Also presumed to occur with the progestin-only pill, contraceptive patch, and vaginal ring.
Management recommendations are indicated by the numbered footnote.
(From Table 3 in Shimp, LA. Contraceptives. RX Consultant. 2006 Apr;XV(4).

hood of this interaction, we recommend possible short-term use of a back-up contraceptive (during antibiotic therapy or for 14 days, whichever is shorter plus an additional 7 days) for a woman taking a 20–35 mcg EE OC who wants to avoid even a small increase in risk of pregnancy. Long-term use of a back-up method is not needed since intestinal flora become resistant to these antibiotics after about 2 weeks.

It is also important to note that some herbs, notably St. John's Wort, interact with the OC.

Key Points for Patient Education
- Women should be counseled about symptoms that may indicate serious health problems potentially associated with OCs. These can be remembered by the mnemonic ACHES: Abdominal pain (gallbladder or liver disease, blood clot), Chest pain (MI, PE), Headaches (stroke, hypertension, migraine), Eye problems (migraine, stroke or TIA, blood clot in the eye), and Severe leg pain (deep venous thrombosis [DVT]).
- Cessation of tobacco smoking should be strongly encouraged and may preclude use of the OC for women > 35 years. The World Heatlh Organization (WHO) suggests that for women >35 years who are light smokers, OCs should be used cautiously but are not contraindicated. For women >40 years, any tobacco use is a contraindication to OC use (15). Whereas the overall effect of oral contracep-

tives on mortality is neutral (rate ratio 0.89; 95% CI, 0.77–1.02), the mortality risk ratio for OC users who smoked 1–14 cigarettes per day was 1.24 (95% CI, 1.03–1.49), and for women smoking 15 or more cigarettes per day was 2.14 (95% CI, 1.81–2.53). This increase in mortality was apparent by age 35–44 years (39).

- Tobacco smoking or use of nicotine-containing products to aid in discontinuing tobacco smoking adversely affects the production of estrogen and increases the metabolism of hormones so use of lower estrogen dose OCs (i.e., 20-mcg pills) may not provide adequate contraceptive efficacy. Increasing the dose of estrogen to offset this effect may increase the risk for adverse effects (e.g., venous thromboembolism) that are primarily the result of hepatic exposure rather than systemic exposure (40).
- In beginning use of the OC, the following methods can be used:
  - Immediate Use—the OC can be started at any time after a negative pregnancy test. If the OC is started mid-cycle vs. during days 1–7 (the first week) of the cycle then a back-up method of contraception should be used for 7 days.
  - First-day start—the OC can be started on the first day of menses. When the OC is begun within the first 5 days after a period begins, contraceptive protection begins immediately and use of a back-up method is not necessary.
  - Sunday start—with this approach, the first OC tablet is taken on the first Sunday following the beginning of menses. A back-up method of contraception should be used for the first 7 days the OC is taken when beginning the OC with a Sunday start.
- Information in Table 27.5 (15) below can be used to manage missed pills.

NON-ORAL COMBINED HORMONE CONTRACEPTIVES

Although the OC is a very effective contraceptive, it does require daily ingestion of the tablet and 47% of users miss one or more pills per month (7). Two newer hormonal contraceptive products, OrthoEvra patch and Nuvaring, were de-signed to avoid the need for daily patient action while maintaining a contraceptive efficacy similar to that of the OC.

Transdermal Patch (Ortho-Evra)

Ortho Evra is a thin transdermal patch that contains EE (20 mcg is released every 24 hours) and norelgestromin (an active metabolite of the norgestimate; 150 mcg released daily). As with the OC, inhibition of ovulation is the primary mechanism of action of the contraceptive patch.

The patch is believed to have similar drug interactions, health benefits, and health risks as the OC (15). However, the FDA recently required the addition of a warning to the labeling for the contraceptive patch due to the possibility of adverse effects from higher estrogen levels. Hormone levels in the body differ between the patch and the OC (41). Unlike the OC, hormones from the patch reach the bloodstream without passing through the liver and thus reach higher levels. Furthermore, in a woman taking the OC, estrogen blood levels are increased for only a portion of the day, particularly 1–2 hours after taking the OC. In contrast, women using the patch are exposed to higher levels continually and these levels may be high enough in some women to increase the risk of blood clotting. A woman using the patch may be exposed to approximately 60% more estrogen than if she were taking a 35-mcg OC. The FDA statement says that it is unknown if a higher risk exist for users of the patch compared to women taking an OC. However, the Associated Press reported that users of the patch die or develop blood clots at a rate 3 times higher than women taking an OC (42). Once the patch is removed hormone levels decrease and are essentially absent after 3 days.

Each patch is used for one week. Patch detachment is uncommon (2%–3% of users). Adequate levels of the hormones to produce a contraceptive effect are achieved about 48 hours after placement of the patch. Efficacy of the patch is shown in Table 27.2. Patches may be less effective for women who weigh more than 198 pounds.

Key Points for Patient Education with Use of the Contraceptive Patch:

- The patch should be applied once a week for 3 weeks; then there is a patch-free week.

TABLE 27.5 Management of Missed Oral Contraceptive Pills

Number of Pills Missed	Week Pills Missed	OC Recommendation	Finish This Pill Pack?	Use of Emergency Contraceptive	Use of 7-Day Back-up Method
1	1	Take 2 pills ASAP	Yes	Yes	Yes
1	2–3	Take 2 pills ASAP	Yes	No	No
1	4	Skip placebo pills	Yes	No	No
2–4	1	Take 2 pills ASAP	Yes	Yes*	Yes
2–4	2	Take 2 pills ASAP	Yes	No	No
2–4	3	Start new pack	N/A	No	No
2–4	4	Skip placebo pills	Yes	No	No
5	Any	Take 2 pills ASAP; start new pack	N/A	Yes*	Yes

* Start emergency contraceptive as soon as possible. No need to double up on pills. Take the next pill on the next day.
From Hatcher RA, Trussell J, Stewart FH, et al. eds. Contraceptive Technology,18th ed. New York, NY: Ardent Media, Inc.; 2004.

- The patch should be applied and changed on the same day each week.
- The patch should be applied to clean dry skin. No lotions or sunscreen should be on the area of skin where the patch is applied. Also, the patch should not be applied to sweaty skin.
- The patch can be applied to the upper outer arms, abdomen, buttocks, or the torso (except for breasts).
- When a patch is removed the next patch should be applied to a different area of the body.
- If a patch becomes detached, it can be firmly pressed back on. If the patch will not stick, it should be removed and another patch should be applied immediately.
- If patch use is begun on the first day of menses, use of a back-up method of contraception will not be necessary. If use of the patch is begun on the first Sunday after menses begins then a back-up method of contraception should be used for the first 7 days of patch use.
- Women switching from the OC to the patch should apply the first patch no later than 5 days after their last active OC tablet. If the patch is applied within this timeframe, use of a back-up method of contraception will not be necessary. However, if the patch is applied the Sunday after the last tablet of the OC pill pack, then a back-up method of contraception should be used for the first 7 days of patch use. Women switching from use of DMPA to the patch should apply the first patch on the day their next injection of DMPA would be given.
- If the patch is missed or applied late, follow the directions in Table 27.6.
- A used patch should be folded to limit leakage of the hormones and should be discarded into the trash (not flushed).

Vaginal Ring (NuvaRing)

NuvaRing is a soft, flexible and transparent ring that releases EE (15 mcg/day) and etonorgestrel (active metabolite of desogestrel; 120 mcg/day). The efficacy, drug interactions, side effects, and risks/benefits of this device are thought to be similar to the OC (15). However, it may also be associated with local side effects such as vaginitis or vaginal discharge (5% of users) or vaginal discomfort (2.4%).

The ring is inserted high in the vagina (exact position is not important) and left in place for 21 days. At the end of 21 days, it is removed and discarded. After 1 week, a new ring is inserted.

Contraceptive action begins the first day of use. Expulsion of the device is uncommon but, if it occurs, the woman should rinse the device with cool or warm water and reinsert it as soon as possible, within 3 hours.

Key Points for Patient Education with Use of the Vaginal Contraceptive Ring

- The vaginal ring should be kept refrigerated until use.
- The vaginal contraceptive ring should be compressed and inserted into the vagina. The ring should be placed high in the vagina but exact placement is not necessary. One ring is left in the vagina for 3 weeks. It is *not* removed for sexual intercourse.
- Use of a back-up method of contraception is necessary for the first 7 days the ring is inserted unless a woman has switched from another hormonal method of contraception (i.e., OC, progestin-only pill [POP], DMPA, or levonorgestrel intrauterine system [LNG-IUS]) to use of the vaginal ring. If another hormonal contraceptive has been used the previous month, a woman should insert the ring as follows:
  - Prior OC–insert the vaginal ring on the day a new pill pack would be started
  - Prior POP–insert the vaginal ring on the day she takes the last progestin-only pill
  - Prior DMPA–insert the vaginal ring on the day she is due for her next injection

TABLE 27.6 Management of Missed or Late Transdermal Contraceptive Patch

When Patch Missed	Management
1st week patch	• If a patch is forgotten or late the first week, give emergency contraception if the woman has had unprotected intercourse. • Tell her to place the patch immediately • She should use a back-up method for 7 days • The woman will change her patch each week on the day of the week she started this new patch from now on.
2nd or 3rd week patch	• *1–2 days late*: the woman must remove the old patch and place a new one immediately. No back-up method or emergency contraception is needed. • *More than 2 days late*: Have her remove the old patch and place a new one immediately. Provide emergency contraception if she has had unprotected intercourse (especially if she is 4 days or more late applying her patch). She should use back-up method for 7 days. Tell her to change the patch each week on the day of the week that she placed this new patch.
4th week patch	• Tell her to remove the patch. • She should place a new one on the usual day. • No back-up method or emergency contraception is needed.

From Hatcher RA, Trussell J, Stewart FH, et al. eds. Contraceptive Technology, 18th ed. New York, NY: Ardent Media, Inc.; 2004.

- Prior LNG-IUS–insert the vaginal ring on the day the IUD is removed
- At the end of 3 weeks, the vaginal ring is removed and there is a ring-free week. Menses will occur during this week.
- The vaginal ring should be discarded in the trash (not flushed).
- The next vaginal ring should be inserted on the same day of the week as the previous ring was inserted even if menses are continuing.
- If expulsion of the vaginal ring occurs, the device should be rinsed in cool or warm water and re-inserted as soon as possible but within 3 hours. Use of a back-up method of contraception will be necessary for 7 days if the ring is out of the vagina for more than 3 hours.
- Tampons, vaginal antifungals, and vaginal spermicides can all be used when the vaginal ring is in the vagina.

PROGESTIN-ONLY CONTRACEPTIVES

Description

There are two progestin-only contraceptives: the progestin-only pill (POP), also known as the minipill, and DMPA (intramuscular medroxyprogesterone acetate; Depo-Provera and DMPA-SC 104, subcutaneous medroxyprogesterone acetate; Depo-subQ Provera 104) (43). DMPA-SC 104 is a low-dose formulation of DMPA that is similar in onset of action, efficacy, and safety to DMPA-IM (44). The slower rate of absorption of the subcutaneous formulation allows for the lower dose of DMPA while still providing concentrations that suppress ovulation over a 3-month interval (44).

Both the POP and DMPA have the advantage of eliminating exposure to estrogen. This makes these contraceptive methods particularly useful for women who have contraindications to the use of estrogen. These methods are also more suitable for women who want to breastfeed as they do not impair lactation.

DMPA-IM is currently used by about 2 million U.S. women and more than 20% of U.S. teens who have been sexually active report current or former use of DMPA (45).

Norplant, an implanted contraceptive, is no longer available. However, a single-rod implanted device, Implanon, is available in Europe and may be introduced into the United States.

Mechanism of Action

As with the OCs, the progestin-only contraceptives act by causing thickening of the cervical mucus blocking sperm from entering the uterus. They also inhibit capacitation (ability of sperm to fertilize the egg), interfere with transport of the egg and sperm, and create an inhospitable endometrium for implantation and may inhibit ovulation.

The POP is a tablet that is taken daily with no interruptions. The POP may also suppress ovulation but it does so inconsistently for most women. Because the thickened cervical mucus is critical to its efficacy, the POP must be taken the same time every day as this effect is lost if the pill is taken 3 or more hours later than its usual administration time.

DMPA is a long-acting contraceptive administered via intramuscular or subcutaneous injection every 3 months. In contrast to the POP, its primary contraceptive action is to inhibit ovulation. Both formulations of DMPA are very effective contraceptives (Table 27.2). For example, DMPA is a useful contraceptive for women taking Accutane® due to its efficacy. DMPA is also associated with a slow return of fertility–on average it takes 10 months after the last injection before a woman can become pregnant.

Efficacy

Efficacy of these contraceptives is shown in Table 27.2. The POP contains a very low progestin dose and is slightly less effective than the OC (43). The POP does not suppress ovulation in all users and the maintenance of thickening of cervical mucus is dependent upon consistent dosing at the same time daily. If the POP is taken 3 hours or more past the usual administration time, use of a back-up method is advised for 48 hours to reestablish thickened cervical mucus. In contrast, DMPA is a high progestin dose contraceptive that is very effective. In 18,681 women-cycles of exposure there were no pregnancies in women using DMPA-SC 104. A substantial number of women in this study were overweight or obese; efficacy of DMPA-SC 104 was not lessened among women with higher body mass index (BMI) (44).

Benefits

Progestin-only contraceptives decrease the risk of endometrial and ovarian cancer and, due to the thickened cervical mucus, they also decrease the risk for pelvic inflammatory disease.

Side Effects and Contraindications

Menstrual irregularity is a common occurrence with the POP and contributes to patient dissatisfaction and discontinuation. Irregular bleeding is more common with the POP than with the OCs (19). In addition, amenorrhea is common among women taking the POP consistently (43).

DMPA has two side effects that can decrease patient satisfaction. First, menstrual cycle disturbances are common and are a frequent reason for discontinuation. After more than a year of use, most users of both formulations of DMPA experience amenorrhea. Some women find this disconcerting while others appreciate this effect. Secondly, weight gain is an expected effect of this contraceptive. Weight gain is likely due to an increase in appetite and can be significant. On average, weight gain can be almost 15 pounds over 4 years of use.

The effect of DMPA on bone mineral density (BMD) has long been a concern about this contraceptive method, particularly when used by adolescents who have not reached peak BMD. In November 2004, the FDA required a black box warning be added to Depo-Provera's labeling regarding this effect (45). The warning states that prolonged use of DMPA may result in significant bone loss and the loss is greater the longer DMPA is used. Further, the bone loss may not be completely reversible and a woman should only used DMPA as a long-term contraceptive method (longer than 2 years) if other methods are inadequate for her. Studies in both adolescent and adult women have demonstrated a loss in BMD among users of DMPA (46, 47), although not all studies have found a decrease in BMD (48). Studies have also found that BMD increases when DMPA is discontinued (46). Despite evidence of BMD loss, cross-sectional data from the WHO, New Zealand, and a U.S. longitudinal study all demonstrated that BMD among former DMPA users was comparable to that of women who had never used DMPA (45).

The reduction in BMD is likely the result of the decrease in ovarian production of estrogen secondary to DMPA. The transient effect of DMPA on BMD has been likened to the effect of lactation on BMD. Lactation causes a 4% loss in BMD over 6 months (a greater decline in BMD than reported for DMPA) but when lactation ceases BMD recovers. Further, among former lactating women, BMD is often higher than in women who had not breastfed their infants. Similarly, one study of teens found that former users of DMPA had higher BMD than teens who had never used DMPA (45).

Some clinicians feel that the black box warning for DMPA is inappropriate and caution that limitations to the use of this very effective contraceptive may lead to an increase in unintended pregnancies and abortions when long-term skeletal health does not appear to be jeopardized among DPMA users (45).

Contraindications for the progestin-only contraceptives include breastfeeding during the first 6 weeks postpartum, multiple risk factors for or presence of arterial cardiovascular disease (e.g., age, smoking, hypertension, ischemic heart disease), current deep vein thrombosis/pulmonary embolism (DVT/PE), migraine headaches with focal neurologic symptoms, diabetes mellitus with complications (presence of nephropathy, neuropathy, retinopathy) or if long-standing (>20 years), liver disease (i.e., active viral hepatitis, severe cirrhosis, benign or malignant tumors), or use of medications that affect liver enzymes (e.g., rifampicin, some anticonvulsants) (36).

Drug Interactions

While the POP is susceptible to drug interactions that impair its effectiveness, DMPA has essentially no drug interactions. Medications known to interact with the POP include barbiturates, hydantions, non-nucleotide reverse transcriptase (NNRT) inhibitors, lamotrigine, and rifamycins. In addition, it would be prudent to consider the potential drug interactions listed in Table 27.4 as potential interactions for the POP because progestins provide the major contraceptive action for the OCs.

Key Points for Patient Education

Women considering the POP should be counseled about their potential effect on menstruation, as they are a leading reason for discontinuation. DMPA users should be counseled about possible weight gain and negative effects on BMD.

The use of progestin-only contraceptive methods is compatible with breastfeeding. Patients should not begin their use sooner than 6 weeks postpartum to avoid early postpartum exposure of the infant to hormones due to the neonate's limited ability to metabolize and excrete drugs and the potential for adverse effects of exogenous hormones on developing organs (49). These contraceptives do not decrease milk volume nor do they have adverse effects on child growth or development (49).

Progestin-Only Pills.

- POPs are taken everyday with no breaks (there is no pill-free week monthly). A tablet should be taken every day until the pill pack is empty, the first tablet from the next pill pack will be taken beginning the next day.
- It is important that the POP be taken at the same time every

day as the contraceptive effectiveness depends on keeping cervical mucus thick.
- A back-up method of contraception is generally recommended for the first 7–28 days of use of the POP.
- If the POP is taken 3 or more hours later than usual, a back-up method of contraception should be used for 48 hours to allow cervical mucus to thicken and create a contraceptive action.
- Missed pills: If *one* POP is missed, take the missed pill as soon as it is remembered or take two tablets at the same time. If the pill is taken more than 3 hours after the usual time use a back-up method of contraception for 48 hours. If two or more POP are missed in a row, use a back-up method of contraception and take two tablets 2 days in a row. If unprotected sexual intercourse has occurred, consider use of the emergency contraceptive.
- It is common for women taking the POP to experience menstrual irregularity including absence of menses (amenorrhea).
- A woman should be instructed to see her physician if she experiences severe lower abdominal pain while taking the POP; this may be caused by an ectopic pregnancy or an ovarian cyst.

DMPA.

- This contraceptive is administered by intramuscular or subcutaneous injection every 11–13 weeks. DMPA-IM is injected into the deltoid or gluteus muscles. DMPA-SQ 104 is injected into subcutaneous fat in the upper thigh or abdomen. DMPA-SC 104 can be self-administered by women, decreasing the need for quarterly clinic visits.
- A back-up method of contraception needs to be used for 1 week after the first injection of DMPA-IM. No back-up method is required for DMPA-SC 104 if the initial injection occurs within the first 5 days of menses (44).
- It is common for women using DMPA to experience menstrual irregularity including unpredictable bleeding, frequent bleeding or absence of bleeding (amenorrhea). About half of women using DMPA will stop having any bleeding after 1 year of use and eventually almost all users stop bleeding. This is not harmful.
- It is common for users of both formulations of DMPA to gain weight. A woman may have an increase in appetite from DMPA. Weight gain with the IM formulation is typically 5 pounds during the first year up to 14 pounds after 4 years of use. Women using DMPA should try to consume a healthy diet and engage in weight-bearing exercise to help maintain a healthy weight.
- During the time DMPA is used, bone density may decrease. To counter this effect, an adequate amount of calcium (usually 1,000 mg per day) should be obtained from the diet or through use of calcium supplements. Weight-bearing exercise also helps to increase bone density and strengthen bone.
- When DMPA is discontinued, it takes a number of months for regular menstrual cycles to return. In addition, women typically cannot get pregnant for about 10 months after their last injection. However, by 12 months after the last injection of both formulations of DMPA about 95% users had a resumption of ovulation.
- If a woman is late for her DMPA injection, she should begin use of a back-up method of contraception immediately. If

she had unprotected sexual intercourse (previous injection 13–14 or more weeks before), she should consider use of the emergency contraceptive.

- A woman should be instructed to see her physician if she experiences severe lower abdominal pain while using DMPA. This may be caused by an ectopic pregnancy. She should also contact her physician if she experiences severe headaches, depression, heavy bleeding or signs of infection (e.g., pus) at the injection site.

HORMONAL EMERGENCY CONTRACEPTIVES

Description

Emergency contraceptives (EC) are methods that can be used after intercourse to prevent pregnancy. The risk for an unintended pregnancy is often apparent such as when contraceptives are forgotten or fail and unprotected sexual intercourse occurs. In these cases, use of EC offers the opportunity to avoid an unintended pregnancy. There are two types of oral EC: the levonorgestrel product Plan B and use of OCs containing EE plus either levonorgestrel or norgestrel (6). In 2006 the FDA approved making Plan B available as a nonprescription product for women 18 years of age and older. Women age 17 years and younger will require a prescription for Plan B. A consumer must obtain the nonprescription Plan B from a pharmacist and must show personal identification showing proof of age.

Mechanism of Action

The primary contraceptive action of the EC is prevention or delay of ovulation or fertilization. Although these regimens have the potential to cause changes in the endometrium, reducing the likelihood of implantation, recent research suggests that this is not likely. Post-ovulatory events (i.e., inhibition of implantation) appear to play little, if any, role in its action (50). Nonetheless, to make an informed choice, it is important for women to know that the EC, like other hormonal contraceptives, has the potential to inhibit implantation of a fertilized egg (6). These agents are not, however, abortifacients as they prevent pregnancy before implantation occurs and they do not disrupt an already established pregnancy. Furthermore, there are no known adverse effects to the fetus from inadvertent exposure to EC during early pregnancy. The EC is also regarded as safe for use in breastfeeding woman after 6 weeks postpartum as the progestin-only contraceptives are regarded as safe for use in these women (6).

Efficacy

The effectiveness of the EC is highly dependent on timing (Figure 27.1). Use of Plan B within 72 hours of unprotected intercourse can reduce the likelihood of pregnancy by 89%. The use of OCs in the Yuzpe regimen has been shown to decrease the likelihood of pregnancy by 75%.

Side Effects and Contraindications

It is common for users of EC to experience nausea and vomiting. About 50% of users of the Yuzpe regimen experience nausea and 20% experience vomiting. Users of Plan B experience only half as much nausea and vomiting. Use of an antiemetic prior to taking the EC may reduce the associated nausea and vomiting. There are no evidence-based medical

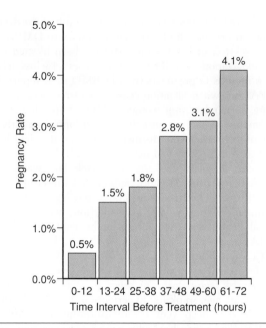

Figure 27.1. • Impact of delay in treatment of ECP effectiveness. (From Figure 12.10 in Hatcher RA, Trussell J, Stewart FH, et al. eds. Contraceptive Technology, 18th ed. New York, NY: Ardent Media, Inc.; 2004:287. Used with permission.)

contraindications to use of the EC (6); however, undiagnosed vaginal bleeding is listed as a contraindication in the prescribing information for Plan B (51).

Drug Interactions

Information about drug interactions with the EC is very limited. The Plan B package insert indicates that interactions with common broad-spectrum antibiotics do not occur. It is unclear if other agents, such as phenytoin or rifampin, which interact with the OCs and POPs will interfere with the effectiveness of the EC (51).

Patient Education

Plan B contains two 750 mcg (0.75 mg) doses of levonorgestrel. The traditional regimen is to take one tablet as soon as possible and to take the second tablet 12 hours later. However, it has been shown that taking both tablets at once (a single 1.5-mg dose) has the same efficacy and no greater side effects than the two-dose regimen (6).

The second form of EC is called the Yuzpe regimen. This regimen uses OCs containing EE plus either levonorgestrel or norgestrel. Norgestrel contains two isomers but only the levonorgestrel is bioactive. Therefore, the dose required of norgestrel is twice that of levonorgestrel. The regimen is two doses of pills taken 12 hours apart over one day of treatment. Each dose contains ≥100 mcg of EE and either ≥1 mg of norgestrel or ≥0.5 mg of levonorgestrel. (Total hormone doses are 200 mcg of EE and either 2 mg of norgestrel or 1 mg of levonorgestrel.) For example, if a prescriber used Alesse (20 mcg EE plus 0.1 mg levonorgestrel), the patient would be instructed to take five tablets for each of the two doses. Using LoOvral, a norgestrel product (30 mcg EE plus 0.3 mg norgestrel), the patient would be instructed to take four tablets for each of the two doses.

Because the EC can delay ovulation, a woman may be at risk of pregnancy following use of the EC. Regular contraception should be initiated or continued after EC use. Also, the EC is less effective at pregnancy prevention than consistent use of other contraceptives. We recommend that providers consider offering EC prescriptions to women at the time of receipt of other forms of contraception.

Key Points for Patient Education
- Take one tablet of Plan B as soon as possible after unprotected sexual intercourse and take the second tablet 12 hours later. Another option is to take both tablets at the same time, as soon as possible after unprotected sexual intercourse. These two ways of taking Plan B are equally effective.
- If an oral contraceptive is used as an emergency contraceptive, the number of tablets per dose will be determined by the amount of hormones in the tablet (your health provider or pharmacist will have to tell you how many tablets to take). Take one dose of the required number of tablets as soon as possible after unprotected sexual intercourse and take the second dose of tablets 12 hours after the first dose. When using an oral contraceptive as an emergency contraceptive, use of two doses is necessary.
- Use of the emergency contraceptive can delay ovulation,therefore the risk/likelihood of pregnancy may be greater than usual just after use of the emergency contraceptive. It is important that a regular method of contraception be started immediately after use of the emergency contraceptive to provide contraceptive action for future acts of sexual intercourse.
- Regular methods of contraception are more effective than the emergency contraceptive at preventing pregnancy. The emergency contraceptive should not be used as a regular contraceptive.
- Common side effects of Plan B and the oral contraceptive when used in doses for emergency contraception include nausea and vomiting. If vomiting occurs within 1 to 2 hours of the dose, the dose should be repeated as soon as possible. Use of a medication to prevent nausea and vomiting such as dimenhydrinate (Dramamine®) or meclizine hydrochloride (Bonine®) should be considered, especially if taking an oral contraceptive as an emergency contraceptive. The anti-nausea medication should be taken one hour prior to the emergency contraceptive.
- Use of an emergency contraceptive may cause a delay in the time of menses; usually this is one week or less. If menses are delayed over 1 week past the usual time or do not occur within 3 weeks after use of the emergency contraceptive, a pregnancy test is advisable.

Intrauterine Device (IUD)
DESCRIPTION
There are two types of IUDs available in the United States: the Copper T-380A (TCu380A; Paragard) and the LNG-IUS (Mirena) (52). Both of these IUDs provide very effective and long-acting but reversible contraceptive action (Table 27.2); the TCU-380A has a 10-year duration of use while the LNG-IUS provides 5 years of use.

MECHANISM OF ACTION
The IUDs contraceptive action is to prevent fertilization of the egg. The TCu380A alters tubal and uterine fluids thus impairing sperm function and preventing fertilization. The LNG-IUS initially releases 20 mcg of levonorgestrel daily which decreases to 10 mcg daily over time. This dose of levonorgestrel is about 10% of that contained in an OC with 150 mcg of levonorgestrel (52). The LNG-IUS has several contraceptive actions including thickening of cervical mucus, inhibiting sperm capacitation and survival, and suppression of the endometrium; in some women it also inhibits ovulation. Importantly, in contrast to common erroneous (consumer) information, IUDs are not abortifacients. In fact, studies have found no fertilized eggs in women using the IUD (52).

EFFICACY
Both IUDs are highly effective with similar, very low failure rates (Table 27.2).

INSERTION
For detailed instruction on placing an IUD, readers can find information in *Contraceptive Technology* (52). Providers are also encouraged to read and follow the manufacturer's instructions on insertion. Prior to insertion and after a discussion of safety and effectiveness, explain the insertion procedure to the patient. Consider administration of an oral analgesic agent at least 30 to 60 minutes before the procedure to minimize pain. The IUD should be inserted slowly and gently.

IUDs may be placed at any time during the menstrual cycle as well as immediately following childbirth (within 10 minutes of expulsion of the placenta) and immediately after or up to 3 weeks after a first trimester abortion. Insertion during menses, at 1–2 days after childbirth, and after a second trimester abortion is associated with higher expulsion rates (52). The traditional reason to insert the IUD during menses was to increase certainty that the woman was not pregnant and to take advantage of the dilation of the cervical os (although the cervical os is equally dilated during midcycle). IUDs can be inserted at any time provided a woman has been using a contraceptive method and is reasonably certain that she is not pregnant or she has not had intercourse since her last normal menses. The IUD may also be inserted 4 weeks to 6 weeks postpartum in a woman who is breastfeeding and has had no menses. The copper IUD may also be used as an emergency contraceptive within 7 days of unprotected intercourse.

There is no consensus on the need for prophylactic antibiotics to prevent infection. There is little risk of infection following correct insertion of an IUD in an otherwise healthy woman and prophylactic antibiotics are generally not needed; ACOG notes that in women who test negative for gonorrhea and chlamydia, prophylactic antibiotics appear to provide no benefit (Strength of Recommendation, SOR = A) (53).

Following the procedure, the woman should be given the IUD user identification card (provided in the IUD packet) including the name of the IUD, date of insertion (completed by the provider), and date of recommended removal. The woman should also be instructed in checking for the IUD string to verify retention.

BENEFITS

IUDs have several contraceptive benefits: high efficacy, no need for contraceptive action once inserted, good safety record, very cost-effective method of contraception, and fertility returns immediately after removal of the IUD. IUDs are an especially good choice for women who cannot use OCs for medical reasons and for women who want long-term contraception but are not candidates for sterilization.

SIDE EFFECTS AND CONTRAINDICATIONS

Both IUDs may cause changes in uterine bleeding, although they differ with regard to their effect. A common adverse effect of the TCu380A is heavy menses and irregular bleeding which are common during the initial 3–6 months of use (19). In contrast, the LNG-IUS tends to cause irregular light bleeding which ceases after several months due to suppression of the endometrium. About 20% of LNG-IUS users develop amenorrhea after a year of use.

With the LNG-IUS a small amount of levonorgestrel may be absorbed and cause systemic side effects (e.g., oily skin, increased appetite — these are general progestin side effects). However, the amount absorbed approximates about 5% of the dose in an OC containing 150 mcg of levonorgestrel and is less than that of a POP (52).

Contraindications for both IUDs include current cervical, endometrial, or ovarian cancer; anatomical abnormalities or fibroids that distort the uterus; current or recent pelvic inflammatory disease (PID)/pelvic infection or sexually transmitted infections (STI) or increased risk of STI/HIV (e.g., multiple partners or partner with multiple partners); AIDS; unexplained vaginal bleeding; and serious liver disease (active viral hepatitis, severe cirrhosis, liver tumors) (36). It is recommended that neither IUD be inserted prior to 4 weeks postpartum. Additional contraindications to use of the LNG-IUS are current DVT/PE, ischemic heart disease, migraines with aura (any age patient), and breast cancer.

New data have shown that two conditions previously linked to IUD use, PID (salpingitis) and tubal infertility, are actually not increased by IUD use. IUDs themselves do not increase the risk of PID, but the insertion process can increase risk for PID. One study found that salpingitis occurred in only about 1 in 1,000 women who had an IUD inserted (52). In addition, the IUD is not contraindicated as a contraceptive method for women with heart valve abnormalities because IUD insertion is not associated with bacteremia.

KEY POINTS FOR PATIENT EDUCATION

Expulsion of the IUDs are uncommon (2%–10% of women) but expulsion is more likely among women who have never been pregnant or who have never carried a pregnancy to term and women with severe dysmenorrhea (52). Patients should be informed that IUDs do not migrate after insertion, although uterine perforation is possible at time of insertion. Women should be instructed to periodically check for the IUD string, particularly over the first few months of use.

A follow-up visit should be planned at about 3–6 weeks following insertion to verify that the IUD is still in place, no infection has occurred, and to address any questions or concerns.

- IUDs are a long-acting very effective method of contraception; the LNG-IUS can be used for 5 years and the Copper T 380A is used for up to 10 years.
- Although the initial cost of an IUD can be expensive, over time the IUD can be very inexpensive.
- Menstrual bleeding patterns are likely to change with IUD use. Users of the Copper T 380A will likely experience an increase in menstrual blood loss. In contrast, users of the LNG-IUS will notice a significant decrease in menstrual bleeding and about 20% of women will experience amenorrhea (52). In addition, during the first few months of IUD use, irregular bleeding is common.
- Cramping and discomfort are common for about 15 minutes after IUD insertion. If cramping continues or is severe, uterine perforation should be considered.
- Expulsion of the IUD occurs in a small number of women. A woman should be told to contact her prescriber if she cannot feel the strings of the IUD, the strings feel long or if she can feel the IUD near the cervix.
- Cramping, pelvic pain, purulent discharge, and/or fever occurring within the first 3 weeks after insertion may indicate uterine infection. The IUD should be removed and the patient treated with appropriate medications.

Barrier Methods

Barrier methods include the diaphragm, cervical cap, contraceptive sponge, and condoms (male and female). The contraceptive action of these methods is achieved by physical and/or chemical (spermicide) barriers to passage of sperm into the uterus and upper reproductive tract. Barrier methods have a higher failure rate than hormonal contraceptives or IUDs. Correct usage is particularly critical to the efficacy of these methods.

DIAPHRAGM AND CERVICAL CAP

Description
The diaphragm and cervical cap (Prentif Cavity-Cervical Cap) are dome-shaped (rim) reusable barrier contraceptives made of latex.

Mechanism of action
Both of these devices act as a physical barrier, covering the cervix, and the spermicide provides a chemical barrier. The diaphragm is inserted so the dome covers the cervix; the cervical cap fits snugly over the cervix to form a seal. Both are used in combination with a spermicide. Spermicide is applied to the diaphragm so that the cup holding the spermicide faces the cervix. One to three teaspoonfuls of spermicide is spread throughout the cup and some additional spermicide is spread around the rim. With the cervical cap, spermicide is applied until it fills about one-third of the cup of the cap. Jelly/gel spermicides are preferred as they adhere best to these contraceptives and are not as easily diluted by cervical secretions.

Efficacy
The most important factor in effectiveness is correct and consistent use. Parity also effects the efficacy for the cervical cap; parous women have almost 3 times the failure rate with perfect use compared to nulliparous women (26% vs. 9%) (54). In contrast, pregnancy rates are similar for parous and nulliparous women who use the diaphragm (Table 27.2).

Fitting and insertion

There are three basic types of diaphragms: arcing, coil, and flat spring. Most providers use the arcing rim style in sizes 60 to 80 mm. An estimate of the correct size is obtained by measuring the distance along the examiner's index finger from the posterior vaginal wall to about 1 cm before the inside of the pubic arch. This distance should correspond to the diameter of the device.

The diaphragm is inserted by pinching the sides together and gently inserting it into the vagina with a small amount of lubricant on the leading edge. Once inserted, it should cover the cervix and fit snugly but comfortably in place with the rim in contact with the posterior and lateral vaginal walls and the anterior edge about one fingerbreadth before the public arch. It should be easily removable by hooking the anterior rim with the index finger and gently pulling the device out of the vagina. The woman (or her partner) should be encouraged to practice insertion and removal in the office, after the fitting, until comfortable with the procedure.

Cervical caps are available in limited sizes (only four) and therefore not all women can be fitted with this device; about 6%–10% of women cannot be fitted (55). The cap is inserted in the same manner by patients and providers by first folding the rim and compressing the dome so that when it is placed over the cervix, the expanding dome creates suction. The cap is then placed over the cervix fitting snugly against the cervix at the fornices, 360 degrees around the rim, so that no gaps are detected. The cap should not become dislodged with gentle attempts of pushing forward or downward with the examining fingers. Once in place, the anterior rim of the cap should be covered by the anterior wall of the vagina and should be as deep as possible from the introitus to avoid dislodgement by the penis. The cap is removed by probing with the index finger, tipping the cap to break the seal, and gently removing.

The diaphragm can be inserted up to 6 hours before intercourse and must remain in place for at least 6 hours afterward but should be removed within 24 hours. If there is more than one act of intercourse, additional spermicide (foam will disperse better) should be inserted into the vagina but the diaphragm should be left in place. The cervical cap provides contraceptive actions for up to 48 hours and additional spermicide is not required if multiple acts of intercourse occur within this period of time. The cap should be inserted about 30 minutes before intercourse (to improve suction) and must remain in place for at least 6 hours after the last act of intercourse. Additional spermicide should be inserted vaginally if intercourse does not occur soon after insertion.

Benefits

The diaphragm and cervical caps may potentially offer some protection of the cervix from exposure to bacteria and viruses, including STIs. There are no data from trials about this potential benefit. However, several studies have found a decreased risk for cervical dysplasia and cancer among women using the diaphragm which was postulated to be due to the cervical protection from HPV (55). The diaphragm is an easily reversible form of contraception, is relatively inexpensive, may permit greater sexual spontaneity, and requires only one visit annually to a healthcare provider (56).

Side Effects and Contraindications

The most common adverse effect of the diaphragm is colonization of the vagina with *Escherichia coli*. This may place a woman at increased risk for bacterial vaginosis and upper genital tract infections. The higher incidence of urinary tract infections (UTI) experienced by diaphragm users may also be partially due to the change in vaginal flora (55). Women who experience frequent UTI should urinate before inserting the diaphragm and after intercourse. It may also be appropriate to have the fit of the diaphragm checked. Similarly, the risk for toxic shock synrome (TSS) is greater among diaphragm users although this is generally limited to cases when the diaphragm is left in place for longer than 24 hours (56).

Women with latex allergy, allergy to spermicides, a history of TSS, or any physical anatomic obstructions to placement of the diaphragm must avoid use. Use of the diaphragm or cervical cap is also contraindicated for women who are at risk or who are HIV infected or have AIDS. Repeated use of the spermicide nonoxynol-9 increases the risk for genital lesions that can increase the risk of acquiring an HIV infection (36).

Key Points for Patient Education

- Women or their partners can insert the diaphragm while standing, squatting, or lying down. Women usually find it easiest to insert the diaphragm by pinching it together with the thumb and third finger of their dominant hand, introducing the device into the introitus, and using the first finger (or opposite hand) to push the back edge inside the vagina. The device should slide easily into place but it may spring out of a woman's hand on initial attempts; she should be warned that this may happen and to not be discouraged. A plastic inserter can also be used to insert the coil and flat spring types of diaphragms.
- The diaphragm is removed by inserting the first finger under the rim and pushing forward or by rotating the wrist (so that the knuckles of the hand are visible) allowing the device to be hooked by the index finger and pulled out of the vagina.
- A diaphragm can be inserted up to 6 hours before intercourse and must remain in position for at least 6 hours after intercourse, but should not remain in the vagina for longer than 24 hours.
- If intercourse occurs more than once during the 6 hours, the diaphragm should be left in place but additional spermicide should be inserted vaginally.
- Women or their partners can insert the cap while standing, squatting, or lying down. The rim of the cap is folded, compressing the dome, so the when it is placed over the cervix, the expanding dome creates suction. The cap is then placed over the cervix fitting snugly against the cervix so that no gaps are detected. Once in place, the anterior rim of the cap should be covered by the anterior wall of the vagina and should be as deep as possible from the introitus to avoid dislodgement by the penis.
- The cap is removed by probing with the index finger, tipping the cap to break the seal, and gently removing.
- Products that can damage latex (e.g., vaginal antifungals, oil-based lubricants such as massage oil, hand lotion or Vaseline) should not be used with the diaphragm or cervical

cap. Use of these devices should be avoided until at least 3 days after use of a vaginal antifungal.

- Both the diaphragm and cervical cap are cleaned with mild soap and water and dried before storage. Prior to each use, these devices should be checked for small holes/leaks (fill cup with water or hold up to light).
- The package labeling states that the diaphragm needs to be replaced every 1–2 years or after pregnancy or a 10 or more pound change in weight; however, weight change does not commonly require a change in diaphragm size (55).

CONTRACEPTIVE SPONGE (TODAY SPONGE)

Description
The contraceptive sponge is a soft, one-size polyurethane foam device containing the spermicide nonoxynol-9. It is a single-use device.

Mechanism of Action
There are three actions that provide a contraceptive benefit: spermicide, sponge absorption of sperm, and physical blocking of sperm (holds spermicide against cervix and blocks cervical opening).

Efficacy
The sponge is more effective for women who have never had a child. The failure rate for nulliparous women (16% failure rate) is half that for parous women (failure rate 32%) (Table 27.2). This device offers no protection against STI.

Benefits
The sponge provides 24-hour protection, can be inserted well before intercourse, and can be used for multiple acts of intercourse. It is a relatively low-cost nonprescription device.

Side Effects and Contraindications
The sponge should not be used while menstruating as this increases the risk of TSS.

Drug Interactions
The sponge should not be used concurrently with a vaginal antifungal as this result in dilution of the spermicide and decreased contraceptive effectiveness.

Key Points for Patient Education
- To use the sponge, moisten with 2 tablespoons of water, squeeze once, and then insert so that dimple is pressed over the cervix; the loop should be away from the cervix.
- The sponge provides a contraceptive action for 24 hours, including multiple acts of intercourse, and can be inserted well before intercourse.
- The sponge should remain in place for at least 6 hours after last act of intercourse but it should be removed within 24 hours. Extended time in the vagina can result in a bad odor and a risk of TSS.
- The sponge is removed by pulling on the loop. When the sponge is removed it should be checked to be sure it is intact; all pieces should be removed from the vagina.
- The sponge should be discarded into the trash.
- The sponge should not be used concurrently with a vaginal antifungal.
- The sponge should not be used during menstruation.

MALE AND FEMALE CONDOMS

Description and Mechanism of Action
The male condom is a sheath that covers the penis and acts as a physical barrier contraceptive. Male condoms are made of three different materials: latex, polyurethane and lamb caecum (natural skin). Useful characteristics of condoms are lubrication (reduces tearing) and a receptacle end to hold the semen. There is no contraceptive advantage to the use of condoms lubricated with spermicide and they are higher in cost, have a shorter shelf life, and have been associated with higher risk of urinary tract infection (UTI) among female partners (57).

The female condom is a device that is comprised of a polyurethane sheath spanning two rings—one to anchor the device internally near the cervix and the other to lie outside the vagina partially covering the labia—that provides a physical barrier. The device is coated on the inside with a lubricant. The female condom is more expensive than the male condom with a typical cost of $3.

Efficacy
The effectiveness of the condom as a contraceptive is highly dependent upon correct use. Although pregnancy occurred in only 2% of couples using the male condom correctly, among couples not using the male condom consistently or correctly 15% became pregnant (57). A similar situation exists for the female condom; with perfect use only 5% of women become pregnant while with inconsistent or incorrect usage 21% of women become pregnant.

Benefits
Latex and synthetic condoms reduce the risk of many bacterial and viral STIs. Latex condoms are superior to polyurethane and natural skin condoms for protection against STI. Natural skin condoms have small pores through which viruses and bacteria can pass; polyurethane condoms are more prone to slippage than the latex condoms. Additionally, STIs are transmitted in two ways—via infected semen and vaginal discharge (e.g., gonorrhea, trichomonas) or via contact with infected skin or mucosal surfaces (e.g., genital herpes, syphilis, HPV). The latex condom provides greater protection against diseases transmitted via discharge than for those STIs transmitted by exposure to infected skin or tissue (58).

Side Effects and Contraindications
Use of a condom along with a spermicide (regularly) may cause skin irritation or tiny abrasions which also has the potential to increase the risk for STI. Some individuals are allergic to latex and may be unable to use latex condoms. Some individuals may also develop contact dermatitis from the lubricant or spermicide component of some condoms. If a reaction occurs, switching to another type of condom may eliminate the problem.

Key Points for Patient Education
- The male condom is applied over the erect penis. It should be unrolled a short distance over a finger to be certain that it is unrolling properly. If the condom does not have a

receptacle/reservoir end, users should pinch the tip of the condom to leave about one-half inch of space at the end when putting the condom on the penis to hold the semen. The condom is gently rolled down the shaft to the base of the penis.

- The penis should be withdrawn soon after ejaculation, while still erect, holding the rim of the condom against the base of the penis to prevent slippage. Remove the condom away from the partner's genitals without spilling the semen, check for visible damage, and discard.
- The female condom is inserted into the vagina by pinching together the upper ring, introducing the device into the vagina, and pushing it into place with the first finger inserted inside the condom to ensure placement over the cervix. It can be inserted up to 8 hours before intercourse. It should not be used in combination with a male condom as the friction between the two condoms may displace one or both.
- Only water-based lubricant products (e.g., K-Y jelly, Astroglide, Replens) should be used along with male condoms; oil-based lubricants (e.g., baby oil, hand lotion, vaseline) and vaginal spermicides can damage latex condoms and reduce their contraceptive effectiveness.
- Female (polyurethane) condoms and male polyurethane condoms are not adversely affected by vaginal spermicides, oil-based lubricants, or vaginal antifungal preparations.
- Latex condom use should be avoided until at least 3 days after use of a vaginal antifungal.
- Some individuals are allergic to latex or have skin reactions to the lubricant or spermicide component of some condoms. Switching to another type of condom may eliminate the problem.
- Condoms should be used before their expiration date and should be stored in a cool dry location to avoid deterioration caused by heat, light, and air.

SPERMICIDE

Description and Mechanism of Action
Spermicides, which contain the agent nonoxynol-9, come in a variety of forms (cream, gel, foam, film, suppository/insert) and can be used alone or in combination with other contraceptives such as diaphragms and condoms. Nonoxynol-9 is a surfactant that destroys the sperm cell membrane.

Efficacy
An adequate amount of spermicide is required for good contraceptive efficacy. Patients should be instructed to use the full amount of spermicide recommended by product labeling and to follow other important instructions (e.g., shaking a foam product as long as recommended). In addition, a spermicide product with at least 100 mg of nonoxynol-9 per dose should be used as lower doses may provide less contraceptive efficacy (59). Spermicides should be inserted close to the time of intercourse to avoid dilution. Some spermicides offer immediate protection (foam, gels), whereas others (suppository and film) must be inserted at least 15 minutes before intercourse so they have time to dissolve and spread. When used alone or with a condom, a foam product is preferred as foams spread more completely and also offer the benefit of bubbles as a physical barrier. Viscous gels can also provide a physical barrier. All forms are effective when inserted less than 1 hour

before intercourse. Women should not wash away the spermicide or douche for at least 6 hours after intercourse.

Benefits
The benefits of spermicides have to do primarily with ease of use; they are available without a prescription, are low cost, and are easily used. These products can also be used in conjunction with condoms to increase contraceptive effectiveness and can be used as a back-up method by women initiating use of another contraceptive such as the oral contraceptive.

Side Effects and Contraindications
Common side effects of spermicides are messiness (excessive lubrication or leakage from the vagina), skin irritation (temporary) and personal dislikes (e.g., taste, having to wait for dissolution prior to intercourse). The spermicides are also associated with changes in vaginal flora that have the potential to increase the risk for *Candida vaginitis* or *Bacterial vaginosis*. However, studies have not found a higher incidence of these vaginal infections in association with spermicide use (60). In contrast, UTIs have been shown to be more common among women using contraceptive methods involving use of spermicides (i.e., in conjunction with a diaphragm or male condom) (60).

The spermicide nonoxynol-9 does not protect against any STIs including HIV (61, 62). In fact, when used frequently (more than 3–4 times daily), nonoxynol-9 causes lesions of the vaginal mucosa that facilitate transmission of HIV (63, 64). According to the WHO, spermicide use is contraindicated among women who are at high risk of HIV or are HIV-infected or who have AIDS (36). However, it is still a viable contraceptive option for women using a spermicidal contraceptive episodically who are at low risk of HIV or other STIs (61, 64).

Drug Interactions
Vaginal lubricants and vaginal antifungal products should not be used at the same time as the vaginal spermicides. Insertion of other vaginal products concurrently will have the effect of diluting the spermicide and may decrease contraceptive effectiveness. The spermicide should provide a lubricating effect for couples desiring this effect.

Key Points for Patient Education
- Prior to inserting a vaginal spermicide, wash hands with soap and water.
- Follow the directions on the package labeling.
- Use of an adequate amount of spermicide is important for contraceptive effectiveness.
  - If shaking of a foam product is required, be sure to shake for the suggested time. Shaking creates bubbles which assist in the contraceptive action.
  - Allow the time for certain spermicides to dissolve or melt before intercourse.
- Insert the spermicide high into the vagina, near the cervix.
- If more than 1 hour has elapsed since insertion of spermicide before intercourse, more spermicide should be inserted vaginally. Additional spermicide should be inserted before each act of intercourse.

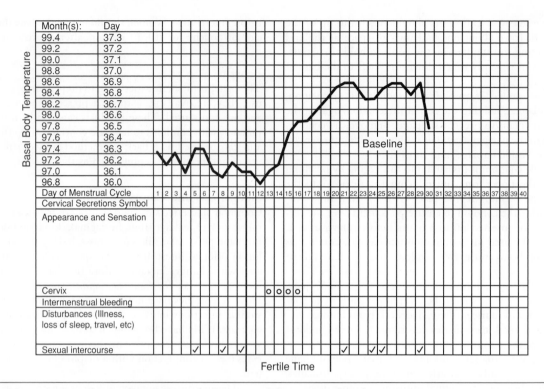

Figure 27.2. • Symptothermal variations during a model menstrual cycle. From Figure 15-3 in Hatcher RA, Trussell J, Stewart FH, et al. eds. Contraceptive Technology, 18th ed. New York, NY: Ardent Media, Inc.; 2004:327. Used with permission.

- The spermicide must remain in the vagina for at least 6 hours after intercourse.
- If your product has a plastic reusable applicator, wash the applicator with soap and water after each use.
- Be sure to have an extra container of spermicide on hand. It is hard to determine when a container is almost empty.

Natural Family Planning/Fertility Awareness Methods

DESCRIPTION

There are several methods of natural family planning (NFP). These methods depend on identifying days during each menstrual cycle when intercourse is most likely to result in pregnancy. In the calendar method, a woman determines her period of fertility based on previous menstrual cycles over 1 year. Fertile days are calculated by subtracting 18 days from the length of the shortest cycle (first fertile day) and 11 days from the longest cycle (last fertile day). Intercourse is avoided or a barrier method is used during these days. High cycle variability makes this method less effective.

The temperature method is based on the rise in basal body temperature (BBT) that occurs just after ovulation (0.4°F to 1.0°F). The mucus method is based on the change in consistency of cervical mucus from thick and dry to clear, thin, and sticky at ovulation. Both are used to predict the time of ovulation; intercourse is avoided or a barrier method is used for several days before and after presumed ovulation.

In the symptothermal method, couples use a combination of two or more fertility indicators. An example of a chart used to document the rise in BBT, cervical mucus changes, and other symptoms that may assist women in determining fertile days is shown in Figure 27.2.

MECHANISM OF ACTION

Based on knowledge of female reproductive physiology—that a woman's egg survives less than 1 day and sperm survive up to 5 days inside the female genital tract—the actual fertile period lasts for about 6 days each cycle (5). By avoiding intercourse for a number of days before and after the time that an individual women is likely to ovulate each month, the couple can avoid pregnancy.

EFFICACY

Among perfect users, the number of women experiencing unplanned pregnancy using these methods varies from 2% (symptothermal method) to 9% (calendar method) (Table 27.2). In actual practice, rates vary from 13%–20%. Authors of a Cochrane review were unable to determine the comparative effectiveness of fertility-awareness based methods due to poor quality of studies and limited continuation rates by subjects (65).

BENEFITS

Cost is minimal, including only charts and a basal body thermometer, unless a barrier method is used during the fertile days instead of abstinence. Use of these methods also increases a couple's knowledge of the woman's reproductive system; this may increase active involvement by both partners and enhance a woman's self-reliance. NFP can also be used to conceive and to detect impaired fertility.

SIDE EFFECTS AND CONTRAINDICATIONS

There are no side effects with NFP, but the method offers no protection against STIs. In addition, to use this method, a woman must have fairly regular ovulatory cycles. Certain conditions may make it difficult to use this method including recent menarche or childbirth, breastfeeding, persistent genital tract infections, time soon after discontinuing a hormonal contraceptive, or perimenopause.

KEY POINTS FOR PATIENT EDUCATION

Couples need careful instruction, often over several sessions with a trained instructor, to use this method effectively.

- A woman should record her basal temperature before rising each morning from bed. A special BBT thermometer is available to assist in documenting the small rise that follows ovulation.
- The cervical mucus should be checked following menses. When the mucus becomes slippery (resembling raw egg white), a woman is entering her most fertile days that continue until 3 days after the last day that the slippery mucus appears. Women may notice other symptoms of ovulation such as adnexal pain (mittelschmerz) or low backache, abdominal bloating, vulvar swelling, spotting, or a widening of the cervical os.
- Test kits to detect the LH surge that triggers ovulation are also available, but these are expensive.
- Intercourse should be avoided from the time that the fertile period begins (first day of slippery mucus) until the third day following the peak day of fertility (day of ovulation, rise in BBT, and/or last day of slippery mucus).
- The safest days for intercourse are when the mucus is dry between menses and the first day of slippery mucus (approximately 4 days) and following the last day of slippery mucus until menses begins (approximately 8 days).
- The days during menses may not be safe in women with short cycles as they may enter their fertile period in the last days of bleeding.
- Couples may engage in noncoital sexual activities during periods of abstinence; knowing that sexual satisfaction may be obtained by alternate means may help couples abstain from intercourse more successfully during the fertile time.

MEDICAL ABORTION

Many women and their partners find themselves facing an unwanted pregnancy. For many years the only option available was aspiration abortion (commonly called surgical abortion). In recent years, women have gained new options.

The availability of legal abortion, since 1973 in this country, has resulted in a large decrease in maternal mortality and morbidity, primarily from a reduction in sepsis, hemorrhage, and trauma (66). However, aspiration abortion is not available to many women. The number of abortion providers declined by 11% between 1996 and 2000 leaving 87% of all U.S. counties without an abortion provider (67). In a 2001–2002 survey of all known abortion providers in the United States, investigators at The Alan Guttmacher Institute found only 37% of them offered services before 5 weeks from the last menstrual period (68). In addition, providers estimated that one-quarter of women having abortions in non-hospital facilities travel 50 miles or more for services. More recently, there have been efforts to integrate abortion care into the primary care setting to allow for improved access, greater privacy, and improved

continuity of care for women and families facing this health crisis (69, 70).

Medical abortion refers to the use of medications to induce an abortion rather than aspiration abortion. Over the past two decades, medical methods have been developed throughout the world and some are currently in use in the United States. Medical abortions account for 5%–6% of the abortions performed in the United States (67). Medical abortion is an option for women who wish to terminate a pregnancy up to 63 days gestation (calculated from the first day of the last menstrual period).

Description

Medications and the regimens currently used in medical abortion are shown in Table 27.7 (71). Administration of mifepristone followed by a prostaglandin analogue (usually misoprostol) is the most commonly used medical abortion regimen.

Mechanism of Action

Mifepristone (RU-486) is a derivative of norethindrone that has a high affinity for progesterone receptors, binding to them and preventing activation (acts a progesterone antagonist). It also stimulates prostaglandin synthesis by cells of the early decidua. It causes decidual necrosis, cervical softening, increased contractility (24–36 hours following its administration), and increased sensitivity to prostaglandins.

Misoprostol is a prostaglandin analogue that causes uterine contractions. It may be given orally or vaginally, the later route of administration causing greater uterine contractility.

Methotrexate is a cytotoxic drug that blocks dihydofolate reductase, an enzyme involved in DNA synthesis. It causes early abortion by blocking the folic acid in fetal cells preventing cell division. It acts on the cytotrophoblast rather than the developing embryo.

Efficacy

The efficacy of these regimens is shown in Table 27.7 and ranges from 88%–99%. Authors of a recent Cochrane review comparing medical with surgical abortion were only able to find six studies, mostly with small sample sizes, comparing four different interventions (72). No information was available on the most common regimen. Prostaglandin used alone seemed less effective and more painful compared to surgical first-trimester abortion. However, there was inadequate evidence to comment on the acceptability and side effects of medical compared to surgical first-trimester abortions.

With respect to the different medical regimens, authors of another Cochrane review found that mifepristone 200 mg shows similar effectiveness in achieving complete abortion compared to 600 mg (4 trials, RR 1.07, 95% CI 0.87 to 1.32) (73). In addition, higher effectiveness, but at higher patient cost, is seen with the combined regimen compared to prostaglandin alone (4 of 5 trials) (73). Administration of 800 mcg of misoprostol vaginally rather than orally also improves efficacy (second regimen listed, Table 27.7) and allows for high completion rates up to 63 days gestational age (71, 73).

Without the use of vaginal or buccal misoprostol, efficacy decreases rapidly with advancing gestational age. For example, using the first regimen listed in Table 27.7 (oral mifepristone and oral misoprostol), efficacy decreases from 96%–98% for pregnancies up to 42 days to less than 85% for pregnancies

TABLE 27.7 Comparison of Common Medical Abortion Regimens

Common Regimens	Overall Success Rates (%)	Advantages and Disadvantages	Gestational Age
Mifepristone, 600 mg orally + misoprostol, 400 μg orally (FDA-approved regimen)	92	Must remain in office or clinic 4 hours after administration	Up to 49 days
Mifepristone, 200 mg orally + misoprostol, 800 μg vaginally (Alternative evidence-based regimen)	95–99	Compared with FDA-approved regimen • More effective • Less time to expulsion • Fewer side effects • Requires vaginal administrationof a medication	Up to 63 days
Methotrexate, 50 mg/m2 IM or 50 mg vaginally, + misoprostol, 800 μg vaginally 3–7 days later	92–96	Compared with mifepristone-misoprostol regimen: • Takes longer for expulsion in 20%–30% of women • Readily available medications • Low drug cost	Up to 49 days
Misoprostol only, 800 μg vaginally repeated for up to three doses	88	• Requires complicated dosing regimens • Significantly higher incidence of side effects than other regimens • Low drug cost	Up to 56 days

Abbreviations: FDA, U.S. Food and Drug Administration; IM, intramuscularly
From: ACOG practice bulletin. Clinical management guidelines of obstetrician-gynecologists. Number 67, October 2005. Medical management of abortion. Obstet Gynecol. 2005;106(4):873.

beyond 49 days (71). Adding a possible second dose of misoprostol was shown to improve efficacy in a Scottish case series, and eliminated the effect of gestation on overall efficacy (74).

Procedure

The FDA approved regimen includes 600 mg of mifepristone orally followed about 48 hours later with 400 micrograms of oral misoprostol. Alternative regimens include 200 mg of oral mifepristone followed by 800 mcg of misoprostol vaginally or bucally administered (or self-administered) anywhere from 6–8 hours to 72 hours afterwards. These regimens have been shown to be more effective with fewer side effects and lower cost (SOR = A) (71).

Recommended laboratory tests prior to medical abortion are hemoglobin or hematocrit and blood typing (71). Anti-D immune globulin should be administered if indicated. Confirmation of pregnancy by ultrasound or pregnancy testing is necessary (SOR = B). Ultrasound confirmation and dating is recommended as all the U.S. trials have used ultrasound; however, results from French trials suggest that selective use of ultrasound is sufficient when patients are managed by highly experienced clinicians (71).

Follow-up in 1–2 weeks is recommended, but there is no consensus on whether an office visit is necessary. Methods to verify abortion include ultrasound, a history of bleeding with uterine involution on physical examination, and human chorionic gonadotropin testing (71). β-hCG should decrease

by 50% within 1 week for regimens including mifepristone or methotrexate and misoprostol administered between 2–5 days afterwards (71). However, a 75% decrease in hCG is needed to assure completed abortion; total disappearance of hCG may take as long as 90 days after the procedure. If hCG remains elevated, consider ectopic pregnancy.

Benefits

Medical abortion can be offered earlier than surgical abortion and affords a woman both privacy and autonomy. Most women will be able to avoid surgical intervention with its small risk of uterine or cervical injury, infection, and the risk of anesthesia. Medical abortions are less painful and may be emotionally easier. In one study, despite a high rate of reported side effects, 64%–95% of women would select the method again (75). In addition, both aspiration and medical abortion in the first trimester are safer than carrying a pregnancy to term.

Side Effects and Contraindications

Medical abortion causes more bleeding than surgical abortion although the amount is rarely clinically significant. Less than 1% of women require emergent curettage because of excessive bleeding (71). Cramping is also part of the process and may be severe. With all medical regimens, there is some degree of waiting and uncertainty (expulsion may take days to weeks) and an extra clinic visit required.

Side effects of medical abortion using mifepristone and misoprostol include nausea (20%–52%), thermoregulatory dysfunction (i.e., warmth, fever, chills, hot flash; 9%–56%), dizziness (12%–37%), headache (10%–37%), vomiting (5%–30%), and diarrhea (1%–27%) (71). Use of vaginal misoprostol decreases the time to expulsion and limits gastrointestinal side effects.

Methotrexate may rarely cause oral ulcers (<1%). Infection has also been reported after medical abortion including 4 deaths from endometritis and toxic shock syndrome associated with *Clostridium sordellii* that occurred within 1 week after medically induced abortions (76); this infection has also been reported in cases of death following childbirth and miscarriage. A review of the literature shows that the overall rate of infection following medical abortion seems very low (0.92%, n = 46,421) (77).

Medical abortion is contraindicated in women whose pregnancies are more advanced than those shown in Table 27.7. Medical abortion is also contraindicated in women with ectopic pregnancy, IUD in place, severe anemia, or known coagulopathy (71). Women on long-term systemic steroids or who have allergy to the medications used in abortion are not candidates. Women with uncontrolled seizure disorder should not receive misoprostol. Women with cardiovascular disease, uncontrolled hypertension, or chronic liver, renal, or respiratory disease have been excluded from clinical trials so less is known about the safety of medical abortion for these women. Medical abortion should not be attempted where there is not immediate access to surgical abortion. Other considerations include a woman's interest in participation in her care, keeping follow-up appointments, and her ability to understand the instructions due to limited cognition or language barrier.

Patient Education

As in all abortion care counseling, patients and couples should include a discussion of whether the woman is certain about her decision to terminate the pregnancy. Once she has made the decision, the method to be used may be selected. Counseling should include benefits and risks of both medical and aspiration procedures (as above) and the woman should be questioned about potential contraindications. If there are no medical or other contraindications (above) and her pregnancy is 63 days or less gestation, she is a candidate for medical abortion.

Definitions of failed medical abortion varies by author and includes the presence of gestational cardiac activity 2 weeks after initiating the procedure or any medical abortion that subsequently involves an aspiration procedure. Women with continuing pregnancies following medical abortion should have their abortion completed by aspiration. Opinions vary with respect to management of persistent gestational sac without cardiac activity in which expectant management or the use of repeated doses of misoprostol is likely to be effective. Other reasons for a subsequent aspiration procedure include heavy bleeding (patients are generally told to monitor for excessive bleeding and if they experience 2 soaked maxi-pads per hour for 2 or more hours in a row, to call and to be evaluated), and patient intolerance of the procedure.

Pain control may be achieved with oral acetaminophen or acetaminophen with codeine. Nonsteroidal anti-inflammatory drugs (NSAIDs) may also be used. NSAIDs do not need to be avoided because, although they reduce the synthesis of endogenous prostaglandins, they do not interfere with the action of already formed prostaglandins.

Anxiety seems to be a common psychological symptom after abortion and providers should create openings for women to discuss their feelings and concerns at follow-up. In addition, in a review of psychological experiences and sexual relationships before and after induced abortion, Bradshaw and Slade found 10%–20% of women experienced sexual problems in the first weeks and months after an abortion, with 5%–20% reporting sexual difficulties a year later (78). There do not seem to be long-term psychological ill affects attributable to abortion. In addition, contraceptive use 1-year post-abortion was found in one small study to be increased (79).

CHOOSING A BIRTH CONTROL METHOD: ASSISTING PATIENTS WITH OPTIMAL DECISION-MAKING

The health provider has an important role in screening for health conditions that may influence the choice of a birth control method or require treatment before initiating contraception. The first visit for this purpose also presents an opportunity to offer periodic health screening services such as genital tract cancer screening or immunization (see Chapter 6, Well Adult Care). During this visit, the following aspects of the history and physical examination will provide useful risk information for patients to consider in choosing an initial birth control method.

Key History

A medial history should be obtained focusing on current and past illnesses such as thrombophlebitis, acute liver disease, genital infections, or breast cancer; allergies to latex or spermicides; and past gynecologic surgeries. Major contraindications to the use of the oral contraceptive are shown in Table 27.3; contraindications for other methods are described within each method's section. Because hormonal methods may alter menstrual patterns, a review of a woman's current menstrual pattern is helpful. Patients should be asked whether they have a new partner and a monogamous relationship with a partner to determine the need for protection against STIs. Other aspects of the sexual history that are helpful to consider include how effective a method needs to be, past successes or failures with methods, frequency of intercourse, and motivation to use a method at the time of intercourse. Figure 27.3 incorporates many of these considerations in an algorithm to guide in the selection of a method.

Physical Examination

A blood pressure measurement should be obtained to identify uncontrolled hypertension, which is a relative contraindication for the combined OC and requires intervention. If blood pressure is elevated, the measurement should be repeated at another visit to confirm hypertension (see Chapter 11, Hypertension). Women should undergo a cardiac examination to rule out valvular heart disease that is a relative contraindication to IUD insertion. A clinical breast examination may be useful in identifying breast cancer (sensitivity 0.92, specificity 0.65,

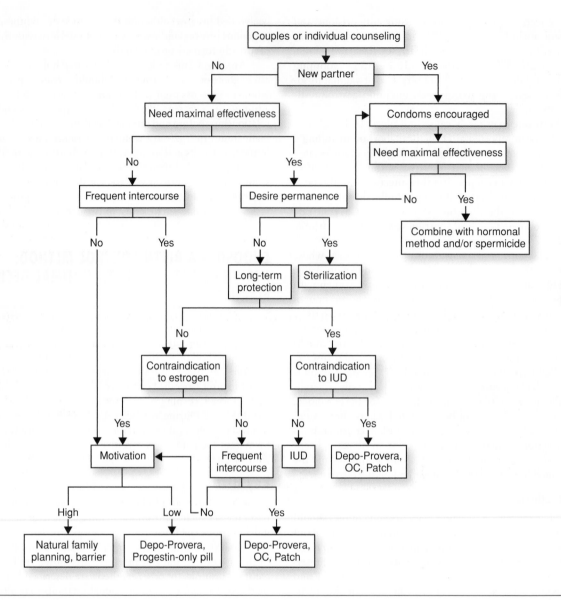

Figure 27.3. • **Algorithm to guide in the selection of a contraceptive method.** (Adapted from Smith MA, Shimp. Family planning. In Smith MA, Shimp LA, eds. Common Problems in Women's Health Care. New York, NY: McGraw-Hill Companies, 2000. Used with permission.)

+LR 2.6, -LR 0.1). This condition precludes use of combined OCs and women should be encouraged to promptly report any self- or partner-identified breast masses for prompt evaluation (see Chapter 26, Breast Problems).

A pelvic examination is performed looking for evidence of STI on the skin, vulva and cervix and for structural abnormalities of the vagina and uterus. Physical findings of common STIs are listed in Table 27.8. The presence of an STI is a contraindication to IUD insertion. Patients with a current or past history of STI should be encouraged to consider methods that protect against STIs (i.e., barrier, spermicide); especially if eradication of the disease is not possible (e.g., some viral STIs) or reinfection is likely. Suspicion or confirmation of AIDS, positive HIV diagnosis, syphilis, gonorrhea, chancroid, lymphogranuloma venereum and granuloma inguinale must

be reported to the local health department within 3 days of the patient visit.

For female adolescents, it may be more important to provide a method of contraception and defer the pelvic examination if the examination itself poses a barrier to initiating contraception. The examination may be performed at a follow-up visit once trust has been established (80)

Ancillary Tests

A Pap smear should be obtained if the woman is sexually active and never had one or has not had one in the past 3 years (see Chapter 6, Well Adult Care). Cultures for gonorrhea and *Chlamydia* should be performed, following informed consent, in women <25 years of age (SOR = A) and encouraged in others based on history and examination findings. Testing

TABLE 27.8 Physical Examination Findings That May Indicate a Sexually Transmitted Infection

Skin
  Maculopapular skin rashes (secondary syphilis)
  Vesicles or ulcers that are painless (primary syphilis, granuloma inguinale) or painful (genital herpes, chancroid) on the anus, mouth, labia, or cervix often with associated inguinal lymphadenopathy
  Flesh-colored to brownish exophytic, hyperkeratotic papules (warts) on the skin of the genital or perianal area (human papilloma virus (HPV))
Genitalia
  Flesh-colored to brownish exophytic, hyperkeratotic papules (warts) on mucosal surfaces of the genital or perianal areas (HPV)
  Nonpurulent (primary genital herpes), frothy (trichomoniasis), or purulent (gonorrhea, chlamydia) vaginal discharge
Pelvic examination
  Inflamed cervix that bleeds easily (gonorrhea, *Chlamydia*)
  Tenderness of the uterus or adnexal areas on examination (gonorrhea, chlamydia, pelvic inflammatory disease)
Rectal examination
  Tenderness or bleeding on rectal examination

From: Smith MA, Shimp LA. Family Planning. In: Smith MA, Shimp LA, eds. 20 Common Problems in Women's Health Care. New York, NY: McGraw-Hill Companies; 2000:21–64.

by genital culture or with serum for VDRL or HIV should be encouraged for patients in non-exclusive relationships and offered to others, particularly if the history is suggestive of risk.

Additional laboratory investigations including liver function, lipid profile, or coagulation profile may be reserved for patients with risk factors.

Algorithm

Selection of a contraceptive method—one the patient is willing to use consistently and correctly and one that is medically appropriate—is critical. In addition, no one method of contraception is likely to be suitable for each woman, man, or couple. Various contraceptive methods may be appropriate for a person during their lifetime. For example, a young woman may select an effective method such as an oral contraceptive but use it in combination with condoms until she is in an established monogamous relationship; then she might use only the OC. After giving birth, she might use a progestin-only pill that will provide good efficacy but not impair breastfeeding. If she determines that she does not want more children, she may opt for sterilization (herself or her partner) or a long-term contraceptive such as an IUD.

When individuals choose a contraceptive method they must choose between a reversible and permanent form (sterilization) of contraception. Almost two-thirds of women of re-

productive age who are using a contraceptive method are utilizing a reversible method (e.g. oral contraceptive, condom) (1).

The algorithm shown in Figure 27.3 can be useful in assisting couples or individuals in selecting a method of birth control. Condoms should be encouraged for new partnerships, teenage partners, patients at high risk of STIs, and for couples where one partner has a viral STI and the other partner is not infected. For those requiring maximal pregnancy protection, methods with the least opportunity for user error should be employed (e.g., IUD and DMPA). Women engaging in frequent intercourse should consider OCs or DMPA; those who have less frequent intercourse or a contraindication to estrogen use might consider vaginal barrier methods or NFP. Finally, the POP is an option for older women with contraindications to estrogen and for lactating women. Patients should be encouraged to consider or choose a second method of contraception in case the chosen method proves unacceptable.

FOLLOW-UP AND MANAGING CONTRACEPTIVE SIDE EFFECTS

Many women experience side effects that require intervention to encourage continued use or identification of an alternative contraceptive method. The following is a list of options for patients who wish to continue use of a chosen method.

Oral Contraceptives (OC)

Of women choosing an OC, approximately 25% experience minor side effects during the first 3 months after initiation (9). Women should be told about common side effects, how to minimize the common side effects that occur, and symptoms (described in the previous section on OCs) that indicate potentially serious adverse effects.

Common side effects include nausea and breast changes. Most women adjust to use of the OC and nausea resolves within the first 3 months of use without the need for changes in OC prescribing; taking the OC with food and/or taking it at bedtime can minimize this side effect. Alternatively, a pill with lower or no estrogen can be used. Breast tenderness also may decrease over time and use of a proper fitting bra can help reduce discomfort and a pill lower in estrogen and/or progestin may decrease this symptom.

Menstrual changes are also common, typically a decrease in menses or amenorrhea. Providers can reassure women that decreased or minimal menses is normal; if a woman is uncomfortable with amenorrhea, an OC with increased estrogen activity, a third-generation progestin pill, or a pill with higher progestin potency may alleviate this side effect. Spotting and bleeding affect up to half of women, particular with use of OCs with low hormone doses during the first several months of OC use. Most women will adjust to the OC and this symptom will disappear after 3 months. Bleeding may occur because of missed pills, erratic timing of administration, or drug interactions. If heavy menstrual bleeding occurs, a NSAID may be used to reduce bleeding. Alternatively, a pill with higher progestin potency, a third-generation progestin pill, or increased estrogen content may be effective.

Women may also notice increases in vaginal discharge in

response to the estrogen component of the OC. Reassure the patient that this is normal. Visual changes or decreased tolerance for contact lens users may indicate a change in the eye with hormone use and an ophthalmic exam is recommended. Weight gain is not common with use of the OC (38) and negative mood changes and decreased libido are uncommon, occurring is less than 20% of users (9).

Transdermal Patch (Ortho-Evra)

To avoid irritation from the patch, women should apply each new patch to a different place on the skin than that used for the previous patch. If skin irritation, redness, or a rash occurs, the patch can be removed and a new patch applied to a new skin location until the next "change day"(41). Single replacement patches are available from pharmacies.

Intrauterine Device (IUD)

Heavy periods associated with the IUD usually decrease over time. NSAIDs, such as ibuprofen (400–600 mg three times daily), can be used during the first few days of menses. Vaginal bleeding with pain should prompt evaluation for ectopic pregnancy.

If the patient becomes pregnant with the IUD in place, confirm that the pregnancy is intrauterine and remove the IUD. Early removal reduces the risk of spontaneous miscarriage or preterm delivery (52). A woman's plans for continuation of the pregnancy and options available to her should be discussed.

Symptoms of IUD expulsion include unusual vaginal discharge, cramping or pain, spotting, dyspareunia or male discomfort during intercourse, absence or lengthening of the IUD string, and presence of the IUD in the cervical os or vagina (52). If the IUD is partially expelled, remove the IUD and consider insertion of a new IUD.

IUD strings may be missing, too short, or too long. If the string is missing and the woman is unaware of expulsion of the IUD, an ultrasound or x-ray may be obtained. If the string is within the canal, it may be brought through the os with a cotton swab or endometrial biopsy instrument. If the IUD is in place, nothing more needs to be done. If the male partner complains of penile discomfort because of the string, strings may be cut shorter.

Condoms and Spermicides

If irritation is experienced, patients should be encouraged to try an alternative product before abandoning these contraceptive methods.

SUMMARY AND FUTURE CONSIDERATIONS

Primary care providers can help to reach the goals for prevention of unplanned pregnancy set forth in Healthy People 2010 by helping women/couples select a birth control method that meets the characteristics they desire, by patient education and counseling about how to most effectively use that method, by discussing the importance of switching to another method if quitting the initial chosen method, and by discussing and providing a prescription for the emergency contraceptive. Medical abortion should also be discussed as an option for women who wish to terminate a pregnancy up to 63 days gestation.

Contraceptive choices will undoubtedly change in the future. Some advances on the horizon are:

- Lybrel® (Wyeth Pharmaceuticals). A non-cyclic oral contraceptive (20 mcg EE and 90 mcg levonorgestrel) that is designed to be taken every day, 365 days per year without a placebo or pill-free interval. Studies have found that the safety profile for Lybrel is similar to that of other OCs and that menstruation resumes quickly following discontinuation of Lybrel (81). The majority (69%) of women using the continuous contraceptive reported no bleeding (i.e., breakthrough bleeding with no need for sanitary protection) by month 6 of use. Resumption of menses or pregnancy occurred within 90 days of discontinuation of Lybrel for 99% of women.

  Absence of menstruation will be desirable for some women (e.g., severe dysmenorrhea or convenience) but disconcerting for others (prefer to have the monthly menstrual cycle and assurance that they are not pregnant). Throughout history women have had many fewer menses than women today because sexually active women were typically either pregnant or lactating. The absense of menses may have health benefits: the greater the number of menses, the greater the risk for ovarian, endometrial and breast cancer (82). An FDA new drug application was submitted.

- Implanon® (Organon USA, Inc.). A single-rod implantable contraceptive that contains 68 mcg of the progestin etonorgestrel (active metabolite of desogestrel). Implanon, inserted subdermally provides contraceptive action for 3 years. Efficacy is very high (no pregnancies within the first 70,000 cycles studied). Contraceptive actions include inhibition of ovulation, thickened cervical mucus, and atrophic endometrium (43). As with other progestin-only contraceptives, the most common reason for discontinuance (13% of users) is bleeding pattern changes. Insertion and removal of the device has been reported as generally without complication; average insertion time—30 seconds and average removal time—4 minutes (83). Return to normal menstrual pattern and fertility after discontinuation is rapid (83). This device has received FDA-approval.

- Protectaid® – (Axcan Pharma Ltd.). A contraceptive sponge. It contains a combination of low-doses of three spermicides: nonoxynol-9 (6.25 mg), benzalkonium chloride (6.25 mg), and sodium cholate (25 mg). The use of low doses of the three spermicides is designed to minimize vaginal and penile irritation. Protectaid provides contraceptive action for 12 hours, even with multiple acts of intercourse. It should be inserted at least 15 minutes before intercourse and remain in place for at least 6 hours after intercourse.84 This device is available as a nonprescription product in Canada and some European countries.

CASE 1 DISCUSSION

In addition to asking about Ms. Baker and her partner's willingness to continue to use a method at the time of intercourse, she should be asked about the presence of any contraindications to oral contraceptive use (Table 27.3). Family history of breast cancer and current concerns about restarting a different oral contraceptive should be solicited. A blood pressure, cardiac examination, and breast examination should be completed and, although she does not need a Pap smear at this time, she should be encouraged to undergo testing for gonorrhea and *Chlamydia* and offered testing for syphilis and AIDS. Options for highly effective methods appropriate for her to consider include condom combined with vaginal spermicide, condom and depot medroxyprogesterone acetate (DMPA) or condom and an OC or patch (possibly changing to just the hormonal contraceptive if and when she believes that she now has a long-term partner and she is satisfied with her adherence to daily pills or weekly patch). If she chooses DMPA, she should be comfortable with the likelihood of menstrual irregularity or amenorrhea and accepting of some weigh gain. If she chooses to restart an oral contraceptive, selection of a 35 mcg EE product will provide greater protection should she miss a pill and should improve her acne. OCs particularly suitable for a patient with acne include low-dose norethindrone products, Ortho-Tricyclen, Estrostep, and Yasmin. Written information should be provided about managing missed pills. If she selects a patch, she should be informed that her risk of blood clots might be increased more than with the pill and written information about the patch should be provided. In either case, information about Plan B AND which she can obtain at a pharmacy since she is over age 18 years or a presciption for an oral contraceptive to use as an emergency contraceptive should be provided with instructions in use in case of condom breakage or if she misses one or more pills. Any concerns about mechanism of action of emergency contraception (primary contraceptive action is prevention or delay of ovulation or fertilization) should be discussed and she should be encouraged to call the office if she has occasion to use it, especially if her next menstrual cycle is more than one week late (pregnancy test indicated).

CASE 2 DISCUSSION

Questions to pose to Mrs. Thompson include her need for a highly effective contraceptive, she and her husband's motivation to use a method at the time of intercourse, and her past experience with contraceptive methods. She should be counseled about smoking cessation based on her stage of change and advised to quit. If she is ready to try smoking cessation, she might be placed on a nicotine patch or bupropion to assist in her quit attempt and follow-up should be arranged.

If she has had normal Pap smears in the past, including the past year, and is comfortable with decreasing the frequency of Pap smears to every 3 years, this test may be omitted. After her focused physical examination (see Chapter 6, Well Adult Care), contraceptive options should be presented including a POP, IUD, or condom and spermicide. If a somewhat less effective method is an option, a diaphragm, male or female condom, or natural family planning method may also be considered. If the patient wishes to continue a combined oral contraceptive, she must be aware of her increased risk for MI and stroke; these risks will be lessened after smoking cessation or with use of a third-generation OC (one containing desogestrel or norgestimate). If she wishes to continue a combined OC, one with 20 mcg EE is preferred to reduce cardiovascular risk and breast tenderness.

REFERENCES

1. The Alan Guttmacher Institute. Contraceptive use. New York, NY; Washington, DC; 2006.
2. The Alan Guttmacher Institute. Looking at Men's sexual and reproductive health needs. New York, NY; Washington, DC; 2002
3. Smith MA, Shimp LA. Family planning. In: Smith MA, Shimp LA, eds. 20 Common Problems in Women's Health Care. New York, NY: McGraw-Hill Companies, 2000:21–64.
4. Abma JC, Martinez GM, Mosher WD, Dawson BS. Teenagers in the United States: sexual activity, contraceptive use, and childbearing, 2002. Vital Health Stat 23. 2004;(24):1–48.
5. Hatcher RA, Namnoun AB. The menstrual cycle. In: Hatcher RA, Trussell J, Stewart FH, et al., eds. Contraceptive Technology, 18th ed. New York, NY: Ardent Media, Inc., 2004:63–72.
6. Stewart FH, Trussell J, Van Look PFA. Emergency contraception. In: Hatcher RA, Trussell J, Stewart FH, et al., eds. Contraceptive Technology. New York, NY: Ardent Media, Inc; 2004:279–303.
7. Herndon EJ, Zieman M. New Contraceptive Options. Am Fam Physician. 2004;69:853–860.
8. The Alan Guttmacher Institute. Preventing unintended pregnancy in the US. New York, NY; Washington, DC; 2004.
9. Seibert C, Barbouche E, Fagan J, et. al. Prescribing oral contraceptives for women older than 35 years of age. Ann Intern Med 2003;138:54–64.
10. US Department of Health and Human Services. Family planning In: Healthy People 2010, Vol. 2, 2nd ed. Washington, DC: U.S. Department of Health and Human Services; 2000. Available at *http://www.healthypeople.gov/Document/pdf/Volume 1/09Family.pdf*. Accessed January 6, 2006.
11. Alan Guttmacher Institute. Facts on induced abortion in the United States. New York, NY; Washington, DC; 2006.
12. Stewart FH, Ellertson C, Cates W. Abortion. In: Hatcher RA, Trussell J, Stewart FH, et al. eds. Contraceptive Technology, 18th ed. New York, NY: Ardent Media, Inc.; 2004: 673–700.
13. American Pharmaceutical Association. Emergency contraception: the pharmacist's role. Washington, DC, 2000.
14. Brown SS, Eisenberg L, Committee on Unintended Pregnancy, Institute of Medicine. The Best Intentions: Unintended Pregnancy and the Well-Being of Children and Families. Washington, DC: National Academy Press, 1995.
15. Hatcher RA, Nelson A. Combined hormonal contraceptive methods. In: Hatcher RA, Trussell J, Stewart FH, et al. eds. Contraceptive Technology, 18th ed. New York, NY: Ardent Media, Inc.; 2004:391–460.
16. American Academy of Pediatrics. Emergency contraception. Pediatrics. 2005;116(4):1026–35.
17. American College of Obstetricians and Gynecologists (ACOG). Emergency oral contraception. Washington, DC: American College of Obstetricians and Gynecologists; 2001 Mar:no. 25.
18. Mosher WD, Martinez GM, Chandra A, et. al. Use of contraception and use of family planning services in the United States 1982–2002. Advance data from vital and health statistics; Hyattsville, MD: National Center for Health Statistics; 2004:no. 350.
19. The Medical Letter, Inc. Treatment guidelines: choice of contraceptives. Med Lett. 2004; 2(24):55–62.

20. Holt VL, Cushing-Haugen KL, Daling JR. Body weight and risk of oral contraceptive failure. Obstet Gynecol. 2002;99:820–827.

21. Walker GR, Schlesselman JJ, Ness RB. Family history of ovarian cancer, oral contraceptive use, and ovarian cancer risk. Am J Obstet Gynecol. 2002;186:8–14.

22. Farley TMM, Meirik O, Chang CL, Poulter NR. Combined oral contraceptives, smoking, and cardiovascular risk. J Epidemiol Community Health. 1998;52:775–785.

23. Rosenberg L, Palmer JR, Rao MS, Shapiro S. Low-dose oral contraceptive use and the risk of myocardial infarction. Arch Intern Med. 2001;161:1065–1070.

24. Curtis KM, Mohallajee AP, Martins SL, Peterson HB. Combined oral contraceptive use among women with hypertension: a systematic review. Contraception. 2006;73(2):179–188.

25. Khader YS, Rice J, Lefant J, Abueita O. Oral contraceptives use and the risk of myocardial infarction: a meta-analysis. Contraception. 2003;68(1):11–17.

26. Tanis B, Van Den Bosch MAAJ, Kemmeren JM, et al. Oral contraceptives and the risk of myocardial infarction. N Engl J Med. 2001; 345(25):1787–1193.

27. Gillum LA, Mamidipudi SK, Johnston SC. Ischemic stroke risk with oral contraceptives. A meta-anlaysis. JAMA. 2000;284:72–78.

28. Chang CL, Donaghy M, Poulter N. Migraine and stroke in young women: case-control study. The World Health Organisation Collaborative Study of Cardiovascular Disease and Steroid Hormone Contraception. BMJ. 1999 Jan 2;318(7175):13–18.

29. Tanis B, Rosendaal C, Frits R. Venous and arterial thrombosis during oral contraceptive use: risks and risk factors. Semin Vasc Med. 2003;3(1):69–84.

30. Kemmeren JM, Algra A, Grobbee DE. Third generation oral contraceptives and risk of venous thrombosis: meta-analysis. BMJ. 2001;323:131–134.

31. Marchbanks PA, McDonald JA, Wilson HG, et al. Oral contraceptives and the risk of breast cancer. N Engl J Med. 2002; 346:2025–2032.

32. Grabrick DM, Hartmann LG, Cerhan JR, et al. Risk of breast cancer with oral contraceptive use in women with a family history of breast cancer. JAMA. 2000;284:1791–1198.

33. IARC. IARC Monograph programme finds combined estrogen-progestogen contraceptives and menopausal therapy are carcinogenic to humans [press release]. Lyon, France: IARC. July 29, 2005, no. 167, IARC. Combined estrogen-progestogen contraceptives. Vol 91; monograph No. 1, Section 5, 3rd draft, rev 3, 2005.

34. Narod SA, Dube MP, Klinj J, et al. Oral contraceptives and the risk of breast cancer in BRCA1 and BRCA2 mutation carriers. J Natl Cancer Inst. 2002;94:1773–1779.

35. Castle PE, Walker JL, Schiffman M, Wheeler CM. Hormonal contraceptive use, pregnancy, and parity, and the risk of cervical intraepithelial neoplasia 3 among oncogenic HPA DNA-positive women with equivocal or mildly abnormal cytology. Int J Cancer. 2005;117:1007–1012.

36. World Health Organization. Medical Eligibility Criteria for Contraceptive Use, 2004. Available at http://www.who.int/reproductive-health/publications. Accessed May 31, 2006.

37. Helms SE, Bredle DL, Zajic J, et al. Oral contraceptive failure rates and oral antibiotics. J Am Acad Dermatol. 1997;36:705–710.

38. Gallo MF, Lopez DA, Grimes KF, et al. Combination contraceptives: effect on weight (Cochrane Review). In: The Cochrane Library. Oxford, England: Update Software; 2006: Issue 1.

39. Vessey M, Painter R, Yeats. Mortality in relation to oral contraceptive use and cigarette smoking. Lancet. 2003;362(9379):185–191.

40. Tansavatdi K, McClain B, Herrington DM. The effects of smoking on estradiol metabolism. Minerva Ginecologica 2004;56(1):105–114.

41. Ortho-Evra® Prescribing Information. Orth-McNeil Pharmaceutical Inc. Raritan, NJ: November, 2005.

42. Associated Press: KaiserNetwork.org. Daily women's health report. Ortho-Evra—new FDA required warning, increased risk of VTE. July 19, 2005. Available at http://www.kaisernetwork.org/daily_reports/rep_repro_recent_reports.cfm?dr_DateTIme=07-19-05%show=yes#31463. Accessed March 10, 2006.

43. Hatcher RA. Depo-Provera injection, implants, and progestin-only pills (minipills). In: Hatcher RA, Trussell J, Stewart FH, et al. eds. Contraceptive Technology, 18th ed. New York, NY: Ardent Media, Inc.; 2004:461–494.

44. Jain J, Jakimiuk AJ, Bode FR, et. al. Contraceptive efficacy and safety of DMPA-SC. Contraception. 2004;70(4):269–275.

45. Kaunitz AM. Depo-Provera's black box: time to reconsider? Contraception. 2005 Sep; 72(3):165–167.

46. Scholes D, LaCroix AZ, Ichikawa LE, et al. Change in bone mineral density among adolescent women using and discontinuing depot medroxyprogesterone acetate contraception. Arch Pediatr Adolesc Med. 2005;159(2):139–144.

47. Clark MK, Sowers MR, Nichols S, Levy B. Bone mineral density changes over two years in first-time users of depot medroxyprogesterone acetate. Fertil Steril. 2004;82(6):1580–1586.

48. Beksinska ME, Smit JA, Kleinschmidt I, et al. Bone mineral density in women aged 40–49 years using depot-medroxyprogesterone acetate, northisterone enaanthate or combined oral contraceptives for contraception. Contraception. 2005; 71(3):170–175.

49. Kennedy KI, Trussell J. Postpartum contraception and lactation. In: Hatcher RA, Trussell J, Stewart FH, et al. eds. Contraceptive Technology, 18th ed. New York, NY: Ardent Media, Inc.; 2004:575–600.

50. Croxatto HB, Ortiz ME, Muller AL. Mechanisms of action of emergency contraception. Steroids, 2003;68(10–13):1095–1098.

51. Plan B® Prescribing Information. Duramed Pharmaceuticals, Inc. Pomona NY, February, 2004.

52. Grimes DA. Intrauterine devices In: Hatcher RA, Trussell J, Stewart FH, et al. eds. Contraceptive Technology, 18th ed. New York, NY: Ardent Media, Inc.; 2004:495–530.

53. American College of Obstetricians and Gynecologists (ACOG). Antibiotic prophylaxis for gynecologic procedures. Washington, DC: American College of Obstetricians and Gynecologists; 2001 Jan:no. 23).

54. Trussell J. Contraceptive efficacy. In: Hatcher RA, Trussell J, Stewart FH, et al. eds. Contraceptive Technology, 18th ed. New York, NY: Ardent Media, Inc.; 2004:773–845.

55. Cates W, Stewart F. Vaginal barriers. In: Hatcher RA, Trussell J, Stewart FH, et al. eds. Contraceptive Technology, 18th ed. New York, NY: Ardent Media, Inc.; 2004:365–389.

56. Allen RE. Diaphragm fitting. Am Fam Physician. 2004;69(1):97–106.

57. Warner L, Hatcher RA, Steiner MJ. Male condoms. In: Hatcher RA, Trussell J, Stewart FH, et al. eds. Contraceptive Technology, 18th ed. New York, NY: Ardent Media, Inc.; 2004:331–353.

58. CDC fact sheet for public health personnel: male latex condoms and sexually transmitted diseases. July 2001. Available at http://www.cdc.gov/nchstp/od/latex.htm. Accessed March 11, 2006.

59. Raymond EG, Chen PL, Luoto J. Contraceptive effectiveness and safety of five nonoxynol-9 spermicides: A randomized trial. Obstet Gynecol. 2004;103(3):430–439.

60. Cates W, Raymond EG. Vaginal spermicides. In: Hatcher RA, Trussell J, Stewart FH, et al. eds. Contraceptive Technology, 18th ed. New York, NY: Ardent Media, Inc.; 2004: 355–363.

61. Wilkinson D, Ramjee G, Tholandi M, Rutherford G. Nonoxynol-9 for preventing vaginal acquisition of sexually transmitted infections by women from men (Cochrane Review). In: The Cochrane Library. Oxford, England: Update Software; 2002:Issue 1.

62. Cates W. Review of Non-hormonal contraception (condoms, intrauterine devices, nonoxynol-9 and combos) in HIV acquisition. J Acquir Immune Defic Syndr 2005;38(suppl 1): S8–S10.

63. Hillier SL, Moench T, Shattock R, et. al. In vitro and In vivo The story of nonoxynol 9. J Acquir Immune Defic Syndr 2005;39(May 1):1–8.

64. World Health Organization. WHO/CONRAD technical consultation on nonoxynol-9, World Health Organization, Geneva, 9–10 October 2001: summary report. Reproductive Health Matters 2002;10(20):175–181.

65. Grimes DA, Gallo MF, Grigorieva V, et al. Fertility-awareness based methods for contraception. Cochrane Database Syst Rev. 2004 Oct 18;(4):CD004860.

66. Singh K, Ratnam SS. The influence of abortion legislation on maternal mortality. Int J Gynaecol Obstet. 1998;63(suppl 1):S213–S219.

67. Finer LB, Henshaw SK. Abortion incidence and services in the United States in 2000. Perspect Sex Reprod Health. 2003; 35:6–15.

68. Henshaw SK, Finer LB. The accessibility of abortion services in the United States, 2001. Perspect Sex Reprod Health. 2003; 35(1):16–24.

69. Gold M. Abortion training in family medicine. Fam Med. 1996;28(4):287–288.

70. Bennett I, Aguirre AC, Burg J, et al. Initiating abortion training in residency programs: issues and obstacles. Fam Med. 2006; 38(5):330–335.

71. ACOG practice bulletin. Clinical management guidelines of obstetrician-gynecologists. Number 67, October 2005. Medical management of abortion. Obstet Gynecol. 2005;106(4): 871–882.

72. Say L, Kulier R, Gulmezoglu M, Campana A. Medical versus surgical methods for first trimester termination of pregnancy. Cochrane Database Syst Rev. 2005 Jan 25;(1):CD003037.

73. Kulier R, Gulmezoglu AM, Hofmeyr GJ, et al. Medical methods for first trimester abortion. Cochrane Database Syst Rev. 2004;(2):CD002855.

74. Ashok PW, Templeton A, Wagaarachchi PT, Flett GM. Factors affecting the outcome of early medical abortion: a review of 4132 consecutive cases. BJOG. 2002;109(11):1281–1289.

75. Winikoff B. Acceptability of medical abortion in early pregnancy. Fam Plann Perspect. 1995;27(4):142–148, 185.

76. Fischer M, Bhatnagar J, Guarner J, et al. Fatal toxic shock syndrome associated with Clostridium sordellii after medical abortion. N Engl J Med. 2005;353(22):2352–2360.

77. Shannon C, Brothers LP, Philip NM, Winikoff B. Infection after medical abortion: a review of the literature. Contraception. 2004;70(3):183–190.

78. Bradshaw Z, Slade P. The effects of induced abortion on emotional experiences and relationships: a critical review of the literature. Clin Psychol Rev. 2003 Dec;23(7):929–958.

79. Kero A, Lalos A. Increased contraceptive use one year post-abortion. Hum Reprod. 2005;20(11):3085–3090.

80. Stewart FH, Harper CC, Ellerston CE, et al. Clinical breast and pelvic examination requirements for hormonal contraception. Current practice vs evidence. JAMA. 2001;285: 2232–2239.

81. New Findings from Two Studies on Lybrel presented at ACOG Media authors (*not* study authors) Candace Steele and Christopher Garland. Available at *http://www.wyeth.com/ news?nav= display&navTo =/wyeth_html/home/news/ pressreleases/2006/1147122267860.html* June, 11, 2006.

82. Neighmond P. National Public Radio. "Continuous contraception" may banish periods. Morning Edition, June 9, 2006). Available at *http://www.npr.org/templates/story/story.php?storyId = 5458926.* Accessed June 11, 2006.

83. Funk S, Miller MM, Mishell DR, et. al. Safety and efficacy of Implanon, a single-rod implatable contraceptive containing etonorgestrel. Contraception. 2005;71(5):319–325.

84. Protectaid product page. Available at *http://www. 77canadapharmacy.com/protectaid.php.* Accessed June 12, 2006.

CHAPTER 28

Dysuria

George R. Bergus

CASE 1

A 28-year-old woman presents with a 24-hour history of dysuria and urinary frequency. She has been forcing oral fluids without improvement. She denies fever, chills, or flank pain. She has been sexually active with one partner for 3 months and uses oral contraceptive pills for birth control.

CLINICAL QUESTIONS

1. Is her dysuria due to infection?
2. If the dysuria is from a urinary tract infection (UTI), does the infection involve the upper or lower urinary tract?
3. Is the UTI an isolated or recurrent episode?

Dysuria is pain or discomfort associated with urination that is localized to the bladder or urethra. This is a common chief complaint in the primary care office setting (1). Approximately 3% of all office visits are in response to this symptom, with associated medical care costs in excess of $1 billion each year (2, 3). Most patients with dysuria will be otherwise healthy women who have an uncomplicated urinary tract infection (UTI) requiring only minimal evaluation and a short course of antibiotics (see Table 28.1). However, physicians need to approach the complaint of dysuria with some sophistication so that the appropriate work-up and treatment can be selected based on location of infection, age and gender of the patient, the patient's underlying health, and any complicated factors signaling a more complicated infection.

UTIs can be divided into four very broad categories: (a) acute uncomplicated lower tract infection in women, (b) recurrent uncomplicated lower tract infection in women, (c) acute upper tract infection (pyelonephritis) in women, and (d) UTIs in children, men, and geriatric patients. Each of these large groups should be further divided into simple and complex infections as there are important differences in their evaluation and treatment.

PATHOPHYSIOLOGY AND DIFFERENTIAL DIAGNOSIS

Pathophysiology

Almost all UTIs are caused by bacteria that normally inhabit the colon; 80% to 90% of community-acquired UTIs in adults and children are from *Escherichia coli (E. coli)* (4, 5). The predominance of a single species of bacterium is important because it allows empiric therapy to have a high probability of success. Other gram-negative organisms (*Proteus* species, *Klebsiella pneumoniae,* and *Pseudomonas aeruginosa*) cause infections but are much less common except in hospitalized patients, immunocompromised patients, or patients who have undergone recent genitourinary catheterization or instrumentation. Gram-positive organisms (*Staphylococcus saprophyticus, Staphylococcus aureus,* group B *streptococcus,* and *Enterococcus faecium*) are also uropathogens, but are much less common causes of UTI. Anaerobic bacteria predominate in the gut but almost never cause UTI.

The usual route of infection is one in which bacteria ascend from the perineum, pass through the urethra, and invade the bladder. Only a small number of *E. coli* strains are typically involved in these infections. These strains have a variety of virulence factors, including adhesive fimbriae, which allow these bacteria to adhere to the uroepithelium and resist the flushing action of urine flow. Infections usually remain within the lower urinary tract, but can sometimes ascend through the ureters to invade the upper urinary tract. When the renal parenchyma becomes infected, the infection is called pyelonephritis. Infections within the urinary tract are only rarely caused by a blood-borne source.

Differential Diagnosis

UTI, the focus of this chapter, is the most common cause of dysuria. Dysuria can also be from other focal inflammation in the vagina, perineal area, prostate, or urethra, however. Common vaginal infections that cause dysuria include bacterial vaginosis, vaginal candidiasis, and vaginal trichomoniasis. Vaginal atrophy, from the loss of estrogen stimulation to the vaginal mucosa and vulvar skin, can also be associated with dysuria. As the epithelium thins, it becomes prone to injury, with resulting dysuria and pruritis.

Urethritis is caused by sexually transmitted infections such as gonorrhea, chlamydia, herpes simplex, or trichomoniasis. Prostate infections can cause dysuria and are typically associated with decreased urine flow, urgency, and hesitancy. Both acute prostatitis and upper tract UTI may present as fever and dysuria. These other causes of dysuria are discussed in the following chapters: vaginitis (Chapter 34), prostate infection (Chapter 31), and sexually transmitted infections (Chapter 33).

Dysuria is sometimes attributed to the poorly understood "urethral syndrome." This syndrome of pain on urination without clearly identifiable cause has been ascribed to trauma, chemical irritation, low levels of urinary pathogens, or infection of periurethral tissue by unknown microorganisms (6).

TABLE 28.1 Differential Diagnosis of Dysuria in Otherwise Healthy Women of Reproductive Age

Diagnosis	Frequency
Lower tract UTI	Very common (70% of women with dysuria)
Vaginitis	Common
Upper tract UTI	Uncommon
Urethritis	Uncommon*
Perineal trauma	Rare

*May be more common in college health centers and reproductive health clinics
UTI, urinary tract infection.

The diagnosis of urethral syndrome is made only after the symptomatic patient has had normal findings on physical examination, and normal urinalysis and culture.

Risk Factors and Clinical Epidemiology

Except for the neonatal period, females have a higher risk for UTI than do males. During the third and fourth decades, this gender difference is at its maximum, with women at 40 to 50 times greater risk of UTI. Young adult women have the highest incidence of UTI of any group, and average one infection every other year (7). Elderly men develop UTI at a rate approaching that observed in elderly women, particularly when they are living in an institutional setting.

Not all women are prone to UTI; only 50% to 60% report ever having an infection. Individuals with certain genetic, physiologic, or behavioral risk factors are more prone to develop UTI. For example, 10% to 20% of women have an epithelium to which uropathogenic *E. coli* adhere more easily. A history of at least two previous UTIs is a marker for this type of epithelium and is a strong predictor of subsequent infections. Another high-risk group are women with colonization of the vagina by uropathogens. The use of a contraceptive cream or jelly with Nonoxynol 9 is associated with this colonization and subsequent UTI. Other risk factors include sexual intercourse, fecal incontinence (7), and a shorter distance from urethra to anus (8). Although urethral length is purported to be a risk factor for UTI, one study found no increase in the risk of UTI with shorter urethral length in women (8). Stasis of urine in the bladder adds to risk by facilitating bacterial multiplication, and incomplete bladder emptying is a common cause of stasis. It should not be surprising that women who use a diaphragm and spermicide for contraception are prone to UTI. The diaphragm can cause urinary stasis (particularly if it is too large); the spermicide promotes colonization of the vagina with uropathogens; and sexual activity increases the chance that uropathogens enter the urinary tract. Although infrequent voiding and wiping front to back after bowel movements have been hypothesized as risk factors, research has not confirmed the associations (9). Risk factors for pyelonephritis in healthy women are very similar to those reported for lower tract infection and include sexual behaviors and a personal or family history of UTI (10).

CLINICAL EVALUATION

The extent of clinical evaluation of urinary symptoms varies and depends largely on the clinical setting of the patient. In some cases, management by telephone may be appropriate, whereas in others, a detailed physical examination supplemented by laboratory investigation is required.

History

UTIs in healthy adults are typically accompanied by urinary frequency, nocturia, pain on urination, and suprapubic discomfort. The clinician can use the history to determine the probability of UTI, and to exclude other causes for symptoms. When a healthy adult woman complains of dysuria and has no vaginal symptoms, there is a 65% to 75% probability that UTI is the cause (11, 12). If the same woman also reports urinary frequency or urgency, the probability of UTI rises to more than 90%. In this setting little further clinical evaluation is needed if there are no risk factors for a complicated infection (13). If vaginal complaints are also present or the dysuria is described as external, a more thorough evaluation is needed to exclude sexually transmitted diseases and vaginitis. When the patient complains of both dysuria and vaginal discharge, the probability of UTI drops to below 20%. In addition, if a woman who previously has had cystitis complains of a recurrence of the symptoms, the probability of UTI is also about 90% (14). It is important to remember the complaint of dysuria is not as diagnostic of UTI in young children, elderly women, or males.

The key elements of the history and physical examination of the patient with dysuria, including test characteristics when known, are listed in Table 28.2. Note that no single element of the history and physical exam is very accurate. Elements of the history that suggest infection of the upper urinary tract (pyelonephritis) include fever, chills, abdominal pain, flank pain, and vomiting. However, in some studies, up to one-third of patients with only lower tract infections have fever or flank pain. Conversely, women with symptoms only suggestive of lower tract infection may have some degree of upper tract involvement.

Risk factors for upper tract involvement (i.e., occult pyelonephritis) include young or geriatric age, dysuria for more than 7 days, an immunosuppressing condition, an episode of acute pyelonephritis within the past year, known anatomic abnormality, a history of recurrent infections, and diabetes mellitus (3). "Red flags" for these more serious infections are summarized in Table 28.3.

Physical Examination

The physical examination in adults with dysuria should be focused, while in children it should be more comprehensive. You will need to obtain the patient's vital signs, palpate the mid and lower abdomen, and percuss the flanks of the patient. Tenderness over a flank or in the mid abdomen suggests upper tract disease; however, suprapubic tenderness with an uncomplicated lower tract infection is common. In men, the penis should be gently milked to elicit a urethral discharge, and a

TABLE 28.2 Key Elements of the History and Physical Examination for Dysuria

Diagnosis	Question or Maneuver	Sensitivity	Specificity	LR+	LR−
UTI					
	Nocturia	0.67	0.62	1.8	0.53
	Dysuria	0.80	0.50	1.6	0.40
	Urgency	0.39	0.71	1.3	0.86
	Frequency	0.87	0.32	1.3	0.41
	Offensive odor of urine	0.20	0.85	1.3	0.94
Pyelonephritis					
	Chills and rigors	0.32	0.87	2.5	0.78
	Fever	0.44	0.80	2.2	0.70
	Nausea and vomiting	0.24	0.84	1.5	0.90
	Flank pain	0.48	0.67	1.5	0.78

UTI, urinary tract infection.
Data are from References 75 and 76

rectal exam performed to feel for a tender or boggy prostate, as these findings suggest urethritis and prostatitis, respectively. You should also perform a vaginal examination on women who complain of vaginal discharge or irritation (see Chapter 34 for more on the management of vaginitis).

Laboratory Tests
COLLECTING A SPECIMEN

Adults and toilet-trained children can provide noncontaminated specimens by catching a midstream specimen of urine in a sterile container (the first few seconds of urine is not collected, as it can contain bacteria from the distal urethra). Giving the patient thorough instructions about cleansing the urethra and genitalia has been stressed in many textbooks, but controlled studies have not demonstrated any advantage to this practice (15, 16).

Catheterization is the most frequently used method for

obtaining urine specimens from infants and young children. This method has a high success rate of obtaining a noncontaminated specimen, and is safe (17). Suprapubic aspiration of the bladder can also be used, but is more invasive, requires more physician time, and is no more successful. A urine sample obtained by placing a plastic collection bag over a child's genitalia often provides confusing data, since contamination of the collected urine with bacteria from the skin is common. A culture from bagged urine is only useful if it shows no bacteria growth.

URINALYSIS

The urinalysis includes a dry reagent test strip (the dipstick) and microscopy of a centrifuged urine sample. The dipstick, which detects blood, nitrite, and leukocyte esterase in the urine, is simple to perform, and takes less than 5 minutes from sample collection to test result. The sensitivity, specificity, and likelihood ratios for dipstick and microscopic urinalysis are summarized in Table 28.4.

The leukocyte esterase (LE) test detects the presence of an esterase from white blood cells and has a 76% reported sensitivity for detecting UTI in a primary care setting (18). It is less sensitive in patients with only mild symptoms and more sensitive in patients with severe symptoms (19). False-positive results can occur because of contamination by vaginal leukocytes or leukocytes from chlamydial urethritis. Additionally, a false positive LE can be caused by high urine pH, high levels of urine glucose, and certain drugs in the urine including tetracycline, cephalexin, gentamicin, imipenem, or clavulanic acid (20).

Nitrite is found in the urine when dietary nitrates are excreted into the urine and converted to nitrite by bacteria. In a primary care setting only about 50% of patients with UTI will have a positive nitrite test (18). There are three reasons why the sensitivity of this test for UTI is not very high. Gram-positive and *Pseudomonas* species will not be detected with this urine test, because these bacteria do not convert urinary

TABLE 28.3 "Red Flags" for a Complicated Infection

- Male gender
- Prepubertal or geriatric age
- Symptoms for more than 7 days
- An immunosuppressing condition
- An episode of acute pyelonephritis within the past year
- Known anatomic abnormality
- Diabetes mellitus
- Fever
- Flank pain or tenderness

Adapted from Johnson JR, Stamm WE. Diagnosis and treatment of acute urinary tract infections. Infect Dis Clin North Am 1987;1(4): 773–791.

TABLE 28.4 Characteristics of Urine Tests for Primary Care Patients with Dysuria[1]

Test	Sensitivity	Specificity	LR+	LR−
Dipstick				
Leukocyte esterase (LE)	0.76	0.46	1.4	0.52
Nitrite	0.49	0.85	4.4	0.60
Either LE or nitrite	0.90	0.65	2.6	0.15
Sediment Microscopy				
1 bacterium/HPFb	0.95	0.85	6.3	0.06
10 bacteria/HPFb	0.85	0.99	85	0.15
5 WBC/HPFc	0.91	0.48	1.7	0.19
10 WBC/HPFb	0.82	0.65	2.3	0.28
5 RBC/HPFa	0.44	0.88	3.7	0.60

HPF, high power field; RBC, red blood count; WBC, white blood count.
[1] Bailey BL. Urinalysis predictive of urine culture results. J Fam Pract 1995;40:45–50.
[2] Deville WL, Yzermans JC, van Duijn NP, Bezemer PD, van der Windt DA, Bouter LM. The urine dipstick test useful to rule out infections. A meta-analysis of the accuracy. BMC Urol. 2004; 4:4.

nitrates to nitrites. Those gram-negative bacteria, including *E. coli*, that do convert nitrates to nitrites need several hours of contact with the urine to complete the conversion. Lastly, patients who excrete few nitrates into their urine, such as vegetarians, are especially likely to have a false negative result. While a negative nitrite test is not very helpful at ruling out UTI (LR- 0.6), a positive nitrite test in a person with dysuria is very suggestive of UTI (LR+ 3.3). Using the leukocyte esterase and nitrate in combination (the dipstick is considered positive if either test is positive and negative only if both tests are negative) is a better predictor of UTI than either test individually.

Blood is detected by a dipstick using the peroxidase-like activity of hemoglobin in the urine. False-positive reactions can occur from the peroxidase-like activity of myoglobin or the presence of bacteria that produce peroxidase. Many patients with UTI do not have blood in the urine, but when present is useful for ruling in the diagnosis.

Direct microscopy of the urinary sediment is used to look for white cells (pyuria), red cells (hematuria), bacteria (bacteriuria), and white cell casts. The sediment is prepared by centrifuging a 10 cc tube of freshly voided urine, decanting the urine, and then resuspending the sediment with the residual urine adhering to the inside of the tube. The microscopy results are influenced by how long the urine is allowed to sit after collection, the duration and speed of centrifugation, the technique used to decant the urine and resuspend the sediment, and the technique of the individual performing the microscopy.

Although the number of leukocytes per high-power field (400× magnification) in the resuspended urine sediment is commonly used to diagnose UTI, there is disagreement about how many leukocytes identify the presence of infection. Some authors have suggested that as few as 2 white blood cells per high-power field (WBC/hpf) can be used to identify infected urine, whereas others maintain that 5, 10, or even 15 WBC/

hpf are more appropriate cutpoints (21, 22). Instead of one rigid criterion, it is appropriate to use the number of WBC/hpf in combination with the patient's probability of UTI before testing (23). For example, in a woman with typical symptoms of UTI and a high probability of UTI, 2 WBC/hpf can be considered positive. In men and children with dysuria, who have a lower risk of UTI, a more stringent cutpoint of 5 WBC/hpf is appropriate to define a positive test. Finally, in a patient without any symptoms, you might use 10 to 15 WBC/hpf as a cut-off for diagnosing UTI. This Bayesian approach will reduce the number of incorrect diagnoses.

The presence of bacteria at high power (400×) is also suggestive of UTI. If no bacteria are found in the sediment, a UTI is ruled out (LR- 0.06), and if 10 or more bacteria are seen per high-power field, the infection is ruled in (LR+ 85). Intermediate bacterial counts are less helpful diagnostically. White cell casts can also be found in the urine sediment and are identified by their tube-like granular appearance. Their presence suggests inflammation within the kidney, with white blood cells collecting within the renal tubules. Infection is the primary cause of these casts, although interstitial nephritis can also produce them.

URINE CULTURE

The reference standard for the diagnosis of UTI is a "positive" urine culture meaning that a urine culture grows at least 100 colony-forming units (cfu) of a pathogenic bacteria per milliliter of urine (24, 25). The definition of a "positive" culture has changed over time. Formerly, growth of 100,000 cfu/mL was required before the culture was thought to indicate infection, but more recent studies demonstrated that a cut-off of 100,000 cfu/mL can miss about half of the women with infections. Low colony count infections do not seem to have any different spontaneous cure rate than high colony count infections (26). In fact, most low colony count infections will progress to high colony count infections if they are not treated.

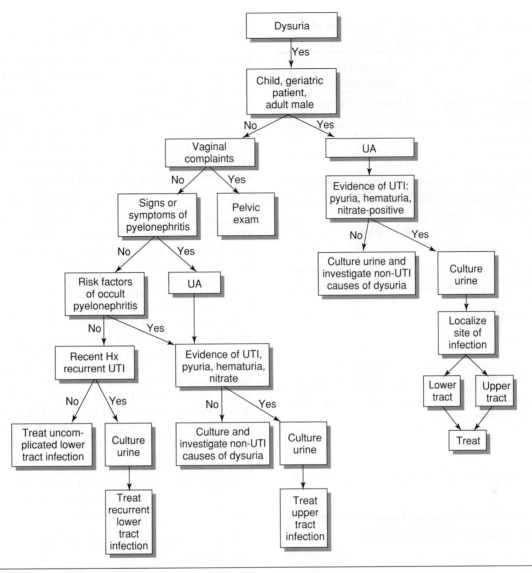

Figure 28.1. • **Algorithm for the management of dysuria.cm**

Urine cultures are useful to confirm the infection, identify the organism and its antibiotic susceptibilities, or confirm successful treatment. However, for a number of reasons, a culture is not typically part of the evaluation of a premenopausal woman with acute dysuria from what appears to be an uncomplicated lower tract infection. First, culture results are not available at the time you prescribe antibiotic therapy and frequently are still not available by the end of the treatment. Second, conventional culture is not a sensitive test for infection (25), and third, cultures have not been found to be highly predictive of the clinical outcome of antibiotic treatment in this group of patients (27). Because of these problems, urine cultures are not cost-effective in the routine care of UTI in healthy women (28). Cultures are necessary when evaluating dysuria in children, men, and older women, and in younger women who have either a significant probability of an upper tract infection, or infection with bacteria not likely to respond to first-line antibiotics.

MANAGEMENT

In managing a patient with UTI, you should tailor the treatment plan to the characteristics of your patient and his or her infection. An algorithm for management appears in Figure 28.1. Because UTI is very common in young, healthy women with dysuria, and because much of the required clinical data about women with dysuria can be collected over the telephone, some health providers and health care organizations manage suspected UTI in selected female patients without an office visit. A small randomized controlled trial found that telephone management was just as good as outpatient management for selected patients (29). A larger prospective study similarly found that this approach decreases laboratory use and overall costs while maintaining or improving the quality of care for patients with acute dysuria (30). This conclusion is also supported by a retrospective study of more than 4,000 women managed through telephone contact, in which only

be given orally if the patient is able to tolerate them (44). Fifteen percent of these patients will have bacteremia, so blood cultures should be obtained prior to starting parenteral antibiotics (38). Intravenous antibiotics should be continued until the patient has been afebrile for 24 hours; the patient can then be switched to an oral agent to complete the 7–14 days of therapy. It is not necessary to observe patients as inpatients for 24 hours after switching to oral antibiotics (46).

When patients do not improve after 72 hours of parenteral therapy, imaging is indicated to identify a perinephric abscess, an intrarenal abscess, an unrecognized anatomic abnormality, or ureteral obstruction; either sonography or computed tomography can be used to identify these complications. Abscess or obstruction is an indication for urologic consultation. Complicated infections should be treated for at least 21 days.

To confirm cure after clinical resolution of pyelonephritis, a follow-up culture should be obtained 2 to 4 weeks after the end of antibiotic treatment. Imaging of the urinary tract after successful treatment is not recommended except in women with more than one episode of pyelonephritis, a slow response to parenteral antibiotics, abnormalities on their follow-up urinalysis, or a history of childhood UTI without previous imaging

SPECIAL CONSIDERATIONS

Adult Men with UTIs

A more extensive evaluation is warranted in men with dysuria because they are more likely to have a complicated infection. As with women, men should be identified as having either an upper tract or a lower tract infection. Other causes of dysuria, including prostatitis (Chapter 31) and urethritis, need to be excluded as causes of urinary symptoms.

The initial choice of antibiotic for men with a suspected lower tract infection is typically a fluoroquinolone. Pretreatment culture is recommended, and antibiotic treatment should be continued for 7 to 10 days. Shorter-duration treatment is not well studied in men. Men with pyelonephritis can be treated as outpatients, with a fluoroquinolone, or in hospital with parenteral antibiotics if their symptoms are more severe. Those managed as outpatients should be treated for 14 days, whereas hospitalized patients should receive a total of 14 to 21 days of antibiotic therapy. After a second lower tract infection or a single episode of pyelonephritis, the adult male patient should undergo imaging to identify an anatomic abnormality or nephrolithiasis. Ultrasonography and plain abdominal radiograph appear to be comparable to intravenous pyelogram (IVP) as the initial imaging study (47).

UTIs in Older Adults

In older patients UTI can present without urinary symptoms but as mental status changes, tachypnea, tachycardia, fever, gait instability, or falls. These symptoms are not specific and can be caused by many other conditions, including other infections, hypoxia, an adverse reaction to medications, or metabolic abnormalities. Diagnosis of UTI in this age group is challenging because the symptoms are nonspecific, and asymptomatic bacteriuria is common, affecting 10% of elderly men and 20% of elderly women (48).

Lower tract UTI in nonfrail elderly women should be treated for at least 3 days (49). Although a duration of 7 to 14 days is traditionally recommended for older women, a recent randomized trial in healthy older women found that 3 days was adequate (50). Urine culture should be obtained before treatment because the organism or its antibiotic sensitivity is not as predictable as in younger women. Pending the culture results, these patients can be started on a fluoroquinolone or TMP/SMX. Older patients with upper tract infections should be treated using the same guidelines given for men in the preceding section.

Some elderly women get repeated UTIs. If these are from documented relapses occurring after short-course therapy, subsequent infections should be treated for 14 days with an oral antibiotic, which is selected based on the culture and susceptibility testing. After frequent relapses the patient should be evaluated for undiagnosed nephrolithiasis and for an abnormally large residual volume after voiding. If one of these predisposing problems is not found, a trial of topical estrogens can be tried to reduce the frequency of UTI. A nightly application of estrogen cream to the vaginal area for 2 weeks followed by biweekly application diminishes vaginal colonization by gram-negative uropathogens and typically reduces episodes of symptomatic UTI (50).

UTIs in Children

Approximately 5% to 8% of girls and 1% to 2% of boys have at least one symptomatic UTI during childhood (51). As with adults, children can be at increased risk for UTI because of perineal colonization by uropathogens or urine stasis in the bladder. Young children are prone to perineal colonization because of fecal incontinence. Several studies have also shown that noncircumcised male infants are at a higher risk for UTIs compared to their circumcised peers, perhaps because they are more likely to harbor E. coli on their genitalia (52). Older children can be prone to urine stasis because of infrequent voiding. Vesicoureteral reflux can also be responsible for incomplete bladder emptying and places children of all age groups at increased risk for UTI.

In young children, UTI is of particular concern due to the 20% incidence of bacteremia associated with these infections as well as the possibility of progressive renal damage as a result of recurrent infection. There remains many unanswered questions about UTI in young children, and these questions are important areas of research. Between 30% and 50% of young children with UTI will have vesico-ureteral reflux (53). This reflux places young children at high risk for recurrent upper tract infections and progressive renal scarring from lower tract infection; progressive scarring is thought to be strongly linked with subsequent development of hypertension and renal failure. Although this chain of events is debated, it is central to current recommendations about the evaluation and treatment of young children with possible UTI.

CLINICAL EVALUATION

You should always perform a thorough history and physical in a child with suspected UTI to exclude other causes of the symptoms. In addition, children can have UTI without the dysuria or other urinary symptoms typically seen in adults. The presence of a UTI should always be considered in infants and young children 2 months to 2 years of age with unexplained fever (54). Neonates with UTI might present only with late-onset jaundice, poor weight gain, irritability, or hypothermia. In infants, diarrhea, vomiting, or failure to thrive might be the only presenting complaint (55). A recent study found that among girls under the age of 2 presenting to the emergency department with fever, approximately 5% had a culture positive UTI as the cause. White race, age <12 months, temperature >39°C, absence of another potential source of fever, and fever for 2 days or longer were independent predictors of UTI. Not having at least two of these predictors made UTI unlikely (LR- 0.16) (56).

Classic urinary symptoms that typify UTI in adults are relatively uncommon in preschool children, with only 10% of UTIs presenting with these complaints. In school-age children, UTI can present with dysuria, but it can also present as abdominal pain or urinary incontinence. Urethral irritation from bubble bath irritation, vaginitis, pin worms, and trauma resulting from masturbation or sexual abuse are more common causes of dysuria in children than is UTI.

LABORATORY TESTS

Urinalysis is not a sensitive test for UTI in infants and young children; the false negative rate is approximately 50% (57). Nor is this test specific for UTI; young children can develop pyuria after viral immunization or with nonurinary foci of infection. Therefore, urine culture is a routine part of the evaluation of infants and young children with possible UTI, regardless of the result of the urinalysis. In older children, the dipstick and microscopic urinalyses are useful tests for assessing infection and have similar sensitivity and specificity as those reported in adults (see Table 28.4).

MANAGEMENT

After 2 months of age, children with lower tract UTI are treated along the same general guidelines as UTIs in men. When symptoms are mild and the urinalysis suggests an infection, 7 to 14 days of oral antibiotics should be prescribed after a urine sample is obtained for culture. However, there is growing evidence that 3 days of therapy are as effective as the longer courses, with fewer adverse events associated with treatment (58). TMP/SMX, amoxicillin/clavulanate, nitrofurantoin, or a third-generation cephalosporin are reasonable first choices for treating these infections. The fluoroquinolones have not been routinely used in children because of their potential toxicity to growing cartilage, although large studies have not confirmed this toxicity (59) (see Table 28.6).

All children less than 2 months of age with UTI need hospitalization and parenteral antibiotics. When a child is past infancy and has the manifestations of an upper tract infection, outpatient therapy is possible as long as the child appears nontoxic, is tolerating oral fluids, does not have a history of severe reflux, and whose follow-up is assured (60). Use of an oral third-generation cephalosporin (e.g., cefixime) as the initial treatment of UTI in nonhospitalized febrile children has been the best studied. Optimal duration of treatment is less well defined. Generally 14 days is used, although some research suggests shorter treatments might be adequate (61). If hospitalization is required because of the age of the child (<2 months old) or the severity of the infection, parenteral ampicillin and gentamicin or a third-generation cephalosporin should be used as initial coverage, with therapy later adjusted based on the

urine culture and sensitivity results. Single daily dosing of gentamicin is safe and effective.

A urine culture should be obtained after completion of therapy in children to confirm successful treatment of the infection. Renal function should also be evaluated by measuring the serum creatinine. Imaging studies to detect anatomic or functional abnormalities, such as vesicoureteral reflux, are indicated for children with UTI with any of the following: any UTI in a child <2 years of age, recurrent lower tract infections in children >2 years of age, or a single episode of pyelonephritis in children >2 years of age. If imaging is indicated, then it is recommended that prophylactic antibiotics be administered pending the test result (53).

Although there are many different recommendations about imaging based on expert opinion, few randomized studies have been done (62). Behind all the recommendations for imaging lies the reasoning that early detection of urologic abnormalities will lead to interventions that will prevent chronic renal damage. The different recommendations are not totally consistent, and researchers have found that imaging is inconsistently used in children. In addition, a recent study has questioned whether any imaging should routinely be undertaken (63).

With this uncertain background some general statements about imaging can be made. Renal sonography can be used to detect urinary tract obstruction. When significant abnormalities are seen on the sonogram, additional information can be obtained using an IVP. Acute pyelonephritis can be confirmed by a technetium-99m dimercaptosuccinic acid (DMSA) renal scan, and renal scarring can be demonstrated if DMSA is used in follow-up. Voiding cystourethrography can be used to define urethral and bladder anatomy, and to assess vesicoureteral reflux. This procedure can be undertaken as soon as it is convenient following the infection (53). Some physicians routinely delay imaging for 3 to 6 weeks after successful treatment of the infection to allow inflammation-related changes to abate, but these residual changes are not clinically significant (64).

Catheter-Associated UTI

Catheter-associated UTI is a common source of iatrogenic gram-negative bacteremia because catheters are frequently used in patients with diminished resistance to infection and provide an easy portal of entry for bacteria. Catheter-related infections can be prevented by removing the urinary catheter as soon as possible, or by not inserting one in the first place. Prophylactic antibiotics may reduce the risk of catheter-related infections in patients who have only a short-term need for a catheter, such as postoperative patients (65, 66) but prophylaxis is not routinely used because of the concern about producing resistant organisms (67).

Prophylaxis does not work with long-term placement of a catheter; almost all catheterized patients will develop bacteriuria within 30 days. Maintaining a closed drainage system, and adhering to appropriate catheter care techniques will limit infection and complications in the short run. But as the duration of catheterization is the principal determinant of infection with long-term indwelling catheters, it is not clear that any interventions can decrease the prevalence of bacteriuria in this setting. Intermittent catheterization will markedly reduce the risk of UTI and is preferable to a chronic, indwelling catheter.

However, many people using intermittent catheterization will develop UTI, and most will develop asymptomatic bacteriuria (68).

Many catheter-associated infections occur in nursing homes because 5% to 10% of residents in these institutions have long-term indwelling catheters. Nearly all of these patients are bacteriuric and will have colonization with multiple organisms. Catheter flushing or daily perineal care does not prevent infection. Patients should be cultured and treated only when they become symptomatic. Antibiotic therapy of culture positive but otherwise asymptomatic patients will only enhance the emergence of resistance in the pathogens that cause urinary infections. Evaluation is a challenge because symptoms may only consist of low-grade fever, decreased appetite, weight loss, increased confusion, or problems with falling.

When the infection is mild, treatment with an oral fluoroquinolone is usually successful, and hospitalization is not necessary. The catheter should be replaced if it has been in place for more than 2 weeks. Bacteria adhere to the surface of the urinary catheters and create a biofilm, which prevents antibiotics from reaching the embedded bacteria. Although there are no studies that define the optimal duration of therapy, 5 to 7 days of therapy are often used. Parenteral antibiotics are indicated for moderately severe infections. In all cases of catheter-associated UTI, it is important to remember that most patients with catheters are elderly or medically compromised, and are usually less able to tolerate an infection than young adults.

Asymptomatic Bacteriuria

Asymptomatic bacteriuria can occur in all age groups but screening for this condition is only recommended in several specific situations. The U.S. Preventive Services Task Force recommends that all pregnant women be screened with a urine culture at 12 to 16 weeks of gestation. The American College of Obstetrics and Gynecology also recommends universal screening at the first prenatal visit (69). Screening in pregnancy is important because 5%–10% of women will have asymptomatic bacteriuria, and these women have a 20- to 30-fold increased risk of developing pyelonephritis during pregnancy compared with women without bacteriuria. Antibiotic treatment reduces this risk of pyelonephritis from 20%–35% to 1%–4% (70). Pregnant women need to be screened by urine culture because the urinalysis alone will miss 25% to 50% of women with asymptomatic bacteriuria (71).

An oral cephalosporin, nitrofurantoin, or TMP/SMX can be used for treatment, although the latter is avoided at term because of the concern that sulfonamides increase the risk of neonatal kernicterus. The duration of antibiotic therapy for asymptomatic bacteriuria is controversial but 3 to 7 days of therapy are widely used (72). Treatment should be followed by culture to confirm successful clearing of bacteriuria. Women with asymptomatic bacteriuria at any point during pregnancy have an increased risk of redeveloping this condition after treatment, and should be repeatedly screened by urine culture. Antibiotic prophylaxis is an option for women who develop recurrent asymptomatic bacteriuria or pyelonephritis during pregnancy.

Screening for asymptomatic bacteriuria is also recommended in children with recurrent UTI (73). The child should bring a urine sample for culture at increasing intervals (e.g.,

1 month, 3 months, 6 months, 12 months, and then yearly) because recurrent infection is common. Alternatively, home nitrite testing of first morning urine samples is an effective way to identify recurrent bacteriuria before the child becomes symptomatic.

Asymptomatic bacteriuria is also common in elderly patients, occurring in 10% of men and 20% of women. A higher prevalence of asymptomatic bacteriuria is found in nursing homes. Although this finding is a marker of poor health and a risk factor for death, there is good evidence that treatment of this condition with antibiotics does not improve health (74). Although the bacteriuria can be eradicated by the use of antibiotics, it tends to recur quickly. Screening is therefore not recommended in this group.

CASE DISCUSSION

The presence of these urinary symptoms in the absence of vaginal complaints makes UTI highly likely in this patient. You should identify whether the patient has risk factors that should warn you of a possible complicated UTI (see Table 28.3). For an uncomplicated UTI in a healthy woman, only limited laboratory investigation, if any, is warranted. Prior to obtaining any tests, the probability of UTI in this patient with dysuria, if she reports frequency but has no vaginal symptoms, is approximately 90%. When empiric therapy is not chosen, a reasonable strategy is to perform a dipstick evaluation of the urine. If this test is positive for blood, leukocyte esterase, or nitrite, you could presume the presence of UTI. If all results are negative, you can perform a microscopic examination of the centrifuged sediment. If the patient has an uncomplicated lower tract infection, she should be treated with 3 days of TMP/SMX (one double-strength tablet, twice daily). Ciprofloxacin 250 mg by mouth, twice a day for 3 days is an option if resistance to TMP/SMX is over 20% in your area. No follow up is needed unless symptoms do not resolve. If the patient is thought to be at risk for having a complicated UTI (despite having symptoms suggestive of only a lower tract infection), she should have a urine culture, receive 7 days of treatment, and be followed to confirm cure.

REFERENCES

1. Stamm WE, Hooton TM. Management of urinary tract infections in adults. N Engl J Med. 1993;329(18):1328–1334.
2. Patton JP, Nash DB, Abrutyn E. Urinary tract infection: economic considerations. Med Clin North Am. 1991;75(2):495–513.
3. Johnson JR, Stamm WE. Diagnosis and treatment of acute urinary tract infections. Infect Dis Clin North Am.1987;1(4):773–791.
4. Wilkie ME, Almond MK, Marsh FP. Diagnosis and management of urinary tract infection in adults. BMJ. 1992;305:1137–1141.
5. Todd JK. Management of urinary tract infections: Children are different. Pediatr Rev. 1996;16(5):190–196.
6. Gittes RF, Nakamura RM. Female urethral syndrome. A female prostatitis? West J Med. 1996;164:435–438.
7. Hooton TM, Scholes D, Hughes JP, et al. A prospective study of risk factors for symptomatic urinary tract infection in young women. N Engl J Med. 1996;335:468–474.
8. Hooton TM, Stapleton AE, Roberts PL, Winter C, Scholes

D, Bavendam T, Stamm WE. Perineal anatomy and urine-voiding characteristics of young women with and without recurrent urinary tract infections. Clin Infect Dis. 1999;29: 1600–1601.

9. Scholes D, Hooton TM, Roberts PL, Stapleton AE, Gupta K, Stamm WE. Risk factors for recurrent urinary tract infection in young women. J Infect Dis. 2000;182:1177–1182.

10. Scholes D, Hooton TM, Roberts PL, Gupta K, Stapleton AE, Stamm WE. Risk factors associated with acute pyelonephritis in healthy women. Ann Intern Med. 2005;142(1):20–27.

11. Berg AO, Heidrich FE, Fihn SD, et al. Establishing the cause of genitourinary symptoms in women in a family practice. JAMA. 1984;251(5):620–625.

12. Komaroff AL, Pass TM, McCue JD, Cohen AB, Hendricks TM, Friedland G. Management strategies for urinary and vaginal infections. Arch Intern Med. 1978;138:1069–1073.

13. Bent S, Nallamothu BK, Simel DL, Fihn SD, Saint S. Does this woman have an acute uncomplicated urinary tract infection? JAMA. 2002;287(20):2701–2710.

14. Gupta K, Hooton TM, Roberts PL, Stamm WE. Patient-initiated treatment of uncomplicated recurrent urinary tract infections in young women. Ann Intern Med. 2001;135(1): 9–16.

15. Bradbury SM. Collection of urine specimens in general practice: to clean or not to clean? J R Coll Gen Pract. 1988;38(313): 363–365.

16. Lifshitz E, Kramer L. Outpatient urine culture: does collection technique matter? Arch Intern Med. 2000;160: 2537–2540.

17. Pollack CV Jr., Pollack ES. Suprapubic bladder aspiration versus urethral catheterization in ill infants: success, efficiency and complication rates. Ann Emerg Med. 1994;23:225–230.

18. Deville WL, Yzermans JC, van Duijn NP, Bezemer PD, van der Windt DA, Bouter LM. The urine dipstick test useful to rule out infections. A meta-analysis of the accuracy. BMC Urol. 2004;4:4.

19. Lachs MS, Nachamkin I, Edelstein PH, Goldman J, Feinstein AR, Schwartz JS. Spectrum bias in the evaluation of diagnostic tests: lessons from the rapid dipstick test for urinary tract infection. Ann Intern Med. 1992;117:135–140.

20. Beer JH, Vogt A, Neftel K, Cottagnoud P. False-positive results for leucocytes in urine dipstick test with common antibiotics. BMJ. 1996;313:25.

21. Alwall N. Pyuria: Deposit in high-power microscopic field—WBC/HPF versus WBC/mm3 in counting chamber. Acta Med Scand. 1973;194:537–540.

22. Wigton RS, Hoellerich VL, Ornato JP, Leu V, Mazzotta LA, Cheng IC. Use of clinical findings in the diagnosis of urinary tract infection in women. Arch Intern Med. 1985;145: 2222–2227.

23. Bergus GR. When is a test "positive"? The use of decision analysis to optimize test interpretation. Fam Med. 1993;25: 656–660.

24. Latham RH, Wong ES, Larson A, Coyle M, Stamm WE. Laboratory diagnosis of urinary tract infection in ambulatory women. JAMA. 1985;254:3333–3336.

25. Stamm WE, Counts GW, Running KR, Fihn S, Turck M, Holmes KK. Diagnosis of coliform infection in acutely dysuric women. N Engl J Med. 1982;307:463–468.

26. Arav-Boger R, Leibovici L, Danon YL. Urinary tract infections with low and high colony counts in young women. Spontaneous remission and single-dose vs multiple-day treatment. Arch Intern Med. 1994;154:300–304.

27. Richards D, Toop L, Chambers S, Fletcher L. Response to antibiotics of women with symptoms of urinary tract infection but negative dipstick urine test results: double blind randomised controlled trial. BMJ. 2005;331(7509):143.

28. Carlson KJ, Mulley AG. Management of acute dysuria. Ann Intern Med. 1985;102:244–249.

29. Barry HC, Hickner J, Ebell MH. A randomized controlled trial of telephone management of suspected urinary track infections in women. J Fam Pract. 2001;50:589–594.

30. Saint S, Scholes D, Fihn SD, Farrell RG, Stamm WE. The effectiveness of a clinical practice guideline for the management of presumed uncomplicated urinary tract infection in women. Am J Med. 1999;106:636–641.

31. Vinson DR, Quesenberry CP Jr. The safety of telephone management of presumed cystitis in women. Arch Intern Med. 2004;164(9):1026–1029.

32. Christiaens TC, De Meyere M, Verschraegen G, Peersman W, Heytens S, De Maeseneer JM. Randomised controlled trial of nitrofurantoin versus placebo in the treatment of uncomplicated urinary tract infection in adult women. Br J Gen Pract. 2002;52(482):729–734.

33. Jepson RG, Mihaljevic L, Craig J. Cranberries for treating urinary tract infections. CRG. Cochrane Database Syst Rev. 2000;(2):CD001322.

34. Hooton TM, Scholes D, Gupta K, Stapleton AE, Roberts PL, Stamm WE. Amoxicillin-clavulanate vs ciprofloxacin for the treatment of uncomplicated cystitis in women: a randomized trial. JAMA. 2005;293(8):949–955.

35. Milo G, Katchman EA, Paul M, Christiaens T, Baerheim A, Leibovici L. Duration of antibacterial treatment for uncomplicated urinary tract infection in women. Cochrane Database Syst Rev. 2005;2:CD004682.

36. Hooton TM, Winter C, Tiu F, Stamm WE. Randomized comparative trial and cost analysis of 3-day antimicrobial regimens for treatment of acute cystitis in women. JAMA. 1995; 273(1):41–45.

37. Ernst EJ, Ernst ME, Hoehns JD, Bergus GR. Women's quality of life is decreased by acute cystitis and antibiotic adverse effects associated with treatment. Health Qual Life Outcomes. 2005;3(1):45.

38. Gupta K, Hooton TM, Stamm WE. Increasing antimicrobial resistance and the management of uncomplicated community-acquired urinary tract infections. Ann Intern Med. 2001; 135(1):41–50.

39. Fihn SD, Johnson C, Roberts PL, Running K, Stamm WE. Trimethoprim-sulfamethoxazole for acute dysuria in women: a single-dose or 10-day course. Ann Intern Med. 1988;108:350–357.

40. Ronald AR, Boutros P, Mourtada H. Bacteriuria localization and response to single-dose therapy in women. JAMA. 1976; 235:1854–1856.

41. Kontiokari T, Sundqvist K, M Nuutinen M, et al. Randomised trial of cranberry-lingonberry juice and Lactobacillus GG drink for the prevention of urinary tract infections in women. BMJ. 2001;322 1571–1575.

42. Eckford SD, Keane DP, Lamond E, Jackson SR, Abrams P. Hydration monitoring in the prevention of recurrent idiopathic urinary tract infections in pre-menopausal women. Br J Urol. 1995;76(1):90–93.

43. Pinson AG, Philbrick JT, Lindbeck GH, Schorling JB. Oral antibiotic therapy for acute pyelonephritis: a methodologic review of the literature. J Gen Intern Med. 1992;7:544–553.

44. Mombelli G, Pezzoli R, Pinoja-Lutz G, Monotti R, Marone C, Franciolli M. Oral vs intravenous ciprofloxacin in the initial empirical management of severe pyelonephritis or complicated urinary tract infections: a prospective randomized clinical trial. Arch Intern Med. 1999;159:53–58.

45. Talan DA, Stamm WE, Hooton TM, Moran GJ, Burke T, Iravani A, et al. Comparison of ciprofloxacin (7 days) and trimethoprim-sulfamethoxazole (14 days) for acute uncom-

plicated pyelonephritis in women: a randomized trial. JAMA. 2000;283:1583–1590.

46. Caceres VM, Stange KC, Kikano EG, Zyzanski SJ. The clinical utility of a day of hospital observation after switching from intravenous to oral antibiotic therapy in the treatment of pyelonephritis. J Fam Pract. 1994;39:337–340.

47. Andrews SJ, Brooks PT, Hanbury DC, et al. Ultrasonography and abdominal radiography versus intravenous urography in investigation of urinary tract infection in men: prospective incident cohort study. BMJ. 2002;324(7335):454–456.

48. Boscia JA, Kobasa WD, Knight RA, Abrutyn E, Levison ME, Kaye D. Epidemiology of bacteriuria in an elderly ambulatory population. Am J Med. 1986;80(2):208–214.

49. Vogel T, Verreault R, Gourdeau M, Morin M, Grenier-Gosselin L, Rochette L. Optimal duration of antibiotic therapy for uncomplicated urinary tract infection in older women: a double-blind randomized controlled trial. CMAJ. 2004;170(4):469–473.

50. Cardozo L, Lose G, McClish D, Versi E, de Koning Gans H. A systematic review of estrogens for recurrent urinary tract infections: third report of the hormones and urogenital therapy (HUT) committee. Int Urogynecol J Pelvic Floor Dysfunct. 2001;12(1):15–20.

51. Stark H. Urinary tract infections in girls: the cost-effectiveness of currently recommended investigative routines. Pediatr Nephrol. 1997;11(2):174–177;discussion 180–181.

52. Wiswell TE, Roscelli JD. Corroborative evidence for the decreased incidence of urinary tract infections in circumcised male infants. Pediatrics. 1986;78(1):96–99.

53. Downs SM. Technical report: urinary tract infections in febrile infants and young children. The Urinary Tract Subcommittee of the American Academy of Pediatrics Committee on Quality Improvement. Pediatrics. 1999;103:e54.

54. American Academy of Pediatrics. Committee on Quality Improvement. Subcommittee on Urinary Tract Infection. Practice parameter: the diagnosis, treatment, and evaluation of the initial urinary tract infection in febrile infants and young children. Pediatrics. 1999;103:843–852.

55. Edelmann CM Jr, Ogwo JE, Fine BP, Martinez A. The prevalence of bacteriuria in full-term and premature newborn infants. J Pediatr. 1973;82:125–132.

56. Gorelick MH, Shaw KN. Clinical decision rule to identify febrile young girls at risk for urinary tract infection. Arch Pediatr Adolesc Med. 2000;154(4):386–390.

57. Crain EF, Gershel JC. Urinary tract infections in febrile infants younger than 8 weeks of age. Pediatrics. 1990;86(3):363–367.

58. Michael M, Hodson EM, Craig JC, Martin S, Moyer VA. Short compared with standard duration of antibiotic treatment for urinary tract infection: a systematic review of randomised controlled trials. Arch Dis Child. 2002;87(2):118–123.

59. Sabharwal V, Marchant CD. Fluoroquinolone use in children. Pediatr Infect Dis J. 2006;25(3):257–258.

60. Bloomfield P, Hodson EM, Craig JC. Antibiotics for acute pyelonephritis in children. Cochrane Database Syst Rev. 2005; 1:CD003772.

61. Michael M, Hodson EM, Craig JC, Martin S, Moyer VA. Short versus standard duration oral antibiotic therapy for acute urinary tract infection in children. Cochrane Database Syst Rev. 2003;1:CD003966.

62. Dick PT, Feldman W. Routine diagnostic imaging for childhood urinary tract infections: a systematic over-view. J Pediatr. 1996;128:15–22.

63. Hoberman A, Charron M, Hickey RW, Baskin M, Kearney DH, Wald ER. Imaging studies after a first febrile urinary tract infection in young children. N Engl J Med. 2003;348(3): 195–202.

64. McDonald A, Scranton M, Gillespie R, Mahajan V, Edwards GA. Voiding cystourethrograms and urinary tract infections: how long to wait? Pediatrics. 2000;105(4):E50.

65. Niel-Weise BS, van den Broek PJ. Antibiotic policies for short-term catheter bladder drainage in adults. Cochrane Database Syst Rev. 2005;3:CD005428.

66. Saint S, Lipsky BA. Preventing catheter-related bacteriuria: should we? Can we? How? Arch Intern Med. 1999;159: 800–808.

67. Rutschmann OT, Zwahlen A. Use of norfloxacin for prevention of symptomatic urinary tract infection in chronically catheterized patients. Eur J Clin Microbiol Infect Dis. 1995; 14(5):441–444.

68. Bakke A, Digranes A, Hoisaeter PA. Physical predictors of infection in patients treated with clean intermittent catheterization: a prospective 7-year study. Br J Urol. 1997;79(1): 85–90.

69. The American Academy of Obstetricians and Gynecologists (ACOG). Antimicrobial therapy for obstetric patients. ACOG Educational Bulletin. March 1998, Number 245.

70. Smaill, F. Antibiotics for asymptomatic bacteriuria in pregnancy. Cochrane Pregnancy and Childbirth Group Cochrane Database Syst Rev. 2005;4.

71. Bachman JW, Heise RH, Naessens JM, Timmerman MG. A study of various tests to detect asymptomatic urinary tract infections in an obstetric population. JAMA. 1993;270(16): 1971–1974.

72. Villar J, Widmer M, Lydon-Rochelle MT, Gülmezoglu AM, Roganti A. Duration of treatment for asymptomatic bacteriuria during pregnancy. Cochrane Database Syst Rev. 2006; 2.

73. Kemper KJ, Avner ED. The case against screening urinalyses for asymptomatic bacteriuria in children. Am J Dis Child. 1992;146:343–346.

74. Abrutyn E, Mossey J, Berlin JA, et al. Does asymptomatic bacteriuria predict mortality and does antimicrobial treatment reduce mortality in elderly ambulatory women? Ann Intern Med. 1994;120:827–833.

75. Dobbs FF, Fleming DM. A simple scoring system for evaluating symptoms, history and urine dipstick testing in the diagnosis of urinary tract infection. J R Coll Gen Pract. 1987;37: 100–104.

76. Österberg E, Aspevall O, Grillner L, Persson E. Young women with symptoms of urinary infection. Prevalence and diagnosis of chlamydial infection and evaluation of rapid screening of bacteriuria. Scand J Prim Health Care. 1996;14: 43–49.

77. Bailey BL. Urinalysis predictive of urine culture results. J Fam Pract. 1995;40:45–50.

CHAPTER 29

Menstrual Syndromes

Elizabeth A. Burns and Louise Parent-Stevens

Menstrual complaints, in general, are common and concerning to women. In a recent study of women in Scotland who were referred to hospital-based gynecology clinics for menstrual issues, the top three complaints were period-type pain with periods (33%), mood changes around periods (32.8%), and the amount of menstrual flow being more than it used to be (29.1%). Other concerns included periods persisting for too many days (25.3%), interrupting daily life (24.3%), feeling unwell/tired (23.4%), experiencing pain before the period (17.5%), complaints associated with hygiene, and concern that something serious might be wrong (1).

These problems present throughout the reproductive years and should be evaluated with care. Physicians should keep in mind that adolescents may present with a complaint of menstrual problems, but other issues, such as contraception, undesired pregnancy, sexually transmitted infection, or sexual assault may be the real reason for the visit (2). A careful history, respecting the privacy of the patient and issues of confidentiality, will enable a patient to tell her story and her concerns accurately.

Three of the most common syndromes related to menstruation will be covered in this chapter. Dysmenorrhea, which may afflict up to 60% of menstruating women (3), can be mild or extremely debilitating and concerning. Premenstrual symptoms affect most women, but the premenstrual syndrome (PMS) affects approximately 30% of women and the premenstrual dysphoric disorder (PMDD) fewer still (4). Abnormal uterine bleeding is a presenting complaint in 20% of gynecology visits and accounts for approximately 25% of gynecologic procedures (5).

Dysmenorrhea

CASE 1

Ms. J. is a 19-year-old African-American woman who relates a 5-year history of severe cramps at the onset of her menses. The pain is so severe that she regularly misses 2 to 3 days of university classes per month; she missed the same number of days while attending high school. Since her menarche at age 10, her menses have been regular and occur every 29 days with a flow of 6 days. The first 2 days of her menses are very heavy with passage of several quarter-sized clots, and during the remaining 4 days she has a moderate flow that decreases to only spotting by day

5. She describes the pain as very intense, colicky in nature, and a level 9 out of 10 on days 1 and 2.

Upon further questioning, she informs you that she has moderate cramping that begins the day before her period starts. She has tried acetaminophen in the past with poor resolution of her symptoms. Her basic health history is otherwise unremarkable. She is quite concerned about the source of her pelvic pain and does not want to continue missing important class and lab time. She is also very active in sports (volleyball and basketball varsity teams) and wants to remain active all month.

She has been sexually active since age 16, has had one sexual partner (her current boyfriend), and is G_0P_0. They use condoms and she has not had any sexually transmitted infections (STIs). Her affect in the office is appropriate and pleasant, and a physical examination (including a pelvic exam) is normal. Because she had a Pap smear 3 months ago, you do not repeat the study.

CLINICAL QUESTIONS

1. What is an appropriate laboratory and radiologic evaluation?
2. What is the best course of treatment for this condition?

Dysmenorrhea, defined as painful menstrual periods, can be classified into primary and secondary types. Primary dysmenorrhea, the more common presentation, is menstrual pain in a patient with normal pelvic anatomy and no underlying pathology. It has a usual onset between menarche and 20 years of age. Pain typically begins 24–36 hours prior to the onset of menses and can continue for the first 3 days of menstruation. The pain is cyclical and often described as crampy. Associated symptoms may include headache, nausea, inner thigh pain, and lower back pain. Secondary dysmenorrhea is associated with underlying pelvic pathology and often has its onset after age 20. The pain of secondary dysmenorrhea is usually progressive with age and is not always synchronous with menses.

PATHOPHYSIOLOGY

The pathophysiology of primary dysmenorrhea is linked to increased prostaglandin (PG) activity in the uterus, which causes uterine contractions and ischemia (6). Both PGF2α and PGE2 are produced by the endometrium during ovulatory cycles. PGF2α mediates pain sensations and simulates smooth muscle contractions and PGE2 is a vasodilator that also inhibits platelet aggregation. Studies have also shown that women with primary dysmenorrhea secrete an increased amount of vasopression, which causes myometrial hyperactivity and vasoconstriction, resulting in uterine ischemia and pain (7, 8).

The pathophysiology of secondary dysmenorrhea varies with the underlying cause. The differential diagnosis for secondary dysmenorrhea is shown in Table 29.1. The etiology in an individual patient depends on her age, history, and physical examination findings.

CLINICAL EVALUATION

The evaluation of a woman with dysmenorrhea should focus on her age, sexual history, clinical presentation, as well as her physical examination. Some patients, especially adolescents, may be reluctant to discuss their sexuality with a health care provider. It is important that patients, including adolescents,

TABLE 29.1 Differential Diagnosis of Menstrual Problems

Category	Diagnosis	Frequency in Primary Care
Primary Dysmenorrhea		Very common
Secondary Dysmenorrhea	Cervical stenosis	Common
	Cervical polyps	Common
	Ovarian cysts	Common
	Pelvic inflammatory disease	Common
	Endometriosis	Common
	Leiomyomas/fibroids	Common
	Intrauterine device complications	Uncommon
	Endometrial cancer	Uncommon
	Imperforate hymen	Rare
	Uterine synechiae	Rare
	Tubo-ovarian abscess	Rare
Premenstrual syndrome		Common
	Major depressive and anxiety disorders	Common
	Chronic medical conditions (e.g., diabetes, thyroid disease, autoimmune disorders)	Common
	Oral contraceptive use	Common
	Substance abuse	Uncommon
	Eating disorders	Uncommon
	Personality disorders	Rare
Abnormal uterine bleeding		Common
	Anovulatory bleeding	Common
	Hormonal medication use	Common
	Intrauterine pregnancy	Common
	Spontaneous abortion	Common
	Ectopic pregnancy	Uncommon
	Molar pregnancy	Rare
	Infections	Uncommon
	Trauma, foreign body	Rare
	Thyroid disease	Fairly common
	Coagulopathies, blood dyscrasias	Uncommon
	Medication (non-hormonal) use	Uncommon
	Systemic disease (adrenal, hepatic, renal)	Rare
	Cervical, uterine cancer	Uncommon
	Vaginal, vulvar cancer	Rare

be questioned in a comfortable and private setting. If legally and ethically possible (e.g., patient is not engaging in dangerous or life-threatening behavior) patient confidentiality should be maintained.

History

The initial evaluation of dysmenorrhea should include a complete menstrual history from menarche, including the type of symptoms experienced, the age of onset, the timing of symptoms in relationship to her menstrual cycle, and the severity and duration of symptoms. A sexual history should be obtained from all women. In a woman with mild to moderate cramps that began before age 20, which occur up to 48 hours before the onset of menses, and in the presence of a normal pelvic and abdominal exam, the most likely diagnosis is primary dysmenorrhea. New onset of pain after age 20 or pelvic pain at times other than the menstrual cycle requires further evaluation for a secondary cause of dysmenorrhea.

Endometriosis, a common cause of secondary dysmenorrhea, should be considered if the patient has pain at the time of ovulation or risk factors for endometriosis, including early menarche, heavy menses, nulliparity or a family history of endometriosis (9). The presence of back pain and diarrhea is suggestive of endometrial implants on the bowel.

A diagnosis of cervical stenosis should be considered in patients with a history of multiple colopscopies and surgical (including cryosurgical) treatments of the cervix. Women who have never had menses and present with severe pelvic pain should be evaluated for imperforate hymen.

Any sexually active woman who presents with pelvic pain, with or without vaginal discharge, should be evaluated for pelvic inflammatory disease (PID). Pelvic pain accompanied by fever, chills or symptoms of systemic illness may be indicative of PID or tubo-ovarian abscess.

Cervical stenosis, leiomyomas and endometrial cancer should be considered in women who are perimenopausal, menopausal or postmenopausal. In a postmenopausal woman with vaginal bleeding, with or without accompanying pain, endometrial cancer must be ruled out. (See Tables 29.2 and 29.3)

Physical Examination

The physical examination for the assessment of dysmenorrhea generally includes an abdominal and pelvic exam. However, in a young woman who has never been sexually active, the pelvic exam can be omitted if her presentation is consistent with a diagnosis of primary dysmenorrhea (7). The abdominal examination should evaluate the uterus and ovaries for enlargement or masses. The pelvic examination should also evaluate the uterus and adnexal areas for masses or areas of tenderness. Findings of pelvic tenderness, cervical motion tenderness, uterosacral nodularity, enlarged ovaries or a fixed uterus are suggestive of endometriosis (10). Exquisite pain on palpation of the adnexal area or an area of adnexal fullness is consistent with tubo-ovarian abscess, especially if accompanied by fever. Unfortunately, physical examination is neither specific nor sensitive for diagnosing endometriosis.

Diagnostic Testing

As the diagnosis of primary dysmenorrhea is based chiefly on history and presentation, confirmatory tests are not necessary.

In the evaluation of secondary dysmenorrhea, tests should be guided by the clinical evaluation. Cultures for sexually transmitted infections (STIs), including gonorrhea and chlamydia, should be done in women with a history of vaginal or cervical discharge, multiple sex partners, unprotected intercourse, or recent onset of symptoms (less than 14 days). If warranted, HIV testing should also be offered to the patient.

Serum CA-125 levels may be elevated in endometriosis and ovarian cancer; however, this test has a low sensitivity and a high false negative rate, especially in early ovarian cancer and is not recommended as a diagnostic test for either condition (10, 11). Patients with pain at time of ovulation should have a transvaginal ultrasound (TVU) that is useful in diagnosing as well as excluding ovarian cysts or tubo-ovarian abscess (11). Magnetic resonance imaging (MRI) has a high sensitivity (90%) and specificity (98%) for the diagnosis of endometrial cysts (12) but a lower sensitivity (69%) and specificity (75%) for the diagnosis of endometriosis. (13) (Table 29.4)

Recommended Diagnostic Strategy

A general approach to the patient with menstual-related pain is outlined in the algorithm in Figure 29.1. The initial goal is to distinguish between primary and secondary dysmenorrhea, as this will guide the management strategy in an individual patient.

MANAGEMENT

When treating a patient with dysmenorrhea, it is important to remember that the perception and experience of pain is highly individual and may not always correlate with clinical findings. The goals of dysmenorrhea management are to identify the cause of the patient's pain, relieve her symptoms, and restore functioning to the greatest extent possible. The strength of recommendation (SOR) rating for different management strategies is listed in Table 29.5.

Primary Dysmenorrhea

Nonsteroidal anti-inflammatory drugs (NSAIDs), the most common initial treatment for primary dysmenorrhea, are effective in 80%–85% of cases (14). (See Table 29.6 for a listing of agents commonly used.) The NSAID should be initiated with the onset of pain or menses and continued on a scheduled regimen for the first 2 to 3 days of the menstrual flow. Although there does not appear to be a significant difference in efficacy between the non-aspirin NSAIDs, there is wide patient variability in response and side effects with any specific NSAID (15). If one NSAID is ineffective at adequate doses, the patient can try an NSAID from a different class. Alternately, you can consider prescribing oral contraceptive (OC); these are effective in 50%–80% of cases. There is no evidence that any one OC is more effective at treating dysmenorrhea than another (16). Use of an NSAID along with an OC provides additional pain relief (17). For patients who prefer nonpharmacologic management, use of a low-level heat patch has been shown to be efficacious (18, 19).

Once treatment of primary dysmenorrhea has been initiated, efficacy of the treatment should be assessed after several months and annually. Once successful treatment has been

TABLE 29.2 Key Elements in the History and Physical Examination for Dysmenorrhea and Abnormal Uterine Bleeding

Question/Maneuver	Diagnosis
Dysmenorrhea	
Information about age, duration and description of symptoms, prior history of dysmenorrhea, prior treatments and response to treatments, previous prescribed and OTC medications for dysmenorrhea, other key medical conditions, general health	Assist in creating and narrowing the differential diagnosis
Look for red flags (see Table 29.3)	Screen for PID, endometrial cancer, ectopic pregnancy, and tubo-ovarian abscess
Dysmenorrhea that is more intense at the time of ovulation or persists as menstrual flow diminishes	Endometriosis
Obtain sexual history, history of STIs	PID, dyspareunia
History of gynecologic surgery	Pelvic adhesions, cervical stenosis
Psychosocial history	Assist in understanding the patient's perception(s) of pain, coping skills, and formulation of a treatment plan
Temperature	Infectious causes
Focused abdominal and pelvic examinations	
Palpable/enlarged uterus	Leiomyomas, pregnancy, malignancy
Cervical stenosis on speculum examination	Cervical stenosis
Thick purulent cervical discharge	Cervicitis, PID
Tender and enlarged adnexal area	PID
Bleeding from cervical os in postmenopausal woman	Malignancy
Abnormal uterine bleeding	
Determine if woman is ovulatory	Determines which diagnostic pathway to follow (Figs. 29.3 and 29.4)
Information about age, OB/GYN history, menstrual history, description of symptoms, rating of pain, response to prior treatments, and general health	Assist in creating and narrowing the differential diagnosis
Look for red flags (see Table 29.3)	Screen for uterine cancer, ectopic pregnancy, threatened or missed abortion
Medications	Warfarin sodium or aspirin
Focused abdominal and pelvic examination: speculum and bimanual examination, observe for petechiae, palpate thyroid	If abnormalities are elicited, focuses examiner on particular differential diagnosis

OB/GYN, obstetric and/or gynecologic; OTC, over the counter; PID, pelvic inflammatory disease; STIs, sexually transmitted infections.

achieved, the patient should be reevaluated if her symptoms recur.

Secondary Dysmenorrhea

The choice of treatment for secondary dysmenorrhea will be dictated by the underlying etiology. Management approaches for several causes are outlined below.

ENDOMETRIOSIS

The management of endometriosis is dependent on the goals of treatment. For control of pain, the patient can be treated with OCs and NSAIDs. OC cycles, given consecutively with-

out a placebo week, can be tried if standard dosing of OCs provides inadequate relief (20). If these interventions are unsuccessful, the patient should be referred to a gynecologist for possible surgical ablation or treatment with other forms of medical management, such as danazol, and GnRH agonists.

If restoration of fertility is the desired outcome, the patient should be referred to a gynecologist as surgical interventions may produce better outcomes (21).

PELVIC INFLAMMATORY DISEASE

Most patients with PID can be treated as outpatients. If the patient appears septic, is pregnant, is unlikely to follow-up

TABLE 29.3 Red Flags Suggesting Progressive or Life-Threatening Disease in Patients with Pelvic Pain or Abnormal Uterine Bleeding

Diagnosis	Red Flags Suggestive of the Disease
Uterine cancer	Any vaginal bleeding in a postmenopausal woman or intermenstrual bleeding in a perimenopausal woman, >5 mm of thickness of endometrium on transvaginal ultrasound, palpable pelvic mass, or endometrial cells on Pap smear
Ectopic pregnancy	Missed period, or abnormal previous period, with unilateral pelvic pain; may have vaginal bleeding; may have adnexal fullness palpated on pelvic examination
Missed or threatened abortion	Missed or abnormal previous period, with severe pelvic cramping/pain and vaginal bleeding
Pelvic inflammatory disease	Fever, purulent vaginal discharge, abdominal or pelvic pain, exquisitely tender on palpation of pelvic organs, malaise, septic appearance
Tubo-ovarian abscess	Fever, malaise, septic appearance, palpable fullness in the adnexa, or exquisite tenderness on pelvic examination

appropriately, or has failed to respond to appropriate oral antibiotics, she should be admitted for IV antibiotic treatment. See Chapter 33 for more complete information on the treatment of PID.

OVARIAN CYSTS AND CERVICAL POLYPS

If ovarian cysts are unilocular, less than 6 cm in diameter on ultrasound, and the CA-125 level is normal, the patient can be managed expectantly or treatment with NSAIDs or OCs can be initiated. If the cysts are larger than 6 cm, multilocular, bilateral, solid or mixed cystic/solid or if the CA-125 is elevated, you should refer the patient to a gynecologist for further evaluation (11).

If cervical polyps are the cause of pelvic pain, referral to a gynecologist should be given if the family physician is not trained in cervical curettage or hysteroscopy.

TUBO-OVARIAN ABSCESS

Tubo-ovarian abscess is a medical emergency and the patient should immediately be stabilized and referred to a gynecologist.

CASE 1 DISCUSSION

Ms. J.'s premenstrual and menstrual history, negative ROS and her completely normal physical examination confirm that this is a case of primary dysmenorrhea. There are no findings in her history to lead you to consider the need for laboratory or radiologic studies. These studies are only needed for evaluation of secondary causes of dysmenorrhea.

The best course of treatment would be a NSAID such

TABLE 29.4 Characteristics of Diagnostic Tests Useful in Patients with Dysmenorrhea and Abnormal Uterine Bleeding

Diagnosis	Test	Sensitivity	Specificity	LR+	LR−
Dysmenorrhea					
Endometrial cysts	MRI (12)	90	98	45	0.1
Endometriosis	MRI (13)	69	75	2.76	0.4
Abnormal uterine bleeding					
Menorrhagia	Low ferritin, clots over 1.1 inch, changing pad every 1–2 hours (34)	60	86	4.28	0.46
Uterine Cancer	Endometrial biopsy-premenopausal women (40)	91	98	45.5	0.09
	Endometrial biopsy-postmenopausal women (40)	99.6	98	49.8	0.004
	TVU endometrial thickness ≥5 mm (no HT) (41)	96	92	12	0.04
	TVU endometrial thickness ≥5mm (on HT) (41)	96	77	4.17	0.05

LR, likelihood ratio; MRI, magnetic resonance imaging

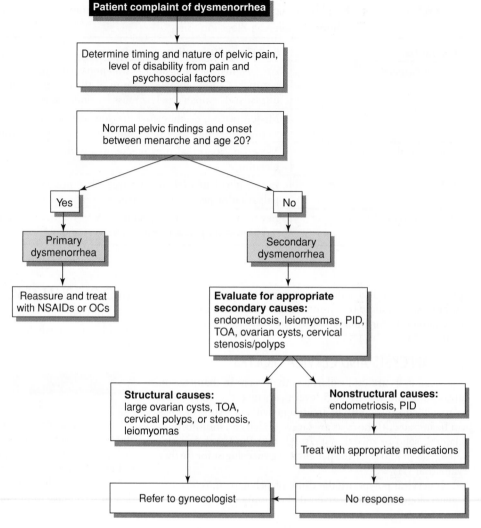

Patient complaint of dysmenorrhea

Determine timing and nature of pelvic pain, level of disability from pain and psychosocial factors

Normal pelvic findings and onset between menarche and age 20?

Yes

No

Primary dysmenorrhea

Secondary dysmenorrhea

Reassure and treat with NSAIDs or OCs

Evaluate for appropriate secondary causes: endometriosis, leiomyomas, PID, TOA, ovarian cysts, cervical stenosis/polyps

Structural causes: large ovarian cysts, TOA, cervical polyps, or stenosis, leiomyomas

Nonstructural causes: endometriosis, PID

Treat with appropriate medications

Refer to gynecologist

No response

Figure 29.1. • General approach to the patient with dysmenorrhea. NSAIDs, nonsteroidal anti-inflammatory drugs; OCs, oral contraceptives; PID, pelvic inflammatory disease; TOA, tubo-ovarian abscess.

as ibuprofen 400–600 mg orally three times daily, at the onset of pain and continued for the first 2 to 3 days of her menses. In the case of individuals with severe cramping, such as this patient, a follow-up phone call after 1 month of treatment is helpful to confirm the efficacy of the treatment and, if appropriate, to discuss other treatment options and the need for office evaluation.

PREMENSTRUAL SYNDROME

CASE 2

Mrs. B., a 43 year-old Hispanic female, presents with a complaint of mood swings. She has been experiencing increasing irritability and crying spells in the week before her menses. She also admits to mild symptoms of bloating (ring and shoe tightness) and increased fatigue during the same time period. The symptoms abate once her menses begin. This has been ongoing for several years but she feels

that it is worsening and is affecting her job as a school secretary as well as her relationship with her husband and three teenage children. Her menses are regular (every 28–30 days) and moderately heavy but she denies menstrual cramps. Her last menses was 24 days ago. Her mother experienced menopause at age 53. She is 5′4″, 135 pounds. She does not smoke, does not take any chronic medications other than a calcium supplement for osteoporosis prevention (600 mg calcium twice daily), and has no known allergies. She admits to a sedentary lifestyle. Mrs. B. has no history of medical or psychiatric conditions and her last physical examination (including a gynecologic exam) was normal. During the visit, she appears moderately anxious and as you interview her, she begins to cry.

CLINICAL QUESTIONS

1. What additional evaluation (clinical, laboratory or radiologic) should be undertaken to confirm her diagnosis?
2. What therapeutic options would be appropriate for the management of this patient?

TABLE 29.5 Management of Dysmenorrhea, Premenstrual Syndrome and Abnormal Uterine Bleeding

Target Disorder	Intervention	Strength of Recommendation*	Comments
Dysmenorrhea	NSAIDs	A	See Table 29.6 for specific agents and dosing
	OCs	A	
Endometriosis	NSAIDs	B	First line for mild-moderate disease
	OCs	A	Continuous (non-cyclic) use may be beneficial
	Medroxyprogesterone acetate	A	
	Danazol	A	Antiestrogenic/androgenic effects
	GnRH agonists	A	Antiestrogenic effects are concern—combination with low-dose estrogen/progestin may limit side effects
PMS	SSRIs	A	See Table 29.7 for specific agents and dosing
	Calcium supplementation	A	1,200 mg/day of elemental calcium
	Other serotonergic antidepressants	B	Not as well studied as SSRIs. See Table 29.7 for specific agents and dosing
	Buspirone	B	Primary effect is to reduce anxiety. See Table 29.7 for dosing
	Alprazolam	B	Primary effect is to reduce anxiety. See Table 29.7 for dosing
	Spironolactone (25)	B	Intermittent dosing during luteal phase. Primary effect is to limit bloating and fluid retention
	Pyridoxine (vitamin B6) (27)	B	Usually 50 mg daily. Primary effect is on depression and generalized symptoms
	Magnesium (28)	B	Generally felt to be safe in the absence of renal or cardiovascular disease
	NSAIDs	B	Mefenamic acid and naproxen best studied. Primary effect is for relief of pain and headache
	Chasteberry (30)	B	Herbal remedy
	Vitamin E	C	Generally felt to be non-toxic
	Lifestyle modifications	C	Low risks and non-PMS benefits
Abnormal uterine bleeding	NSAIDs (46)	B	As effective as other alternatives; taken during menstrual flow

(continued)

TABLE 29.5 Management of Dysmenorrhea, Premenstrual Syndrome and Abnormal Uterine Bleeding (*continued*)

Target Disorder	Intervention	Strength of Recommendation*	Comments
Abnormal uterine bleeding	NSAIDs (46)	B	As effective as other alternatives; taken during menstrual flow
	OCs, cyclic progesterone, HT (46)	B	Effective for AUB; need to caution about side effects and proper administration; may take several cycles to be effective
	Levonorgesterol intrauterine device (47)	A	Effective in decreasing AUB
	Endometrial ablation (48)	A	Effective in decreasing AUB; not for women who wish to maintain fertility; many methods now available, but no evidence to recommend one over another

AUB, abnormal uterine bleeding; GnRH, gonadatropin releasing hormone; HT, hormone therapy; NSAIDs, nonsteroidal anti-inflammatory drugs; OCs, oral contraceptive pills; PMS, premenstrual syndrome; SSRIs, selective serotonin reuptake inhibitors.

*A = consistent, good-quality patient-oriented evidence; B = inconsistent or limited-quality patient-oriented evidence; C = consensus, disease-oriented evidence, usual practice, expert opinion, or case series. For information about the SORT evidence rating system, see *http://www.aafp.org/afpsort.xml*.

TABLE 29.6 NSAIDs for the Treatment of Dysmenorrhea

Drug	Contraindications (CI)/Cautions/ Adverse Effects (AE)	Dosage	Relative Cost*
Dysmenorrhea			
Traditional NSAIDs	CI: Aspirin-induced bronchospasm AE: gastric irritation/ulceration, exacerbation of HTN, renal disease		
Diclofenac		50 mg 3 times/d or 100 mg stat then 50 mg 3 times/d, max 150 mg/d	$$ $
Ibuprofen		200–800 mg q 4–6 hrs, max 3,200 mg/d	$
Ketoprofen		12.5–50 mg q 6–8 hrs, max 300 mg/d	$
Meclofenamate		100 mg tid (not to exceed 6 days), max 400 mg/d	$$$
Mefenamic acid		500 mg stat, then 250 mg q 4 hrs (not to exceed 1 week)	
Naproxen		500 mg stat, then 250 mg q 6–8hrs, max 1,250 mg/d	$
Naproxen sodium		440–550 mg stat, then 220–275 mg q 6–12 hrs	$–$$
COX-2 selective NSAIDs			
Celecoxib†	CI: sulfa allergy	400 mg stat, then 200 mg 2 times/d	$$$
Mild-moderate pain†			
Etodolac		200–400 mg q 6–8 hrs, max 1000 mg/d 64(180)	$$
Fenoprofen		200 mg q 6–8 hrs, max 3200 mg/d	$$$

d, daily; tid, three times a day; q, every.
*Relative cost: $, <$33.00; $$, $34.00–$66.00; $$$, >$67.00
†Do not use as first-line treatment—may be used as alternates if first-line NSAIDs are ineffective or not tolerated.

Premenstrual syndrome (PMS) is the term for a constellation of physical, emotional, and behavioral symptoms that occur during the luteal phase of the menstrual cycle. Premenstrual dysphoric disorder (PMDD), defined as a severe form of PMS, significantly affects a patient's ability to function. (For the purposes of this chapter, the term PMS will be inclusive of both PMS and PMDD unless otherwise specified.) The presentation of PMS varies significantly between women and can also vary from cycle to cycle in an individual woman. The most common and distressing symptoms are emotional lability, anger, irritability, anxiety, depression and "feeling out of control." Other common symptoms include fluid retention, edema, breast tenderness, headaches, and dietary cravings (22). By definition, symptoms begin during the luteal phase and must abate with the onset of menses. The patient must be symptom free during the follicular phase and the symptoms cannot be attributable to other physical or psychological causes.

The etiology of PMS is unclear and numerous theories have been postulated and then discarded. Currently, research suggests that in susceptible women, the normal hormonal fluctuations of the menstrual cycle trigger an altered sensitivity to the neurotransmitter serotonin (22, 23).

Surveys show that approximately 85% of menstruating women experience at least one symptom associated with PMS, whereas PMDD is reported to occur in 5% to 20% of the menstruating female population (4, 22).

DIFFERENTIAL DIAGNOSIS

Many medical and psychiatric conditions may be exacerbated by the hormonal fluctuations of the menstrual cycle, causing symptoms that mimic PMS. Table 29.1 lists some of the conditions for the differential diagnosis of PMS.

CLINICAL EVALUATION

PMS is a diagnosis of exclusion; therefore a thorough history and focused physical examination are vital to making an appropriate diagnosis.

History

Initially, the interview should focus on the patient's symptoms, including age at onset, onset and severity in relation to her menstrual cycle, and when, if ever, the symptoms abate. The patient should be asked to what degree her symptoms cause distress or impair her functioning. If the patient does not experience a symptom-free interval during the follicular phase, menstrual exacerbation of a chronic condition should be considered rather than a diagnosis of PMS.

A thorough medical history should be taken to assess for medical conditions that may mimic PMS symptoms. A patient with rheumatoid arthritis who complains of increased fatigue and joint pains during the luteal phase is experiencing an exacerbation of her underlying disease rather than true PMS. The patient should be questioned about any personal or family history of depressive/anxiety disorders as these may predispose to PMS. However, these conditions may also be exacerbated

during the luteal phase so a clear history of absence of symptoms during the follicular phase should be elicited prior to making a diagnosis of PMS. A history of similar symptoms during pregnancy, the post-partum period, or while on hormonal contraception is suggestive of PMS (4).

Physical Examination

In an otherwise healthy woman, there are no physical abnormalities associated with PMS. If a patient has no specific physical complaints related to her symptoms, the physical exam may be brief, however, the patient should be up to date on her gynecologic exam. Presence of symptoms that may indicate a medical condition, such as joint pains, should be assessed.

Diagnostic Testing

There are no laboratory or imaging tests that confirm the diagnosis of PMS. If the patient has symptoms of or risk for a medical condition, such as thyroid disease or an autoimmune disease, which may be exacerbated premenstrually, appropriate diagnostic testing should be done prior to a diagnosis of PMS. In women over age 40, a follicle-stimulating hormone (FSH) level should be measured to assess if perimenopause is a factor in the patient's symptoms (4).

Recommended Diagnostic Strategy

Several entities, including the American College of Obstetricians (ACOG) and the American Psychiatric Association (APA) have published diagnostic criteria for PMS and PMDD, however, there is not consensus on this issue (4). Both sets of criteria require that symptoms occur during the luteal phase, remit during the follicular phase, and cause some degree of dysfunction. The ACOG criteria for PMS are broad, requiring a sole symptom while the APA's criteria for PMDD, published in the DSM-IV and commonly utilized for research purposes, are more strict, requiring a minimum of 5 symptoms, one of which must be dysphoric in nature (4, 24).

For an accurate diagnosis of PMS, the patient should ideally log her daily symptoms for a minimum of 2 menstrual cycles. Although the patient can record her symptoms on a calendar or in a notebook, use of a standardized daily symptoms calendar can facilitate the process. Examples of such tools include as the Daily Symptom Report (DSR), the Daily Record of Severity of Problems (DRSP), the Calendar of Premenstrual Experience (COPE) or the Prospective Record of the Impact and Severity of Menstruation (PRISM) (4, 22). (See *http://www.mckinley.uiuc.edu/handouts/pre_menstrual_syndrome/pre_menstrual_syndrome.html* for an example of a menstrual diary.) A record which shows a pattern of moderate to severe symptoms during the luteal phase which are absent or significantly minimized during the follicular phase is consistent with a diagnosis of PMS. In reality, it may be difficult to for patients to provide such a log. Less cumbersome diagnostic strategies may include use of abbreviated monitoring forms or having the patient schedule an evaluation during the late luteal phase at which time she is most likely to be experiencing her symptoms (4).

Given the lack of diagnostic agreement and the difficulty in obtaining good prospective data, failure of an individual to meet the strict criteria for PMDD, as outlined in DSM-IV, should not preclude a clinical diagnosis of PMDD and initiation of appropriate therapy.

MANAGEMENT

Although most ovulating women have some degree of premenstrual discomfort or mood change, women who seek medical attention because their symptoms interfere with normal work, personal activities, or relationships should be offered therapeutic intervention. The focus of therapy should be guided by the patient's specific symptoms, with emphasis on the symptom(s) that cause the patient the most distress. The patient should understand that no single therapy is effective for all symptoms and that identifying the best treatment may require the trial of several agents for several months each. Many treatment modalities have been suggested for PMS, however, there are few well-controlled clinical trials. The treatment recommendations for PMS and the strength of recommendation supporting their use are listed in Table 29.5.

Non-Pharmacologic Management

Education and supportive measures are important in the management of PMS and have been reported to improve symptoms and a patient's sense of control. Lifestyle modifications, including relaxation techniques, regular aerobic exercise, sodium and caffeine restriction and increased intake of complex carbohydrates, are widely recommended for PMS management. Despite lack of evidence to support effectiveness, the limited risks and other benefits of these interventions warrant their use (25). In patients with mild symptoms, a 2-month trial of lifestyle modification is reasonable. For women with moderate to severe symptoms, addition of a pharmacologic agent to lifestyle modification is appropriate.

Pharmacologic Therapy
DIETARY SUPPLEMENTS

Calcium supplementation (1,200 mg/day) has been shown in one large study to improve the physical and mood symptoms of PMS (26) (SOR = A). Although this effect has not been confirmed by additional studies, the relative safety and importance of calcium in the prevention of osteoporosis justifies its routine use in women with PMS (25).

Pyridoxine (vitamin B6) has been widely studied in PMS. A systematic review of these studies suggests that pyridoxine may provide some benefit for irritability, breast tenderness, fatigue and bloating (27) (SOR = B). Due to the risk of neurotoxicity with chronic use of higher doses, pyridoxine dose should be limited to 50mg/day. Magnesium, 200–360 mg/day may provide improvement in symptoms (SOR = B) but there is inadequate data to support a recommendation for the use of vitamin E (25, 28) (SOR = C).

PSYCHOTHERAPEUTIC AGENTS

There is good clinical evidence that SSRIs are effective at improving mood symptoms related to PMS (SOR = A). Fluoxetine, sertraline, and paroxetine carry an FDA-approved indication for the treatment of PMS. Limited clinical trial data support a similar effect with other SSRIs and non-SSRI serotonergic antidepressants (see Table 29.5).

Intermittent treatment (dosing during the luteal phase only) has been shown to be equally efficacious to daily dosing and is preferred due to fewer side effects and lower cost (29). Because of the data supporting their efficacy, these agents are considered first line therapy in patients with significant psychological symptoms of PMS.

If anxiety is the primary complaint and the patient has not responded to an appropriate trial of a serotonergic antidepressant, an anxiolytic can be tried. Luteal phase dosing of either buspirone or alprazolam has been shown in small trials to be effective in managing anxiety related to PMS (SOR = B). Due to concerns regarding the addictive potential of alprazolam and the relative lack of data on use of these agents in PMS, they are considered second-line therapy after the SSRIs (23). Dosing information is provided in Table 29.7.

Treatment of Physical Symptoms

Some women experience marked fluid retention and bloating during the premenstrual period. Spironolactone, a mild diuretic with antiandrogenic properties, has been shown in clinical trials to improve the subjective symptom of bloating (22, 25) (SOR = B). It is dosed at 100 mg daily during the luteal phase. Other diuretics have not been well studied in the management of PMS. NSAIDs are useful for the management of menstrual headaches and the joint and muscle aches that can occur with PMS.

HERBAL MEDICINE

Patients commonly use herbal preparations for PMS-related complaints but there is very little good clinical data on the majority of these agents. Chasteberry, in some but not all studies, has been shown to reduce symptoms of PMS (30, 31) (SOR = B). Evening primrose oil has not been shown to be of benefit (31).

HORMONAL THERAPY AND MENSTRUAL CYCLE MODULATION

The effect of oral contraceptives on PMS is unclear. Some studies suggest an increased risk for PMS in women taking OCs while others report an improvement in PMS symptoms. If a woman with PMS desires to use OCs for contraception, she should monitor her symptoms closely and consider switching to alternate contraception if an exacerbation is noted. Despite a theory that PMS is caused by progesterone deficiency, studies do not support a beneficial effect of progesterone therapy in PMS (25).

Elimination of the hormonal fluctuations of the menstrual cycle has been shown to improve PMS and the condition generally abates once menopause occurs. Bilateral oophorectomy and drugs that eliminate menstrual cyclicity, such as danazol and the GnRH agonists, have been shown to effectively treat PMS but are associated with significant risks (22). Patients with severe PMS who have failed other therapies should be referred to a gynecologist for discussion of these interventions.

CASE 2 DISCUSSION

Mrs. B.'s clinical presentation (symptoms, timing of onset and remission), negative medical and psychiatric history, and normal physical exam are consistent with a diagnosis of PMS. There are no laboratory or radiologic tests for diagnosing PMS. To confirm the clinical diagnosis, a prospective rating of daily symptoms for several cycles is appropriate, however, given the patient's distress, empiric therapy can be initiated. Patient education, lifestyle modifications (aerobic exercise, sodium restriction) and continuation of calcium supplementa-

TABLE 29.7 Psychotropic Drugs for the Management of PMS

Drug	Contraindications (CI)/Cautions (C)/Adverse Effects (AE)	Dosage*	Relative Cost†
PMS			
SSRIs	CI: MAOI use AE: anxiety, insomnia, decreased libido		
Citalopram (Celexa)		20 mg daily or 10–30 mg intermittently	$$
Fluoxetine (Prozac, Serafem)		20 mg daily or 20 mg intermittently	$
Fluvoxamine (Luvox)		100 mg daily	$$
Paroxetine (Paxil, Paxil CR)		5–30 mg daily 12.5–25 mg daily (CR) or 12.5–25 mg CR intermittently	$
Sertraline (Zoloft)		50–150 mg daily or 100 mg intermittently	$$
Other serotonergic antidepressants			
Nefazodone	CI: MAOI use C: multiple drug interactions AE: Hepatoxicity, constipation	200–600 mg daily	$$
Venlafaxine (Effexor)	CI: MAOI use AE: HTN	50 mg daily	$$
Tricyclic antidepressants	CI: MAOI use C: H/O seizures, narrow angle glaucoma, CV disease AE: Sedation, urinary retention		
Clomipramine		25–75 mg daily or 25–75 mg intermittently	$
Nortriptyline		50–125 mg daily	$
Anxiolytic			
Alprazolam	C: Drug interactions; taper the dose over 2 days after the onset of menses AE: Drowsiness, dependence	1–2 mg intermittently	$
Buspirone	CI: MAOI use AE: Drowsiness, dizziness	25–60 mg intermittently	$$

*Intermittent dosing begins on day 14 of cycle and continues until onset of menses.
†Relative cost: $, <$33.00; $$, $34.00–$66.00; $$$, >$67.00

tion should be encouraged for their possible effect on PMS symptoms as well as their non-PMS benefits. Because her mood swings are her greatest concern, a trial of an SSRI, such as sertraline given during the luteal phase only, should be offered to this patient. She should be encouraged to follow up after 2 months for evaluation of treatment efficacy.

ABNORMAL UTERINE BLEEDING

CASE 3

Mrs. W. is a 50-year-old Caucasian woman who presents to your office concerned about changes in her menstrual pattern. For the past 6 months, she has had either very heavy menstrual flow lasting up to 10 days, or very light spotting. She has not had a period in 2 months. She has been married for 30 years, and had three normal vaginal deliveries. She has had no major medical illnesses, no surgeries, and no STIs. Menarche was at age 12. Her weight is stable and she takes no medications or herbal supplements. Her mother went through menopause at age 55. Her family history is negative for cancer and endocrine disease. Her ROS is negative. Her physical examination, including pelvic and bimanual exam, was completely normal.

CLINICAL QUESTIONS

1. What is the next step in your evaluation of her symptoms?
2. What is the best approach to management of this patient to control her bleeding episodes?

DEFINITIONS

It is important to have an understanding of what is normal, or at least the range of normal, when it comes to a woman's menstrual cycle. Variability in the menstrual cycle has been noted at the beginning and end of a woman's reproductive life. An analysis of menstrual records from over 1,000 women reveals that most women set their own menstrual interval by age 19 and that the length and variability change imperceptibly between ages 19 and 49 years (32). Between the 5th and 95th percentiles, the menstrual cycle ranges from 24 to 42 days. The majority of women will have cycles between 21 and 35 days, but only about 15% have an actual cycle length of 28 days (33). Bleeding days range from 4 to 8 days within the 5th to 95th percentile group. Between ages 15 and 43, most women will have no more than a three-day variation in cycle length. Variability increases to 4–5 days after age 44 for the majority of menstruating women (32).

The traditional definitions of abnormal menstrual patterns are as follows (33):

- Oligomenorrhea—intervals greater than 35 days
- Polymenorrhea—intervals less than 24 days
- Menorrhagia—regular normal intervals with excessive flow or duration
- Metrorrhagia—irregular intervals with excessive flow or duration

Analysis of menstrual patterns in women, defining abnormal patterns as those falling outside the 5th to 95th percentile suggest that infrequent bleeding be defined as fewer than two bleeding episodes in a 90-day period. Frequent bleeding episodes are defined as more than 4 bleeding episodes in a 90-day period. Prolonged bleeding (95th percentile) is an episode lasting 10 days or more (32). Menorrhagia has been difficult to determine quantitatively in the clinical setting. Traditionally defined as blood loss of ≥80 mL per bleeding episode, methods to measure or approximate this degree of blood loss have been cumbersome and impractical. A recent study reported a model for determining menorrhagia based on clot size (over 1.1 inch in diameter), low ferritin level, and rate of change of sanitary protection (every 1–2 hours or more frequently). This model correctly identified 76% of women with measured menstrual blood flow of ≥80 mL and supports the idea that the subjective judgment of the patient, long thought to be unreliable, should be used in the assessment of heavy menstrual bleeding (34) (SOR = A). Menorrhagia occurring in the absence of structural uterine disease is referred to as dysfunctional uterine bleeding (DUB).

PATHOPHYSIOLOGY

Normal uterine bleeding is the result of cyclic, sequential stimulation of the endometrium by estrogen and progesterone, and occurs after withdrawal of the hormonal effect. This pattern is mimicked pharmacologically by OCs and some HT (hormone therapy) regimens. Abnormal uterine bleeding (AUB) can result from hormonal disturbances such as estrogen withdrawal (estrogen only HT, missed pill) or unopposed estrogen with breakthrough bleeding (anovulatory cycles). Women on progesterone only medications (contraceptive pill, implants, injections) can have abnormal bleeding patterns due to progesterone withdrawal or breakthrough bleeding (33).

Anovulatory cycles can be due to many etiologies including PCOS (polycystic ovary syndrome), eating disorders, endocrinopathies (i.e., thyroid disease or prolactinoma), obesity, or the suppression of ovulation due to weight loss or excessive exercise. A recent review of menstrual abnormalities in women with thyroid disease revealed that AUB is less frequent than traditionally believed. In a recent study of women with hyperthyroidism, 21.5% reported menstrual irregularities compared to the 50%–60% in older series. 23.4% of women with hypothyroidism reported menstrual irregularities compared to 50%–70%. The most common complaint in both groups was oligomenorrhea (35). Anovulation is also seen at the extremes of a woman's reproductive life. In reproductive age women, anovulatory bleeding and hormonal medication use represent the most common causes of non-cyclic bleeding (5, 33).

Other possible causes of abnormal uterine bleeding include pregnancy and pregnancy-related conditions such as an ectopic pregnancy, miscarriage, placenta previa, placental abruption, trophoblastic disease, or retained products of conception. Benign lesions of the uterus (polyps, adenomyosis, leiomyomata), genital tract infections, and malignant lesions of the reproductive tract may also cause AUB. Risk factors for endometrial cancer include age (over 40), anovulatory cycles, obesity, nulliparity, diabetes, and tamoxifen therapy. Endometrial cancer has been reported in women under age 40 and women with chronic anovulation and obesity who present with abnormal bleeding should be considered at risk (36).

Medications such as antipsychotics, anticoagulants, SSRIs, corticosteroids, and tamoxifen have been known to cause AUB, as have certain herbal supplements (i.e., ginseng, ginkgo, soy). Renal, hepatic, adrenal, and thyroid disease, and blood dyscrasias may cause AUB. Other causes for AUB include foreign objects, including IUDs, trauma, and congenital (Mullerian) structural abnormalities (5,37). Coagulopathies, once thought to be a rare cause of abnormal bleeding, have been shown to be present in 13% of women with heavy uterine bleeding (38).

Some etiologies of abnormal uterine bleeding will vary with age. The incidence of structural lesions and endometrial cancer increases with age. Pregnancy-related causes occur during the reproductive years. Anovulation can occur throughout the reproductive years as well. Table 29.1 lists a differential diagnosis of AUB by frequency.

CLINICAL EVALUATION

While many women presenting for an evaluation of a menstrual problem will give a straightforward history, clinicians should remember that, for the adolescent, such a complaint may be an acceptable way to obtain a medical evaluation. The adolescent may be concerned about pregnancy, contraception, sexually transmitted infections, or sexual assault (2). The pelvic exam can be very traumatic to adolescent patients coming for a first evaluation or for women who have a history of sexual assault. The patient's cultural background or personal comfort level may also result in a limited (abdominal only) exam. In these cases, the history and further laboratory and pelvic ultrasound investigations can assist in identifying the most likely diagnosis.

History

The initial evaluation of AUB should include a complete menstrual history from menarche, in order to understand if this is a chronic or newly acquired pattern of bleeding. The bleeding episodes should be quantified and characterized. A history of clots over 1.1 inch and a report of changing sanitary pads or tampons every 1 to 2 hours or more frequently supports a diagnosis of menorrhagia (34). Cyclical periods associated with premenstrual symptoms suggestive of a progesterone effect (breast tenderness, dysmenorrhea) provide over a 95% probability that the woman is ovulating (5). Timing of the bleeding episodes (postcoital, intermenstrual, mid-cycle) should be noted. A history of pregnancy symptoms and/or abdominal pain, even in the presence of reported previous period-like bleeding, should raise suspicion that the patient is having a complication of pregnancy. Inquiring about associated symptoms and complaints, such as dyspareunia, galactorrhea, and hirsutism will help complete the patient's history of the presenting complaint.

A sexual history, reproductive history, and a careful review of current medications, including OTC supplements and herbals, are also essential to making a diagnosis. A review of systems should help evaluate for systemic diseases (adrenal, renal, hepatic, thyroid) or coagulopathies. A screening test developed to detect underlying coagulation disorders includes the following: a history of excessive menstrual bleeding since menarche; or history of one of the following—postpartum hemorrhage, surgery related bleeding, or bleeding associated with dental work; or a history of two or more of the following—bruising greater than 5 cm once or twice a month, epistaxis once or twice a month, frequent gum bleeding, family history of bleeding symptoms (SOR = B). These symptoms occur statistically more often in women with von Willebrand disease and a positive screen will help determine further workup (39).

In addition, the woman's past medical and surgical history and previous exam findings and evaluations may help in establishing the etiology of AUB.

Physical Examination

To evaluate the severity of bleeding, patients should be screened for orthostatic hypotension and an elevated pulse rate. Other vital signs of importance are pain, weight, and body mass index (BMI). The patient should be observed for signs of systemic disease (bruising, petechiae, jaundice). The physical exam, based on the history, should be performed. The thyroid gland should be examined. Careful attention should be given to the abdominal and pelvic exam, to evaluate for hepatosplenomegaly and uterine enlargement due to fibroids or pregnancy.

On pelvic exam, evidence of infection, trauma, foreign body, IUD string, cervical polyps or neoplasia may help identify the source of the bleeding. Trauma or foreign bodies may indicate sexual assault or self-mutilation. Cervical cultures, a pap smear and a biopsy of any visible lesion should be done at the time of the initial exam if possible. Uterine size, shape, and consistency should be assessed. Adenomyosis is strongly suspected in a uterus that is enlarged, diffusely tender, and soft to boggy to palpation. Irregular contours are more likely with fibroids. The adnexal exam can help identify any masses or localized pain suggestive of an ectopic pregnancy or abscess. A recto-vaginal exam may be helpful in assessing structural abnormalities (5).

Testing

Laboratory testing should be systematic and based on the information from the history and the physical exam. Initial testing should be directed at eliminating life-threatening or serious conditions, such as pregnancy (serum hCG) or severe anemia (hemoglobin or hematocrit). Thyroid stimulating hormone (TSH) and prolactin levels should be obtained if history (oligomenorrhea, galactorrhea) or physical exam (enlarged thyroid, galactorrhea) is suggestive. Women with known or suspected systemic illness should have appropriate laboratory evaluation (5, 37). If a coagulopathy is suspected, hemostasis testing should be done in consultation with a hematologist, as the accurate diagnosis of von Willebrand disease is dependent on appropriate testing conditions. Tests, beyond the initial hemoglobin and platelet count, include a PT, APTT, VWF antigen, ristocetin cofactor, Factor VIII, ABO type, Ivy bleeding time and/or platelet function analyzer-100 closure time. Iron studies should be obtained for the anemic patient (39).

For women with suspected PCOS (the most common cause of oligomenorrhea in adolescents), a GTT and fasting insulin level can be obtained to assess insulin resistance. Serum testosterone, DHEA-S, and 17-α hydroxyprogesterone should be obtained in patients with hirsutism and hyperandrogenism (2).

The next step in the evaluation of AUB is to determine the need for further investigation, such as an endometrial biopsy, TVU, or hysteroscopy, to evaluate for endometrial cancer and structural abnormalities. Which investigation is chosen to begin with may be a matter of what is available and acceptable to the patient. A meta-analysis of studies to assess the accuracy of endometrial sampling devices showed that the Pipelle had the best detection rate for endometrial cancer in both pre- (91%) and post- (99.6%) menopausal women (see Table 29.4). The detection rate for atypical hyperplasia was 81%. The specificity was over 98% (40) (SOR = A). A meta-analysis of TVU studies showed that when a thickness of greater than 5 mm was used to define abnormal uterine thickening, the sensitivity was 96% for women with cancer and 92% for women with endometrial disease (SOR = A) (Table 29.4). This did not vary with HT use. Specificity did vary with HT use; it was 92% off HT, but 77% on HT (41).

A recent study compared biopsy (Pipelle or Tao brush), hysteroscopy with biopsy, and ultrasound (including TVU) to determine the optimal work-up for AUB (42). In the high-risk (postmenopausal bleeding) group, hysteroscopy was marginally more cost effective than ultrasound; biopsy alone was most cost effective in the moderate risk group (premenopausal 40 years or older/under 40 with risk factors for endometrial cancer); and, ultrasound was most cost effective in the low-risk (premenopausal under 40 years) group (SOR = B). Cost differences were relatively small, however. Note was made that the Tao brush was more effective in obtaining adequate biopsy samples in postmenopausal women (42). A randomized

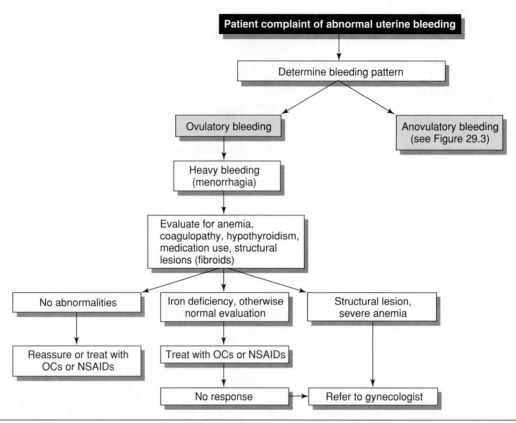

Figure 29.2. • **General approach to the patient with abnormal uterine bleeding.** NSAIDs, nonsteroidal anti-inflammatory drugs; OCs, oral contraceptives. (Reprinted with permission from Wathen PI, Henderson MC, Witz CA. Abnormal uterine bleeding. Med Clin North Am. 1995;79:329–344.)

trial comparing biopsy alone with hysteroscopy and biopsy in a group of premenopausal women with AUB showed that outpatient hysteroscopy was acceptable to patients and they were significantly happier with this level of investigation (SOR = A). However, the procedure had little influence on clinical management and increased the cost of care (43).

Ultrasound is more likely to identify structural abnormalities that would be missed with the biopsy alone or hysteroscopy approach. It was also more acceptable to patients. A recent cost analysis comparing various models demonstrated that starting with TVU was most cost effective in pre-and peri-menopausal women where the prevalence of benign disease is so much greater. However, 5%–10% of the time, the endometrium cannot be visualized. This would need to be followed up by biopsy and hysteroscopy or saline infusion sonography (42, 44, 45). MRI and saline infusion sonography can be used to further evaluate patients for leiomyomata and adenomyosis (5).

MANAGEMENT

Once life-threatening complications have been ruled out, management can proceed according to the etiology for the bleeding. As described above, women who are over 35, or who are at increased risk for endometrial cancer, or who have abnormal findings on exam require further testing. Although

algorithms have fallen out of favor with some (5), they still present a way to conceptualize the workup in a systematic fashion (see Figures 29.2 and 29.3). Detection of structural abnormalities, such as an endometrial stripe over 5 mm, endometrial atypia or adenocarcinoma will usually result in a referral to a gynecologist for further evaluation. The clinician's challenge, once the initial diagnosis is made, is to effectively get the bleeding under control with the minimum of side effects. This can be done using medications, a levonorgestrel-releasing IUD (LNG IUS), or surgical interventions.

Medications have been shown to effectively control AUB, both by regulating the menstrual cycle (i.e., OCs, cyclical progesterone) and decreasing the amount of blood flow (i.e., NSAIDs, oral luteal progesterone, OCs, Danazol, tranexamic acid, ethamsylate, LNG IUS) (see Table 29.5). NSAIDs have been shown to be less effective than tranexamic acid or Danazol, but the latter medications are less frequently used due to risks, side effects, and cost. There were no statistical differences between naproxen and mefenamic acid, or between NSAIDs and oral luteal progestogens, LNG IUS, ethamsylate, and OCs (46) (SOR = B).

In a study of LNG IUS compared to cyclical 21-day oral progesterone therapy for menorrhagia, the LNG IUS was more effective, had greater patient satisfaction, and its use led to a higher proportion of deferred surgery when compared with oral medication use (47) (SOR = A). In a study comparing medical and surgical therapy, surgery reduced menstrual

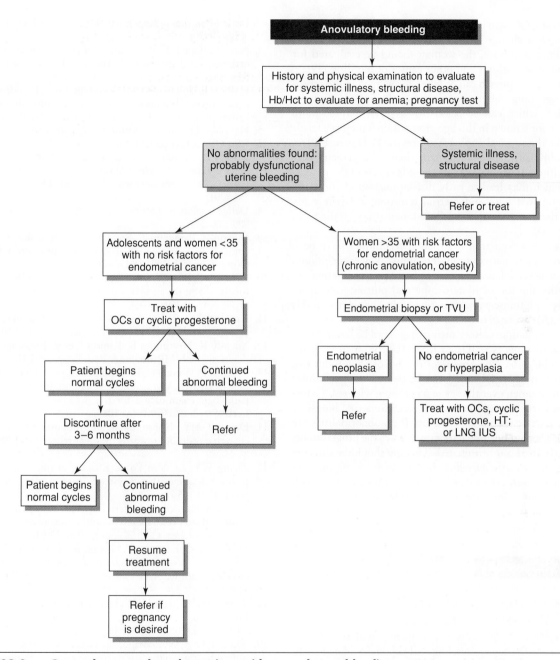

Figure 29.3. • General approach to the patient with anovulatory bleeding. Hb, hemoglobin; Hct, hematocrit; HT, hormone therapy; LNG IUS, levonorgestral releasing IUD (intrauterine device); OCs, oral contraceptives. (Adapted with permission from Wathen PI, Henderson MC, Witz CA. Abnormal uterine bleeding. Med Clin North Am. 1995;79:329–344.)

bleeding more than most medical treatments, but the LNG IUS appeared equally effective in improving quality of life (48) (SOR = A).

In adolescents with anovulatory menorrhagia (DUB), OCs, if not contraindicated, will effectively control the bleeding and have the added advantage of establishing a predictable bleeding pattern and providing contraception. For those women unable to tolerate cyclical hormonal (estrogen/progesterone or progestin only) therapy, NSAIDs at the time of the menstrual flow will decrease the bleeding and may be an acceptable alternative (see Table 29.6).

Consideration should be given to the evaluation for medi-

cal causes of anovulatory cycles. Some of the testing for von Willebrand disease should be done before the patient is placed on OCs (39). Adolescents with PCOS will have their menorrhagia controlled by OCs, but issues of obesity and insulin resistance must also be addressed and treated (2).

If there is no response to the treatment for menorrhagia after 3 months, further evaluation should be undertaken, either at the primary care office or through gynecological referral. Irregular bleeding/spotting may occur in the first 3 months of OC use, especially with progestin-only pills, so care should be taken to provide counseling on how to take the medication (same time every day). Intermenstrual spotting in women using OCs can be treated with NSAIDs, supplemental estrogen, or a change in the pill formulation. However, if the bleeding continues, the woman should be evaluated for structural abnormalities and other causes of bleeding (49).

The same approach can be taken for women in the reproductive age range after appropriate evaluation. Use of the LNG IUS, which can be placed for 5 years, may be more acceptable for women in this age group. It does preserve fertility, unlike the surgical approaches, and the IUD is cost-effective. Additionally, insertion can be done in a primary care office. Although women do note the side effects of the progestogen, which may lead to early discontinuation of the IUD, when compared with endometrial resection, a 3-year study showed that both treatments reduced menstrual bleeding (50) (SOR = A).

Surgical endometrial destruction techniques have been developed as alternatives to hysterectomy. Newer techniques (such as balloon ablation, bipolar radiofrequency ablation) do not require the use of hysteroscopy and outcomes compare favorably with transcervical resection of the endometrium (51) (SOR = A).

Women with ovulatory menorrhagia can be treated with hormonal therapy, NSAIDs, or LNG IUS. Women with an-ovulatory bleeding who are under the age of 35 without risk factors for endometrial cancer can be treated using a similar approach. Women over the age of 35 or those with risk factors for endometrial cancer should have an endometrial biopsy or TVU as part of the initial work up. If no abnormalities are detected, a trial of hormonal therapy (OC, cyclic progesterone, HT, LNG IUS) can be initiated. Therapy should be directed toward control of the bleeding. If there is no or minimal response in 3 months, re-evaluation (with additional studies such as hysteroscopy, saline infusion sonography) should take place.

CASE 3 DISCUSSION

Given this woman's age, history and physical findings, the next step is an endometrial biopsy, which shows hyperplasia without atypia. A diagnosis of peri-menopausal anovulatory AUB is made. Patient counseling and expectant management can be used if the patient does not wish HT. If she would like to control the regularity and amount of bleeding, her initial treatment options would be cyclical or daily estrogen/progesterone, cyclical progesterone or a progestogen IUD. She chooses a 3- to 6-month trial of cyclical progesterone and close follow-up.

Acknowledgment

Barbara Supanich, RSM, MD, was the author of this chapter in the Fourth Edition.

REFERENCES

1. Warner PE, Critchley HOD, Lumsden MA et al. Menorrhagia II: Is the 80-mL blood loss criterion useful in management of complaint of menorrhagia? Am J Obstet Gynecol. 2004; 190:1224–1229.
2. Hickey M, Balen A. Menstrual disorders in adolescence: investigation and management. Hum Reprod Update. 2003; 9(5):493–504.
3. Nasir L, Bope ET. Management of pelvic pain from dysmenorrhea or endometriosis. J Am Board Fam Pract. 2004;17: S43–S47.
4. Halbreich U. The diagnosis of premenstrual syndromes and premenstrual dysphoric disorder-clinical procedures and research perspectives. Gynecol Endocrinol. 2004;19:320–334.
5. Hatasaka H. The evaluation of abnormal uterine bleeding. Clin Obstet Gynecol. 2005; 48(2):258–273.
6. Durain D. Primary dysmenorrhea: assessment and management update. J Midwifery Womens Health. 2004;49:520–528.
7. French L. Dysmenorrhea. Am Fam Physician. 2005;71: 285–291.
8. Deligeoroglou E. Dysmenorrhea. Ann NY Acad Sci. 2000; 900:237–244.
9. Vigano P, Parazzini F, Somigliana E, et al. Endometriosis: epidemiology and aetiological factors. Best Pract Res Clin Obstet Gynecol. 2004;18:177–200.
10. Kennedy S, Bergqvist A, Chapron C, et al. ESHRE guideline for the diagnosis and treatment of endometriosis. Hum Reprod. 2005;10:2698–2704.
11. Knudsen UB, Tabor A, Mosgaard B, et al. Management of ovarian cysts. Acta Obstet Gynecol Scand. 2004;83:1012–1021.
12. Itogashi K, Nishimura K, Kinura I, et al. Endometrial cysts: diagnosis with MR imaging. Radiology. 1991;180(1):73–78.
13. Stratton P, Winkel C, Premkumar A, et al. Diagnostic accuracy of laparoscopy, magnetic resonance imaging, and histopathologic examination for the detection of endometriosis. Fertil Steril. 2003;79:1078–1085.
14. Dawood MY. Nonsteroidal anti-inflammatory drugs and changing attitudes towards dysmenorrhea. Am J Med. 1988; 84:23–29.
15. Zhang WY, Li Wan Po A. Efficacy of minor analgesics in primary dysmenorrhea: a systematic review. Br J Obstet Gynaecol. 1998;105:780–789.
16. Milsom I, Sundell G, Andersch B. The influence of different combined oral contraceptives on the prevalence and severity of dysmenorrhea. Contraception. 1990;42:497–506.
17. Jacobson J, Lundstrom V. Nilsson B. Naproxen in the treatment of OC-resistant primary dysmenorrhea: a double-blind cross-over study. Acta Obstet Gynecol Scand Suppl. 1983; 113:87–89.
18. Akin MD, Weingard KW, Hengehold DA, et al. Continuous low-level topical heat in the treatment of dysmenorrhea. Obstet Gynecol. 2001;97:343–349.
19. Akin M, Price W, Rodriguez Jr G, et al. Continuous low-level topical heat wrap therapy as compared to acetaminophen for primary dysmenorrhea. J Reprod Med. 2004;49:739–745.
20. Vercellini P, Fontino G, DeGiorgi O, et al. Continuous use of an oral contraceptive for endometriosis-associated recurrent dysmenorrhea that does not respond to a cyclic pill regimen. Fertil Steril. 2003;80:560–563.
21. Falcone T, Goldberg JM, Miller KF. Endometriosis: medical and surgical intervention. Curr Opin Obstet Gynecol. 1996; 8:178–183.
22. Dickerson LM, Mazyck PJ, Hunter MH. Premenstrual syndrome. Am Fam Physican. 2003;67:1743–1752.
23. Bhatia SC, Bhatia SK. Diagnosis and treatment of premenstrual dysphoric disorder. Am Fam Physician. 2002;66: 1239–1248.
24. American Psychiatric Association: Premenstrual dysphoric disorder. In: Diagnostic and Statistical Manual of Mental Disorders, 4th ed. Washington, DC: American Psychiatric Association; 1994:715.
25. Douglas S. Premenstrual syndrome: evidence-based treat-

ment in family practice. Can Fam Physician. 2002;48: 1789–1797.

26. Thys-Jacob S, Starkey P, Bernstein D, et al. Calcium carbonate and the premenstrual syndrome: effects on premenstrual and menstrual symptoms. Am J Obstet Gynecol. 1998;179: 444–452.

27. Wyatt PM, Dimmock PW, Jones PW, Shaughn O'Brien PM. Efficacy of vitamin B6 in the treatment of premenstrual syndrome: systematic review. BMJ. 1999;318:1375–1381.

28. Bendich A. The potential for dietary supplements to reduce premenstrual syndrome (PMS) symptoms. J Am Coll Nutr. 2000;19:3–12.

29. Dimmock PW, Wyatt PM, Jones PW, O'Brien PM. Efficacy of selective serotonin-reuptake inhibitors in premenstrual syndrome: a systematic review. Lancet. 2000;356:1131–1136.

30. Girman A, Lee R, Kligler B. An integrative medicine approach to premenstrual syndrome. Clin J Women's Health. 2002;2:116–127.

31. Stevinson C, Ernst E. Complementary/alternative therapies for premenstrual syndrome: a systematic review of randomized controlled trials. Am J Obstet Gynecol. 2001;185: 227–235.

32. Belsey EM, Pinol APY, and Task Force on Long-Acting Systemic Agents for Fertility Regulation. Menstrual bleeding patterns in untreated women. Contraception. 1997;55:57–65.

33. Speroff L, Fritz MA. Clinical Gynecologic Endocrinology and Infertility, 7th ed. Philadelphia, PA: Lippincott Williams & Wilkins; 2005:547–571.

34. Warner PE, Critchely HOD, Lumsden MA et al. Menorrhagia I: Measured blood loss, clinical features, and outcome in women with heavy periods: A survey with follow up data. Am J Obstet Gynecol. 2004;190:1216–1223.

35. Krassas GE. Thyroid disease and female reproduction. Fertil Steril. 2000;74(6):1063–1070.

36. Pellerin GP, Finan MA. Endometrial cancer in women 45 years of age or younger: A clinicopathological analysis. Am J Obstet Gynecol. 2005;193:1640–1644.

37. Albers JR, Hull SK, Wesley RM. Abnormal uterine bleeding. Am Fam Physician. 2004;69:1915–1926.

38. Munro MG, Lukes AS. Abnormal uterine bleeding and underlying hemostatic disorders: Report of a consensus process. Fertil Steril. 2005;84:1335–1337.

39. Kouides PA, Conard J, Peyvandi F, et al. Hemostasis and menstruation: appropriate investigation for underlying disorders of hemostasis in women with excessive menstrual bleeding. Fertil Steril. 2005;84:1345–1351.

40. Dijkhuizen FPHLJ, Mol BWJ, Brolmann HAM, et al. The accuracy of endometrial sampling in the diagnosis of patients with endometrial carcinoma and hyperplasia. A meta-analysis. Cancer. 2000;89:1765–1772.

41. Smith-Bindman R, Kerlikowske K, Feldstein VA, et al. Endovaginal ultrasound to exclude endometrial cancer and other endometrial abnormalities. JAMA. 1998;280: 1510–1517.

42. Critchley HOD, Warner P, Lee AJ, Brechin S, Guise J, Graham B. Evaluation of abnormal uterine bleeding: comparison of three outpatient procedures within cohorts defined by age and menopausal status. Health Technol Assess. 2004;8(34): iii-iv, 1–139.

43. Bain C, Parkin DE, Cooper KG. Is outpatient diagnostic hysteroscopy more useful than endometrial biopsy alone for the investigation of abnormal uterine bleeding in unselected premenopausal women? A randomized comparison. Br J Obstet Gynaecol. 2002;109:805–811.

44. Medverd JR, Dubinsky TJ. Cost analysis model: US versus endometrial biopsy in evaluation of peri- and postmenopausal abnormal vaginal bleeding. Radiology. 2002; 222(3):619–627.

45. Dubinsky TJ. Value of sonography in the diagnosis of abnormal vaginal bleeding. J Clin Ultrasound. 2004;32:348–353.

46. Lethaby A, Augood C, Duckitt D. Nonsteroidal anti-inflammatory drugs for heavy menstrual bleeding (Cochrane Review). In: The Cochrane Library. Oxford, England: Update Software; 1998:Issue 3.

47. Lethaby AE, Cooke I, Rees M. Progersterone or progestogen-releasing intrauterine systems for heavy menstrual bleeding (Cochrane Review). In: The Cochrane Library. Oxford, England: Update Software; 2005:Issue 4.

48. Marjoribanks J, Lethaby A, Farquhar C. Surgery versus medical therapy for heavy menstrual bleeding (Cochrane Review). In: The Cochrane Library. Oxford, England: Update Software; 2003:Issue 2.

49. Schrager S. Abnormal uterine bleeding associated with hormonal contraception. Am Fam Physician. 2002;65:2073–2080.

50. Rauramo I, Elo I, Istre O. Long-term treatment of menorrhagia with levonorgestrel intrauterine system versus endometrial resection. Obstet Gynecol. 2004;104:1314–1321.

51. Lethaby A, Hickey M, Garry R. Endometrial destruction techniques for heavy menstrual bleeding (Cochrane Review). In: The Cochrane Library. Oxford, England: Update Software; 2005:Issue 4.

CHAPTER 30

Promoting Health for Women at Menopause

Linda French and Cathleen Abbott

CASE

Mrs. G. is a 48-year-old woman who complains of hot flashes that wake her up at night. She also finds that daytime hot flashes are not only uncomfortable, but also can be quite embarrassing. Her menstrual periods have been irregular for about 2 years, and the last was 2 months ago.

QUESTIONS

1. What additional history would you obtain?
2. Assuming that she has normal physical examination results, what treatment options would you offer her?
3. What other preventive services would you offer her?

Menopause is defined as permanent amenorrhea in a previously cycling woman. Natural menopause is the permanent cessation of menstrual cycles caused by the exhaustion of the ovaries. Medical intervention that removes or terminates ovarian function also leads to menopause. If a premenopausal woman has a hysterectomy without oophorectomy, her ovaries may still produce hormonal cycles. In this case she is generally considered to be premenopausal until ovarian cycles stop.

According to the World Health Organization, "The term perimenopause should include the period immediately prior to the menopause (when the endocrinologic, biological, and clinical features of approaching menopause commence) and the first year after the last menstrual period." It usually begins with an increase in menstrual irregularity. Climacteric is another term referring to the period around menopause, and begins with the onset of any symptoms attributed to the menopausal transition. Common climacteric symptoms, in order of frequency, are: vasomotor symptoms (hot flashes), mood disturbances, sleep disturbances, decreased libido, and vaginal dryness. Of women with symptoms, 50% can be expected to consult a physician regarding menopause.

In addition to the menopause, there are other changes that affect women in the middle years. These include personal issues of sexuality and aging, the "empty nest" response generated by children becoming fledgling adults, aging parents who may be ill or disabled, and health problems of friends and spouses. These developmental life changes can provoke symptoms similar to those of menopause or aggravate ones that already exist. On the other hand, there are many women who find "menopausal zest." Their children are out of the home, financial security may be reached, and there no longer is a fear of pregnancy.

NATURAL HISTORY

Beginning gradually, usually in the early to middle 40s, a woman's hormonal rhythm changes. There is a progressive decrease in ovarian mass and decreased production of ovarian hormones, including inhibin. Reduced levels of inhibin, even without a corresponding reduction in estrogen level, may cause the follicle-stimulating hormone (FSH) level to rise. Ovarian production of progesterone diminishes as the corpus luteum, formed after ovulation, decreases in size. Menstrual cycles become somewhat shorter, and estrogen changes are more variable. Levels are sometimes even higher than in former years because of recruitment of more ovarian follicles by higher FSH levels, which can increase estrogen production. Estrogen tends to predominate over progesterone, promoting fibroid changes in the uterus and breasts.

Before menopause, the ovary produces most of the body's circulating estrogen, which consists of three types: estriol (E3), estradiol (E2), and estrone (E1). Total estrogen decreases by about 60% after menopause, and the major reduction is in E2. The proportion of E1, which is primarily produced by fat cells, increases. Obese women have higher postmenopausal estrogen levels for this reason. This may contribute to the higher-than-average risk for endometrial and ovarian cancers in obese women.

The mean age at menopause in the United States is 51.3 years (1). Smokers experience menopause 1.8 years earlier than nonsmokers (age 50.2 vs. 52.0). Perimenopausal menstrual irregularity begins around age 47.5, typically lasting 4 years, with the majority of women in the range of 1 to 7 years. For 10% of women, menses simply cease without previous menstrual irregularity. Premature menopause is defined as cessation of menstrual periods before 40 years of age. About 10% of women are menopausal by age 46, 30% to 35% by age 50, and 90% by age 56. There is a familial tendency toward similarity in age at menopause.

Hysterectomy is an important cause of menopause in the United States, with over 600,000 surgeries performed annually. About 30% of US women have undergone hysterectomy by age 65, but the rate is decreasing as alternative therapies for some conditions gain acceptance. The rate is still more frequent than in European countries, where 6% to 20% of women undergo hysterectomy. The peak age for hysterectomy for US women is in their 40s. Fibroids are the most common reason for hysterectomy in women ages 45 to 54, endometrial hyperplasia for women ages 55 to 64, and uterine prolapse for women older than 65 years. Only about 10% of hysterectomies performed are because of cancer. Climacteric symptoms are

455

generally more severe for women who have undergone hysterectomy with oophorectomy before their natural menopause. More vasomotor complaints are noted, and bone loss is more severe. Postoperative memory losses have also been demonstrated, and sexual satisfaction can also be impaired. Routine oophorectomy at the time of hysterectomy for women 40 to 50 years old appears to be decreasing (2).

History

The patient-centered medical history can be divided into three areas: menstrual, urogenital, and climacteric symptoms. Key items include:

- Menstrual history: last menstrual period (LMP), last normal menstrual period, length of cycles, regularity of cycles, amount of bleeding, associated symptoms (such as dysmenorrhea, premenstrual symptoms, breast tenderness), and contraception (past and current)
- Urogenital: change in sexual activity and libido, dyspareunia, urinary frequency or incontinence, symptoms of cystitis and vaginitis
- Climacteric: hot flashes (frequency, timing, triggering stimuli, successful relief measures), mood, sleep patterns, skin and hair texture
- Health maintenance issues: exercise, weight and appetite, recreation, alcohol, smoking, drug habits, diet and vitamin supplements, occupation, Papanicolaou (Pap) smears and mammograms, social support
- Relevant past medical history: risk factors for osteoporosis, heart disease, and cancer
- Relevant family history: familial history of menopause and current health status of family members

Physical Examination

The physical examination focuses on evaluation of general appearance, and breast and pelvic examinations.

- General appearance: evidence of dry skin or fatigue; condition of hair and nails; affect; weight and distribution of fat; height and spine (change in height, kyphosis, or cervical hump)
- Neck examination: thyroid, cervical lymph nodes
- Breast examination: texture, masses, tenderness, discharge, axillary lymph nodes
- Pelvic examination: genitalia, urethra, vagina (atrophy, discharge), cervix (friability, discharge), uterus (size, mobility), adnexae (should not be palpable by the time women reach menopause)

DIAGNOSIS OF MENOPAUSE

Menopause is traditionally diagnosed retrospectively—1 year after the LMP. Increasingly, menopause is diagnosed based on a FSH level over 40 mIU/mL. In women receiving estrogens, either as oral contraceptives or for treatment of perimenopausal symptoms, FSH levels should be measured 7 to 10 days after stopping estrogens. A high FSH may not be reliable to diagnose menopause because the level can drop again, accompanied by further ovulatory cycles. Further ovulatory cycles are not expected if FSH is over 60 mIU/mL (3).

Vasomotor Symptoms

Vasomotor symptoms or hot flashes are the most common symptom associated with the menopause transition. Hot flashes are sensations of warmth, frequently accompanied by skin flushing and perspiration. A chill may follow. This is the consequence of a sudden change in the hypothalamic control of temperature regulation, although the precise triggers have not been elucidated. Estimates are that 50% to 80% of women experience these symptoms beginning several years before menopause.

Hot flashes occur commonly among women in their thirties and forties who have regular menstrual cycles. In one prospective study of women in Massachusetts (1), the prevalence of hot flashes peaked at 50% in the year that menses ceased. By 4 years after the final menstrual period, 20% of women still had hot flashes. In another study, the incidence of hot flashes was 25% in premenopausal women, 69% in perimenopausal women, and 39% in late postmenopausal women (>4.5 years) (4). Fifteen years after menopause, 10% of women may continue to have moderate to severe hot flashes. Vasomotor symptoms beginning in perimenopause can be lifelong.

Hot flashes are more common in certain population subgroups: African-American women (5), women with a maternal history of hot flashes (6), and premenopausal women with premenstrual syndrome and other menstrual cycle abnormalities (7). Factors associated with a decreased risk of vasomotor symptoms are higher education (college degree vs. less), and abrupt cessation of menses (without perimenopausal menstrual irregularity). Obesity has been more often associated with an increased rather than a decreased likelihood of hot flashes. Exercise has been associated with less likelihood of hot flashes in observational studies, but a well-designed clinical trial showed no benefit (7).

Treatment of Vasomotor Symptoms

Numerous well-controlled studies have shown the effectiveness of oral or transdermal estrogen-containing therapy for hot flashes, with 70%–90% of women experiencing good relief (8, 9). Low-dose estrogen plus testosterone has been shown to be more effective than low-dose estrogen only, and as effective as high-dose estrogen only (10). However, evidence of safety is lacking for the long-term use of testosterone in postmenopausal women. The weight of evidence regarding phytoestrogens is that they are not effective therapy (11, 12).

Alternatives to estrogen for treatment of hot flashes include gabapentin, venlafaxine, paroxetine, clonidine, and megestrol acetate (see Table 30.1). Gabapentin at a sufficient dose (300 mg three times daily) reduces hot flashes by about half, whereas low doses (100 mg three times daily) are no different than placebo (13). A 20% reduction in hot flashes can be expected with clonidine (14), but this agent may impair sleep quality (15). Transdermal progesterone cream alone may improve vasomotor symptoms, although concerns about increased breast cancer risk limits use. Megestrol appears to be nearly as effective as estrogen with a 70% reduction in symptoms (16). Although long-term use of megestrol acetate by cancer survivors for the treatment of hot flashes has been shown to be effective and well tolerated (14), it is not custom-

TABLE 30.1 Nonestrogen Treatments for Vasomotor Symptoms

Generic (Trade)	Side Effects with More Than 10% Incidence	Usual Dose	Relative Cost per Month*
Gabapentin (Neurontin, generic)	Somnolence Dizziness Fatigue	300 mg three times daily	$$
Paroxetine (Paxil, generic)	Insomnia Somnolence Dizziness Tremor	20 mg daily	$$
Venlafaxine (Effexor)	Nausea Headache Somnolence Dry mouth Dizziness Insomnia	75 mg daily or 37.5 mg twice daily	$$$
Clonidine (Catapres, generic)	Dry mouth Somnolence Dizziness Constipation	0.1 mg twice daily	$
Megestrol (Megace, generic)	Weight gain Caution: small risk of thromboembolism	20 mg twice daily	$
Black cohosh (Remifemin, generic)	Not documented	40 mg twice daily	$

*Relative cost: $ = <$33.00; $$ = $34.00 – $66.00; $$$ = >$67.00

ary to use it for other women at menopause. Small studies (17) of relaxation techniques have also shown symptom reduction.

Mood Disturbances

Irritability and mood swings are common climacteric complaints. Women often compare them with what they experienced previously as premenstrual symptoms. However, studies of depressive symptoms in menopausal women indicate that menopause is not associated with increased rates of major depression. Women with previous history of postpartum depression may be at increased risk for recurrence of depression in perimenopause. Stressful life context and poor health status appear to be more important risk factors for depression than symptoms of menopause in climacteric women.

In a meta-analysis of 26 studies of the effect of hormone therapy (HT) on depressed mood (18), estrogen showed limited effectiveness in improving depressed mood. The addition of synthetic progestins reduced the estrogen effect. Androgens alone or with estrogen had the greatest effect for improving depressed mood. Other reviews have concluded that estrogen therapy (ET) or combined hormone therapy (CHT) has little effect in the treatment of psychological symptoms (including anxiety, and cognitive and affective symptoms). It is not effective as monotherapy for major depression. As an adjuvant to psychotropic therapy, it may have limited effect. There is insufficient evidence to support prophylactic HT to prevent depression in women whose medical history includes prior postpartum depression. Estrogens do not affect the ability of

a woman with moderate to severe vasomotor symptoms to cope with stress.

Women with mild psychological and predominantly vasomotor symptoms may benefit from a trial of HT before using psychotropic medication. For important dysphoric symptoms, antidepressants are indicated. Androgens may be helpful, but safety with long-term use has not been established.

Sleep Disturbance

Many perimenopausal women complain of poor sleep, often attributed to nocturnal hot flashes. Subjective impairment of sleep quality that is associated with climacteric vasomotor symptoms did not manifest as abnormalities in polysomnographic sleep recordings (19). High body mass index and increased age are associated with polysomnographic abnormalities. Treatment, as described above for vasomotor symptoms, may improve poor sleep that is attributed to night sweats. Other standard approaches to insomnia, such as sleep hygiene measures and progressive relaxation techniques, also can be used. If sleep apnea is suspected, a sleep study may be indicated.

Urogenital Symptoms

Urogenital symptoms are reported by up to 40% of postmenopausal women, although some studies estimate that only 20% of them seek treatment. Premenopausal vaginal tissues are normally elastic and rugated with a high glycogen content, which helps maintain the bacterial flora dominated by *lactoba-*

cilli and a vaginal pH between 3.5 and 4.5. After the decline in estrogen postmenopausally, the mucosa thins with loss of collagen support and fibrous transformation of the elastic fibers. As the glycogen content declines the *lactobacilli* become less prominent leading to an increase in the vaginal pH, typically to 5.5–6.8. The result is vaginal dryness and gradual atrophy of the genital tract. The labia shrink, the mucosa loses its rugae and becomes smooth and pale, the introitus and vagina may contract, and a urethral caruncle may be noted. Women who smoke and those who have never given birth vaginally tend to have more marked atrophy. Atrophic vaginitis refers to associated symptoms of vaginal discomfort, including dryness, burning, and itching. Urinary symptoms may coincide, such as frequency, urgency, dysuria, and stress incontinence. Some women develop recurrent urinary tract infection (UTI) or symptomatic bacterial vaginosis.

Low-dose topical estrogen is effective treatment for atrophic vaginitis (see Table 30.2). Estrogen may be used locally in the form of creams, tablets, pessaries, or vaginal rings; they appear to be equally effective. Serum estrogen levels with topical therapy are approximately one tenth that of systemic therapy. A clinical trial of topical estrogen for women who developed recurrent UTI postmenopausally showed mean reduction in recurrences from 6 to less than 1 annually (20). Topical estrogen may also improve stress incontinence in the presence of vaginal atrophy.

Another class of treatment shown to be effective is vaginal lubricants including liquid and gel products to coat and moisturize the vaginal epithelium. There is some evidence that the gel product (Replens) used three times weekly may be as effective as a topical estrogen. Vitamins D and E have also been studied and may be helpful (21). Several other "natural remedies" have been suggested, but controlled trials to demonstrate efficacy and safety are lacking.

Continuing sexual activity is associated with maintaining elasticity and lubrication. A causal relationship is difficult to determine because better elasticity may allow some women to continue intercourse. On the other hand semen may help to maintain lower pH.

Sexual Function

Women's sexual interest usually declines gradually during the late reproductive years with an additional drop at the time of menopause (22). Dyspareunia is also a frequent complaint related to genital dryness and involution. For sexual dysfunction caused by urogenital atrophy, a low dose of intravaginal estrogen generally gives good symptom relief within 6 months without altering the endometrium. In a systematic review of HT for climacteric symptoms related to sexual function (23), vaginal dryness improved with ET in seven of eight studies; dyspareunia improved in only one of six studies (with transdermal 17-β-E2); orgasm increased in only one (using ethinyl estradiol) of five studies; and sexual interest increased in none of seven studies using conjugated estrogens. However, testosterone and dehydroepiandrosterone (DHEA) seem to increase sexual interest when added to estrogen therapy. Use of androgens to treat female sexual dysfunction in premenopausal and postmenopausal women is the subject of current research in an attempt to establish long-term safety. In one study of sildenafil (Viagra) there was no benefit to middle-aged women with sexual arousal difficulties (24).

OSTEOPOROSIS PREVENTION AND TREATMENT

Maximum bone density is attained in young adulthood. Women then typically lose 50% of cancellous and 30% of trabecular bone mass over their remaining lifetime. (Men lose 30% and 20%, respectively.) Cancellous bone is concentrated in the spine and ends of long bones. Bone loss begins in the premenopausal years and accelerates in the early postmenopausal years. Increased osteoclastic activity in the immediate postmenopausal period causes an imbalance between bone resorption and formation. This is more damaging than that caused by decreased osteoblastic activity. The net result is that bone turnover increases, with more resorption than formation of bone.

Poor intake of calcium and vitamin D, sedentary lifestyle, low body fat, and Caucasian race (especially Northern European ancestry) increase the risk of osteoporosis (see Table 30.3). Smoking is a significant risk for osteoporotic hip fractures (19% of current smokers vs. 12% of those who have never smoked, with a dose-response gradient) (25). Certain medical conditions and medications, such as excess thyroid hormone (whether endogenous or exogenous) and long-term oral glucocorticoid (e.g., prednisone) treatment, cause bone loss. Prolonged functional amenorrhea, brought on by competitive athletic training or excessive weight loss, and other ovulatory disturbances can also contribute to bone loss in younger women.

Prevention is the least costly approach to osteoporosis and should begin in youth (see Table 30.4.). Primary prevention should include smoking cessation, weight-bearing exercise, and sufficient intake of calcium and vitamin D. Although ET has been shown to decrease risk of osteoporosis (strength of recommendation = B), progesterone alone is not an effective therapy. Screening for osteoporosis is recommended routinely at age 65 by the US Preventive Services Task Force and at 60–64 years with risk factors. The most appropriate way to diagnose osteoporosis is by dual-energy x-ray absorptiometry of both spine and femur. If bone density is less than 2.5 standard deviations (SD) below the mean for young women (T-score), a diagnosis of osteoporosis is confirmed. If bone mineral density (BMD) is less than 1 SD but not less than 2.5 SD below the mean for young women, a diagnosis of osteopenia is made and measures for prevention of further bone loss should be instituted. Testing intervals less than 2 years are too short for assessing interval change.

Pharmacologic Treatments

Estrogen produces a dose-response gradient for bone maintenance in postmenopausal women (see Table 30.2). HT decreases fractures while treatment continues. Combined regimens of estrogen and testosterone (e.g., Estratest) maintain bone mass better than estrogen alone. Discontinuation leads to a phase of accelerated bone loss like that following natural menopause. Protection against fractures is lost within 5 years after cessation of HT (26). Concerns about cardiovascular and breast cancer risks of CHT have led to a decrease in use of HT for prevention and treatment of osteoporosis. Most recently, ultra low-dose estrogen-only therapy has been studied and found to improve bone density without endometrial stimulation (27, 28).

TABLE 30.2 Hormone Preparations for Perimenopausal Women (Estrogens)

Generic (Trade)	Form	Doses Available	Usual Dose	Relative Cost*
Estrones				
Conjugated estrogen (Premarin, generic)	Oral	0.3, 0.45, 0.625, 0.9, 1.25	One tablet daily, lower doses most commonly used	$$
	Vaginal cream	0.625mg/g	1/2–1 applicator	$$$
Esterified estrogens (Menest)	Oral	0.3, 0.625, 1.25, 2.5 mg	0.3–1.25 mg	$–$$
Estropipate (Ogen, Ortho-est, generic)	Oral	0.625, 1.25, 2.5, 5 mg	0.625–1.25 mg	$
Ogen vaginal	Vaginal	1.5 mg/g	1\2–1 applicator	$
Estradiols				
Micronized estradiol (Estrace, generic)	Oral	0.5, 1, 2 mg	0.5–1 mg	$$
	Vaginal cream	0.1 mg/g	1/2–1 applicator	$$
Estradiol	Oral	0.45, 0.5, 0.9, 1, 1.5, 1.8, 2 mg	One tablet daily	$
Conjugated B estrogen (Enjuvia)	Oral	0.625, 1.25 mg,	One tablet daily	$$$ (? not marketed yet)
17β-estradiol	Transdermal	0.025, 0.05, 0.075, 0.1 mg/ 24 h patches		$
Climara	Transdermal	0.025, 0.0375, 0.05, 0.06, 0.075, 0.1 mg/d	Once weekly	$$
Alora	Transdermal	0.025, 0.05, 0.075, 0.1 mg/d	Twice weekly	$$
Vivelle/Vivelle Dot	Transdermal	0.025, 0.0375, 0.05, 0.075, 0.1 mg/24 h	Twice weekly	$$
Menostar	Transdermal	0.014 mg/24 h	Once weekly	$$
Estradiol Topical Emulsion (Estrasorb)	Transdermal	1.74 g pkg with 2.5 mg estradiol hemihydrate/g	One pkg to each leg daily	$$
Gel 0.06% (Estrogel)	Transdermal	1.25 g per pump with 0.75 mg estradiol	One pump once or twice daily	$$
Estradiol ring (Estring)	Vaginal ring	7.5 mcg/24 h for 90 d	One ring every 90 d	$$$
(Femring)		50 or 100 mcg/ 24 h for 90 days		$$$
Estradiol vaginal tablet (Vagifem)	Vaginal tablet	0.025 mg	1 tablet twice weekly	$$
Progestins				
Micronized progesterone (Prometrium)	Oral	100 mg, 200 mg	200 mg/d	$$$
Medroxyprogesterone acetate (Provera, generic)	Oral	2.5, 5, 10 mg	2.5 mg daily, or cyclic use of higher doses	$
Combined estrogen and progestin				
Conjugated estrogens plus medroxyprogesterone acetate (Prempro Premphase)	Oral	0.625/5 mg, 0.45/1.5 mg, 0.3/1.5 mg	Once daily	$$
	Oral	0.625 mg 0.625/5 mg	Day 1–14 Day 15–28	$$

(continued)

TABLE 30.2 Hormone Preparations for Perimenopausal Women (Estrogens) (*continued*)

Generic (Trade)	Form	Doses Available	Usual Dose	Relative Cost*
17β-Estradiol plus norethindrone acetate (CombiPatch)	Transdermal	0.05 mg estradiol plus 0.14 or 0.25 mg norethindrone acetate	Twice weekly	$$
Ethinyl estradiol/ norethindrone acetate (FemHRT)	Oral	2.5 **mcg** ethinyl estradiol/ 0.5 mg **norethindrone** acetate or 5 **mcg** ethinyl estradiol/1 mg norethnindrone acetate	Once daily	$$
Estradiol plus Norgestimate (Prefest)	Oral	1 mg estradiol in all tablets plus norgestimate 0.09 mcg pulsed (3 tablets with, then 3 tablets without)	Once daily	$$
Androgens				
Testosterone	Transdermal			
1% gel (Androgel, Testim)	Transdermal	2.5, 5 g tube or packet	0.5 g daily (5 mg)	$$$
Combination estrogen and androgen				
Esterified estrogens and methyltestosterone (Estratest, or Estratest HS)	Tablet	1.25 mg E/2.5 mg M	1 per day	$$
	Tablet	0.625 mg E/1.25 mg M	1 per day	$$

*Relative cost: $ = <$33.00; $$ = $34.00–$66.00; $$$ = >$67.00

Other pharmacologic treatments available for treatment of osteoporosis are presented in Table 30.5. They include bisphosphonates, salmon calcitonin, and a human parathyroid hormone analog. Sufficient intake of calcium (1,500 mg elemental calcium daily) and vitamin D (800 IU daily or 50,000 IU every 2 months) should be concurrent with the administration of any of these drugs.

Bisphosphonates are the most commonly used therapies for osteoporosis. They are potent inhibitors of bone resorption. Several are approved for treatment of osteoporosis. This class of medications is also effective in the treatment of bone diseases such as Paget's disease, myeloma, and bone metastases.

Alendronate (Fosamax) was the first bisphosphonates approved by the US Food and Drug Administration (FDA) for the treatment of post-menopausal osteoporosis. It is taken orally on an empty stomach (with clear fluids while standing or sitting), 5 mg daily or 35 mg weekly for prevention, 10 mg daily or 70 mg weekly for treatment. It reduces the incidence of vertebral and nonvertebral fractures by about half. Gastroesophageal reflux is a common adverse effect. Esophageal ulcer, myalgia, and arthralgia are also possible adverse drug events. Treatment lasting at least 5 years is recommended for osteoporosis, but the optimal duration of treatment has not been established. Alendronate can also be used on a quarter-year cycle, 14 days on and 76 off, as preventive treatment for high-risk or osteopenic women.

Risedronate (Actonel) reduces vertebral and nonvertebral fractures over a 3-year period in women with osteoporosis (29). Adverse effects are similar to those of alendronate, but may be milder. BMD improves from baseline less than with alendronate, but a difference in incidence of fracture between the two has not been demonstrated (30).

Ibandronate (Boniva) has also been shown effective and

TABLE 30.3 Risk Factors for Osteoporosis

Genetic predisposition
    Caucasian, especially Northern European
Lifestyle factors
    Smoking
    Sedentary
    Poor calcium intake
    Poor vitamin D intake
Reproductive history
    Early premenopausal vasomotor symptoms
    History of functional amenorrhea
    Ovulatory disturbances (oligomenorrhea)
    Premature ovarian failure
    Premenopausal hysterectomy
    Premenopausal oophorectomy
Medications
    Glucocorticoids (e.g., prednisone)
    Excess thyroid hormone
    Depo-medroxyprogesterone acetate
    Chemotherapeutic agents

TABLE 30.4 Preventing Osteoporosis

Intervention	Strength of Recommendation*	Comments
Smoking cessation	A	
Weight-bearing exercise	A	
Calcium	A	1,000 mg or more daily
Vitamin D	A	400 IU for all women, 800 IU for elderly
Estrogen or bisphosphonate therapy	B	Especially in high-risk women
Testosterone	C	Evidence of long-term safety is lacking
Dehydroepiandrosterone	C	Evidence of efficacy is lacking

*A = consistent, good-quality patient-oriented evidence; B = inconsistent or limited-quality patient-oriented evidence; C = consensus, disease-oriented evidence, usual practice, expert opinion, or case series. For information about the SORT evidence rating system, see *http://www.aafp.org/afpsort.xml*.

TABLE 30.5 Pharmacological Therapies for Osteoporosis

Generic (Trade)	Formulations	Usual Dosing	Relative Monthly Cost*
Bisphosphonates			
Alendronate (Fosamax)	5 mg, 10 mg 35 mg, 40 mg, 70 mg 70 mg/75 ml oral solution	10 mg daily or 70 mg weekly Prevention: 5 mg daily or 35 mg weekly (40 mg dosage recommended for treatment of Paget's)	$$$
Alendronate +cholecalciferol (Fosamax Plus D)	70 mg + 2,800 IU	70/2,800 once weekly	$$$
Ibandronate (Boniva)	2.5 mg, 150 mg	2.5 mg daily or 150 mg once monthly, treatment or prevention	$$$
Risedronate (Actonel)	5 mg, 30 mg, 35 mg	Prevention and treatment 5 mg daily or 35 mg weekly (30-mg dosage recommended for treatment of Paget's)	$$$
Risedronate and calcium (Actonel with calcium)	35 mg + 1250 mg calcium carbonate	Once weekly	$$$
Others			
Salmon Calcitonin (Miacalcin)	2 ml bottles of 15 activations, 200 IU per activation for intranasal use	One activation daily in alternating nostrils for treatment but not prevention, also effective for pain management of osteoporotic fracture	$$$
Raloxifene (Evista)	60 mg tablet	One daily for prevention or treatment	$$$
Human parathyroid hormone (Forteo)	750 mcg/3ml pen injector device	20 mcg subcutaneously daily	$$$

*Relative cost: $, <$33.00; $$, $34.00–$66.00; $$$, >$67.00

can be given once monthly at a dosage of 150 mg, or daily dose of 2.5 mg. One study suggested that the once monthly regimen of this drug was preferred by 75% of the women compared with alendronate weekly dosing, based on convenience and less frequent side-effects (31).

Pamidronate (Aredia) 30–60 mg intravenously every 6 months is occasionally used but is not FDA approved for osteoporosis. Zoledronic acid (Zometa) is another bisphosphonate that is used for malignant bone disease.

Three other classes of medications may be used to treat osteoporosis. Raloxifene, a selective estrogen receptor modulator (SERM), has been shown in short-term studies to prevent vertebral fractures. Intranasal calcitonin (Miacalcin) may also be used. Data on fracture incidence with this treatment are not available. Human parathyroid hormone, teriparatide (Fortéo), is the first approved drug for osteoporosis treatment that acts by stimulating osteoblastic activity. It can be used to treat severe osteoporosis, but is quite expensive. It is generally given in a daily dosage of 20 mcg subcutaneously for up to 2 years. It increases bone density and decreases back pain associated with recurrent vertebral fractures. Interestingly, the combination of teriparatide with alendronate does not increase bone density more than either one alone, although their mechanisms of action differ (32).

MENOPAUSAL HORMONE THERAPIES

The once popular term "hormone replacement therapy" has been largely dropped in the medical literature following release of results from the Women's Health Initiative study (WHI) in 2002 (33), when it was realized that it is not acceptable practice to routinely treat menopause as a hormone deficient state. The favored terms are HT, which may be divided into ET or CHT. HT continues to be prescribed frequently for symptomatic relief as described above.

A woman without a uterus can take ET continuously. To reduce the risk of endometrial cancer, a woman with a uterus should receive CHT, with progestin to protect against the endometrial cancer risk with unopposed estrogen. CHT may be taken either continuously or cyclically as described below; the latter allowing for withdrawal bleeding. To avoid unpredictable uterine bleeding, a woman should generally be at least 3 years postmenopause to use a continuous regimen. Table 30.2 lists options for hormone preparations.

There are several ways of prescribing CHT, with the most commonly used progestin, medroxyprogesterone (Provera). It can be taken cyclically in a 5- to 10-mg daily dose for 10 to 14 days per 28- or 30-day cycle, or continuously in a 2.5- to 5-mg daily dose. For women who complain of symptoms on the days off of estrogen with cyclic treatment, estrogen can be given continuously, adding progestin for 10 to 14 days each month. Continuous estrogen, with use of progestin for 14 days each quarter, (i.e., every 3 months) has also been shown to provide adequate endometrial protection (34). Micronized progesterone is approved for cyclic administration only, with a usual dose of 200 mg daily for 14 days in each cycle.

Several combination products are on the market. These are generally less costly than prescriptions for an estrogen and progestin separately. One of these (Ortho-Prefest) is a pulse regimen that includes estrogen daily and alternating norgesti-mate—3 days on and 3 days off, equivalent to a continuous treatment.

Some vendors promote "bioequivalent" HT giving the impression that it is safer. Usually women provide saliva samples for customization of dosing. However, there is no evidence to suggest that it is safer, and saliva samples are a poor method of determining systemic levels.

Cardiovascular Effects

The WHI was conducted with a principle objective to answer the question of whether HT was cardioprotective as suggested by observational data. To the contrary, there were small increases in the CHT group of myocardial infarctions, strokes, and venous thromboembolism, with a mean of 5.2 years follow-up (see Table 30.6). The most common adverse effect was venous thromboembolism affecting 0.9% of women with 5 years of treatment. The ET portion of the study reported in 2004 had almost 2 years longer follow-up. It showed no increase in myocardial infarctions and similar increases in stroke and venous thromboembolism.

There are some metabolic differences between oral and transdermal routes of administration of HT. However, a small clinical trial of transdermal estrogen for secondary prevention of coronary events showed no benefit (35).

Risk of Breast Cancer

The WHI study of CHT was stopped when the increase in risk of breast cancer with active treatment became statistically significant, with a mean duration of treatment of about 5 years. Previous studies of CHT showed similar increases. There is still some uncertainty whether ET increases breast cancer risk. If so, it is of much smaller magnitude than with CHT. The WHI showed a nonsignificant decrease in breast cancer with almost 7 years ET use (36). A meta-analysis of large observational studies suggests an increase in breast cancer risk of smaller magnitude than with CHT (37).

Memory

Although observational studies suggested benefit of HT for cognitive function, the WHI showed a slight increase in risk of the diagnosis of Alzheimer's disease as well as a more important risk of at least a 2-point decline in mini-mental status exam score (38, 39). Another clinical trial showed no benefit from adjunctive treatment with estrogen in women with Alzheimer's disease (40). ET did not slow Alzheimer's disease progression or improve global cognitive or functional outcomes for women with mild to moderate disease.

Other Effects

There is a small increase in risk of gall bladder surgery of about 1% of women with 5 years use of HT (41). In addition, about one in eight women has worsening of urinary incontinence with use of HT (42). Ethanol causes a delay in the initial degradation of sex hormones. Appropriate dosing for women with regular alcohol consumption may be less than that for nondrinkers (43). Grapefruit juice also delays the degradation of estrogen (44). Several studies have documented that there is not an increase in weight or body fat with use of HT in perimenopausal women.

TABLE 30.6 Risks and Benefits of Combined Hormone Therapy in the Women's Health Initiative Study

Outcome	NNH* for 1 Year	NNH for 5 Years
Myocardial infarction	1,429	286
Stroke	1,250	250
Venous thromboembolism	555	111
Deep venous thrombosis	1,000	200
Pulmonary embolism	1,250	250
Breast cancer	1,250	250
Balance of risks versus benefits	500	100

Outcome	NNT† for 1 Year	NNT for 5 Years
Hip fracture	2,000	400
Vertebral fracture	2,000	400
Colon or rectal cancer	1,667	333

*NNH means "number needed to harm." It stands for the number people getting treatment when one person gets the harmful effect.
†NNT means "number needed to treat." It stands for the number of people getting treatment when one person gets the beneficial effect.

Androgens

Endogenous production of testosterone decreases gradually during a woman's reproductive years. Exogenous testosterone has a beneficial effect on bone density and libido in perimenopausal women (45). However, long-term safety data are lacking and caution with use is warranted. Testosterone is available either alone or in combination with conjugated estrogen (Estratest and Estratest HS) at a daily dose of 1.25–2.5 mg of testosterone. It is also available in a topical gel formulation intended for men (Androgel). Alternatively it can be compounded in a cream and used topically on the skin or vulva.

The adrenal glands are the main source of endogenous androgens in postmenopausal women. The principal hormones are DHEA and dehydroepiandrosterone sulfate. Higher-dose oral estrogen treatment significantly reduces the bioavailability of endogenous androgens by increasing sex hormone-binding globulin, thereby creating a hypoandrogenic state. A review of 11 studies (46) suggests that 50 mg per day of DHEA may be helpful treatment for sexual dysfunction; risks should be assessed for individual patients. DHEA is available as a dietary supplement.

SERMs

SERMs are a subject of active investigation. These compounds act differently at estrogen receptors in various organs. On some receptors they may have an estrogen-like effect, and on others an antiestrogen effect. There are currently three products available in the United States: tamoxifen, raloxifene, and toremifene. The last is only approved for treatment of metastatic breast cancer and will not be reviewed here. Approval for tibolone, available in many other countries, was expected about the time WHI results were published, and has been delayed.

The FDA has approved the use of tamoxifen for the prevention of breast cancer in high-risk women. The evidence of efficacy for this use comes from the National Cancer Institute/National Surgical Adjuvant Breast and Bowel Cancer Prevention Trial (47). This was a 5-year study of more than 13,000 women at high risk for breast cancer. It showed a 45% decrease in relative risk of breast cancer in the tamoxifen-treated group. The number needed to treat to prevent one case of invasive breast cancer was 77 patients treated for 5 years (or 385 per year), which would cost $400,000 to $500,000 for each case prevented. The long-term protection from breast cancer after such treatment is unknown. Two smaller European studies showed no protective effect.

There are some risks associated with the use of tamoxifen. The risk of deep vein thrombosis (DVT) is about three times the normal risk and is similar to the increased risk associated with estrogen replacement therapy. Tamoxifen has an estrogenic effect on endometrium. Studies have found endometrial hyperplasia, abnormal uterine bleeding, and an increased risk of endometrial cancer. Hot flashes are a common and often unpleasant adverse event. Moderate to severe vasomotor symptoms occur in about 17% of women. Although a protective effect on bone density has been noted in postmenopausal women, this effect is less than that of estrogen, and premenopausal women experience bone loss. A significant increase in clinically evident depression has also been observed. Tamoxifen has a positive effect on the lipid profile of postmenopausal women. However, data are lacking regarding the effect of tamoxifen on cardiac events. There is a slight increase in risk of stroke.

Women with a defined 5-year projected risk of breast cancer that equals or exceeds 1.66% (according to the Gail model, which is available in the public domain) may be offered tamoxifen 20 mg/d for up to 5 years as an option to reduce that risk. The US Preventive Services Task Force estimates that for a 55-year-old woman with a uterus the risks of tamoxifen outweigh the benefits, unless the breast cancer risk for the next 5 years is more than 4%. A discussion of the risks and benefits is necessary. There has been no demonstrated benefit for overall health, breast cancer–specific survival, or overall survival. These uncertainties should also be explained.

Raloxifene has been approved for treating osteoporosis, although it is less effective than estrogen or alendronate (48). To date, raloxifene has been proven helpful in preventing vertebral fractures, but not fractures of the hip, ankle, or wrist. The study of Tamoxifen and Raloxifene (STAR) showed that raloxifene is as effective as tamoxifen for breast cancer risk with adverse events. Therefore, raloxifene is likely to replace tamoxifen for this purpose (49).

Other SERMs are in development and testing. The hope is to find drugs that are tailored to produce a better balance of estrogenic and antiestrogenic effects, thus providing the benefits of estrogen while reducing its risk to the breast and uterus, and minimizing side effects. The publication of results from the WHI has led to greater caution in the introduction of such drugs.

Phytoestrogens

There are several classes of plant substances that are functionally similar to E2, including isoflavones (legumes), lignins (linseed), coumestans, and resorcylic acid lactones. Known as phytoestrogens, they include at least 20 compounds from 300 plants. They are weaker than natural estrogens, and are not stored in tissues. Common phytoestrogen-containing foods are parsley, garlic, soybeans, wheat, rice, dates, pomegranates, cherries, and coffee. Phytoestrogens are also found in the herbs licorice, red clover, thyme, turmeric, and hops verbena. Soy is the legume highest in isoflavones. Some phytoestrogens have been isolated and are sold over the counter. For example, two isoflavonoids derived from soy—genistein and daidzein—have estrogen-like activity. A synthetic phytoestrogen—ipriflavone—is also available.

Women report fewer menopausal symptoms in parts of the world where the staple diet includes foods high in phytoestrogens. The incidence of breast and other cancers, as well as coronary artery disease, is lower for Japanese women, who excrete far more isoflavonoids in their urine than do European or American women. It has been hypothesized that the lower rates of climacteric vasomotor symptoms among Japanese women may be attributable to soy consumption. Phytoestrogens may be among the dietary factors affording protection against cancer and heart disease in vegetarians in general. There is some evidence that isoflavones do not increase endometrial thickness. However, the effect of pharmacological doses of isolated isoflavones on breast and endometrial cancer risks are uncertain, and caution is warranted.

There have been several well-designed, randomized controlled trials of phytoestrogens in menopausal women. Most trials have failed to find a significant effect of soy or isoflavones on vasomotor symptoms versus placebo (11, 12). The common pattern is that hot flashes improve over time in both active

treatment and placebo arms, and any improvement of the isoflavone-treated group improvement over placebo is small and neither clinically nor statistically significant. Another trial assessing effects of isoflavones on cognitive function, bone mineral density, and plasma lipids found no differences versus placebo after 1 year of treatment, with good adherence (50).

Black cohosh is an herbal preparation often used for treating menopausal symptoms. In Germany, a standardized preparation is approved for short-term (6 months) use. A systematic review (51) of herbal preparations for treating menopausal symptoms found that the available studies were too few and too weak to provide clear evidence of benefit. One small study compared a 40 mg dose of isopropanolic extract of black cohosh with 25 mcg E2 transdermally and showed equivalent benefit on hot flash frequency over the 3-month duration of the trial (52).

EDUCATIONAL INTERVENTIONS

In a British trial (53) of small-group educational interventions to prepare for menopause, beliefs about menopause were less negative in the intervention group. In another randomized trial (54) of education to prepare for menopause, groups were given either written information; guided lecture–discussion; or a personalized, decision-support exercise. The lecture–discussion was marginally better than the written information, and the personalized decision-support approach was least effective. The investigators concluded that carefully written information is effective in promoting knowledge, adherence, and satisfaction among well-educated, interested women.

There are many books available for the lay public about menopause. Any that have not been updated after 2002 are out of date. The quality of information about pharmacotherapy and non-pharmacotherapy options is variable. Many publications promote herbal products that are not effective or for which evidence of benefit is lacking. Two books with objective information are *A Woman's Guide to Menopause and Perimenopause* by Minkin and Wright, and *The Greatest Experiment Ever Performed on Women* by Seaman. The latter traces the history of menopausal hormone use through the results of the WHI. Other resources are listed in Table 30.7.

CASE DISCUSSION

The history should include the patient's reproductive, menstrual, and sexual history; past medical and surgical history; and social history including smoking and alcohol use. Her family history is especially important regarding breast cancer. It is also important to elicit her opinions and beliefs regarding both menopause and her health in general to guide the decision-making process regarding treatment.

If the patient does not have contraindications, the risks and benefits of cyclic CHT should be discussed as well as alternative approaches. Measuring the FSH level before initiating treatment is not necessary. Continuous HT would not be a good choice because unpredictable bleeding beyond 6 months of use is likely without well-established menopause. If she has important concerns about breast cancer risk, espe-

TABLE 30.7 Resources for Patient Education Regarding Menopause

Organization	Contact Information	Description
North American Menopause Society	*www.menopause.org*	Menopause guidebook *Menopause: A New Beginning* (5th grade reading level) Web site also has list of frequently asked questions and answers, and suggested reading list
American Academy of Family Physicians	1-800-944-0000	*Menopause: What to Expect When Your Body is Changing* *Osteoporosis: Keeping Your Bones Healthy and Strong*
American College of Obstetricians and Gynecologists	1-800-410-ACOG	Brochures *Midlife Transitions: A Guide to Approaching Menopause* *The Menopause Years* *Preventing Osteoporosis*
Office on Women's Health, US Department of Health and Human Services	*www.4woman.gov/owh/pub/ menoguide.htm*	Resource guide including agencies, institutions, reports, and books

cially if there is a family history of breast cancer in a first-degree relative, she may not want to pursue this option.

If the patient is still at risk for unintended pregnancy, she might consider the use of a progesterone intrauterine device. In that case, she would be eligible to use ET and avoid excess breast cancer risk.

Micronized progesterone could be offered along with estrogen for its more favorable effect on lipids and lack of evidence of increase in breast cancer risk (although it has not been shown to be safer in long-term studies). Other choices that are worth considering in this case are gabapentin, proxetine, and venlafaxine. An androgen (low-dose testosterone or DHEA 25–50 mg/d) for short-term use may be considered if there is an insufficient response to the initial-dose regimen of HT (including 0.625 mg of conjugated estrogen or 1 mg of E2) or if lack of libido is an issue. If testosterone is used, consider monitoring serum level to assure that dosing is not excessive.

If she smokes, HT should be avoided and smoking cessation counseling is the most important preventive service that can be offered to her to prevent cardiovascular disease, smoking-related cancers, lung disease, and osteoporosis. Other preventive services that should be offered at this time are a Pap smear every 3 years, or more often if risk factors for cervical cancer are present; a mammogram every 1 to 2 years; checking cholesterol level every 5 years; and tetanus booster every 10 years. It would be a good time to advise her to start screening for colon cancer and to obtain a flu vaccine annually starting at age 50. She should be counseled for prevention of osteoporosis through adequate weight-bearing exercise and calcium and vitamin D intake.

REFERENCES

1. McKinlay S, Brambilla PJ, Posnere JG. The normal menopause transition. Maturitas. 1992;14:103–115.
2. Parker WH, Broder MS, Liu Z, Shoupe D, Farquhar C, Berek JS. Ovarian conservation at the time of hysterectomy for benign disease. Obstet Gynecol. 2005;106(2):219–226.
3. Landgren BM, Collins A, Csemiczky G, Burger HG, Baksheev L, Robertson DM. Menopause transition: Annual changes in serum hormonal patterns over the menstrual cycle in women during a nine-year period prior to menopause. J Clin Endocrinol Metab. 2004;89(6):2763–2769.
4. Barentsen R, Groeneveld FP, Bareman FP, et al. Women's opinion on withdrawal bleeding with hormone replacement therapy. Eur J Obstet Gynecol Reprod Biol. 1993;51:203–207.
5. Grisso J, Freeman EW, Maurin E, Garcia-Espans B, Berlin JA. Racial differences in menopause information and the experience of hot flashes. J Gen Intern Med. 1999;14:98–103.
6. Staropoli C, Flaws JA, Bush TL, Moulton AW. Predictors of hot flashes. J Womens Health. 1998;7:1149–1155.
7. Barnhart K, Freeman E, Grisso JA, et al. The effect of dehydorepiandrosterone supplementation to symptomatic peimenopausal women on serum endocrine profiles, lipid parameters, and health-related quality of life. J Clin Endocrinol Metab. 1999;84:3896–3902.
8. Bachmann GA. Vasomotor flushes in menopausal women. Am J Obstet Gynecol. 1999;180(3 Pt 2):S312–316.
9. Washburn S, Burke GL, Morgan T, Anthony M. Effect of soy protein on serum lipoproteins, blood pressure, and menopausal symptoms in perimenopausal women. Menopause. 1999;6:7–13.
10. Notelovitz M, Cassel D, Hille D, et al. Efficacy of continuous sequential transdermal estradiol and norethindrone acetate in relieving vasomotor symptoms associated with menopause. Am J Obstet Gynecol. 2000;182:7–12.
11. Tice JA, Ettinger B, Ensrud K, Wallace R, Blackwell T, Cummings SR. Phytoestrogen supplements for the treatment of hot flashes: the Isoflavone Clover Extract (ICE) study: a randomized controlled trial. JAMA. 2003;290(2):207–214.
12. Secreto G, Chiechi LM, Amadori A, et al. Soy isoflavones and melatonin for the relief of climacteric symptoms: a multicenter, double-blind, randomized study. Maturitas. 2004; 47(1):11–20.
13. Pandya KJ, Morrow GR, Roscoe JA, et al. Gabapentin for

hot flashes in 420 women with breast cancer: a randomised double-blind placebo-controlled trial. Lancet. 2005;366(9488): 818–824.

14. Greendale G, Lee NP, Arriola ER. The menopause. Lancet. 1999;353:571–580.

15. Pandya K, Raubertas RF, Flynn PJ, et al. Oral clonidine in postmenopausal patients with breast cancer experiencing tamoxifen-induced hot flashes: A University of Rochester Cancer Center Community Clinical Oncology Program study. Ann Intern Med. 2000;132:788–793.

16. Quella S, Loprinzi CL, Sloan JA, et al. Long term use of megestrol acetate by cancer survivors for the treatment of hot flashes. Cancer. 1998;82:1784–1788.

17. Nedstrand E, Wijma K, Wyon Y, Hammar M. Applied relaxation and oral estradiol treatment of vasomotor symptoms in postmenopausal women. Maturitas. 2005;51(2):154–162.

18. Zweifel J, O'Brien WH. Meta-analysis of the effect of hormone replacement therapy on depressed mood. Psychoneuroendocrinology. 1997;22:189–212.

19. Polo-Kantola P, Erkkola R, Irjala K, Helenius H, Pullinen S, Polo O. Climacteric symptoms and sleep quality. Obstet Gynecol. 1999;94:219–224.

20. Raz R, Stamm WE. A controlled trial of intravaginal estriol in postmenopausal women with recurrent urinary tract infections. N Engl J Med. 1993;329(11):753–756.

21. Bygdeman M, Swahn ML. Replens versus dienoestrol cream in the symptomatic treatment of vaginal atrophy in postmenopausal women. Maturitas. 1996;23(3):259–263.

22. Dennerstein L, Dudley E, Burger H. Are changes in sexual functioning during midlife due to aging or menopause? Fertil Steril. 2001;76:456–460.

23. McCoy N. Sexual issues for postmenopausal women. Top Geriatr Rehab. 1997;12:28–39.

24. Modelska K, Cummings S. Female sexual dysfunction in postmenopausal women: systematic review of placebo-controlled trials. Am J Obstet Gynecol. 2003;188(1):286–293.

25. Law M, Hackshaw AK. A meta-analysis of cigarette smoking, bone mineral density and risk of hip fracture: recognition of major effect. BMJ. 1997;315:841–846.

26. Barrett-Connor E, Wehren LE, Siris ES, et al. Recency and duration of postmenopausal hormone therapy: effects on bone mineral density and fracture risk in the National Osteoporosis Risk Assessment (NORA) study. Menopause. 2003;10(5): 412–419.

27. Johnson SR, Ettinger B, Macer JL, Ensrud KE, Quan J, Grady D. Uterine and vaginal effects of unopposed ultralow-dose transdermal estradiol. Obstet Gynecol. 2005;105(4): 779–787.

28. Ettinger B, Ensrud KE, Wallace R, et al. Effects of ultralow-dose transdermal estradiol on bone mineral density: a randomized clinical trial. Obstet Gynecol. 2004;104(3):443–451.

29. Harris S, Watts NB, Genant HK, et al. Effects of risedronate treatment of vertebral and nonvertebral fractures in women with postmenopausal osteoporosis: A randomized controlled trial. JAMA. 1999;282:1344–1352.

30. Rosen CJ, Hochberg MC, Bonnick SL, et al. Treatment with once-weekly alendronate 70 mg compared with once-weekly risedronate 35 mg in women with postmenopausal osteoporosis: a randomized double-blind study. J Bone Miner Res. 2005;20(1):141–151.

31. Emkey R, Koltun W, Beusterien K, et al. Patient preference for once-monthly ibandronate versus once-weekly alendronate in a randomized, open-label, cross-over trial: the Boniva Alendronate Trial in Osteoporosis (BALTO). Curr Med Res Opin. 2005;21(12):1895–1903.

32. Black DM, Greenspan SL, Ensrud KE, et al. The effects of parathyroid hormone and alendronate alone or in combina-

tion in postmenopausal osteoporosis. N Engl J Med. 2003; 349(13):1207–1215.

33. Writing Group for the Women's Health Initiative Investigators. Risks and benefits of estrogen plus progestin in healthy postmenopausal women: Principal results for the Women's Health Initiative Randomized Controlled Trial. JAMA. 2002; 288:321–333.

34. Odmark IS, Bixo M, Endlund D, et al. Endometrial safety and bleeding pattern during a five-year treatment with long-cycle hormone therapy. Menopause. 2005;12:699–707.

35. Clarke SC, Kelleher J, Lloyd-Jones H, Slack M, Schofiel PM. A study of hormone replacement therapy in postmenopausal women with ischaemic heart disease: the Papworth HRT atherosclerosis study. BJOG. 2002;109(9):1056–1062.

36. Women's Health Initiative Steering Committee. Effects of conjugated equine estrogens in postmenopausal women with hysterectomy. JAMA. 2004;291:1701–1712.

37. Shah NR, Borenstein J, Dubois RW. Postmenopausal hormone therapy and breast cancer: a systematic review and meta-analysis. Menopause. 2005;12(6):668–678.

38. Rapp SR, Espeland MA, Shumaker SA, et al. Effect of estrogen plus progestin on global cognitive function in postmenopausal women: The Women's Health Initiative Memory Study: a randomized controlled trial. JAMA. 2003;289(20): 2663–2672.

39. Shumaker SA, Legault C, Thal L, et al. Estrogen plus progestin and the incidence of dementia and mild cognitive impairment in postmenopausal women: The Women's Health Initiative Memory Study: a randomized controlled trial. JAMA. 2003;289(20):2651–2662.

40. Mulnard R, Cotman CW, Kawas C, et al. Estrogen replacement therapy for mild to moderate Alzheimer's disease: a randomized controlled trial. JAMA. 2000;283:1007–1015.

41. Cirillo DJ, Wallace RB, Rodabough RJ, et al. Effect of estrogen therapy on gallbladder disease. JAMA. 2005;293(3): 330–339.

42. Grady D, Brown JS, Vittinghoff E, Applegate W, Warner E, Snyder T. Postmenopausal hormones and incontinence: The Heart and Estrogen/Progestin Replacement Study. Obstet Gynecol. 2001;97:116–120.

43. Ginsburg J, Prelevic GM. Lack of significant hormonal effects and controlled trials of phyto-estrogens. Lancet. 2000; 355:163–164.

44. Schubert W, Cullberg G, Edgar B, Hedner T. Inhibition of 17B-estradiol metabolism by grapefruit juice in ovariectomized women. Maturitas. 1995;20:155–163.

45. Goldstat R, Briganti E, Tran J, Wolfe R, Davis SR. Transdermal testosterone therapy improves well-being, mood, and sexual function in premenopausal women. Menopause. 2003; 10(5):390–398.

46. Cutler W, Genovese-Stone E. Wellness in women after 40 years of age: the role of sex hormones and pheromones. Dis Mon. 1998:423–546.

47. Fisher B, Constantino JP, Wickerham DL. Tamoxifen for prevention of breast cancer: report of the National Surgical Adjuvant Breast and Bowel Project P-1 Study. J Natl Cancer Inst. 1998;90:1371–1388.

48. Ettinger B, Black DM, Mitlak BH, et al. Reduction of vertebral fracture risk in postmenopausal women with osteoporosis treated with raloxifene: results from a 3-year randomized clinical trial. JAMA. 1999;282:637–645.

49. Vogel VG, Constantino JP, Wickerham DL, et al. Effects of tamoxifen vs. raloxifene on the risk of developing invasive breast cancer and other disease outcomes: the NSABP Study of Tamoxifen and Raloxifene (STAR) P-2 trial. JAMA 2006; 295:2727–2741.

50. Kreijkamp-Kaspers S, Kok L, Grobbee DE, et al. Effect of soy protein containing isoflavones on cognitive function, bone mineral density, and plasma lipids in postmenopausal women: a randomized controlled trial. JAMA. 2004;292(1): 65–74.

51. Huntley AL, Ernst E. A systematic review of herbal medicinal products for the treatment of menopausal symptoms. Menopause. 2003;10(5):465–476.

52. Nappi RE, Malavasi B, Brunda b, Facchinetti F. Efficacy of Cimicifuga racemosa on climacteric complaints: a randomized study versus low-dose transdermal estradiol. Gynecol Endocrinol. 2005;20(1):30–35.

53. Liao K, Hunter MS. Preparation for menopause: prospective evaluation of a health education intervention for mid-aged women. Maturitas. 1998;29:215–224.

54. Rothert M, Holmes-Rovner M, Rovner D, et al. An educational intervention as decision support for menopausal women. Res Nurs Health. 1997;20:377–387.

CHAPTER 31

Men's Health Concerns

Anthony J. Viera and Larissa S. Buccolo

BENIGN PROSTATIC HYPERPLASIA

CASE 1

Mr. J. is a 61-year-old man being seen for a blood pressure check after recently being started on 25 mg of hydrochlorothiazide daily. You note that his blood pressure remains elevated. He also complains of some difficulty emptying his bladder and is particularly bothered by having to get up several times in the night to void. He was told by a physician at his last checkup 1 year ago that his prostate was slightly enlarged, but he was not bothered by urinary symptoms at that time. He mentions that his neighbor goes to a urologist and asks if he should see a urologist.

CLINICAL QUESTIONS

1. How do you make the diagnosis of benign prostatic hyperplasia (BPH)?
2. What factors should you take into consideration when managing BPH?
3. When should a man with BPH be referred to a urologist?

Benign prostatic hyperplasia (BPH) refers to neoplastic, nonmalignant proliferation of the prostatic tissue surrounding the urethra. BPH is a condition that occurs in aging men as the prostate gland undergoes exposure to androgenic and estrogenic stimulation over time (1). While a genetic component to development of BPH exists, only increasing age and androgenic stimulation are well-established as etiologic factors. Smoking, diet, sexual activity, and vasectomy have not been shown to be associated with BPH. Race and socioeconomic status are also not associated with BPH (2). The prevalence of BPH is estimated to be 8% in men in their 30s, 50% in men in their 50s, and 80% in men older than 80 years (3). These estimates correlate with histologically-defined BPH discovered at autopsy (4). BPH is clinically important when it leads to lower urinary tract symptoms (LUTS) or bladder outlet obstruction (BOO). Potential complications of BOO include renal failure, urinary retention (acute and chronic), recurrent urinary tract infections (UTIs), bladder calculi, and bladder dysfunction.

Per year, acute urinary retention (AUR) develops in 1%–2% of men with symptoms of BPH (5). However, the symptoms of BPH do not necessarily progress in every man who initially presents with LUTS or AUR. In one study of 212 men who presented with either LUTS or AUR and were followed for 4 to 7 years, 48 percent of those who did not have surgery no longer had symptoms of BPH (6). In another study, 52% of men who did not have surgery had no change in their BPH symptoms over 5 years, 32% had improvement, and only 15% developed worsening symptoms (6). In addition to increasing age, three risk factors seem to be most predictive of those men whose BPH will be progressive: change in size and force of urinary stream, sensation of incomplete emptying, and enlarged prostate on digital rectal examination (7).

The symptoms of BPH result from a combination of factors. The increased tone of the richly innervated prostatic smooth muscle fibers creates a dynamic (reversible) obstruction. As the prostate itself enlarges, it creates a mechanical (fixed) obstruction as it encroaches on and impinges the urethra. The bladder, in response to the increased outlet resistance, begins to increase the force of its contractions. Eventually, the detrusor muscle develops hypertrophy and fibrosis. Collagen deposition in the bladder wall leads to loss of bladder elasticity and compliance. Loss of normal control over the reflex detrusor response can ensue and, left untreated, can progress to severe bladder dysfunction.

Symptoms that may develop throughout this process are shown in Table 31.1. These symptoms are not specific for BPH, however, and not all patients with BPH develop LUTS. Patients with LUTS attributable to BPH usually have some combination of irritative and obstructive symptoms.

Other disorders can cause LUTS or BOO and thus mimic BPH. These include other diseases of the prostate such as prostate cancer or prostatitis; disorders of the bladder such as tumor, calculus, or neurogenic bladder; and disorders of the urethra such as urethritis or stricture.

INITIAL EVALUATION

The goals of the history are to clarify symptoms consistent with BPH and exclude other conditions that mimic BPH. Ask the patient if he has a history of prostate problems or other urologic disease. Note any recent or remote urethral or bladder trauma (including instrumentation). Ask about the symptoms described in Table 31.1, but also ask questions to help in excluding other conditions that might cause LUTS (see previous paragraph). Other neurologic symptoms should raise your suspicion for neurogenic bladder. A history of UTI may support a diagnosis of BPH (caused by retained urine), but

TABLE 31.1 Lower Urinary Tract Symptoms

Primarily Irritative
  Urinary frequency
  Urinary urgency
  Nocturia
  Urge incontinence
Primarily Obstructive
  Decreased force and caliber of urinary stream
  Hesitancy getting urinary stream started
  Straining to void
  Interruption of urinary stream
  Terminal dribbling
  Prolonged urination (due to decreased flow rate)
  Sensation of incomplete bladder emptying

may also be indicative of other problems, such as prostatitis or bladder tumor. Inquire about sexually transmitted diseases. Hematuria may be secondary to BPH, but such a history may also signify bladder tumor, urolithiasis, or other urinary tract pathology. A history of erectile dysfunction (ED) is also important to consider for both diagnostic as well as therapeutic considerations. Pelvic pain, back pain, or weight loss are not due to BPH.

The examination for suspected BPH focuses on the abdomen, genital area, and rectum. Bladder distension can sometimes be detected by palpating and percussing the suprapubic region. Digital rectal examination (DRE) is performed to assess the size, consistency, and shape of the prostate. Ability to estimate prostate size might be improved by training using a three-dimensional prostate model (8). A tender, boggy prostate is more consistent with prostatitis (see Prostatitis). In BPH, the prostate typically feels enlarged and rubbery. However, the size of the prostate does not correlate with BPH symptoms. Any area of firm induration, nodularity, or asymmetry is suggestive of malignancy. At the conclusion of the DRE, note the anal sphincter tone. A decreased tone suggests a neurogenic disorder. Note the patient's gait and lower extremity neuromuscular function.

DIAGNOSTIC TESTING

The only essential laboratory test needed in the initial evaluation of men suspected of having BPH is a urinalysis. The presence of hematuria should prompt consideration for referral for cystoscopy. The presence of white blood cells might signify infection (cystitis or prostatitis). A serum creatinine is no longer recommended in the initial evaluation of BPH because there are no data demonstrating a relationship between severity of LUTS and impaired renal function, and baseline renal insufficiency is no more common in men with BPH than similarly aged men in the general population (9, 10). A serum prostate specific antigen (PSA) test is an optional test in men with LUTS thought to be secondary to BPH. The PSA test should be discussed and ordered just as it would in any man 50 years and older, with at least a 10-year life expectancy who elects to be screened (see section on Prostate Cancer). In discussing PSA with men as part of BPH evaluation,

consider whether knowledge of the PSA level or the presence of prostate cancer would change management. It is important to remember that 25% of men with BPH have an elevated PSA.

Other optional tests in the evaluation of BPH include urine cytology, post-void residual (PVR) volume, and a maximal urinary flow rate. Urine cytology may be a useful option in men with predominantly irritative voiding symptoms who have a history of smoking or other risk factors for bladder cancer. A large PVR volume (e.g., greater than 350 mL) may be associated with bladder dysfunction and predict a less favorable response to treatment. Although a PVR can be determined in the family physician's office by simple in-out catheterization or a bladder scanner, maximal urinary flow rate and tests such as uroflowmetry (uroflow) studies are generally performed in a specialist's office. A uroflow test is used to estimate the volume urinated as well as duration and velocity of urination. Such tests are probably most useful in men contemplating invasive treatment options.

MANAGEMENT

American Urologic Association Symptom Score

The American Urologic Association (AUA) Symptom Score is a valid and reliable tool to evaluate the severity of BPH symptoms once the diagnosis is made (see Table 31.2). It consists of seven items and can be self-administered or interviewer-administered. In addition to documenting initial severity of BPH, it can be used to guide treatment decisions, monitor treatment effectiveness, and track progression. Neither BPH symptoms nor the AUA Symptom Score correlate with prostate size (11).

The rates of transurethral surgery for BPH declined significantly from the mid 1980s to the mid 1990s (12). This decline was partly from increasing availability of effective medical therapies. As a result, family physicians and other primary care providers have an important role in helping men make informed decisions regarding treatment. The management of BPH is guided by symptoms. Men without bothersome symptoms are best managed by a strategy of watchful waiting. Men bothered by moderate to severe symptoms (AUA Symptom Score ≥8) could opt for watchful waiting, medical treatment, minimally invasive therapy, or surgery. Figure 31.1 illustrates a management algorithm.

Watchful Waiting

A management strategy in which a patient is monitored but receives no active treatment is called watchful waiting. Men with mild BPH symptoms and men who are not particularly bothered by symptoms—even if categorized by AUA Symptom Score as moderate or severe—are appropriate candidates for watchful waiting. Also, men for whom the risk of side effects outweighs the potential symptom improvement are appropriate candidates for watchful waiting. General measures that might be helpful include avoiding caffeinated and alcohol-containing beverages and eliminating medications that can exacerbate urinary symptoms (e.g., diuretics, anticholinergics, tricyclic antidepressants). Men opting for a strategy of watchful waiting are usually re-evaluated yearly.

TABLE 31.2 American Urological Association Symptom Score for Benign Prostatic Hyperplasia*

CIRCLE THE ONE BEST ANSWER TO EACH QUESTION

Questions	Never	<1 time in 5	<half the time	About half the time	>half the time	Almost always
Over the past month, how often have you had the feeling that you did not empty your bladder completely after you finished urinating?	0	1	2	3	4	5
Over the past month, how often have you had to urinate again less than 2 hours after you finished urinating?	0	1	2	3	4	5
Over the past month, how often have you found that you stopped and started again several times when you urinated?	0	1	2	3	4	5
Over the past month, how often have you found it difficult to postpone urination?	0	1	2	3	4	5
Over the past month, how often have you had a weak urinary stream?	0	1	2	3	4	5
Over the past month, how often have you had trouble getting your urine stream started?	0	1	2	3	4	5
Over the past month, how many times have you averaged getting up to urinate from the time you went to bed at night until the time you got up in the morning?	None	One time	Two times	Three times	Four times	Five times

Total score: _____ (sum of circled numbers)

Key: 0–7, absent/mild symptoms; 8–19, moderate symptoms; 20+, severe symptoms
*Modified from Barry MJ, Fowler FJ, O'Leary MP, et al. The American Urological Association Symptom Index for benign prostatic hyperplasia. J Urol. 1992;148:1549–1557.

Pharmacotherapy
ALPHA-BLOCKERS

Alpha-adrenergic blockers have been well-studied and are generally the first-line medications used for BPH (see Table 31.3). They reduce LUTS by relieving the dynamic component of bladder outlet obstruction. The currently used alpha-blockers are similarly effective and produce on average a 4- to 6-point improvement in the AUA Symptom Score (10). The effects of doxazosin, tamsulosin, and terazosin are dose-dependent, and doses should be titrated gradually as side effects (e.g., orthostatic hypotension, dizziness) are also dose-dependent. Alfuzosin does not require titration. Because of increased incidence of side effects, neither the short-acting alpha blocker prazosin (Minipres) nor the non-selective alpha-blocker phenoxybenzamine are recommended.

5-ALPHA-REDUCTASE INHIBITORS

The 5-alpha-reductase inhibitors suppress the conversion of testosterone to dihydroxytestosterone, which plays an important role in prostate growth. Thus, these medications reduce LUTS by relieving the fixed component of BOO and are an option for men with BPH who have demonstrable prostatic enlargement. They are not effective—and thus not appropriate—for men who do not have enlarged prostates. They also must be taken for 3 to 6 months before a benefit is likely to be observed. The combination of an alpha-blocker with a 5-alpha reductase inhibitor is particularly effective in delaying the progression of BPH in men bothered by LUTS, who have demonstrably enlarged prostates. The best studied combination is doxazosin with finasteride. In one study of 3,047 men 50 years or older, with a mean AUA Symptom Score of 16.9, who were followed for 5 years, compared to placebo, mono-

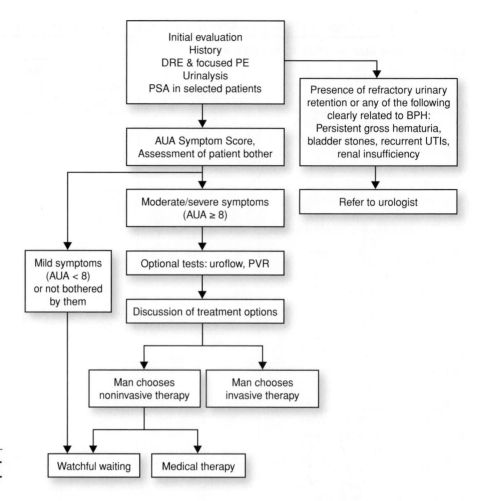

Figure 31.1 • Benign prostatic hyperplasia (BPH) diagnosis and treatment.

therapy with doxazosin reduced clinical progression of BPH by 39%, and monotherapy with finasteride reduced clinical progression by 34%. The combination of the two medications reduced clinical progression of BPH by 66% compared to placebo (13). Added cost and potentially more adverse effects are obviously issues when a 5-alpha reductase inhibitor is added to an alpha-blocker.

PLANT EXTRACTS

Plant extracts (phytotherapies) have been a popular form of therapy for BPH in Europe and, consistent with overall enthusiasm for complementary and alternative medicine, have gained popularity among men in the United States. Although many herbal remedies have been touted as beneficial for BPH or "prostate health," few have been well-studied. A systematic review of 18 randomized, controlled trials of saw palmetto preparations showed that self-rated improvement of BPH was 1.7 times more likely among men taking saw palmetto than among men taking placebo (14). Other plant extracts that may have some short-term benefit include pygeum africanum and B-sitosterol (15, 16). The lack of standardization of herbal products must be taken into consideration when discussing them with patients. Dosages vary and adverse effects are generally mild. The current AUA guideline does not recommend plant extracts for treatment of BPH.

Indications for Urologic Referral

Transurethral resection of the prostate (TURP) is considered the gold-standard surgical treatment for BPH. Symptom reduction is generally quite substantial. A large Veterans Administration study comparing TURP to watchful waiting showed a nearly 10 point reduction in symptom score in the TURP group compared to a 5.5 point reduction in the watchful waiting group. There was also a significant increase in urinary flow rate in men undergoing TURP (17).

Other surgical or invasive options include transurethral incision of the prostate (TUIP), transurethral needle ablation (TUNA), electrovaporization, and several techniques of laser prostatectomy. TUIP is an outpatient procedure generally limited to prostates of smaller size. TUNA is minimally invasive and performed under local anesthesia but is less effective than TURP. Both TUIP and TUNA are associated with high rates of secondary procedures. Prostatic stents can be used in certain high-risk patients with urinary retention but are associated with significant complications. Open prostatectomy is rarely performed in the United States for BPH and would generally be reserved for men with excessively large prostates. Men with bothersome symptoms who are considering invasive therapy, either as an initial therapeutic option or because of symptoms refractory to medical management, should be re-

TABLE 31.3 Medications for Benign Prostatic Hyperplasia*

Alpha-blockers
  Alfuzosin (Uroxatral)
    Dose: 10 mg daily; take with food
    Common adverse effects: orthostatic hypotension, dizziness, headache, weakness, rhinitis
    Comments: May have less cardiovascular effects than doxazosin and terazosin
    Cost for 1-month supply: $76.49
  Doxazosin (Cardura)
    Dose: Start 1 mg at bedtime; titrate to 8 mg
    Common adverse effects: orthostatic hypotension, dizziness, headache, weakness, rhinitis
    Comments: May be useful in men with concomitant hypertension
    Cost for 1-month supply: $21.56 for 4mg tablets (generic)
  Tamsulosin (Flomax)
    Dose: Start 0.4 mg daily; titrate to 0.8 mg
    Common adverse effects: orthostatic hypotension, dizziness, headache, weakness, rhinitis
    Comments: May have less cardiovascular effects than doxazosin and terazosin
    Cost for 1-month supply: $75.19
  Terazosin (Hytrin)
    Dose: Start 1 mg at bedtime; titrate to 10 mg
    Common adverse effects: orthostatic hypotension, dizziness, headache, weakness, rhinitis
    Comments: May be useful in men with concomitant hypertension
    Cost for 1-month supply: $13.99 for all strengths (generic)
5α-Reductase Inhibitors
  Dutasteride (Avodart)
    Dose: 0.5 mg daily
    Common adverse effects: erectile dysfunction, decreased libido, decreased ejaculate volume
    Comments: Consider checking prostate specific antigen (PSA) after 3 to 6 months for new baseline
    Cost for 1-month supply: $92.39
  Finasteride (Proscar)
    Dose: 5 mg daily
    Common adverse effects: erectile dysfunction, decreased libido, decreased ejaculate volume, gynecomastia, orthostatic hypotension
    Comments: Consider checking PSA after 3 to 6 months for new baseline
    Cost for 1-month supply: $92.99

*Prices from www.drugstore.com, accessed February 16, 2007. Actual prices will vary depending on dose, formulation, local conditions, co-pays, and other factors.

ferred to a urologist. Men who develop acute urinary retention should be referred for consideration of definitive therapy. Additional indications for referral are shown in Table 31.4. The evidence for pharmacologic and surgical treatments is summarized in Table 31.5.

DISCUSSION CASE 1

The diagnosis of BPH is made by a combination of history, focused physical examination, and a urinalysis. Once the diagnosis is made, the AUA Symptom Score can be used to gauge severity. Ultimately, the patient will tell you how bothered he is by the symptoms, and this will assist in guiding management after a discussion about risks and benefits. If Mr. J.'s symptoms are moderately or severely bothersome, a referral to a urologist might be indicated so that invasive treatment options can be discussed. However, Mr. J.'s symptoms at this point are proba-

TABLE 31.4 Indications for Referral

Acute urinary retention (especially if failed attempt at catheter removal)
Bladder stones (although rarely due to BPH)
Diagnosis is uncertain
Man requests referral
Recurrent gross hematuria
Recurrent urinary tract infections
Renal insufficiency (especially if responds to period of bladder catheterization)
Symptoms refractory to medical management (most common reason)

BPH, benign prostatic hyperplasia

TABLE 31.5 Strength of Recommendation for BPH Treatments

Intervention	Efficacy	Strength of Recommendation*	Comment
TURP	10 point reduction in AUA Symptom Score	A	Surgical risks
Alpha-blocker	4 to 6 point reduction in AUA Symptom Score	A	First-line medication
5α-Reductase Inhibitor	Combined with alpha-blocker, 6 point reduction in AUA Symptom score; combination reduces progression by up to 66% compared to placebo	A	Only in men with enlarged prostates

AUA, American Urologic Association; BPH, benign prostatic hyperplasia; TURP, transurethral resection of the prostate
*A = consistent, good-quality patient-oriented evidence; B = inconsistent or limited-quality patient-oriented evidence; C = consensus, disease-oriented evidence, usual practice, expert opinion, or case series. For information about the SORT evidence rating system, see *http://www.aafp.org/afpsort.xml*.

bly mild or moderate, in which case a trial of no diuretics might be considered before initiation of an alpha-blocker (which would also help control his blood pressure).

PROSTATITIS

CASE 2

Mr. S. is a 35-year-old married man who complains of painful ejaculation, a dull ache in his scrotum, and low back pain for 3 weeks. The symptoms were mild at first but have increased in severity. He denies any history of sexually transmitted infections. When asked, he does say that he has occasional discomfort when urinating. He is otherwise healthy. In clinic, he is afebrile, and his prostate examination is normal. A urinalysis reveals trace leukocyte esterase but is otherwise negative.

CLINICAL QUESTIONS

1. How do you distinguish between the different prostatitis syndromes?
2. How does the management of the prostatitis syndromes differ?

Prostatitis is a common problem that tends to affect young and middle-aged men. Acute prostatitis is generally caused by ascending infection of the urinary tract and is the most easily recognized but least common of the prostatitis syndromes (see Table 31.6). Approximately 7% of men with prostatitis have chronic bacterial prostatitis. It may occur as a complication of acute prostatitis or may manifest as recurrent UTIs. Chronic prostatitis/chronic pelvic pain syndrome (CP/CPPS) may present with similar symptoms, with no demonstrable bacterial source. It is the most common of the prostatitis syndromes.

The man with acute prostatitis will usually complain of urinary symptoms (irritative and obstructive), perineal or pelvic pain, and fever. Acute cystitis rarely occurs in men who have normal urinary tract anatomy and function. Thus, lower UTI in a man should suggest prostatitis as the diagnosis. A

DRE usually reveals a tender, boggy prostate. Prostatic massage for purposes of obtaining expressed prostatic secretions is not indicated (18). If urinalysis reveals leukocytes, a urine culture should also be ordered.

Acute prostatitis is treated with antimicrobials active against common infecting organisms, typically Gram-negative rods (e.g., *Escherichia coli*, *Proteus spp.*), but also Gram-positive cocci (e.g., enterococcus). Broad spectrum antibiotics are begun while the urine culture is pending. Nonsteroidal anti-inflammatory drugs (NSAIDs), if not contraindicated, may be useful for pain relief. Infection of the prostate gland, particularly if early treatment is not initiated, can be a source of severe systemic infection, or sepsis. Such an acutely ill patient requiring hospitalization and parenteral therapy would rarely present to a primary care office. A man who cannot tolerate oral antimicrobials would also require hospitalization.

A man who has recurrent UTIs not attributable to bladder catheterization or another urinary tract abnormality may have underlying chronic bacterial prostatitis. Such a patient may have had preceding acute bacterial prostatitis or may present *de novo* with urinary symptoms (e.g., dysuria, frequency) or low back, perineal, or groin discomfort. However, there is no evidence of acute bacterial prostatitis (e.g., no fever and normal DRE). Antibiotics are prescribed for a minimum of 6 weeks.

CHRONIC PROSTATITIS /CHRONIC PELVIC PAIN SYNDROME

CP/CPPS encompasses both the disorders previously referred to as nonbacterial (or abacterial) prostatitis and prostatodynia. The etiology is unknown, and studies do not support causative roles of infectious agents such as chlamydia, ureaplasma, or mycoplasma. Furthermore, it is not clear that the prostate is involved in all cases of CP/CPPS. Symptoms are similar to those of chronic bacterial prostatitis, but there is no identifiable source of infection. The "four-glass test," which includes postprostatic massage analysis of expressed prostatic secretions and urine, has been described for use in diagnosing CP/CPPS. However, its clinical usefulness is minimal (19). Treatment is with alpha-blockers and anti-inflammatory drugs.

TABLE 31.6 Prostatitis Syndromes

Diagnosis	Symptoms	Physical examination and laboratory tests	Management
Acute prostatitis	Acute onset of fever, chills, dysuria, pelvic or perineal pain	Tender, boggy, warm prostate. Urinalysis reveals pyuria, bacteriuria, occasionally hematuria.	Avoid prostatic massage and urethral catheters. Order urine culture, and consider gonorrhea/chlamydia testing. Order blood cultures and hospitalize if systemically ill. Intravenous antibiotic options include ampicillin/sulbactam or ampicillin plus an aminoglycoside (gentamicin or tobramycin), or a fluoroquinolone. Oral antibiotic options include TMP/SMX DS or a fluoroquinolone. Treat for 4 to 6 weeks. NSAIDs may help relieve pain and inflammation.
Chronic bacterial prostatitis	Gradual onset of mild to moderate urinary symptoms, pain in lower back, perineum, lower abdomen or genitals, painful ejaculation or hematospermia	Minimally tender or normal prostate exam. Urinalysis consistent with UTI.	Order urine culture. Consider gonorrhea/chlamydia testing. Treat with TMP/SMX DS or fluoroquinolone for 6 to 12 weeks. In event of recurrence, treat with a second course of antibiotics (and for longer duration if the first course was six weeks).
Chronic prostatitis/chronic pelvic pain syndrome (CPPS)	Similar to symptoms of chronic bacterial prostatitis.	Prostate is normal or minimally tender. Urinalysis is not consistent with UTI.	Order urine culture (should be negative). Consider gonorrhea/chlamydia testing. Treat with alpha-blockers (e.g., terazosin) for minimum of six months. NSAIDs and/or sitz baths may help alleviate pain.

NSAIDs, nonsteroidal anti-inflammatory drugs; TMP/SMX DS, double-strength trimethoprim/sulfamethoxazole; UTI, urinary tract infection

DISCUSSION CASE 2

Mr. S.'s gradual onset of symptoms suggests that he has either chronic bacterial prostatitis or CPPS. The absence of fever or other acute signs, and the normal prostate exam make acute bacterial prostatitis unlikely. A urine culture should be ordered, and a trial of antibiotics is probably warranted pending the culture result. If the urine culture is negative, he probably has CPPS. The treatment would then consist of NSAIDs and alpha-blockers for a minimum of 6 months.

PROSTATE CANCER

CASE 3

Mr. B. is a 49-year-old African-American male who presents to your clinic at the insistence of his wife after they viewed a video at their church encouraging men to get tested for prostate cancer. He currently feels well and just asks for a prostate cancer check. His digital rectal examination is normal. You discuss the risks and benefits of prostate cancer screening and proceed with a DRE (which is normal), and order a PSA. One week later, the man returns to your office to discuss his PSA result of 3.1 ng/mL.

CLINICAL QUESTIONS

1. Does screening for prostate cancer reduce morbidity and mortality?
2. Why is there no ideal cutoff of PSA level for screening men for prostate cancer?
3. What would you include in your discussion with a man who asks about prostate cancer screening? What would you include in your discussion if the man is diagnosed with localized prostate cancer?

Excluding nonmelanoma skin cancer, prostate cancer continues to be the most common cancer in American men, and is second only to lung cancer as the leading cause of cancer death in men. The cause of prostate cancer is unknown. Of the most important known risk factors (see Table 31.7), only diet is mutable.

Prostate cancer is generally slow-growing, which contributes to the complexity of prostate cancer screening and the adage, "Many more men die *with* prostate cancer than *from* prostate cancer." Autopsy series have shown that among men who die from something other than prostate cancer, up to a quarter of those 50 to 59 years old have prostate cancer, and two-thirds of men over 80 years old have prostate cancer (20). Whereas an American man's lifetime risk of developing pros-

TABLE 31.7 Risk Factors for Prostate Cancer

Age
—Rarely diagnosed before age 45; risk increases with age
Race/Ethnicity
—More common in African-American men than whites or Hispanics
Genetic Factors
—Men with a first-degree relative with prostate cancer have a two-fold increased risk
—BRCA mutations may increase risk
Diet
—Diets high in animal fat or low in vegetables increase risk

BRCA, breast cancer susceptibility gene

tate cancer is 17%, his risk of dying from prostate cancer is 3% (21).

Occasionally, prostate cancer is diagnosed as a result of evaluation for symptoms such as difficulty urinating, new onset erectile dysfunction, or back or hip pain (advanced prostate cancer can metastasize to bone). Patients diagnosed in this manner are more likely to have advanced disease.

Most prostate cancer, however, is diagnosed as a result of measuring blood levels of PSA in asymptomatic men. PSA is an enzyme secreted by the outer coating of the prostate gland and the periurethral glands. It aids in release of spermatozoa from the seminal vesicles. PSA was isolated and purified in 1979, and a test to measure its level in the blood was developed in 1980 (22). A PSA >4.0 ng/mL is generally considered abnormal. Some experts recommend repeating PSA before proceeding to biopsy, since PSA levels tend to fluctuate (23, 24). As would be expected, men with higher PSA values (PSA

>10 ng/mL) are much more likely to have prostate cancer diagnosed than men whose PSA levels are in the intermediate range (between 4.0 and 10 ng/mL). Prostate cancer detected as a result of PSA levels >10 ng/mL is also more likely to be at an advanced (extracapsular) stage. It is also important to recognize that prostate cancer is by no means a rare occurrence in men with a PSA level of <4.0 ng/mL. In one study in which 2,950 men with PSA levels <4.0 ng/mL and normal DREs for 7 years underwent prostate biopsy, 15% had prostate cancer, including high-grade cancers (25). The test characteristics for various levels of PSA are shown in Table 31.8 (26).

Several strategies have been developed to try to enhance diagnostic specificity of PSA in the intermediate range (4 to 10 ng/mL). A high percentage of free PSA (e.g., >25%) in a man with a total PSA between 4.0 to 10 ng/mL may signify a lower risk of prostate cancer (27). Age-specific PSA ranges and PSA velocity have also been used, although these have not proved to be superior to simple PSA testing. A validated clinical decision rule (Figure 31.2) uses age, DRE, and PSA (with or without free PSA) in a nomogram to estimate a man's risk of having prostate cancer detected by biopsy (28). The nomogram without free PSA has an area under the receiver operating characteristic curve of 0.69, whereas the nomogram with free PSA has an area under the receiver operating characteristic curve of 0.77. For comparison, the area under the receiver operating characteristic curve for values of PSA alone in the range of 4.0 to 10 ng/mL may be as low as 0.51 (no better than random guessing) (29).

SCREENING FOR PROSTATE CANCER

Before the advent of PSA, a test known as prostatic acid phosphatase (PAP) was used as a marker to follow patients with advanced prostate cancer. Because of PAP's poor sensitivity, it was never considered for use as a screening test (22). Similarly, the earliest clinical studies of PSA also had implications

TABLE 31.8 Operating Characteristics of the PSA for the Detection of Prostate Cancer

PSA (ng/mL)	Any Cancer vs. No Cancer				Gleason Score ≥8 vs. GLEASON Score <8 or No Cancer			
	Sensitivity	Specificity	LR +	LR −	Sensitivity	Specificity	LR +	LR −
1.1	83.4	38.9	1.36	.43	94.7	35.9	1.48	.15
1.6	67.0	58.7	1.62	.56	89.5	53.5	1.92	.20
2.1	52.6	72.5	1.91	.65	86.0	65.9	2.52	.21
2.6	40.5	81.1	2.14	.73	78.9	75.1	3.17	.28
3.1	32.2	86.7	2.42	.78	68.4	81.0	3.6	.39
4.1	20.5	93.8	3.30	.85	50.9	89.1	4.67	.55
6.1	4.6	98.5	3.07	.97	26.3	97.5	10.5	.75
8.1	1.7	99.4	2.83	.99	10.5	99.0	10.5	.90
10.1	0.9	99.7	3.00	.99	5.3	99.5	10.6	.95

PSA, prostate specific antigen
Adapted from: Thompson IM, Ankerst DP, Chi C, et al. Operating characteristics of prostate-specific antigen in men with an initial PSA level of 3.0 ng/ml or lower. JAMA. 2005;294(1):66–70. LRs calculated from sensitivity and specificity.

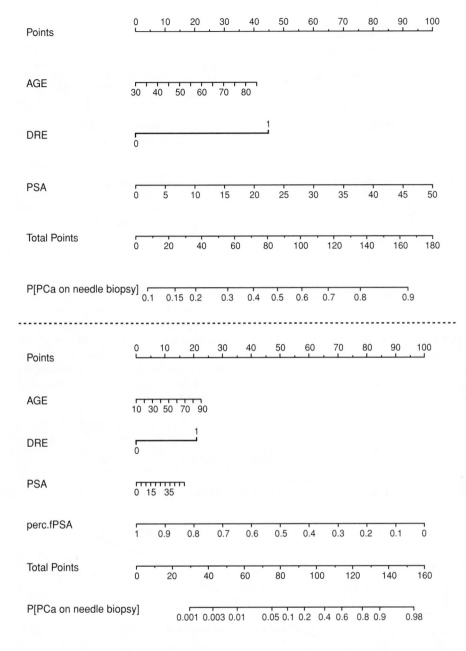

Figure 31.2 • Nomograms for predicting probability of positive prostate biopsy. Find the patient's age, DRE, and PSA (and free PSA if applicable). For each variable, draw a vertical line up to "points" at the top of the nomogram. Sum the points and draw a line from "total points" to the bottom of the nomogram to find probability of positive prostate biopsy. From: Karakiewicz PI, Benayoun S, Kattan MW, et al. Development and validation of a nomogram predicting the outcome of prostate biopsy based on patient age, digital rectal examination and serum prostate specific antigen. J Urol. Jun 2005; 173(6): 1930–1934. Palm US based version available at www.auq.org

for its use as a marker to follow patients with prostate cancer, and interestingly, early researchers actually denounced the potential of PSA as a screening test because of poor specificity (30). Those who suggested using PSA as a screening test originally proposed much higher cutpoints than the one currently used. Receiver operator characteristic curve analysis of PSA demonstrates that there is no cutpoint that has simultaneous high sensitivity and high specificity for use in screening asymptomatic men for prostate cancer (26).

PSA may also be elevated for a number of reasons not related to prostate cancer. BPH, a condition that is also very common in older men, may cause elevations in PSA. Prostatitis and prostate or lower genital tract procedures may also elevate PSA. While a DRE may lead to minimal transient elevations in PSA, measurement of PSA may be conducted immediately following DRE.

Abnormal prostate findings on the DRE include nodules or induration. Asymmetry of the prostate gland is abnormal but can also be due to BPH. Further limitations of the DRE as a prostate cancer screening test include its lack of sensitivity, estimated to be 59% (31). Prostate cancer diagnosed by DRE is usually more advanced than prostate cancer diagnosed solely as a result of PSA screening.

The controversy surrounding prostate cancer screening stems not from whether prostate cancer can be *detected* at an earlier stage but rather from whether *treatment* of prostate cancer at an earlier stage is better than treatment at a later stage. Studies of screening for prostate cancer using PSA have been observational and thus have generally suffered from two major biases—lead-time bias and length-time bias.

Lead-time bias occurs when people whose disease was diagnosed by screening appear to have longer survival than those whose disease was diagnosed because of symptoms or signs, even if actual years of life were not prolonged (see Fig-

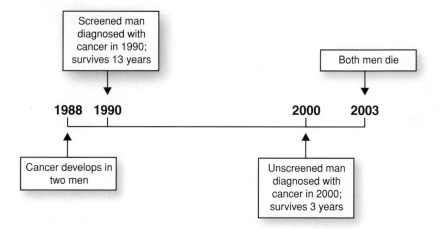

Figure 31.3 • Lead time bias. Screening gives the appearance that the man diagnosed in 1990 survived longer when in fact both men lived 13 years after they developed cancer. Adapted from: Bhatnager V, Kaplan RM. Treatment options for prostate cancer: evaluating the evidence. Am Fam Physician. May 15, 2005; 71(10):1915.

ure 31.3). This apparent discrepancy occurs because "survival" is measured from time of diagnosis. Hence, a person who is screened may be diagnosed earlier than a person who is not screened. Length-time bias occurs because screening tends to detect more indolent cases of cancer, whereas rapidly-growing cancers are less likely to be detected by screening because they are in the presymptomatic phase for a much shorter time (see Figure 31.4). Therefore, men who are screened will appear

to have a better prognosis because they have cancers that inherently have a better prognosis. The way to mitigate these two important biases is to perform randomized controlled trials of screening. Two such trials are underway at the time of this writing. However, even if the trials demonstrate a reduction in prostate cancer mortality attributable to PSA screening, the problem of whether such benefits outweigh the harms and costs (to individual men and society) will remain.

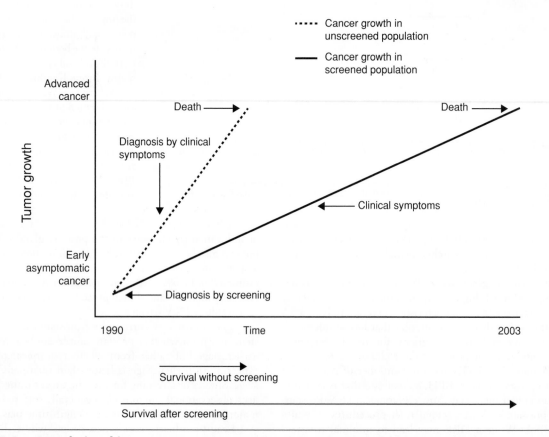

Figure 31.4 • Length-time bias. Aggressive cancers are less likely to be detected by screening than slow-growing cancers. Thus, screening appears favorable because it detects cancers that have a more favorable prognosis. Adapted from: Bhatnager V, Kaplan RM. Treatment options for prostate cancer: evaluating the evidence. Am Fam Physician. May 15, 2005; 71(10):1915.

Current Screening Recommendations

Given the limitations in our knowledge of screening for prostate cancer using PSA, several major organizations have issued similar recommendations. The American Cancer Society (ACS) recommends that prostate cancer screening should be offered annually, beginning at age 50, to men who have at least a 10-year life expectancy. The ACS recommends that men at high risk (African-American men, and men with a strong family history of one or more first-degree relatives diagnosed at an early age) should be offered testing beginning at age 45 (21). Even in high-risk groups, however, the same uncertainties about screening apply (32).

The AUA recommends that the decision to undergo PSA testing should be individualized. Patients should be informed of the known risks and the potential benefits (33). Risks include the problems of potential treatment (impotence and incontinence) that might result from initiation of the screening cascade. Other potential treatment problems include bowel troubles, breast swelling, and hot flashes (32). Screening risks include the anxiety about the test and its results, as well as the potential for false reassurance. That is, some men with normal PSA levels will still have underlying prostate cancer (25). The American College of Physicians has recommended that informed consent (similar to consent before a surgical procedure) be obtained prior to PSA testing (34). The American Academy of Family Physicians (AAFP) agrees with the recommendation that PSA testing be a shared or informed decision and provides decision support tools on their Web site (35).

The US Preventive Services Task Force (USPSTF), widely accepted as the authority on preventive services, found good evidence that PSA screening can detect early-stage prostate cancer but mixed and inconclusive evidence that early detection improves health outcomes (32). Because screening is associated with important problems, including frequent false-positive results and unnecessary anxiety (36), biopsies, and potential complications of treatment of some cancers that may never have affected a patient's health, the Task Force concluded that evidence is insufficient to determine whether the benefits outweigh the harms for a screened population (32).

What Should Clinicians Do?

Despite the absence of firm evidence of effectiveness, prostate cancer screening is common in clinical practice. However, given the uncertainties surrounding prostate cancer screening, the USPSTF concluded that clinicians should not order screening without first discussing with patients its potential but uncertain benefits and possible harms (32). Clinicians should inform men of the gaps in the evidence and should help them to consider their personal preferences and risk profile before deciding whether to be tested.

Shared decision making (SDM) is an intervention that occurs in the clinical setting, in which the patient and the clinician collaborate in decision making (37). SDM is predicated on the fact that some decisions regarding health care involve considerable uncertainty. In SDM regarding prostate cancer screening using PSA, the clinician and the patient would discuss the options and their risks/benefits. This would be a two-way dialogue in which both the patient and the clinician would share information. The expected outcome is a mutually agreeable decision that reflects the health preferences of the patient (38). Decision aids have been developed to facilitate SDM (39, 40).

Similarly, informed decision making (IDM) interventions can help people understand the issues involved in prostate cancer screening. IDM and SDM are mutually supportive. IDM is said to have occurred when a person understands the disease being addressed and comprehends what the clinical service involves, including its risks, benefits, limitations, alternatives, and uncertainties; has considered his or her values and preferences and makes a decision consistent with them; and believes he or she has participated in decision making at the level desired (41).

DIAGNOSIS OF PROSTATE CANCER

Diagnosis of prostate cancer is made by transrectal ultrasound (TRUS) guided biopsy usually performed in the urologist's office. A minimum of six samples (a sextant biopsy) from the prostate are taken. If an initial biopsy is negative in a man with a persistently elevated PSA or a suspicious DRE, some urologists will perform a repeat biopsy. In one study of 820 men with PSA levels between 4.0 and 10 ng/mL who underwent a second biopsy, prostate cancer was found in 10% (42). Complications of prostate biopsy include pain (25%), hematuria (23%), hematospermia (50%), and rectal bleeding (1%) (43).

MANAGEMENT

Staging of Prostate Cancer

The main objective of staging is to determine whether prostate cancer is organ-confined or has spread outside the prostate gland. The tumor-node-metastasis (TNM) staging system is shown in Table 31.9. Assignment of stage based on clinical or pathological criteria is sometimes denoted by a "c" or "p."

The Gleason histologic grading system is shown in Table 31.10. The Gleason score is useful because of its prognostic value. To derive a Gleason score, the two most predominant glandular patterns of the prostate tumor are assigned a grade from 1 (most highly differentiated) to 5 (most poorly differentiated). These two grades are combined for a total score, with scores of 4 or higher carrying a worse prognosis (44). Additional tests that might be used to assist in clinical staging in those with higher Gleason scores and/or TNM stages include radionuclide bone scans, computed tomography (CT) scans of the abdomen/pelvis, and magnetic resonance imaging (MRI) of the prostate gland and surrounding structures.

Advanced Prostate Cancer

Five percent of men with prostate cancer already have distant metastases at the time the diagnosis is made (21). Treatment of such metastatic prostate cancer is primarily by androgen deprivation therapy (ADT). The goal of treatment at this stage is palliative—mainly to decrease bone pain, which it does in 80% to 90% of patients (45). There are several methods of ADT including bilateral orchiectomy, continuous luteinizing hormone releasing hormone (LHRH) agonists (e.g., leuprolide), and nonsteroidal antiandrogens (e.g., flutamide). Side

TABLE 31.9 Tumor-Node-Metastasis (TNM) Staging of Prostate Cancer

Primary tumor

TX	Primary tumor cannot be assessed		
T1	Clinically inapparent tumor neither palpable nor visible by imaging	a	Incidental finding in ≤5% of tissue resected
		b	Incidental finding in >5% of tissue resected
		c	Identified by needle biopsy (e.g., because of elevated PSA
T2	Tumor confined within the prostate	a	Involves ≤half of one lobe
		b	Involves >half of one lobe but not both lobes
		c	Involves both lobes
T3	Tumor extends through the prostatic capsule	a	Extracapsular extension (unilateral or bilateral)
		b	Tumor invades seminal vesicle(s)
T4	Tumor is fixed or invades adjacent structures other than seminal vesicles: bladder neck, external sphincter, rectum, levator muscles, and/or pelvic wall		

Nodes

NX	Regional lymph nodes not assessed		
N0	No regional node metastasis		
N1	Metastasis in regional node(s)		

Metastasis

M0	No distant metastasis		
M1	Distant metastasis	a	Nonregional lymph nodes
		b	Metastasis in bone(s)
		c	Other site(s) with or without bone disease

PSA, prostate specific antigen
Greene FL, Page DL, Fleming ID, et al, eds. AJCC Cancer Staging Manual, 6th ed. New York, NY, Springer-Verlag; 2002.
Used with the permission of the American Joint Committee on Cancer (AJCC), Chicago, Illinois. The original source for this material is the AJCC Cancer Staging Manual, Sixth Edition (2002) published by Springer-Verlag New York. Available at *www.springeronline.com*.

effects are substantial and include hot flashes, ED, gynecomastia, and bone loss. Because bone loss (and consequent fractures) can be substantial, men undergoing ADT should receive calcium and vitamin D supplements. Men with locally advanced prostate cancer are usually offered external beam radiation therapy in addition to ADT.

Early Prostate Cancer

Options for treatment of early, or localized, prostate cancer include watchful waiting, radiation therapy (RT), or surgery.

The efficacy of these three management options remains uncertain. Radiation and surgical options pose risks of treatment complications (see Screening for Prostate Cancer). Although the risk is substantial in both groups, men treated by radical prostatectomy may be more likely to develop urinary incontinence (15% vs. 4%) or ED (79% vs. 64%) than men treated by RT (46).

In discussions with men regarding watchful waiting versus treatment options, factors to consider include expected remaining lifespan and whether the cancer was detected as

TABLE 31.10 Gleason Scoring of Prostate Cancer

Gleason Score	Interpretation	10-Year Disease Specific Survival*
2 to 4	Well-differentiated or low-grade	90%
5 to 7	Moderately differentiated	80%
8 to 10	Poorly differentiated or high-grade	45% to 65%

*Lu-Yao GL, Yao SL. Population-based study of long-term survival in patients with clinically localized prostate cancer. Lancet. 1997; 349:906–910

a result of symptoms versus detected by screening. In one randomized trial comparing radical prostatectomy to watchful waiting for moderately or well-differentiated prostate cancer (95% of which was detected by symptoms), disease-specific mortality was lower in the radical prostatectomy group (9.6% vs. 14.9%; p = 0.01), with a number needed to treat (NNT) of 19 (47). All-cause mortality was also lower in the men who underwent radical prostatectomy (27% vs. 32%; p = 0.04). The benefit was noted primarily in men who had longer duration of follow-up, i.e., those less than 65 years of age (47). In men with a remaining lifespan of 10 years or less, watchful waiting may be preferred as it poses less risk of ED and urinary incontinence and is associated with no change in all-cause mortality or quality of life, even in men whose prostate cancer was detected by symptoms (48). It may also be useful to consider quality-adjusted life years (QALYs) when discussing treatment options with men. One study estimated differences in QALYs between management options based on Gleason score (49). Taking into account the effects of lead-time, for Gleason scores of 2 to 4, QALYs were greater with watchful waiting. For Gleason scores 7 to 10, treatment (prostatectomy or RT) resulted in greater QALYs. For Gleason scores of 5 to 6, QALYs varied depending on the assumptions used in the model.

PREVENTION OF PROSTATE CANCER

Men interested in potential ways to decrease their risk of prostate cancer should consider decreasing their dietary intake of animal fat (particularly red meat and dairy products), and increasing their intake of fruits and vegetables to at least 28 servings per week (50). Supplementation with selenium may provide additional benefit, but further study is required (26). Finasteride, which inhibits the conversion of testosterone to dihydrotestosterone, may decrease a man's overall risk of developing prostate cancer (from 24% to 18%), but may increase the risk of high-grade disease (from 5.1% to 6.4%) (51); thus, it is not currently recommended for prevention of prostate cancer. Men taking finasteride for BPH should be advised of this potential risk.

DISCUSSION CASE 3

You should inform Mr. B. of the known risks and benefits of prostate cancer screening, including the fact that we do not know if prostate cancer screening reduces morbidity or mortality. Ideally, you would use a decision aid such as the one available on the AAFP Web site at *http://www.aafp.org/x19519.xm*. Many men will still choose to undergo PSA testing after an informed discussion, and some will not. It is important to document the discussion regardless of the man's decision. Mr. B.'s PSA of 3.1 ng/mL, while below the cutoff of 4.0 ng/mL, does not necessarily mean that he does not have prostate cancer. If you estimate Mr. B.'s pretest probability of having prostate cancer based on prevalence studies, you can then use the information in Table 31.7 to estimate his post-test probability of having cancer. Alternatively, using the algorithm in Figure 31.2, Mr. B. has approximately a 15% probability of

having prostate cancer detected on biopsy. If he is referred to a urologist and a prostate biopsy reveals early (localized) cancer, a discussion of the risks and benefits of the treatment options would be the next step.

ERECTILE DYSFUNCTION

CASE 4

Mr. M. is a 44-year-old white man who, during an employer-mandated physical exam, asks you for a prescription for Viagra®. He is currently married and reports that he and his wife have a good relationship. He reports no medical problems, but a review of his chart shows that his blood pressure was elevated on his last three visits. He has smoked one pack of cigarettes per day for 28 years and drinks a "few beers" on the weekends. His blood pressure today is 172/100 mm Hg. He is obese, has a few spider angiomas on his trunk, a slightly enlarged liver, and an elevated aspartate aminotransferase and gammaglutamyl transferase on laboratory evaluation.

CLINICAL QUESTIONS

1. What history and physical examination items suggest an organic etiology for a man with erectile dysfunction (ED)?
2. Which tests should you consider for a man being evaluated for ED?
3. What are the available treatments for ED?

ED was once thought to be an inevitable consequence of advancing age, and was rarely addressed in the primary care setting. Now that a variety of effective treatments are available and widely advertised in magazines and on television, it is seen as a common medical disorder, with significant quality of life implications; consequently, more men are seeking treatment.

The Massachusetts Male Aging Study (MMAS) was a landmark study in determining the prevalence of sexual dysfunction among American men. The MMAS was a large cohort study of 1,709 men ages 40–70 from 1987–1989, with a follow-up phase in 1995–1997 (52). This study demonstrated age-specific declines in sexual functioning, specifically in erectile function, libido, and ejaculatory function. Forty percent of men in their 40s admitted to some level of sexual dysfunction, and this increased approximately 10% with each decade advance in age. Overall, 35% of men had moderate to complete ED (53). The follow-up study confirmed these age-associated declines and demonstrated that these changes were nonlinear, meaning that the magnitude of change was larger with increasing age in all areas of sexual functioning (52). This included frequency of intercourse, erectile function, sexual desire, satisfaction with sex, and frequency of orgasm; notably, not all these variables are physically demanding, so there is no simple explanation for this decline (52).

This age-associated decline in sexual dysfunction was further confirmed in a prospective study in 31,742 men ages

TABLE 31.11 Relative Risk of Lifestyle Variables and Comorbid Conditions Associated with Sexual Dysfunction

Variable	Relative Risk	95% Confidence Interval
Physical activity[a]	0.7	0.6–0.7
Obesity[b]	1.3	1.2–1.4
Smoking	1.3	1.1–1.4
Television viewing time[c]	1.2	1.1–1.3
Diabetes	1.5	1.2–1.9
Nonprostate cancer	1.4	1.1–1.6
Stroke	1.4	1.0–1.9
Antidepressant use	1.7	1.2–2.2
B-blocker use	1.2	1.1–1.5

a = >32.6 metabolic equivalent hours (METs) per week (equivalent of running 3 hours per week)
b = body mass index >28.7 kg/m^2
c = >20 hours per week

Data from: Bacon CG, Mittleman MA, Kawachi I, Giovannucci E, Glasser DB, Rimm EB. Sexual function in men older than 50 years of age: results from the Health Professionals Follow-up Study. Ann Intern Med. 2003;139161–139168.

53–90, 33% of whom (after men with prostate cancer were excluded) admitted to ED in the preceding 3 months. Other aspects of sexual functioning, such as sexual desire and ability to achieve orgasm, were again shown to sharply decline each decade after age 50 (54).

Several modifiable health factors have also been linked with ED. Smoking, inactivity, and obesity are all associated with an increased risk of sexual dysfunction (Table 31.11) (54). Interestingly, alcohol intake did not appear to be a negative risk factor, and moderate intake appeared to be beneficial (relative risk 0.9) (54). Common comorbidities, such as diabetes, hypertension, and hypercholesterolemia, and medications including alpha-blockers, beta-blockers, thiazide diuretics, and finasteride, also had a negative effect on sexual functioning (54).

Laumann et al analyzed data from the 1992 National Health and Social Life Survey of adults aged 18–59. Men in the study had a 31% prevalence of sexual dysfunction; thus, problems with sexual functioning are not confined to the older population. Positive risk factors in this study were history of a sexually transmitted disease, stress, recent decrease in household income, non-marital status, history of same-sex activity, and history of adult-child sexual contact (55).

NORMAL PHYSIOLOGY

Normal penile erection is a vascular event that is triggered by neurologic stimuli in the presence of appropriate hormonal and psychologic influences. A penile erection begins with neural stimulation, which includes tactile and psychologic stimuli. Neural impulses stimulated by sexual images in the brain enter the spinal cord and then proceed via the parasympathetic pathway to the pelvic vascular bed, allowing for increased blood flow into the corpus cavernosa of the penis. A sacral reflex arc is activated by tactile stimulation, which also allows for

redirection of blood flow into the penis. Psychogenic erections are more common in younger men, whereas most erections in older men are the result of tactile stimuli (56, 57).

With the proper stimuli, acetylcholine and nitric oxide (NO) are released by the nerves innervating the smooth muscle of the corpus cavernosum. NO enters the smooth muscle cells and, through a pathway involving cyclic guanosine monophosphate (cGMP), causes relaxation of the smooth muscle of the corpus cavernosum. The smooth muscle of the penile arteries also relaxes, allowing for increased arterial blood flow from the hypogastric artery into the penis. As the lacunar spaces within the corpus cavernosum fill with blood, they expand and pressure within the penis builds. This increase in pressure inhibits venous outflow. The perineal muscles also contract, further increasing penile pressure above that of the abdominal aorta. This trapping of blood in the penis produces an erection. Detumescence is mediated by sympathetic pathways and occurs when NO levels decrease, and the enzyme phosphodiesterase type 5 (PDE5) metabolizes cGMP (58, 59).

Testosterone is not only an important factor in sexual desire, but is also thought to have a local effect on the penis. Testosterone receptors are present on the smooth muscle of the corpus cavernosum and appear to aid in maintaining NO levels in the penis. Thus, an adequate androgen supply is also necessary for an erection to occur (59).

CAUSES OF ERECTILE DYSFUNCTION

ED is defined as the inability to acquire or maintain an erection sufficient to have intercourse more than 75 percent of the time (56). The cause is usually multifactorial and can involve disruption anywhere in the spectrum of the vascular, neurologic, hormonal, and psychologic mediators of normal erectile physiology. It is important to remember that ED is not the sole manifestation of sexual dysfunction. Frequency of intercourse, sexual desire, ability to achieve orgasm, and overall satisfaction with sex are all important for the quality of an individual's sexual functioning.

An estimated 70% of cases of ED are vascular in origin (58). Normal arterial blood flow is an absolute requirement to sustain an erection. Failure to store blood in the venous system can also cause vasculogenic impotence. Many of the risk factors and comorbidities associated with ED (see Table 31.12) are also factors associated with poor circulation.

Along with sufficient arterial blood flow, relaxation of the smooth muscle of the corpus cavernosum is the other event that is necessary to achieve an erection. Smokers, diabetics, and patients with testosterone deficiency have lower levels of NO synthetase in their corpus cavernosum (56). There are many intricacies involved in smooth muscle relaxation of the corpus, including NO activity and adrenergic stimulation, and problems in this area are likely multifactorial.

Depression was discovered by the MMAS to be the second most common risk factor for ED (53). Other psychogenic factors, such as interpersonal conflict, stress, and anxiety, also play a role in ED. Again, it becomes apparent that many of the risk factors for ED are also risk factors for depression, and vice versa. These include obesity, sedentary lifestyle, increasing age, and smoking, as well as chronic medical conditions such as diabetes and ischemic heart disease (58). Psychologic factors can further exacerbate the problem. Experiencing ED can be very depressing for a man, and performance anxiety is common after a man experiences even one episode of ED. Sex then becomes an anxiety provoking experience, and much of the man's focus becomes whether or not he will be able to perform. Adrenergic release caused by stress during intercourse further perpetuates the problem because of its effect on smooth muscle in the penis.

A complicating issue is that many of the medicines used to treat the risk factors for ED can themselves cause ED. Antidepressants, particularly selective serotonin reuptake inhibitors (SSRIs) are one of the most common culprits and can cause problems with libido and ejaculatory function as well as ED (58). After antidepressants, antihypertensives are probably the next most common class of drugs causing ED, particu-

TABLE 31.13	Medications Associated with Erectile Dysfunction
Alpha-blockers	
Antidepressants	
Beta-blockers	
Cimetidine	
Clonidine	
Finasteride	
Ketoconazole	
Methadone	
Methyldopa	
Nicotine	
Spironolactone	
Thiazide diuretics	

larly thiazide diuretics. Table 31.13 lists substances commonly associated with ED.

INITIAL EVALUATION

The evaluation of any man with ED begins with a careful history and physical exam. Discussion of sexual function often needs to be initiated by the physician. In one survey, 71% of patients thought their doctor would dismiss their sexual concerns if brought up, and 68% thought that discussing the problem with their doctor would embarrass the physician (60). Screening questionnaires, including questions about sexual dysfunction, given at well-male visits can be useful tools in identifying men who are having sexual issues; they also can provide the physician with a way of broaching the subject. More specific questionnaires, such as the Sexual Health Inventory for Men, can also help with history intake in a less embarrassing manner for the patient (55). A careful history and physical exam has been shown to have a 95% sensitivity for diagnosing organic ED (although only a 50% specificity) (61). Important questions in the history include the timing of the

TABLE 31.12	Risk Factors for Erectile Dysfunction
Age	Ischemic heart disease
Androgen deficiency	Medication use
Anxiety	Metabolic syndrome
Chronic renal failure	Multiple sclerosis
Cycling (prolonged pressure on pudendal and cavernosal nerves)	Obesity
	Peripheral vascular disease
Depression	Prostate surgery
Diabetes mellitus	Sedentary lifestyle
Dyslipidemia	Substance abuse
Genitourinary trauma	Tobacco use
Herniated discs	Unresolved patient/partner conflict
Hyperprolactinemia	
Hypertension	
Hyperthyroidism	
Hypothyroidism	

problem (rapid vs. gradual), ability to achieve an erection and orgasm during masturbation, the presence of morning erections, and whether or not there are any marital problems. Sudden loss of erectile function with every attempt is almost always psychogenic in origin. ED that gradually increases in frequency can be organic or psychogenic. The presence of nocturnal and morning erections means that neurologic reflexes and penile blood flow are intact; therefore, presence of these usually points to a psychogenic cause. The physician must also be sure to assess for the presence of risk factors for ED.

A physical examination, including examination of the genitourinary system, is obligatory. Evaluation should include assessment of secondary sexual characteristics, a testicular exam, noting size and any masses or other abnormalities, assessment for normal penile anatomy, and a prostate exam to evaluate for evidence of prostatitis or malignancy (59). The physician should also be sure to note any evidence of poor circulation elsewhere in the body, the presence of gynecomastia, and any neurologic signs that could point to a pituitary tumor or spinal cord lesion.

The results of the history and physical examination should be used to guide the remainder of the evaluation. Laboratory studies may be done to assess for risk factors such as diabetes, hypercholesterolemia, hypogonadism, and endocrine abnormalities (59). One study of 1,455 men with ED found abnormalities on laboratory testing in 28% of the patients (62). Low plasma testosterone was found in 6.9% of subjects, hyperprolactinemia in 1.2%, elevated random glucose in 9.3%, elevated ferritin in 1.6%, and hypercholesterolemia in 15%. Although glucose and lipid testing had the highest yield in this study, therapy was more effective for the conditions identified by the lower-yield tests (testosterone and prolactin).

If history, physical exam, and laboratory testing fail to reveal an etiology, further testing is available but will usually require referral to a urologist. Nocturnal penile tumescence (NPT) testing can be useful, particularly if the patient or his partner is unable to give a good history of nocturnal and morning erections. Portable devices such as the Rigi-Scan can be used to quantify the number and rigidity of nighttime erectile episodes. Rigi-Scan is up to 93% accurate at classifying ED as organic versus psychogenic, although there is a 12% false negative rate (61). Other special tests such as duplex ultrasound, angiography, and penile plethysmography are much less common and should be left to the discretion of the consulting urologist. Typically these tests would be reserved for those patients who failed conservative management and were considering an invasive procedure.

MANAGEMENT

Of the 30 million American men currently estimated to suffer from ED, only 3 million are being treated (59). Treatment of any patient with ED should follow a step-wise approach, beginning with the least-invasive therapies, and continuing until an effective treatment is found. Lifestyle modifications, such as weight loss, smoking cessation, and personal or marital counseling when indicated, should be considered a first-line therapy. Modification of drug therapy when an offending agent could be present is also an initial step. Treatment for

comorbid conditions and androgen replacement should also be performed when indicated. A study by Esposito et al showed that increased physical activity and reduction in body mass index independently improved ED in obese men ages 35–55 years (63). Of men in the intervention group, 31% had regained sexual function after 3 years of lifestyle changes. If lifestyle changes are either ineffective or not feasible, the next line of treatment is usually oral medications. Figure 31.5 shows an algorithm that can guide evaluation and management.

Pharmacotherapy
ORAL MEDICATIONS

The release of sildenafil (Viagra®) in 1998 revolutionized the treatment of ED by providing an effective, noninvasive therapy for ED that patients could obtain from their primary care physician. The PDE5 inhibitors, sildenafil (Viagra®), tadalafil (Cialis®), and vardenafil (Levitra®) have been successful for the treatment of ED in 85% of cases (58). PDE5 inhibitors selectively inhibit the catabolism of cGMP, allowing the erectile response to occur only in the presence of appropriate stimulation (64). It is important to emphasize to patients that PDE5 inhibitors work to enhance an erection rather than cause one. Therefore, sexual stimulation is required for the NO release in the corpus cavernosum, which then works through cGMP to cause smooth muscle relaxation. Because the PDE5 inhibitors work through preventing the breakdown of cGMP, they cannot cause an erection without stimulation first.

Side effects of the PDE5 inhibitors are generally mild, and include flushing, dyspepsia, headache, and rhinitis. These medications seem to be effective regardless of the etiology of the sexual dysfunction, although certain populations, such as diabetic men, have lower success rates (64). All of the PDE5 inhibitors are contraindicated in patients taking nitrates. Nitrates act as a donor of NO, which increases cGMP. Because PDE5 inhibitors prevent the breakdown of cGMP, the combination can cause an overload of cGMP, and subsequently significant vasodilation and hypotension (65). A washout period for sildenafil and vardenafil of 24 hours (48 hours for tadalafil) is recommended before nitrate administration (65). Table 31.14 compares the currently available PDE5 inhibitors.

Sildenafil was the first of the PDE5 inhibitors to be released, and thus has the most data on efficacy and safety. Although the onset of erection after sildenafil administration can be anywhere from 15 to 60 minutes, optimal response is usually seen at 60 minutes. Response is also best at least 2 hours after a meal, since fatty foods can interfere with absorption. There is a dose-response effect to sildenafil, and patients may not achieve success with the first few trials. Men should allow 6–8 trials to assess adequacy of treatment. Headache and flushing are the most common side effects. About 3% of patients taking sildenafil may also experience blue vision caused by concomitant inhibition of PDE6 present in the retina. This side effect is less common with the other PDE5 inhibitors. A transient decrease in blood pressure has been observed after taking sildenafil. In many patients with ED, reducing vascular resistance may actually be of some benefit. No adverse cardiac effects have been observed with sildenafil.

Vardenafil, which the US Food and Drug Administration (FDA) approved in 2003, was the second PDE5 inhibitor made available. It has a very similar structure to sildenafil

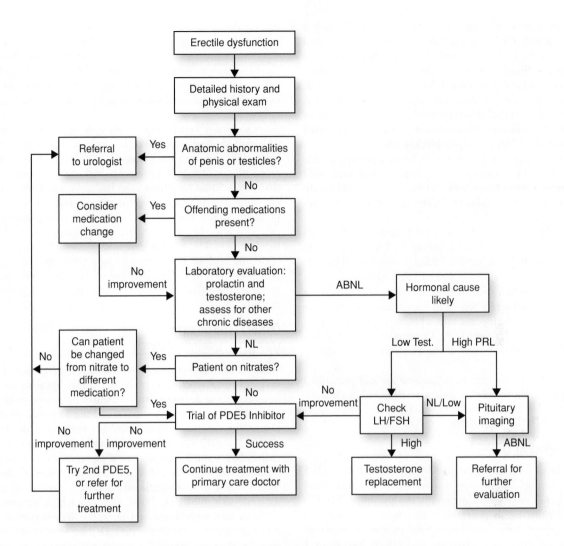

Figure 31.5 • Algorithm for management and treatment of erectile dysfunction.   PRL, prolactin; LH, luteinizing hormone; FSH, follicle stimulating hormone; Test, testosterone; NL, normal; ABNL, abnormal. Adapted from: Miller TA. Diagnostic evaluation of erectile dysfunction. AM Fam Physician 2006;61(1):95–104, 109–110 and Jackson G. Erectile dysfunction: a management algorithm. Int J Clinical Practice 2004; 58(8):733–734.

TABLE 31.14   Comparison of the PDE5 Inhibitors

	Sildenafil	Tadalafil	Vardenafil
Doses (mg)	25, 50, 100	5, 10, 20	2.5, 5, 10, 20
Onset (minutes)	14–30	16–45	20–30
Duration (hours)	4	36	4
Active metabolite	Yes	No	Yes
Half-life (hours)	3–4	17.5	4–5
Cost (10 tablets)	$91–$94	$95–$102	$88–$95

Adapted from Carson CC. Erectile dysfunction: evaluation and new treatment options. Psychosomatic Medicine. 2004;66: 664–71. Cost information from *www.drugstore.com*. Accessed on 11/29/05.

and exhibits many of the same properties. Vardenafil also has a half-life of about 4 hours, and absorption may be affected by high-fat meals. Unlike sildenafil, however, there is no dose-response curve. Similar side effects are observed as with sildenafil, although blue vision is much less common. A very modest decrease in blood pressure and increase in heart rate has been observed with use, although this has not shown to be of any cardiac significance. Nevertheless, because of potential hypotension, the FDA lists alpha-blocker use as a contraindication to taking vardenafil (59, 65). Efficacy rates are similar to sildenafil, although one study demonstrated that vardenafil was effective in 60% of men who did not respond to sildenafil (66). Thus, if a patient fails one PDE5 inhibitor, he may respond to another.

Tadalafil is the newest of the PDE5 inhibitors. Tadalafil is unique in its long half-life, allowing for efficacy of up to 36 hours; food does not seem to affect absorption. The side effect profile is similar to the other PDE5 inhibitors, except for a higher frequency of back pain (6%–7%). The back pain is usually mild and rarely results in discontinuation (59). The cardiac profile again appears safe, although a mild drop in blood pressure has been noted (65). Concomitant use of alpha-blocker should be avoided, with the exception of tamsulosin (59).

Alpha-antagonists such as yohimbine are still prescribed by some physicians for the treatment of ED. Although some benefit has been reported in meta-analysis, controlled trials have shown lack of benefit (58).

TRANSURETHRAL DRUGS

After a patient has undergone an adequate trial of the PDE5 inhibitors, second-line therapy is usually either transurethral drugs or penile injections. Intraurethral alprostadil (MUSE) is prostaglandin E1 in pellet form that is inserted with an applicator about 3 cm into the urethral meatus. It is placed 5–10 minutes prior to intercourse, and effects last about 1 hour. A randomized controlled trial of 1,511 men with various organic causes of ED showed successful intercourse in 43% versus 12% of the placebo group. Of the responders, 7 out of 10 applications resulted in successful intercourse. Eighty-eight percent of men did not think that application of the pellet was uncomfortable. Side effects, the most common of which was penile pain, were mild and rarely resulted in discontinuation (67).

Unlike the oral agents, alprostadil will cause an erection even without sexual stimuli. Prostaglandin E1 works by stimulating intracellular production of cyclic adenosine monophosphate (cAMP). The combination of alprostadil plus sildenafil may be effective in patients who do not respond to monotherapy, but this should only be done under the recommendation of a urologist (58).

PENILE INJECTIONS

Intracorporeal injection therapy (ICI) is self-injection of prostaglandin E1, papaverine, or papaverine plus phentolamine into the corporeal body of the penis 10 minutes prior to intercourse. Prostaglandin E1 injections, as with the transurethral suppositories, work by direct stimulation of cAMP, causing smooth muscle relaxation. Although injections are generally painless, this therapy is usually limited by the man's fear of

self-injection, and occasionally prolonged dull pain in the penis. Only one injection should be done in 24 hours (58).

Papaverine is a phosphodiesterase inhibitor that also works by smooth muscle relaxation. It is rarely used as a single agent because of high rates of penile scarring. It is more often combined with phentolamine, which is a direct alpha-1-antagonist (58).

One study comparing 22 men on ICI and 31 men on sildenafil showed equal patient satisfaction with both treatments (68). Another study showed a 97.6% positive response rate with one of four ICI protocols, including combinations of drugs (69). Some men have even had a return of spontaneous erections after long-term treatment with ICI, particularly alprostadil. In one study, 85% of men were having spontaneous erections after 12 months of treatment, compared to 37% at baseline (70). The most feared side effect of ICI is priapism, occurring in about 11% of men using papaverine and 1% using alprostadil (71, 72). The first dose of ICI, therefore, is often given in the office to monitor the patient for a prolonged erection.

Other Treatments
VACUUM-ASSIST DEVICES

After the above treatments have failed, vacuum-assisted erection devices are often the last step before invasive therapy. Several of these devices exist, which are engineered to increase arterial flow by vacuum pressure, and use a tourniquet device to prevent venous outflow. Problems with these devices include a low patient satisfaction rate and high rate of discontinuation. In one study 129 patients with organic ED were given training on the device and followed for a mean of 37 months. There was a 65% discontinuation rate, including all of the patients with mild ED. There was also a high dropout rate (70%) in men with complete ED, so the highest continuation rate was in men with moderate ED. The most common reasons for stopping were that it was not effective, it was too painful, or too cumbersome. Overall, 35% of the patients were satisfied with the device and continued use (73). Problems with the device include interference with ejaculation because of the tourniquet component, a hinge-effect at the base of the penis, and a maximum safe use of up to 1 hour.

PENILE PROSTHESES

Surgically placed prosthetic devices include malleable rods and inflatable prosthetics. These are usually reserved for last resort treatments. Once a patient has failed oral agents, referral to a urologist is appropriate to determine further therapy. The evidence for these treatments of ED is summarized in Table 31.15.

DISCUSSION CASE 4

First, a more detailed history should be obtained to define the exact nature of the sexual dysfunction. Patients may request Viagra® when their problem is actually related to libido or problems achieving orgasm rather than ED. Mr. M. has several risk factors for ED, including obesity, untreated hypertension, and tobacco use. He also has the stigmata of heavy alcohol use. Although alcohol use per se is not well linked to ED, he

TABLE 31.15 Strength of Recommendation for Treatments of Erectile Dysfunction

Intervention	Efficacy	Strength of Recommendation*	Comment
PDE5 inhibitor	60%–95% for all-cause ED	A	Similar for all agents; less effective for certain etiologies
Intraurethral alprostadil	43% overall; 67% among initial in-office responders	A	Efficacy rate for at home coitus
Intracorporeal injection therapy	Up to 97.6%	A	Depends on agent used; efficacy rate includes drug combinations
Vacuum-assist device	35% overall; includes high drop-out rate; up to 89% in adherent patients	B	For rigidity only; no evidence for effect on orgasm
Penile Prosthetic Surgery	64%–93%	C	Limiting factor is mechanical dysfunction; for erection only, not orgasm or overall satisfaction

*A = consistent, good-quality patient-oriented evidence; B = inconsistent or limited-quality patient-oriented evidence; C = consensus, disease-oriented evidence, usual practice, expert opinion, or case series. For information about the SORT evidence rating system, see *http://www.aafp.org/afpsort.xml*.

is certainly likely to have difficulty getting an erection while he is intoxicated, which may be the majority of the time. These lifestyle issues need to be addressed with Mr. M. before treating his ED with medication. He needs to be educated that smoking cessation and weight loss can help restore erectile function. At the very least, his blood pressure needs to be adequately controlled, and then sexual function reassessed to see if he is still a candidate for a PDE5 inhibitor. A further laboratory workup should also be done for other chronic diseases such as diabetes.

PERFORMANCE-ENHANCING SUPPLEMENTS

CASE 5

B.B. is a 16-year-old male who presents for a preparticipation sports physical to play football. As part of your conversation, you bring up the topic of performance-enhancing supplements. B.B. tells you that he is using creatine to help him "bulk up."

CLINICAL QUESTIONS
1. How common is the use of performance-enhancing supplements?
2. What do you tell patients who ask about or use performance-enhancing supplements?

As many as 4% of American adults report using a sports supplement at least once, and 1.2 million report regular use (74). These "performing-enhancing supplements" range from ana-

bolic steroids to hormonal and dietary supplements such as androstenedione, dihydroepiandrosterone (DHEA), growth hormone, and creatine. These substances are marketed to aid in weight loss, increase lean body mass, build muscle, and increase strength.

Nutritional supplements are often thought to be safe because they are "natural." However, these substances are not regulated, and some have caused serious adverse effects, including death. The 1994 US Dietary Supplement Health and Education Act made it legal to sell substances labeled as "dietary supplements" without FDA approval, if the substance is not labeled to treat, prevent, or cure a specific disease. These substances do not undergo safety and efficacy evaluation and do not have to meet any quality control standards. Use of supplements is not limited to college and professional athletes; androgen use has been reported in up to 6% of boys as young as age 13 (75). In a cross-sectional survey of approximately 1,000 athletes, 29% of adolescent boys admitted to use of creatine, amino acids and other protein supplements, DHEA, and hydroxyl-beta-methylbutyrate (HMB) (76).

We will review some of the more common forms of sports supplements, purported benefits, evidence for efficacy, and adverse effects. While addressed in this chapter on men's health concerns, it must be remembered that much of this information applies to women as well.

ANDROGENS

Androgens taken for performance enhancement include injectable testosterone esters (the same as used for medical supplementation), oral 17-alpha-alkylated androgens (the so-called "anabolic steroids"), and androgen precursors (androstenedione and DHEA). Athletes use androgens hoping to promote muscle growth by increasing serum testosterone.

TABLE 31.16 Adverse Effects of Androgens

Androgenic
- Acne
- Alopecia
- Decreased levels of sex hormone-binding globulin
- Decreased sperm count (often reversible)
- Decreased testicular size
- Gynecomastia
- Hirsutism
- Increased risk of prostate diseases
- Premature epiphyseal closure with diminished adult height
- Suppresses endogenous testicular function
- Virilization (women, children)

Cardiovascular
- Cardiomyopathy
- Decreased high density liproprotein
- Increased risk of thromboembolism, acute myocardial infarction, stroke, or pulmonary embolus

Hepatic (particularly with 17-alkylated steroids)
- Cholestatic jaundice
- Elevated liver enzymes
- Peliosis hepatic
- Tumors

Hematopoietic
- Erythrocytosis (direct stimulation of erythropoiesis)

Psychologic
- Addiction
- Aggressive behavior
- Depression
- Dysphoria and rage
- Increased libido
- Psychosis
- Withdrawal

Needle sharing
- Cellulitis
- Endocarditis
- Hepatitis
- HIV

Adapted from Table 1 in: Rogol AD. Sex steroid and growth hormone supplementation to enhance performance in adolescent athletes. Curr Opin Pediatr. 2000;12(4):382–7.

However, no high-quality evidence is available to suggest that these supplements actually work, yet harmful effects do exist (see Table 31.16).

The 17-alpha-alkylated androgens were developed to have a primarily anabolic effect, thus receiving the name anabolic steroids. By having a higher ratio of anabolic to androgenic activity, they could build lean body mass and decrease body fat, while minimizing the androgenic activity that causes bothersome side effects. Further benefit is achieved from the anti-catabolic effects of these substances, which may allow for rapid recovery after intense training sessions. However, none of these substances are really devoid of androgenic effects (77), so bothersome and potentially harmful side effects are still a problem despite what the manufacturer may claim. The Anabolic Steroids Control Act of 1990 made androgenic-anabolic steroids Schedule III controlled substances (78); nevertheless, the 17-alpha-alkylated androgens, along with testosterone esters, are still used for performance enhancement. These substances taken by athletes are usually obtained illegally and are commonly "counterfeit" substances, often not even containing the expected ingredients. One study in Germany showed by gas chromatography and mass spectrometry that 15 of 42 products obtained on the black market did not contain the ingredients claimed (79).

Lifetime use of anabolic steroids has been reported in 4.9% of men (80). Studies have proven the anabolic benefits of exogenous testosterone in men with normal baseline testosterone levels, with increases in muscle mass and strength, particularly with simultaneous exercise. However, dosages used by athletes far exceed those recommended for testosterone replacement. The study by Bhasin et al used 600 mg of the testosterone enanthate weekly, which is six times the replacement dose used for hypogonadism (81).

Perhaps far more common than androgenic-anabolic steroids is the use of androgen precursors, androstenedione, and DHEA. These substances are widely available in over-the-counter preparations. These "natural" alternatives to anabolic steroids are thought to be converted to testosterone in the body, thereby increasing serum testosterone levels and promoting muscle growth during resistance training. Androstenedione is naturally produced in the adrenal glands and testes, but a form derived from plants is sold in tablets with a recommended dose of 100 to 300 mg daily. There are no large randomized controlled trials studying the true physiologic effects of androstenedione, and the few small studies that exist fail to show any benefits of increased muscle mass or strength. The largest study examining both short- and long-term effects of androstenedione was done with 20 men ages 19–29, and compared 300 mg/day of androstenedione to placebo (82). No difference was found in muscle strength, histological exam of type II muscle fibers, lean body mass percentages, or serum free and total testosterone concentrations. Serum estradiol and estrone concentrations were higher, however, after 2 weeks of androstenedione use compared to baseline levels. High-density lipoprotein (HDL) cholesterol levels were decreased by 12% in the study group. Although patients were studied for only 8 weeks, this observation leads to the assumption that androstenedione may increase cardiovascular risk, as well as estrogenic side effects, such as gynecomastia. Although other studies have shown increases of blood hormone levels after taking androstenedione, no performance-enhancing benefits were shown in these cases. A study in 30- to 56-year-old men showed elevated serum levels of androstenedione, free testosterone, and dihydrotestosterone after taking 300 mg/day of androstenedione (83). However, serum total testosterone did not increase, and a 68% increase in estradiol levels was noted. This study also confirmed a significant decrease in HDL with use of the supplement. A study of 42 men aged 20–40 did show an increase in serum testosterone concentrations by 34%, with 300 mg/day of androstenedione use, but also had a concomitant increase in serum estrone and estradiol levels by 196%. Furthermore, testosterone levels had returned to normal by the following day, making any anabolic benefits questionable (84).

DHEA, produced in the body by the adrenal cortex, is another precursor to both androgens and estrogens. Although banned as a prescription drug by the FDA in 1996, DHEA has since been labeled as a nutritional supplement, and is now being sold over-the-counter (85). No randomized studies have been done evaluating anabolic benefits of DHEA. One small study of 14 men using DHEA for 6 months showed serum increases in DHEA and levels of DHEAS, but no resultant increase in serum testosterone (85).

Insulin-like growth factor-1 (IGF-1), growth hormone, and human chorionic gonadotropin (hCG) have also been used to increase circulating testosterone levels. HCG acts like luteinizing hormone to stimulate the Leydig cells of the testes to secrete testosterone. IGF-1 has a theoretical anabolic benefit, but no studies have shown it to be of benefit on strength, exercise capacity, or muscle strength, and large doses can cause hypoglycemia. In growth-hormone deficient individuals, supplementation can increase strength and lean body mass, but these effects have never been shown to occur in athletes with normal baseline growth hormone levels (77).

Although the USPSTF does not recommend routine screening for steroid use, it is an important topic to broach with young patients as part of the routine assessment. Most of supplement users' knowledge comes from their peers and information obtained on product labeling, and is often incorrect or misleading. Only 18% of adolescents using anabolic steroids in Colorado said that they were informed about steroid use by a physician (86).

NUTRITIONAL SUPPLEMENTS

Creatine

Creatine is the most common supplement used by athletes. Among football players alone, up to 30% in high school and 71% of Division I players have reported using creatine (87, 88). A non-essential amino acid, half of the body's daily requirement of creatine is synthesized endogenously in the liver, kidneys, and pancreas, while half is obtained from diet (highest abundance is in meat and fish). The phosphorylated version of creatine, creatine phosphate, acts as a phosphate donor for the production of adenosine triphosphate (ATP) from adenosine diphosphate (ADP) in skeletal muscle cells. The amount of creatine phosphate in the body has been shown to be enhanced by 10%–30% with creatine supplementation (89, 90). Increasing the amount of creatine phosphate in skeletal muscle allows for faster regeneration of ATP, which in turn theoretically leads to enhanced muscle strength and power, and an increase in lean body mass (91). This becomes important in high-intensity, repetitive, short-duration exercise (74) such as weight-lifting, in which aerobically produced ATP is insufficient (92). In one study of Division I collegiate athletes, 89% of the 80 athletes using creatine perceived a positive benefit (93). Other studies have specifically demonstrated an increase in maximum weight lifted on a bench press (94, 95) and a higher number of bench press repetitions (96). Aerobic activity, however, is unlikely to be affected by excess creatine phosphate, as fat and glucose breakdown is able to supply the energy needed for aerobic activity. In addition to energy production, creatine phosphate aids in the buffering of intracellular acidosis and the activation of glycogenolysis. The recommended loading dose for creatine supplementation is 20–30 g per day for 5–7 days, with a maintenance of 2–4 g per day (97).

Most of the side effects of creatine are related to the large osmotic load it supplies to the body. Dehydration is likely to occur as intravascular fluid volume is depleted. The movement of fluid into extravascular spaces can also lead to gastrointestinal complaints, muscle soreness, heat intolerance, electrolyte imbalances, and weight gain from fluid retention. Another potential problem is side effects related to contaminants that are present in some supplements (98). In the same study of Division I college athletes mentioned above, 38% of those using creatine reported significant side effects (93). Although there have been a few reports of renal impairment related to creatine (99, 100), creatine is unlikely to be particularly nephrotoxic (101). The fact remains that much about the long-term use of creatine supplementation is not known.

54. Bacon CG, Mittleman MA, Kawachi I, Giovannucci E, Glasser DB, Rimm EB. Sexual function in men older than 50 years of age: results from the Health Professionals Follow-up Study. Ann Intern Med. 2003;139:161–168.
55. Laumann EO, Paik A, Rosen RC. Sexual dysfunction in the United States: prevalence and predictors. JAMA. 1999; 281:537–544.
56. Spark RF. Overview of male sexual dysfunction. UpToDate. September 29, 2004. Available at *www.uptodate.com*. Accessed October 17, 2005.
57. Lue TF. Sexual Function and Dysfunction: Physiology of Penile Erection and Pathophysiology of Erectile Dysfunction and Priapism. In: Walsh PC, ed. Campbell's Urology. 8th ed. Philadelphia, PA: Saunders;2002:1589–1618.
58. Melman A, Christ GJ. The hemodynamics of erection and the pharmacotherapies of erectile dysfunction. Heart Disease. 2002;4:252–264.
59. Carson CC. Erectile dysfunction: evaluation and new treatment options. Psychosomatic Medicine. 2004;66:664–671.
60. Marwick C. Survey says patients expect little clinician help on sex. JAMA. 1999;281(23):2173–2174.
61. Davis-Joseph B, Tiefer L, Melman A. Accuracy of the initial history and physical examination to establish the etiology of erectile dysfunction. Urology. 1995;45(3):498–502.
62. Earle CM, Stuckey BGA. Biochemical screening in the assessment of erectile dysfunction: what tests decide future therapy? Urology. 2003;62:727–731.
63. Esposito K, Giugliano F, Di Palo C, et al. Effect of lifestyle changes on erectile dysfunction in obese men. JAMA. 2004; 291(24):2978–2984.
64. Goldstein I, Lue TF, Padma-Nathan H, Rosen RC, Steers WD, Wicker PA. Oral sildenafil in the treatment of erectile dysfunction. N Engl J Med. 1998;338(20):1397–1404.
65. Kloner RA. Cardiovascular effects of the 3 phosphodiesterase-5 inhibitors approved for the treatment of erectile dysfunction. Circulation. 2004;110:3149–3155.
66. Carson CC, Hatzichristou D, Carrier S, Lording D, Young J. Vardenafil as efficacious in men with erectile dysfunction unresponsive to prior sildenafil therapy: results of a Phase III clinical trial—patient response with vardenafil in sildenafil non responders. Int J Impot Res. 2003(Suppl 14):72.
67. Padma-Nathan H, Hellstrom WJ, Kaiser FE, et al. Treatment of men with erectile dysfunction with transurethral alprostadil. Medicated Urethral System for Erection (MUSE) Study Group. N Engl J Med. 1997;336(1):1–7.
68. Rajpurkar A, Dhabuwala CB. Comparison of satisfaction rates and erectile function in patients treated with sildenafil, intracavernous prostaglandin E1 and penile implant surgery for erectile dysfunction in urology practice. J Urol. 2003; 170(1):159–163.
69. Baniel J, Israilov S, Engelstein D, Shmueli J, Segenreich E, Livne PM. Three-year outcome of a progressive treatment program for erectile dysfunction with intracavernous injections of vasoactive drugs. Urology. 2000;56(4):647–652.
70. Brock G, Tu LM, Linet OI. Return of spontaneous erection during long-term intracavernosal alprostadil (Caverject) treatment. Urology. 2001;57(3):536–541.
71. Secil M, Arslan D, Goktay AY, Esen AA, Dicle O, Pirnar T. The prediction of papaverine induced priapism by color Doppler sonography. J Urol. 2001;165(2):416–418.
72. Linet OI, Ogrinc FG. Efficacy and safety of intracavernosal alprostadil in men with erectile dysfunction. The Alprostadil Study Group. N Engl J Med. 1996;334(14):873–877.
73. Dutta TC, Eid JF. Vacuum constriction devices for erectile dysfunction: a long-term, prospective study of patients with mild, moderate, and severe dysfunction. Urology. 1999;54(5): 891–893.
74. Lawrence ME, Kirby DF. Nutrition and sports supplements: fact or fiction. J Clin Gastroenterol. 2002;35(4): 299–306.
75. DuRant RH, Rickert VI, Ashworth CS, Newman C, Slavens G. Use of multiple drugs among adolescents who use anabolic steroids. N Engl J Med. 1993;328(13):922–926.
76. Gardiner P, Wornham W. Recent review of complementary and alternative medicine used by adolescents. Curr Opin Pediatr. 2000;12(4):298–302.
77. Rogol AD. Sex steroid and growth hormone supplementation to enhance performance in adolescent athletes. Curr Opin Pediatr. 2000;12(4):382–387.
78. Blue JG, Lombardo JA. Nutritional aspects of exercise: steroids and steroid-like compounds. Clin Sports Med. 1999; 18(3):667–689.
79. Musshoff F, Daldrup T, Ritsch M. Anabolic steroids on the German black market. Arch Kriminol. 1997;199(5–6): 152–158.
80. Yesalis CE, Barsukiewicz CK, Kopstein AN, Bahrke MS. Trends in anabolic-androgenic steroid use among adolescents. Arch Pediatr Adolesc Med. 1997;151(12):1197–1206.
81. Bhasin S, Storer TW, Berman N, et al. The effects of supraphysiologic doses of testosterone on muscle size and strength in normal men. N Engl J Med. 1996;335(1):1–7.
82. King DS, Sharp RL, Vukovich MD, et al. Effect of oral androstenedione on serum testosterone and adaptations to resistance training in young men: a randomized controlled trial. JAMA. 1999;281(21):2020–2028.
83. Brown GA, Vukovich MD, Martini ER, et al. Endocrine responses to chronic androstenedione intake in 30- to 56-year-old men. J Clin Endocrinol Metab. 2000;85(11): 4074–4080.
84. Leder BZ, Longcope C, Catlin DH, Ahrens B, Schoenfeld DA, Finkelstein JS. Oral androstenedione administration and serum testosterone concentrations in young men. JAMA. 2000;283(6):779–782.
85. Acacio BD, Stanczyk FZ, Mullin P, Saadat P, Jafarian N, Sokol RZ. Pharmacokinetics of dehydroepiandrosterone and its metabolites after long-term daily oral administration to healthy young men. Fertil Steril. 2004;81(3):595–604.
86. Tanner SM, Miller DW, Alongi C. Anabolic steroid use by adolescents: prevalence, motives, and knowledge of risks. Clin J Sport Med. 1995;5(2):108–115.
87. LaBotz M, Smith BW. Creatine supplement use in an NCAA Division I athletic program. Clin J Sport Med. 1999; 9(3):167–169.
88. McGuine TA, Sullivan JC, Bernhardt DT. Creatine supplementation in high school football players. Clin J Sport Med. 2001;11(4):247–253.
89. Hultman E, Soderlund K, Timmons JA, Cederblad G, Greenhaff PL. Muscle creatine loading in men. J Appl Physiol. 1996;81(1):232–237.
90. Febbraio MA, Flanagan TR, Snow RJ, Zhao S, Carey MF. Effect of creatine supplementation on intramuscular TCr, metabolism and performance during intermittent, supramaximal exercise in humans. Acta Physiol Scand. 1995; 155(4):387–395.
91. SB R. Creatine supplementation and athletic performance. J Ortho Sport Phys Ther. 2003;33(10):615–621.
92. Nemet D, Wolach B, Eliakim A. Proteins and amino acid supplementation in sports: are they truly necessary? Isr Med Assoc J. 2005;7(5):328–332.
93. Greenwood M, Farris J, Kreider R, Greenwood L, Byars A. Creatine supplementation patterns and perceived effects in select Division I collegiate athletes. Clin J Sport Med. 2000;10(3):191–194.
94. Earnest CP, Snell PG, Rodriguez R, Almada AL, Mitchell

TL. The effect of creatine monohydrate ingestion on anaerobic power indices, muscular strength and body composition. Acta Physiol Scand. 1995;153(2):207–209.

95. Dempsey RL, Mazzone MF, Meurer LN. Does oral creatine supplementation improve strength? A meta-analysis. J Fam Pract. 2002;51(11):945–951.

96. Volek JS, Kraemer WJ, Bush JA, et al. Creatine supplementation enhances muscular performance during high-intensity resistance exercise. J Am Diet Assoc. 1997;97(7):765–770.

97. Schwenk TL, Costley CD. When food becomes a drug: nonanabolic nutritional supplement use in athletes. Am J Sports Med. 2002;30(6):907–916.

98. Bizzarini E, De Angelis L. Is the use of oral creatine supplementation safe? J Sports Med Phys Fitness. 2004;44(4):411–416.

99. Bolotte CP. Creatine supplementation in athletes: benefits and potential risks. J La State Med Soc. 1998;150(7):325–327.

100. Pecci MA, Lombardo JA. Performance-enhancing supplements. Phys Med Rehabil Clin N Am. 2000;11(4):949–960.

101. Poortmans JR, Francaux M. Long-term oral creatine supplementation does not impair renal function in healthy athletes. Med Sci Sports Exerc. 1999;31(8):1108–1110.

102. Rubinstein ML, Federman DG. Sports supplements. Can dietary additives boost athletic performance and potential? Postgrad Med. 2000;108(4):103–106, 109–112.

103. Evans GW. The effect of chromium picolinate on insulin controlled parameters in humans. Int J Biosocial Med Res. 1989;11:163–180.

104. Hasten DL, Rome EP, Franks BD, Hegsted M. Effects of chromium picolinate on beginning weight training students. Int J Sport Nutr. 1992;2(4):343–350.

105. Lukaski HC, Bolonchuk WW, Siders WA, Milne DB. Chromium supplementation and resistance training: effects on body composition, strength, and trace element status of men. Am J Clin Nutr. 1996;63(6):954–965.

106. Trent LK, Theiding-Cancel D. Effects of chromium picolinate on body composition. J Sports Med Phys Fitness. 1995;35:273–280.

107. Cerulli J, Grabe DW, Gauthier I, Malone M, McGoldrick MD. Chromium picolinate toxicity. Ann Pharmacother. 1998;32(4):428–431.

108. Shimomura Y, Murakami T, Nakai N, Nagasaki M, Harris RA. Exercise promotes BCAA catabolism: effects of BCAA supplementation on skeletal muscle during exercise. J Nutr. 2004;134(Suppl 6):1583S–1587S.

109. Andraws R, Chawla P, Brown DL. Cardiovascular effects of ephedra alkaloids: a comprehensive review. Progress in Cardiovascular Diseases. 2005;47(4):217–225.

110. Haller CA, Jacob P, 3rd, Benowitz NL. Enhanced stimulant and metabolic effects of combined ephedrine and caffeine. Clin Pharmacol Ther. 2004;75(4):259–273.

CHAPTER 32

Relationship Issues

Sandra C. Clark and Timothy P. Daaleman

One of the joys of family medicine is the privilege of working with families. To follow a couple through pregnancy and delivery, and then to care for their growing family—helping them to manage acute and chronic illnesses, celebrating their successes, and guiding them through the various psychosocial stresses that inevitably arise during their individual and family life cycles—is satisfying and beneficial for both family and care provider. As a consequence of continuity of care through multiple life cycle episodes, the bonds of mutual trust and affection increase exponentially. Most experienced primary care providers will agree that the most comprehensive and effective way to treat illness and stress in an individual is to understand the dynamic it has created within the patient's family.

In the past, the term "family" was restricted to married couples and their children; now we apply the term to those individuals who serve as someone's primary interpersonal network. The American Academy of Family Physicians defines family as a group of individuals with a continuing legal, genetic, and/or emotional relationship. This definition recognizes the fact that families now come in all shapes and sizes. Using children as the reference point, census data find that only about two thirds of children live in what was considered a traditional family—a family with children and their married parents. This is not to say that both parents are the biologic parents. In 2000, 4.6% of children lived with a stepparent creating the "blended family"; almost a quarter of children live with a single unmarried parent, usually with a single mother; and approximately 6% lived in an unmarried partner household. Five percent of children lived with neither parent; the majority of these children are being raised by grandparents (1). Increasing trends towards domestic and international adoption, couples choosing not to have children, and homosexual couples who raise children also affect the composition of today's family. Additionally, according to the 2002 National Health Care Statistics, approximately 9% of women do not expect to have children (2). It is a necessary challenge for the primary care provider to keep up with the evolving family as it grows, branches, and divides. Devoting a section of the medical chart or the electronic medical record to a family description or genogram can be extremely helpful.

The intent of this chapter is to explore issues relevant to primary care providers as they follow families coming together, expanding, breaking apart, and regenerating. The number and variety of relationship issues that present in the family care provider's office is vast; thus, in this chapter we will discuss some of the more common problems; further information is available in the recommended readings.

SEXUALITY AND SEXUAL IDENTITY

CASE 1

J.L. is a 33-year-old Latino man who left Mexico 5 years ago to come to the United States to work in the computer industry. Freed from the influence of his very traditional family and a strong cultural bias against homosexuality in his country of origin, he began a relationship with another man a few years ago. He now presents to you because his partner has tested positive for HIV. He is understandably anxious. He states that he has not told his family back home that he is gay, and that he is not even sure that he is gay.

CLINICAL QUESTIONS

1. In addition to the medical work up, how should this patient be counseled?
2. Is it possible that he is not gay?
3. Should he tell his family?

Sexual exploration and the struggle for sexual identity are important steps towards establishing a stable relationship. In the 2002 National Survey of Family Growth, 12,571 men and women aged 15–44 years of age were surveyed using audio computer-assisted self-interviewing. Their findings provide normative data about sexual behavior:

- Multiple partners over the life span is common. Men aged 30–44 reported a median of 6–8 female sexual partners in their lifetimes; the median for women was about 4.
- Oral sex without vaginal intercourse is more common than previously thought in heterosexual teenagers (13% of young men and 11% of young women at ages 15–17).
- Same-sex activity is not uncommon. Six percent of men reported having had anal or oral sex with another man (2.9% in the preceding 12 months); for women, 11 percent reported having a sexual experience with another woman (4.4% in the preceding 12 months). The proportion who considers themselves homosexual and bisexual is lower than the proportions who report ever having same-sex experiences. Among adults aged 18–44, 2.3% of men consider themselves homosexual, and 1.8% bisexual; for women, the corresponding proportions are 1.3% and 2.8%, respectively (3).

These data reflect both a certain amount of confusion and openness to experimentation on the part of teens and young adults regarding sexuality. When a young adult presents to a primary care practice, sexuality needs to be explored in a sensitive, nonjudgmental manner, with an emphasis on confidentiality. Also keep in mind that many teens and young adults do not include touching and fellatio in the category of "sex." The primary care provider should be comfortable discussing the possibility of sexual experimentation and the risks that experimentation might carry in terms of sexually transmitted diseases and anxiety. Birth control and emergency contraception need to be a part of any discussion about sexuality. Patients may also need support and guidance if they plan to discuss their homosexuality or bisexuality with family and friends.

It is important to ask about a history of rape or childhood sexual abuse as part of a discussion on sexuality. A recent survey showed a prevalence rate of 13.5% for women and 2.5% for men for sexual abuse, either by rape or molestation. Rape and childhood sexual abuse are strong predictors of depression, anxiety, substance abuse and post-traumatic stress disorder (4). In addition, a history of rape or molestation, especially when penetration is involved, is a strong predictor of sexual dysfunction, including conditions such as anorgasmia, pelvic pain, or hypoactive sexual desire. These patients may benefit from psychotherapy (5).

For a homosexual teen or young adult, coming out to friends and family is probably one of the most stressful events of his or her life. Family reactions tend to vary widely, from acceptance to banishment from the family. Studies have shown that some parents go through a grief process when they discover that their child is homosexual, which parallels the grief process for death—shock, denial, sadness, anger, and eventual acceptance. Some parents will attempt to bargain with their child, withholding love or financial resources until he or she "changes back" to a heterosexual orientation.

Nevertheless, most experts agree that coming out is a way to maintain honesty and intimacy within a family, and that admitting to a homosexual orientation ultimately benefits both the homosexual's family and his or her future relationships. Patients who anticipate coming out to their family should be given anticipatory guidance. Primary care providers should caution patience and restraint in the face of their parents' initial reaction. For example, if a parent's initial response to his or her son's homosexuality is anger and rejection of his lifestyle, he should avoid responding with more anger. Calmly reaffirming his position, or giving his parents more time to reconsider their position, would be a far better response. In cases where parents react in an extreme manner, the provider should work to get the patient and his or her family into therapy (6).

DISCUSSION CASE 1

J.L. tests positive for HIV. He is devastated. He has been talking with his partner, with whom he has decided to stay, and they will both be managed at a private infectious disease clinic. He plans to return home over Christmas, but does not feel he is ready to discuss his homosexuality or his HIV status with his family.

Immigrant populations are a particularly vulnerable group of patients. As illustrated in the above case, single men and women coming to the United States are at high risk for sexual experimentation, sexually transmitted diseases, and unwanted pregnancy, especially if they come from a country where there is a strong cultural bias against homosexuality and having sex outside of marriage.

THE INFERTILE COUPLE

CASE 2

M.R. is a 28-year-old Caucasian woman who comes to your office with her partner requesting a physical exam. She has unsuccessfully been trying to conceive for the past 6 months. Her current partner has fathered a child with another woman. She has a long history of irregular menses that come every 3–6 months and are very heavy in quantity. Family history is unremarkable except for a maternal grandmother with diabetes. On exam she is noted to be overweight with a body mass index of 32, and has mild hirsuitism. The exam is otherwise unremarkable.

CLINICAL QUESTIONS

1. How would you manage this couple at the first office visit?
2. Which aspects of an infertility evaluation can be performed by the family care provider?
3. At what point is referral to a specialist warranted? And if so, what kind of specialist?

Humans are genetically and culturally programmed to form family units, to procreate, and to raise our young. Though some choose to not have children, most couples will attempt to conceive. For couples wanting children, infertility can be a devastating blow to their view of who they are and what they want to achieve in life. Studies show that infertile women are significantly more depressed than their fertile counterparts, with depression and anxiety levels equivalent to those of women with heart disease, cancer, or HIV-positive status. In one study, 11% of infertile women studied met the criteria for major depressive episode.

Infertility is defined as 12 months of appropriately timed intercourse that does not result in conception. Only 20% of couples actively trying to conceive will be successful in a given month, but 85% will become pregnant within a year. Thus, by definition, the infertility rate for couples is 15%. The likelihood of infertility increases the later a woman decides to try to get pregnant; by the time a woman is 35 years of age, the live birth rate is half that of the younger population (7).

The family care provider can play a very active role in the work-up of infertility, especially in the early stages. Some problems, such as metabolic syndrome, can be entirely managed by the primary care provider. For persistent fertility problems, however, the primary care provider and the patient need to negotiate the point at which specialty care is needed. At this point, the primary care provider can continue to offer psychosocial support to the family, and help them with decision making.

When one considers all of the factors that must be in place and working to achieve conception, it is a wonder that the infertility rate is so low. A male needs an adequate quantity of good-quality sperm, which demands a functioning pituitary-gonadal axis and normal male anatomy. A woman needs functioning ovaries, good-quality ova, patent fallopian tubes, a receptive uterus, and a functioning pituitary-gonadal axis. In up to 40% of infertile couples, the cause is found to be at least partly caused by a male factor. Female pelvic conditions (endometriosis, tubal disease, pelvic adhesions) account for 30%–40% of cases; ovulatory dysfunction and cervical factors each contribute another 10%–15%. Roughly 10% of infertility cases remain unexplained after a thorough work-up (7).

An infertility work-up initially consists of a careful history and examination of both partners. Table 32.1 provides an overview of infertility history (8). Although women frequently present to the office alone to discuss infertility, having both partners present will provide much more useful information for the provider, including direct observation of how the couple is interacting.

The physical examination of the man should include: estimate of the volume of the testes (should be greater than 10mL); an examination for varicoceles (best done with the patient standing and performing the valsalva maneuver); and, if appropriate, screening tests for sexually transmitted disease. The examination of the woman should include a full pelvic exam looking for anatomic abnormalities, evidence of infection, and adnexal tenderness that might indicate endometriosis or ovarian pathology. A screening endocrine examination should also be done, including the thyroid, breasts (looking for galactorrhea), and the skin and hair (looking for evidence of excess androgen) (9).

Initial laboratory evaluation of the man should include a semen analysis. No blood tests are mandatory; instead, they should be performed only if suggested by abnormalities on the history and physical exam. If genetic disorders are suspected, chromosomal testing should be done. Klinefelter syndrome is one such disorder; it is found in approximately one in 700–1,000 men, and arises from meiotic nondisjunction of the X chromosome creating an XXY karyotype. These patients usually have small, firm testes, low serum testosterone levels, and azoospermia (9).

A woman who has never had a menstrual cycle carries the diagnosis of primary amenorrhea, and should be referred to an endocrinologist or gynecologist. Women with secondary amenorrhea or irregular menses should have serum levels of thyroid stimulating hormone and prolactin tested. To assess for hypogonadism, a progestational challenge can be done with 10 mg of medroxyprogesterone acetate daily for 13 days. If there is menstrual bleeding at the end of the progesterone therapy, estrogen production is adequate. A negative result (i.e., no withdrawal bleeding) suggests premature ovarian failure; a follicle stimulating hormone and estrogen level would confirm this diagnosis. Women with clitoromegaly, hirsutism, and acne should be tested for congenital adrenal hyperplasia, with a dihydroepiandrosterone sulfate level (9).

A common cause of anovulation is polycystic ovary syndrome (PCOS), defined as the presence of oligo or anovulation in combination with hyperandrogenism. It has been estimated that 5%–7% of women of reproductive age suffer from this disease. The syndrome is suggested by findings of truncal obesity, hirsutism, male pattern baldness, or acanthosis nigrans. Laboratory findings suggestive of PCOS include elevations of testosterone, leuteinizing hormone, and the glucose:

TABLE 32.1   Highlights of History-Taking for an Infertile Couple

Family History	Is there a family history of genetic disorders?
	Is there a family history of diabetes?
Sexual History	What is the timing of intercourse with the fertility period?
	Does the patient know when her fertility period is?
	Is there a history of erectile dysfunction or ejaculatory dysfunction?
	Is intercourse painful?
	Is there a history of sexually transmitted diseases?
Menstrual History	Are the patient's menstrual periods regular?
	Are her menses heavy or painful?
Toxin Exposure	Has the patient been exposed to radiation?
	Does the patient use marijuana or alcohol? How much?
	Does the patient smoke?
Social History	How important is conception to both partners?
	How strong is the relationship at this point?
	How has the inability to conceive so far affected your relationship?
	What diagnostic testing or assisted reproductive technologies would you be willing to try?

Source: Trantham P. The infertile couple. Am Fam Physician. 1996;54(3):1001–1010.

insulin ratio. The diagnosis is made based on the history and physical, when other diseases have been ruled out. Endovaginal ultrasound can be helpful, especially if the patient has pelvic pain or a palpable ovary on exam, but it is not necessary to make the diagnosis of PCOS. Ultrasound will typically show ovaries with multiple small cysts.

Clomiphene and metformin are the most common treatments used by family care providers to treat ovulatory dysfunction. They can be used alone or in combination. Clomiphene is usually started at 50 mg per day for five days on days 3–7 of the menstrual cycle; the cycle either coming on its own, or induced using a progesterone withdrawal as described above. Clomiphene induces ovulation in 8%–30% of cases. A home ovulation kit can help guide the timing of intercourse. Metformin at doses as high as 2,000 mg per day is another option, especially when PCOS is suspected. Recent studies have shown that a combination of clomiphene and metformin increases ovulation rates to 75%–90% (10).

Women with a history of normal menses can be assumed to ovulate. Their workup should be directed toward anatomic problems, such as tubal patency, endometrial receptivity, the presence of scar tissue or endometriosis involving the pelvic organs, or inhospitable cervical mucus. This work-up is usually done by a gynecologist. Performing a hysterosalpingogram (HSG) involves injecting dye through the cervix and into the endometrial cavity; from which it passes into the fallopian tubes. The HSG gives useful information regarding the shape and lining of the uterus, and the patency of the fallopian tubes. Hysteroscopy is used to directly view the endometrial lining to look for irregularities, such as scar tissue or polyps. Laparoscopy is used to visualize the pelvic organs. For most young couples with normal histories and exams, it is reasonable to get a semen analysis, document ovulation with a home kit, and wait up to 2 years before beginning more extensive testing. Couples with unexplained infertility have a pregnancy rate of 60%–70% within 3 years. Because of their declining fertility rate, women who present at age 35 for infertility require immediate evaluation and management. Couples that are taking clomiphene, metformin, or both should be given a 3- to 6-month trial before referral to an infertility specialist for more aggressive therapies. Intrauterine insemination generally has a success rate of 17% per cycle, and *in vitro* insemination has a success rate of 44% per cycle (11).

Throughout the infertility work-up the primary care provider needs to follow the mental health of the couple. How are they managing as a couple and individually? Is there a perception of blame by one partner towards the other? How is their sex life? Are they both in agreement with the work-up, and the increasingly expensive options for conception? Would they consider adoption, and at what point? There are no easy answers for these questions, but the primary care provider can serve as an important facilitator for these discussions. The presence of marital stress and depression needs to be assessed and managed in the office, or by referral to a mental health specialist.

DISCUSSION CASE 2

M.R. had a normal laboratory workup, with the exception of a high low-density lipoprotein of 160 and a low high-density lipoprotein of 20 on her lipid profile. She was given the presumptive diagnosis of metabolic syndrome and placed on high-dose metformin therapy. Within 2 months of starting the medicine, her menses became regular, and within 3 months she successfully conceived.

This case describes an effective, inexpensive intervention in a couple with infertility. In the presence of typical physical examination findings and suggestive labs, a working diagnosis was made. Medical therapy was initiated and resulted in a successful conception.

THE CHILD WITH SPECIAL CARE NEEDS

CASE 3

C.R. is the 6 lb, 5 oz male product of a term delivery to a 38-year-old with three healthy children. His exam is significant for folded ears, epicanthal folds, and transverse palmar creases. His heart exam is normal, and he is taking formula well. You order an echocardiogram and request a genetics consultation. You inform the parents that you suspect that their child has Down's syndrome.

The parents are upset and angry. They point out that the mother had a reassuring level 2 ultrasound and normal alpha fetal protein. How could this have happened to their child? You answer their questions as best you can, tell them about the studies you have ordered, and make plans to visit with them again in the hospital the following day.

CLINICAL QUESTION

1. Beyond listening and expressing empathy, what can you do to help these parents?

American parents tend to have high expectations of their children. More than many other cultures, American parents sacrifice, plan, and obsess about their children's futures. We clog their schedules with school, sports, and lessons, with the goal of creating children who will develop into successful and self sufficient adults. So how do family care providers deal with the families of children with special needs, the "imperfect" children?

Children with special health care needs (CSHCN) are defined as having medical, behavioral, or other health care needs for more than 1 year. According to the 2002 National Survey of CSHCN, almost 13% of US children meet this definition, including 4% who have chronic emotional, behavioral, or developmental problems (12).

In dealing with CSHCN, the concept of the "medical home" is critical. A medical home is an office or clinic where a patient can receive routine sick and well care, can identify a personal doctor or nurse as his or her own, has no difficulty in obtaining needed medical referrals, can get needed care coordination, and can have family-centered care. According to the National Survey, only half of CSHCN receive care that meets all five of the components established for medical home, and access to a medical home is significantly affected by race and ethnicity, and poverty (13). The family care provider is ideally suited to provide the medical home for CSHCN. Because family care providers and their office staff can provide ongoing relationships with an entire family, the family practice office is in an excellent position to help parents adjust to the grief and the altered circumstances that having a CSHCN can bring, and to make medical care a supportive part of their parenting of the child. Family-oriented health care providers can help coordinate and explain the results of the specialty care that is necessary. This is particularly true of families with cultural and language barriers.

Caring for CSHCN requires that the primary care provider be well trained in detecting developmental and emotional problems at an early stage. Age appropriate pediatric exam sheets or templates, which list developmental milestones for particular ages, should be available at the time of exam. Also, the primary care provider should be knowledgeable about the resources available in his or her area, and how to access these resources. Practices that deal with a large number of children may want to consider on-site psychological services or having a social worker on-call to assist them with coordinating the care for CSHCN.

DISCUSSION CASE 3

The following day you see the parents of C.R. in the hospital. The mother is still tearful but much more engaged in the care of their child. They have spoken with the genetics team, and a karyotype is pending. The echocardiogram was normal. The mother states that her biggest fear for her child is that he will suffer. You empathize with her fear and begin to discuss local resources that are available to the family and child. The patient is scheduled to see you in your office in 2 days. Follow-up is also scheduled at a specialty pediatric clinic at the hospital for children with Down's syndrome.

INTIMATE PARTNER VIOLENCE

CASE 4

Y.W. is a 32-year-old female who appears in your office for the first time because of a recent fall. The patient states she tripped down some stairs and hurt her shoulder. Her affect is flat, and she has alcohol on her breath. On exam she has an obvious deformity over her distal left clavicle and several bruises of varying ages. You tell her that her injury and exam are suspicious for domestic violence. She denies that she has been hit or raped by her partner. You put her in a sling and send her for an x-ray, which confirms a distal clavicle fracture. Over the next two visits Y.W. continues to deny domestic violence but allows you to discuss safety in the home. Six months later she calls you to say that her husband has beaten her up, and she wants to be seen.

CLINICAL QUESTION

1. What should you include in your evaluation?

Intimate partner violence (IPV) is defined as actual or threatened physical or sexual violence or emotional or psychological abuse by a current or former spouse or dating partner (14). It is the most extreme manifestation of relationship dysfunction, and is one of the more frustrating problems facing the primary care provider. Screening for and managing IPV is time consuming, requires frequent follow up, and often has an unsatisfactory outcome. But one has only to get past the front page headlines of the local newspaper to see the consequences of IPV. Each year it is estimated that 1,200 women die as a consequence of IPV (15). This figure does not include the far greater number of victims who live in constant fear.

The victims of IPV are overwhelmingly female, women being abused 4.3 more often than men (14, 16). One in four women in the United States has reported being physically and/or sexually abused by a current or former partner, and 1.5% report being abused within the last year (17). A recent study of four community-based primary care internal medicine clinics confirms these figures, and stresses the need for screening. In that study, 21.4% of women who completed the self administered survey in the clinic reported having experienced domestic violence sometime in their adult lives, and 5.5% had experienced domestic violence in the year before presentation (18). The study administered several psychological tests to women who had recently been abused, and to women who had not been abused. In comparison with women not recently abused, currently abused women were more likely to be younger than 35; single or separated; had more physical symptoms (e.g., headache, back pain); had higher scores on measures of depression, anxiety, and somatization; were more likely to be abusing drugs and alcohol; and were more likely to have attempted suicide (18). Pregnancy is a particularly susceptible time for women to be abused, with estimates as high as 17% of women being physically or sexually abused at this time (19).

Clinicians must be familiar with the typical cycle of abuse. The cycle begins with a gradual increase in tension between the victim and the abuser. This can take the form of name calling, increasing jealousy, suspicion of infidelity, and/or controlling behavior. The tension mounts until the victim is physically or sexually assaulted. A period of remorse on the part of the abuser then follows during which time he/she will ask forgiveness and promise change; the victim will frequently forgive and take back the abuser. A variable period of relative stability will ensue, followed by increasing tension as before. Not all IPV follows this cycle, however, as some abuse will end after the first cycle; for others the violence is either unpredictable or not mitigated by periods of tranquility.

All women should be screened for IPV. It is reasonable to screen during annual exams and during urgent visits that involve injuries consistent with IPV, multiple somatic complaints, or depression. However, it is dangerous for a victim of IPV to be asked about domestic violence when the abusing partner (or someone who might report to the abusing partner) is present. Therefore, all screenings, whether written or oral, must be done with only the patient present. Getting the patient alone should, however, be approached with caution, creativity, and diplomacy, as a controlling partner will often not let the patient out of sight in a clinic, for fear that they will admit to abuse.

There are several screening tools available to detect IPV in a primary care setting:

- The Conflict Tactics Scale (CTS) and the Index of Spouse Abuse (ISA) are the gold standards of detection, but are time consuming and impractical in an office setting; the ISA consisting of 30 items on a scale of 1 to 5, and the CTS consisting of 19 items on a 7-point ordinal.
- The Partner Violence Screen (PVS) consists of the following four questions: 1) Have you been hit, kicked, punched, or otherwise hurt by someone within the past year?; 2) If so, by whom?; 3) Do you feel safe in your current relationship?; and 4) Is there a partner from a previous relationship who is making you feel unsafe now? The PVS shows sensitivity of 71.4% and specificity of 84.4 (20).
- A second screen, Abuse Assessment Screen, is designed to assess IPV in pregnancy and consists of the following three questions: 1) Within the last year have you been hit, slapped, kicked, or otherwise physically hurt by someone?; 2) Since you've been pregnant have you been hit, slapped, kicked, or otherwise physically hurt by someone?; and 3) Within the past year, has anyone forced you to have sexual activities? This questionnaire also has a body map for marking injuries (19).
- The Hurt, Insulted, Threatened, and Screamed (HITS) scale is a paper and pencil instrument that comprising the following four items that are scored on a 5-point scale: How often does your partner physically **H**urt you, **I**nsult you or talk down to you, **T**hreaten you with harm, and **S**cream and curse at you? One study has shown a sensitivity of 96% and a specificity of 91%, using a cut-off of greater than 10.5 as indicative of abuse (21).

Once the primary care provider determines that a patient is the victim of IPV, the next step is to assess the acuity of the situation. Is it safe for the patient to go home? Should the police be called? Currently, six states require reporting domestic violence: Kentucky, California, Colorado, New Hampshire, Rhode Island, and New Mexico; however, reporting is controversial. Some opponents state that it discourages some women from seeking treatment for IPV, and that it increases the risk of retribution by the abusing partner. Proponents feel that it takes the burden of the decision from an often conflicted victim, and that it leads to more arrests and treatment of abusing partners (22).

If a patient is thought to be in imminent danger of further abuse, whether or not the police are involved, the provider and patient should negotiate a safety plan by placing her in a shelter for battered women, a hotel, or with a trusted relative or friend. If the patient decides to return home, prompt follow up by office visit or phone call should be completed.

Once the acuity of the situation is resolved, the provider needs to perform a thorough history, and a focused exam. The history should include:

- **Time frame:** When did the abuse start?
- **Manner:** How is the partner being abused?
- **Frequency:** How often is the patient being abused?
- **Past Plan:** What are the actions and resources that the victim has used in the past to **deal** with the abuse?
- **Future Plan:** Does the patient have a **plan** for dealing with future abuse?
- **Safety:** Are there others in the home, particularly children, who are at risk for abuse?

If the patient presents with physical evidence of abuse, the mechanism of injury must be fully detailed. A body map or photograph demonstrating the location and severity of the injuries is a very useful supplement to written notes.

One of the most important roles that a primary care provider can play when dealing with a victim of IPV is to listen. Admitting to abuse is often painful and embarrassing. Many victims blame themselves for the abuse. It is important to dispel this myth. Simply stating "nobody ever deserves to be abused by their partner" can be very powerful and affirming for the patient. The primary care provider needs to have a good understanding of community resources to discuss options, such as alternative living situations or local shelters. Handouts with important numbers, including crisis hotlines, legal resources, and emergency shelters, should be given. Close follow-up is important.

In addition to dealing with IPA issues, comorbidities should be addressed. Alcohol, drug addiction, and depression are frequently present in abused women. Both conditions impair the victim's ability to make decisions and plan for the future, and treatment can make a tremendous difference in their ability to cope (18).

Finally, primary care providers need to consider the management of IPV as an ongoing process. Many women will repeatedly return to an abusive situation, often for years, before leaving their partners; some women never leave; and sometimes the abuse stops with or without intervention. The provider needs to constantly reassess the situation and guide the patient towards a safe and positive outcome. It is also critical to realize that women are particularly susceptible to abuse when they leave a relationship. In fact, many women will refuse to leave an abusive partner for fear of retaliation. In a 2003 study of women who survived a homicide attempt by an intimate partner, two-thirds of the attempts happened around the time of a relationship change, and half of the women did not realize that their lives were in danger. Thus primary care providers need to make sure patients have a safety plan when they intend to leave their abusive partner (23).

DISCUSSION CASE 4

You work Y.W. into your schedule that day. She admits to a long history of physical and sexual abuse by her present partner. On exam she is covered with bruises to her face, arms, and abdomen. She allows you to photograph her bruises. She is screened for depression but decides against medicine. You give her written resources, including emergency numbers, domestic violence counseling programs, and information on obtaining a restraining order. The next time you see her in clinic she has left her partner and has started to work on her substance abuse problem.

The case above illustrates the need for patience in dealing with IPV. It took time for Y.W. to trust her primary care provider, and even longer for her to leave her abusive partner. What helped the process along was offering help and resources despite the fact that she was denying abuse. Y.W. ultimately responded to this concern by admitting to IPV and dealing with her abusive relationship as well as her alcoholism.

INFIDELITY

CASE 5

B.B. is a 50-year-old church organist and music director who presents with an irritating vaginal discharge for the past several weeks. She has been married for 20 years to the same man. She denies infidelity but admits that her husband drinks too much and has appeared aloof recently. Her pelvic exam reveals a greenish/yellow discharge and a mild cervicitis. You take cultures and confirm her contact information. Two days later her culture comes back positive for chlamydia.

CLINICAL QUESTIONS

1. How will you discuss the results of B.B.'s testing with her?
2. How will you counsel her?

Infidelity is a common challenge faced by couples, which has lasting effects on a relationship because once discovered, it causes mistrust and a reevaluation of the core values shared by the couple. It is estimated that between 20%–25% of Americans will have sex with someone other than their spouse while they are married. In the past, the male partner was more likely to engage in extramarital sex (EMS), but as women have entered the workforce the difference between the sexes has narrowed. Studies have shown that, compared to faithful partners, perpetrators of EMS are less satisfied with their marriage, have a higher level of education and socioeconomic status, and were married at a younger age. Infidelity occurs most often when one partner works, and the other is unemployed (24).

EMS most often presents in primary care in the context of a sexually transmitted disease (STD). Whether or not the infection is suspected, discussing the implications of an STD is akin to walking through a mine field—one never knows when or if an explosion will occur. Therefore, first and foremost, do not discuss the implications of an STD with a patient until you have the results in hand. Many relationships have been ruined based on the suspicion of an STD, which later turned out to be a nonsexually transmitted infection. Discussing a positive test for an STD should preferably be done face-to-face with the infected patient—alone. The implication of infidelity should be frankly but tactfully discussed. If the patient is the perpetrator, discussions need to center around informing all partners involved, so that they will also seek treatment. If the patient is the "victim" of EMS, guiding the patient through the basics of how to confront his or her partner can be very helpful. The safety of both the accusing party and the accused needs to be assessed.

Primary care providers should routinely ask about infidelity during physical exams. "How strong is your relationship with your current partner?" will occasionally elicit a discussion on actual or suspected EMS. A more telling question is "Would you like to be tested for sexually transmitted diseases as part of the exam?" A positive answer should be followed up and discussed.

Not surprisingly, infidelity frequently leads to long-term problems within a relationship. In one sampling of psychotherapists, 34% of couples seeking treatment where EMS was involved ended up divorcing, and only about 15% of relationships remained intact and were characterized by improvement and growth (25). Couples therapy or individual therapy should be encouraged to guide patients through decisions about recommitting to versus ending their relationship.

DISCUSSION CASE 5

B.B. was asked by the office nurse to come in for a visit to "explain her results." The patient was then informed of the positive result of her chlamydia testing. The patient was surprised but did not appear overly upset. Prescriptions were written for both her and her husband. She stated she felt safe in her home and did not anticipate any problems when she informed her husband of his need for treatment. She did not return to the clinic for several months. When she did finally come in for treatment of a cold, she stated that she was still married but was emotionally separated from her husband.

MARITAL SEPARATION AND DIVORCE

CASE 6

M.A. is a 25-year-old who comes alone to discuss her marriage. She has two young daughters. Last summer her husband temporarily moved the family across the country to take a 3-month job. To save money, they moved in with his parents, who lived near the temporary job.

Separated from the support system she had come to know and rely on, M.A. was overwhelmed with caring for their two children, the cramped living quarters, and a less than ideal relationship with her husband's family. She decided to come back home early, find a job, and be close to her side of the family. Her husband was unhappy with the decision, but M.A. expected that they would work out their differences when he returned home. He ended up staying at the job longer than expected and when he came for a visit, stated that he was no longer in love with her, and that her decision to leave early was the end of their marriage. M.A. is a devout Catholic and wants to stay married.

CLINICAL QUESTIONS

1. How would you counsel M.A.?
2. How can the primary care provider anticipate and guide young couples early in a relationship?
3. How does divorce impact families?

Throughout the family cycle, the primary care provider needs to be aware of the usual stresses that marriages go through, and provide anticipatory guidance. For example, the years after the first child is born tend to be looked back on as some of the best years of a couple's life, but they are also stressful for the parents, and place a strain on the marriage. A newborn brings many sleepless nights, adjustments of work schedules and careers, constant negotiation and relegation of parental duties, and less intimacy. Mothers and fathers who decide to quit their jobs to stay at home with the baby may feel underappreciated and socially isolated. During this critical time, the provider might initiate a conversation by asking how the couple is dealing with the demands of having a baby, and then, depending on the response, the provider could discuss proper communication techniques, the need for a part-time baby sitter on a regular basis, or local resources for stay-at-home parents. Other examples of stresses that may occur within a family include job changes, illness, or financial issues. Table 32.2 provides a number of communication tips that can be provided as part of a well adult visit or a premarital exam, or in counseling couples who are having difficulty (26). Table 32.3 lists tips for physicians working with couples.

The scope of divorce in the United States is far-reaching. Consider these statistics from the 2001 article by Charles Bryner, "Children of Divorce":

- Approximately 45% of marriages end in divorce.
- Only 50% of single parent households headed by the mother have child support agreements from the father, and of those, only 50% receive the full amounts due.
- An employed mother in a two-parent home is in contact with the children 25 hours a week. After the divorce, this number decreases to 5.5 hours a week. A housewife spends 45 hours a week with her children; after divorce she spends 11 hours a week with them.
- The employed father predivorce spends an average of 20 hours a week with his children, but only 2 hours a week after the divorce.

TABLE 32.2 Tips on Effective Communication for Couples

- Schedule or choose a time to talk when there will be little distraction.
- Keep your discussions private; avoid having them in front of family or friends.
- Start with a positive statement. For example: "I love you and I see that you have been working very hard to help me, but I am feeling . . . "
- Use "I" statements instead of "YOU" statements. For example: "I" get upset when I'm not consulted on how we should handle our finances" instead of "You never include me in big financial decisions."
- Do not walk out in the middle of a conversation, unless you feel that you are on the verge of doing or saying something you will regret. If you do leave a discussion, try to continue it as soon as possible.
- It is okay to initiate a difficult or complicated conversation with a letter, but the letter must be followed with face-to-face conversation.
- Discussions are not "won" or "lost." Both parties should feel they have gained something.

Source: Starling BP, Martin A. Improving marital relationships: strategies for the family physician. J Am Board Fam Pract. 1992;5(5):511–516.

TABLE 32.3 Tips for Primary Care Providers on Working with Couples

- Try to understand and accept their belief system and values; don't impose yours on them. Many couples and families may function quite harmoniously with a very different concept from yours of how a family should work. Focus on the problem that they specifically bring to you.
- Do not take sides.
- Try to give patients an easy, concrete task to complete before the next visit. For example, if the couple was arguing about how to divide up child care responsibilities, for the next visit have them separately draw up a list of things they would be willing to do.

- Five years after a divorce, one of three children found themselves still embroiled in the ongoing bitterness of their two battling parents. At 10 years, half of the women and a third of the men studied were still intensely angry at their former spouses (27).

These are grim statistics, and they take a toll on both the parents and the children. Divorce usually involves the betrayal of an ideal for marriage followed by a breakdown in effective communication. What once was a relationship built on trust and shared goals becomes a dysfunctional and angry set of individuals (28).

Children also suffer before, during, and after divorce. Parents in a high conflict relationship often have no emotions or time left over for their children, and they frequently project their anger and frustration towards their partner onto their children. Children are often witnesses to verbal and at times physical abuse. They will often be drawn into alliances with one parent against the other and begin distancing themselves from one parent. As a result studies have shown that children of divorce have more behavioral, academic, and conduct problems than children with intact families. In fact, approximately half of these problems are detectable as early as 4 years before parents actually separate. The conflict in the home, therefore, rather than the actual separation and divorce, is often the cause of many of the problems that children have. In these families, divorce might actually be better for the children, rather than staying in a high conflict situation (29).

Several recent studies have been done that support the trend towards joint custody. Children spend more time with both parents in this situation. When both parents continue in the parenting role—helping with homework and setting limits for example, instead of using their time for special trips and entertainment—children appear to adjust better. Children whose parents decide on mediation instead of a prolonged and occasionally ugly legal battle tend to do better as well.

Half of divorced persons remarry within 5 years (27). If one or both of the parents bring children into the new relationship, a "blended" family begins. Living in a blended family requires flexibility and many adjustments by everyone in the family. Depending on custody arrangements, children may or may not be in the home at any given time. New alliances have to be established, and the prickly issues of respect and authority have to be negotiated.

Primary care providers are ideally positioned to help a struggling family. As discussed earlier, interventions early in the conflict, done in the office or by a family therapist, should be aimed at reestablishing effective communication. The "Ten Commandments of Divorce" (Table 32.4) is a helpful tool that can be provided as part of primary care-based counseling (27).

Throughout a separation or divorce, comorbidities such as depression and insomnia need to be addressed, and the family, separately or together, should be followed closely for problems related to the conflict. It is crucial for the family care provider to recognize that the parents' psychological health and the strength of the parent-child bond are important factors for a family in this transition.

DISCUSSION CASE 6

M.A. asked her husband to join her in marital therapy. He refused. She then wrote her husband a letter reasserting her commitment to the marriage. At this point she was treated for depression because she began losing patience with her children and felt like she was crying all the time. When her husband returned he admitted that he had begun seeing another woman, again stating that M.A. was to blame for the end of their relationship. At this point M.A. decided to take her children and move in with her relatives. The couple is now pursuing a divorce.

This case illustrates that often the primary care provider will see only half of a conflicted couple, making effective interventions difficult. If only one of the partners has been treated, the other partner may feel at a disadvantage coming in for treatment or therapy. In this case a family therapist might be a better option, if the couple will agree to it. If either partner refuses to engage in meaningful communication, the marriage has little chance at success.

THE IMPACT OF DISABLING CHRONIC ILLNESS ON FAMILY RELATIONSHIPS

CASE 7

D.B. and his wife J.B. have been patients of yours for several years. D.B. is a 75-year-old man with a history of diabetes, hypertension, and renal insufficiency. Two years ago he suffered an embolic stroke. Though he recovered physically from the stroke, he has become increasingly confused and distant since that time. His behavior has also been somewhat disinhibited. His most recent Mini-Mental State Examination yielded a score of 16, consistent with dementia. In an office visit for her chronic neck pain, his wife J.B. breaks down in tears, saying that she is overwhelmed with looking after her husband in the home, and that she has lost her best friend of 40 years, and is mourning the loss. Her weight has dropped 15 pounds over 6 months, and she is unable to sleep.

CLINICAL QUESTIONS

1. What are your clinical roles and responsibilities to both J.B. and D.B.?
2. How should you screen for family stress or any emotional fallout in D.B. or other family caregivers, as chronic illnesses progress?
3. What clinical interventions and approaches to caring for D.B.'s illness are inclusive of family caregivers?

TABLE 32.4 The Ten Commandments for Divorcing Parents

1. Inform the children of the divorce, and explain the reason for the divorce in terms that are appropriate for the ages of the children, and are neutral. Both parents should be present, and all children should be told at the same time, unless it is impossible.
2. Reassure the children (especially the younger children) that the divorce is not their fault. Repeat this explanation over and over and over.
3. Except for cases of abusive relationships or concerns of immediate safety, inform the children well in advance of anyone moving out of the house.
4. Clearly inform the children of the expected family structure after the divorce, and who will live where. Discuss visitation clearly.
5. Do not make children be adults.
6. Do not discuss money. Children do not comprehend money or the true costs of maintaining a household. If they ask, do not lie, but be aware that $200 seems like a small fortune to a school-aged child.
7. Children need rules. Be consistent in this area, even if it is the only area in your entire life that is consistent.
8. Children must never be forced into taking sides. Both parents love them, and they can love both parents.
9. Belittling your ex-spouse should be avoided within earshot of the children. They believe everything you say, even when it is out of anger or frustration. But do not lie to cover up irresponsible behavior by the other parent. Children will see through it quickly, and your credibility will suffer in other areas.
10. Never, ever put your children in the middle between you and your spouse. They are not buffers or pawns or messengers or prizes to divide like property. They are your children. They are the most precious things in the world to any parent. They are the one best thing that came out of the marriage.

Source: Bryner CL. Children of divorce. J Am Board Fam Pract. 2001;14:201–210.

Epidemiology

Chronic diseases, such as heart disease, stroke, cancer, and dementia are among the most prevalent and serious health conditions today, accounting for 70% of all deaths in the United States (30, 31). These diseases disproportionately affect older adults; approximately 80% of elders have at least one chronic condition resulting in pain, loss of function, or limited activity (32). The scope of care delivered to these patients by family members is staggering: an estimated 27.6 million family caregivers provide care to patients, and the economic value of their care is estimated to be $196 billion (33). There is wide variation in the amount of care needed depending on the disease. For example, annual care costs for patients with Alzheimer's disease are estimated at $65 billion; for depression, however, these costs total only $9 billion (34, 35). Patients with Alzheimer's disease are dependent on caregivers for long periods of time, greatly impacting family caregivers' time and taxing their financial resources (36, 37).

Caregiving generally connotes informal and unpaid care, which is usually provided by family members, and goes beyond the support provided in social relationships (38). The primary family caregiver is most often the spouse (70%), followed by an adult child (20%), and friends or distant relatives (10%); 70% of caregivers are women (39, 40).

Evaluation

Caregiving exerts a substantial strain, so primary care providers should be attentive to stressors that impact the emotional and physical health of family caregivers. The patient-provider continuity in a long-standing provider-family relationship offers the provider familiarity with the patient's social and cultural context, which impacts the illness trajectory (41). With this understanding as a foundation, clinicians can gauge the impact of illness on family caregiving by monitoring stressors and resources (33). Stressors include caregiving tasks and conflicts (e.g., family conflict, employment strains, financial burdens) that occur as a result of caregiving (36). Providers should be attentive to physical complaints that may indicate caregiver burden or burnout. Poor sleep, increased irritability, and depressed mood or affect can be indicators of worsening emotional strain (36). Community-based resources, such as area agencies on aging and faith communities, can provide respite and other supportive services to help reduce the physical and emotional burden of caregiving.

Management of Family Relationships in the Context of Chronic Illness

A family-focused approach to chronic illness emphasizes several areas: 1) defining and assessing the relational context in which care takes place; 2) including the caregiver, other family members, and friends as potential targets for interventions; 3) addressing the relational, personal, and educational needs of the patient and family members; 4) viewing disease as an ongoing process that requires continuity of care between the health care team and the family; and 5) including the patient, caregiver, and other family members in outcomes assessment (41). Interventions to help manage family relationships and reduce potential negative outcomes for the family system include support groups, addressing family relationships, and psychotherapy (41). Support groups target coping, decision making, and problem solving among family members. Family relationship interventions use a variety of behavioral and educational techniques to foster emotional expression and collaboration among family members. Psychotherapy is usually reserved for families with severe dysfunctional relationships caused by the disease burden or preexisting family dynamics (41).

It is inevitable that as caregiver patients get sicker, primary care providers will increase their interaction with caregivers. Providers can help caregivers:

- Obtain health care power of attorney. This is especially important if the caregiver is not the patient's spouse. When many decisions need to be made quickly, a family needs one voice, and legally that voice is the person with the health care power of attorney.
- Know the patient's end-of-life wishes and help caregivers feel comfortable carrying out those wishes.
- Know about existing community resources to help care for the patient at home.
- Consider in advance, at what point, if any, the caregiver would wish to have the patient placed in an alternative living situation.
- Determine how the caregiver is faring with the stress.

Another tool the primary care provider can use to help a family understand and better care for an ill family member is the family meeting. When done properly, the family meeting serves to update the family on the patient's condition, discuss the course of the patient's disease, and answer questions about past and future testing and therapies. It is also a great opportunity to observe how the family interacts, to mediate differences in opinion, and to negotiate a path that hopefully is agreeable to all. Ultimately, the family meeting is most helpful to the primary caregiver who will feel more supported and less overwhelmed with the patient's ongoing care. The primary care provider can encourage this process by asking each family member or friend how they can help the caregiver and patient.

Death, Dying, and Bereavement

Chronic illness often leads to a transition from active care to palliative care. Primary care providers need to keep in mind four major areas in providing palliative care: effective communication and establishment of care goals; coordination of care; pain and symptom care; and social, spiritual, and bereavement support (42).

Providers should initiate and seek to maintain an open-ended and ongoing discussion about the type of care that patients and family members wish to receive, and their overall goals of care. Advance care planning builds on these open-ended discussions. When discussing advance care planning, providers should outline the patient's preferences in the event of several potential clinical scenarios (e.g., hospitalization, home care) regarding disease progression. Once a care plan has been established, several copies of the advance directive should be made for the medical record; family members and the provider's pager number and direct phone line to the clinic should be given.

A primary goal in palliative care is the relief of symptoms that contribute to suffering, such as pain, nausea, and dyspnea (43). Regular, standardized assessment is the foundation for effective treatment. Professional and family caregivers should direct their routine assessments toward specific symptoms (e.g., dyspnea, constipation) and away from medical parameters such as vital signs for patients who have elected palliative care (44).

Patients approaching death and their family members have needs that cut across psychological, social, and spiritual domains. Dying is a time of tremendous stress but also offers important opportunities for growth, intimacy, reconciliation, and closure within relationships. Family care providers who care for these patients should be attentive for various cues that indicate depression, familial conflict, or spiritual distress, and consider resources, such as hospice and palliative care services, that can provide care and support in these areas (43).

DISCUSSION CASE 7

A family meeting is called to discuss the long-term care of D.B. The meeting consists of D.B., his wife, and two of their three children. His wife is adamant that she wants to keep him in their home as long as possible. Their daughter agrees to watch D.B. at least once a week so that her mother can have time to shop or be with friends. D.B's son is angry and thinks that more testing needs to be done to be sure of the diagnosis. He thinks that his father is overmedicated, and it is causing his confusion. You address his concerns by acknowledging his frustration, and then you review all of the medicines that D.B. takes for his hypertension and diabetes, and discuss the reasons he takes them, and the consequences of stopping them. You offer them the phone number of a home

health agency that might have nursing aids available to help in the home.

On a separate visit with D.B.'s wife, you screen for depression and give her the titles of several books that deal with relatives with dementia.

CONCLUSION: PRACTICING EFFECTIVE BEHAVIORAL MEDICINE IN PRIMARY CARE

Keeping up with the latest developments in primary care is an ongoing challenge. In reviewing the literature, it is clear that acute and chronic diseases receive far more attention than do problems of human relationships. Thus, studies of the care and prevention of chronic diseases, such as diabetes and congestive heart failure, are abundant, usually with large scale, prospective, randomized trials to back the recommendations. In contrast, there are far fewer trials of the common behavioral interventions discussed in this chapter, such as screening and counseling for domestic violence, or of primary care provider counseling for marital dysfunction. Table 32.5 summarizes some of the best evidence, and as the reader can see, it is rather modest.

Behavioral research is harder to conduct than randomized trials of a new drug. Results tend to rely on intangibles, such as the level of trust between provider and patient, and the skill of the provider in conveying information in a manner that is acceptable and easily understood. Studies tend to be small in scale as well. Furthermore, there is no analog to the

TABLE 32.5 Summary of Key Evidence-Based Recommendations Regarding Management of Relationship Issues

Recommendation	Strength of Recommendation*
Sexuality	
Screening annually for chlamydia in adolescents	A
Screening for HIV, **RPR, GC** annually in adolescents	B
Counseling adolescents on birth control	C
Counseling homosexuals on coming out	C
Infertility	
Metformin for the use of polycystic ovary disease	B
Clomiphene for the use of ovulatory dysfunction	B
Assisted technologies for couples with infertility	C
Intimate Partner Violence	
Screening women for domestic violence	C
Divorce	
Counseling on effective communication between couples	C
Self-Management of Chronic Illness	
Effectiveness of using self-management in chronic illness	B

*A = consistent, good-quality patient-oriented evidence; B = inconsistent or limited-quality patient-oriented evidence; C = consensus, disease-oriented evidence, usual practice, expert opinion, or case series. For information about the SORT evidence rating system, see *http://www.aafp.org/afpsort.xml*.

pharmaceutical industry pumping funding into research on interventions related to relationship issues. Thus, the strength of the recommendations for these topics tends to be less than that for chronic diseases. Nevertheless, the data and recommendations presented in Table 32.5 are based on good-quality studies, and represent areas of consensus within the behavioral medicine field.

Yet the modest attention to behavioral issues in the primary care literature is misleading, for relationships and their problems are everywhere in medicine. Furthermore, it is in the area of relationships that primary care providers can often be the most effective: by knowing the patient, the family, and the human life cycle; by being able to read subtle signs in a patient's body language, vocal intonation, or symptoms; by recognizing when it's important to take an extra few minutes to allow a patient's story to unfold; and by knowing how to effectively respond when a behavioral problem presents itself. The rewards of such effort are immense. Providers who are comfortable exploring and assisting in relationship issues find that, through their patients, the workday reveals with increasing depth the richness and variety of human experience.

REFERENCES

1. Lugaila T, Overturf J. Children and the households they live in: 2000. Washington, DC: US Census Bureau, 2004.
2. Centers for Disease Control and Prevention. Fertility, family planning, and reproductive health of US Women: Data from the 2002 National Survey of Family Growth. National Center for Health Statistics. Series 23, Number 25. Hyattsville, MD: US Department of Health and Human Services; 2005
3. Mosher W, Chandra A, Jones J. Sexual behavior and selected health measures: men and women 15–44 years of age, United States, 2002. Adv Data. 2005;362:1–55.
4. Monlar BE, Buka S, Kessler R. Child sexual abuse and subsequent psychopathology: results from the National Comorbidity Survey. Am J Public Health. 2001;91(5):753–760.
5. Sarwar D, Durlak J. Childhood sexual abuse as a predictor of adult female sexual dysfunction: a study of couples seeking sex therapy. Child Abuse Negl. 1996;20(10):963–972.
6. LaSala M. Lesbians, Gay men, and their parents: family therapy for the coming-out crisis. Fam Process. 2000;39(1):67–79.
7. Whitman-Elia G, Baxley E. A primary care approach to the infertile couple. J Am Board Fam Pract. 2001;14(1):33–45.
8. Trantham P. The infertile couple. Am Fam Physician. 1996;54(3):1001–1010.
9. Frey K, Patel K. The evaluation and management of infertility by the primary care physician. Mayo Clin Proc. 2004;79(11):1439–1443.
10. Barbieri R. Metformin for the treatment of polycystic ovary syndrome. Obstet Gynecol. 2003;101(4):785–793.
11. Andrews M, Gibbons W, Oehninger S, et al. Optimizing use of assisted reproduction. Am J Obstet Gynecol. 2003;189(2):327–332.
12. Centers for Disease Control and Prevention. Mental health in the US: health care well being of children with chronic emotional, behavioral, or developmental problems—United States, 2001. MMRW Morb Mortal Wkly Rep. 2005;54(39):985–989.
13. Strickland B, McPherson M, Weissman G, Van Dyck P, Huang ZH, Newacheck P. Access to the medical home: results of the National Survey of Children with Special Health Care Needs. Pediatrics. 2004;113(5):1485–1492.
14. Craft C (ed). National Center for Injury Prevention and Control Injury Fact Book 2001–2002. Atlanta, GA: Centers for Disease Control and Prevention; 2004.
15. US Bureau of Justice Statistics. Bureau of Justice Statistics Crime Data Brief. Intimate partner violence, 1993–2001. Washington, DC: US Department of Justice.; 2003. US Department of Justice Publication No.19838.
16. Krug EG, Dahlberg LL, Mercy JA. World report on violence and health. Biomedica. 2002;2:327–336.
17. Tjaden P, Thoennes N. Full report of the prevalence, incidence, and consequences of violence against women. Washington, DC: National Institute of Justice, 2000.
18. McCauley J, Kern D, Kolodner K, et al. The "Battering Syndrome": prevalence and clinical characteristics of domestic violence in primary care internal medicine practices. Ann Inter Med. 1995;123(10):737–746.
19. McFarlane J, Parker B, Soeken K, Bullock L. Assessing for abuse during pregnancy. JAMA. 1992;267(23):3176–3178.
20. Feldhaus K, Koziol-McLain J, Amsbury H, Norton L, Lowenstein S, Abbott J. Accuracy of 3 brief screening questions for detecting partner violence in the emergency department. JAMA. 1997;277(17):1357–1361.
21. Sherin KM, Sinacore JM, Li XQ, Zitter RE, Shakil A. HITS: a short domestic violence screening tool for use in a family practice setting. Fam Med. 1998;30(7):508–512.
22. Iavicoli L. Mandatory reporting of domestic violence: the law, friend or foe? Mt Sinai J Med. 2005;72(4):228–231.
23. Nicolaidis C, Curry MA, Ulrich Y, et al. Could we have known? A qualitative analysis of data from women who survived an attempted homicide by an intimate partner. J Gen Intern Med. 2003;18(10):788–794.
24. Atkins DC, Jacobson NS, Baucom DH. Understanding infidelity: correlates in a national random sample. J Fam Psychol. 2001;15(4):735–749.
25. Charny IW, Parnass S. The impact of extramarital relationships on the continuation of marriages. J Sex Marital Ther. 1995;21(2):100–115.
26. Starling BP, Martin A. Improving marital relationships: strategies for the family physician. J Am Board Fam Pract. 1992;5(5):511–516.
27. Bryner CL. Children of divorce. J Am Board Fam Pract. 2001;14(3):201–210.
28. Weiss RS. Coping with loss: separation and other problems that threaten relationships. Br Med J. 1998;316(7136):1011–1013.
29. Kelly JB. Children's adjustment in conflicted marriage and divorce: a decade review of research. J Am Acad Child Adolesc Psychiatry. 2000;39(8):963–973.
30. Bauserman R. Child adjustment in joint-custody versus sole-custody arrangements: a meta-analytic review. J Fam Psychol. 2002;16(1):91–102.
31. Bodenheimer T, Wagner EH, Grumbach K. Improving primary care for patients with chronic illness. JAMA. 2002;288(14):1775–1779.
32. Coleman MT, Newton KS. Supporting self-management in patients with chronic illness. Am Fam Physician. 2005;72(8):1503–1510.
33. Bodenheimer T, Lorig K, Homan H, Grumbach K. Patient self-management of chronic disease in primary care. JAMA. 2002;288(19):2469–2475.
34. Fisher L, Weihs KL. Can addressing family relationships improve outcomes in chronic disease? Report of the National Working Group on Family-Based Interventions in Chronic Disease. J Fam Pract. 2000;49(6):561–566.
35. Schulz R, Beach SR, Lind B, et al. Involvement in caregiving and adjustment to death of a spouse: findings from the caregiver health effects study. JAMA. 2001;285(24):3123–3129.
36. Teno JM, Clarridge BR, Casey V, et al. Family perspectives

on end-of-life care at the last place of care. JAMA. 2004; 291(1):88–93.

37. Scholte op Reimer WJ, de Haan RJ, Rijnders PT, Limburg M, van den Bos GA. The burden of caregiving in partners of long-term stroke survivors. Stroke. 1998;29(8):1605–1611.

38. Lee S, Colditz GA, Berkman LF, Kawachi I. Caregiving and risk of coronary heart disease in US women: a prospective study. Am J Prev Med. 2003;24(2):113–119.

39. Van den Heuvel ET, de Witte LP, Schure LM, Sanderman R, Meyboom-de Jong B. Risk factors for burn-out in caregivers of stroke patients, and possibilities for intervention. Clin Rehabil. 2001;15(6):669–77.

40. Grant I, Adler KA, Patterson TL, Dimsdale JE, Ziegler MG, Irwin MR. Health consequences of Alzheimer's caregiving transitions: effects of placement and bereavement. Psychosom Med. 2002;64(3):477–486.

41. Dracup K, Evangelista LS, Doering L, Tullman D, Moser DK, Hamilton M. Emotional well-being in spouses of patients with advanced heart failure. Heart Lung. 2004;33(6): 354–361.

42. Fisher L, Lieberman MA. Alzheimer's disease: the impact of the family on spouses, offspring, and inlaws. Fam Process. 1994;33(3):305–325.

43. Garrand L, Dew MA, Eazor LR, DeKosky ST, Reynolds CF. Caregiving burden and psychiatric morbidity in spouses of persons with mild cognitive impairment. Int J Geriatr Psychiatry. 2005;20(6):512–522.

44. Haley WE, LaMonde LA, Han B, Narramore S, Schonwetter, R. Family caregiving in hospice: effects on psychological and health functioning among caregivers of hospice patients with lung cancer or dementia. Hospice J. 2001;15(4):1–18.

CHAPTER 33

Sexually Transmitted Infections

Karl E. Miller

CASE

A 23-year-old woman comes to the office complaining of a discharge from the vagina. The patient had been in a monogamous relationship until recently and admits to having three different sexual partners within the last few weeks. Her main concern is that she may have a sexually transmitted infection. On physical examination you note that she has a purulent discharge from the cervix and the remainder of the pelvic examination is normal. You perform a test on the cervical discharge for *Chlamydia* and gonorrhea and sample the discharge to perform a microscopic examination. Because your suspicion for a sexually transmitted infection (STI) is high, you initiate antibiotic therapy and schedule the patient for a follow-up visit.

CLINICAL QUESTIONS

1. What symptoms are present in women who may have pelvic inflammatory disease (PID)?
2. What are the best tests to diagnose *Chlamydia* and gonorrhea?
3. What strategies have been shown to improve prevention of STIs?

STIs can cause a broad range of symptoms, from no or few symptoms to those that can be life-threatening. To reduce the morbidity and mortality related to STIs, the Centers for Disease Control and Prevention (CDC) and other organizations have established guidelines for the diagnosis and management of these infections. This chapter addresses the most common and important STIs, including *Chlamydia*, gonorrhea, HIV, human papillomavirus (HPV), and herpes simplex. Other infections can be transmitted sexually including hepatitis (see Chapter 23, Chronic Liver Disease) and trichomonasis (see Chapter 34, Vaginitis).

INITIAL EVALUATION

The general approach to a patient with an STI begins by obtaining detailed information about his or her presenting complaint. In women this should include information about any vaginal discharge, the character of that discharge and any odor, vaginal bleeding particularly after intercourse, pelvic or abdominal pain, information concerning their menstrual cycles, any possibility she may be pregnant, and the presence of any painful or painless genital lesions or ulcers. In men the history should include the following: presence and character of any penile discharge, dysuria, pain in the scrotum or testicles, and the presence of any painful or painless genital lesions or ulcers. For both men and women, information about generalized symptoms such as fevers, chills, sweats, myalgias, fatigue, and rash can provide insight into the severity of the STI.

Specific information about the sexual history and potential contact information should be addressed. This needs to be performed in a straight-forward nonjudgmental manner and should include information concerning recent or remote sexual contacts. It also should include a risk assessment for STIs. This includes asking about multiple sexual partners, recent change in partners, patient's assessment of their partner's sexual habits, history of any STI, and patient's and partner's substance abuse history, particularly intravenous drugs. To be nonjudgmental, questions should be simple and, when possible, answered with one or two words. The following are some examples: Are you currently sexually active? (You may have to define what this means to some patients.) If you are, is it with men, women, or both?

The physical examination of the genital region in men and women needs to be approached with care. Chaperones should be present when you are performing this examination. The patient should be informed when you are going to perform certain aspects of the exam such as: "You will feel me touch you here."

Women who may have an STI should have a pelvic examination. This includes observing the external genitalia, peri-rectal area, inner aspects of thighs and suprapubic areas for any lesions or ulcers and any visible discharge. The speculum examination should include observing the appearance of the cervix and any discharge from the cervix itself and the presence of any vaginal discharge or lesions. A swab in the cervix is used to obtain the specimen for *Chlamydia* and gonorrhea screening. The bimanual examination should include an assessment of tenderness with cervical motion, tenderness over the uterus or ovaries, and enlargement or mass in the adnexal area.

The genital examination in men includes observation of the penis, scrotum, peri-rectal, inner thigh, and suprapubic areas to assess for any lesions or ulcers or penile discharge. It is important in men who are not circumcised or those with some foreskin present to retract the foreskin and observe the area around the glans of the penis. Palpation of the penis and scrotum for any tenderness or mass is performed next. In addition, the inguinal canal should be palpated for any lymphadenopathy. If there is a penile discharge present or the patient has had a recent STI exposure, a screen for *Chlamydia* and gonorrhea should be performed. This is best done if the penis is milked starting at the base of the penis before the sample is obtained.

Different states have different requirements for which STIs are reportable to the health department. Even though most laboratories report positive tests for STIs it is still the responsibility of physicians to report these infections. When dealing with patients and STIs it is important to have a follow-up visit during which the results of the test can be discussed with the patient. Providing this information over the phone or via the mail should be avoided when possible. Most states have specific rules for testing and reporting HIV-positive tests that may differ from other STIs. Patients who have been tested for HIV should be seen in person and results discussed. In patients who are negative this should include information for reducing their risk for contracting HIV. Most of the time no information about STIs can be legally shared with partners or other individuals unless the patient specifically gives you permission (preferably in writing). An exception is cases where the health department is following up on potential exposures or there is an issue concerning occupational exposure.

DIAGNOSIS AND TREATMENT OF COMMON INFECTIONS

Chlamydia

Chlamydia trachomatis causes a significant number of sexually transmitted infections (STIs). This organism is an obligatory intracellular bacteria that predominately infects the columnar cells of the genital tract. The incubation period ranges from 1 week to 1 month. In 2004 there were more than 900,000 new cases of *C. trachomatis* reported to the CDC (1). This is a rate of 319.6 cases per 100,000 and is an increase in the rate of 5.9% compared to 2003 (1). The majority of this increase was believed to be secondary to better screening in certain populations and the use of more sensitive *Chlamydia* tests.

CLINICAL EVALUATION

Presenting symptoms vary depending on gender, age and site of infection. Lower genital tract infections in women caused by *C. trachomatis* occur in the endocervix and usually cause a mucoid vaginal discharge with no odor or external pruritus. In fact, a significant number of women with *Chlamydia* infections of the lower genital tract will have no or minimal symptoms (2). Physical findings include cervicitis (an inflammation of the cervix) with a yellow or cloudy mucoid discharge from the os. The cervix is friable; that is, it tends to bleed easily when rubbed with a swab or scraped with a spatula. Symptoms alone cannot be used to predict if women do or do not have a *Chlamydia* infection so clinical microscopy and the amine test (significant odor release with addition of potassium hydroxide to vaginal secretions) can be used to help differentiate *Chlamydia* infection from other infections such as urinary tract infection (see Chapter 28, Dysuria), bacterial vaginosis, and trichomoniasis (3). An important aspect of *Chlamydia* infections in the lower genital tract is that they do not cause vaginitis. If vaginal discharge is present without a discharge

from the cervix, this usually indicates a different diagnosis or co-infection.

Women can also develop urethritis because of *C. trachomatis* infections. Symptoms may consist of dysuria without frequency or urgency. A urethral discharge can be elicited by compressing the urethra during the pelvic examination. Urinalysis will typically show more than 5 white blood cells per high-power field (WBCs/HPF) but urine cultures will not grow any organisms.

Urethritis and occasionally epididymitis occur in men with infections secondary to *C. trachomatis*. In fact, approximately 30%–40% of urethritis in males is secondary to *C. trachomatis* and the prevalence decreases as men age (2). Symptoms can be absent or may include a mild to moderate, clear to white urethral discharge. The discharge is best observed in the morning before the patient voids. In order to observe the discharge the penis may need to be milked by applying pressure from the base of the penis to the glans.

The diagnosis of nongonococcal urethritis can be confirmed by the presence of a mucopurulent discharge from the penis, a Gram stain of the discharge with more than 5 WBCs/HPF (oil immersion), and no intracellular Gram-negative diplococci (3). Another test that can be used to confirm the diagnosis of urethritis is a positive leukocyte esterase test on first-void urine or microscopic examination of first-void urine that has 10 or more WBCs/HPF (3).

Untreated *Chlamydia* infections can occasionally spread to the epididymis in men. This infection causes unilateral testicular pain with scrotal erythema tenderness, or swelling over the epididymis. Males age 35 and younger who have epididymitis are more likely to have *C. trachomatis* as etiologic agent than those older than age 35.

DIAGNOSTIC TESTING

C. trachomatis infections can be detected using culture and nonculture techniques. Culture techniques are considered the gold standard but according to the CDC nonculture techniques can replace cultures in some instances. The newest nonculture technique is nucleic acid amplification tests (NAAT). These tests have good sensitivity (85%) and specificity (94–99.5%) for endocervical and urethral samples when compared to cultures (4). The NAAT techniques can be used to diagnose *Chlamydia* in women with urogenital disease by either an endocervical sample or a urine specimen. The urine sample technique has been shown to be effective and may eliminate the need for a pelvic examination (5).

Diagnosis of *C. trachomatis* in males with suspected urethritis is best done by using NAAT technique (4). The test should be performed to detect both *Chlamydia* and gonococcal infections.

Because of the significant number of co-infections any patient receiving testing for *Chlamydia* infection should also receive a test for gonorrhea (2). This recommendation was supported by a recent study that found 20% of men and 42% of women had infections with both *Chlamydia* and gonorrhea (6).

Testing for *Chlamydia* infection in neonates who develop ophthalmia neonatorum can be done by either culture or nonculture techniques (2). When collecting a specimen the eyelid needs to be everted and the sample obtained from the inner aspect of the eyelid. Sampling the exudates decreases the likelihood of obtaining an adequate sample and increases the risk for a false-negative test (2).

Infants suspected of having pneumonia caused by *Chlamydia* can be tested by obtaining a sample from the nasopharynx. Nonculture techniques can be used in these cases but they are less sensitive and specific for nasopharyngeal specimens than for ocular specimens (2). If tracheal aspirates or lung biopsies are being collected for pneumonia in this age group the samples should be tested for *C. trachomatis* (2). Findings on chest radiographs include hyperinflation and bilateral diffuse infiltrates. Peripheral eosinophilia can sometimes be present in infants with *Chlamydia* pneumonia.

TREATMENT OF *CHLAMYDIA*

The treatment for *C. trachomatis* infections depends on several factors. These include the site of the infection, the age of the patient, and whether the infection is complicated or uncomplicated. Treatment in women who are pregnant is discussed later.

Evidence-based guidelines from the CDC for the treatment of uncomplicated genital *Chlamydia* infections are shown in Table 33.1 (2). Recommended treatment regimen for uncomplicated genital *Chlamydia* infections include azithromycin 1 g orally in a single dose or doxycycline 100 mg orally twice per day for 7 days (2). Either regimen is acceptable since they have the same cure rates and adverse effects (7). Azithromycin provides the benefit of being able to provide the patient with the one-time dose, which can be witnessed while they are still in the office. If patients vomit the azithromycin within 1 to 2 hours after taking the medication, an

alternative treatment should be considered. Recommended and alternative regimens are shown in Table 33.1 for patients who are unable to tolerate azithromycin or doxycycline (2).

Follow-up of patients with urethritis is only necessary if symptoms persist or recur after completion of the antibiotic course. If symptoms are present that suggests recurrent or persistent urethritis, the CDC recommend treating this with metronidazole 2 g orally in a single dose, plus erythromycin base 500 mg twice per day for 7 days or erythromycin ethylsuccinate 800 mg orally 4 times per day for 7 days (2). This recommendation is to provide treatment for other bacterial causes. Patients receiving treatment should be advised to abstain from sexual intercourse until 7 days after treatment was started. In addition, exposure information for the last 60 days should be obtained and screening for other STIs such as HIV testing should be discussed (2).

The CDC currently does not recommend reculturing or repeating the nonculture test for *Chlamydia* after completion of the antibiotic course unless the patient has persistent symptoms or is pregnant (2). Because re-infection is a common problem, the CDC recommends that women with *Chlamydia* infections should be rescreened 3 to 4 months after antibiotic completion. Women who present within 12 months after their initial infection who have not been screened should be reassessed for infection regardless of whether the patient believes their sex partner was treated or not (2).

CHLAMYDIA INFECTIONS IN CHILDREN

Neonates who develop conjunctivits (ophthalmia neonatorum) from *C. trachomatis* exposure during the delivery have

TABLE 33.1 Treatment Regimens for Uncomplicated Urogenital *Chlamydia* Infections in Men and Women

Medication	Dosage	Frequency and Duration	Cost
Recommended regimens			
Azithromycin	1 g	A single dose	$$
Doxycycline	100 mg	2 times/d for 7 days	$
Alternative regimens			
Erythromycin base	500 mg	4 times/d for 7 days	$
Erythromycin ethylsuccinate	800 mg	4 times/d for 7 days	$
Ofloxacin	300 mg	2 times/d for 7 days	$$$
Levofloxacin	500 mg	Once per day for 7 days	$$$
Recommended regimens–pregnant Patient			
Erythromycin base	500 mg	4 times/d for 7 days	$
Amoxicillin	500 mg	3 times/d for 7 days	$
Alternative regimens– pregnant patients			
Erythromycin base	250 mg	4 times/d for 14 days	$
Erythromycin ethylsuccinate	800mg	4 times/d for 7days	$
Erythromycin ethylsuccinate	400 mg	4 times/d for 14 days	$
Azithromycin	1 gm	A single dose	$$

Adapted from: Workowski KA, Levine WC. Sexually transmitted diseases treatment guidelines 2002. Centers for Disease Control and Prevention. MMWR. 2002;51(RR-6):1–80.

swelling in one or both eyes with mucopurulent drainage. The infection usually occurs within 5–12 days of birth but may develop up to 1 month of age (2). The prophylaxis with silver nitrate or antimicrobial ointment used to reduce the risk of eye infections in neonates does not reduce their risk of *Chlamydia* infections of the conjunctiva.

Chlamydia pneumonia can develop in infants age 1–3 months that are exposed to *C. trachomatis* during delivery. The characteristics of *Chlamydia* pneumonia in this age group include a protracted onset of symptoms, a staccato cough usually with no wheezing and no temperature elevation (2).

Ophthalmia neonatorum is treated with erythromycin base or ethylsuccinate 50 mg/kg/day orally divided in 4 doses per day for 14 days total (2). The cure rate for both is only 80% so a second course of therapy may be necessary (2). *O. neonatorum* does not respond to topical treatment, so its use is inadequate and should not be used in conjunction with systemic treatment.

Pneumonia in children secondary to *C. trachomatis* is also treated with erythromycin base or ethylsuccinate 50 mg/kg/day orally divided into 4 doses per day for 14 days (2). As with ophthalmic infection, a second course of therapy may be necessary.

CHLAMYDIA INFECTION IN PREGNANCY

Pregnant women with *C. trachomatis* infection cannot be treated with doxycycline, ofloxacin or levofloxacin because these are contraindicated during pregnancy. Recommended regimens include erythromycin base or amoxicillin (1) (see Table 33.1). Amoxicillin is more effective and tends to have fewer side effects than erythromycin when treating antenatal *Chlamydia* infection (7, 8). In addition, because amoxicillin is better tolerated than erythromycin, compliance should be better (7). Preliminary data suggest that azithromycin is an effective and safe alternative (2).

Testing for cure in pregnant patients with *C. trachomatis* infection should be performed 3 weeks after completion of treatment and the preferred testing method is by culture technique (2). If risk for re-exposure is high during the pregnancy, repeat screening may be indicated throughout the pregnancy.

REITER'S SYNDROME

Individuals with *Chlamydia* infections can develop a reactive arthritis. This occurs in approximately 1% of men with *Chlamydia* infection and is even less common in women, with a male to female ratio of 5:1 (2). The onset of the arthritis is 1–3 weeks after the beginning of a *Chlamydia* infection. The joints involvement is asymmetrical with multiple joints affected but the arthritis has predilection for the lower extremities. In addition to the joint involvement, individuals with this disease will have urethritis in men and women or cervicitis in women, conjunctivitis, and painless mucocutaneous lesions. The mucocutaneous lesions are papulosquamous eruptions that tend to occur on the palms of the hands and the soles of the feet. The initial episode usually lasts for 3 to 4 months but in rare cases the synovitis may last for one year. This combination of disease processes is more commonly known as Reiter's syndrome.

Gonorrhea

Neisseria gonorrhoeae is one of the more common sexually transmitted diseases in the United States with approximately 800,000 new cases reported annually (9, 10). These infections can cause a broad range of symptoms from their total absence to those that are potentially life-threatening. The urogenital tract is the most common site for *N. gonorrhoeae* infections but it can also infect the anorectal area, pharynx and conjunctiva. Severe cases of this infection can lead to disseminated gonococcal infections, endocarditis, and meningitis, and in women, pelvic inflammatory disease (PID).

CLINICAL EVALUATION

Gonorrhea infections in the lower genital tract in women occur in the endocervix. Common symptoms include an odorless vaginal discharge, vaginal bleeding (particularly after intercourse), and dyspareunia. The presence or absence of symptoms cannot be used to predict the presence of *N. gonorrhoeae* (2). Physical findings include cervicitis with a mucopurulent drainage from the os. The cervix is friable and tends to bleed easily when rubbed with a swab. Gonorrhea infections do not cause vaginitis but vaginal findings may be caused by other co-infections.

A potential complication of gonorrhea infections in females is an ascending infection that causes acute salpingitis with or without endometritis, also known as pelvic inflammatory disease (PID). This occurs in 10%–20% of women who have endocervical gonorrhea (9).

Unlike women with urogenital gonorrhea, men tend to be symptomatic. The normal incubation period after exposure is 2–6 days at which time men develop a purulent discharge from the penis and dysuria. On physical examination, the penis may have a yellowish, purulent discharge present at the meatus and the meatus may be erythematous. If there is no discharge noted, it may be expressed by milking the penis.

Although usually caused by other bacteria, epididymitis in men may also be caused by *N. gonorrhoea, particularly in younger men*. Symptoms include unilateral testicular pain without the discharge or dysuria. The patient may or may not have a fever. On examination the epididymis is swollen and tender to palpation.

Gonorrhea infections can be present in the rectal area in men and women. In women it can occur because of perianal contamination from a cervical infection or a direct infection from anal intercourse. In men this infection occurs because of direct exposure through anal intercourse. Most individuals with rectal gonococcal infections have few if any symptoms. If symptoms are present, they consist of anal pruritus and a mucopurulent anal discharge that is usually seen with a bowel movement and on the stool. Rectal pain, tenesmus, and bleeding may be present in some cases with this occurring more commonly in men who have sex with men. In severe cases of gonococcal rectal infection, it is sometimes difficult to differentiate this infection from inflammatory bowel disease such as ulcerative colitis.

Pharyngeal infections caused by *N. gonorrhoeae* usually occur after orogenital exposure to another individual with this infection. Symptoms tend to be mild or may be absent. The pharynx may be erythematous or may have some exudates present. Anterior cervical lymphadenopathy may also be present. Most cases will spontaneously resolve with no treatment and do not usually result in any adverse sequelae but treatment should be initiated to reduce the transmission risk (2).

Gonorrhea in Children

Gonococcal infections occur in children and are categorized by the age of children at the onset of the infection. During the neonatal period and the first year gonorrhea infections can cause conjunctivitis (ophthalmia neonatorum), pharyngitis, and rectal infections and in rare cases pneumonia. These infections usually develop within 2–5 days after birth because of the neonate's exposure to infected cervical exudates. After age 1, almost all gonococcal infections are due to child abuse.

Other causes of *ophthalmia neonatorum* are more common than *N. gonorrhoeae* but identifying and treating gonorrhea is important because left untreated it can cause perforation of the globe of the eye and blindness. Those infants at risk for developing gonococcal conjunctivitis include those neonates who do not receive ophthalmic prophylaxis, whose mother has had no prenatal care, or whose mother has a history of STIs or substance abuse. Common findings in the neonate include inflammation of the conjunctiva and mucopurulent discharge from the eye.

The most common cause of gonococcal infections in preadolescent children is from sexual abuse (2). The usual presentation is a child with symptoms of vaginal discharge. Pharyngeal and rectal infections may also be present and usually do not cause symptoms.

Disseminated Gonococcal Infection

Disseminated gonococcal infection is a rare complication of *N. gonorrhoeae* infections that occurs in 1%–3% of adults who do not receive treatment for gonorrhea. In this infection the organism is disseminated to other areas in the body by septic emboli. The septic emboli cause polyarticular tenosynovitis and dermatitis (2). Symptoms may be mild with slight joint pain, few skin lesions, and no fever to severe with overt polyarthritis and high fever. Patients with disseminated gonorrhea tend to have no symptoms of urogenital infection.

The skin lesions are usually few in number and are limited to the extremities. They start as papules and progress to pustules with a hemorrhagic component. Bullae, petechiae or necrotic lesions may also be present. Once the infection evolves into the septic arthritis phase of the infection the skin lesions are usually resolved. Cultures from the skin lesion and blood are usually negative for *N. gonorrhoeae*.

The wrist, ankles, hands, and feet are most common joints involved with disseminated gonorrhea. The axial skeleton is rarely involved in this infection. Initial aspiration of the joint may be negative for any infection. Left untreated the joint involvement will develop into a septic arthritis which is most likely to involve the elbow, wrist, knee, or ankle. Once the joints become septic they are swollen, red, and warm to touch.

The severe adverse effects of disseminated gonorrhea have declined substantially over the last few years with the advent of antibiotic therapy. These include bacterial endocarditis, meningitis, and myocarditis. Gonococcal endocarditis usually affects the aortic valve which it tends to destroy it rapidly. This destruction leads to an abrupt onset of congestive heart failure.

DIAGNOSTIC TESTING

Both culture and nonculture methods for detecting *N. gonorrhoeae* are available. Although the culture techniques are considered the gold standard, they have been replaced in some instances by the nonculture techniques, in particular the nucleic acid amplification tests (NAAT). These tests have good sensitivity (92%–96%) and specificity (94%–99%) when compared with cultures (4). In women with urogenital disease the NAAT techniques can be used to diagnose gonorrhea by either an endocervical sample or urine specimens. Urine samples have a lower sensitivity and therefore a higher false negative rate than endocervical samples (4). The testing for men with suspected urogenital gonorrhea infection can be performed by either culture or nonculture techniques such as NAAT (4). If the sample is obtained by using a urethral swab, the sample is best obtained by milking the penis first. NAATs can be used on urine samples in men to detect urogenital gonorrhea.

Preliminary data suggest that NAATs can be used to detect rectal gonorrhea infections (4). However, the CDC still recommends that culture should be used to establish the diagnosis in any person suspected of having rectal gonorrhea (2). Similarly, the current CDC recommendations for testing patients with suspected pharyngeal gonorrhea is cultures with appropriate transport media (2).

Gonorrhea in Children

Testing for *N. gonorrhoeae* in children should be performed using a culture method (2). Nonculture techniques should not be used alone because they are not approved by the FDA for use in children. This could result in a positive test being discounted if child abuse is suspected. Specimen samples from the vagina, pharynx, urethra, or rectum should be plated on selective media for isolating *N. gonorrhoeae*.

Testing for *N. gonorrhoeae* in neonates who have ophthalmia neonatorum include an initial Gram stain of the conjunctival exudates (2). If intracellular Gram-negative diplococci are identified, the presumptive diagnosis on *N. gonorrhoeae* is made and treatment initiated. Gonococcal cultures are performed at the same time to make the definitive diagnosis (2).

Disseminated Gonococcal Infection

Patients with suspected disseminated gonococcal infection should be assessed by aspirating fluid from a joint. The joint fluid will usually have more than 40,000 leukocytes/mm^3 and a Gram stain will show Gram-negative intracellular diplococci. The joint fluid should also be cultured for *N. gonorroeae* but in most cases the cultures will be negative (2).

TREATMENT

Despite the fact the CDC has published guidelines in the diagnosis, treatment and prevention of sexually transmitted diseases, compliance with these guidelines is low. In one recent study of an emergency department, compliance with these guidelines ranged from 14% to 79% with respect to history taking, physical examination, diagnostic testing, treatment, and counseling about safe sex (12). Less than one-third of the cases in this study received the CDC recommended antibiotics. In order to reduce the incidence of this infection and its long-term consequences, physicians should have ready access to CDC guidelines (available online at *www.cdc.gov/mmwr/preview/mmwrhtml/rr5106a1.htm*) and utilize these guidelines in their practices (2). When treating patients with gonococcal

TABLE 33.2 Treatment Guidelines for Uncomplicated Gonococcal Infections of the Cervix, Urethra, and Rectum in Men and Women

Medication	Dose and Route	Cost
Cefixime*	400 mg orally in a single dose	$
Ceftriaxone	125 mg intramuscularly in a single dose	$$$
Ciprofloxacin	500 mg orally in a single dose	$
Levofloxacin	250 mg orally in a single dose	$
Ofloxacin	400 mg orally in a single dose	$

* This medication has not been available at times.
Note: certain areas of the country have fluoroquinolone-resistant organisms so this class should not be used in those areas or in patients who may have contracted gonorrhea from that are.
Adapted from: Workowski KA, Levine WC. Sexually transmitted diseases treatment guidelines 2002. Centers for Disease Control and Prevention. MMWR Recomm Rep. 2002;51(RR-6)1–78.

infections it is also important to consider treating for *Chlamydia* infection (see Table 33.1) because 10%–30% of patients with gonorrhea will have a concomitant *Chlamydia* infection (2).

Treatment recommendations by the CDC for uncomplicated gonococcal infections of the cervix, urethra, and rectum include oral and parenteral options (see Table 33.2) (2). Fluoroquinolones have been shown to provide similar cure rates when compared to ceftriaxone (8) but there has been an increasing incidence of fluoroquinolone-resistant *N. gonorrhoeae* in certain areas. This has led the CDC to advise against using fluoroquinolones in individuals who live in Asia, the Pacific Islands (including Hawaii), and in California (2). Recently the CDC also noted that there was a substantial increase of fluoroquinolone-resistant *N. gonorrhoeae* in men who have sex with men and no longer recommend fluoroquinolones as first-line treatment in these individuals (13). Other areas with concerns about fluoroquinolone-resistant *N. gonorrhoeae* include England, Wales, and Canada (14, 15). When treating patients with gonorrhea it is important to obtain a travel history in order to assess their risk for having fluoroquinolone-resistant *N. gonorrhoeae* (2).

Pharyngeal gonococcal infections are more difficult to eradicate than urogenital or anorectal infections because few antibiotic regimens can reliably cure this infection. Because ceftriaxone 125 mg intramuscularly in a single dose or ciprofloxacin 500 mg orally in a single dose have been proven to be effective against pharyngeal gonorrhea, these are the only regimens recommended by the CDC (2). The same concerns about fluoroquinolone-resistant *N. gonorrhoeae* is present with pharyngeal infections as mentioned above.

Treatment of Gonorrhea in Children

The treatment for ophthalmia neonatorum or suspected gonococcal infections in children is ceftriaxone 25–50 mg/kg intravenously or intramuscularly in a single dose (2). The dose given should not exceed 125 mg total. Fluoroquinolones should be avoided in this age group until they weigh 45 kg or more because of the concern this group of medications may damage their articular cartilage (2).

Treatment of Disseminated Infections

Patients with suspected disseminated gonococcal infections should be hospitalized for their initial treatment (2). The initial evaluation should include examining for any clinical signs of endocarditis or meningitis. The current CDC recommendation is for ceftriaxone 1 g intramuscularly or intravenously every 24 hours (2). Other alternative therapies are listed in Table 33.3. Parenteral antibiotics should be continued for 24–48 hours after clinical improvement begins and then switch to oral regimens (see Table 33.3) that need to be continued for a total of 7 days (2).

Treatment of Gonorrhea in Pregnancy

Fluoroquinolones and tetracyclines are contraindicated in women who are pregnant. If a gonococcal infection is present

TABLE 33.3 Treatment Regimens for Disseminated Gonococcal Infections

Recommended parenteral
- Ceftriaxone 1 gm IM or IV q24h
  Alternative parenteral
- Cefotaxime 1 gm IV q8h
- Ciprofloxacin 400 mg IV q12h
- Levofloxacin 250 mg IV daily
- Spectinomycin 2 g IM q12h
Oral Regimen*
- Cefixime 400 mg twice daily
- Ciprofloxacin 500 mg twice daily
- Ofloxacin 400 mg twice daily
- Levofloxacin 500 mg once daily

*Can be started 24–48 hours after improvement begins and at least one week of combined parenteral and/or oral antimicrobial therapy needs to be completed.
Adapted from: Sexually transmitted diseases treatment guidelines 2002. Centers for Disease Control and Prevention. MMWR Recomm Rep. 2002;51(RR-6)1–78.

in a pregnant patient she should receive the recommended or alternative cephalosporin (2). If the patient cannot tolerate or is allergic to cephalosporins, the alternative is a single 2-g dose of spectinomycin intramuscularly. Both of these alternative regimens have similar cure rates (16).

Pelvic Inflammatory Disease

Women with *Chlamydia*, gonorrhea or other infections in the lower genital tract may develop an ascending infection that causes acute salpingitis with or without endometritis, also known as PID. In 2003 there were an estimated 168,837 women ages 15 to 44 who were diagnosed with PID in emergency departments and over 100,000 seen initially in physicians' offices with PID (1).

CLINICAL EVALUATION

Symptoms tend to have a subacute onset and usually develop during menses or the first 2 weeks of the menstrual cycle (2). Symptoms may range from being absent in some to severe abdominal pain with high fevers. Other symptoms include dyspareunia, prolonged menses, and intramenstrual bleeding. Women who develop PID have a 20% chance of becoming infertile, 18% chance of developing pelvic pain, and 9% lifetime chance of a tubal pregnancy (2).

The CDC recommends that physicians should maintain a low threshold for diagnosing PID (2). Because of the substantial adverse impact untreated PID can have in women, the CDC recommends empiric treatment for PID in women at risk for STDs if they have uterine/adnexal tenderness and/or cervical motion tenderness and no other causes can be identified (2). The sensitivity and specificity of history, physical and diagnostic testing to determine the presence or absence of PID are noted in Table 33.4 (17–22).

DIAGNOSTIC TESTING

The initial diagnosis of PID based on signs and symptoms needs to be confirmed with further diagnostic testing. Laboratory evaluation of women with PID includes either a sedimen-

tation rate or c-reactive protein, a complete blood count, and testing for the presence of *Chlamydia* and gonorrhea. Although nonspecific, elevation in the sedimentation rate and c-reactive protein suggests the presence of inflammation. A white blood cell count that is elevated indicates the infection has created a systemic reaction. The presence of *Chlamydia* and/or gonorrhea infections does not confirm the diagnosis of PID.

Diagnostic imaging such as transvaginal ultrasound or MRI can be used to evaluate PID in patients who have a adnexal mass in palpation, if the diagnosis is uncertain, or if inpatient treatment is necessary because of the severity of the infection. Abnormal findings include thickened, fluid filled tubes, with or without free pelvic fluid or a tubo-ovarian complex (2).

Two diagnostic tests that should be considered for patients with PID who are not responding to therapy or are severely ill are endometrial biopsy and laproscopic examination of the pelvis. Both are specific in the diagnosis of PID but carry the risks of any invasive procedure (2).

TREATMENT

PID treatment in the outpatient setting has been shown to be as effective as inpatient treatment (23). The CDC has published guidelines for when it is appropriate to initiate therapy as an inpatient (see Table 33.5 (2). The options for outpatient treatment include two regimens that are equally effective (2) (see Table 33.6). If patients with PID meet any of the criteria for hospitalization and parenteral antibiotic therapy is indicated the preferred regimen is cefotetan 2 gm IV every 12 hours, or cefoxitin 2 gm IV every 6 hours plus doxycycline 100 mg orally or IV every 12 hours. Doxycycline should be given orally when ever possible because it causes sclerosis and obliteration of venous access.

Human Immunodeficiency Virus

HIV is a retrovirus that produces a broad spectrum of disease from the asymptomatic state to acquired immunodeficiency

TABLE 33.4 History, Physical and Diagnostic Data for Establishing the Diagnosis of Pelvic Inflammatory Disease (PID) (17, 22)

	Sensitivity	Specificity	LR+	LR−
Elevated C-reactive protein (21, 22)	85	80	4.3	0.19
Gonorrhea/ *Chlamydia* culture-any site (21)	77	77	3.3	0.3
Endometrial biopsy (22)	77	77	3.3	0.3
Sed rate >20 mm/hr (17)	70	69	2.3	0.43
Palpable mass (18, 19)	48	76	2	0.7
Temperature >38°C (18, 19)	32	82	1.8	0.8
Pain >4 days V (17)	78	54	1.7	0.41
Fever/chills (18, 19)	37	77	1.6	0.82
Purulent vaginal discharge (20)	74	42	1.3	0.6
Not useful				
History of IUD use (17)	35	75	1.4	0.87
Urinary symptoms (18, 19)	19	79	0.9	1.03
Irregular menses (18, 19)	38	58	0.9	1.1

TABLE 33.5   Criteria for Hospitalization Patients with Pelvic Inflammatory Disease (PID)

- Nonresponse to oral antimicrobial therapy
- Patient is pregnant
- Severe illness such as nausea and vomiting or high fever
- Surgical emergencies cannot be excluded
- Tubo-ovarian abscess present
- Unable to follow or tolerate outpatient oral regimen

Adapted from: Workowski KA, Levine WC. Sexually transmitted diseases treatment guidelines 2002. Centers for Disease Control and Prevention. MMWR. 2002;51(RR-6):1–80.

syndrome (AIDS). The transition from initial HIV infection to AIDS takes a median of ten years. During this time, viral replication occurs and then accelerates as the immune system deteriorates. Most transmission of the virus occurs through sexual contact but other modes of transmission include any exchange of blood or other infected body fluids. This includes intravenous drug use, maternal to child transmission, and accidental exposure to contaminated blood or blood products. Detection of HIV is important because early treatment can slow the decline of the immune system, may impact the treatment of other STIs, and provides physicians and other healthcare workers an opportunity to provide counseling and other support services to reduce the risk for HIV transmission to others (2).

The annual rate of HIV/AIDS diagnosis is 20.7 per 100,000 (24). This is not a significant increase from data reported in 2001 (24). Although the overall rate did not increase, the rates for blacks and Asian/Pacific Islanders did increase from 2001 to 2004 (24). The most common route of infection for men was through male-to-male sexual contact and for women it was though high-risk heterosexual contact (24).

CLINICAL EVALUATION

Although most individuals with HIV infection are asymptomatic, a portion of newly infected individuals will develop an acute retroviral syndrome. Presenting symptoms include fever, pharyngitis, weight loss, adenopathy, and nausea/vomiting. The difficulty with this acute illness is that testing for HIV may be negative because it takes from 3 weeks to 6 months for individuals to develop detectable HIV antibodies.

HIV progresses over time although with the newer treatments the disease has changed from uniformly causing death to more of a chronic disease state. Individuals who do not respond to treatment or fail to get treatment will progress to AIDS. This is defined as having two or more opportunistic infections or having a CD4 count less than 200 cells/mm^3. The

TABLE 33.6   CDC Recommended Pelvic Inflammatory Disease (PID) Treatment Regimens

Outpatient Regimens (All Oral Regimens Need to be for 14 Days)
Oral regimen A
  • Ofloxacin 400 mg orally BID
    - or -
  • Levofloxacin 500 mg once daily
    -with or without -
  • Metronidazole 500 mg BID
Oral regimen B
  • Ceftriaxone 250 mg IM in a single dose
    - or -
  • Cefoxitin 2 gm IM plus Probenecid 1 gm orally in a single doses
    - and -
  • Doxycycline 100 mg orally BID
    - with or without -
  • Metronidazole 500 mg BID
Inpatient regimens*
Parenteral regimen A
  • Cefotetan 2 gm IV every 12 hours
    - or -
  • Cefoxitin 2 gm IV every 6 hours
    - plus -
	• Doxycycline 100 orally or IV every 12 hours
	Parenteral regimen B
	  • Clindamycin 900 mg IV every 8 hours
	    - plus -
	  • Gentamicin loading dose IV or IM (2 mg/kg of body weight) followed by maintenance dose (1.5 mg/kg) every 8 hours
	(alternatively a single daily dose may be substituted)
	Alternative parenteral regimen
	  • Ofloxacin 400 mg IV every 12 hours
	    - or -
	  • Levofloxacin 500 mg IV once daily
	    - with or without –
	  • Metronidazole 500 mg IV every 8 hours
	    - or -
	  • Ampicillin/Sulbactam 3 gm IV every 6 hours plus doxycycline 100 mg orally or IV every 12 hours

* Note that inpatient regimens may be discontinued 24 hours after the patient shows clinical improvement with continuation of an oral regimen for total antibiotic course of at least 14 days.
Adapted from: Workowski KA, Levine WC. Sexually transmitted diseases treatment guidelines 2002. Centers for Disease Control and Prevention. MMWR. 2002;51(RR-6):1–80.

presenting symptoms of patients with AIDS vary depending on which opportunistic infection is present and what system it impacts.

DIAGNOSTIC TESTING

Because individuals with HIV can be asymptomatic, the CDC states that testing should be recommended and offered to all persons who seek an evaluation and treatment for STIs (2). Informed consent should be done before the test and results provided only in person. Negative results should be followed with education about reducing risky sexual behaviors (2). Individuals with positive results must receive initial counseling about the implications of a positive test and receive behavioral, psychosocial, and medical evaluation as well as future monitoring services.

Initial testing for HIV is performed using an enzyme immunoassay for antibodies to HIV (2). If the initial test is positive, confirmatory tests using the Western blot or an immunofluoroscence assay needs to be performed. If the confirmatory test is positive, the patient is considered to have HIV and should be considered capable of transmitting the virus.

The current guidelines for initial laboratory evaluation of patients with newly diagnosed HIV disease include CD4 cell count, plasma HIV RNA (viral load), complete blood count, liver and renal functions, and urinalysis. The following tests should be performed to identify opportunistic infections: 1) Rapid Plasma Reagin (RPR) or Venereal Disease Research Laboratory (VDRL) tests; 2) tuberculin skin test unless a history of previous tuberculosis or positive skin test; 3) *Toxoplsma gondii* IgG; 4) hepatitis A, B and C serologies; 5) Pap smears in women (25). A fasting blood glucose and lipid panel may be performed for baseline levels prior to initiating antiretroviral therapy because certain regimens can cause elevation of blood glucose and abnormal changes in lipids (25).

TREATMENT

The current recommendation is to start antiretroviral therapy in all patients with a history of an AIDS-defining illness or severe HIV infection regardless of the CD4 count and in those whose CD4 counts are less than 200 cells/mm^3 (25). Patients should be offered antiretroviral therapy if they are asymptomatic and have CD4 counts of 201–350 cells/mm^3. If patients with HIV have CD4 count of over 350 cells/mm^3 and HIV RNA of less than 100,000 copies/mL, antiretroviral therapy should be deferred unless they develop an AIDS-defining illness (25).

Treatment of HIV and AIDS has changed dramatically over the last few years. This change has occurred so quickly that current treatment recommendations by the National Institute of Health (NIH) are kept at its website *(http://AIDSinfo.nih.gov)* and not in a printed document (25).

Human Papillomavirus

Human papillomavirus (HPV) is a common sexually transmitted infection. In the general population it is more commonly known as genital warts. There are many viral types of HPV; types 16, 18, 31, 33 and 35 are associated with the development of cervical dysplasia and cancer and other external genital squamous intraepithelial lesions (2). HPV types 6 and 11 lesions are usually visible but are rarely associated with invasive carcinoma of the lower genital tract. Since HPV is not a reportable disease the prevalence can only be estimated. Current data that are available only on the prevalence of the high-risk HPV type estimate that 29% of the general population is infected with the virus (1). The prevalence is highest in the 14–19 year old age group (1).

CLINICAL EVALUATION

Most individuals with HPV have no symptoms and have subclinical disease present. Any symptoms are usually related to local irritation of the lesions. Lesions can be small flat or verucus (elevated with hyperkeratosis) type warts. The sites that are commonly infected with HPV include the penis, scrotum, vulva, perineum and perianal skin. Other potential infected sites include the cervix, vagina, urethra, anus, and mouth. Intra-anal HPV lesions occur mainly in those who have receptive anal intercourse while those in the perianal area can occur without any history of anal intercourse.

HPV can be transmitted easily with simple contact between infected individuals and their partners. Condoms reduce the risk of transmission but because HPV tends to be present in multiple different sites condoms do not prevent the transmission of this virus. The infection tends to be transient with a significant number of individuals having spontaneous resolution of the virus without any treatment.

DIAGNOSTIC TESTING

The diagnosis of HPV is usually a clinical diagnosis based on appearance of the lesions and their locations. Cervical HPV can be diagnosed by Pap smear with the typical koiliocytic changes (circumnuclear halo) present on the slide. The Pap smear with HPV present will usually be reported as low grade squamous intraepithelial lesion. (LSIL). Viral typing is not performed on Pap smears unless there are atypical changes of undetermined significance. At that time, a DNA probe can be used to determine the presence or absence of high risk HPV types. If a lesion is present and the diagnosis uncertain, a biopsy of the site can confirm if the lesion is HPV.

TREATMENT

Treatment of HPV is individualized. Because no studies have shown that treatment reduces infectivity, treatment is often limited to symptomatic lesions (2). Treatment options are shown in Table 33.7. Success of treatment does not depend on the regimen utilized but on the number and size of warts (2).

The management of individuals with HPV does not necessarily include examination of their sexual partners (2). Discovering and/or treating partners' HPV has not been shown to reduce transmission or play any role in recurrences (2). However, sexual partners may benefit from an evaluation for other STIs and counseling concerning the implications of their partner having HPV (2). Also, women who have a history of HPV should have Pap smears on a regular basis because of the increased risk for cervical cancer.

Herpes Simplex Virus

Herpes simplex virus (HSV) has two serotypes (HSV-1 and HSV-2). HSV-2 is more likely to be associated with genital herpes but HSV-1 can also cause genital infections. There are three HSV genital infection syndromes: 1) first-episode

TABLE 33.7 Treatment for External Genitalia Human Papillomavirus

Medication/Modality	Instructions	Comments	Cost
Patient applied			
Podofilox 0.5% solution or gel	Patient applies to warts 2 times/d for 3 days followed by 4 days of no therapy. May repeat for up to 4 cycles	• Total area treated should not exceed 10 cm^2 or total volume used per day not greater than 0.5 ml. • Safety not proven during pregnancy	$$$
Imiquimod 5% cream	Patient applies to warts once daily at bedtime, three times per week for up to 16 weeks.	• Treatment area should be washed with soap 6–10 hours after application. • Safety not proven during pregnancy	$$$
Provider-administered			
Cryotherapy with liquid nitrogen or cryoprobe	Follow appropriate directions based on system utilized	• Repeat application usually needed every 1–2 weeks • Must be trained in technique because over- or undertreatment can reduce the efficacy or increase complication rates	$$
Podophyllin resin 10%–25% in a compound tincture of benzoin	• Small amount applied to each wart and allowed to air dry • Weekly treatments until resolution	• Total area treated should not exceed 10 cm^2 or total volume used per day not greater than 0.5 ml. • Safety not proven during pregnancy.	$$
Trichloroacetic acid (TCA) or bichloroacetic acid (BCA) 80%–90%	• Apply small amount only to warts and allow to dry • Treatment may be repeated weekly until resolved	Easy to apply excessive amounts and cause skin irritation	$$
Surgical removal	Tangential scissor or shave excision, curettage, or electrosurgery	• Advantage of warts being eliminated in one treatment • Disadvantage is the potential complication from surgery	$$$
Intralesional interferon	• Interferon injected directly into warts • Repeat treatment usually necessary	Causes significant systemic adverse effects so not recommended for routine treatment	$$$
Laser surgery	• Based on equipment. • Usually only requires one treatment	Reserved for more extensive lesions because of potential complications	$$$

Adapted from: Workowski KA, Levine WC. Sexually transmitted diseases treatment guidelines 2002. Centers for Disease Control and Prevention. MMWR. 2002;51(RR-6):1–80.

primary infection, 2) first-episode nonprimary infection, and 3) recurrent episodes. In 2004 the total number of physician office visits for genital HSV infection was estimated to be 269,000 (1).

CLINICAL EVALUATION

First-episode primary HSV genital infection occurs in patients who have never had genital herpes before and usually causes significant symptoms. These symptoms include a prodrome prior to the breakout of any cutaneous lesions which consists of fever, malaise, headache, myalgia, and genital parasthesias. Cutaneous lesions will develop in 1–3 days after the prodrome and the lesions are multiple, painful bilateral vesicles in the genital or perianal area. As the infection progresses these le-

sions will become ulcerated. The lesions continue to develop into week two of the infection and painful inguinal lymphadenopathy is usually present. Viral shedding can occur during the prodrome and as long as there are open lesions. The majority of genital herpes is secondary to HSV-2 but up to 30% of first-episode infections are caused by HSV-1 (2). This has important implications because patients with HSV-1 genital infections are less likely to have recurrent episodes than those with HSV-2 infections.

The first-episode nonprimary genital HSV infection occurs in individuals who have previous unrecognized HSV infections. Patients with this syndrome tend to have less severe symptoms, fewer lesions, heal faster and have a shorter period of viral shedding.

Recurrent HSV infection is defined as any episode of this infection after the first episode. There is usually a prodrome prior to breakout of the lesions which consists of tingling, pruritus, or dysthesias. The lesions will erupt in the same site as the primary episode and will crust over in 4 to 5 days. Viral shedding can occur at anytime during this process. In addition, viral shedding can occur at times with no symptoms so patients are unaware that they may spread the infection (2).

DIAGNOSTIC TESTING

According to the CDC HSV cell culture is still the preferred virologic test for patients with genital ulcers (2). The sensitivity of HSV culture however declines as the lesions heal so it needs to be performed in the first few days of a breakout. There are polymerase chain reaction (PCR) assays for HPV DNA that are more sensitive but their use in the diagnosis of genital HSV is still being debated (26).

TREATMENT

The treatment regimen for patients with genital HSV infections depends on if the episode is the first, recurrent, or if preventing recurrence is the goal. All individuals with genital herpes can use saline washes to keep the area clean and analgesia for pain. Topical anesthetic agents should be used cautiously because of the potential for sensitization (26).

First-episodes of genital HSV should be treated within five days of the start of the infection and while new lesions are still forming (26). Anti-viral medications have been shown to reduce the severity and duration of the first-episode but have not been shown to alter the natural history of the disease (26). The current recommendations include acyclovir 200 mg five times per day or 400 mg three times per day, famciclovir 250 mg 3 times per day, or valaciclovir 1,000 mg twice per day, all given for 7 to 10 days (2). A recent guideline from the National Guideline Clearinghouse concerning the treatment of first-episode HSV recommends that the antivirals not be used for more than 5 days because prolonged treatment has not been shown to be effective (26). The current recommendation did suggest that it may be necessary to continue for longer than ten days if lesions are still appearing (26). The topical antiviral agent is less effective than the oral medications and there is no benefit to using both topical and oral treatments. Patients who are immunocompromised may require ten days of therapy (26).

Recurrent episodes of HSV genital lesions are common after the first episode but tend to diminish over time. These recurrent breakouts can be treated with episodic or suppressive therapy. Episodic therapy is used when individuals start to have recurrent symptoms. This therapy should be patient-initiated and patients should be provided with a prescription for the antiviral medication. The recommended therapy for episodic treatment includes acyclovir 800 mg twice per day, 400 mg three times per day, or 200 mg five times per day, famciclovir 125 mg twice per day, or valacyclovir 500 mg twice per day or 1.0 g once per day (2). All of these should be given for 5 days. Selection of the regimen should be based on ease of administration and cost because the regimens appear to provide similar response rates (2).

Long-term suppressive therapy has been shown to reduce the frequency of recurrent HSV infections in patients who have more than six episodes per year (26). Suppressive therapy may be effective in those patients with six or fewer outbreaks per year but the data are lacking to support this therapy (26). The recommended suppressive therapy includes acyclovir 400 mg twice per day, famciclovir 250 mg twice per day, or valicyclovir 500 mg or 1.0 g once per day (2). Patients with more than 10 recurrent episodes per year may not respond as well to 500 mg of valicyclovir so the other regimens should be utilized (2). In one study various doses of valicyclovir (500 mg or 1 gm daily or 250 mg twice daily) were all effective in reducing recurrent episodes and were equally well tolerated (27).

Because the natural course of recurrent HSV infection is to have fewer outbreaks over time, suppressive therapy could be discontinued after one year of therapy (2). This should be done after discussing the issue with the patient. If two recurrent breakouts occur, suppressive therapy should be re-instituted.

Asymptomatic viral shedding can occur in some individuals with genital HSV infections. This is more likely to occur in individuals who have HSV-2 infections, during the first year after the first-episode and if they have frequent symptomatic recurrences (26). If individuals who shed HSV without any symptoms could potentially infect someone at high risk for HSV infection (i.e., pregnant or with HIV disease), the viral shedding can be reduced by acyclovir 400 mg twice per day (26).

Because of the significant adverse effect of neonatal herpes infections, various strategies are being studied to reduce this potentially deadly infection. In one study, prophylactic acyclovir 200 mg four times per day or 400 mg three times per day starting at 36 weeks' gestation reduced the number of cesarean deliveries (28). In addition, these two regimens decreased the recurrence of clinically apparent genital herpes lesions and reduced viral shedding at the time of delivery (28).

A prevention strategy for HSV infection is to provide immunization against the virus in individuals at high risk for contracting this infection. In a recent study, the new HSV-2 vaccine was effective in reducing the attack rate of this infection in women whose partners were newly diagnosed with genital HSV-2 (23). The number needed to treat (NNT) was 11 but the vaccine has limited use because it was shown only to be effective in women who were HSV-1 and HSV-2 seronegative (23).

Syphilis

Syphilis is a systemic STI that is caused by the spirochete *Treponema pallidum* and the presenting symptoms are related to the stage of the infection (primary, secondary, tertiary and latent). In theory the organism that causes syphilis in the latent and tertiary phases is replicating at a slower rate so any treatment would require a longer duration. In addition, there is less risk for transmission of this STI during these phases but it is still possible. The number of new cases of primary and secondary syphilis increased to 7,980 in 2004 with a rate of 2.7 cases per 100,000 population (1). The majority of this increase was in men (1).

CLINICAL EVALUATION

The primary infection causes a painless solitary genital ulcer (chance). The ulcer is raised with an indurated base, well-defined, and clean. Along with the chancre, nontender inguinal lymphadenopathy will be present.

Secondary syphilis infection occurs approximately 4 to 10 weeks after the primary infection. The secondary infection causes a non-pruritic maculopapular rash that is present on the trunk and limbs. It is one of the few rashes that also can be present on the palms of the hands and soles of the feet. Other symptoms can include muscle and joint aches, fatigue, low-grade fever and generalized lymphadenopathy.

Left untreated, the symptoms related to secondary syphilis will spontaneously resolve in 3 to 12 weeks and lead to the latent phase. During this phase patients will have no signs or symptoms of syphilis. If the primary syphilis infection has occurred within 1 year the phase is called early latent phase, whereas those over 1 year are called late latent phase. Left untreated approximately one-third of these patients will develop tertiary syphilis. During this phase patients can develop cardiac, neurological, auditory abnormalities, and gummatous lesions (a small, rubbery granuloma with a necrotic center and enclosed by a fibrous capsule).

DIAGNOSTIC TESTING

The definitive diagnosis of early syphilis is done using a dark-field examination and direct fluorescent antibody tests of exudates from a lesion or tissue. However, this requires that a lesion be present and a sample obtained from the base of the lesion. There are two classes of test available to make a presumptive diagnosis of syphilis, nontreponemal and treponemal tests. The nontreponemal tests are the VDRL and the RPR. The treponemal tests include fluorescent treponemal antibody absorb (FTA-ABS) and *T. pallidum* particle agglutination (TP-PA). In order to establish the diagnosis of syphilis a confirmatory test using a treponemal test needs to be performed because of the number of false positive nontreponemal tests (2).

Nontreponemal tests antibody titers that usually correlate with disease activity. A fourfold change in titer is necessary in order to consider the change significant (2). Also, the repeat nontreponemal tests needs to be the same initial tests and preferably done by the same laboratory (2). Nontreponemal tests usually over time will become nonreactive after treatment but in some patients low titers of antibodies can persist for long periods of time.

Patients who have positive treponemal tests will have positive tests for the remainder of their lives regardless of disease activity (2). Treponemal antibody titers do not correlate well with disease activity and should not be used to assess treatment response.

Evaluation of patients with neurosyphilis includes a spinal tap to assess the cerebrospinal fluid. Testing on the fluid in patients with suspected neurosyphilis should include glucose, protein, VDRL and FTA-ABS (2). The VDRL-CSF is considered the standard for diagnosing neurosyphilis but in some cases the test may be negative. The addition of the FTA-ABS can be used to confirm these negative results. If both the VDRL-CSF and CSF FTA-ABS are negative than neurosyphilis can be excluded (2).

TREATMENT

Benzathine penicillin G given intramuscularly has been shown through randomized controlled trials to be effective in treating syphilis (2). The dosage and the length of treatment is based on the stage of the infection (see Table 33.8). Oral penicillin and combinations of benzathine and procaine penicillins are not considered appropriate therapy for syphilis (2).

Syphilis transmission can only occur when the mucocutaneous lesions are present. In order to reduce the likelihood of continued transmission of this STI the CDC has established guidelines for managing sexual partners of individuals with

TABLE 33.8 Treatment Recommendations for Syphilis

Stage	Age Group	Medication
Primary and secondary	Adult	Benzathine penicillin G 2.4 million units IM in a single dose
Primary and secondary	Children	Benzathine penicillin G 50,000 units/kg IM, up to the adult dose (2.4 million units) in a single dose
Early latent	Adult	Benzathine penicillin G 2.4 million units IM in a single dose
Early latent	Children	Benzathine penicillin G 50,000 units/kg IM, up to the adult dose (2.4 million units) in a single dose
Late latent or unknown duration	Adult	Benzathine penicillin G 2.4 million units IM at one-week intervals for three doses
Late latent or unknown duration	Children	Benzathine penicillin G 50,000 units/kg IM, up to the adult dose (2.4 million units) in a single dose at one-week intervals for three doses
Tertiary	Adult	Benzathine penicillin G 2.4 million units IM at one-week intervals for three doses

Adapted from: Workowski KA, Levine WC. Sexually transmitted diseases treatment guidelines 2002. Centers for Disease Control and Prevention. MMWR. 2002;51(RR-6):1–80.

syphilis. Individuals who are exposed within 90 days preceding the diagnosis of primary, secondary or early latent syphilis should be treated presumptively (2). If the exposure occurred more than 90 days before the diagnosis, presumptive treatment should be given if follow-up care is uncertain (2). Presumptive treatment of sexual partners should also be performed if the contact person has high treponemal serologic titers if duration of syphilis is unknown. Long-term partners of individuals with latent syphilis do not require presumptive treatment but should receive a clinical and serological evaluation for syphilis (2).

SCREENING AND PREVENTION OF STIS

The CDC has published guidelines on the prevention and control of STIs based on five major concepts (2) (see Table 33.9). Primary prevention starts with changing risky sexual behaviors that increase individuals risks for STIs (2). Secondary prevention consists of detecting and treating STIs in a standardized fashion (29, 30).

An STI prevention message that is individualized and based on patients' stages of development and understanding of sexual issues is the best prevention strategy (31). This message should be delivered in a nonjudgmental fashion. Physicians should also address misconceptions about STD protective behavior in adolescents and young adults (e.g., that virgins cannot become infected). Performing counseling and discussing behavior interventions have been shown to reduce the likelihood of STD and reduce risky sexual behavior (32). In addition, intensive behavior counseling has been shown to prevent one case of Chlamydia or gonorrhea over one year for every 12 women enrolled (31).

The CDC and the US Preventive Services Task Force (USPSTF) do recommend screening certain populations for STDs. According to the CDC all sexually active women age 24 and younger should receive annual screening for Chlamydia and gonorrhea infection, as well as women over age 24 if they are at risk (i.e,. a new sexual partner or a history of multiple

sexual partners) (2). The USPSTF strongly recommends that all women age 25 and younger should receive routine screening for Chlamydia and gonorrhea (33, 34). Screening for Chlamydia and gonorrhea infections is not recommended for males, even men who have sex with men (35, 36). The USPSTF have found insufficient evidence to recommend for or against routine screening of asymptomatic men (33).

Potential benefits of screening selected populations for HIV include educating HIV positive patients about transmission of the virus, initiating antiretroviral therapy during pregnancy to reduce the potential transmission to the fetus or newborn, and initiating antiretroviral therapy early to improve overall outcomes in these individuals (37, 38). The USPSTF recommends that all adolescent and adults who are at increased risk for HIV should be screened for the disease (37). Those at risk include men who have sex with men; men and women having sex with multiple partners; men and women who exchange sex for money or drugs or have partners who do; past or present injecting drug users; individuals who past or present partners were HIV-infected, bisexual, or injection drug users; persons being treated for STIs; and persons who received blood transfusions between 1978 and 1985 (37). Individuals who request HIV testing should also be considered high risk and screened. Also, patients who seek healthcare at high-risk settings such as STI clinics, correction facilities, homeless shelters, tuberculosis clinics, clinics serving men who have sex with men, and adolescent clinics where the HIV prevalence is high should be screened for HIV regardless of their reported risk factors (37). There are inadequate data to support screening all adolescent and adults for HIV (37).

One of the fastest growing groups of persons with newly diagnosed HIV is women. This fact has major implications when considering the potential of mother-to-child transmission during pregnancy, labor and delivery, and after delivery. Because of these factors and the reduction of transmission when antiretrovirals are used, the USPSTF recommends universal screening of all pregnant women (38).

CASE DISCUSSION

The initial case brings together the various issues that physicians face when dealing with a patient that has a potential STI. The patient is 23 years old and is in the age group that has the highest risk for STIs, in particular Chlamydia and gonorrhea. Her sexual behaviors also increase her risk because of the multiple sexual partners. The purulent discharge from the cervix makes the diagnosis of Chlamydia and/or gonorrhea more likely but other causes are possible.

The case also points out an important aspect when dealing with potential STIs. Sometimes it is necessary to initiate empirical antibiotic therapy prior to having the results of the Chlamydia and gonorrhea tests. This is necessary because of the potential for losing the patient to follow-up and reducing the likelihood of the patient exposing her partners to an STI.

Even if the evaluation of the patient does not discover an STI, this encounter provides an excellent opportunity to screen for STIs and to discuss behaviors that will reduce the likelihood of future issues with STIs. This provides physicians

---

TABLE 33.9 Five Major Concepts for Prevention of STIs

1. Education and counseling concerning safer sex behavior in those at risk
2. Identification of asymptomatic infected persons and of symptomatic persons unlikely to seek diagnostic and treatment services
3. Effective diagnosis and treatment of infected individuals
4. Evaluation, treatment and counseling of sex partners whose partners are infected with STDs
5. Pre-exposure immunizations for vaccine-preventable STIs

Adapted from: Workowski KA, Levine WC. Sexually transmitted diseases treatment guidelines 2002. Centers for Disease Control and Prevention. MMWR. 2002;51(RR-6):1–80.

with the true "teachable moment" during the time spent with this patient.

REFERENCES

1. Centers for Disease Control and Prevention. STD Surveillance 2004. September 2005. Available at *http://cdc.gov/std/stats/04pdf/2004Surveillance-all.pdf*. Accessed December 30, 2005.
2. Workowski KA, Levine WC. Sexually transmitted diseases treatment guidelines 2002. Centers for Disease Control and Prevention. MMWR. 2002;51(RR-6):1–80.
3. Landers DV, Wiesenfeld HC, Heine RP, Krohn MA, Hillier SL. Predictive value of the clinical diagnosis of lower genital tract infection in women. Am J Obstet Gynecol. 2004;190:1004–1010.
4. Centers for Disease Control and Prevention. Screening tests to detect *Chlamydia trachomatis* and *Neiserria gonorrhoeae* infections—2002. MMWR. 2002;51(RR-15):1–38.
5. Shafer MAB, Pantell RH, Schachter J. Is the routine pelvic examination needed with the advent of urine-based screening for sexually transmitted diseases? Arch Pediatr Adolesc Med 1999;153:119–125.
6. Lyss SB, Kamb ML, Peterman TA, et al. *Chlamydia trachomatis* among patients infected with and treated for *Neisseria gonorrhoeae* in sexually transmitted disease clinics in the United States. Ann Intern Med. 2003;139:178–185.
7. Lau CY, Qureshi AK. Azithromycin versus doxycycline for genital *Chlamydia* infections: a meta-analysis of randomized clinical trials (Structured abstract) (Cochrane Review). In: The Cochrane Library. Oxford, England: Update Software; 2004:Issue 2.
8. Turrentine MA, Newton ER. Amoxicillin or erythromycin for the treatment of antenatal *Chlamydia* infection: a meta-analysis (Structured abstract) (Cochrane Review). In: The Cochrane Library. Oxford, England: Update Software; 2004:Issue 2.
9. Institute of Medicine, Division of Health Promotion and Disease Prevention. The hidden epidemic: confronting sexually transmitted diseases. Eng TR, Butler WT, eds. Washington, DC: National Academy Press; 1997.
10. Weinstock H, Berman S, Cates W. Sexually transmitted infections in American youth: incidence and prevalence estimates, 2000. Persp Sexual Reprod Health. 2004;36:6–10.
11. Koumans EH, Johnson RE, Knapp JS, St Louis ME. Laboratory testing for *Neisseria gonorrhoeae* by recently introduced nonculture tests: a performance review with clinical and public health consequences (Structured abstract) 1998. (The Database of Abstracts of Reviews of Effectiveness (DARE)). (Cochrane Review). In: The Cochrane Library. Oxford, England: Update Software; (Cochrane Review). In: The Cochrane Library. Oxford, England: Update Software; 2004:Issue 2.
12. Kane BG, Degutis LC, Sayward HK, D'Onofrio G. Compliance with the Centers for Disease Control and Prevention recommendations for the diagnosis and treatment of sexually transmitted diseases. Acad Emerg Med. 2004;11(4):371–377.
13. Brocklehurst P, Rooney G. Interventions for treating genital *Chlamydia* trachomatis infection in pregnancy (Cochrane Review). In: The Cochrane Library. Oxford, England: Update Software; 2004:Issue 2.
14. Fenton KA, Ison C, Johnson AP, et al. Ciprofloxacin resistance in *Neisseria gonorrhoeae* in England and Whales in 2002. Lancet. 2003;361:1867–1869.
15. Sarwal S, Wong T, Sevigny C, Ng L-K. Increasing incidence of ciprofloxacin-resistant *Neisseria gonorrhoeae* infection in Canada. CMAJ. 2003;168(7):872–873.
16. Brocklehurst P. Antibiotics for gonorrhea in pregnancy (Cochrane Review). In: The Cochrane Library. Oxford, England: Update Software; 2004:Issue 2.
17. Wolner-Hanseen P, Svensson L, Mardh PA, Westrom L. Laproscopic findings and contraceptive use in women with signs and symptoms suggestive of acute salpingitis. Obstet Gynecol. 1985;66:233–238.
18. Jacobson L, Westrom L. Objective diagnosis of acute pelvic inflammatory disease. Diagnostic and prognostic value of routine laproscopy. Am J Obstet Gynecol. 1969;105:1088–1098.
19. Hadgu A, Westrom L, Brooks CA, et al. Predicting acute pelvic inflammatory disease: a multivariate analysis. Am J Obstet Gynecol. 1986;155:954–960.
20. Wasserheit JN, Bell TA, Kiviat NB, et al. Microbial causes of proven pelvic inflammatory disease and efficacy of clindamycin and tobramycin. Ann Intern Med. 1986:104:187–193.
21. Lehtinen M, Laine S, Heinonen PK, et al. Serum C-reactive protein determination in acute pelvic inflammatory disease. Am J Obstet Gynecol. 1986:154:158–159.
22. Paavonen J, Aine R, Teisala K, Heinonen PK, Punnonen R. Comparison of endometrial biopsy and peritoneal fluid cytology testing with laproscopy in the diagnosis of acute pelvic inflammatory disease. Am J Obstet Gynecol. 1985;1515:645–650.
23. Ness RB, Soper DE, Holley RL, et al. Effectiveness of inpatient and outpatient treatment strategies for women with pelvic inflammatory disease: results from the Pelvic Inflammatory Disease Evaluation and Clinical Health (PEACH) Randomized Trial. Am J Obstet Gynecol. 2002;186:929–937.
24. Centers for Disease Control and Prevention. Trends in HIV/AIDS diagnoses—33 states, 2001–2004. MMWR. 2005;54:1149–1153.
25. Department of Health and Human Services. Guidelines for the use of antiretroviral agents in HIV-1 infected adults and adolescents. October 6, 2005. Available at *http://AIDSinfo.nih.gov/guidelines/AA_100605.pdf*. Accessed October 6, 2005.
26. National Guideline Clearinghouse. 2002 national guideline for the management of genital herpes. Availble at *http://www.guidelines.gov/summary/summary.asp?view_id = 1& doc_id = 3035*. Accessed August 25, 2005.
27. Reitano M, Tyring S, Wang W, et al. Valacyclovir for the suppression of recurrent genital herpes simplex virus infection: A large-scale dose range-finding study. J Infect Dis. 1998;178:603–610.
28. Sheffeld JS, Hollier LM, Hill JB, Stuart GS, Wendel GD. Acyclovir prophylaxis to prevent herpes simplex virus recurrence at delivery: a systematic review. Obstet Gynecol. 2003; 102:1396–1403.
29. Sangani P, Rutherford G, Wilkinson D. Population-based interventions for reducing sexually transmitted infections, including HIV infection. (Cochrane Review). In: The Cochrane Library. Oxford, England: Update Software; 2004:Issue 2.
30. Kane BG, Degutis LC, Sayward HK, D'Onofrio G. Compliance with the Centers for Disease Control and Prevention recommendations for the diagnosis and treatment of sexually transmitted diseases. Acad Emerg Med. 2004;11:371–377.
31. Shier LA, Ancheta R, Goodman E, Chiou VM, Lyden MR, Emans SJ. Randomized controlled trial of a safer sex intervention for high-risk adolescent girls. Arch Pediatr Adolesc Med. 2001;155:73–79.
32. Shain RN, Piper JM, Holden AE, et al. Prevention of gonorrhea and *Chlamydia* through behavioral intervention: results of two-year controlled randomized trial in minority women. Sex Transm Dis. 2004;31:401–408.

33. US Preventive Service Task Force. Screening for *Chlamydia* infection. 2001. Available at *http://www.ahrq.gov/clinic/uspstf/uspschlm.htm*. Accessed October 5, 2005.

34. US Preventive Services Task Force. Screening for Gonorrhea in Guide to Clinical Preventive Services, 2nd ed. Available at *http://www.ncbi.nih.gov/books/bv.fcgi?rid = hstat3.section.10931*. Accessed May 19, 2005.

35. Nelson HD, Saha S, Helfand M. Screening for *Chlamydia* infection (Structured abstract) (Cochrane Review). In: The Cochrane Library. Oxford, England: Update Software; 2004: Issue 2.

36. Cook RL, George K, Silvestre AJ, et al. Prevalence of *Chlamydia* and gonorrhea among a population of men who have sex with men. Sex Transm Infect. 2002;78:190–193.

37. US Preventive Service Task Force. Screening for HIV for the US Preventive Services Task Force. 2001. Availble at http://*www.ahrq.gov/clinic/uspstf05/hiv/hivrs.htm*. Accessed August 25, 2005.

38. US Preventive Service Task Force. Prenatal screening for HIV for the US Preventive Services Task Force. 2001. Availble at *http://www.ahrq.gov/clinic/uspstf05/hiv/hivprenat.htm*. Accessed August 25, 2005.

CHAPTER 34

Vaginitis

Barbara D. Reed

CASE

Mrs. C. is a 25-year-old woman, married for 6 months, who calls in to request treatment for her "yeast infection." She has noted increased discharge for the past 2 weeks that is white with a faint yellow tinge, and she has mild vulvar itching. She had a yeast infection 2 years earlier that she self-treated and her symptoms resolved, but she wants to get a prescription medication this time so that it will be covered by her insurance. Mrs. C is taking oral contraceptives, smokes 1/2 pack per day, and does not have diabetes.

CLINICAL QUESTIONS

1. How likely is the diagnosis of *Candida* vulvovaginitis in this woman?
2. Does her use of oral contraceptives and her previous response to over-the-counter (OTC) antifungals make you more certain of her current diagnosis?
3. Should she be encouraged to try OTC antifungals and come into the office if her symptoms persist?

Vaginal symptoms are very common among postpubertal women. Although rarely progressive or life threatening in the acute, symptomatic phase, these symptoms lead to large health-related costs due to the resulting morbidity, medical expenses, and time taken from work for evaluation and treatment. In addition, two of the most common vaginal syndromes—bacterial vaginosis (BV) and *Trichomonas* vaginitis (TV) — are associated with adverse pregnancy outcomes (1–4), although treatment during pregnancy has not been consistently beneficial (5, 6). Unfortunately, the evaluation of vaginal symptoms is too often insufficient to correctly identify the diagnosis and rule out more serious disease.

The availability of nonprescription medication for the treatment of *Candida* vulvovaginitis (CVV) has led to self-diagnosis and misdiagnosis. Women presenting with vaginal symptoms are now more likely to have already self-diagnosed and possibly self-treated prior to being seen for their symptoms. Therefore, the probability of vaginal symptoms representing something other than vulvovaginal candidiasis has increased.

PATHOPHYSIOLOGY AND DIFFERENTIAL DIAGNOSIS

Pathophysiology

Vaginal symptoms such as increased discharge, itching, odor, swelling, or irritation may occur in any woman — partnered or single, sexually active or not, premenopausal or postmenopausal. Although children can present with similar symptoms, these symptoms are less common prior to menarche, and symptoms in the pediatric age groups will not be addressed here.

The normal vaginal milieu consists of clear or white vaginal fluid that on microscopic examination demonstrates desquamated vaginal nonkeratinized epithelial cells. The bacterial flora of the vagina consists predominantly of *Lactobacillus acidophilus* (a gram-positive, facultative long rod) although diphtheroids, *Staphylococcus epidermidis*, beta-hemolytic streptococci, and coliforms are also present. The normal pH is 4.5 or less. White blood cells are not part of the normal vaginal fluid contents; when present, they reflect vaginal or cervical inflammation, although a specific cause cannot always be determined. The presence of copious discharge or discharge that is curd-like, foamy, or discolored suggests vaginal infection, as does a fishy odor of the discharge or swelling of the genital tissues (often identified as shiny, smoother skin in the vestibule or vagina). Erythema of the tissues suggests inflammation or an allergic reaction, while ulcers, papules, warts, pigmentary changes, or dystrophic changes suggest a nonvaginitis etiology.

Symptoms of vaginal infection reflect alterations in the normal protective vaginal flora, overgrowth of organisms not typically predominant in the vagina (*Gardnerella vaginalis*, *Mobiluncus* anaerobes, *Trichomonas vaginalis*) and/or overgrowth or reactions to organisms occasionally found in the vagina in an asymptomatic state (*Candida* vulvovaginitis). Vaginal symptoms may also be unrelated to vaginal infection, and may be of neuropathic, dermatologic, or allergic origins. Symptoms of vaginitis may be related to an inflammatory reaction, the altered acidity of the vaginal contents, an invasion of organisms into the vaginal lining, or the response of the tissues to toxic byproducts of altered flora or pathologic organisms.

BACTERIAL VAGINOSIS

Bacterial vaginosis (BV), the most common infection-related vaginal syndrome, is present in at least one-third of women with vaginal symptoms and in about one-fifth of all women regardless of symptoms (7, 8). The etiology of BV is not clearly understood, but women with this entity are more likely to have one or more of the following in the vaginal discharge: *Gardnerella vaginalis* (a facultative gram-variable coccobacillary, or short-rod organism), *Mobiluncus* (an anaerobic, curved gram-variable, motile short rod), *Mycoplasma hominis*, or one or more types of anaerobes such as Bacteroides and Peptostreptococcus. Subsequently, women with BV have an "abnormal" background flora observed on normal saline microscopic examination, characterized by a lack of long rods typical of lactobacilli and with a predominance of short rods, curved rods, or coccobacilli. Women lacking lactobacilli in the vagina, or those with H_2O_2-negative lactobacilli, are prone to developing BV (but not *Candida* vulvovaginitis or *Trichomonas* vaginitis) (9).

Whether BV is sexually transmitted remains controversial, and research is hampered by the lack of a clinical correlate to BV in the male. Treatment trials of women with BV and their male sexual partners show conflicting results (10, 11). However, a study on lesbian women suggests that BV concordance among monogamous women partners is high (72.7%) (12). Furthermore, studies suggest that BV is associated with an increased risk of other STIs, including *Chlamydia trachomatis*, *Neisseria gonorrhoeae*, herpes, and syphilis, and with preterm delivery (2).

CANDIDA VULVOVAGINITIS

Candida vulvovaginitis (CVV) is present in roughly one-quarter of women with vaginal symptoms. However, not all women have symptoms and/or signs when *Candida* is present.

A number of factors are associated with *Candida* vulvovaginitis, such as use of oral contraceptives, use of the contraceptive sponge, use of the intrauterine device (IUD) or barrier methods, recent use of antibiotics, gastrointestinal carriage of *Candida*, a diet rich in sugars or yeasts, and the presence of diabetes (13). Unfortunately, none of these risk factors is consistently associated with symptomatic *Candida* vulvovaginitis (8, 13–15). Data clearly support an association between the presence of *Candida* species in the vagina and presence in the rectum and oral cavity of the woman and in the penis, semen, rectum, and oral cavity of her sexual partner (16–18), as well as an association between cunnilingus and *Candida* vulvovaginitis in women (19–21). However, there is no evidence that eradication of these other sources of *Candida* decreases the likelihood of recurrence of symptomatic *Candida* vulvovaginitis (22, 23), and presence of Candida in the male partner (tongue, urine, semen, or feces) is not associated with an increased risk of recurrence in the female partner (18).

The significance of asymptomatic *Candida* colonization of the vagina, recognized in approximately 20% of women, is unknown. Therefore, screening or treatment of asymptomatic cases has not been recommended (8, 24).

TRICHOMONAS VAGINITIS

Trichomonas vaginitis (TV) is present in 20% or fewer of women with vaginal symptoms (7, 8), and is caused by a flagellated protozoan. It is the only cause of vaginitis that is clearly sexually transmitted, and is more common in women who have had multiple sexual partners or who have recently had a new partner. However, the presence of *Trichomonas* vaginalis may be overlooked for years—by both the patient and her medical provider—and hence this diagnosis does not necessarily imply a recent exposure. Approximately 30% or more of women with *Trichomonas* vaginitis have other STIs (25), and this coinfection may increase the risk of upper genital tract disease (26). Thus, women with *Trichomonas* vaginitis should be routinely tested for sexually transmitted infections (STIs) that are easily missed (e.g. *Chlamydia trachomatis*, cervical changes associated with human papillomavirus (HPV), HIV disease, and *Neisseria gonorrhoeae*).

TABLE 34.1 Differential Diagnoses in Women with Vaginal Symptoms

Diagnosis	Frequency (if available)
Very common	
Bacterial vaginosis	33%–52%
Candida vulvovaginitis	20%–25%
Common	
Trichomonas vaginitis	7%–14%
Cervicitis	
Vulvodynia	3%–8%
Uncommon	
Allergic vaginosis	
Atrophic vaginitis	
Genital ulcers: herpes simplex, syphilis, and chancroid	
Lichen sclerosus	
Lichen planus	
Lichen simplex chronicus	
Vulvar intraepithelial neoplasia	
Pelvic inflammatory disease (PID)	
Lactobacillosis	

Differential Diagnosis of Vaginal Symptoms

Two of three women with vulvovaginal complaints have candidal vulvovaginitis, BV, or TV. Roughly one-third of cases (and more in postmenopausal women) (27), are caused by other diagnoses, such as lichen sclerosus, atrophic vaginitis, vulvodynia, less common bacterial infections, and other entities not yet characterized (see Table 34.1) (8, 28). These other diagnoses may be associated with long-term complications, symptoms, pregnancy risk, or progression of disease. Treatment should be guided by the diagnosis; a shotgun approach, although sometimes effective in decreasing the symptoms, is unlikely to adequately address the problem if the diagnosis is unclear or erroneous.

CLINICAL EVALUATION

The clinical evaluation of a woman with vulvovaginal complaints includes a careful history (including an assessment of risk factors for vaginitis and symptoms of other genital problems), a physical examination with a pelvic evaluation, an office laboratory assessment, and central laboratory tests when indicated (see Figure 34.1).

History and Physical Examination

The physical examination findings associated with the most common causes of vaginal symptoms are listed in Table 34.2. While these findings may identify a group of women at in-

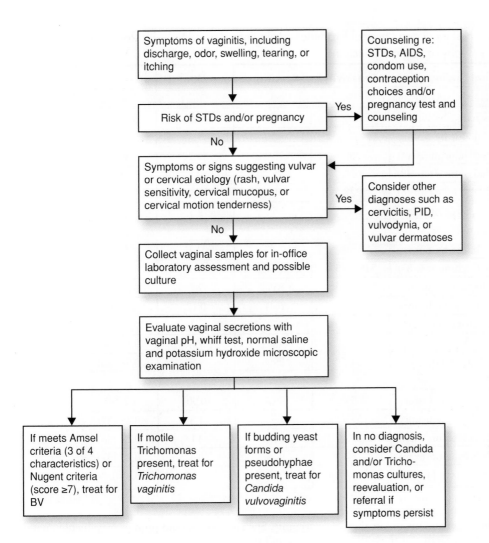

Figure 34.1 • General approach to the evaluation of vaginal symptoms. BV, bacterial vaginosis; PID, pelvic inflammatory disease; STD, sexually transmitted disease.

creased risk for a specific infection and may be useful in suggesting the need for further studies, no finding on examination is pathognomonic of a specific infection. In caring for individual patients, overreliance on risk-factors may lead to misdiagnosis.

BACTERIAL VAGINOSIS (BV)

Women with BV often complain of a "fishy" odor from the vaginal area, and this odor may become accentuated after exposure to semen during intercourse. Although not typical of BV, itching may occur, but it is usually not as severe as in women with *Candida* vulvovaginitis or even *Trichomonas* vaginitis. Approximately one-half of women with BV are asymptomatic.

On examination, the patient with BV has an increased quantity of creamy white, yellow, green, or gray discharge. It is unusual to have signs of inflammation such as marked erythema, swelling of the labia or vagina, or excoriations from scratching. The clinician may note a fishy odor, but its absence does not rule out BV. When present, a gray discharge is useful for suggesting the diagnosis (LR+ 22).

CANDIDA VULVOVAGINITIS (CVV)

The signs and symptoms of CVV range from florid, thick, curd-like white discharge clinging to the vaginal and cervical mucosa with marked erythema of the vaginal and/or vulvar lining and edema of the tissues, to a fairly normal appearing genital examination with minimal discharge. Many women complain of vaginal itch. Small sensitive mucosal tears, with a "paper-cut" appearance, occasionally occur on the vulva.

TRICHOMONAS VAGINITIS (TV)

Women with TV may complain of an increased vaginal discharge that is often thin or foamy in texture and discolored. Other symptoms overlap with the other causes of vaginitis, including odor and itching that may be mild to severe. In severe cases, lower abdominal pain and occasionally fever may be present.

On examination, the discharge of *Trichomonas* vaginitis is typically copious, thin, discolored (green, gray, tan), and occasionally foamy in consistency. A fishy odor may be appreciated but is not typically noted. In practice, however, the majority of women with *Trichomonas* infection have a nonde-

TABLE 34.2 Historical and Physical Examination Findings Associated with Common Types of Vaginal Infections

History and Physical Finding	Sensitivity	Specificity	LR+	LR−
Bacterial vaginosis				
Increased discharge by history	59%	67%	1.8	0.61 (82)
Malodor by history	97%	40%	1.6	0.07 (82)
"High Cheese" odor on exam	78%	75%	3.2	0.30 (83)
Increased discharge on exam (8)	62%	75%	2.5	0.51 (83)
Gray discharge on exam (8)	22%	99%	22	0.8
Yellow discharge on exam	60%	85%	4.1	0.46
Candida vulvovaginitis				
Cheesy discharge by history	65%	73%	2.4	0.48 (14)
Vaginal itching (84, 85)	51%–75%	78%–82%	2.8–4.2	0.3–0.5
"External" dysuria	33%	85%	2.2	0.79 (86)
Watery discharge by history	4%	63%	0.12	1.5 (14)
White curdy discharge on exam	16%	97%	6.1	0.86 (24)
Vulvar edema	17%	98%	7.8	0.85 (86)
Vulvar erythema	54%	79%	2.5	0.58 (86)
Trichomonas vaginitis				
Any discharge by history	65%	29%	0.90	1.2 (87)
Itching by history	35%	76%	1.5	0.85 (87)
Yellow discharge on exam	89%	93%	14	0.12 (88)
Erythema or edema on exam	18%	97%	6.4	0.85 (87)
Strawberry cervix (89–91)	2%–44%	99%	2.0–43.0	0.6–0.99

script discharge that is white and homogenous, not unlike that characteristic of BV. A "strawberry" appearance of the cervix is suggestive of *Trichomonas* infection but is an infrequent finding.

Diagnostic Criteria

The diagnosis of bacterial vaginosis is made clinically during the office visit and does not require central laboratory confirmation. No culture result, including that of *Gardnerella vaginalis*, is diagnostic of bacterial vaginosis. The Amsel criteria have been used to make this diagnosis over the past decade and correlate well with symptomatology and response to treatment (29). More recent data on the accuracy of the Gram stain diagnosis of BV suggest this may be used as well (30), and may be more sensitive than the Amsel criteria (31). Table 34.3 summarizes these criteria.

CVV is diagnosed in a symptomatic woman by identifying the organism — either on the KOH microscopic preparation in the office, by culture (in the office or at a referral laboratory), or by DNA or antigen detection methods. The presence or absence of risk factors and other clinical findings may be suggestive of the diagnosis, but these are inaccurate and are often misleading.

Diagnosing *Trichomonas* vaginitis depends on identifying the organism — either on the normal saline microscopic examination, on culture, or on molecular DNA testing. Identifying *Trichomonas* on a cytology smear (Papanicolaou test) is inaccurate. Such a report should prompt reevaluation, not diagnosis and treatment.

Recent evidence indicates that patient-obtained vaginal specimens, using a cotton-tipped swab in the distal vagina, results in similar sensitivity for the diagnosis of vaginitis as physician-collected specimens for *Trichomonas* (32, 33), BV (34), and CVV (32).

Laboratory Tests

Office testing should precede central laboratory testing; the latter is recommended if the diagnosis remains unclear (7, 8, 35). Table 34.4 lists the available laboratory tests and their use as first- or second-line evaluations when the diagnosis is uncertain or the patient has persistent symptoms or prompt recurrences.

OFFICE TESTING

Four tests are central to the laboratory evaluation of vaginal secretions.

pH Assessment

To conduct this test, apply a drop or two of vaginal discharge to a small piece of pH paper that changes color in the desired pH range (4.0 to 5.5 is adequate). The pH of vaginal secretions is increased (>4.5) in most cases of bacterial vaginosis and *Trichomonas* vaginitis, while in *Candida* vulvovaginitis, the pH is usually normal (≤4.5.)

TABLE 34.3 Amsel and Nugent Criteria for Diagnosing BV.

Give 1 Point for Each Symptom; A Score of 3 or More is 70% Sensitive and 94% Specific for BV	
Sign	**Points**
Homogenous vaginal discharge	1
Elevated pH of vaginal secretions (>4.5)	1
Positive amine (whiff) test	1
Clue cells	1
Total:	

Nugent criteria. Score as indicated below; a score of 7 or more is 89%–100% sensitive and 83%–97% specific for BV.		
Microscopic Findings	**Number**	**Score**
Lactobacillus morphotypes (0 to 4)	Many	0
	None	4
Gardnerella and *Bacteroides* species (0 to 4)	None	0
	Many	4
Curved gram-variable rods (0 to 2)	None	0
	Many	2
	Total:	

Amine Test (Whiff Test)

Place a small amount of vaginal discharge on a microscope slide and add a drop or two of 10% KOH (potassium hydroxide) solution. The release of aromatic amines (described as a "fishy" odor) indicates the increased presence of anaerobes. This finding is associated with bacterial vaginosis and *Trichomonas* vaginitis.

Normal Saline (NS) Microscopic Evaluation

At the bedside, mix a drop of vaginal discharge with a small amount of non-bacteriostatic normal saline. Place a drop of the solution on a microscope slide at the time of microscopic evaluation. First look for motile *Trichomonas vaginalis*. If at low power you notice motile organisms that are approximately the size of white blood cells (as opposed to sperm, which are much smaller), use high power to confirm the presence of beating flagella and the typical teardrop yet fluctuating shape of motile *Trichomonas* vaginalis.

Next, look for clue cells, white blood cells, and atypical background flora. Clue cells are epithelial cells covered with bacteria that obscure the typical smooth border expected of normal epithelial cells. Typical background flora consist of epithelial cells with a largely clear cytoplasm, few or no surrounding white blood cells, and most of the surrounding bacterial flora consisting of long rods. A lack of long-rod predominance and/or the presence of a large proportion of short rods, cocci, or curved rods suggests an "abnormal background flora," which is independently associated with bacterial vaginosis (see Table 34.4). In women with *Candida* vulvovaginitis or *Trichomonas* vaginitis, white blood cells may be abundant; however, in many (milder) cases they may be present only in low numbers.

Potassium Hydroxide (KOH) Microscopic Preparation

Perform this test with the same slide used for the amine ("whiff") test, on which a sample of undiluted vaginal discharge (or swabbing of the moist vaginal walls if no discharge is observed) has been streaked directly to a microscope slide. After adding one to two drops of 10% KOH to the slide, perform the whiff test and allow the slide to sit (during examination of the NS prep) for several minutes, after which the slide should be scanned at low power looking for hyphal or budding yeast components, with confirmation by high power. Although as single spore forms yeast may occur, diagnosis based on single yeast forms is less accurate than that based on the identification of budding yeast forms (two or more forms still connected together while budding) or of pseudohyphae (consisting of branching filaments with budding yeast forms attached along the edge). Although the majority of *Candida* strains causing vulvovaginitis are *C. albicans*, 7% to 16% of cases are associated with Torulopsis glabrata—a nonhyphae-forming fungus (36).

CENTRAL LABORATORY TESTING

If the physical examination and office testing fail to clarify the diagnosis, further laboratory information may be required. This will be true in a sizable proportion of cases (8, 28).

Cervicitis

If cervicitis is suspected, test for *Chlamydia trachomatis* and *Neisseria gonorrhoeae* by culture or by molecular means, including immunologic or DNA identification techniques. The molecular tests do not require viable organisms for diagnosis, resulting in easier specimen handling and transport. A specimen taken from the cervical os, including discharge and cells,

TABLE 34.4 Tests Used to Diagnose Vaginitis

Diagnostic Test References	1st line	2nd line	Sensitivity	Specificity	LR+	LR−	Relative Cost
Bacterial vaginosis							
Whiff test (8, 92)	X		29%	95%	5.8	0.75	$
3 of 4 Amsel criteria (93)*	X		70%	94%	11.7	0.32	$
Abnormal background flora on Gram stain (93, 94)†	X	X	89%–100%	83%–97%	5.2–33.3	0.0–0.1	$
Symptoms (35)	X		47%	79%	2.2	0.67	$
Clue cells (microscopy) (8, 93–95)	X		37%–97%	79%–92%	1.8–12.1	0.03–0.80	$
PH>4.5 (8, 35, 93, 94, 96)	X		67%–89%	49%–77%	1.3–3.9	0.14–0.67	$
Clue cells (cytology) (94)		X	88%	99%	88.0	0.12	$$
Culture-*Gardnerella* (95)			88%	86%	6.3	0.14	$$
Proline amino-peptidase assay (97)		X	93%	91%–93%	2.5–13.3	0.08–0.14	$$
PCR—*Gardnerella* (28, 98)			91%–95%	60%–63%	2.3–2.6	0.08–0.15	$$$
***Candida* vulvovaginitis**							
KOH (8, 85, 93, 99, 100)	X		22%–61%	77%–94%	1–10	.41–1.0	$
PH of secretions ≤4.5 (92, 101)	X		82%–100%	9%–32%	1–1.5	0.0–2.0	$
Cytology (42)		X	80%	99%	80.0	0.2	$$
Molecular testing— Immunologic or PCR (28)		X	75%	96%	18.8	0.3	$$
Candida culture (symptomatic women) (102, 103)		X	93%–100%	83%	5.4–5.9	0.0–0.1	$$
Slide latex agglutination (14, 99, 103, 104)		X	65%–81%	59%–98%	1.6–40.5	0.2–0.6	$$
***Trichomonas* vaginitis**							
Normal saline Prep (28, 41, 105–108)	X		17%–80%	96%–99%	4.3–85	0.2–0.9	$
NS prep and spun Urine (109)	X		85%	Low	NA	NA	$
Trichomonas cultures		X	80%	100%	80–0	0–2	$$
Enzyme-linked Immunosorbent (106, 107)		X	77%–93%	98%–100%	38.5–93.0	0.1–0.2	$$
Molecular testing (Immunologic, PCR) (40, 41, 87, 99, 110)		X	90%–100%	94%–100%	15.0–1800	0.0–0.1	$$
Cytology (87, 108, 111)			35%–64%	55%–99%	0.8–64	0.4–1.2	$$
Trichomonas vaginitis or BV							
Lactoferrin (112)		X	79%	83%	4.6	0.3	$$

*Using Gram stain as reference standard
†Using Amstel criteria as reference standard

should be inoculated into specific transport media for these tests. See (Chapter 33, Sexually Transmitted Infections).

Gardnerella or *Mobiluncus* Evaluation

The diagnosis of bacterial vaginosis is based on clinical criteria, such as the Amsel criteria or the abnormal Gram stain (Nugent criteria), and no central laboratory confirmation is recommended.

Candida culture

Because only 50% of cases of *Candida* vulvovaginitis will have a positive KOH preparation that clearly indicates pseudohyphae or budding yeast forms, an accurate diagnosis may require *Candida* culture. The vaginal specimen should be transported in a medium used for bacterial specimens, or it may be directly inoculated onto a fungal growth media such as Sabouraud CG or Nickerson's media or placed in Diamond's

Media Modified and incubated up to 48 hours. Typical white domed-shaped colonies (2- to 3-mm diameter) on solid agar suggest yeast growth, which can be confirmed by microscopic evaluation of a sample of the growth. Liquid Diamond's Media Modified also can be examined microscopically to determine yeast (or trichomonal) growth (37).

Trichomonas Culture

Only half of women with Trichomonas infection will have vaginal discharge with enough Trichomonas actively swimming on the normal saline preparation to allow an accurate diagnosis. Therefore, a Trichomonas culture may be beneficial in women with persistent symptoms. Culture media, such as liquid Diamond's Media Modified, can be used to culture these organisms (38). A small sample of vaginal discharge is inoculated into the liquid at room temperature, and the medium is incubated at approximately 35°C for 3 to 10 days. A drop from deep in the tube (a more anaerobic environment) can be removed for microscopic evaluation every 1 to 3 days. Other Trichomonas culture media is now available commercially as well (39).

Molecular Testing for *Candida* Species or *Trichomonas* Vaginalis

Molecular tests for identifying *Trichomonas vaginalis, Gardnerella vaginalis*, and *Candida* species, include direct immunofluorescence, enzyme immunoassay, and DNA identification using DNA probes. All are more sensitive than wet smear alone, although they are also more expensive. A DNA-probe test for *Trichomonas* vaginalis (Affirm VP Microbial Identification Test) is 80% to 90% sensitive and 99.8% to 100% specific compared to culture in women with high numbers of organisms present (40, 41). *Gardnerella* vaginalis can also be identified by this test. The accuracy is similar to that obtained by clue cell evaluation microscopically, suggesting that it might serve as a surrogate test for clue cell evaluation (40).

Cytology Smear (Papanicolaou)

Diagnoses reported on cytology examinations can be helpful in some cases (*Candida* infection) but are less accurate with others (*Trichomonas vaginalis* or *Chlamydia trachomatis* infection). The presence of budding yeast forms or pseudohyphae on cytology indicates yeast, but the absence of such findings cannot rule out this infection, owing to a sensitivity of only 80% (42).

Self-Diagnosis of *Candida* Vulvovaginitis by Women

Over-the-counter antifungal medications are now available for the treatment of *Candida* vulvovaginitis. This implies to women that they should be able to self-diagnose this disorder and treat themselves without risk. However, studies show that women with and without a previous history of *Candida* vulvovaginitis are inaccurate in diagnosing a "classic case" of *Candida* vulvovaginitis 66% and 89% of the time, respectively. Also, women with a prior history of CVV were more likely to think CVV was present when they were presented with scenarios describing pelvic inflammatory disease, bacterial vaginosis, urinary tract infection, and *Trichomonas* vaginitis than were women without such a history (43). This poor diagnostic accuracy is expected in light of the high proportion of cases of *Candida* vulvovaginitis that are not "classic" in symptoms and presentation, and is congruent with the data indicating that physicians cannot make the diagnosis in the majority of cases using history alone (7).

MANAGEMENT

Protocols for treating acute bacterial vaginosis, *Candida* vulvovaginitis, and *Trichomonas* vaginitis are listed in Table 34.5. Common or important adverse effects of drugs used to treat these infections include hepatotoxicity (oral antimycotics), a disulfiram-like effect with alcohol use (oral metronidazole), and gastrointestinal upset (oral metronidazole, clindamycin, tinidazole, and antimycotics). Natural and herbal treatments for BV and CVV have been described (44) and are used frequently by patients (45). However, data are lacking on their efficacy.

Treatment of Bacterial Vaginosis

Treatment of acute bacterial vaginosis consists primarily of metronidazole or clindamycin, either intravaginally or orally. Several other regimens have also been suggested (see Table 34.5). Treatment is effective more than 80% of the time when an accurate diagnosis is made. Meta-analysis of the data on oral metronidazole regimens for the treatment of BV suggests that a 2 g stat dose is as effective as the 500 mg twice daily dose for 7 days, although recurrences may be slightly more common (46, 47).

Recurrent infection and persistence of BV can occur with any of the regimens and has been noted in as many as one-third of women within 1 to 3 months of therapy (48). All patients with recurrent or persistent infection should be evaluated for other diagnoses such as CVV, because multiple diagnoses occur commonly in women with recurrent disease. *Mobiluncus* species, recognized as curved rods on the normal saline preparation in some women with BV, may be less susceptible to metronidazole than to clindamycin; hence, this may guide original therapy or therapy for recurrences.

Recurrent or resistant BV can be treated with a change to a different recommended therapy, or with prolonged courses (14 days or more) of the oral or intravaginal metronidazole or clindamycin regimens or of amoxicillin/clavulanate 500 mg by mouth three times daily, with continuation until the microscopic examination normalizes (49, 50). Other newer options include use of tinidazole, 2 g orally (51), or formulation of intravaginal ovules containing metronidazole and Nystatin (see Table 34.5).

Attempts to re-colonize H_2O_2-producing *Lactobacillus acidophilus* in the vagina have been made, with little evidence of efficacy in preventing post-antibiotic candidal colonization (52). Treatment of sexual partners of women with BV is controversial and is not routinely recommended. It might be considered in cases of recurrent BV (10, 53).

TREATMENT OF BV IN PREGNANCY

Although BV during pregnancy is associated with adverse pregnancy outcomes, controversy exists regarding whether screening and treatment during pregnancy changes these outcomes (3). The use of oral clindamycin, 300 mg by mouth

TABLE 34.5 Treatment for Bacterial Vaginosis, *Candida* Vulvovaginitis, and *Trichomonas* Vaginitis

Medication	Strength	Dosage	Efficacy	OTC	Relative Cost
Bacterial vaginosis					
Acute cases					
Metronidazole	500 mg tablet	1 PO BID for 7 d	84%–97%	No	$
Clindamycin	2% vaginal cream	1 applicatorful in vagina Q HS for 7 d	72%–94%	No	$$
Metronidazole	0.75% vaginal gel	1 applicatorful in vagina daily or BID for 5 d	75%–79%	No	$$
Alternate treatment					
Metronidazole	500 mg tablets	4 by mouth 1 time	79%	No	$
Clindamycin	300 mg tablets	1 PO BID for 7–14 d	94%	No	$$
Clindamycin ovule	100 mg ovule	1 in vagina Q HS for 3 d	54%	No	$$
Resistant or recurrent cases					
Acute regimens above	See above	Extend the course to 14 d or change to alternate therapy	Little data available	No	$–$$
Tinidazole	500 mg tablet	4 tablets PO one time	84%	No	$
Intravaginal metronidazole and nystatin	500 mg metronidazole and 100,000 U Nystatin per ovule	1 ovule intravaginally Q HS for 5–7 nights	93%	No	Requires compounding pharmacy
***Candida* vulvovaginitis**					
Acute cases					
Miconazole	200 mg suppository	1 Q HS for 3 days;	66%	Yes	$$
	2% vaginal cream	1 applicatorful in vagina q hs for 7 days;	No data available	Yes	$
	100mg vaginal suppository	1 in vagina Q HS for 7 d	No data available	Yes	$
Clotrimazole	100 mg suppository	1 in vagina Q HS for 7 days;	52%–72% long-term 72%–77% short-term 50%–65% long-term	Yes	$
	1% vaginal cream	1 applicatorful in vagina Q HS for 3 d;		Yes	
	500 mg suppository	1 in vagina once		No	
Butaconazole	2% vaginal cream	1 applicatorful in vagina Q HS for 3 d	81%–92%; may be useful in non-*C.albicans* species	Yes	$
Terconazole	80 mg suppository	1 in vagina Q HS for 3 d;	See below	No	$$
	0.8% vaginal cream	1 applicatorful in vagina Q HS for 3 d;	In vitro, less effect in non-*C. albicans*	No	$
	0.4% vaginal cream	1 applicatorful in vagina Q HS for 7 d	No data available	No	$$

Drug	Formulation	Dosing	Efficacy	Partner treatment	Cost
Tioconazole	6.5% vaginal ointment	1 applicatorful in vagina once	Ointment base will melt or dissolve condoms. Avoid intercourse with condoms for 3 d after use.	Yes	$
Fluconazole	150 mg tablet	1 tablet orally once	56%–98%	No	$
Itraconazole	100 mg tablet	2 tablets PO QD for 3 d	74%–85% short term and 51%–85% long term	No	$$
Persistent or recurrent cases					
Topical treatments Above	See above	Prolong the course to 14–21 d	Varies	Varies	See above
Oral regimens above	See above	Extended dosing regimens	No data available	No	See above
Fluconazole	150 mg	1 tablet on day 1 and 1 tablet on day 4	88%	No	$
Boric acid	600 mg in vaginal suppository	1 intravaginally BID for 14 d	77%–81%	No	$ (must be compounded)
Flucytosine	5 mg suppository	1 in vagina Q HS for 14 d	93%	No	Unknown
Maintenance regimens for recurrent disease					
Miconazole	100 mg suppository	2 times/week	No data found	Yes	$$
Clotrimazole	500 mg suppository	1 intravaginally per week	86% over 6 months	No	$
Terconazole	0.8% vaginal cream	Weekly applicatorful in vagina	Decreased to 4 episodes per 10 women over 6 months	No	$
Boric acid	600 mg suppository	1 in vagina twice a week	No data found	No	$ (must be compounded)
Ketoconazole	100 mg tablet	1 PO daily	95% during 6 month treatment. 48% recurred after discontinuation.	No	$
Fluconazole	150 mg tablet	1 PO Weekly	50% reduction in recurrences while on drug	No	$
Itraconazole	100 mg tablet	1 daily or 400 mg monthly	No data found	No	$
***Trichomonas* Vaginitis**					
Acute cases					
Metronidazole	500 mg tablet	2 g = 4 tablets PO once patient and partner(s)	80%–96%	No	$
Metronidazole	500 mg tablet	1 tablet PO BID for 7 d	90%–95%	No	$
Tinidazole	500 mg tablet	2 g = 4 tablets PO once	84%	No	$

(continued)

CHAPTER 35

Ankle and Knee Pain

James VanHuysen, Derrick Blackwell, and Henry C. Barry

CASE 1

A 26-year-old athlete limps into your office complaining of right ankle pain. The ankle was injured while playing soccer: he jumped for a head ball and came down on another athlete's foot. There was no pop, but the ankle was painful over the lateral aspect and began to swell. The athlete was able to limp off the field. On examination you observe swelling and ecchymosis over the lateral malleolus, but find no bony tenderness. Anterior draw test shows the same amount of movement as the opposite ankle. The squeeze test is negative.

CLINICAL QUESTIONS

1. Would you x-ray the ankle?
2. What do you tell the athlete who wants a radiograph?
3. What initial course of treatment would you recommend?

CASE 2

A 43-year-old limps into your office complaining of pain and swelling of the right knee. The knee was injured yesterday while playing soccer. Although not sure of the order of events as the injury occurred quickly, she thinks the knee was twisted when she planted for a turn. The knee swelled immediately, and the patient was initially unable to bear weight but is walking now. The knee is still swollen and bruised. On examination, you observe a puffy knee, and the patella appears to be "floating." There is moderate ecchymosis. The range of motion appears normal, but there is a lot of spasm and guarding. You find no tenderness of the patella or the head of the fibula. You find no joint line tenderness, but on Lachman testing, the knee slides forward 1 cm and feels like it would keep sliding. The degree of guarding is such that you are unable to do a McMurray test.

CLINICAL QUESTIONS

1. Would you X-ray the knee?
2. What initial course of treatment would you recommend?
3. What is the most important course of action to take?

ANKLE PAIN

Ankle pain is among the most common and important musculoskeletal complaints seen by primary care physicians, accounting for more than 750,000 outpatient visits each year (1). Additionally, ankle injuries are the most common injuries in sports, accounting for over one third of all acute injuries (2). Ankle pain may be caused by acute injury, overuse injury, or other conditions such as arthritis.

Ankle pain can be either traumatic or nontraumatic. The painful ankle may be acute, chronic, or a combination of both. Traumatic disorders include sprains, strains, dislocations, fractures, and overuse syndromes, such as tendinitis and stress fractures. Nontraumatic disorders include arthritis, osteomyelitis, and neoplasms.

DIFFERENTIAL DIAGNOSIS/ PATHOPHYSIOLOGY/ANATOMY

The ankle joint, depicted in Figure 35.1, includes the distal fibula, talus, and distal tibia. The mortise (combined joint structure) formed from these bones is stabilized on the lateral side by the anterior talofibular ligament, the calcaneal fibular ligament, the posterior talofibular ligament, and the peroneus longus and brevis. The anterior talofibular ligament is part of the lateral joint capsule, running from the anterior distal fibula to the neck of the talus. In the frontal plane, the anterior tibiofibular (ATFL) and posterior tibiofibular ligaments stabilize the mortise and allow minimal motion between the distal tibia and fibula. The tibia and fibula are also joined with a syndesmosis, a thickened sheet of interosseous membrane, further stabilizing the mortise. On the medial side, the deltoid ligament is composed of a superficial and deep layer of ligaments, which makes the ankle quite resistant to eversion stress. The mortise of the ankle joint allows dorsiflexion, plantar flexion, and internal and external rotation. The subtalar joint formed by the talus and calcaneus allows true inversion, eversion, and internal and external rotation. Finally, the Achilles tendon attaches at the posterior portion of the calcaneus, assisting in plantar flexion.

Acute injuries to the ankle can result in tears of the lateral or medial ligaments or the tibiofibular ligaments and syndesmosis, tendinous injuries to the ankle or forefoot, or fractures of the ankle or midfoot. Approximately 90% of ankle injuries result from forced inversion with the ankle in plantar flexion (2). The ATFL is the most commonly injured ligament. The ATFL is vulnerable during plantar flexion because it is

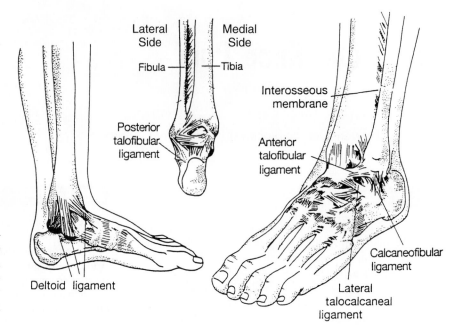

Figure 35.1 • Anatomy of the ankle joint. (Adapted from Leach RE. A nonsurgical approach to early mobility: acute ankle sprain, treat vigorously for best results. J Musculoskel Med. 1983; 1[1]:69.)

aligned vertically (parallel to the fibula) and is under tension. One common ATFL injury occurs when one basketball player lands on another player's foot and inverts the ankle. In fact, the majority of individuals can accurately describe the mechanism of trauma.

Achilles tendinitis is a common, often chronic condition, which can cause ankle pain. The mechanism is repetitive eccentric microtrauma that stresses the peritendinous structures, resulting in inflammation and even partial tendon rupture. Training errors, running in improper shoes, running on hills, and running on uneven or hard surfaces are common causes of Achilles tendonitis (3). Achilles tendon rupture is a common hazard in jumping sports and can be a complication of steroid injections (4) and fluoroquinolone antibiotics (5). The differential diagnosis of ankle pain is summarized in Table 35.1.

CLINICAL EVALUATION

You should perform a careful history and physical examination in all patients with ankle pain. It is especially important to address potential red flags (see Table 35.2). These conditions are serious and require early referral. Finally, you should ask all patients about their treatment and activity goals. For instance, an elderly patient with severe arthritis may wish only to be independent in transferring out of bed and in getting to the bathroom. Others may desire return to full contact sports. Management should be individualized and congruent with the patient's goals.

History and Physical Examination

The history should address the location, duration, character, and intensity of pain. It should also include a description of potential contributing mechanisms, ameliorating or exacerbating factors, previous injury, and current treatment. The mechanism of injury is the single most important element of the

history in patients with possible ankle sprains. You should also inquire about the chronicity of the symptoms and about changes in the level of activity, such as an increase in the number of miles or an increase in the intensity of workouts. Further history should concentrate on previous injuries, whether a "snap" or "pop" was felt (suggesting ligament rupture), the time delay from injury to the onset of symptoms, and the initial treatment given. Symptoms such as an inability to bear weight immediately after the injury or a feeling that the ankle "gives way" are especially worrisome; the former is an important factor in distinguishing sprain from fracture (see Figure 35.2, Ottawa Ankle Rules [OAR]). The Achilles tendon can also cause ankle pain. Typically, the person will complain of pain in the posterior portion of the ankle.

A solid knowledge of the functional anatomy of the ankle is imperative. Besides palpation, stress testing should be performed (see Figure 35.3). The talar tilt test evaluates the calcaneofibular ligament (CFL) and is performed by stabilizing the distal lower leg in one hand while grasping each side of the foot at the talus with the examiner's thumb on one side and forefingers on the other side. Varus stress is applied, and any qualitative difference between ankles suggests instability. The anterior drawer test is performed with the ankle slightly externally rotated and plantar flexed; a 3 mm difference between ankles suggests disruption of the ATFL.

To help distinguish an ankle sprain from a fracture, you should palpate the posterior edge and the tip of each malleolus and the base of the fifth metatarsal. You should also have the patient take four steps. This information is used in the OAR, and can be used to determine the need for radiography (see Figure 35.2).

The squeeze test compresses the tibia and fibula together above the midpoint of the calf. Pain indicates a syndesmosis sprain. The Cotton test for syndesmosis sprains is performed like the talar tilt test, except mediolateral force is applied, and any degree of motion over 3 mm is considered abnormal. Side-

TABLE 35.1 Differential Diagnosis of Ankle and Knee Pain

Diagnosis	Frequency in Primary Care	Frequency in Emergency Department
Ankle		
Inversion sprain	Very common	Very common
Avulsion fracture	Common	Very common
Achilles tendonitis	Common	Common
Eversion sprain	Uncommon	Uncommon
Fibular fracture	Uncommon	Common
Syndesmosis sprain	Uncommon	Uncommon
Trimalleolar fracture	Rare	Rare
Knee		
Anterior knee pain*	Very common	Very common
Osteoarthritis	Common	Common
Patellar tendonitis	Common	Common
MCL/LCL strain or tear	Common	Common
Meniscal tear	Common	Common
ACL strain or tear	Common	Common
Patellar dislocation	Uncommon	Uncommon
Fracture	Uncommon	Uncommon

*Also known as patellofemoral dysfunction or chondromalacia patellae.

to-side comparisons should be performed in both of these tests. Injuries to the deltoid ligament result from dorsiflexion-eversion trauma, are relatively rare, and are often associated with fractures. Clinically, the components of the deltoid ligament are inseparable.

A visible defect in the Achilles tendon may occur in cases of complete or partial rupture. Palpation of the Achilles ten-

TABLE 35.2 Red Flags Suggesting Progressive or Life-Threatening Disease in Patients with Ankle or Knee Pain

Red Flag	Diagnosis Suspected
Hemarthrosis	Internal derangement
Knee pain and limp	Hip disorder (e.g. Legg-Perthes, in child with slipped capital femoral epiphysis, normal knee examination)
Poor response to treatment	Internal derangement, malignancy (rare)
Bony swelling	Tumor
Fever	Osteomyelitis, septic arthritis
Rash, joint swelling	Collagen vascular disorders, gonococcal arthritis

don may reveal crepitus, tenderness, swelling, or a gap. The Thompson test (or midcalf compression test) assesses if the Achilles tendon is intact. The gastrocnemius and the soleus are compressed and if the foot plantar flexes, the test is negative or normal. If not, the test is positive, indicating complete or near complete rupture of the tendon.

Ankle sprains are classified by grade according to the degree of instability and functional disability. This classification is important because it guides therapy. Grade I injuries have minimal swelling and partial ligament tearing, but no clinical instability. Grade II injuries usually result from a complete tear of the ATFL and often have a positive anterior drawer test, ecchymosis, and swelling. This is also the most common type of injury diagnosed by physicians. Grade III injuries result from complete ligamentous disruption of the ATFL and CFL, with frank instability on stress testing. If a complete tear of the deltoid ligament is felt on eversion testing, radiographs should be ordered immediately to look for fracture.

Diagnostic Testing

Less than 10% of patients presenting with ankle injury in the family practice setting have a significant ankle fracture. The risk is somewhat higher in the emergency department. To reduce unnecessary use of radiographs and make the treatment of ankle injuries more cost effective, the OAR (see Figure 35.2) have been developed and prospectively evaluated. Prospective multicenter evaluation of the OAR has yielded 93% to 100% sensitivities compared with 69% and 76% clinical

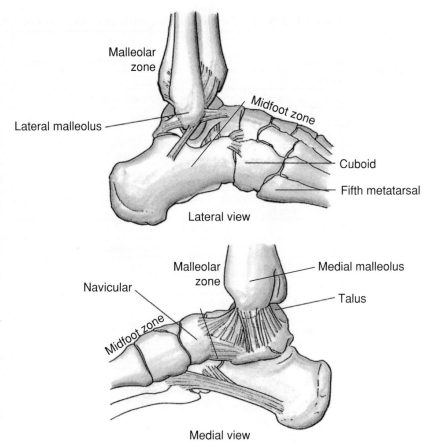

Figure 35.2 • Ottawa ankle rules for radiographic series in acute injuries.
You should perform a radiograph if the patient has pain in the malleolar or midfoot zone and one of the following:

• Bony tenderness at posterior edge or tip of either malleoli
• Bony tenderness over the navicular
• Bony tenderness at the base of the fifth metatarsal
• Inability to bear weight both immediately and in the emergency department (four steps), i.e., patient is unable to transfer weight twice onto each foot regardless of limping

(Text adapted from Stiell IG, McKnight RD, Greenberg GH, et al. Implementation of the Ottawa ankle rules. JAMA. 1994;271. Illustration reprinted with permission from Moore KL, Agur AMR. Essential Clinical Anatomy. Baltimore, MD: Williams & Wilkins; 1995: 276.)

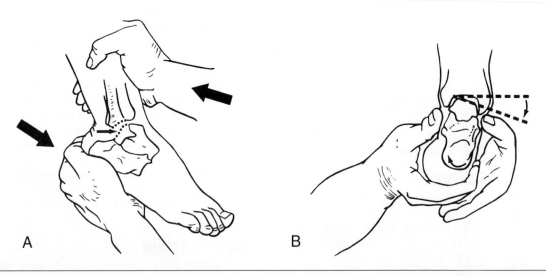

Figure 35.3 • Stress testing of the ankle. **A.** Positive anterior drawer sign (small arrow). The anterior drawer sign test is used to evaluate the intactness of the anterior talofibular ligament. **B.** Test to evaluate the stability of the anterior talofibular and calcaneofibular ligaments. The ankle is unstable if the anterior talofibular and calcaneofibular ligaments are torn. (Reprinted with permission from American Osteopathic Association. Foundations for Osteopathic Medicine. Baltimore, MD: Williams & Wilkins; 1997:638.)

TABLE 35.3 Key Elements of the History and Physical Examination in Patients with Ankle or Knee Pain

Ankle pain					
Diagnosis	**Test**	**Sensitivity**	**Specificity**	**LR +**	**LR −**
Sprain versus fracture	Ottawa ankle rule	1.00	0.39	1.64	~0.01
Knee pain					
Diagnosis	**Test**	**Sensitivity**	**Specificity**	**LR +**	**LR −**
Fracture (33)	Ottawa Knee Rule (see Table 35.7)	1.00	0.49	2	~0.01
ACL tear (28)	Lachman test	0.60–1.0	0.92	25.0	0.1
Meniscus injury (28)	Joint line tenderness McMurray test	0.79 0.53	0.91 0.59	0.9 1.3	1.1 0.8

examination sensitivities for ankle and midfoot fractures, respectively (see Table 35.3) (6, 7). Thus, no more than 1 in 300 family practice patients with acute ankle injury and a negative evaluation using the OAR will have a fracture. Additional validation of the OAR shows that the sensitivity of these rules for ankle fractures remains above 95% (8), but the sensitivity for midfoot fractures is slightly lower and more variable (9). In the emergency department setting, the percentage of patients with ankle injury for whom radiographs were ordered was reduced from 83% to 60%. The OAR are also valid in children with ankle injuries (8).

Keep in mind that the decision rule applies to an acutely injured ankle. You may wish to obtain radiographs when you find bone pain in the absence of injury, when the patient experiences night pain, or when symptoms do not fit conventional diagnoses or respond to treatment. These symptoms may indicate more serious conditions (see Table 35.2). Although radiographic stress testing, arthrography, and arthroscopy have been used in some centers to assess injury severity, the results of such testing rarely change the conservative treatment given, and they are not recommended.

Ultrasound (10–12) and magnetic resonance imaging (MRI) (11, 13–15) have been used to evaluate suspected Achilles tendinitis or Achilles tendon rupture. Although ultrasound is reported to be fairly sensitive and specific, there is no accepted gold standard, and the published studies have not included a wide spectrum of case severity. MRI has typically been studied in patients undergoing surgery. Most importantly, neither study is known to add significantly to the clinical examination. Nevertheless, the MRI, by demonstrating the extent of the defect, particularly for young athletes in high demand sports, can help with prognosis and the decision to allow the athlete to return to play.

MANAGEMENT

As with many other conditions, management of ankle pain begins with an assessment of goals. You should then proceed to address symptom relief, as that is usually the reason the patient seeks care, and then restoration of function. Table 35.4 summarizes some treatment options and the level of evidence for the interventions, and Table 35.5 summarizes commonly used pharmacotherapy for ankle pain.

Ankle Sprains
INITIAL MANAGEMENT

Nonsteroidal anti-inflammatory drugs (NSAIDs) are commonly used in all sprains for analgesia and to aid in reducing inflammation (see Table 35.5). The cyclooxygenase-2 (COX-2) agents rapidly became the most commonly prescribed drugs in the NSAID class because of claims of reduced gastrointestinal toxicity. The claim of reduced gastrointestinal complications is not proven with long-term use or concurrent use of aspirin. The COX-2 inhibitors are comparable to other NSAIDs and acetaminophen for analgesia. Further, the US Food and Drug Administration pulled the COX-2 rofecoxib in September 2004 due to an increased risk of heart attack and stroke with long-term use.

Grades I and II lateral ankle sprains usually heal in approximately 8–15 days, respectively. Grade I sprains are treated symptomatically with ice, compression wraps, and elevation. Contrary to intuition, these sprains do not require immobilization. Early mobilization improves function, reduces pain and swelling and speeds return to work and sports (15, 16). Grade II sprains should be treated with ice, compression, and elevation for 48 to 72 hours, along with immobilization in a lace-up splint for 2 to 7 days (17). Crutches will help the patient avoid putting weight on the injured ankle.

The management of grade III lateral ankle sprains is similar, although recovery is longer, and some patients may require surgery. The management of syndesmosis sprains follows that of third-degree sprains. Healing time is 6 to 8 weeks, and a longer period of immobilization is needed. Removable splints (i.e., posterior splint, pneumatic splint, or a Bledsoe brace) or casting facilitates progressive weight-bearing. Progressive weight-bearing, as tolerated, should be allowed, and analgesics should be prescribed. Passive range-of-motion exercises (e.g., tracing the alphabet, drawing circles, etc. with the foot), especially dorsiflexion, should begin within a week of the injury. Although one systematic review (18) suggests that patients with severe sprains do better with surgery, a more critical review suggests that the methods to support this conclusion are too flawed (19).

TABLE 35.4 Management of Ankle Sprain

Treatment	Efficacy	Strength of Recommendation*	Comment
Early mobilization (15, 16)	Compared with those treated with bracing, patients treated with early mobilization are twice as likely to return to sport; return to activity 5 days sooner; 2.6 times less likely to experience instability; and 1.8 times more likely to be satisfied with their outcome.	A	Systematic review of clinical trials have found no studies showing harm, reduced function, or pain and most show improvement in patient-oriented outcomes with early mobilization.
Lace-up ankle brace (17)	Compared with semi-rigid braces, lace-up braces are 4 times less likely to experience swelling	A	
Semi-rigid brace (17)	Compared with elastic bandage, patients return to activity 4 days sooner.	A	
Physiotherapy (20)	Prevents subsequent sprains	B	

*A = consistent, good-quality patient-oriented evidence; B = inconsistent or limited-quality patient-oriented evidence; C = consensus, disease-oriented evidence, usual practice, expert opinion, or case series. For information about the SORT evidence rating system, see *http://www.aafp.org/afpsort.xml*.

LONG-TERM MANAGEMENT

Rehabilitation of the ankle joint is important in preventing future sprains, although the data are limited (20). Rehabilitation includes strengthening exercises, proprioception training, and functional exercises. The removable splints should be worn until the individual has been pain-free for at least 2 weeks. Patients with sprains treated only by cast immobilization take longer to return to full activity and have worse outcomes unless patients receive intensive rehabilitation and are closely monitored. To speed recovery and minimize time off from work or sport, the use of physical therapy is strongly recommended. Recurrent ankle sprains and chronic pain after an ankle sprain are usually the result of inadequate rehabilitation. These individuals should receive more extensive supervised therapy. If pain persists after an injury despite adequate rehabilitation, occult fracture should be suspected, especially talar dome fractures.

Ankle supports such as semi-rigid orthoses or air-cast braces have been shown to prevent ankle sprains during high-risk sporting activities (e.g., soccer, basketball) (21).

Ankle Fractures

Many fractures can be managed in the office without referral. Avulsion or chip fractures are the most common and can occur at the distal fibula below the level of the mortise, the distal portion of the tibial plafond, and the anterior surface of the talus. Regardless of size, these usually can be treated according to the degree of the associated ankle sprain. If the fragments are displaced more than 2 mm, immobilize the patient in a cast or posterior splint and refer to an orthopedic surgeon. Avulsion fractures of the peroneus brevis insertion from the fifth metatarsal head will heal without treatment but should be immobilized until weight-bearing can be tolerated. Non-displaced navicular and cuboid fractures should be casted.

Fractures of the talus within the mortise, the fibula at or above the joint or mortise surface, the tibial plafond near the joint line, and bimalleolar, trimalleolar, and any displaced fractures should be immobilized and referred. You should refer patients with fractures of the base of the fifth metatarsal (Jones' fracture) and of the growth plate (Salter-Harris fractures) to an orthopedic surgeon. Do not forget to provide analgesics for your patient (see Table 35.5).

Achilles Tendinitis

The evidence to support various management options for Achilles tendinitis is insufficient to suggest a specific best approach (22). Conservative management until better data come along makes reasonable sense: relative rest, rehabilitation of the gastrocnemius and soleus muscles, ice, heel lifts, and analgesics. Rehabilitation of the calf muscles begins with progressive stretching and range-of-motion exercises followed by strength training. NSAIDs may be helpful in reducing pain and inflammation (see Table 35.5). Steroid injection has been advocated by some, but is controversial (22). Attempts should also be made to correct biomechanical abnormalities. Surgery is recommended only for patients who fail conservative therapy and desire to continue running, and those with Achilles tendon ruptures. The rate of rerupture is about 13% in patients treated conservatively compared with about 4% in those treated surgically (number needed to treat = 11; 95% confidence interval [CI], 7–29). However, complications such as adhesions, altered sensation, keloids, and infection appeared in one third of patients treated surgically and in fewer than 3% of patients treated nonoperatively (number needed to treat to harm = 4; 95% CI 2–5). These complications were less common when the repair was percutaneous than with open repair. Given the downside, casting may be reasonable in sedentary patients.

TABLE 35.5 Pharmacotherapy for Ankle or Knee Pain*

Drug	Dosage	Contraindications/Cautions/Adverse Effects	Relative Cost
Acetaminophen	325–650 mg Q 4–6 hrs, up to maximum of 4000 mg daily	History of current ETOH abuse, liver dysfunction	$
Aspirin	Up to 4,000 mg/day (Q 4–6 hr)	NSAID allergy; third trimester of pregnancy; active ulcer; varicella or influenza infection in children and teenagers; caution in pregnancy, lactation, asthma, elderly, impaired renal or liver function, GI ulcers; Adverse effects—prolonged bleeding time, life-threatening allergic reactions, salicylism	$
Ibuprofen	Up to 3200mg/day (TID to QID)	All NSAIDs have the same contraindications as aspirin.	$
Naproxen	250–550mg BID-TID), maximum of 1500 mg/day		$
Tolmetin	600–1,800 mg/ day (TID), maximum 180 mg/day		$$$
Diclofenac	100–150 mg/day (BID-TID) maximum 200 mg/day bid		$
Indomethacin	25–150 mg BID - QID; maximum 200 mg/day	History of proctitis, rectal bleeding (suppository form); late pregnancy; adverse effects: frontal headache, fluid	$
Oxaprozin	1,200 mg once daily, maximum 1800 mg/day	Avoid use in the elderly	$$$
Piroxicam	20 mg once daily	Depression; Parkinson's disease; epilepsy; sepsis	$
Etodolac	600–1,200 mg/day (BID-QID), maximum 1,200 mg/day		$$
Nabumetone	1,000–2,000 mg/day (QD or BID)	Slow onset of action; most useful for chronic pain	$$
Celexicob	100–200mg QD -BID	Caution when used with patients with cardiovascular disease†, reduced gastrointestinal bleeding (7%) in select populations, but it still can occur	$$$
Etodolac	600–1,200 mg/day(BID-QID), maximum 1,200 mg/day		$$
Nabumetone	1,000–2,000 mg/day (QD or BID)	Slow onset of action; most useful for chronic pain	$$
Celexicob	100–200mg QD -BID	Caution when used with patients with cardiovascular disease†, reduced gastrointestinal bleeding (7%) in select populations, but it still can occur	$$$

Abbreviations: ETOH, alcohol; GI, gastrointestinal; NSAID, nonsteroidal anti-inflammatory drugs.
*$ = <$33, $$ = $34–$66, $$$ > $67.
*The degree of analgesic effect does not vary significantly among acetaminophen, nonsteroidal anti-inflammatory drugs, and COX-2 inhibitors.
†COX II inhibitors have been linked with increased risk of thrombotic events resulting in some having been withdrawn from the market (48).

1. Would you x-ray the ankle?

According to the Ottawa Ankle Rules (OAR), the patient does NOT need x-rays of the injured ankle. He exhibited no focal bony tenderness over the navicular bone or either malleolus and ambulated immediately post-injury and four steps in the office.

2. What would you tell the athlete who wants a radiograph?

Explain to the athlete in understandable terms that the likelihood of fracture is extremely low when the OAR are negative. Inform the athlete that the expected clinical course is approximately 8 days to resolution for a grade I sprain, and that any pain persisting beyond that would be an indication for radiographs.

3. What initial course of treatment would you recommend?

The player presents with a grade I ankle sprain. Thus, the focus of treatment would be symptomatic relief. Symptomatic treatment would include ice, compression wraps, elevation, nonsteroidal anti-inflammatory drugs for analgesia and anti-inflammatory effects, and weight-bearing to patient tolerance. You should counsel the patient on expected course of healing (approximately 8 days). No immobilization is indicated in grade I ankle sprains.

KNEE PAIN

Although ankles are the most commonly injured joint in sports, patients see a physician twice as frequently for knee pain, accounting for nearly 2 million visits to family physicians annually (1). Similar to ankle pain, knee pain is most commonly caused by acute injury, overuse, or more commonly from degenerative joint disease. The differential diagnosis for knee pain is summarized in Table 35.1.

The demands of sports and recreation have created stresses for knees that are vulnerable to rotation, direct contact, and repetitive load. Although the history provides major clues to the diagnosis, knowledge of the anatomy and a careful examination of the knee are essential. Primary care physicians can manage most knee injuries. Some acute knee injuries require surgery to restore function and allow return to work or play; this underscores the importance of an accurate diagnosis and knowledge of the appropriate criteria for referral.

The knee joint (see Figure 35.4) consists of the patella, tibia, and femur. The patella is a sesamoid bone with a keel-shaped undersurface that fits between the medial and lateral femoral condyles. The primary stabilizers of the knee are the anterior and posterior cruciate ligaments (ACL and PCL), the medial and lateral collateral ligaments (MCL and LCL), the menisci, the joint capsule, and the medial and lateral retinacula that attach to the patella. Secondary stabilizers of the knee include the iliotibial band (tensor fascia lata) and the quadriceps, hamstrings, and popliteus muscles.

The knee acts as a hinge that allows forward translation and internal rotation of the tibia during leg flexion and rearward translation and external rotation during extension. While the knee is flexed, the MCL and LCL provide stability to medially and laterally directed stress, respectively. The

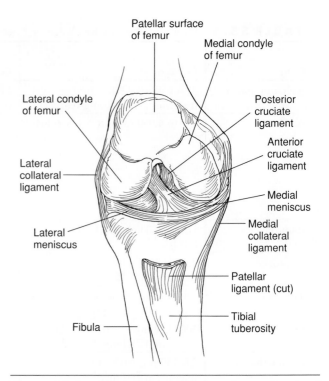

Figure 35.4 • Knee joint, anterior view. (Reprinted with permission from Rucker LM. Essentials of Adult Ambulatory Care. Baltimore, MD: Williams & Wilkins; 1997:556.)

MCL and LCL also limit external and internal rotation during knee extension and flexion. The ACL is the only structure that prevents anterior movement of the tibia on the femur. It also helps the MCL stabilize the knee during lateral stress when the knee is flexed. The PCL resists posterior movement of the tibia on the femur. The crescent-shaped medial and lateral menisci act primarily as shock absorbers but also stabilize the knee during movements such as pivoting. The popliteus muscle holds the lateral meniscus back during knee flexion, locks the knee in full extension, and unlocks the knee during the initiation of flexion.

Injuries to the knee ligaments and cartilage are common, although the exact frequency depends upon the population and activity. For example, skiers have approximately four ACL injuries per 100,000 skier days (23), while soccer players have about 0.1 injuries per 1,000 player hours (24). Women are 2 to 8 times as likely as men to sustain ACL injuries (25). Isolated meniscus tears are the most frequent acute knee injury in an athletic population. Nordic skiers have a high rate of knee injury (2.1 injuries per 1,000 skier days), even though many people consider this activity to be "easy on the knees." Most (58%) of these injuries, however, are to the MCL (26).

DIFFERENTIAL DIAGNOSIS

AKP (a catch-all term that includes common conditions such as patellar tendonitis, patellofemoral dysfunction, chondromalacia patellae, etc.) and osteoarthritis (OA) of the knee are other common causes of knee pain and are seen in athletes and nonathletes alike. Osgood-Schlatter's disease should also be considered when pubescent children present with AKP.

Acute traumatic injuries to the knee include tears of the ACL, MCL, LCL, and menisci. Other examples of acute trauma include dislocation or subluxation of the patella and fractures of the patella, tibial plateau, femoral condyles, and fibular head. Common chronic traumatic injuries include patellar tendonitis and chondromalacia patellae. AKP is a heterogeneous group of disorders, but has become synonymous with chondromalacia patellae. Chondromalacia patellae is also called patellofemoral dysfunction (PFD), because the underlying cause of chondromalacia is thought to be poor tracking of the patella between the femoral condyles.

The mechanism of injury is an important clue to the specific diagnosis. Collateral ligament injuries result from medially or laterally directed stress to a planted knee, such as in football or skiing. Posterior cruciate injuries are rare and usually occur in a motor vehicle accident when a flexed knee hits a dashboard. The ACL can be injured by many mechanisms such as: an external force applied to a planted knee (e.g., during a football tackle); hyperextension and internal rotation (e.g., a basketball or volleyball player landing on somebody's foot); sudden deceleration with a flexed knee that pivots or rotates (e.g., a skiing fall); landing and pivoting or cutting (e.g., in soccer); or falling backward with a ski boot, displacing the tibia anteriorly. These mechanisms are not specific for ACL injuries, as sudden twisting or pivoting can also injure the menisci or cause patellar dislocation.

Chronic knee pain may be a long-term sequela of previous injury, especially if it was incompletely rehabilitated. Chronic knee pain is often associated with weak quadriceps muscles from disuse, resulting in PFD or AKP. The causes of OA are multiple. The primary problem may, in fact, be genetic, traumatic, or obesity rather than overactivity or exercise (27).

CLINICAL EVALUATION

When evaluating a patient with knee pain, you should ask about the location, duration, character, and intensity of pain. You should also obtain a description of potential contributing mechanisms, the position of the knee at the time of the injury, ameliorating or exacerbating factors, previous injury, and current treatment. Potential red flags, which are serious and may require early referral, are summarized in Table 35.2. Finally, you should determine the patient's treatment and activity goals, so management can be individualized.

History and Physical Examination

The mechanism of injury and the presence of hemarthrosis are the two strongest indicators of internal derangement of the knee. Patients with hemarthrosis are likely to complain of sudden swelling (less than 24 hours after the injury) and bruising. Hearing or feeling a "pop" suggests an ACL tear, whereas locking of the knee is typically associated with meniscus injuries or a loose joint body (usually cartilage). Inability to bear weight and persistent giving way of the knee indicate internal derangement but are not specific for any one injury. Patients with AKP often experience pain with specific actions

such as climbing up or down stairs, squatting, or prolonged sitting with the knees flexed. They may also report snapping, popping, clicking, or catching sensations in the knee. Patients with OA typically complain of stiffness with inactivity and pain with weight-bearing activity. In contrast to the stiffness associated with rheumatoid arthritis, the stiffness of OA often improves after a few minutes of activity. Swelling of the knee is not common in OA except during an acute flare-up or in the presence of severe OA associated with bony changes.

A thorough and complete knee examination for meniscus or ligamentous injury is better at diagnosis than any one specific maneuver (28). Table 35.3 summarizes the accuracy of various elements of the knee examination. The Lachman test is very good at ruling in and ruling out anterior cruciate ligament tears (likelihood ratio [LR]+, 25.0; LR-, 0.1) in experienced hands (28). The Lachman test is performed with the knee flexed to 20° to 30°; the top hand stabilizes the femur while the lower hand wraps around the inside of the proximal tibia, with the thumb on top directing anterior and slightly outward force. When the leg is too large or the hands too small, place a knee or other firm support under the thigh, and with both hands placed near the tibial plateau, determine the amount of anterior translation and the firmness of the end point. A 3-mm side-to-side difference or the absence of a distinct stop (also called an "endpoint") indicates an ACL tear. Before the Lachman test is performed, flex the knee to 90 degrees and push the tibia in a posterior direction (posterior drawer) to ensure PCL integrity. If the PCL is torn, the Lachman test is still accurate but must be done more carefully.

The presence of hemarthrosis suggests a significant knee injury that will require surgery. Patients with hemarthrosis usually have significant effusions and ecchymosis. Although it is difficult to distinguish between effusion and hemarthrosis without aspirating the joint, the presence of ecchymosis and the onset of swelling in less than 24 hours will favor hemarthrosis. Approximately 70% of knee injuries with hemarthrosis are ACL tears (29). Osteochondral fractures are seen in about 10% of knee injuries with hemarthrosis. Although many studies report the prevalence of derangement in a series of subjects with hemarthrosis, one cannot calculate likelihood ratios without knowing about the other injured patients who did not have hemarthrosis. This is a common problem in the orthopedic literature.

Joint line tenderness (JLT) is not very reliable for diagnosing meniscus tears (LR+, 0.9; LR-, 1.1) (28). Posterolateral or posteromedial pain that occurs at the extremes of flexion or extension suggests meniscal injury. In a patient with anterior JLT, pain with squatting suggests chondromalacia rather than a meniscus tear. The McMurray test (see Figure 35.5) is another physical examination maneuver used to detect meniscal damage. To perform this test, place the knee in full flexion. Using a combination of external rotation and valgus stress with the fingers along the lateral joint line and the lower hand cupping the heel, the knee is slowly brought into extension. (Varus stress bows the lower leg medially; valgus stress bows the lower leg laterally.) A palpable click suggests a lateral meniscus tear. With the fingers along the medial joint line, the same maneuver is performed with internal rotation and varus stress to detect medial meniscus tears. If the range of motion of the knee is restricted, a McMurray test cannot be

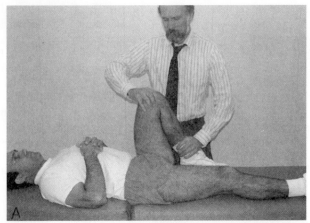

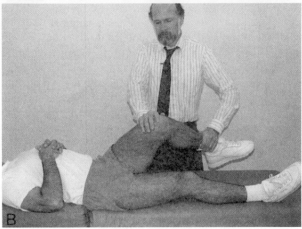

Figure 35.5 • McMurray test. **A.** Starting position. **B.** Extension of the leg with valgus and internal rotation evaluates the medial meniscus, while extension of the leg with varus force and external rotation evaluates the lateral meniscus. (Reproduced with permission from Hyde TE, Gengenbach MS. Conservative Management of Sports Injuries. Baltimore, MD: Williams & Wilkins; 1997:392.)

performed accurately. By itself, the McMurray test is neither sensitive (53%) nor specific (59%) (28).

When a patient's history suggests a collateral ligament injury, the severity is determined by the physical examination. Side-to-side comparisons are essential. Pathologic laxity is graded according to the amount of joint opening during Lachman's test, and is classified as grade 1 (less than 5 mm), grade 2 (5 to 8 mm), grade 3 (8 to 11 mm), and grade 4 (more than 11 mm) (30). Grade I and grade II tears have definite end points, but grade III tears have soft or mushy end points.

When diagnosing meniscal and/or ligamentous injuries of the knee, it is important to complete a comprehensive knee exam rather than using individual knee exams separately. When evaluating ACL tears, a composite assessment of the knee had a LR+ of 25.0 and LR- of 0.04. Evaluation of meniscal lesions using a composite assessment produced LR+ of 2.7 and LR- of 0.4. A combination of clinical exam maneuvers along with detailed history are better at diagnosing meniscal and ligamentous injuries of the knee rather than the use specific individual physical exam tests separately, although for

meniscal injuries, even the composite examination has only modest diagnostic accuracy (28).

If the diagnosis is uncertain (e.g., the patient is guarding too much or swelling prohibits adequate testing), application of ice, temporary immobilization, and the use of analgesics are common techniques for reducing the swelling and pain. The patient should return within a week for repeat evaluation.

Examination of the knee in patients with AKP often reveals atrophy of the quadriceps and crepitus with manipulation of the patella. Several clinical tests for AKP have been reported such as patellar apprehension, patellar compression, and patellar laxity. These are qualitative tests, and their accuracy has not been quantified. In the patellar apprehension test, the examiner applies inferiorly directed pressure at the superior portion of the patella. In the patellar compression test, the examiner firmly holds the patella in place while the patient contracts the quadriceps muscle. In either the patellar apprehension test or the patellar compression test, if the patient winces, grabs the knee, or otherwise voices displeasure, the test is considered positive. Patellar laxity is tested by manipulating the patella and determining the degree of movement in comparison with the opposite knee.

Diagnostic Testing

The accuracy of imaging studies for the evaluation of the injured knee is shown in Table 35.6. Stiell developed and validated the Ottawa Knee Rules (see Table 35.7) to assist in the evaluation of acute knee injuries, in patients 18 years of age and older (31, 32). He found that the rule is 100% sensitive for fracture, but other investigators have found somewhat lower sensitivity (85% to 97%). The rule is easy to use, and clinicians correctly interpret it 96% of the time (33). If the rule is negative, there is less than 1% risk of fracture. The Pittsburgh knee rules, another clinical decision tool for acute knee injures, is about 99% sensitive and 60% specific (34). The Pittsburgh knee rules recommend that radiography is ordered for patients with pain caused by a fall or blunt trauma, and who are less than 12 years of age or over 50 years old. For patients of other ages, x-rays are necessary only if patients are unable to walk four full weight-bearing steps.

In adolescents with open growth plates, a more conservative approach should be taken because no clinical prediction rules have been validated in this population. Also keep in mind that the decision rule applies only to an acutely injured knee. You may wish to obtain radiographs when you find bone pain in the absence of injury, when the patient experiences night pain, or when the patient's symptoms do not fit conventional diagnoses or respond to treatment. These symptoms may indicate the presence of more serious conditions (see Table 35.2).

In the absence of fracture, radiographs rarely alter the management of an acute knee injury. If internal derangement of the knee is suspected, the question of performing MRI arises. Although MRI is sensitive and specific for ACL tears, several studies have found it to be less accurate than the clinical examination (35–37). The literature on diagnostic testing suffers from many flaws, including the lack of an accepted gold standard, the absence of a wide spectrum of injury severity, and failure to adequately account for the potential effect of examiner experience.

MRI should not be used to diagnose a suspected isolated

TABLE 35.6 Characteristics of Diagnostic Tests in Patients with Knee Pain

Diagnosis	Test	Sens	Spec	LR +	LR −
"Internal derangement"	MRI	0.82	0.87	6.3	0.2
"Acute meniscus tear"	MRI*	0.89	0.92	11	0.1
Chondromalacia patellae	MRI†	0.29	0.97	9.6	0.7
	MR arthrogram	0.69	0.99	70	0.3
	CT arthrogram	0.65	0.99	65	0.3

Abbreviations: CT, computed tomography; MR, magnetic resonance; MRI, magnetic resonance imaging.
*Reported range of sensitivity 0.82 to 0.95, specificity 0.87 to 0.95.
†Reported range of sensitivity 0.19 to 0.38.

ACL tear. If an examiner is not certain that there is an ACL tear, referral to a physician with greater experience is usually more cost effective than ordering an MRI (35). MRIs have been used to search for associated meniscal lesions or bone contusions because the presence of these lesions is a relative indication for surgical ACL repair. This approach is being abandoned because most ACL tears usually are repaired. An exception is the patient who initially elects not to have surgery for an ACL tear. If meniscal damage is seen on the MRI along with the ACL tear, surgical repair should be strongly encouraged.

MRI will also detect meniscal lesions. The sensitivity and specificity vary from 82% to 95% and 87% to 95%, respectively. An MRI can be helpful if a patient with a strongly suggestive history and persistent pain has a negative clinical examination and poor response to conservative therapy (several weeks of rest followed by physical therapy). However, as many as 16% of asymptomatic patients may have meniscal abnormalities on MRI (38, 39)! This emphasizes the importance of taking a good history and using clinical signs to determine a mechanism for injury and then deciding if an MRI is warranted.

Although AKP is best diagnosed clinically, several radiographic procedures, such as plain radiography, MRI, computed axial tomography (CT) scan, sonography, and scintigraphy, are also available. None are needed in most patients with AKP. Imaging should be reserved for those who fail to respond to therapy or if the diagnosis is in doubt. The characteristics of these tests are summarized in Table 35.6. Although radiographs using Merchant's views have been a standard among some specialists for years, the findings rarely alter the initial conservative management. Merchant's views are performed with the knees flexed 45 degrees and the X-ray beam declined 30 degrees. More than 16 degrees of subluxation is considered abnormal.

Gagliardi (40) compared MRI, MR arthrography, and CT arthrography to surgical findings in patients with AKP ranging from mild to severe. MRI was relatively insensitive (19% to 38% depending upon severity) but very specific (97%). MR arthrography was more sensitive (69%) and was also specific (99%). CT arthrography was most sensitive (65%), and had 100% specificity. Thus, each procedure was very good at ruling in disease if positive (LR +, 7 to 14 for MRI, and 60 to 70 for CT or MR arthrography) but was less helpful when normal (LR-, 0.3 to 0.8).

All of the following results may be found on radiographs of patients with OA: normal findings; sclerotic joint margins; asymmetric joint space narrowing; subchondral cyst formation; osteophytes; and bone destruction. None of these findings are specific, and they may be found in many other arthritides.

MANAGEMENT

Begin by assessing the patient's goals and current level of function. Symptom relief should then be addressed, as that is usually the reason the patient seeks care, followed by helping the patient return to function. Table 35.8 summarizes the available treatment options and the level of evidence to support them; medications commonly used for management of knee pain are listed in Table 35.5.

There are five major reasons to refer a patient for knee surgery, which include the following: hemarthrosis or rapid fluid accumulation; ACL or meniscus tears; third-degree collateral ligament injuries; uncertainty about the diagnosis; or poor response to conservative treatment. Appropriate surgical referral, therefore, depends on the ability of the primary care physician to perform an accurate and complete history and physical examination of the patient with knee pain.

Initial Management of Knee Injuries

The initial management of an acute knee injury depends on the type and severity of the injury. Fractures should be immo-

TABLE 35.7 The Ottawa Knee Rules

Obtain a radiograph of the knee if the patient has any of the following characteristics:

- Age 55 years or older
- Tenderness at the head of the fibula
- Isolated patella tenderness
- Inability to flex to 90 degrees
- Inability to bear weight both immediately and in the emergency department (four weight transfers onto each leg, regardless of limping)

Adapted from Stiell IG, Greenberg GH, Wells GA, et al. Derivation of a decision rule for the use of radiography in acute knee injuries. Ann Emerg Med. 1995;26:405–413.

TABLE 35.8 Management of the Most Common Causes of Knee Pain

Diagnosis	Treatment	Strength of Recommendation*	Comments
Knee pain (49)	Exercise: NNT = 13 to reduce pain by greater than 50%	B	2-year exercise program
Anterior cruciate ligament tear	Surgery: unclear benefit(41)	C	
Meniscus tear	Surgery	C	
Osteoarthritis	Glucosamine (Rotta preparation), NNT = 5 to improve pain		
	Intra-articular corticosteroid injection(46): NNT = 5 for improved pain at 6 months	A	
Severe osteoarthritis	Arthroscopic debridement is no more effective than sham surgery	B	
Anterior knee pain	Patella taping (compared with sham taping, pain is reduced 1.9 points on 10 point scale)(43)	B	

Abbreviation: NNT, number needed to treat

*A = consistent, good-quality patient-oriented evidence; B = inconsistent or limited-quality patient-oriented evidence; C = consensus, disease-oriented evidence, usual practice, expert opinion, or case series. For information about the SORT evidence rating system, see *http://www.aafp.org/afpsort.xml*.

bilized in a long leg splint, patients referred immediately to an orthopedic surgeon, and appropriate analgesia given. Collateral ligament tears, whether grade I or grade II, should be treated with a knee immobilizer and crutches until the pain has subsided enough to permit weight-bearing. Ice, compression, and elevation also help reduce pain and swelling. When unable to adequately examine an acutely injured knee, you should begin symptomatic therapy and reexamine within a week. To prevent weakness of the quadriceps and secondary AKP, the patient should begin isometric and leg raise exercises (one leg at a time) while wearing the immobilizer. As the pain dissipates, range-of-motion exercises should be started, followed by a progression of stationary bicycle riding and resistance exercises before returning to sports-specific training. Grade I sprains usually heal in a week or less, whereas grade II injuries may take 2 to 3 weeks to heal. Grade III injuries generally should be referred to an orthopedic surgeon. These injuries are usually treated with a brace that allows 30 degrees of flexion for 2 weeks; the brace is then unlocked to allow 30 to 90 degrees of flexion. Return to full activity may take up to 9 weeks.

The initial management of an ACL tear is immobilization and referral to an orthopedic surgeon. Factors associated with a greater likelihood of success with surgical reconstruction of the ACL include isolated injury (vs. multiple derangements), younger patient age, and activities that do not include jumping or cutting. Reduced likelihood of success may occur with greater degree of displacement of the tibia on the femur, physically demanding work activity or sports, and poor compliance with a rehabilitation program. Surgery is also indicated in an individual who initially elects not to have surgery but has repeated episodes of the knee "giving out" or is unable to perform daily activities.

The initial management of meniscus tears is controversial. In most cases, rest and protected weight-bearing combined with a short course of physical therapy comprise the initial treatment. If locking, pain, or inability to return to usual activities persists beyond 3 to 4 weeks, the patient should be referred.

Patellar dislocations are treated both surgically and conservatively, although the redislocation rate may be as high as 25% to 35% with conservative treatment. There may be an associated tear of the medial retinaculum or of the insertion of the vastus medialis. Conservative therapy consists of a brief period of immobilization, ice, and compression, followed by bracing the patella with a lateral buttress knee sleeve and starting a functional rehabilitation program. Patients usually are able to return to full activity after recovery.

Long-Term Management of Knee Disorders

For adult patients, it is unclear if the outcome of surgery for ACL tears is better than conservative treatment (41). Physical therapy is usually indicated for individuals undergoing casting or surgical procedures. Although physical therapy to strengthen the quadriceps and hamstrings in the ACL-deficient knee can allow the individual to return to sports or full activity, several prospective longitudinal studies have shown that the incidence of meniscal tears, degenerative arthritis, pain, and disability are significantly greater in those who elect conservative treatment. This is particularly true for those who have meniscus tears associated with the initial ACL tear. Prophylactic bracing has not been shown to stabilize the anterior cruciate deficient knee, or prevent these unsuccessful outcomes (42).

AKP generally should be managed conservatively, with analgesics (see Table 35.5), quadricep-strengthening exercises, patellar taping (43), and ice. Particularly useful are eccentric exercises that strengthen the quadriceps near the patellar insertion (44). These are performed by having the patient stand on one leg and then squat partially. Surgical intervention is usually not needed, and is reserved for patients who fail conservative therapy or have anatomic defects, such as patella alta or severe genu varum.

OA is a chronic, degenerative condition. NSAIDs are commonly prescribed, but no studies have evaluated their impact on functional outcomes or disease progression. As OA is not an inflammatory condition, NSAIDs may be no better than acetaminophen for long-term management of OA. A short NSAID course (1 to 2 weeks) may be beneficial during an acute flare-up.

Glucosamine, a form of amino sugar that occurs naturally in the body, is used to treat OA. It comes in two preparations, Rotta and non-Rotta. Only the Rotta preparation has shown any benefit for pain and function in patients with symptomatic OA (45). Corticosteroid injections are rarely indicated. Although intra-articular steroids may provide pain relief (46), the effect is brief and does not alter the course of the disease, and recurrent steroid use can damage articular cartilage. Physical therapy and flexibility and strength training may help to maintain function. Patients with refractory pain, impaired mobility, and severe OA on radiograph should be referred to an orthopedic surgeon for possible joint replacement, or intra-articular injection of viscous biosynthetic cartilage precursors (hyaluronic acid). However, arthroscopic debridement of the knee is no better than sham surgery in improving long-term pain and function (47). See Chapter 36 for a detailed discussion of OA.

CASE 2 DISCUSSION

This unfortunate patient has an acute injury with what appears to be a hemarthrosis and marked laxity of the anterior cruciate ligament. There is a high probability of acute rupture of the anterior cruciate ligament. The degree of guarding prevents you from being able to tell if there are other derangements, such as meniscal tears. The spasm and guarding are normal and should not divert your attention from a serious injury. The Ottawa Knee Rule is negative, so a radiograph is not necessary. This person needs to have the knee immobilized and should be on crutches. Give her appropriate medication for pain and arrange for orthopedic evaluation.

REFERENCES

1. National Ambulatory Medical Care Survey. Hyattsville, Maryland: National Center for Health Statistics; 2000.
2. Liu SH, Jason WJ. Lateral ankle sprains and instability problems. Clin Sports Med. 1994;13(4):793–809.
3. Nichols AW. Achilles tendinitis in running athletes. J Am Board Fam Pract. 1989;2(3):196–203.
4. Read MT, Motto SG. Tendo Achillis pain: steroids and outcome. Br J Sports Med. 1992;26(1):15–21.
5. Kowatari K, Nakashima K, Ono A, Yoshihara M, Amano M, Toh S. Levofloxacin-induced bilateral Achilles tendon rupture: a case report and review of the literature. J Orthop Sci. 2004;9(2):186–190.
6. Stiell IG, Greenberg GH, McKnight RD, et al. Decision rules for the use of radiography in acute ankle injuries. Refinement and prospective validation [see comments]. JAMA. 1993; 269(9):1127–1132.
7. Stiell IG, McKnight RD, Greenberg GH, et al. Implementation of the Ottawa ankle rules [see comments]. JAMA. 1994; 271(11):827–832.
8. Bachmann LM, Kolb E, Koller MT, Steurer J, ter Riet G. Accuracy of Ottawa ankle rules to exclude fractures of the ankle and mid-foot: systematic review. BMJ. 2003;326(7386): 417.
9. Pigman EC, Klug RK, Sanford S, Jolly BT. Evaluation of the Ottawa clinical decision rules for the use of radiography in acute ankle and midfoot injuries in the emergency department: an independent site assessment. Ann Emerg Med. 1994; 24(1):41–45.
10. Hartgerink P, Fessell DP, Jacobson JA, van Holsbeeck MT. Full- versus partial-thickness Achilles tendon tears: sonographic accuracy and characterization in 26 cases with surgical correlation. Radiology. 2001;220(2):406–412.
11. Kayser R, Mahlfeld K, Heyde CE. Partial rupture of the proximal Achilles tendon: a differential diagnostic problem in ultrasound imaging. Br J Sports Med. 2005;39(11):838–842; discussion 838–842.
12. Kainberger FM, Engel A, Barton P, Huebsch P, Neuhold A, Salomonowitz E. Injury of the Achilles tendon: diagnosis with sonography. AJR Am J Roentgenol. 1990;155(5): 1031–1036.
13. Haims AH, Schweitzer ME, Patel RS, Hecht P, Wapner KL. MR imaging of the Achilles tendon: overlap of findings in symptomatic and asymptomatic individuals. Skeletal Radiol. 2000;29(11):640–645.
14. Karjalainen PT, Soila K, Aronen HJ, et al. MR imaging of overuse injuries of the Achilles tendon. AJR Am J Roentgenol. 2000;175(1):251–260.
15. Nash CE, Mickan SM, Del Mar CB, Glasziou PP. Resting injured limbs delays recovery: a systematic review. J Fam Pract. 2004;53(9):706–712.
16. Kerkhoffs GM, Rowe BH, Assendelft WJ, Kelly K, Struijs PA, van Dijk CN. Immobilisation and functional treatment for acute lateral ankle ligament injuries in adults. Cochrane Database Syst Rev. 2002;3:CD003762.
17. Kerkhoffs GM, Struijs PA, Marti RK, Assendelft WJ, Blankevoort L, van Dijk CN. Different functional treatment strategies for acute lateral ankle ligament injuries in adults. Cochrane Database Syst Rev. 2002;3:CD002938.
18. Pijnenburg AC, Van Dijk CN, Bossuyt PM, Marti RK. Treatment of ruptures of the lateral ankle ligaments: a meta-analysis. J Bone Joint Surg Am. 2000;82(6):761–773.
19. Kerkhoffs GM, Handoll HH, de Bie R, Rowe BH, Struijs PA. Surgical versus conservative treatment for acute injuries of the lateral ligament complex of the ankle in adults. Cochrane Database Syst Rev. 2002;3:CD000380.
20. Thacker SB, Stroup DF, Branche CM, Gilchrist J, Goodman RA, Weitman EA. The prevention of ankle sprains in sports. A systematic review of the literature. Am J Sports Med. 1999; 27(6):753–760.
21. Handoll HH, Rowe BH, Quinn KM, de Bie R. Interventions for preventing ankle ligament injuries. Cochrane Database Syst Rev. 2001;3:CD000018.
22. McLauchlan GJ, Handoll HH. Interventions for treating acute and chronic Achilles tendinitis. Cochrane Database Syst Rev. 2001;2:CD000232.
23. Koehle MS, Lloyd-Smith R, Taunton JE. Alpine ski injuries and their prevention. Sports Med. 2002;32(12):785–793.
24. Bjordal JM, Arnly F, Hannestad B, Strand T. Epidemiology of anterior cruciate ligament injuries in soccer. Am J Sports Med. 1997;25(3):341–345.

25. Toth AP, Cordasco FA. Anterior cruciate ligament injuries in the female athlete. J Gend Specif Med. 2001;4(4):25–34.

26. Pigman EC, Karakla DW. Skiing injuries during initial military Nordic ski training of a U.S. Marine Corps Battalion Landing Team. Mil Med. 1990;155(7):303–305.

27. Sarzi-Puttini P, Cimmino MA, Scarpa R, et al. Osteoarthritis: an overview of the disease and its treatment strategies. Semin Arthritis Rheum. 2005;35(1 Suppl 1):1–10.

28. Solomon DH, Simel DL, Bates DW, Katz JN, Schaffer JL. The rational clinical examination. Does this patient have a torn meniscus or ligament of the knee? Value of the physical examination. JAMA. 2001;286(13):1610–1620.

29. Lundberg M, Odensten M, Thuomas KA, Messner K. The diagnostic validity of magnetic resonance imaging in acute knee injuries with hemarthrosis. A single-blinded evaluation in 69 patients using high-field MRI before arthroscopy. Int J Sports Med. 1996;17(3):218–222.

30. Lerat JL, Moyen BL, Cladiere F, Besse JL, Abidi H. Knee instability after injury to the anterior cruciate ligament. Quantification of the Lachman test. J Bone Joint Surg Br. 2000;82(1):42–47.

31. Stiell IG, Greenberg GH, Wells GA, et al. Derivation of a decision rule for the use of radiography in acute knee injuries. Ann Emerg Med. 1995;26(4):405–413.

32. Stiell IG, Wells GA, McDowell I, et al. Use of radiography in acute knee injuries: need for clinical decision rules. Acad Emerg Med. 1995;2(11):966–973.

33. Stiell IG, Greenberg GH, Wells GA, et al. Prospective validation of a decision rule for the use of radiography in acute knee injuries. JAMA. 1996;275(8):611–615.

34. Seaberg DC, Yealy DM, Lukens T, Auble T, Mathias S. Multicenter comparison of two clinical decision rules for the use of radiography in acute, high-risk knee injuries. Ann Emerg Med. 1998;32(1):8–13.

35. Gelb HJ, Glasgow SG, Sapega AA, Torg JS. Magnetic resonance imaging of knee disorders. Clinical value and cost-effectiveness in a sports medicine practice. Am J Sports Med. 1996;24(1):99–103.

36. Liu SH, Osti L, Henry M, Bocchi L. The diagnosis of acute complete tears of the anterior cruciate ligament. Comparison of MRI, arthrometry and clinical examination. J Bone Joint Surg Br. 1995;77(4):586–588.

37. Terry GC, Tagert BE, Young MJ. Reliability of the clinical assessment in predicting the cause of internal derangements of the knee. Arthroscopy. 1995;11(5):568–576.

38. Bhattacharyya T, Gale D, Dewire P, et al. The clinical importance of meniscal tears demonstrated by magnetic resonance imaging in osteoarthritis of the knee. J Bone Joint Surg Am. 2003;85-A(1):4–9.

39. Boden SD, Davis DO, Dina TS, et al. A prospective and blinded investigation of magnetic resonance imaging of the knee. Abnormal findings in asymptomatic subjects. Clin Orthop Relat Res. 1992(282):177–185.

40. Gagliardi JA, Chung EM, Chandnani VP, et al. Detection and staging of chondromalacia patellae: relative efficacies of conventional MR imaging, MR arthrography, and CT arthrography. AJR Am J Roentgenol. 1994;163(3):629–636.

41. Linko E, Harilainen A, Malmivaara A, Seitsalo S. Surgical versus conservative interventions for anterior cruciate ligament ruptures in adults. Cochrane Database Syst Rev. 2005; 2:CD001356.

42. Beynnon BD, Johnson RJ, Abate JA, Fleming BC, Nichols CE. Treatment of anterior cruciate ligament injuries, part 2. Am J Sports Med. 2005;33(11):1751–1767.

43. Hinman RS, Crossley KM, McConnell J, Bennell KL. Efficacy of knee tape in the management of osteoarthritis of the knee: blinded randomised controlled trial. BMJ. 2003; 327(7407):135.

44. Heintjes E, Berger MY, Bierma-Zeinstra SM, Bernsen RM, Verhaar JA, Koes BW. Exercise therapy for patellofemoral pain syndrome. Cochrane Database Syst Rev. 2003;4: CD003472.

45. Towheed TE, Maxwell L, Anastassiades TP, et al. Glucosamine therapy for treating osteoarthritis. Cochrane Database Syst Rev. 2005;2:CD002946.

46. Arroll B, Goodyear-Smith F. Corticosteroid injections for osteoarthritis of the knee: meta-analysis. BMJ. 2004;328(7444): 869.

47. Moseley JB, O'Malley K, Petersen NJ, et al. A controlled trial of arthroscopic surgery for osteoarthritis of the knee. N Engl J Med. 2002;347(2):81–88.

48. Bresalier RS, Sandler RS, Quan H, et al. Cardiovascular events associated with rofecoxib in a colorectal adenoma chemoprevention trial. N Engl J Med. 2005;352(11): 1092–1102.

49. Thomas KS, Muir KR, Doherty M, Jones AC, O'Reilly SC, Bassey EJ. Home based exercise programme for knee pain and knee osteoarthritis: randomised controlled trial. BMJ. 2002;325(7367):752.

CHAPTER 36

Arthritis and Rheumatism

John R. Gimpel

CASE

Mr. G., a 71-year-old Caucasian male who is working part-time as a manufacturer's representative, called the family practice office 3 weeks before his scheduled annual physical, asking if it would be advisable to try glucosamine for some occasional stiffness and pains in the joints of both of his hands. The symptoms had begun gradually over the past month, with stiffness noted also in the low back, legs, and one shoulder. Prior to this, his only joint complaints were occasional mild pain or stiffness in one of his knees. Mr. G. was advised that he could try glucosamine, but that results should not be expected for about a month, and this could be followed up on at his annual physical. He was also advised to try acetaminophen as needed for pain, and to call should symptoms worsen.

Upon arriving for his annual physical a few weeks later, further history is discussed. There has been no improvement with joint pain using glucosamine or acetaminophen. Mr. G. now notes that over the past 10 days he has had worsening fatigue, myalgias, and arthralgias, in addition to a decreased appetite. Morning stiffness in the upper and lower extremities lasts about 20–30 minutes, and his right hand has frequently swelled in the past week. His right ankle is swollen today for the first time. There is no headache, visual change, or jaw claudication, and he has not experienced fever.

During the past year, Mr. G. has noticed some fine shaking of his upper extremities when holding a coffee cup or writing. His son-in-law (a neurologist) suggested that he may have essential tremor, as well as the onset of some osteoarthritis. Being a golfer and living in an area endemic for Lyme disease, Mr. G. is concerned about the possibility of this condition, but is unaware of any tick bite or "bulls-eye" erythema migrans rash. He is also concerned as this is the busy time in his golf season, and he is unable to play with his sales clients at all now. Mr. G. is being treated with metformin for type 2 diabetes mellitus, as well as atorvastatin for dyslipidemia and metabolic syndrome, and enalapril/hydrocholothiazide for hypertension. There is no significant family history of arthritis or rheumatic conditions.

On physical examination, Mr. G. is afebrile, with a body mass index of 26.1% (reflecting five pounds of weight loss in the preceding three weeks), and a blood pressure of 170/70 mmHg. He appears to be mildly disheveled and somewhat anxious, which is unusual for him as he is usually well-dressed, well-groomed, and neat in appearance.

There is no evidence of skin rash or lesions, other than a few areas of actinic damage on his face. He has a mild intention tremor of both upper extremities, with no cog-wheeling rigidity or focal neurological deficits. There is mild redness and swelling noted in the metacarpophalangeal joints bilaterally, as well as mild swelling and tenderness of the right ankle. He has mild limitation of range of motion, with some tenderness of the right shoulder, and good range of motion of the knees bilaterally but with some joint enlargement and crepitus of one knee. His temporal arteries are nontender.

CLINICAL QUESTIONS

1. What is the differential diagnosis?
2. What initial diagnostic and therapeutic strategies would be most beneficial and cost effective?

Rheumatic diseases are the most prevalent chronic conditions in the United States, and a leading cause of disability (1). In addition to the high prevalence of arthritic diseases, many other common disorders present with signs and symptoms attributable to the joints and the musculoskeletal system. Over 43 million Americans were affected by arthritis and rheumatic conditions by the late 1990s, at a cost that is equivalent to 2.5% of the gross national product (2). In general, women suffer more frequently from rheumatic complaints than men, and the incidence of arthritic disorders increases rapidly above the age of 50 years. Globally, 20% of all visits to outpatient facilities worldwide are for musculoskeletal conditions (3). In the United States, musculoskeletal complaints rank first in the number of visits to physicians, and collectively disorders of the musculoskeletal system are the number one cause of chronic impairment. With the advancing age of the United States and world populations, the prevalence of musculoskeletal conditions will continue to increase over time.

Most patients with rheumatic complaints are seen first by primary care physicians. The term rheumatism has its roots in early medical practice and was used to describe syndromes involving stiffness and pains in joints and/or muscles. There are more than 100 rheumatic diseases and conditions; however, many of these often cannot clearly be categorized or distinguished from each other (4). The definitive diagnosis may become apparent only after symptoms have been present for some time. The most common problems include degenerative osteoarthritis (OA); soft tissue syndromes such as bursitis, myofascial trigger points, and fibromyalgia; rheumatoid ar-

TABLE 36.1 Prevalence of Rheumatic Disorders per 1,000 Population

Soft Tissue Rheumatic Conditions	Prevalence per 1,000 Population
Nonarticular	132
Bursitis, tendonitis, synovitis	11
Shoulder syndromes	7
Humeral epicondylitis	4
Fibromyalgia	30 women 5 men
Somatic Dysfunction	200
Osteoarthritis (all ages)	
Any joints	250
Hip	13
Knee	35
Osteoarthritis (age >65 y)	
Any joints	750
Knee	95
Hip	55
Gout or pseudogout	3
All ages	3
Age >50 y	15
Inflammatory arthritis	
Rheumatoid arthritis	25
Systemic lupus erythematosus	0.04
Polymyalgia rheumatica (age >50 y)	0.2–0.7
Giant cell arteritis (age >50 y)	0.05–0.1

thritis (RA), and gout (see Table 36.1). Connective tissue diseases such as polymyositis and dermatomyositis, Sjögren's syndrome, and systemic lupus erythematosus (SLE) are encountered rarely (4, 5). Diseases related to infectious causes, such as reactive arthritis, Lyme disease, parvovirus B19, and septic arthritis, are also encountered on a periodic basis in the family practice setting, depending on region of the country or associated patient risk factors. There are many other dysfunctions of the structure and function of the musculoskeletal system (e.g., strains and sprains, somatic dysfunction) that are commonly encountered in primary care practice. Though not generally classified as a rheumatic condition, the diagnosis and treatment of somatic dysfunction will be briefly described in this chapter.

INITIAL EVALUATION

History

When evaluating a patient with joint or musculoskeletal pain, you should determine whether the pain is acute, subacute or chronic, articular (involving a joint or joints themselves) versus nonarticular, and inflammatory versus noninflammatory. Rheumatic presentations can often be classified as regional or generalized, symmetric or asymmetric, peripheral or central,

and progressive or nonprogressive. Are there symptoms suggestive of inflammation or damage to musculoskeletal structures? Is there any evidence, e.g., fever, rash or weight loss, which may indicate a systemic process? Consider whether there are any extra articular features, and attempt to determine functional loss or disability as well as the impact of the problem on the patient's life and well-being. An acute onset of symptoms over fewer than 4 weeks may suggest septic arthritis, gout, or possibly tendonitis, whereas a more chronic and insidious onset suggests OA, RA, or a collagen vascular disease. Articular symptoms suggest OA, RA, gout, or a collagen vascular disease, whereas nonarticular symptoms are associated with soft tissue syndromes such as fibromyalgia, tendonitis, and bursitis. Finally, more diffuse (and even systemic) inflammatory symptoms suggest RA or a collagen vascular disease (see Table 36.2).

The specific location or region of a musculoskeletal problem often is the most important clue to identifying the specific cause. Although there can be overlap, regional syndromes typically affect a single joint or periarticular structure, or an extremity or body region. A regional pain syndrome may also be from referred pain, in which the painful area is distant to the actual source of the disorder (e.g., gallbladder disease or apical lung mass presenting as shoulder pain). Specific arthropathies have a predilection for involving specific joint areas. For example, symmetric involvement of the wrists and

TABLE 36.2 Nonarticular Features of Rheumatic Disorders

Feature	Possible Diagnosis
Skin and/or nail changes	Psoriasis, scleroderma, systemic lupus erythematosus, Reiter's syndrome, Lyme disease (erythema migrans)
Cutaneous/subcutaneous nodules	Gout, rheumatoid arthritis
Conjunctivitis/uveitis/dry eyes	Rheumatoid arthritis, Sjögren's syndrome, Reiter's syndrome
Chest pain, cough, dyspnea	Rheumatoid arthritis, systemic lupus erythematosus
Diarrhea/abdominal pain	Scleroderma, rheumatoid arthritis, Reiter's syndrome, arthritis of inflammatory bowel disease
Dysuria/urethral discharge	Reiter's syndrome

proximal small joints of hands and feet may implicate the diagnosis of RA. Psoriatic arthritis often involves the distal joints of hands and feet, and gout classically presents as an acutely painful and swollen great toe.

The mode of onset and duration of symptoms can also help in making the diagnosis; most chronic rheumatic diseases present with an onset that is subacute—weeks to months rather than hours to days, as compared to gout, Lyme disease, and septic arthritis, where there is typically an acute crescendo of symptoms within hours. In fibromyalgia, the pain typically has spanned years with episodic exacerbations. In inflammatory joint diseases such as RA, the cardinal joint signs and symptoms classically include redness (rubor), warmth or heat (calor), pain (dolor), and swelling (tumor). In RA, when inflammation involves the synovial membranes (synovitis), the patient will experience joint stiffness after immobility, though this symptom can also be present in OA. Typically with degenerative diseases such as OA, joint stiffness and pain will exacerbate with joint use. Although most rheumatic diseases involve morning stiffness, the duration of morning stiffness is a semiquantitative measure of degree of articular inflammation. Early-morning stiffness takes quite a bit longer to dissipate (45 to 60 or more minutes) in inflammatory arthritidies such as RA, than in patients with OA (15 to 30 minutes).

Whereas many rheumatic patients will report generalized weakness in response to pain from articular or perarticular inflammation (e.g., RA and polymylagia rheumatica), patients who present with actual weakness may lead you to suspect muscular pathology. In patients with primary myopathic processes with weakness (e.g., myopathy), muscle weakness is typically symmetrical and involves the proximal muscles most severely. In those with neuropathic processes (e.g., multiple sclerosis, Charcot-Marie-Tooth disease), the distal muscles are more commonly involved (6). Abnormal joint function and disuse also lead directly to muscle wasting.

Patients with arthritic complaints should be questioned about constitutional and systemic symptoms. You may find fatigue, weight loss, anorexia, or low-grade fever with any systemic inflammatory process. Recent genitourinary symptoms and asymmetric oligoarthopathy in the lower extremity suggests reactive arthritis, and the same articular pattern associated with recurrent abdominal pain and bloody diarrhea might also suggest reactive arthritis or the arthopathy of inflammatory bowel disease. A review of systems should include

questions about rashes, tick bites, or skin changes, photosensitivity, mouth ulcers, and dryness of eyes and mouth. Ask about Raynaud's phenomenon, where patients complain of cold hands and feet that are associated with bouts of skin pallor and subsequent cyanosis of the digits. These symptoms are triggered by exposure to cold temperatures or emotional stress, and involve vasospasm of the muscular digital arteries. Primary Raynaud's phenomenon occurs in 5%–15% of the population, typically with an onset between ages 15–25; symptoms are generally mild. Causes of secondary Raynaud's, characterized by attacks that are more intense and associated with ischemic tissue change, include connective tissue disorders such as polymyositis and dermatomyositis, systemic sclerosis, and SLE (6). Fever may indicate sepsis, acute RA, SLE, gout, viral arthritis (e.g., parvovirus B19), or Lyme disease. Some weight loss is often associated with RA, SLE, and scleroderma. Other important aspects of the history include performance of activities of daily living, type of employment and work capacity, sexual function, quality of sleep, and the patient's emotional state. Key elements of the history and physical examination are shown in Table 36.3.

Genetics and Family History

An important aspect of the patient's history includes a family history of the same or similar symptoms (e.g., OA before 40 years of age, gout, and rheumatoid arthritis), and a family history of other autoimmune diseases (e.g., diabetes mellitus, thyroid disorders). Most of the common rheumatic diseases, including autoimmune diseases, result from the interaction of genetic and nongenetic factors. However, aggregation in families for most autoimmune diseases is rather modest; those with RA or SLE may not have a close relative with the same illness. For example, the relative risk for RA in siblings is 2%–17%, and in monozygotic twins is 12%–60% (7). Most of the attention in rheumatic diseases is focused on the major histocompatibility complex (MHC) on chromosome 6, which includes the primary genes that determine immune response patterns and encode the human leukocyte antigens (HLA). However, other genes outside the MHC, such as the tumor necrosis factor (TNF) cytokine pathway, contribute to autoimmune and inflammatory disorders. While the association of HLA with disease provides a classic example of how to develop evidence that a particular allele confers risk for a disease, the relative risks (RR) are generally less than 10, with the

TABLE 36.3 Key Elements of the History and Physical Examination for the Patient with Joint Pain

History

　Specific: joint pain, weakness, stiffness, fatigue

　Joint pattern: number affected, symmetric/asymmetric involvement

　Morning stiffness (15–30 minutes in osteoarthritis, 45–60 minutes in inflammatory arthritis)

　Trajectory: speed of onset, migratory (i.e., Lyme disease), intermittent (i.e., gout), progressive (i.e., rheumatoid arthritis, osteoarthritis)

　Function: assess activities of daily living, assess psychosocial impact of illness

Physical

　Screening musculoskeletal examination, motion/strength testing, examination of normal/abnormal joints, check skin and other systems

Red flags

　Fever, chills, and a monoarticular presentation suggest septic arthritis (especially in prosthetic joint or immunocompromised host)

　Weight loss suggests malignancy with metastases to bone or rheumatoid arthritis

　Constitutional along with multiorgan system signs and symptoms suggests systemic lupus erythematosus, collagen vascular disorder

　Headaches, loss of vision, scalp tenderness, and/or jaw claudication suggest giant cell arteritis

exception of HLA B27 and the spondyloarthropathies, where the RR values approach 100 for ankylosing spondylitis (6).

Physical Examination

The physical examination should start with a general observation of the patient and a review of the patient's vital signs. Fever can suggest an infectious cause but can also be present in acute gout or pseudogout, RA, and immunocompromised patients (8). A screening musculoskeletal examination should include visual inspection, palpation, and the evaluation of joint motion. Observe the patient's general appearance and gait, when possible, and determine static findings such as spinal curves, posture, and general anatomical landmarks. Look for anatomic and functional symmetry (e.g., shoulder heights, scapulae, thenar muscle masses, etc.). With individual joints, look for evidence of articular inflammation, including redness, joint line tenderness, pain on motion, and intra-articular swelling or effusion. Swelling of an arthritic joint can be further exaggerated by adjacent muscle wasting, and is caused by diffuse and usually symmetric enlargement of the synovial membrane. A careful hands-on physical examination can help determine when the soft tissues around a joint are the source of pain, e.g., in olecranon bursitis or prepatellar bursitis (8).

Inspect the hands for muscular atrophy (hollowing of the spaces between metacarpals), and alignment of digits relative to wrist and forearm. Ulnar deviation of the digits is associated with RA. Examine the nails for onycholysis or psoriatic pitting. The presence of redness and telangiectatasia of the nail fold capillaries with close inspection or with magnification indicates a connective tissue disease, such as SLE, scleroderma, or dermatomyositis. Sclerodactyl, or visible and palpable tightening of the skin around the digits, is also typical of scleroderma as is the presence of ulcers in the pulp of digits. Inspect the joints and periarticular structures for swelling, deformity,

erythema, and nodules. Heberden's and Bouchard's nodes are the articular swelling of the distal interphalangeal (DIP) and proximal interphalangeal (PIP) joints, respectively, and are typical of OA. Dactylitis, which is the diffuse swelling and redness of a whole digit, suggests spondyloarthropathy (e.g., psoriatic or reactive arthritis).

Effusions are collections of fluid within the joint caused by inflammation or trauma. The joint capsule is distended, and the fluid can be moved to different parts of the joint by external pressure. Irregular bony enlargement can coexist with synovial swelling and occurs most often in OA of the knee and interphalangeal joints of the hand. Local areas of tenderness over the joint or soft tissue usually indicate inflammation. In acute inflammatory arthritis, the skin overlying the joint may be reddened or even edematous. Palpate any affected joints or muscle areas. You may elicit tenderness or detect warmth over a joint that may be proportionate to the degree of inflammation. Synovial swelling has a jelly-like feel and is often tender and warm to the touch, but may not be painful when the joint is moved passively. Rheumatic disease can also present with discrete nodules under the skin on tendon sheaths or in bursae.

You may be able to feel tissue texture abnormalities over a joint or in muscular and soft tissue structures, such as increased humidity or moisture over an inflamed structure, or a ropy, fibrotic thickened feel to a chronically contracted muscle. Palpate for crepitus, a grinding sensation that is most often caused by the motion of eroded cartilage and adjacent bone surfaces in OA. Crepitus can also be felt in inflamed tendon sheaths. An algorithm to distinguish different rheumatic and connective tissue disorders is shown in Figure 36.1.

Next, proceed with range of motion (ROM) testing. Regional screening can help to identify individual joints for fur-

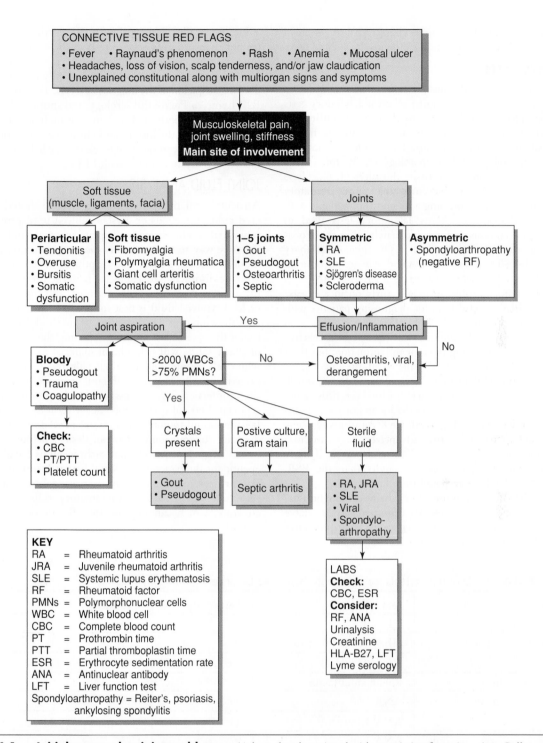

Figure 36.1 • Initial approach to joint problems. (Adapted and reprinted with permission from American College of Rheumatology, Ad Hoc Committee on Clinical Guidelines. Guidelines for the initial evaluation of the adult patient with acute musculoskeletal symptoms. Arthritis Rheum. 1996;39:1–8.)

ther evaluation. Involved joints should first be moved actively if possible by the patient, and then passively by the examiner. Restriction of joint ROM has major implications for rehabilitation, function, and prognosis, and can be caused by intra-articular factors such as cartilage damage, loose fragments, excess synovial membrane, or substantial effusions. Extra-articular causes of limited ROM include contractures of the joint capsule, shortened tendons, and muscle spasm secondary to pain or somatic dysfunction. Passive motion testing is the best indicator of joint damage because this maneuver excludes the complicating contributions of associated muscular and periarticular problems. Some joints may be hypermobile because of instability caused by: 1. dislocation or subluxation; 2. weakening or damage to ligaments; or 3. muscle wasting. This often leads to the permanent deformities characteristically seen in RA (wrists, fingers, and feet) and OA (hands, knees, and feet).

Laboratory Tests

In rheumatic disorders, the history and clinical examination are the keys to effective diagnosis, whereas laboratory tests and radiographs are used mainly to clarify and confirm an already strong suspicion of a specific diagnosis. Specific historical, clinical, and laboratory criteria have been developed by the American College of Rheumatology (ACR) for a wide range of joint and connective tissue disorders (4, 6). These criteria are considerably more accurate than either laboratory testing or imaging in establishing a diagnosis in patients with musculoskeletal disorders. Many laboratory tests used in rheumatologic diagnosis perform adequately when the probability of disease is high, but are much less useful in the primary care office where diseases such as RA and SLE are uncommon (6, 9–11). Clinically obvious arthritis is often associated with a normal laboratory profile, especially early on in a disease process. Potentially useful tests for diagnosing patients with joint pain are shown in Table 36.4.

The erythrocyte sedimentation rate (ESR) and C-reactive protein (CRP) are screening tests for inflammation, but their specificity is quite low. Up to the age of 50, the upper limit of normal for the ESR in most laboratories is 15–20 mm/h in men and 25–30 mm/h in women (12). However, ESR values generally increase by 5 mm/h every decade in normal patients over the age of 40. A very high ESR (>90 mm/h) is typically associated with giant cell arteritis, advanced collagen vascular disease, and septic arthritis. The CRP level may be a more timely indicator of current disease activity than the ESR, which changes slowly in response to inflammation.

Immunologic tests are used to evaluate certain unusual connective tissue disorders (4, 5). Commercially available rheumatic screening panels have a poor positive predictive value, especially in the primary care setting. Serial testing (rather than ordering several tests at the same time) reduces false-positive diagnoses and halves errors of classification. Consequently, tests should be ordered only if there already is a strong suspicion of the diagnosis (9–11). Tests such as HLA-B27, Lyme, or Parvovirus serology, and antiphospholipid antibodies are only indicated if there is a high suspicion for the disease based on the history and physical examination. Serum measurement of complement levels may be helpful in assessing disease activity in patients with SLE.

JOINT FLUID ANALYSIS

An acutely inflamed monoarticular arthritis should be considered either infectious or crystal-induced until proven otherwise. Arthrocentesis, with adequate synovial fluid analysis, is the only way to unequivocally diagnose infection or crystal-induced disease, and can be helpful in differentiating other arthritic disorders (see Table 36.5). Sterile precautions during the aspiration procedure are essential, and fresh (2 hours old or less) synovial fluid is best for analysis. Access is easiest at sites showing capsular distention. If no fluid can be aspirated (often the case in acute gout), irrigating the joint with 2 mL of sterile saline will help obtain material for crystal analysis, white cell counts, and bacterial culture. If infection is suspected clinically, cultures of blood, urine, or another primary site of infection (e.g., abscess) may be helpful in diagnosis, as synovial fluid cultures may be negative in early infection (8). It is important to note that a crystal-proven diagnosis of gout does not rule out joint infection. Besides helping to rule out infection, gout, or pseudogout, arthrocentesis can also be therapeutic for the patient. In cases of hemarthrosis or inflammation, arthrocentesis can help by decreasing intra-articular pressure and by removing inflammatory cells and activated enzymes, which can increase the efficacy of intra-articular steroids.

TABLE 36.4 Diagnostic Tests for Different Rheumatic Disorders Among Symptomatic Patients

Disease	Test	Sensitivity	Specificity	LR +	LR −
Reiter's syndrome	HLA-B27	50%–80%			
Ankylosing spondylitis	HLA-B27 (white patients)	92%	92%	12	0.1
	HLA-B27 (black patients)	50%	98%	25	0.5
Rheumatoid arthritis	Rheumatoid factor	70%–80%			
Rheumatoid arthritis	ANA 1:40	49%	68%	1.5	0.8
	ANA 1:160	14%	95%	2.8	0.9
Systemic lupus erythematosus	ANA 1:40	97%	68%	3.0	0.0
	ANA 1:160	95%	95%	19	0.1
Sjögren's syndrome	ANA 1:40	84%	68%	2.6	0.2
	ANA 1:160	74%	95%	15	0.3
Scleroderma	ANA 1:40	100%	68%	3.1	0.0
	ANA 1:160	87%	95%	17	0.1

Reprinted with permission from Tan EM, Feltkamp TEW, Smolen JS, et al. Range of antinuclear antibodies in "healthy" individuals. Arthritis Rheum. 1997;40:1601–1611.
Abbreviations: ANA, antinuclear antibody; LR, likelihood ratio.

TABLE 36.5 Findings in Synovial Fluid

Diagnosis	White Cell Count	PMN (%)	Color/Clarity	Other
Normal	0–200	0–25	Clear/yellow	None
Trauma	5,000	50	Red/opaque	RBC + +
Osteoarthritis	500–2,000	<25	Clear to slightly cloudy/ yellow-white	Cartilage debris, Mucin clot firm
Acute rheumatic fever	2,000–15,000	50	Yellow/white	None
Gout	2,000–100,000	75	Yellow-white/translucent or opaque	Urate crystals
Pseudogout	2,000–100,000	75	Yellow-white/translucent or opaque	Pyrophosphate crystals
Septic arthritis	50,000–100,000, maybe > 100,000	>95	Yellow-white/opaque	Positive culture in 80%, positive Gram stain in 70%, Mucin clot friable
Rheumatoid arthritis	2,000–100,000	>50	Yellow-white/translucent-opaque	Mucin clot, often xanthochromic,

Abbreviations: PMN, polymorphonuclear leukocytes; RBC + +, red blood cell.

Imaging Studies

Radiographs can be helpful in establishing objective criteria for making a diagnosis, but often fail to confirm arthritic disease, and changes occur later in the usual disease course than a positive history or physical examination (13). Characteristic findings are shown in Table 36.6. Radioisotope bone scans can be useful for excluding osteomyelitis, metastases, infarcts, or necrosis, although in general their specificity is poor. Magnetic resonance imaging (MRI) is helpful in looking at soft tissues, such as ligaments and tendons, in problems related to the shoulders or knees, or in spinal cord impingement caused by disc disease or spinal stenosis.

GENERAL APPROACH TO MANAGEMENT

Most patients presenting with joint pain in primary care practice will have transient or limited episodes involving one to three joints. Less commonly, patients will present with disabling and severely decompensating rheumatic complaints. Broad goals of management include the following:

- Symptom relief—medication, rest, splinting
- Restoration/maintenance of motion and function—physical therapy/occupational therapy/manipulative treatment
- Prevention/correction of deformities—physical therapy, surgery
- Suppression of symptoms—medication
- Emotional health—education, social work, physical conditioning, counseling on employment and sexuality.

The family physician should be able to identify the major rheumatic disorders, arrange a program of pain relief (physical modalities, injections, and analgesics), advise on appropriate rest and disease-specific therapy, and provide patient education and appropriate exercise programs as indicated. Referral to a rheumatologist is indicated when the diagnosis is unclear,

TABLE 36.6 Typical Radiographic Findings in Arthritic Conditions

Disease	Finding
Rheumatoid arthritis	Osteopenia, joint surface erosions, subchondral bone cysts
Systemic lupus erythematosus	Minimal nonspecific changes
Gout	Bone cysts, punched out erosions on joint surfaces
Ankylosing spondylitis	Bilateral sacroiliitis, squaring of lumbar vertebrae, irregular bone erosion and sclerosis at the corners of the vertebrae, vertical syndesmosphytes and loss of definition of apophyseal joints, juxta-articular osteoporosis, joint fusion
Osteoarthritis	Nonuniform joint space loss (may be minimal and reflect the only finding early in OA), osteophyte formation, calcification of cartilage, cyst formation, and subchondral sclerosis

the disease is severe or progressive, dangerous and complex therapy is needed, or special studies and procedures are required. Referral to an orthopedic surgeon is indicated when the patient might benefit from joint replacement or reconstructive surgery. Use of other professionals (e.g., physical therapists, occupational therapists) may be an important adjunct to treatment for certain patients.

Pharmacotherapy

Medications can help relieve the symptoms of arthritis in four ways: relieving pain, controlling inflammation, attacking hypertrophic synovial tissues, or inhibiting the autoimmune response. In most cases, oral analgesic medication can be used in combination with rest and local heat. Acetaminophen and nonsteroidal anti-inflammatory drugs (NSAIDs), including aspirin, can be quite effective for analgesia; higher doses of the latter produce an anti-inflammatory effect. Aspirin is still widely prescribed, although some NSAIDs are better tolerated. There is no evidence that any one NSAID is better than another, although patients may empirically respond well to a particular product. Adverse effects include blood loss, renal impairment, and hepatic dysfunction. Monitoring potential adverse effects of NSAIDs requires a baseline complete blood count (CBC), serum creatinine, and liver enzyme tests, followed by an annual CBC and liver enzyme testing (9, 10, 14). Gastrointestinal (GI) adverse effects (e.g., NSAID-induced gastric ulcers) can be countered by prescribing misoprostol, an analogue of prostaglandin E, given 200 μg four times daily. Histamine-2 blockers and proton pump inhibitors are alternatives when misoprostol cannot be tolerated, (e.g., pregnancy as misoprostol can cause abortion or birth defects). Selective cyclooxygenase 2 (COX-2) inhibitors (e.g., celecoxib, rofecoxib) are associated with fewer bleeding complications than other NSAIDs (0.5% versus 1.2% over 1 year of treatment); however, rofecoxib was withdrawn from the market after it was shown that long-term use (greater than 18 months) could be associated with increased risk of heart attack and stroke (15). In addition, COX-2 inhibitors are significantly more expensive than other NSAIDs (16).

Systemic corticosteroids are used predominantly in RA, connective tissue disease, and inflammatory muscle disorders (polymyalgia rheumatica, polymyositis) (5, 17, 18). There are a variety of steroid regimens, most designed to avoid or reduce the adverse effect of adrenal suppression. They can also be used in joint injections, as adjunctive management when one or two joints are not responding to systemic therapy, or for the local injection tender points in myofascial and periarticular syndromes. Corticosteroids should not be injected into a joint until infection can be ruled out (8).

Complementary and Alternative Therapies

Because of the chronic, debilitating nature of arthritis and the lack of a cure, as many as 84% of patients with chronic musculoskeletal complaints use complementary or alternative therapies to improve function and reduce their suffering. Manual medicine or manipulative treatment provided by osteopathic physicians, chiropractors, or physical therapists, as well as massage therapy, are widely used in the United States and many other countries. Other remedies include copper

bracelets, static magnets, acupuncture, reflexology, spa therapy, ginger, green tea, cat's claw, turmeric, vinegar, vitamins B and C, fatty acids (borage, flax seed, and evening primrose oil), methylsulfonylmethane, S-adenosyl-methionine (SAMe), dimethyl sulfoxide, dehydroepiandrosterone, shark cartilage, glucosamine, and chondroitin (19, 20). Consistent and good-quality patient-oriented evidence is lacking to support some of these interventions. Individual case series (particularly with manipulative and manual treatments, food/antigen avoidance, and fasting) report that some patients respond dramatically after more conventional treatment has failed (21). Manipulation, for example, has been validated in the treatment of acute low back pain (22). Glucosamine and chondroitin treatment has also been shown to be effective in the treatment of OA (20). Care must be undertaken with certain herbal and dietary regimens, as there is increasing evidence that adverse effects and drug interactions can occur with a number of oral supplements.

OA (DEGENERATIVE JOINT DISEASE)

OA is the most common arthritic disorder, and is considered to be more degenerative than inflammatory. Risk factors include: age greater than 50, injury to a joint, obesity, prolonged occupational or sports stress (especially competitive contact sports), and heredity. Most healthy asymptomatic people will have developed some evidence of this degenerative process by the age of 55. Biomechanical and immune damage to the articular cartilage, bone, and synovium are thought to be the mechanism. Bone and cartilage are worn away in conjunction with synovial thickening. Bony spurs (osteophytes) form at the articular edges, with local (and generally mild) inflammation involving the joint capsule and adjacent ligaments.

Clinical Evaluation

OA usually presents in middle-aged or older individuals as mild, dull, aching pain in one or a limited number of joints. Pain typically worsens with activity, improves with rest, and can be aggravated by damp, cold weather. There are no systemic symptoms or signs. Stiffness comes from inactivity but commonly improves after about 15 minutes of exercise. Morning stiffness lasts less than 30 minutes (23). Patients may have joint instability or buckling. The patient complains of pain and reduced function and, in the case of knee and hip disease, difficulty walking and climbing stairs. Usually the symptoms will wax and wane over time, with increasing involvement of more joints. However, the patterns and trajectory of the disease are highly variable and often cannot be predicted.

The distribution of joints affected (DIP and PIP) in the hands and feet in OA is different from that in RA, and it is more likely than other arthritides to affect large joints such as the knee or hip, and often involves the hands and the spine as well. There are often boney enlargements and limitation of the ROM of affected joints. The joint will be swollen and cool, and motion may be limited. Crepitus is a common and sensitive criterion for the disease. There may be effusions in large joints. OA of the wrists, ankles, and shoulders is often

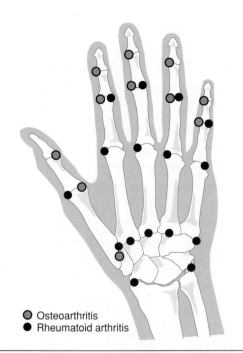

○ Osteoarthritis
● Rheumatoid arthritis

Figure 36.2 • Distribution of joint involvement in rheumatoid arthritis and osteoarthritis.

the result of trauma or other secondary causes. Specific clinical signs include:

- hands—enlargement of the DIP and/or PIP joints; carpometacarpal joint of the thumb often with some deviation of the phalanges; pain on motion (see Figure 36.2)
- feet—swelling (possibly with bunion deformity) of the big toe and DIP joints
- knees and hips—pain and crepitus on passive motion; tenderness to palpation at the joint line; muscle atrophy. Hard swelling is caused by bone spurs, whereas soft swelling comes from effusions. There is significant limitation of ROM on active and passive testing.
- spine—degenerative change is common, often with associated somatic dysfunction leading to limited motion and stiffness of the neck or lower back. Osteophytes (bony spurs) at the facet joints can produce local pain and compression of spinal nerve roots, causing neuropathy (weakness and sensory loss). When disc degeneration and osteophyte formation are severe, spinal canal stenosis can cause direct injury to the spinal cord in the neck or lumbar spine areas (see Chapter 37, Low Back Pain, and Chapter 38, Neck Pain). Spinal stenosis can present with symptoms that mimic claudication.

Laboratory Tests and Imaging Studies

Synovial fluid analysis is useful in ruling out possible inflammatory arthritis (see Table 36.5), but is often not necessary in patients with OA. The ESR is normal except in rare cases of erosive OA or primary generalized OA, which may have an inflammatory presentation much like RA. Radiologic imaging is useful primarily in monitoring disease progression rather than making a diagnosis; osteoarthritic changes are routinely found in asymptomatic patients (see Table 36.6). Computed

tomography (CT) and MRI can be helpful to evaluate possible cervical or lumbar spinal stenosis.

Management

Twice-daily exercise programs and low-impact aerobic conditioning produce increased strength and pain reduction. Activity that causes pain lasting longer than two hours should be avoided. The use of braces, attention to supportive shoes, and other orthotics can relieve pain from asymmetric walking patterns. Exercise to the muscle group or groups that support particular affected joints (e.g., quadriceps for the knees) can be beneficial to reduce the wear and tear on the affected joints. Obese patients should lose weight, especially before orthopedic surgery for joint replacement; weight loss can improve long-term progression (Strength of Recommendation (SOR) = B [23]). Glucosamine sulfate, which is derived from oyster and crab shells, may show some improved efficacy in relieving painful symptoms in some studies when compared to placebo, though it demonstrates limited value after 2–4 months in others (24, 25). It is thought to provide substrate for proteoglycan synthesis and to be mildly anti-inflammatory. However, there is limited information on the long-term efficacy and toxicity of glucosamine. The usual dosage is 1,500 mg daily in three divided doses. Short-term use of glucosamine seems to be well tolerated, with the most common adverse effect of GI discomfort occurring less than with NSAIDs (23).

Chondroitin sulfate, made from shark and cow cartilage, may provide some anti-inflammatory effect similar to glucosamine. Chondroitin sulfate may be superior to placebo in reducing pain of OA (SOR = A [23]). Like glucosamine, chondroitin is also well tolerated by patients, with a somewhat slower onset of action but possibly a longer duration than NSAIDs in OA. Therefore, chondroitin sulfate or glucosamine should be taken for at least 1 month before any symptom relief can be expected. The usual dose of chondroitin sulfate is 1,200 mg daily in three divided doses. There is little evidence that the combination of glucosamine and chondroitin sulfate is better than using either alone, but studies are underway.

Nonrandomized trials with SAM-e have shown some efficacy in OA, but the cost may be prohibitive for most patients. There is little evidence that the use of ginger is beneficial in OA. The use of oral avocado and soybean unsaponifiables in 300 mg daily provided some symptom relief in patients with OA of the hip (24).

Medication can be given for pain relief. Acetaminophen, up to 4000 mg/d, is clearly superior to placebo, and has a similar safety profile, so it is generally considered first-line medical therapy for OA. At higher doses, acetaminophen can cause some GI symptoms, and massive overdosages or use with excessive alcohol (three drinks daily) has been associated with hepatotoxicity. Acetaminophen may not be as effective as NSAIDs for pain reduction in people with OA of the knee and hip, but may be equal in improving function (22, 26, 27). If there is an unacceptable response to acetaminophen, NSAIDs can be either added or substituted, basing the dose on the patient response. The use of topical capsaicin (0.025% cream applied four times daily for OA affecting the knee, ankle, finger, wrist, or shoulder) may be beneficial, with the minor side effect of a localized burning sensation (23); care should be taken to avoid contact with the eyes. It is postulated

TABLE 36.7 Level of Evidence for Different Therapies

Intervention	Strength of Recommendation*
Osteoarthritis	
Nonsteroidal anti-inflammatory drugs	A
Topical analgesics	A
Cyclooyxgenase-2 inhibitors	A
Arthroscopy with joint lavage	A
Intra-articular hyaluronate	A
Glucosamine and chondroitin	B
Acupuncture	B
Intra-articular steroids	B
Opioids	B
Aerobic exercise	B
Occupational interventions	B
Arthroplasty	B
Weight loss	B
Joint replacement	B
Rheumatoid arthritis	
Nonsteroidal anti-inflammatory drugs	A
Disease-modifying agents	A
Minocycline	B
Self-help education, monthly telephone contact with counseling	A
Three months of physical therapy	A
Walking/conditioning program	A
Weight loss	C

*A = consistent, good-quality patient-oriented evidence; B = inconsistent or limited-quality patient-oriented evidence; C = consensus, disease-oriented evidence, usual practice, expert opinion, or case series. For information about the SORT evidence rating system, see *http://www.aafp.org/afpsort.xml*.

to act as an irritant–counter-irritant. In the same fashion, topical analgesic creams (salicylate cream) may be effective for focal joint pain, and can be applied four times daily (23). Tramadol, a nonopioid centrally acting analgesic, can be added to NSAID therapy for short-term use to help with severe pain (23). Intra-articular steroid injections can be used for joints with effusion and inflammation. Another option is to use intra-articular lavage with sterile saline, which has been shown to be more effective, although more costly, than standard medical therapy (28).

Viscosupplementation is now widely used particularly for OA of the knees (29), with relatively low risks of adverse reactions. These viscous agents are injected into the joint space to replace depleted hyaluronic acid (a natural substance essential for maintaining joint fluid viscosity). Sodium hyaluronate (Hyalgan) and Hylan G-F20 (Synvisc) are given in two to five injections (2 mL) over 2 to 4 weeks. Adverse effects (e.g., pain, swelling, allergic reaction) occur in 5% of cases. Studies have confirmed short-term relief of pain and good patient-oriented evidence with viscosupplementation for OA of the knee.

However, costs of the injection series are significant ($600–$800 per course), and long-term effectiveness has not been fully established.

Patients with severe OA who are not responding to medication and those with intractable pain or serious functional impairment should be referred to an orthopedic surgeon for osteotomy or arthroplasty. Fewer than half of patients with OA who undergo arthroscopic debridement (simple lavage or abrasion arthroplasty) will have sustained pain reduction. Long-term outcomes for joint replacement/arthroplasty are good (30, 31).

Table 36.7 lists the level of evidence for different therapies for OA.

PREVENTION

In both primary and secondary prevention of OA, the most important factor in protecting weight-bearing joints is maintaining an appropriate body weight (32). Exercise, especially for supporting joints (quadriceps for knees, abdominal muscles for lumbar spine), has an important role. Patients also should be advised to maintain an adequate vitamin D intake (SOR = C).

RHEUMATOID ARTHRITIS

RA is a chronic inflammatory polyarthritis that primarily affects peripheral joints and related periarticular tissues. It usually starts as an insidious symmetric polyarthritis, often with nonspecific symptoms. Diagnostic criteria include arthritis lasting longer than 6 weeks (though evidence suggests that 12 weeks may more specific), a positive rheumatoid factor (RF), and radiologic damage (4). Although RA is a systemic disease, it mostly affects the synovial membrane of joints. It is approximately three times more frequent in women than in men, and commonly (70% of cases) begins between 25 and 50 years of age. Its prevalence is 0.5%–1.5% of the population in industrialized countries (33).

The exact cause of RA is unknown, but is likely multifactorial in people with a certain genetic susceptibility (HLA-DR shared epitope). Smoking is the major known environmental risk factor for RA, though little is known about the mechanisms involved. It is clear that persistent immune stimulation changes the synovial cell phenotype into one that invades articular cartilage and adjacent tissues. In the affected joint, the synovium forms a pannus of granulomatous tissue that erodes cartilage, ligaments, tendons, and eventually bone. These granulomas can also form subcutaneous nodules (rheumatoid nodules) and affect other organs such as lungs, heart, and bowel. Effusions may be present in joints, and surrounding muscles atrophy from disuse. Severe musculoskeletal deformities can eventually occur, ending in fibrous fusion (ankylosis) of joint surfaces. In the hands, these can be characterized by ulnar deviation, hammer fingers, boutonnière and swan-neck deformities of the fingers, and sometimes tendon rupture in the extremities (see Figure 36.3). The disease can cause flexion deformities of the toes, valgus deviation of the foot, and fixation of the ankle joint. Entrapment neuropathies in arms or legs are common (carpal, ulnar, and tarsal tunnel syndromes). Vasculitis and granulomas can lead to skin ulcers, scleritis in the eye, pleuritis, pulmonary nodules and fibrosis, pericarditis, osteoporosis, and splenomegaly. Sjögren's syndrome (dry eyes and mouth) occurs in 20% of cases.

The differential diagnosis is extensive (see Figure 36.1), and nonrheumatologic causes of the joint pain and swelling, myalgia, fatigue, fever, and weight loss must also be considered. The American College of Rheumatology has produced a set of criteria to promote diagnostic accuracy. When all are present, there is a sensitivity of 90% and specificity of 89% in making the diagnosis (likelihood ratio [LR]+ = 8.9; LR− = 0.11) (4, 34) (see Table 36.8).

Clinical Evaluation

Initially, there are aches and pains in the muscles and joints, sometimes accompanied by a low-grade fever, early morning stiffness (lasting more than 1 hour), fatigue, and weight loss in 70% of patients. Subsequently, there is symmetric joint swelling, usually involving the PIP and metacarpophalangeal or metatarsophalangeal (MTP) joints of the hands or feet respectively (see Figure 36.2). Wrists, knees, and ankles may also be affected. Rarely is only one joint involved. Activities of daily living are usually impaired. The patterns of progression and joint involvement are quite variable and include the following:

- Episodic—lasting a few months, then resolving only to return at shorter intervals
- One or two joints remain inflamed for several months before others are affected
- Morning stiffness and fatigue for many months, but with no pain
- Malaise, fever, weight loss for several months preceding joint involvement
- Progressive subtle swelling of the joints
- Severe onset, getting progressively worse without relief

Some patients suffer from RA for some years, and then the disease becomes inactive or "burned out." Patients may develop signs and symptoms of nonarticular involvement that lead to pulmonary, cardiac, and bowel symptoms (see Table 36.2).

Physical examination findings can include weight loss, fever, joint swelling, tenderness to palpation, loss of motion, an enlarged spleen, effusions, muscle atrophy, inflammation of the tendons and tendon sheaths, and deformities in 20% of cases. Rheumatoid nodules can be found on the extensor aspects of the forearm and elbow area in 25% of patients with RA. Vasculitis can cause peripheral neuropathy in the legs or arms. Similar neuropathy can occur from nerve entrapment by inflammatory tissue. Cardiac arrhythmias, pericarditis, and pleurisy are other results of vasculitis. Finally, a global assessment of function and emotional status should be undertaken (35).

Laboratory Tests and Imaging Studies

RF test results only become positive some time (weeks to months) after the onset of RA. Up to 40% of patients with RA are seronegative early in the course of the disease, when they are also often likely to present to their physician. In fact, 25% of patients with RA never have a positive RF test result.

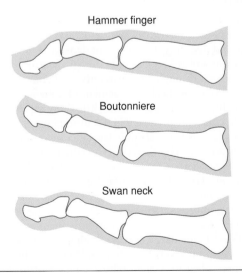

Figure 36.3 • Finger deformities in rheumatoid arthritis.

TABLE 36.8 Diagnostic Criteria for Gout and Rheumatoid Arthritis

Disease	Criteria	Interpretation
Rheumatoid arthritis	Morning stiffness for at least 1 hour	90% sensitive, 89% specific. If pretest probability is 10%, patients meeting criteria have 70% chance of RA.
	At least three joints involved in soft tissue swelling or effusion (joints: PIP, MCP, wrist, elbow, knee, MTP)	
	At least one joint affected in wrist/MCP/PIP distribution	
	Symmetric involvement of the same joint, both sides of body	
	Nodules found subcutaneously or over bony points	
	Rheumatoid factor positive	
	Bone changes (erosions/decalcification) in hand/wrist radiographs	
Gout	In patients with more than one attack of acute arthritis and maximum inflammation within 24 hours	The presence of 6 of 11 of these criteria confirms gout (98% sensitive and 95% specific; LR+, 20; LR−, 0.02) (2).
	Monoarthritis	
	Redness over joints	
	First MTP joint involved	
	Unilateral first MTP joint attack	
	Unilateral tarsal joint attack	
	Tophus identified	
	Hyperuricemia	
	Asymmetric swelling in joint on radiograph	
	Subcortical cysts on radiograph	
	Urate crystals in joint fluid	
	Joint fluid culture negative	

Abbreviations: LR, likelihood ratio; MCP, metacarpophalangeal; MTP, metatarsophalangeal; PIP, proximal interphalangeal; RA, rheumatoid arthritis.

A positive RF titer is generally considered significant at 1:160, and is more predictive of inflammatory disease at 1:320 (9, 10). A number of other rheumatic and nonrheumatic conditions are associated with positive RF. Nonrheumatic conditions associated with a positive RF include bacterial endocarditis, tuberculosis, sarcoidosis, and malignancies. Elderly patients in the general population may have a positive RF 10% of the time, though usually at a very low titer—1:40 or less. Apart from the variable results of RF, antinuclear antibody, ESR, and C-reactive protein tests described earlier (Table 36.4), in RA there is usually a hypochromic anemia with a normal white blood cell count, unless splenomegaly (causing leukopenia) is present. Joint fluid will show typical inflammatory changes (Table 36.5). Radiographic changes are specific but not sensitive. Over half of patients have no detectable erosions in the first 6 months, with the most rapid progression occurring over the first 2 years (36). Baseline studies include both hands and wrists on the same film, and both feet while standing. Early findings show periarticular demineralization and swelling close to the joints. Joint spaces become narrowed, and erosions develop close to articular surfaces. Later changes show subluxation and deformities.

Management
PHARMACOTHERAPY

The major treatment goals are to relieve symptoms (pain, swelling, fatigue), improve joint function, and reduce joint damage and disability. Because joint damage begins 6 months after the onset of RA, continued efforts to control the inflammatory process through disease modifying therapy has become the mainstay of medical management of patients with RA.

The first-line agents in acute disease are aspirin or other NSAIDs, which are preferred in RA to acetaminophen despite higher risks of side effects (37). Consideration must be given to the risks of NSAID therapy, especially in the elderly or in those patients with a history of upper GI bleeding or renal dysfunction. To reduce joint damage and disability, disease modifying antirheumatic drugs (DMARDs) are generally added early in the course of the disease. Methotrexate, a dihydrofolate reductase inhibitor, is currently the most commonly used DMARD for RA. There is a high withdrawal rate with methotrexate, however, because of side effects, and it should not be prescribed to women who are pregnant or anticipate being pregnant (38). TNF receptor blockers are now being widely used early in RA treatment (see below), but at significant cost. Other DMARDs include antimalarials (hydroxychloroquine), sulfasalazine, gold salts, D-penicillamine, and azathioprine. Corticosteroid treatment options include low-dose, pulsed intravenous/intramuscular, or intermittent high-dose regimens (39). Auranofin (oral gold) has been shown to reduce disease activity, but not to significantly impact radiologic progression or long-term functional status, and therefore may be less effective than other DMARDs (40). Leflunomide, an inhibitor of pyrimidine syntheses, has a different mechanism of action than other DMARDS, and is a newer treatment option. Leflunomide has similar efficacy (SOR = A [41]) and incidence of adverse effects as methotrexate, and it is more effective than, and as safe as, sulfasalazine, but its long-term safety profile is unclear. The costs of leflunomide treatment are also higher than treatment with methotrexate or sulfasalazine (41). Combination treatment with several DMARDs may enhance the efficacy over single-drug treatment, but balance of benefit and potential harm must be continually revaluated.

Uncertainty remains concerning therapeutic protocols for RA, but there are three current approaches: the pyramid, the step-down bridge, and the saw-tooth regimen (39). Each approach has evolved with the emergence of new disease modifying agents.

Pyramid
Initially, all patients are started on a program of patient education, which should include family members. A multifaceted program that includes exercise, possibly physical and occupational therapy, and psychological support should be negotiated with the patient early on in the disease process, and be tailored to address specific patient needs throughout the course of the disease. Particular attention to health maintenance, including vaccination (influenza, pneumococcal), smoking cessation, and management of comorbid conditions (diabetes, osteoporosis) is essential. If NSAIDs are not contraindicated, they are started primarily for symptom control, and may be discontinued in the asymptomatic patient. If the patient has not significantly improved in 2 to 3 weeks, treatment with a DMARD is initiated, usually with sulfasalazine (Level A) or hydroxychloroquine, methotrexate alone, or in combinations. All DMARDs have significant potential adverse effects (some which can be countered by the use of folic acid), and careful monitoring is required (see Table 36.9). Low-dose oral corticosteroids are often used to bridge the time period in which the peak response is developing to DMARDs. If DMARDs are ineffective, high-dose corticosteroids may be needed (see Table 36.10). TNF receptor blockers are now being used earlier in the course of RA.

Step-down Bridge
For very aggressive disease, treatment can be initiated with high-dose oral corticosteroids (60 mg prednisone daily), together with hydroxychloroquine, sulfasalazine, and methotrexate, along with folic acid. Medications are then withdrawn sequentially, and the corticosteroids tapered gradually, as control improves.

Saw-tooth
In this regimen, single or combined DMARDs are given, possibly including tumor necrosis factor receptor blockers, and agents are substituted if control deteriorates. Local joint flare-ups can be treated with intra-articular injections of corticosteroids.

Glucocorticoids
Corticosteroids are effective and widely used in rheumatic diseases, but 30% to 50% of patients on long-term steroids will develop osteoporosis (40). The most rapid bone mineral loss occurs in the first 6 to 12 months of therapy. When the oral dose is over 30 mg/d, there is a 2%–50% reduction in bone mineral density (BMD) (42). When the dose is less than 10 mg/d, there is only a 10% reduction in BMD.

To prevent bone loss, use the lowest dose of steroids for the shortest period of time, administer calcium (1,500 mg of elemental calcium/d) and vitamin D (400 to 800 IU/d), and consider hormone replacement therapy, (e.g., estradiol or selective estrogen receptor modulator therapy, such as raloxifene) for postmenopausal women. Bisphosphonates such as alendronate (10 mg daily though weekly or monthly regimens are now available) are effective in preventing and treating bone loss.

Azathioprine, cyclosporine, and cyclophosphamide all have been shown to provide some short-term and/or long-term benefits in patients with RA, but the severity and frequency of toxicity limit their use. There is evidence to suggest that treatment with parenteral gold or with penicillamine is effective in RA (SOR = A), but their use is also limited by their toxicity and potentially serious side effects.

BIOLOGIC RESPONSE MODIFIERS

The use of biologic response modifiers has now become prevalent in the treatment of RA. These agents interfere with human TNF, which is believed to play a major role in promoting inflammation of joint tissues. These agents produce substantial short-term improvement (30% to 50%) and may slow RA progression. They are indicated for moderate or severe active RA patients who have an inadequate response to DMARDs (42, 43). Three products, infliximab, etanercept, and more recently, abatacept, have been approved by the US Food and Drug Administration for use by intravenous infusion or subcutaneous injection. Etanercept has an enhanced effect in improved symptoms and reduction of disease activity and inflammation when given with methotrexate (SOR = A [43]). In patients who are newly diagnosed with RA, the use of etanercept injected subcutaneously twice weekly (25 mg) for 12 months worked as well as methotrexate and was more effective in slowing the damage to joints. Infliximab (3mg/kg or 10mg/kg every 4–8 weeks by infusion) for 6 to 12 months also decreases RA symptoms better than methotrexate alone, with significant reduction of radiographic progression (SOR = A [44]). Long-term safety is still unclear. Common side effects include site soreness, as well as headache, colds, and GI symptoms similar to that with methotrexate. The risks of tuberculosis and lymphoma still need to be studied further. As tuberculosis, invasive fungal infections, and other opportunistic infections have been reported during therapy with these agents, treatment should be discontinued with any sign of infection, and all patients should undergo screening for tuberculosis (PPD testing) prior to initiation of treatment.

TABLE 36.9 Treatment Regimens for Rheumatoid Arthritis

Drug	Peak Response	Maintenance Dose	Laboratory Checks
Antimalarials (hydroxychloroquine, chloroquine)	2–3 mo	Hydroxychloroquine: start with 200 mg orally twice daily; after good response, long-term: decrease back to 200 mg orally daily	Ophthalmic check every 6–12 months, LFT, creatinine every 6 months
Sulfasalazine	4–5 mo	500 mg/d with weekly increase to 2–3 g daily in two divided doses	LFT, CBC, creatinine every 3 months
Methotrexate	3–6 wk	7.5 mg orally every week, increasing to 20 mg every week. Daily folic acid to reduce oral & GI side effects	LFT, CBC, creatinine every 4–8 weeks
Gold salts (sodium thiomalate, aurothioglucose)	5–8 mo	IV/IM 50 mg/week, then monthly	Urine, CBC, LFT every 4 months
Oral auranofin		6 mg daily, may increase after 4–6 months to 9 mg daily. If no response after 3 months at 9 mg then discontinue	
Azathioprine	4–6 mo	1 mg/kg per day; may increase by 0.5 mg/kg at 4 week intervals to a maximum of 2.5 mg/kg	CBC, differential every 2 months
Tumor necrosis factor receptor blockers			PPD screening before initiating treatment monitor for CHF
etanercept		25 mg injected twice weekly (72–96 hours apart)	
infliximab		3 mg/kg infusion, repeated after 2 and 6 weeks, then every 8 weeks	
leflunomide	3–6 wk	100 mg/daily for 1–3 days, then 20 mg a day	LFT, CBC, creatinine Monitor blood pressure

Abbreviations: CBC, complete blood count; CHF, congestive heart failure; GI, gastrointestinal PPD, purified protein derivative; IM, intramuscularly; IV, intravenously; LFT, liver function test.

COMPLEMENTARY AND ALTERNATIVE THERAPY

Alternative treatments similar to those employed for OA are commonly sought out by RA patients. Superficial moist heat and cryotherapy as palliative therapy as well as the use of paraffin wax baths with or without therapeutic exercise have shown short-term benefits, but there is inconsistency in the evidence. Likewise, balneotherapy and spa therapy, and bathing in warm water with or without minerals, have shown some positive results in patient symptoms in small studies, but the evidence is limited by the poor methodological quality of the studies.

Low-level laser therapy has been advocated as an alternative and noninvasive treatment for RA and has demonstrated short-term relief of pain and morning stiffness in small studies, with no side effects. The dosing, the length of treatment time, and the long-term effects are controversial (45).

There is considerable variability in the evidence on the effects and the use of acupuncture, electroacupuncture, transcutaneous electrical nerve stimulation units, or therapeutic ultrasound in RA. The herbal supplement gamma-linolenic acid (GLA) has shown promising effects for RA symptoms, but studies regarding GLA and other herbal products for RA are limited. One herbal product used by RA patients that has shown significant toxicity is tripterygium wilfordii hook F (46).

Table 36.7 lists the level of evidence for different therapies for RA.

LONG-TERM CARE

Randomized controlled studies show that DMARDs and low-dose steroids are 30% to 40% more effective than placebo in improving symptoms and controlling progression of the disease in the short term. Long-term effectiveness has not been established (47); there are limited long-term outcome studies of the various treatment regimens for RA (48).

For long-term RA care, every follow-up visit should include a patient-centered assessment of progress, a review of medications and adverse effects, consideration of health promotion and disease prevention, and a review of functional abilities. Physical examination can be directed to affected

TABLE 36.10   Regimens for Corticosteroid Therapy*

Preparation	Schedule	Usual Dosage	Indication
Prednisone	Daily low dose	7.5 mg	Maintenance therapy
Prednisone	Short-term	20–30 mg/d (1–2 wk) with taper over 7–10 d	Short flare
Prednisone	Maintenance	Alternating 5–10 mg four times daily	
Prednisone	High dose	60 mg daily	Severe, acute illness
Methylprednisolone sodium succinate** (Solu-Medrol)	Intravenous pulse	500–1,000 mg/d for 3 d	Severe flare
Triamcinolone	Intramuscular pulse	80 mg on alternate days 2 times	Severe flare
Methylprednisolone acetate†	Intra-articular Interphalangeal Wrist, ankle, Elbow Knee, shoulder	50–10 mg 10–40 mg 40–80 mg	25-gauge needle 20- to 22-gauge needle 16- to 24-gauge needle

*Adverse effects: skin—thinning, striae, acne, hirsutism, bruising; cardiovascular—hypertension, edema; musculoskeletal—osteopenia, myopathy; personality—mood disorder, insomnia, euphoria; Gastrointestinal—ulcer, bleeding; ophthalmic—glaucoma, cataract; endocrine—adrenal suppression, perforation, pancreatitis; metabolic—diabetes, obesity, menstrual disorders, hyperlipidemia.
†A variety of articular steroid preparations with different half-lives and costs are available.

joints per the patient's complaints, as well as to common areas of systemic involvement (e.g., lungs, heart, skin) or sites of medication side effects. In addition, monitoring the progress of the disease and response to therapy requires repeated measures of joint involvement (inflammation, motion limitation, stiffness, deformity), pain level, results of acute-phase reactant tests (ESR or CRP), and radiographic evidence of damage.

Surgical intervention includes synovectomy to reduce further damage to the joint, resection arthroplasty, joint fusion, and joint replacement (49, 50). Synovectomy is primarily palliative, with relief lasting only 1 to 3 years. Tenosynovectomy involves debriding tendon sheaths to improve motion. Resection arthroplasty removes the damaged part of a nonweight-bearing joint, and arthrodesis relieves pain by fusing the joint. Joint replacement using Silastic® prostheses has been the major innovation in arthritis care in recent years, leading to significant pain relief and improved function; long-term outcomes are not known however.

SUPPORTIVE MANAGEMENT

Physical and occupational health specialists play an important role in helping patients with RA function at home and at work. Dynamic exercise therapy at an appropriate intensity for approximately 3 months has been shown to improve aerobic capability, muscle strength, and joint mobility without increasing pain, joint damage, or disease activity. Manipulative treatment, especially for secondary areas of somatic dysfunction, may assist with symptoms and patient function (51). Supportive care includes splinting to preserve joint function (especially of the wrists), and to protect and rest inflamed joints. There is no evidence that this ultimately reduces deformities, however, and may in fact reduce hand movement. Extra-depth shoes or insoles may be helpful, but there is some conflicting evidence supporting their use and results in the reduction in pain and deformity (52). Occupational therapy can assist patients by teaching them adaptive techniques for daily chores and functional ability (SOR = A). Assistive devices and modification of the home can help patients remain independent for a longer time.

Patients suffering from chronic arthritis often have significant psychosocial problems involving body image, depression, social interactions, and sexuality. Individual and group therapy may be useful, and treatment for depression may be needed; it is essential that the physician maintain an open and caring approach to these patients and their families.

Prognosis

The course of RA is highly variable and unpredictable. Some patients experience flares and remissions, and others have a progressive course. RA has been associated with a shortened life expectancy (6). About 5% of patients will be in remission within 2 years of the first attack, 15% to 25% will have progressive disease despite maximal therapy, and the remainder will follow a varying course. Almost 90% of the joints affected in patients are involved during the first year of the disease. In patients who do not undergo a spontaneous remission (usually within 1 to 2 years of onset), structural joint damage may occur, leading to articular deformities and functional impairment. This damage and the prognosis seem to depend on the severity of the synovial inflammation. About half will be unable to work in 10 years (6). A poor prognosis is indicated by a high-titer RF result (a strongly positive RF result predicts 60% mortality at 8 years, compared with 18% mortality for patients with a negative RF result), rheumatoid nodules, extra-articular involvement, persisting acute phase reactants, more than 20 joints involved, psychological helplessness, and significant functional disability within 1 year of onset. If the ESR remains at approximately 30, the risk ratio of total joint replacement is 2.7, but this increases to 4.8 if the ESR remains above 60. Interestingly, RA commonly goes into remission during pregnancy.

TABLE 38.1 Differential Diagnosis for Neck Pain

Mechanical	**Multiple myeloma**
Nontraumatic	Chondrosarcoma
Neck strain	Glioma
Postural	Syringomyelia
Tension	Neurofibroma
Torticollis (acquired)	Infectious
Spondylosis* (degenerative arthritis)	Osteomyelitis
Myelopathy*	Discitis
Cervical fracture* (see neoplasm)	Meningitis
Traumatic	Herpes zoster
Whiplash syndromes*	Lyme disease
Disc herniation*	Neurologic
Cervical fracture*	Peripheral entrapment
Neck sprain	Brachial plexitis
Sports (stinger*)	Neuropathies
Nonmechanical	Reflex sympathetic dystrophy
Rheumatologic/inflammatory	Referred
Rheumatoid arthritis	Thoracic outlet syndrome
Ankylosing spondylitis	Pancoast tumor
Fibromyalgia	Esophagitis
Polymyalgia rheumatica	Angina
Reiter's syndrome	Vascular dissection
Psoriatic arthritis	Carotidynia
Neoplastic	**Miscellaneous**
Osteoblastoma	Sarcoidosis
Osteochondroma	Paget's disease
Giant cell tumor	
Metastases	
Hemangioma	

*With or without radiculopathy.

the paraspinous sites in the thoracic spine without dermatomal radiation.

Neurogenic pain is caused when nerve roots within the cervical foramina are involved. The sensory and motor nerve roots of the spinal cord join just after passing through the intervertebral foramen. Pressure on the nerve root causes paresthesia, hypesthesia, or hypalgesia but usually not direct pain. Ischemia or mechanical pressure to the capillaries or venules within the dural sheath of the nerve root is now considered the cause. Ischemia affecting the sensory (dorsal) nerve root produces pain in a dermatomal distribution. Stimulation of the motor (ventral) nerve root is thought to produce a deep unpleasant boring sensation in the region of the muscle group innervated by that specific root.

Pain receptors have also been found in the zygapophyseal (facet) joints, spinous ligaments, and neck muscles. Degenerative changes within the cartilage of the facet joints are thought to cause pain, but these changes are usually asymptomatic until trauma has occurred. Administration of local anesthesia within the facet joints produces immediate relief that lasts for the duration of the anesthetic. The method by which mobilization or manipulation of these joints relieves pain is unclear. The striated extensor and flexor muscles of the neck have

pain receptors. Trauma from stretch or compression is an obvious cause of edema and microscopic or macroscopic hemorrhage. Pain at the myofascial periosteal junction can also cause pain when a muscle forcibly contracts. The mechanism of pain with sustained muscle tension, myofascial syndrome, is less well understood. Sustained isometric muscle contractions from stress, poor posture, or sleeping position are thought to occlude arterial flow. These contractions are associated with a buildup of metabolic products, causing further irritation, sustained contraction, and decreased vascular flow. The cycle of ischemia, contraction, metabolic irritants, and further contraction produces pain. Trigger points may be local specific areas of this phenomenon.

Cervical Spondylosis

Cervical spondylosis is degenerative change in the cervical spine. The term is used synonymously with degenerative disc disease or degenerative spondylitis. It is clear that degenerative changes are normal in the aging process. Autopsy studies report spondylosis in 60% of women and 80% of men by the age of 49. By the age of 79, 95% of both sexes have degenerative changes. These changes include narrowed disc height, osteophytes in the disc margins, and arthritic changes in the facet joints (10).

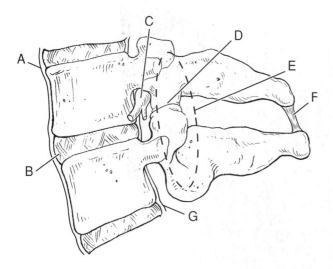

A. Anterior longitudinal ligament
B. Outer annulus of disc
C. Dura
D. Facet capsule
E. Muscle
F. Ligament
G. Posterior longitudinal ligament

Figure 38.1 • Pain receptor sites in the lower cervical spine.

Cervical Spondylotic Myelopathy

Cervical spondylotic (or spondylitic) myelopathy is a condition in which arthritic changes, primarily the development of osteophytes and thickening of the ligamentum flavum, cause direct compression of the spinal cord, resulting in myelopathy. Symptoms develop when the cord has been impinged by 30% or more. Motion can aggravate spinal cord damage by stretching the cord over protruding osteophytes in flexion or by pressure from a thickened bulging ligamentum flavum in extension.

Whiplash

The term whiplash was first coined in 1928 by Dr. Harold Crowe. It is typically defined as an injury to the cervical spine resulting from acceleration (hyperextension) and deceleration (hyperflexion) and of the head during a rear-impact motor vehicle accident. Any external force that results in a violent stretch or tear in the paracervical muscles can cause the injury. It is estimated that a rear impact injury from a car traveling between 9 and 15 mph can generate a force to the neck of 5 Gs (5 times gravitational force). A mild hyperextension of the lower cervical segment can cause strain and trauma to the muscles of the neck. A more significant stress can injure the anterior longitudinal ligament, the nerve roots, and the disc annulus, and most importantly, can force the zygapophyseal joints to impact posteriorly on each other. Diagnostic blocks of the zygapophyseal joints have confirmed that pain in these joints is the most common cause of chronic neck pain after whiplash (11). The symptoms often do not occur for 12 to 24

hours. The delay in symptoms may be from the edema that develops after microscopic hemorrhage and injury. Inflamed edematous muscles will frequently undergo contraction, that is, spasm that results in decreased blood flow and ischemia (as above). There may be subjective or objective evidence of nerve root radiculopathy with whiplash; it implies more significant injury. Because by definition the radiculopathy is a posttraumatic neurologic deficit, whiplash with radiculopathy requires imaging and consideration of referral.

CLINICAL EVALUATION

Although the differential diagnosis of neck pain is broad and includes multiple serious causes, most cases of neck pain seen in the family physician's office are diagnosed using a basic patient-oriented history and physical examination. Learning to differentiate dangerous causes of neck pain using red flag questions and a few diagnostic maneuvers should identify cases of neck pain requiring immediate referral.

History and Physical Examination

The history establishes the character of the pain (sharp, dull, boring, aching, radiating), location (neck, occiput, arm, upper back), mechanism and timing of onset (spontaneous, traumatic, after sleeping, after studying), duration (<3 months = acute; >3 months = chronic) and clinical course (improving or worsening, the presence of aggravating or alleviating symptoms). Radiating symptoms should be described. Is there radiation of pain, numbness, tingling, or weakness? Does the patient have functional limitations? Can he drive? Has he dropped things? What treatment measures have worked or failed in the past? And importantly, what psychosocial stresses or mental health problems may be present?

The physical examination should begin with assessment of the patient's general appearance, posture, stance, and gait. The easiest way to assess the patient's range of motion in the cervical area is to position the patient so that he or she may easily observe the examiner's motions and simply mimic flexion, extension, side-bending, and rotation. This is fast and simple, and reminds the examiner of the normal expected range of motion. The patient may remain seated for neurologic testing. Motor strength, deep tendon reflexes, sensory changes, and long track signs should be checked. Cervical radiculopathy attributable to one nerve root can generally be diagnosed clinically, although there is some variation in individual patients (see Table 38.2).

Three clinical tests can be used to aid the diagnosis of cervical disc herniation. The Spurling test (also known as the Spurling maneuver), or neck compression test, is performed by having the patient side-bend to the side of radicular pain and extend his or her head. In a positive test result, pressure exerted downward on the patient's head will create or intensify radicular symptoms. The Spurling test has been shown to have a positive likelihood ratio (LR+) of 4.3 and a negative likelihood ratio (LR-) of 0.75 (12). This suggests it is useful when positive, but not much help if it is negative. In the axial manual traction test, the examiner pulls up on the head to momentarily decrease the pressure on the cervical root. The arm abduction test is performed by elevating the affected arm

TABLE 38.2 Clinical Findings of Neck Pain with Radiculopathy

Nerve Root	Level	Motor Weakness (Follows Myotomal Pattern)	Sensory Loss (Follows Dermatomal Pattern)	Paresthesia	Referred Pain	Reflex Loss	Subjective Pain
C5	C4/5	Deltoid, shoulder, biceps	Lateral upper arm	None in digits	Shoulder and upper lateral arm	Biceps	Shoulder (but relatively pain free)
C6	C5/6	Biceps, brachioradialis	Thumb and forearm proximal to thumb	Thumb	Radial aspect of forearm	Brachioradialis and biceps	Deltoid, rhomboid muscle areas
C7	C6/7	Triceps	Middle ring finger	Middle finger	Dorsal aspect of forearm	Triceps	Dorsolateral upper arm, superomedial angle of scapula
C8	C7/T1	Finger intrinsic	Inner forearm, little finger	Ring and little finger	Ulnar aspect of forearm and little finger	Triceps or none	Scapula, ulnar side of upper arm

Note: The numbered cervical root passes through the foramen above the numbered cervical vertebra (e.g., the C6 spinal nerve exits in the foramen between the C5 and C6 vertebrae).

over the head of the seated patient. This too decreases the traction on the cervical root. The relief of pain with either test is considered a positive result for cervical root compression. The positive predictive value or likelihood ratios of these last two tests is unknown. There is significant overlap in the physical examination of the neck and shoulder. Please see Chapter 39 for a discussion of the shoulder examination.

Muscular atrophy of the shoulder, arms, or hands could suggest chronic nerve injury. Unsteady gait, lower extremity weakness, hyperreflexia, and L'hermitte's sign (shooting pain down the back with axial head compression) suggest cervical myelopathy.

DIAGNOSTIC TESTING

Laboratory studies are indicated when the history and physical examination suggest systemic disease, inflammatory arthritis, or bone damage. Most nontraumatic cervical problems, including prolapsed intervertebral disc, improve within 4 weeks. Expensive tests have little utility in the initial evaluation phase unless surgery is being considered.

If there is no neurologic deficit, electrodiagnostic tests would be inappropriate because their main use is to assess neurologic function. If neurologic deficit is present, and a reasonable trial of nonsurgical therapy has not been successful, specific anatomic testing (computed tomography [CT] or magnetic resonance imaging [MRI]) might be useful if surgery is becomes an option. A reasonable trial of nonsurgical therapy would be based on the patient's pain and functional limitations, but consideration by the physician of the poor evidence for long-term relief with surgery would be appropriate.

Table 38.3 lists red flags in the history or physical examination of neck pain. If red flags are present or if there is deterioration, uncontrolled pain, progressive disability, or continual weakness for more than 4 weeks, the physician should consider further evaluation. Patients who are older, younger, or frail may deserve an evaluation sooner. However, the natural course of neck pain suggests that most patients will improve in 4 to 8 weeks. Patients with signs of infection or inflammation should have an erythrocyte sedimentation rate, blood count, and screening calcium/metabolic studies.

Radiographs are useful for detecting bony metastases, Paget's disease, myeloma, and ankylosing spondylitis. Radiographs of the neck area should include anteroposterior, lateral, and oblique views to show the foramina of the vertebrae. If occult fracture is ruled out, it may also be useful to request views in flexion and extension to show whether there is any spondylolisthesis (anterior shifting of one vertebral body onto the other). However, the significance of spondylolisthesis without neurologic signs or symptoms is unclear. CT scanning and MRI are much more useful but costly tools in diagnosing nerve root compression, disc disease, and other soft tissue pathology in the neck. MRI may be the study of choice in evaluating disc prolapse, but as in the lumbar spine, false-positive cervical MRI results are common. In patients without neck complaints, MRIs show disc degeneration in 17% of all discs imaged. This finding occurred in at least one disc in 12% of women in their 20s, and in over 80% of men and women over age 60! Approximately 8% of subjects (most over age 50) had posterior disc protrusion and foraminal stenosis (13).

A large prospective cohort trial compared two decision rules used to guide the ordering of cervical-spine xrays in patients with trauma (14). The Canadian C-Spine Rule (CCR, Figure 38.2) was shown to be more sensitive and specific (99.4%, 45.1% with LR+ = 1.8 and LR- = .55). The rule was evaluated in emergency rooms, not the outpatient setting, so should be used with caution.

MANAGEMENT

Initial Management

There is unclear or conflicting evidence on most of the commonly used therapies for uncomplicated neck pain (15–18). There is insufficient evidence on the effects of most treatments; heat or cold, traction, biofeedback, spray and stretch, acupuncture, and laser, to substantiate their effectiveness in patients with uncomplicated neck pain. Table 38.4 provides a long list of unproven treatments evaluated by systematic reviews (15). However, the evidence of negative outcomes is also clearly lacking. The critically thinking physician may continue to prescribe these treatments but should recognize the lack of evidence in their efficacy.

A flow sheet for the management of neck pain is presented in Figure 38.3. This recommended management plan is based on a consensus guideline produced from the Florida Agency for Health Care Policy (19). A list of evidence based treatment options is included in Table 38.5. In patients who are without red flag history, symptoms, or physical findings, it is reasonable to continue symptomatic therapies for up to 4 weeks before further evaluation. If cervical radiographs are negative or show only spondylosis, it is reasonable to continue conservative therapies for up to 8 weeks.

Strengthening exercise may be helpful in chronic mechanical neck pain. Any course of physical therapy should include strengthening exercise as opposed to mobilization or stretching only.

Although the evidence based options for the practitioner are slim, our patients will continue to need our best advice. In the absence of contradictions, certain conservative therapies still seem reasonable. They include: 1) usual activity, with or without the use of a cervical collar (unless a patient's usual activity is unusually physical or dangerous); 2) physical therapy that includes strengthening exercises; 3) nonsteroidal anti-inflammatory drugs (NSAIDs) and/or topical analgesic medication; and 4) mobilization or manipulation plus exercise. Muscle relaxants for acute spasm or opiates on a time-limited course for severe pain may be tried if the need arises.

The rationale for using NSAIDs for neck pain is based on the evidence that they are somewhat effective in treatment of low back pain and osteoarthritis of the knee and hip. NSAID medications have not been shown to be of benefit in neck pain in a systematic review. There is scant information on the effectiveness of any drug therapy for neck pain (18).

Manipulation is a controversial issue. Clinicians who have been trained in manipulation and millions of their patients attest to its value, but the evidence to support manipulation is inconclusive. The latest systematic review reports no signifi-

TABLE 40.4 Strength of Recommendation for Treatment of Bacterial Infections of the Skin*

Site	Infection	Treatment	Strength of Recommendation†
Epidermis	Impetigo Ecthyma (impetigo with ulceration) Bullous impetigo	Topical mupirocin or oral antibiotic that covers GABHS and *S. aureus** (consider CA-MRSA coverage)	A A A
Dermis	Erysipelas Cellulitis (dermis and subcutaneous tissue also)	Oral or intravenous antibiotic* based on severity (consider CA-MRSA coverage)	A A
Dermal appendages (hair follicle, nail fold)	Folliculitis Carbuncle, furuncle Paronychia Abscess	Topical or oral antibiotic* I&D I&D I&D (consider antibiotic for CA-MRSA coverage)	C B B B
Subcutaneous tissue/fascia	Necrotizing fasciitis	Hospitalize Intravenous antibiotic Debridement	B

CA-MRSA coverage, community-acquired methicillin-resistant *S aureus*; GABHS, Group A Beta-hemolytic streptococci; I & D, Incision & Drainage; *S. aureus, Staphylococcus aureus*

*Oral antibiotics must cover *Group A Beta-hemolytic streptococci* and *Staphylococcus aureus*: 1st line—dicloxacillin, cephalexin, 2nd line—clindamycin for severe penicillin allergy

†A = consistent, good-quality patient-oriented evidence; B = inconsistent or limited-quality patient-oriented evidence; C = consensus, disease-oriented evidence, usual practice, expert opinion, or case series. For information about the SORT evidence rating system, see *http://www.aafp.org/afpsort.xml*.

and believe that they have been bitten by a spider. Be wary of so-called "spider bites" especially when the patient has not seen the spider do the biting. CA-MRSA has been reported in athletes of all ages secondary to trauma, close contact, and sharing whirlpools (2).

Fortunately, community-acquired MRSA has a different resistance pattern than the hospital-acquired MRSA and can be treated by a number of older antibiotics including trimethoprim-sulfamethoxazole, clindamycin, tetracycline and doxycycline (3). Patients with recurrent MRSA skin abscesses should be empirically treated for nasal carriage of MRSA using mupirocin ointment to the nares twice daily for 5 days.

Topical antibiotics should only be used as monotherapy for the most mild and superficial bacterial skin infections. Mild cases of impetigo or minor wound infections can be treated with mupirocin (Bactroban) (4, 5). Bacitracin, Polysporin, or Neosporin are not sufficiently effective to be used alone in the treatment of established skin infections. Furthermore, Neosporin should be avoided because it frequently causes contact dermatitis.

IMPETIGO

This condition is a superficial skin infection often characterized by honey crusts. It can also be vesicular or bullous. Impetigo in children often occurs around the nose and mouth. Homeless persons are prone to impetigo because of lack of hygiene and lifestyle risks. Impetigo should be treated for 7 to 10 days with antibiotics that cover *S. pyogenes* and *S. aureus,* such as cephalexin or dicloxacillin (6) (strength of recommendation [SOR] = A). It may help to remove the crusts with warm soaks, and to apply dressings with antibiotic or petrola-

tum ointment to keep the lesions clean, moist and comfortable while the systemic antibiotic is working.

Two variations of impetigo are ecthyma and bullous impetigo. Ecthyma has an ulcerated punched-out base and bullous impetigo is often caused by *S. aureus*. Community-acquired MRSA can present as bullous impetigo in children. Staphylococcal-scalded skin syndrome (SSSS) is a life-threatening, more severe variation of bullous impetigo. In SSSS, the bullae are caused by exfoliating toxin, and the patient is systemically ill. Patients who have SSSS need emergent hospitalization for intravenous antibiotics, fluids, and supportive therapy.

CELLULITIS AND ERYSIPELAS

This condition is an acute infection of the skin that involves the dermis and subcutaneous tissues. Cellulitis is usually caused by β-hemolytic streptococci and *S. aureus*. Erysipelas is a specific type of superficial cellulitis with prominent lymphatic involvement causing lesions that are raised above the level of the surrounding skin with a clear line of demarcation between involved and uninvolved tissue. It is almost always caused by β-hemolytic streptococci and is seen most commonly on the extremities (6).

Cellulitis often begins with a break in the skin caused by trauma, a bite, or an underlying dermatosis (e.g., tinea pedis). It is usually seen on the legs and arms. The severity of the cellulitis, the systemic symptoms, and host factors determine whether oral or parenteral antibiotics are indicated. Crusted lesions from CA-MRSA can progress to celluliti (7).

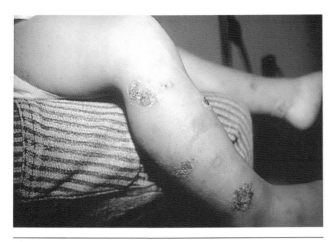

Figure 40.1 • Impetiginized flea bites.

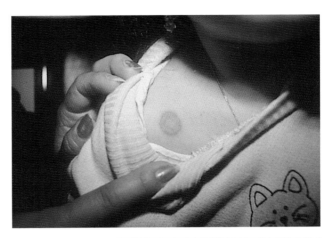

Figure 40.4 • Tinea corporis.

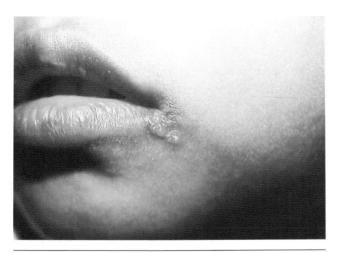

Figure 40.2 • Herpes simplex virus.

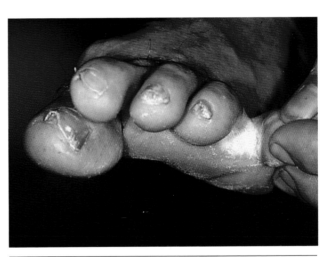

Figure 40.5 • Tinea pedis and onychomycosis.

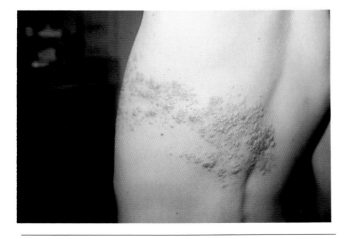

Figure 40.3 • Herpes zoster.

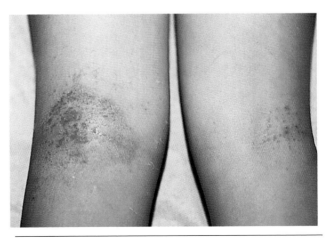

Figure 40.6 • Atopic dermatitis (acute) in the popliteal fossa.

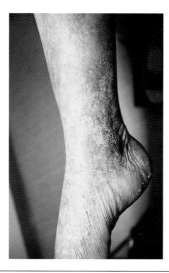

Figure 40.7 • Chronic dermatitis (lichen simplex chronicus).

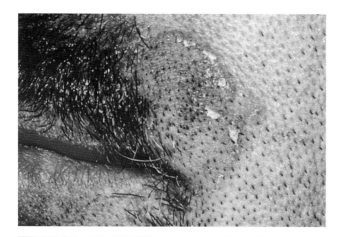

Figure 40.8 • Seborrhea.

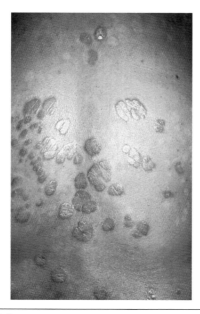

Figure 40.9 • Psoriasis.

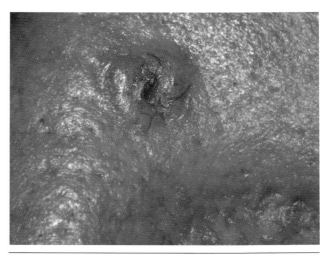

Figure 40.10 • Basal cell carcinoma. (From Goodheart HP. Goodheart's Photoguide of Common Skin Disorders, 2nd ed. Philadelphia, PA: Lippincott Williams & Wilkins, 2003.)

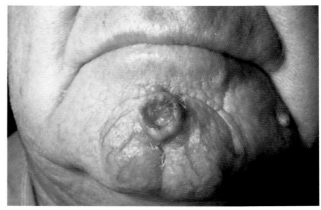

Figure 40.11 • Squamous cell carcinoma. (From Weber J, Kelley J. Health Assessment in Nursing, 2nd ed. Philadelphia, PA: Lippincott Williams & Wilkins, 2003.)

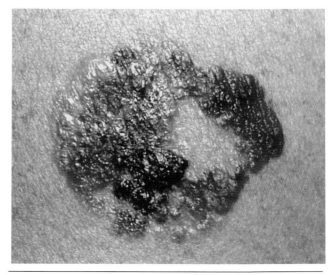

Figure 40.12 • Melanoma. (Courtesy of the Skin Cancer Foundation, New York, NY.)

FOLLICULITIS

Folliculitis is an infection or inflammation of the superficial portion of the hair follicle. Although it is usually caused by *S. aureus*, it can be caused by other bacteria, yeast, or occlusion. Its presentation can include perifollicular erythema, papules, or pustules. Magnification during the skin examination will reveal that the lesions are associated with hair follicles. Hot-tub folliculitis is caused by pseudomonas; folliculitis also can be caused by *Pityrosporum* yeast or occlusion of hair follicles with tight fitting clothing. Treatment ranges from avoiding occlusive clothing and contaminated hot-tubs to the use of topical or oral antibiotics, or antifungals.

ABSCESS

An abscess is defined as a localized collection of pus; abscesses that occur in or directly below the skin include furuncles, carbuncles, and the abscesses around fingernails (acute paronychia). A furuncle or boil is an abscess that starts in a hair follicle or sweat gland. A carbuncle occurs when the furuncle extends into the subcutaneous tissue. Epidermal inclusion cysts often become inflamed and infected and form a skin abscess; skin abscesses can occur anywhere on the body. Most skin abscesses are caused by *S. aureus* with CA-MRSA becoming a more common pathogen (2, 7). Other organisms that can cause abscesses of the skin include *Streptococcus* species, gram-negative bacteria, and anaerobes.

Incision and drainage (I&D) is the preferred treatment for all types of abscesses. The pus must be drained so that the lesion can heal. Systemic antibiotics, whether parenteral or oral, do not adequately penetrate an abscess to cure the infection. If there is significant surrounding cellulitis, systemic antibiotics may be needed as an adjunct to the I&D.

Diagnosis may be easy when the skin overlying the abscess is red, warm, tender, swollen, and fluctuant. When you are uncertain whether a red, warm, swollen area of the skin is cellulitis or an abscess, do a diagnostic needle aspiration. If you get pus from the aspiration, the abscess should be fully opened with a no. 11 scalpel. Because of the high prevalence of CA-MRSA, it is recommended to send a sample of the purulent material to the lab for culture. This can help guide the use of antibiotics, if these are needed and will help your community track the local resistance patterns of *S. aureus*.

NECROTIZING FASCIITIS

Necrotizing fasciitis, or "flesh-eating bacteria," is a deep infection of the subcutaneous tissues and fascia. It often presents with diffuse swelling of the arm or leg, followed by the appearance of bullae with clear fluid that may become violaceous in color. The patient has marked systemic symptoms. Necrotizing fasciitis may be caused by a single organism or be polymicrobial.

Cases of necrotizing fasciitis that occur after varicella or minor injuries, such as scratches and insect bites, are almost always from *S. pyogenes*. In the polymicrobial form, there is an average of five pathogens in each wound, with most of the organisms originating from the bowel flora (e.g., coliforms and anaerobic bacteria) (6).

Necrotizing fasciitis, which at first may look like cellulitis, can lead to cutaneous gangrene, myonecrosis, shock, and death. It is crucial to not miss necrotizing fasciitis because it is life- and limb-threatening and requires surgical debridement

along with intravenous antibiotics. Several clinical features suggest the presence of a necrotizing infection of the skin and its deeper structures: 1. severe, constant pain; 2. bullae; 3. skin necrosis or ecchymosis (bruising) that precedes skin necrosis; 4. gas in the soft tissues, detected by palpation or imaging; 5. edema that extends beyond the margin of erythema; 6. cutaneous anesthesia; 7. systemic toxicity, manifested by fever, delirium, and renal failure; and 8. rapid spread, especially during antibiotic therapy (6).

Viral Infections
WARTS

Warts are caused by more than 100 subtypes of human papillomavirus (HPV). Warts commonly occur on the hands, feet, and genitals. The appearance of the wart is strongly related to its location. Warts on the hands (verruca vulgaris) are usually raised and hyperkeratotic. Warts on the soles of the feet (plantar warts) are flat, disrupt skin lines, have dark dots visible in them, and may be quite painful. Flat warts (verruca plana) are flat and usually seen in groups on the face or legs. Genital warts (condylomata acuminata) often have a cauliflower appearance and are transmitted sexually. Ninety percent of genital warts are caused by HPV 6. High-risk HPV types (HPV 16, 18) generally do not cause visible genital warts and have been associated with cervical intraepithelial neoplasia and cervical cancer (8). New vaccines to prevent transmission of high-risk HPV types have shown promise in decreasing the incidence of cervical cancer in the future (8).

The natural history is for most warts to eventually regress; and there are many treatments for warts. Some warts do not respond to treatment, or recur within a short period of time. A comparison of treatment options for warts is found in Table 40.5. In office practice, the following treatments are generally considered first-line therapy for these conditions:

- Verruca vulgaris: salicylic acid or cryosurgery
- Plantar warts: salicylic acid or cryosurgery
- Flat warts: salicylic acid, topical tretinoin (Retin-A), cryosurgery
- Condylomata acuminata: podophyllin resin, podofilox (Condylox), trichloroacetic acid, cryosurgery, or imiquimod (Aldara)

HERPESVIRUSES

The major herpesviruses that affect the skin are herpes simplex (HSV) types 1 and 2 and varicella-zoster virus (VZV). A major characteristic of herpes infection is that the virus lies dormant in dorsal root ganglia, leading to recurrences. All herpetic skin infections are characterized by vesicular eruptions with surrounding erythema, which progress to ulcers and/or crusts and then reepithelialize over the course of days or weeks. Infections caused by herpes viruses include:

- Herpes gingivostomatitis or labialis (cold sores): caused by HSV (most commonly type 1, but sometimes type 2). A primary episode can affect the entire mouth (gingivostomatitis) and can be accompanied by fever, chills, and malaise. Recurrent episodes often occur on the lips (labialis) and are milder, sometimes asymptomatic, but accompanied by viral shedding (Color Plate Fig. 40.2).
- Genital herpes: caused by HSV (most commonly type 2, but sometimes type 1). This sexually transmitted infection

TABLE 40.5 Comparison of Therapies for Human Papillomavirus Infection[a–c]

Treatment Modality	Average Number of Treatments	Success Rate[d] (%)	Recurrence Rate Within 6 mo (%)	Relative Cost to Patient ($)[+]	Strength of Recommendation[*]
Cryotherapy	1.9	83	28	$$	A
Podophyllin resin	4.2	65	39	$$$	A
Podofilox (Condylox) (patient applied)	10.5	61	34	$$	A
Trichloroacetic acid	4	81	36	$$$	B
CO_2 laser	1.3	89	8	$$	A
Electrocautery	1.4	93	24	$$	B
LEEP	1	90	ND	$	B
Excision	1.1	93	24	$	A
Topical fluorouracil (patient applied)	6.6	71	13	$$	A

LEEP, loop electrosurgical excisional procedure; ND, no data or not recorded.
[+]Relative cost: $ = <$300.00; $$ = $300–$600; $$$ = >$600
[a]This table is based on the author's best estimate as compiled from data from the available literature. Very small studies, studies with results that fell 2 standard deviations beyond the mean, and very poorly designed studies were excluded.
[b]Modified from Mayeaux EJ, Harper MB, Barksdale W, Pope JB. Noncervical human papillomavirus genital infections. Am Fam Physician. 1995;52(4): 1137–1147 (20).
[c]Based on hypothetical patient with 6 initial warts and 2 retreatment warts.
[d]Defined as clearance of all condylomata at the end of healing from therapy.
A = consistent, good-quality patient-oriented evidence; B = inconsistent or limited-quality patient-oriented evidence; C = consensus, disease-oriented evidence, usual practice, expert opinion, or case series. For information about the SORT evidence rating system, see *http://www.aafp.org/afpsort.xml*.

presents as herpetic lesions on the genitals, anus, or buttocks. As in gingivostomatitis, first episodes are often more severe; subsequent episodes range from moderate to asymptomatic but are accompanied by viral shedding and the possibility of transmission to sexual partners. Genital herpes can be spread between active episodes of disease because infected persons can shed the virus asymptomatically. Active ulcers create a higher risk of acquiring HIV during sexual contact with HIV-positive individuals.

- Chickenpox: This is the initial infection of VZV. It typically consists of a few days of fever and respiratory symptoms with the characteristic herpes rash lesions that begin on the trunk and over several days spread more centrifugally. Fortunately, the varicella vaccine has diminished the incidence of chickenpox.
- Herpes zoster (shingles): This is a reactivation of dormant VZV along a skin dermatome (see Color Plate Fig. 40.3). The outbreak is usually unilateral and vesicular.

Most infections with HSV and VZV are acutely painful, uncomplicated, and resolve spontaneously in 1 to 2 weeks. Complications include encephalitis and disseminated infections; these occur especially in infants or immunosuppressed individuals. One prolonged and painful after-effect of the infection is postherpetic neuralgia that presents as chronic pain in the dermatome previously infected with herpes zoster.

There are no cures for HSV or VZV; the goals of therapy, therefore, are to diminish pain, viral shedding, and duration of symptoms, and to prevent recurrences. In HSV, prophylactic daily oral medication can prevent or reduce recurrences;

in zoster, early antiviral treatment may prevent postherpetic neuralgia.

Antiviral agents with proven effectiveness against herpes simplex and herpes zoster are acyclovir, famciclovir, and valacyclovir (SOR = A). These antiviral agents can be used to treat primary and recurrent herpes simplex and herpes zoster, and to prevent recurrent herpes simplex. Acyclovir is the only one also approved to treat acute varicella (chickenpox). Most importantly, we should use the varicella vaccine for primary prevention.

Fungal Infections

Fungal infections of the skin occur at many sites and are most often caused by dermatophytes, *Candida*, or *Pityrosporum* species. The dermatophytes cause tinea infections that are commonly called ringworm, although no worm is involved in ringworm. The typical dermatophyte infection of the body (tinea corporis) has an annular appearance with central clearing, redness, and scale on the perimeter of this well-demarcated lesion (Color Plate Fig. 40.4). Tinea versicolor is caused by an inflammatory reaction to the yeast-like *Pityrosporum* species rather than a dermatophyte. *Candida* thrives on wet mucosal surfaces but also affects the skin; it causes thrush, balanitis, vaginitis, and rashes in the groin and under the breast.

Common dermatophyte infections are:

- Tinea capitis (tinea of the head) causes patchy alopecia (hair loss) with broken hairs and some scaling. Because the hair shaft and follicle are involved, topical antifungals are not effective. Oral antifungal medications include griseofulvin,

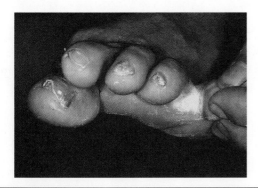

Figure 40.5 • Tinea pedis and onychomycosis.

itraconazole, and terbinafine for 4 to 8 weeks. A meta-analysis found a 2- to 4-week course of terbinafine to be at least as effective as a 6- to 8-week course of griseofulvin for treating *Trichophyton* infections of the scalp. Griseofulvin was likely to be superior to terbinafine for the rare cases of tinea capitis caused by *Microsporum* species (9).

- Tinea corporis (tinea of the body) can occur on almost any part of the body. Small areas may respond well to topical antifungals. Topical over-the-counter (OTC) antifungals (miconazole, clotrimazole) should be first-line agents. Large areas may require treatment with oral antifungals (griseofulvin, terbinafine, itraconazole) for 2 to 4 weeks.
- Tinea cruris (tinea of the groin) may be red and scaling without the central clearing seen in tinea corporis. It should be differentiated from candidal infection, which often is redder and has satellite lesions, and erythrasma, a superficial bacterial infection that may be pink or brown and has coral-red fluorescence under ultraviolet light. Topical or systemic antifungals may be used for tinea cruris depending upon the severity of involvement. If you are uncertain if there is *Candida* involvement, it is best to choose an antifungal agent that covers both dermatophytes and *Candida* (e.g., not tolnaftate [Tinactin] or naftifine [Naftin]).
- Tinea pedis (tinea of the feet) may be seen as macerated white areas between the toes (see Color Plate Fig. 40.5) or as dry red scaling on the soles or sides of the feet (moccasin distribution). A third, less common presentation causes vesicles on the feet. It can be treated with the same topical or oral antifungals used for tinea corporis or cruris. Griseofulvin, terbinafine, or itraconazole may be used when the lesions are not responding to topical agents. A Cochrane review suggests that terbinafine is more effective than griseofulvin (10).

A skin scraping treated with KOH and analyzed using a microscope can be diagnostic when classic hyphae or yeast forms are detected. KOH with DMSO will help to dissolve the cell membranes of the epithelial cells for easier viewing and eliminates the need to heat the slide. False-negative results are common when specimen collection is inadequate, when the patient has started OTC antifungals, or when the slide is read by an inexperienced viewer. Fungal cultures can be expensive and may take a long time to grow, but they can provide the most definitive evidence of fungal infection while providing you with the identity of the fungus.

Onychomycosis is a fungal infection of the nails. Topical antifungal agents do not work well, and oral antifungal agents (itraconazole, terbinafine) are expensive and may cause liver toxicity. These agents can be given continuously for 3 to 4 months or as pulse therapy 1 week a month for 3 to 4 months. It is important to establish a definitive diagnosis of onychomycosis before starting treatment with oral antifungals, because there are other causes for dystrophic nails such as psoriasis, lichen planus, and trauma. The three most useful methods for diagnosis are a KOH preparation from subungual scrapings, a nail culture, or a distal nail clipping sent in formalin for periodic acid-Schiff (PAS) staining by a pathologist. The sensitivities and specificities of each of the techniques are as follows: KOH: 80% and 72%; culture: 59% and 82%; PAS: 92% and 72% (11). A meta-analysis of randomized controlled trials (RCTs) found that continuous terbinafine of 250 mg daily for 16 weeks is the most effective treatment for onychomycosis (number needed to treat [NNT] = 3) (12).

DERMATITIS

Dermatitis is a nonspecific term that means inflammation of the skin. There are many causes and patterns of skin inflammation including eczema, contact dermatitis, and atopic dermatitis. Eczema is the most common type of skin inflammation; it can occur in three stages: acute, subacute, and chronic. Color Plate Figure 40.6 provides an example of acute dermatitis, and Color Plate Figure 40.7 illustrates chronic eczema (lichen simplex chronicus). Common forms of dermatitis are described below:

- Eczema is frequently seen on the hands or feet but can occur on any part of the body. Acute eczema is typically vesicular and red, whereas subacute eczema lacks the vesicles and has prominent scaling and dry, cracking skin. Chronic eczema includes lichenification (thickened plaque with accentuation of the skin lines).
- Nummular eczema is coin-shaped (nummus = coin).
- Contact dermatitis is an allergic response to an allergen such as the chemical found in the poison ivy or poison oak plant (rhus dermatitis). These lesions are often linear and vesicular. Other contact allergens include nickel in jewelry and belt buckles and chemicals in deodorants.
- Atopic dermatitis is a type of eczematous eruption that is itchy, recurrent, and symmetric and often found on flexural

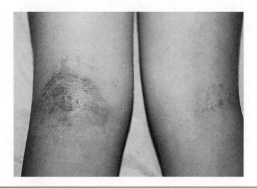

Figure 40.6 • Atopic dermatitis (acute) in the popliteal fossa.

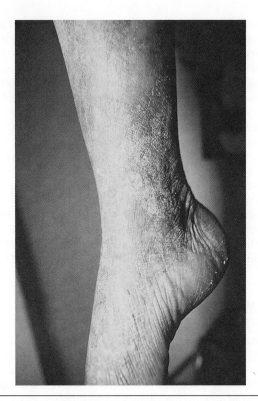

Figure 40.7 • Chronic dermatitis (lichen simplex chronicus).

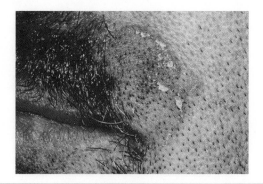

Figure 40.8 • Seborrhea.

surfaces (see Color Plate Fig. 40.6). These patients often have either a personal or a family history of asthma, allergic rhinitis, or conjunctivitis. In infancy, atopic dermatitis often appears on the face. After infancy, the dry, scaling, and red lesions are found in flexural areas such as the antecubital or popliteal fossa. Most atopic dermatitis is not caused by specific allergens, but develops from a number of trigger factors in patients who have a strong genetic predisposition to develop eczematous eruptions.

Treatment for all types of dermatitis has basic principles. First, to avoid drying the skin and increasing the pruritus and inflammation, avoid skin irritants (e.g., drying soaps), bathing too long, and bathing in water that is too hot. Second, use emollients or moisturizers to moisten the skin. Third, treat inflammatory components with a topical steroid, choosing the strength and vehicle based on diagnosis, chronicity, and location. Fourth, because itching is a prominent feature of many types of dermatitis, efforts should be made to stop the scratch-itch cycle. This is especially true for atopic dermatitis and lichen simplex chronicus. Lichen simplex chronicus often needs potent topical steroid ointments to penetrate the thick plaque and moisturize the cracked pruritic skin. There is little evidence that antihistamines improve the outcomes in atopic dermatitis but oral sedating antihistamines are often used to stop itching, especially at night (13).

Finally, any type of dermatitis may develop a secondary bacterial infection. This may take the form of impetigo or weeping and crusting (see Color Plate Fig. 40.6). Signs of infection should lead to treatment with an antibiotic that covers *S. pyogenes* and *S. aureus*.

New topical immunomodulators tacrolimus and pime-crolimus are indicated to treat atopic dermatitis and eczema for adults and children 2 years of age and older. These agents have similar effectiveness when compared with topical steroids without the risk of skin atrophy. However, new concerns about risks for cancer has prompted the US Food and Drug Administration to publish an advisory that states tacrolimus and pimecrolimus should only be used as second-line agents for short-term and intermittent treatment of atopic dermatitis in patients, 2 years and older, unresponsive to, or intolerant of, other treatments.

Seborrhea

Seborrhea is a superficial inflammatory dermatitis. It is a common condition that is characterized by patches of erythema and scaling (Color Plate Fig. 40.8). The typical distribution of seborrhea includes the scalp (dandruff); eyebrows and eyelids; nasolabial creases; behind the ears; eyebrows; forehead; cheeks; around the nose; under the beard or mustache; over the sternum; axillae; submammary folds; umbilicus; groin; and the gluteal creases. These areas are the regions with the greatest number of pilosebaceous units producing sebum.

The prevalence of seborrhea is approximately 3% to 5% in young adults. Its incidence increases with age, and it is especially common in persons with Parkinson's disease and in persons who are HIV-positive. Although the cause of seborrhea is not entirely clear, it is thought to involve an inflammatory hypersensitivity to epidermal, bacterial, or yeast antigens. Persons with seborrhea have a profusion of *Pityrosporum ovale* on the skin. Although this yeast can be a normal skin inhabitant, persons who have seborrhea appear to respond to its presence with an inflammatory reaction.

Seborrhea is characterized by remissions and exacerbations. The most common precipitating factors are stress and cold weather. The treatment of seborrhea should be directed at the inflammation and the *Pityrosporum*.

Seborrhea is highly responsive to topical steroids, so a low-potency steroid is usually adequate. To avoid atrophy, it is especially important to use a low-potency steroid for the treatment of seborrhea on the face; 1% hydrocortisone cream or lotion works well. Prescribe lotion or solution for seborrhea in hair-covered areas because it is easier and less messy to apply than a cream. If scalp seborrhea is severe, you may prescribe a higher-potency steroid solution such as fluocinonide (Lidex) solution or clobetasol propionate (Temovate) scalp

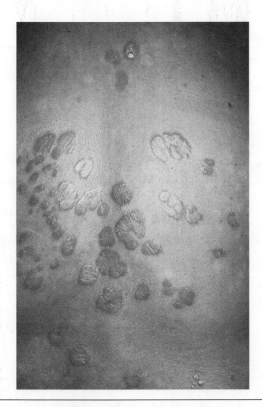

Figure 40.9 • Psoriasis.

application, as the risk of atrophy on the scalp is less than on the face.

To reduce the profusion of *Pityrosporum*, you should direct the patient to apply antifungals to the affected areas. For seborrhea of the scalp, the antifungal shampoos that are most effective contain selenium sulfide, zinc pyrithione, ketoconazole, or coal tar derivatives. For seborrhea of the skin, ketoconazole cream is an effective antifungal preparation.

Patients should understand that these treatments are not curative, and seborrhea may return when they are under stress or they stop using the antiseborrheic shampoos. The antifungals can be used to prevent exacerbations, but the steroids should be applied only to active areas of inflammation.

Psoriasis

Psoriasis is a chronic condition characterized by alterations in the immune system that lead to epidermal proliferation and inflammation. The lesions are well-circumscribed, red, scaling patches, with white thickened scales (Color Plate Fig. 40.9). Areas affected can include the scalp, nails, and extensor surfaces of limbs, elbows, knees, the sacral region, and the genitalia. Psoriasis lesions may also be guttate as in water drops, inverse when found in intertriginous areas such as the inguinal and intergluteal folds, or volar when found on the palms or soles. Psoriatic nail changes occur in 10% to 40% of persons with psoriasis. These nail changes include pitting, onycholysis, and subungual keratosis.

Treatment options for psoriasis include emollients, topical steroids, topical vitamin D (calcipotriene), anthralin, topical tar and tar shampoo, intralesional steroids, ultraviolet light, methotrexate, and topical and oral retinoids. The most com-

mon treatments of psoriasis involve using high-potency topical steroids. Combination therapies are helpful to patients with psoriasis. One RCT demonstrated that a topical combination product of calcipotriene and betamethasone is more effective than either agent used alone in the treatment of psoriasis (NNT = 2) (14). While such a combination product is not commercially available, calcipotriene can be used daily with a daily topical steroid. Tazarotene, a new topical retinoid, is effective for treating plaque psoriasis but may cause local irritation. Combining tazarotene with topical steroids can increase the effectiveness of both agents and reduce the incidence of local adverse effects (15) (SOR = B).

Systemic steroids are contraindicated in psoriasis; they can precipitate severe flares and generalized pustular disease. When using potent topical steroids for chronic therapy in psoriasis (or eczema), it helps to use pulse therapy on weekends to avoid side effects and loss of efficacy. Tacrolimus and pimecrolimus are effective in treating facial and intertriginous psoriasis and can be used to avoid steroid adverse effects (16) (SOR = B).

Acne

Acne is an inflammatory disease of the pilosebaceous unit (sebaceous glands and their associated small hairs). The glands produce sebum, which is a complex lipid mixture, to maintain hydration of the skin. Acne involves blockage of the pilosebaceous unit with sebum and desquamated cells, accompanied by an overgrowth of *Propionibacterium acnes* (*P. acnes*) in the follicle.

Noninflammatory lesions of acne are open comedones (blackheads) and closed comedones (whiteheads). When there is disruption of the follicle wall, *P. acnes*, sebum, hair, and cells extrude into the dermis. This causes inflammation and leads to the formation of papules, pustules, nodules, and cysts. The causes or exacerbating factors for acne are genetics; androgens; stress; excessive friction on the skin (e.g., with sweat bands and helmet straps); cosmetics; and medications, including corticosteroids, lithium, isoniazid, and hormonal contraception with increased androgenicity.)

Table 40.6 summarizes the strength of evidence for acne treatments, and Table 40.7 summarizes treatments based on acne severity. Use morphology to distinguish between noninflammatory (comedonal, obstructive) and inflammatory acne. Determine the distribution and severity of the case and base therapy on the type and severity of the acne. Mild comedonal acne responds to topical retinoids or azelaic acid. More severe inflammatory acne often requires oral antibiotics in combination with topical retinoids and benzoyl peroxide. If this fails, and acne is scarring, consider isotretinoin (Accutane). Isotretinoin is the most potent medication for acne but has many potential side effects, including birth defects. Isotretinan requires prescribers demonstrate competence in selecting and treating patients. The medication should not be prescribed or dispensed to any woman without two negative pregnancy tests and two forms of birth control. When prescribing topical retinoids, explain to the patient that redness and scaling may occur, and that the acne may worsen during the first 2 to 4 weeks before an improvement is seen. Because retinoids increase sun sensitivity, the patient should be warned about sun safety measures.

When starting topical retinoid therapy, it helps to begin

TABLE 40.6 Strength of Recommendation for Medications for Acne Therapy

Topical
- Benzoyl peroxide - antimicrobial effect (gel, cream, lotion) (2.5, 5, 10%) B
- Topical antibiotics - clindamycin and erythromycin B
  - Erythromycin - solution, gel
  - Clindamycin - solution, gel, lotion
- Combination topicals
  - BenzaClin gel – clindamycin 1%, Benzoyl peroxide 5%, B
  - Benzamycin gel - Erythromycin 3%, Benzoyl peroxide 5%, B
- Retinoids
  - tretinoin (Retin-A) gel, cream, liquid, micronized A
  - adapalene (Differin) gel A
  - tazarotene (Tazorac) gel A
- Azelaic acid (Azelex) B

Systemic
- Oral Antibiotics—A
  - Tetracycline 500 mg qd-bid - inexpensive, need to take on an empty stomach; avoid within 2 hours of calcium or calcium containing products
  - Doxycycline 100 mg qd-bid - inexpensive, well tolerated, increases sun sensitivity
  - Minocycline 50mg - 100 mg qd-bid - expensive, less resistance of P. acnes
  - Erythromycin 250mg –500mg bid- inexpensive, frequent GI disturbance
- Estrogen dominant birth control pills – women only - B
- Isotretinoin (Accutane) for cystic and scarring acne that has not responded to other therapies -A

TABLE 40.7 Acne Therapy by Severity

Comedonal Acne—Obstructive acne
- Retinoids
- Azelaic acid
- No place for oral antibiotics

Mild Papulopustular
- Topical antibiotics and benzoyl peroxide
- Retinoids
- Azelaic acid
- May add oral antibiotics if topical agents are not working

Papulopustular or Nodulocystic Acne—Moderate and inflammatory
- May start with topical antibiotic, benzoyl peroxide, and oral antibiotic
- Oral antibiotics are often essential at this stage
- Retinoids
- Consider stopping oral antibiotics when topical agents are working well

Severe Cystic or Scarring Acne
- Isotretinoin

Estrogen dominant birth control pills—can be used for any type of acne in women only, especially if the pill is desired for birth control too.

with the formulations that cause the least inflammation. These include lower potency tretinoin (Retin-A) and adapalene gel (Differin). For oily skin and more severe acne, it may help to use the strongest preparations, such as tretinoin gel, adapalene gel, or tazarotene gel. In a meta-analysis of five randomized trials, adapalene 0.1 % gel was found to be just as efficacious as tretinoin 0.025 % gel, worked faster, and was less irritating and less drying than tretinoin gel (17) (SOR = A). Tazarotene is a potent retinoid that demonstrated greater effectiveness in acne than adapalene in a number of measures (18) (SOR = B). However, tazarotene was associated with transiently greater levels of burning, pruritus, erythema, and peeling compared with adapalene,

Useful combination products for the treatment of acne combine benzoyl peroxide with clindamycin or erythromycin. Benzoyl peroxide has a direct toxic effect on *P. acnes* and defers development of *P. acnes* resistance to antibiotics. The least expensive prescription products for acne include oral tetracycline or doxycycline and topical erythromycin. Patients who cannot afford the very expensive combination products can use these products with OTC benzoyl peroxide.

Sun Damage and Precancers

Sun damage to the skin can be seen in photoaging, which results in mottled hyperpigmentation and wrinkling. Sun damage can lead to precancers such as actinic keratosis and lentigo maligna.

The most common skin cancers are:

- basal cell carcinoma (BCC) 80%
- squamous cell carcinoma (SCC) 16%
- melanoma 4%

Sun exposure is the most important risk factor; other risk factors include a positive family history and fair skin type. The incidence of these cancers increases with age, probably because of cumulative sun exposure.

BCCs are the most common skin cancer and occur 85% of the time on the head and neck. There three major morphologic types are nodular, superficial, and morpheaform (sclerosing). The typical nodular BCC is pearly and raised with telangiectasias (see Color Plate Fig. 40.10). As it expands, its center may ulcerate, bleed, and become crusted. Superficial BCCs look like SCC—red or pink, flat, scaling plaques that may have erosions or crusts. Sclerosing BCCs are rare (1% of BCCs), flat, and scar-like. SCCs can look like a superficial BCC or can be more elevated and nodular; SCCs are frequently hyperkeratotic and bleed easily (see Color Plate Fig. 40.11).

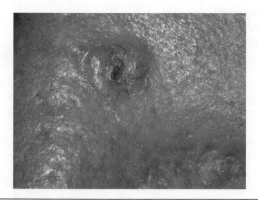

Figure 40.10 • Basal cell carcinoma. (From Goodheart HP. Goodheart's Photoguide of Common Skin Disorders, 2nd ed. Philadelphia, PA: Lippincott Williams & Wilkins, 2003.)

Actinic keratoses (AKs) are premalignant and have a 2% risk of becoming SCC if untreated. Recognizing and treating AKs is a secondary method of skin cancer prevention. There is a spectrum of skin cancer disease—from actinic keratosis to Bowen's disease (SCC *in situ*) to SCC. When a lesion is more thickened or indurated than a typical AK, it is necessary to biopsy it. Otherwise, AKs can be treated easily with cryotherapy or 5-fluorouracil.

Melanoma in the United States has been increasing in the last few decades. Early detection and treatment can prevent deaths and morbidity. Table 40.8 presents "ABCDE" guidelines for the diagnosis of melanoma, and Color Plate Figure 40.12 provides a photograph of a melanoma that meets all the ABCDE criteria. Many benign growths can resemble melanoma, so a suspicious growth should receive a full-depth biopsy to make a definitive diagnosis.

BENIGN GROWTHS THAT CAN BE CONFUSED WITH SKIN CANCERS

Family physicians should have a working knowledge of the most common benign growths. Some benign pigmented lesions that may be confused with melanoma include nevi, con-

TABLE 40.8 ABCDE Guidelines for Diagnosis of Melanoma
Asymmetry. Most early melanomas are asymmetrical—a line through the middle would not create matching halves. Common moles are round and symmetrical.
Border. The borders of early melanomas are often uneven and may have scalloped or notched edges. Common moles have smoother, more even borders.
Color. Common moles usually are a single shade of brown. Varied shades of brown, tan, or black are often the first sign of melanoma. As melanomas progress, the colors red, white, and blue may appear.
Diameter. Early melanomas tend to grow larger than common moles, generally to at least the size of a pencil eraser (about 6 mm or 1\4″ in diameter).
Elevation. Malignant melanoma is almost always elevated, at least in part, so that it is palpable.

genital nevi, seborrheic keratoses, dermatofibromas, and lentigines. It is important to learn the appearance and characteristics of these benign lesions so that you can differentiate them from melanoma. When there is a reasonable suspicion that the lesion is malignant and not one of these benign lesions, a biopsy should be performed.

Sebaceous hyperplasia may look like a BCC. These benign lesions are raised and can have pearly borders and telangiectasias like a BCC. When you are uncertain of the diagnosis, a shave biopsy can remove the lesion and determine whether it is malignant. Completely benign-appearing sebaceous hyperplasia is a cosmetic issue that can be treated electively if desired.

Seborrheic keratosis can mimic melanoma. These lesions develop with age and are often large and pigmented with irregular borders. Although they usually are verrucous and have a stuck-on appearance, they can be flat and irregular. When uncertain of the diagnosis, get a consult or perform a biopsy.

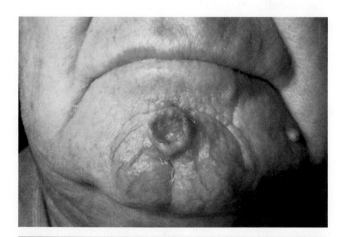

Figure 40.11 • Squamous cell carcinoma. (From Weber J, Kelley J. Health Assessment in Nursing, 2nd ed. Philadelphia, PA: Lippincott Williams & Wilkins, 2003.)

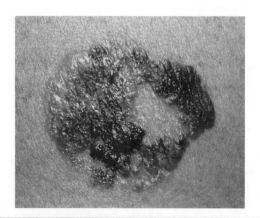

Figure 40.12 • Melanoma. (Courtesy of the Skin Cancer Foundation, New York, NY.)

CONCLUSION

This chapter presents an approach to the diagnosis and treatment of common skin conditions. The focus of treatment has been medical rather than surgical.

Skin surgery is essential for the diagnosis and treatment of skin cancers. A skin biopsy can provide important information when you have some confidence in your differential diagnosis. A biopsy should be performed only if you are fairly certain of the type of lesion involved. The type of biopsy type is determined by the suspected diagnosis. For example, a shave biopsy may not be deep enough for a suspected melanoma, and an elliptical excision may be unnecessarily large for a suspected BCC that turns out to be benign (19). When the lesion is benign, an experienced clinician may be able to diagnose an unknown case without a biopsy, thereby saving the patient from an invasive procedure.

Diagnosing skin conditions often involves learning and recognizing patterns. It is helpful to spend time examining pictures of skin conditions in dermatology atlases and textbooks to learn these patterns. There are also an increasing number of very useful dermatology sites and atlases on the Internet.

Although the skin is the largest organ of the body, it is highly responsive to the psychologic state of the patient. Many skin conditions (acne, seborrhea, psoriasis, eczema) are exacerbated by stress. Therefore, it is important to take into account the whole patient when treating skin conditions. Some skin conditions result from sexually transmitted infections or sun exposure; in such cases it is not enough to prescribe a medicine or cut out a cancer. Instead, you should address the lifestyle changes necessary to prevent recurrence.

Finally, optimal treatment and adherence depend on the patient having a good understanding of the diagnosis and treatment. Therefore, good health care to patients with skin conditions often requires a comprehensive approach to the patient, taking into account the principles of counseling for health education, prevention, psychosocial stressors, and attention to the role of the family.

CASE DISCUSSION

CASE 1

Diagnosis: Flea bites with secondary impetigo infection.

Treatment: Cephalexin suspension by mouth three times daily for 10 days; warm soaks to remove the crusts atraumatically; ongoing flea treatment for the cat; and extermination of the house (if needed).

CASE 2

Diagnosis: Recurrent herpes labialis.

Treatment: Options include: 1. no treatment; 2. oral acyclovir, valacyclovir, or famciclovir; or 3. penciclovir cream.

Prevention: Use sunscreen because sun exposure can precipitate a recurrence. Although stress is a known risk factor for recurrence, there is no evidence that stress management prevents recurrence. The severity and location of this case does not warrant the use of oral antiviral medica-

---

BOX 40-1

Interactive Dermatology Atlas *http://www.dermatlas.net*

The Interactive Dermatology Atlas contains more than 1,000 photographs, a sophisticated search tool, quiz mode, and more than 60 interactive cases. The interactive cases are based on real patient visits and simulate the diagnosis and treatment of patients. There are two sets of family medicine clerkship cases designed for medical students, who are encouraged to take a history, view the images, and perform laboratory tests and biopsies as needed. Students can choose a diagnosis and learn the real diagnosis before deciding upon treatment. Visual comparisons are available to compare the user's diagnosis with the real diagnosis. At the end of each case, information is provided on the recommended management of the patient. Developed by Drs. Richard Usatine and Brian Madden.

Other valuable atlases on the Internet include:

1. DermAtlas — *http://dermatlas.org/*
2. Dermnet *dermnet.com*
3. DermIS (Derm Information Systems) — *http://dermis.net*

Dermmeister — is a dermatology photo atlas for your personal digital assistant featuring more than 500 high-resolution photos of 66 common skin disorders. Developed by Drs. Richard Usatine and Andrew Schechtman. Available free at:
http://www.meistermed.com/MoreMeister/dermmeister/

---

tions for prophylaxis (unlike severe recurrent herpes genitalis).

CASE 3

Diagnosis: Herpes zoster (shingles).

Treatment: No antiviral treatment is indicated because the lesions have been there for 5 days. Treatment has proven to be effective only if begun within 3 days of onset. Symptomatic treatment for pain or pruritus may be given as needed.

Prevention: None. This is unlikely to occur again for this patient, but if disseminated herpes zoster develops or there are risk factors for HIV, perform an HIV test.

CASE 4

Diagnosis: Tinea corporis. Ultraviolet light showed green fluorescence. A skin scraping was done; KOH was added and microscopic analysis revealed branching hyphae. The main differential diagnosis is nummular eczema; central clearing and positive test results for fluorescence and hyphae make the diagnosis of tinea corporis certain.

Treatment: Apply an over-the-counter antifungal cream (clotrimazole or miconazole) twice a day for 2 weeks or until lesion resolves. If initial topical treatment fails, try a second topical antifungal before considering an oral antifungal. (The area involved is too small to warrant systemic treatment.)

Prevention: Take the cat to the veterinarian for treatment.

References

1. Berg AO. Screening for skin cancer: recommendations and rationale. American Journal of Preventive Medicine. 2001;20: 44–46.
2. Kazakova SV, Hageman JC, Matava M, et al. A clone of methicillin-resistant *Staphylococcus aureus* among professional football players. N Engl J Med. 2005;352:468–475.
3. Naimi TS, LeDell KH, Como-Sabetti K, et al. Comparison of community- and health care-associated methicillin-resistant *Staphylococcus aureus* infection. JAMA. 2003;290:2976–2984.
4. Kraus SJ, Eron LJ, Bottenfield GW, Drehobl MA, Bushnell WD, Cupo MA. Mupirocin cream is as effective as oral cephalexin in the treatment of secondarily infected wounds. J Fam Pract. 1998;47:429–433.
5. Koning S, Verhagen AP, van-Suijlekom-Smit LWA, Morris A, Butler CC, van-der-Wouden JC. Interventions for impetigo. Cochrane Database Syst Rev. 2003;2:CD00326.
6. Stevens DL, Bisno AL, Chambers HF, et al. Practice guidelines for the diagnosis and management of skin and soft-tissue infections. Clin Infect Dis. 2005;41:1373–1406.
7. Zetola N, Francis JS, Nuermberger EL, Bishai WR. Community-acquired methicillin-resistant *Staphylococcus aureus*: an emerging threat. Lancet Infect Dis. 2005;5:275–286.
8. Harper DM, Franco EL, Wheeler C, et al. Efficacy of a bivalent L1 virus-like particle vaccine in prevention of infection with human papillomavirus types 16 and 18 in young women: a randomised controlled trial. Lancet. 2004;364: 1757–1765.
9. Fleece D, Gaughan JP, Aronoff SC. Griseofulvin versus terbinafine in the treatment of tinea capitis: a meta-analysis of randomized, clinical trials. Pediatrics. 2004;114:1312–1315.
10. Bell-Syer SE, Hart R, Crawford F, Torgerson DJ, Tyrrell W, Russell I. Oral treatments for fungal infections of the skin of the foot. Cochrane Database Syst Rev. 2002;CD003584.
11. Weinberg JM, Koestenblatt EK, Tutrone WD, Tishler HR, Najarian L. Comparison of diagnostic methods in the evaluation of onychomycosis. J Am Acad Dermatol. 2003;49: 193–197.
12. Crawford F, Young P, Godfrey C, et al. Oral treatments for toenail onychomycosis: a systematic review. Arch Dermatol. 2002;138:811–816.
13. Klein PA, Clark RAF. An evidence-based review of the efficacy of antihistamines in relieving pruritus in atopic dermatitis. Arch Dermatol. 1999;135:1522–1525.
14. Papp KA, Guenther L, Boyden B, et al. Early onset of action and efficacy of a combination of calcipotriene and betamethasone dipropionate in the treatment of psoriasis. J Am Acad Dermatol. 2003;48:48–54.
15. Lebwohl M, Poulin Y. Tazarotene in combination with topical corticosteroids. J Am Acad Dermatol. 1998;39:S139–S143.
16. Lebwohl M, Freeman AK, Chapman MS, Feldman SR, Hartle JE, Henning A. Tacrolimus ointment is effective for facial and intertriginous psoriasis. J Am Acad Dermatol. 2004;51: 723–730.
17. Cunliffe WJ, Poncet M, Loesche C, Verschoore M. A comparison of the efficacy and tolerability of adapalene 0.1% gel versus tretinoin 0.025% gel in patients with acne vulgaris: a meta-analysis of five randomized trials. Br J Dermatol. 1998; 139 Suppl 52:48–56.
18. Webster GF, Guenther L, Poulin YP, Solomon BA, Loven K, Lee J. A multicenter, double-blind, randomized comparison study of the efficacy and tolerability of once-daily tazarotene 0.1% gel and adapalene 0.1% gel for the treatment of facial acne vulgaris. Cutis. 2002;69(2 Suppl):4–11.
19. Usatine R, Moy R, Tobinick E, Siegel D. Skin Surgery: A Practical Guide. St. Louis, MO: Mosby; 1998.
20. Mayeaux EJ Jr, Harper MB, Barksdale W, Pope JB. Noncervical human papillomavirus genital infections. Am Fam Physician. 1995;52:1137–1150.

Skin Wounds: Contusions, Abrasions, Lacerations, and Ulcers

Richard Usatine and Wayne A. Hale

CASE

A 79-year-old patient comes to your office after falling at home. Her left deltoid has a 3-cm-diameter hematoma, and there is a 4 × 3-cm triangular-shaped superficial skin tear of the left forearm. There is a 5-cm-long, full-thickness laceration of the dorsum of her left hand, with exposed but intact tendons. Her left leg has a 4 × 6-cm abrasion on the lower lateral region that is oozing blood and serum. The surrounding skin has the typical hyperpigmentation and skin changes associated with chronic venous insufficiency. Her last tetanus booster was 6 years ago.

CLINICAL QUESTIONS

1. How should you anesthetize, clean, and dress these injuries?
2. How should each of the injuries be treated?
3. Which area is most likely to be susceptible to delayed healing?
4. What are the typical causes and presentations of contusions, abrasions, lacerations, and ulcerations?

Family physicians frequently treat skin injuries. This chapter discusses treatment of the most common skin wounds, including contusions, abrasions, lacerations, and ulcerations.

CLINICAL EVALUATION

History and Physical Examination

In all situations, begin with a good history and physical exam, including a pain assessment. If the skin injuries are secondary to trauma, start with an overall assessment of the patient before focusing on the skin wounds. Assure that the patient's circulatory and respiratory systems have been stabilized if they have been compromised, and control bleeding before any repair is initiated. (The assessment of major trauma is beyond the scope of this chapter, which focuses on the care of skin injuries in patients who are otherwise stable.) Figure 41.1 outlines a general approach to evaluation and treatment of skin injuries.

It is helpful to describe and draw a diagram of the injuries in the chart. Electronic medical records now allow for easy attachments of photographs, which may be preferable to hand drawings. The key to evaluating skin wounds is to think carefully about the type of injury that occurred and the nearby structures that might be affected. Table 41.1 lists red flags that suggest a complicated wound. During your examination, palpate for a foreign body or fracture. Consider the possibility of injury to vital structures near the wound, such as nerves, tendons, or ducts (e.g., the parotid duct). Deep penetration by an injuring object may make open exploration necessary. Wounds involving electrical, thermal, or chemical injury require special evaluation and care, as do bites and puncture wounds. In limb injuries, rule out injury to peripheral motor and sensory nerves by performing and documenting a neurological exam of the involved extremities.

Examine the surrounding skin for evidence of preexisting pathology. For example, skin discoloration, edema, or atrophy may indicate venous, lymphatic, or arterial insufficiency. Loss of sensation, however, may allow the injury to go undetected at first. Muscle weakness or skeletal deformity may have contributed to the accident, and these problems can interfere with the healing process or produce recurrent injury. Explore the possibility of substance abuse or physical abuse if injuries are recurrent, or there are physical findings inconsistent with the history provided.

Diagnostic Testing

Plain radiographs or other imaging modalities should be used if deeper foreign bodies are suspected. Testing for immunity or exposure to communicable disease (e.g., HIV, hepatitis B) may be indicated if exposure to those conditions results from the injury. This is of particular concern for health care workers who sustain workplace injuries.

MANAGEMENT

Pain

Keep in mind that patients who have had physical injuries and skin wounds are often in pain. Ask about pain and administer analgesics as needed to make the patient comfortable while you evaluate and treat the wounds. Often acetaminophen or a nonsteroidal anti-inflammatory drug (NSAID) may be adequate. If active bleeding is a problem, stay away from aspirin and NSAIDs initially. For more painful injuries, discuss the benefits and risks of opiate analgesics, such as hydrocodone/acetaminophen. Patients may need to go home with a limited prescription for an opiate analgesic depending on the extent of the injury. If the patient is in recovery from a history of substance abuse, discuss the risks of relapse and develop a plan to help the patient avoid relapse while still providing

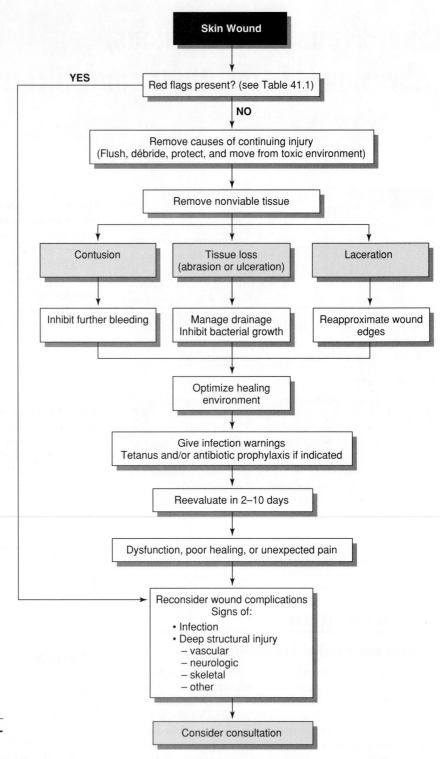

Figure 41.1 • Wound treatment algorithm.

adequate pain control. Do not withhold pain medication simply because the patient has an addiction history.

Tetanus Immunization

Any time one treats patients whose skin has been injured, remember to inquire about tetanus immunization status and give any indicated immunization. For tetanus-prone wounds (characterized by the presence of contamination, devitalized

tissue, puncture, muscle involvement, or more than 24 hours old), give a tetanus booster if the patient has not had one within 5 years; for clean wounds, the time allowance is 10 years. If the patient has not had a primary tetanus immunization series, also administer tetanus immune globulin for tetanus-prone wounds. Advise those patients lacking previous immunization (e.g., the elderly) to have a tetanus booster in 1 month and again in 6 to 12 months (1).

TABLE 41.1 Inspection of Red Flags in Skin Wounds

Sign	Check For
Deformity, severe swelling, increased pain on stressing bone	Fracture
Inability to visualize wound extent	Injury to deep structure
Difficulty controlling bleeding	Injury to large vessel
Altered function	Injury to nerve or musculoskeletal structures

CLINICAL EVALUATION AND MANAGEMENT OF SPECIFIC INJURIES

Contusions

A contusion (also known as a bruise or ecchymosis) results from trauma that injures underlying soft-tissue structures while leaving the epidermis intact. Cellular, vascular, and lymphatic damage causes blood and other fluids to leak into the tissue, producing swelling and discoloration. A hematoma occurs when enough extravasated blood collects to produce a palpable knot.

Large bruises can take weeks to resolve, particularly if there is accompanying hematoma formation. The area of ecchymosis will gradually change from blue or purple to yellow-brown as the blood is converted to hematin and reabsorbed. These ecchymoses may travel to more dependent areas. Hematomas around the knee or calf, for example, will often lead to ecchymoses of the ankle or foot. Hematomas usually clot and become quite firm; they may become red, warm, and tender as the clot liquefies. At this stage they may appear to be infected, although this is seldom the case. To reduce their concerns during healing, instruct patients about the sequential changes they can expect.

Initially, minimize hemorrhage and edema by elevating the affected part and applying pressure and ice. In general, do not aspirate or otherwise drain hematomas because they may recur, or you may introduce infection or both. Consider an underlying hemostatic disorder if the amount of bleeding seems out of proportion to the injury, but remember that tissue fragility normally increases as people age, and that many people take aspirin and NSAIDs on a regular basis; both aspirin and NSAIDs will inhibit platelet function.

Recommend applying cold for 5 to 30 minutes several times daily until swelling has stopped, usually for at least 48 hours after the injury (strength of recommendation [SOR] = C). Depending on the area involved, give instructions on using an ice water bath, massaging with water frozen in a Styrofoam cup, or using an ice pack. Refreezable chemical gel ice packs are commercially available, but bags of crushed ice or frozen vegetables work equally well. Advise the patient that hematomas generally will be resorbed over several weeks if there is no reinjury. Rarely, hematomas in muscle will develop myositis ossificans with calcification of the involved tissue.

Abrasions

Abrasions are caused by scraping trauma that removes epidermis. For example, accidents that cause a person to slide on pavement are frequent causes of severe abrasions. These injuries tend to be quite painful because many nerve endings are exposed. As in a second-degree burn, the loss of epidermis causes the skin to lose water through weeping and evaporation. These injuries are often over joint surfaces, and the scab that forms tends to crack open when the joint moves.

All abrasions should be cleaned with soap and water or another cleansing agent. Adequate cleaning of more severe abrasions may require anesthesia. Apply topical anesthetic agents for superficial abrasions, and use an injectable anesthetic (e.g., lidocaine) for deep or dirty wounds. Avoid using epinephrine-anesthetic combinations in the digits or penis, as they are associated with ischemia of the distal tissues. Next, irrigate with sterile saline or a mild antiseptic solution. Use forceps or gauze to remove ground-in dirt or asphalt to prevent tattoo formation. One method for preventing a "road-rash tattoo" is to wrap petrolatum (i.e., Vaseline) gauze or gauze with Bacitracin around the fingers and wipe off the asphalt and other foreign material embedded in the skin (2).

Once the abrasion is clean, your goal is to keep the wound moist and free of infection until it has reepithelialized. Direct the patient to apply petrolatum or a topical antibiotic such as Bacitracin or Polysporin. This can be covered with any type of clean nonstick dressing (3). Alternatively, semiocclusive, transparent wound coverings that hasten reepithelialization by retaining moisture while allowing oxygen to reach the wound are available over-the-counter and in many office settings. If the abraded area is extensive, see the patient every day or two until infection seems unlikely. Systemic antibiotic prophylaxis is generally not indicated, but if the exudate becomes frankly purulent or there is spreading erythema, obtain a culture and start an appropriate antibiotic.

Lacerations

The goals of laceration repair are:

1. Hemostasis
2. Prevention of infection
3. Preservation of function
4. Restoration of appearance
5. Minimization of patient discomfort (2)

When repairing skin, it is helpful to understand the three phases of wound healing. These phases include:

Phase 1 (initial lag phase, days 0 to 5)
No gain in wound strength
Phase 2 (fibroplasia phase, days 5 to 14)
Rapid increase in wound strength occurs
At 2 weeks, the wound has achieved only 7% of its final strength

Phase 3 (final maturation phase, day 14 until healing is complete)
Further connective tissue remodeling
Up to 80% of normal skin strength (2)

Nonabsorbable skin sutures or staples are used to give the wound strength during the initial two phases. After the nonabsorbable skin sutures are removed, wound-closure tapes or previously placed deep, absorbable sutures may play an important role in the final phases of wound healing.

Indications for immediate wound closure include:

- Lacerations that are open and less than 18 hours old (less than 24 hours old on the face)
- Bite wounds in cosmetically important areas (close follow-up recommended)

Contraindications to immediate wound closure include:

- Wounds greater than 18 hours old (greater than 24 hours old on the face)
- Animal and human bite wounds—exceptions include facial wounds and large wounds from dog bites
- Puncture wounds

Each laceration needs to be evaluated to determine if it requires closure and which closure method will be work best. Choices include sutures, staples, tapes, or glue (tissue adhesive). Tapes such as Steri-Strips or a tissue adhesive may be adequate when the laceration is superficial and/or the patient is a child who would need sedation for a surgical repair. Table 41.2 lists the essentials for wound assessment.

A Cochrane Systematic Review demonstrated that tissue adhesives are an acceptable alternative to standard wound closure for repairing simple traumatic lacerations. They offer decreased procedure time and less pain compared to standard wound closure with sutures. A small but statistically significant increased rate of dehiscence (wound opening) with tissue adhesives is observed (4). Staples are also faster to place than sutures and are particularly good for closing scalp lacerations (5). Both staples and tissue adhesives are often more expensive than standard sutures and therefore may not be available in all medical settings.

Inspection, evaluation, cleaning, and treatment of larger lacerations requires adequate anesthesia. Young children may need sedation. Lidocaine in 1% or 2% concentration is the most commonly used anesthetic solution. Before injection, ask the patient if he is allergic to the medication or any other topical or local anesthetics. Although it is permissible to administer up to 4.5 mg/kg (body weight) of lidocaine (the 1% solution contains 10 mg/mL), use the minimum amount necessary to avoid toxicity. Preparations that combine lidocaine with epinephrine can be used to decrease bleeding, minimize the risk of lidocaine toxicity and prolong anesthesia. Epinephrine should be avoided in areas in which its vasoconstrictive effects might cause gangrene, such as the fingers, toes, earlobes, or penis. Adequate anesthesia is generally produced in 10 minutes.

To minimize the pain of injecting local anesthetic:

- Use a small-gauge needle (27- or 30-gauge)
- Inject slowly
- Inject directly into the dermis through the open wound (not through intact skin)
- Warm anesthetic to body temperature
- Buffer the anesthetic with sodium bicarbonate, although this is optional (2)

In some areas, a nerve block may be more effective than local injection. Circumferential blocks work well for injuries of the ear and nose. Block of the mental nerve produces good anesthesia to the lower lip and chin. Usually a digital block of a finger or toe is used. This is accomplished by anesthetizing the dorsal and ventral nerve branches on each side of the affected digit. To perform a digital block, use 3 cc of 1% or 2% lidocaine without epinephrine, and a 27- or 30-gauge needle. Inject at the base of the digit and as you direct the needle toward the plantar surface inject 1 mL of lidocaine (no epinephrine) around both branches of the digital nerve and repeat with 1 cc on the other side. It is helpful to add an additional 1 cc of lidocaine across the top of the digit to prevent pain carried by the smaller digital nerves that traverse this area.

Once adequate anesthesia is obtained, the wound can be inspected and cleaned. An antiseptic solution, such as povidone-iodine (Betadine) or chlorhexidine (Hibiclens), may be used for initial cleaning of the surrounding skin, but not in the wound. If significant contamination with bacteria or chemicals is suspected, flush the wound profusely with sterile saline. Cleaning of the wound should be done by irrigation with normal saline. This can be accomplished by attaching an 18-gauge angiocatheter or a commercially available splash shield to a 30-mL syringe. At least 200 cc of irrigation is recommended (SOR = C). Alternatively, an intravenous bag with a compression device can be used to provide a high-pressure stream through an angiocatheter or needle. Debride severely contaminated or nonviable tissue, but be especially sparing on the face, where significant tissue loss can result in deformity. Clipping hair from around the laceration can make

TABLE 41.2 Essentials of Wound Assessment (2)

Mechanism of injury	Sharp versus blunt trauma, bite
Dirty versus clean	Barnyard versus kitchen sink
Time since injury	Suture up to 18 hr after injury; 24 hr after injury on face
Foreign body	Explore and obtain radiograph for metal or glass
Functional examination	Neurovascular, muscular, tendons
Need for prophylactic antibiotics	If needed, give as soon as possible and cover *S. aureus*

TABLE 41.3 Basic Supplies for Laceration Repair

Equipment	Uses
Gauze sponges	Absorbing blood and dressing wounds
Sterile gloves and eye protection	Protecting physician and patient from transfer of infectious organisms
Sterile drapes	Sterile field that sutures and instruments may contact
Adequate lighting	Complete visualization of wound
Toothed Adson forceps	Gentle grasp of tissues and foreign materials
Small hemostats	Closing bleeding vessels and grasping tissue
Smooth Adson forceps	Less traumatic grasp of tissues
Needle holder	Grasping the suture needle
Small Iris scissors	Cutting and undermining tissue
Scalpel with blade (no. 15)	Cutting tissue
Suture material and needle	Drawing wound edges together
Skin hooks (optional)	Pulling wound edges without damaging the surface

suturing easier, but avoid shaving the skin, which can increase the risk of infection.

After the initial assessment and administration of local or regional anesthetic, wounds should be thoroughly inspected for foreign bodies, deep tissue layer damage, and injury to nerve, vessel, or tendon. A radiograph should be obtained to look for remaining glass or metal in wounds sustained with broken glass or metal. Complex wounds, or those in cosmetically important areas, should be closed by an experienced practitioner.

The timing of wound closure is important. The risk of infection is lowest if a laceration is repaired soon after injury, although cleaned wounds generally do well if closed within 18 hours (6). If the wound is more than 18 to 24 hours old, it should simply be cleaned, inspected, and then dressed; suturing would promote infection by introducing foreign material and preventing drainage. If there is no sign of infection by the third to fifth day and approximation of wound edges is desirable, then the wound may be sutured.

PREPARING FOR WOUND REPAIR

Having inspected and cleansed the wound and decided that it is appropriate to close the wound surgically, make certain that all potentially necessary instruments and supplies are at hand. Table 41.3 lists basic supplies for laceration repair. Table 41.4 suggests suture sizes for various body locations.

A number of suture materials are available, and each has its advantages. These include:

- Monofilament nylon (Ethilon, Dermalon) or polypropylene (Prolene) sutures produce less skin reactivity and fewer infections. These are nonabsorbable and are used for closing most lacerations.
- Braided sutures (Vicryl, Mersilene) cause less discomfort on mucosal surfaces (such as the lip or tongue) than the stiffer monofilaments.
- Absorbable materials (chromic gut, Vicryl, Dexon) are used for subsurface or mucosal repair.

Attached to the suture is a curved needle, the size and shape of which are generally shown on the package. A reverse-cutting, plastics grade needle (labeled P) is appropriate in most circumstances. Grip it with a needle holder approximately one third of the way from the blunt end. The proper grasp (see Figure 41.2) and following the curve of the needle when placing the suture will minimize needle bending.

After the wound is anesthetized and cleaned, and you have positioned the patient and your instruments, you are ready to put on sterile gloves and drape the wound. At this point, examine the wound carefully and plan your repair. Trim wound edges so that they are parallel, only if this can be done without removing essential tissue. When making an incision to straighten a wound margin, first mark the incision with the scalpel, then use scissors to cut perpendicular to the skin surface. Make excisions in hair-bearing skin parallel to the hair shafts to avoid damage to the follicles. After evaluating the wound, if you do not believe you can perform an

TABLE 41.4 Guidelines for Suture Selection and Timing of Suture Removal

Location	Suture Size for Skin Closure	Days to Removal
Face	5–0 or 6–0	4–5
Scalp	3–0 or 4–0	5–7
Trunk and extremities	4–0 or 5–0	7–10
Over joint surfaces	3–0 or 4–0	10–14

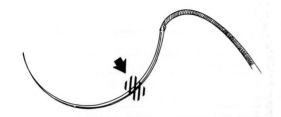

Figure 41.2 • Correct position for grasping a suture needle. This position provides enough length to rotate the needle through soft tissues, but is far enough forward to minimize bending.

optimum repair, consult a surgeon who has the necessary skills.

SUTURING TECHNIQUES

Appropriate closure technique varies according to the depth of the laceration and the body area involved.

- Single-layer closure is used for superficial wounds and in areas with little subcutaneous tissue, such as the digits and backs of the hands. It is also useful on the scalp, where hemostasis can be a problem.
- Layered repair is better for deeper wounds, particularly in cosmetically sensitive areas such as the face.

Principles of proper suture placement are shown in Figure 41.3. The goal is to gently evert the skin for better wound healing and cosmesis. This is done by creating a loop that is as wide at the bottom as near the skin surface. You can facilitate this by pulling back on the edge of the skin with forceps or skin hooks while pushing the needle through the skin at a 90-degree angle to the surface. Next, rotate your wrist to bring the needle up through the opposite wound edge, going wider in the deeper tissue. This can be facilitated by putting pressure on the skin with the tip of the forceps before puncturing up through the skin.

Usually sutures are placed as far apart as they are wide. In areas of skin tension, however, place sutures closer together

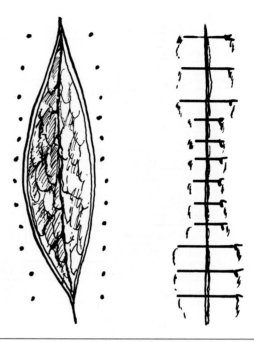

Figure 41.4 • Closure of an ellipse. Suturing is begun at one end of the wound. As the middle is approached, sutures are placed closer to each other and closer to the wound edge to minimize tension on each stitch.

and closer to the wound edge. Figure 41.4 shows this principle in the closure of an ellipse. A wound can be closed by halving it or starting at one end and working toward the other end.

A valuable method in lacerations with widely separated edges is to place deep sutures first or use a vertical mattress suture (see Figure 41.5). The deep stitches will hold the dermis together for weeks, with suture that will dissolve over time. The alternative is to use vertical mattress sutures that provide greater strength and better approximation of tissue. Because they tend to heal leaving visible suture marks, alternate them with simple sutures. The mattress sutures can then be removed early, leaving the simple sutures for support.

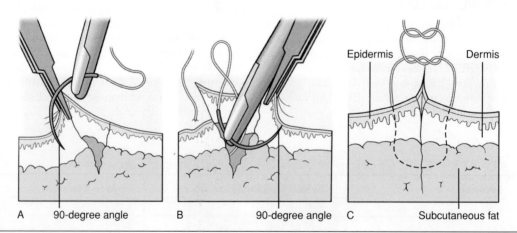

Figure 41.3 • Proper skin suture technique. **A.** Perpendicular insertion of the needle is aided by pulling back on the skin with the forceps. **B.** The reloaded needle is inserted upward through the fat and dermis to come out at a 90 degree angle to the epidermis. **C.** The final suture path has a modified flask shape to promote eversion of the skin edges and improved healing.

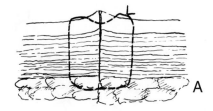

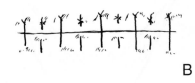

Figure 41.5 • Repair using vertical mattress sutures. **A.** Placement of vertical mattress suture. **B.** Wound closure with simple sutures alternating with vertical mattress sutures.

The best technique for reducing tension on a wound is to place buried or deep sutures with absorbable material (see Figure 41.6). Placement of deep sutures is aided by undermining the tissue below the layer being closed. In part A of Figure 41.6, undermining has been performed in the fatty layer. It is best to use the scissors in a spreading motion to minimize vascular and nerve disruption, then place sutures so that the knots are buried. After the wound edges are brought together with the first layer of buried sutures the second layer of closure is accomplished with simple interrupted sutures or a running stitch.

V-shaped lacerations are repaired with the technique shown in Figure 41.7 or by using tissue adhesive, to minimize risk of compromise to the blood supply at the tip of the flap. The dog's ear deformity results when you have more skin on one side than the other toward the end of the wound, despite efforts to separate sutures by equal distances on both sides. The longer side tends to rise, making it difficult to approximate the edges without bunching on that side. Repair is performed as shown in Figure 41.8. Make the wound edges equal again by extending the wound with an incision at a 45-degree angle toward the side with excess length. After undermining, excise the overlapping dog's ear and suture the incision. If some excess still remains on that side, repeat the process.

AREA-SPECIFIC CONSIDERATIONS

The character of skin and subcutaneous tissue over the body varies greatly. Suturing techniques and materials, therefore, vary from site to site, as shown in Table 41.4.

Lacerations of the scalp often are caused by blows that split the skin to, and sometimes through, the galea. If the galea is lacerated, close it as a layer, after palpating to detect signs of skull fracture. The remaining closure is best performed as a single layer, using a large needle and 3–0 or 4–0 suture material (skin staples are a good alternative here). This generally provides adequate hemostasis if occasional large bleeders are clipped with a hemostat and coagulated or tied off (exercising care not to injure nerves or other vital structures). After the repair, rinse as much blood as possible out of the patient's hair because it can be difficult to remove later.

Facial lacerations require particular care to minimize scarring. Using tissue scissors, trim the wound edges so they are smooth and follow natural skin lines, if this can be done by removing only a small amount of tissue. Use the layered skin closure shown in Figure 41.6, which will minimize tension on the surface. For surface suturing, use thin (6–0) monofilament sutures and remove them early, replacing with adhesive strips (Steri-Strips). Mark landmarks, such as the vermilion border of the lips, before they are obscured by injecting the anesthetic. The first suture can then be placed to assure correct alignment.

Lacerations of the tongue do not require repair, unless they are very large or bleed persistently despite application of ice and pressure. Similarly, lacerations of the oral mucosa usually heal well without suturing. Lacerations that penetrate from the skin into the oral cavity should include repair of the skin and muscle only, unless the mucosal defect is large. Leav-

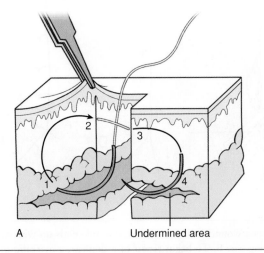

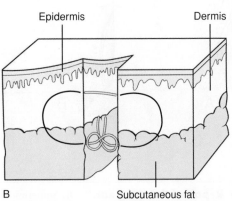

Figure 41.6 • Deep or buried suture technique. **A.** The needle enters the undermined area (1) and exits at the dermal-epidermal junction (2). The needle holder is reloaded and the needle is inserted at the dermal-epidermal junction to exit below in the subcutaneous fat. **B.** The tied knot is buried below the skin surface.

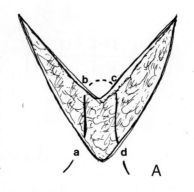
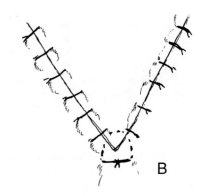

Figure 41.7 • Repair of a flap laceration. **A.** The needle is inserted on one side of the wound apex (*a*), passed through the subcuticular tissue of the flap (*b–c*), and then brought out on the opposite side of the wound apex (*d*). **B.** Simple sutures are then placed far enough away from the apex to prevent compromise of circulation to the tip.

ing the mucosal surface open to heal secondarily reduces the chance of infection.

AFTERCARE

Petrolatum or antibiotic ointment is useful in nonbandaged wounds to promote healing by keeping the epithelium moist and reducing bacterial colonization (7). For draining wounds, apply a nonadherent material, such as Telfa, under a layer of cotton gauze. Tell patients to keep sutured wounds dry for 24 hours, after which showering is permitted. In areas of skin stretch, support lacerations by splinting the affected part until adequately healed.

Infection is the biggest threat to wound healing. As noted earlier, aggressive wound cleaning and tetanus prophylaxis are most effective at preventing infection. Antibiotics are not indicated for simple wounds (8), but many experts recommend their use when a bone, tendon, or joint space has been penetrated, and for heavily contaminated wounds (SOR = C)

When cosmetically important, selected animal bites may be closed after careful cleansing (9). Human bites require par-

ticularly careful cleaning and observation because of the large number of bacteria in saliva; generally these wounds should be treated as infected from the onset.

Whether antibiotics are used or not, inform the patient about signs of infection, which include: progressive swelling, redness, heat or pain, and increased drainage. Because infection typically takes 1 to 3 days to become apparent, recheck high-risk lacerations at 48 to 72 hours. Written instructions regarding wound care can be quite helpful because patients often are distressed and will remember little of the verbal advice they receive.

Timing of suture removal varies with the location and type of wound. Table 41.4 lists suture removal times. The goal is to leave sutures in long enough to prevent wound dehiscence, but not so long as to cause suture marks. If infection occurs, you may need to remove some sutures early to allow drainage and to prevent abscess formation.

To remove a suture, elevate the knot with forceps, cut one side of the loop near the skin, and then put gentle traction on the knot. Do not cut the knot off both sides of a loop

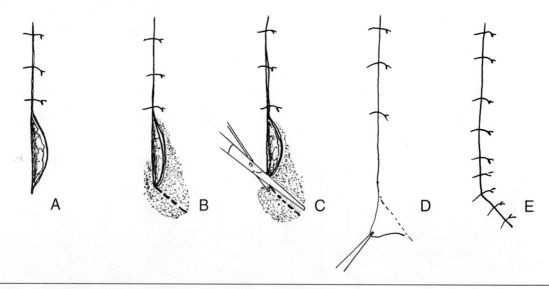

Figure 41.8 • Repair of the "dog ear." **A.** Sometimes, as a wound is being sutured, one side ends up with more remaining tissue than the other, which creates an unsightly bulge called a dog ear. **B.** To begin repair of a dog ear, a marking incision is made 45° from the end of the wound toward the longer side. **C.** Scissors are used to cut along the marking, and then used to undermine the shaded area. **D.** The longer skin edge is pulled across the incision line, and the resulting triangle of skin is excised along the line of overlap. **E.** The even skin edges can now be easily sutured.

TABLE 41.5 Injury Care Instructions for Patients

1. Keep the injured area raised above the heart as much as possible to decrease swelling.
2. Apply ice to sprains and deep bruises frequently for 1–2 days. For small areas, freeze water in a Styrofoam cup, then peel back the top edge. For larger areas, use an ice pack or a bag of frozen vegetables. A layer of cloth will prevent frostbite to the skin.
3. Inspect wounds daily for signs of infection (fever, swelling, or spreading redness and tenderness). If signs of infection develop or the wound starts to pull apart return for evaluation.
4. Keep any splints or pressure dressings on until instructed to remove them.
5. Return to our office to have your wound(s) checked in _____ days. Return to our office for suture removal in _____ days.

because the free ends may retract into the skin and be difficult to retrieve. To reinforce the wound, apply sterile adhesive strips, preparing the wound edges with tincture of benzoin to promote adhesion. These strips come off when soaked, so advise patients to keep them dry for a few days before washing them off. Warn the patient about infection symptoms (Table 41.5) and that the natural healing process may cause the wound to look red and swollen over the first few months, but within 6 months, it will have improved.

Skin Ulcers

Acute skin ulcerations may be caused by accidental trauma, but also by excessive scratching in a patient with pruritus. Many skin ulcers are caused by pressure in patients that are immobilized or have impaired sensation. These include decubitus ulcers in the elderly and in patients with spinal cord injuries. Diabetic foot ulcers are caused by lack of protective sensation and occur in areas of wounds or increased pressure. Ulceration caused by systemic illness (e.g., ischemic emboli from vasculitis or disseminated infection) is treated by addressing the underlying disorder.

Ulceration produces skin defects that are not amenable to simple surgical approximation; healing requires growth of epidermal tissue into the damaged area. This growth occurs most rapidly in oxygen-rich, moist environments where leukocytes are allowed to accumulate. Frequent cleansing, particularly with cytotoxic solutions such as povidone-iodine (e.g., Betadine) or chlorhexidine (e.g., Hibiclens), only delays healing.

Venous stasis dermatitis can result in particularly refractory ulcerations of the lower legs. Venous congestion results from damage to the deep veins draining the lower legs. It occurs after injury or, more commonly, after deep vein thrombosis. Treatment of these ulcers requires a huge expenditure of medical resources worldwide. Table 41.6 shows the evidence supporting various treatments.

Effective treatment of venous stasis ulcers requires compression to reduce tissue edema. Care must be taken to avoid wrapping so tightly that arterial circulation is compromised. Layered wraps have not been proven more effective than single-layer Unna wrappings using zinc paste-impregnated gauze (10); however, absorptive layers may be necessary to prevent frequent dressing changes caused by excessive exudate. Medication with pentoxyphylline (Trental) has been associated with more rapid healing (11). Elastic compression stockings, elevation, and protection from trauma help to prevent recurrence after ulcers are healed.

CASE DISCUSSION

An ice pack and pressure should be applied to the left deltoid hematoma intermittently for 24 to 48 hours. After cleaning the skin tear with sterile saline, the intact skin flap may be laid back over the wound base and held in place with some occlusive transparent wound covering. The laceration of the dorsum of the left hand should be flushed profusely with normal saline solution after anesthetizing with injected lidocaine. Because no tendon injury is noted, the wound can be closed with simple sutures or skin staples. No further tetanus immunization is needed for this clean wound, but prophylactic antibiotics are indicated because of the tendon exposure. The left lower leg abrasion can be treated with antibiotic ointment and a nonstick dressing; however, a chronic ulcer may result because of the preexisting venous stasis dermatitis.

TABLE 41.6 Evidence for Treatment Recommendations for Venous Stasis Ulcers

Treatment Strategy	Strength of Recommendation*	Recommendations/Comments
Compression bandaging	A	Higher pressure is better, as long as arterial compression is avoided
Layered compression bandaging	B	No data to prove better than single-layer bandage
Oral pentoxifylline	B	No cost-effectiveness data
Cultured skin grafts	C	Very expensive
Recombinant growth factor (Regranex)	C	Indicated in diabetic ulcers, very expensive

*A = consistent, good-quality patient-oriented evidence; B = inconsistent or limited-quality patient-oriented evidence; C = consensus, disease-oriented evidence, usual practice, expert opinion, or case series. For information about the SORT evidence rating system, see *http://www.aafp.org/afpsort.xml.*

Therefore, the left lower leg abrasion is most susceptible to delayed healing.

REFERENCES

1. Recommendations of the Immunization Practices Advisory Committee (ACIP) on diphtheria, tetanus, and pertussis: recommendations for vaccine use and other preventive measures. MMWR. 1991;40(suppl RR-10):1–28.
2. Usatine R. Coates W. Laceration repair. In: Pfenninger JL, Fowler GC, eds. Procedures for Primary Care Physicians, 2nd ed. St. Louis, MO: Mosby; 2003.
3. Smack DP, Harrington AC, Dunn C, et al. Infection and allergy incidence in ambulatory surgery patients using white petrolatum vs. bacitracin ointment. JAMA. 1996;276: 972–977.
4. Farion K, Osmond MH, Hartling L, et al. Tissue adhesives for traumatic lacerations in children and adults. Cochrane Database Syst Rev. 2002;(3):CDOO3326.
5. Kanegaye JT, Vance CW, Chan L, Schonfeld N. Comparison of skin stapling devices and standard sutures for pediatric scalp lacerations: a randomized study of cost and time benefits. J Pediatr. 1997;130(5):808–813.
6. Berk WA, Osbourne DD, Taylor DD. Evaluation of the "golden period" for wound repair: 204 cases from a third world emergency department. Ann Emerg Med. 1988;17: 496–500.
7. Dire DJ, Coppola M, Dwyer DA, Lorette JJ, Karr JL. Prospective evaluation of topical antibiotics for preventing infections in uncomplicated soft-tissue wounds repaired in the ED. Acad Emerg Med. 1995;2:4–10.
8. Cummings P, Del Beccaro MA. Antibiotics to prevent infection of simple wounds: a meta-analysis of randomized studies. Am J Emerg Med. 1995;13:396–400.
9. Chen E, Hornig S, Shepherd SM, Hollander JE. Primary closure of mammalian bites. Acad Emerg Med. 2000;7(2): 157–161.
10. Cullum N, Nelson EA, Fletcher AW, Sheldon TA. Compression for venous leg ulcers (Cochrane Review). In: The Cochrane Library. Chichester, UK: John Wiley and Sons, Ltd; 2005: Issue 1.
11. Jull AB, Waters J, Arroll B. Oral pentoxifylline for treatment of venous leg ulcers. The Cochrane Database of Syst Rev. In: The Cochrane Library. Oxford, England: Update Software; 2000: Issue 4.

CHAPTER 42

Cognitive Impairment

John P. Langlois and Soo Borson

CASE STUDY (PART 1)

Mrs. H., a 68-year-old female, presents to your office complaining of "memory problems." Over the past year she has noted increasing difficulty recalling the names of friends and acquaintances, and she reports occasional trouble thinking of the proper words to express her thoughts. The day before her appointment she found herself in the garage, car keys in hand, unable to remember why she was there or where she intended to go. "I'm worried that I'm losing my memory, and that I have Alzheimer's disease," she says.

CLINICAL QUESTIONS

1. What are the causes of cognitive complaints in previously normal patients?
2. What are the diagnostic tests and techniques that differentiate normal aging changes from cognitive impairment and distinguish between its causes?
3. Are there effective methods to prevent, reverse, or slow the progression of cognitive impairment?

Complaints about cognitive problems, such as memory loss, slowed thinking, or reduced mental capacity, are common among older persons. Some slowing in mental processing and function are a normal part of aging; however, the incidence of diseases causing progressive cognitive losses also increases with advancing age. Therefore, the family physician must be prepared to:

- thoroughly and efficiently screen for cognitive losses and evaluate cognitive complaints;
- determine when a patient's cognitive changes appear to be consistent with normal aging, reassure and counsel them appropriately, and provide ongoing monitoring; and
- diagnose and manage dementia and other causes of progressive cognitive impairment.

Cognitive impairment is defined as a reduction in cognitive functioning from a previously stable baseline. The most common cause of cognitive impairment in the elderly is dementia—a syndrome that may be temporary and reversible, or permanent and progressive. The prevalence of dementia among persons aged 65 and older is between 4%–7% (1). Dementia increases dramatically with age, so that the frequency of dementia among persons over 85 may exceed 45% (2). It is not entirely a disease of the elderly, however; its prevalence among persons aged 45 to 65 is between 67 to 81 per 100,000

(3). Diagnostic criteria for dementia include: a) impairment in memory; b) impairment in abstract thinking, judgment, or other higher cortical functions, or personality change; and c) impairment severe enough to interfere significantly with work, usual social activities, or relationships with others (4). The most common cause of dementia is Alzheimer's disease.

Not all cognitive complaints reflect dementia. Indeed, the majority of older persons who present in primary care with complaints about their memory or other cognitive symptoms will not have dementia. On the other hand, people with dementia are often unaware of or minimize their symptoms. Therefore, the family physician must systematically evaluate cognitive complaints. A first step is to identify whether complaints appear to suggest normal memory lapses or dementia (see Table 42.1). The challenge is that the onset of dementia is insidious, and the transition from normal cognition with lapses to diagnosable dementia is gradual and, therefore, a challenge to detect early.

Assessing cognitive impairment and diagnosing and managing the impact of dementia will be a growing part of every family practice. Normal aging is associated with more reported memory problems and small declines in objective tests of memory (5); the family physician must be adept at assessing and following patients who have mild cognitive symptoms, to identify those who develop a significant and progressive dementia. A typical family physician manages several patients with dementia; in addition, early dementia is frequently undiagnosed, and may occur in up to 5.7% of older primary care patients (6). Since the population over age 65 will grow in coming decades, the importance of this problem in family medicine will only increase.

DIFFERENTIAL DIAGNOSIS

Alzheimer's disease is the most common cause of progressive dementia, causing an estimated 60%–70% of dementias in the United States. Pathological changes consist of diffuse cortical atrophy, loss of neurons, amyloid plaques, and neurofibrillary tangles. Memory loss is an early and prominent symptom. In addition, Alzheimer's patients have difficulty learning new information and remembering it for more than a few minutes, with loss of more distant memories occurring later in the disease. As the disease progresses, more cognitive problems develop, including disorientation, aphasia, apraxia, impaired judgment, and visuospatial dysfunction. These changes result in progressive difficulties with activities of daily life (ADLs). Managing medications and home finances, driving safely and without getting lost, and planning and preparing meals can be

TABLE 42.1 Tips on Differentiating Normal Cognitive Lapses From Dementia

Domain of Cognitive Function	Examples of Behaviors Suggesting. . . .	
	Normal Lapses	**Moderate Stage Dementia**
Memory in daily tasks	Forgetting an acquaintance's name	Unexplained confusion in familiar situations
Performance of familiar tasks	Leaving the kettle on to boil	Forgetting to serve a meal just prepared
Language	Trouble finding the right word	Forgetting simple words or substituting inappropriate words
Orientation	Forgetting the day or date	Getting lost in own neighborhood
Judgment	Choosing to wear a light sweater on a cold night	Wearing a bathrobe to the store; wearing two blouses at once
Abstract thinking	Making a mistake in balancing the checkbook	Inability to do basic calculations
Misplacing objects	Temporarily misplacing car keys or glasses	Putting the iron in the freezer, or the wristwatch in the sugar bowl
Mood and behavior	Getting the blues in a sad situation	Rapid mood swings or irritability for no apparent reason
Personality	Gradual perceptible change with age and changing circumstances	Sudden, dramatic change from baseline, especially new suspiciousness or mood swings
Initiative	Occasionally getting tired of housework and social obligations	Sustained lack of interest, involvement in usual pursuits

Adapted from: Alzheimer's Association, "What are the warning signs?" *http://www.alz.org*. Accessed September 1998.

progressively impaired in mild to moderate dementia. Social conversation, interaction, and relationships can be remarkably well maintained, as can memory for emotionally salient events, making close questioning and objective assessment important in uncovering the true level of global functioning.

In moderate to severe disease, more basic activities, such as dressing, eating, speech, and bowel and bladder continence, are lost. Behavioral changes are common, including anxiety, irritability, depression, and personality changes. Additional problems, such as hallucinations, delusions, aggressive behavior, and wandering, can develop and make home care difficult. The course of Alzheimer's disease varies from person to person but often follows a fairly predictable sequence of changes (see Table 42.2).

The differential diagnosis of Alzheimer's disease is fairly long. Table 42.3 identifies some of the more important alternative diagnoses; the subsequent sections of this chapter discuss many in detail.

Vascular dementia comprises approximately 15%–20% of dementia cases in the United States. Patients often have multiple risk factors for cerebrovascular disease (e.g., diabetes, hyperlipidemia, smoking), and a history of hypertension is common. They may have a known history of stroke and/or transient ischemic attacks or may not have had clinically recognized events. Computerized axial tomography (CAT) and magnetic resonance imaging (MRI) of the brain will show multiple areas of ischemic damage. Typically, these patients will show a stepwise decline in cognitive and neurological functioning as additional vascular events occur, as opposed to

the steadier progressive decline seen in Alzheimer's disease, although the stepwise pattern in patients with only repeated microvascular events may be too subtle for patients and family members to clearly identify. A history of strokes alone is not sufficient to establish cerebrovascular disease as the cause of dementia; it should be accompanied by focal motor and sensory neurologic impairments, consistent findings on neuroimaging, and a stepwise pattern of progression. Approximately 10%–20% of patients with dementia have clinical and pathologic findings of both Alzheimer's disease and vascular dementia, i.e., have *mixed dementia*.

The remaining causes of dementia comprise approximately 10% of diagnoses. These include the following:

- *Lewy body dementia*. The distinct presentation of this dementia includes Parkinsonian rigidity and postural instability, psychosis (typically visual hallucinations, often nonthreatening to the patient), prominent fluctuation in attention and often in behavior, other psychiatric complications, and neurogenic orthostatic hypotension (7). Most authorities now consider the *dementia of Parkinson's disease* to be Lewy body dementia, although some patients have Alzheimer's disease, cerebrovascular disease, or mixtures of several pathological types. Typically the dementia symptoms occur late in the course of the disease, after the major neurologic abnormalities (and usually the diagnosis of Parkinson's disease) have been present for a number of years.
- *Frontotemporal dementia*, an increasingly recognized cause of dementia, occurs in several variants. The most familiar,

TABLE 42.2 Stages of Dementia

Categories of Cognitive Function	Common Symptoms and Signs by Stage		
	Mild Dementia	**Moderate Dementia**	**Severe Dementia**
Orientation	Disorientation to date	Disoriented to date, place Getting lost in familiar areas	Loses recognition of close family
Language	Naming difficulties (anomia)	Expression and comprehension difficulties (aphasia)	Nearly unintelligible verbal output
Judgment and competency	Decreased insight but usually able to give informed consent	Can state opinion on simple or basic issues	Very little insight; generally need proxy consent
Recent memory	Significant problems	Severe problems	Absent
Long-term memory	Generally intact	Significant problems	Severe problems, or absent memory
Other neurological tests	Difficulty copying figures or doing clock drawing	Severely impaired calculating skills	
Activities of daily living (ADLs)	Problems with dressing and grooming	Urinary "accidents" progressing to incontinence Gait instability	Develops need for assistance with feeding and repositioning
Instrumental ADLs	Problems managing finances	Unable to cook, shop, or bank	Unable to do any
Mood and behavior	Social withdrawal Irritability, mood change Need for reminders Repetition of stories and questions	Delusions, agitation, aggression Restless, anxious, depressed	Resists caregivers, withdrawn when not stimulated, self-stimulation (e.g., hollering) common
Mini-Mental State Examination (MMSE) Score *	20–28	10–19	0–9

*These ranges apply to persons who have a high school education or greater; persons with less education may have lower threshold scores.

Pick's disease, occurs most frequently between ages 45 and 65, but other forms of frontotemporal dementia, including some familial variants, may occur later (8). It is characterized by relatively prominent personality changes (apathy, agitation, aggression, disinhibition, depression, and inappropriate affect), impaired reasoning and insight, and compulsive behaviors. These unusual personality changes are often mistaken for primary psychiatric disease at first, before the global loss of cognitive abilities becomes obvious. Neuroimaging can be helpful when it shows atrophy of the frontal and anterior temporal lobes; functional imaging, using single-photon-emission computed tomography or positron-emission tomography, may be required to show the typical regional pattern and distinguish it from other causes of dementia, but these findings may be absent early in the evolution of the disease.

- *Nondegenerative, often potentially reversible, disorders.* There are several uncommon but important causes of a dementia-like syndrome that are believed to be reversible or to stabilize with treatment. These include delirium, depression, hypothyroidism, vitamin B12 deficiency, neurosyphilis, treatable brain tumors, normal pressure hydrocephalus and subdural hematomas. The approach to diagnosing and rul-

ing out these entities is discussed in more detail later in this chapter.

Mild Cognitive Impairment

A recent and evolving area of research and controversy relates to a relatively new diagnostic category called mild cognitive impairment (MCI). Diagnosis of dementia requires cognitive losses in two or more areas sufficient enough to impair everyday function. MCI is diagnosed when a patient is found to have clear, testable and reproducible deficits in one area of cognitive function (e.g., short-term memory) but does not meet the criteria for dementia because cognitive deficits are relatively mild, and everyday function is generally preserved (9).

Because of difficulties in operationalizing this consensus definition, studies of patients diagnosed with MCI over time have found variable risk of progression to dementia. Recent studies suggest that a subset of patients with MCI—those with a "pure memory" form (e.g., who cannot name any of three objects at 5 minutes)—progress rapidly to dementia (41% in 1 year; 64% after 2 years) (10). However, in population-based studies, up to half of patients with MCI revert to normal

TABLE 42.3 Differential Diagnosis of Cognitive Impairment

Disease Category	Diagnoses
Neurodegenerative	Alzheimer's disease
	Diffuse Lewy body disease
	Dementia caused by Parkinson's disease
	Progressive supranuclear palsy,
	Multi-system atrophy and other "Parkinson plus" syndromes
	Frontotemporal dementias
	Huntington's disease
Metabolic/ Deficiency	Vitamin B12 deficiency
	Thyroid disease
	Alcohol-related
Vascular	Multi-infarct dementia
	Chronic subdural hematoma
	Post-subarrachnoid hemmorrhage
	"Strategic" infarcts (e.g., thalamus)
Infectious	Neurosyphilis
	HIV-related
	Cryptococcal meningitis
	Herpes simplex encephalitis
	Postencephalitic
	Creutzfeld-Jakob disease
Structural	Brain tumor
	Normal pressure hydrocephalus
Epileptiform	Partial complex status epilepticus
	Absence states
Other	Major depression
	Delirium
	Posttraumatic
	Postsurgical
	Heavy metal toxicity
	Multiple sclerosis
	Hypoxic

cognition after a year, and rates of progression to dementia have been lower.

Currently, the boundaries are fuzzy between MCI and normal cognition on one end of the spectrum and MCI and dementia on the other. Thus, more research and more easily applied diagnostic and prognostic criteria are needed. In the meantime, patients with MCI, when identified in the primary care setting, should be followed longitudinally for signs of progression to dementia.

INITIAL EVALUATION

The first step in assessing patients with cognitive complaints—or noncomplaining patients whose behavior suggests

a problem—is to perform a thorough initial evaluation with a carefully honed history and physical. Screening and diagnostic tools are used to help determine if their problems fall within the range of normal. If a significant loss of cognitive function is present, then it is crucial to search for treatable or reversible causes. Once a clear diagnosis is made, education, support, and medical management can help produce the best outcome possible for the patient, the family, and caregivers.

The diagnosis of dementia is a clinical one, made primarily on the basis of the history and physical, and the use of appropriate clinical tools. Whereas the differential diagnosis of cognitive impairment is long (see Table 42.3), the diagnosis and probable etiology of dementia can be determined in most cases from basic clinical data alone. Lab work and imaging are mainly helpful in the search for potentially reversible

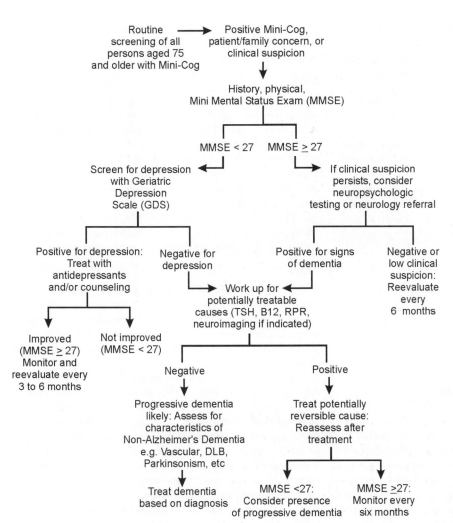

Figure 42.1 • Diagnostic approach to cognitive impairment.

causes, or where the initial clinical assessment suggests an atypical cause. Figure 42.1 provides an overview of the diagnostic approach to cognitive complaints.

History and Physical Examination

A clinical cognitive history should be obtained from both the patient and a knowledgeable informant, usually a family member. Patients with dementia typically underreport the extent and impact of their deficits, most often because of the effects of brain disease itself, at times exaggerated by denial due to embarrassment or fear. If the patient typically comes to appointments alone, ask for permission to contact a close family member; ideally, have the patient bring the family member with them to the next appointment.

The history should include questions about common functional lapses that occur early in dementia, such as:

- forgetting names, events, and important occasions;
- having difficulty finding words to express thoughts;
- taking less initiative;
- falling behind on everyday responsibilities previously done without difficulty (e.g. not paying bills, or paying the same bill twice);
- having difficulty sorting and organizing paperwork;
- getting lost in familiar places; and

- having difficulty learning to use a new household gadget or forgetting how to use a familiar one.

In addition to specific cognitive function probes such as these, patients and families should be asked about personality, mood, or behavior change, and encouraged to mention any other concerns they might have. Particularly important for primary care are questions related to the ability to follow recommended treatments. Ask the patient to name all of his/ her medications and what they are for. Find out from family members whether the patient is able to manage medications without help or requires reminders or setup.

A thorough physical exam, with a special focus on the neurologic exam, is important. Some important physical findings to look for, and their implications, include:

- The patient with uncomplicated mild to moderate Alzheimer's disease should have a normal neurologic examination.
- The presence of Parkinsonian signs would suggest dementia with Lewy bodies, the evolution of dementia in a previously diagnosed patient with Parkinson disease, or one of the "Parkinson plus" diseases such as progressive supranuclear palsy, to which paresis of vertical gaze is an important clue.
- Asymmetry of strength or reflexes, gait impairment, and mild increases in neuromuscular tone, in the presence of

cognitive impairment, suggest cerebrovascular disease (or the rare corticobasal degeneration).

- Poor balance may be found in a number of neurodegenerative and cerebrovascular diseases, but may also occur in the patient with orthostatic hypotension, a common complication of dementia caused by an impaired sense of thirst, a voluntary reduction of fluid intake to avoid urinary urgency, or overtreated hypertension.
- Resting tremor is most suggestive of a Parkinson-related disease, while action tremors may suggest cerebellar degeneration or drug effects.
- Peripheral neuropathy is most often idiopathic; however, if present, it should trigger evaluation for B12 deficiency, toxic causes (e.g., chemotherapy), or alcohol-related central nervous system (CNS) dysfunction (if associated with cerebellar ataxia).

Diagnostic and Screening Tools

Formal evaluation of cognitive status allows the family physician to uncover hidden and unexpected problems at an early stage, where diagnostic and therapeutic interventions may be most valuable. These same strategies and tools can provide a useful initial evaluation of patients complaining of memory problems or other cognitive symptoms.

Routine screening of older adults for cognitive impairment has been addressed by the United States Preventive Services Task Force (11). Their critical review of the literature concluded that no randomized trials have been conducted to assess the effects of screening for dementia, and that, lacking such data, there is no basis for recommending either for or against screening. On the other hand, large health systems with incentives to manage costs, such as Kaiser Permanente, recommend screening at any age when cognitive impairment is suspected, and routine screening for the very old, where rates of dementia are high.

Several easy-to-use tools are available to assess cognition. Because they are well established and complement each other, we are presenting the following cognitive screening instruments: the Mini-Mental State Examination (MMSE), the Mini-Cog, and the Functional Activities Questionnaire (FAQ). Later in this section, we will present formal tools that rapidly screen for delirium and depression, two reversible illnesses that often are mistaken for dementia.

MMSE

The most widely used short cognitive assessment tool is the MMSE. This familiar tool has a series of questions and tasks that the physician or a well-trained assistant administers to the patient. These tasks test a variety of mental and cognitive functions including orientation, registration and recall, short-term memory, naming, spatial relations, and others. Based on the patient's response or performance, each item is individually scored and totaled, resulting in an overall score from 0–30 points. The test typically takes 8–15 minutes to administer. Many clinicians feel this is too long for routine screening and efficient use in the routine primary care office visit. Figure 42.2 lists the MMSE items.

Interpreting the MMSE score is not straightforward. The traditional cutoff (23 points) misses many patients with early dementia; a screening test cutoff of approximately 27 is proba-

bly better. The MMSE is sensitive to education; so persons who have completed eighth grade or less may score up to 5 points lower than common cutoffs and still be normal.

MINI-COG

The Mini-Cog, taking no more than 2–4 minutes, fits easily within the time constraints of primary care visits. It is at least as effective as the MMSE in both population-based (12) and multi-ethnic community samples (13). The Mini-Cog uses recall of three unrelated words and a clock drawing task. Scores vary from 0 (worst) to 5 (best). It detects cognitive impairment and dementia earlier than patients' own physicians in a community study (14).

Figure 42.3 describes the Mini-Cog and its interpretation. Many other short screens are available for use in primary care, each with their own strengths and weaknesses (15).

FAQ

The FAQ assesses 10 everyday cognitive functions and preferably is rated by someone who knows the patient well, rather than by the patient (16). Figure 42.4 provides the FAQ questions. Higher scores indicate greater need for help; scores above 9 (out of a possible 30) are considered suspicious for dementia.

The FAQ has several limitations. As a functional evaluation tool, it has a "floor" effect in that by the time patients have reached moderate dementia, they tend to score at or near 30. It also lacks items particularly important for primary care practice, such as questions about medication use and other health behaviors that are likely to be affected. For patients with established dementia, functional assessment should also include basic ADLs, such as bathing, dressing, ambulation, eating, and toileting. Nonetheless, the FAQ is sensitive to change over time and can be useful to monitor patients in whom early dementia is suspected.

Searching for Treatable Causes and Contributing Factors

If the initial evaluation indicates the presence of cognitive impairment, the physician should then search for potentially treatable or reversible causes of this problem. This step is vital in differentiating patients where therapeutic interventions may reverse some loss or slow progression significantly, from the chronic dementias of aging, which have a generally poorer prognosis and a higher likelihood of progression. Table 42.4 lists and describes the common red flags suggesting that a patient may have one of the treatable causes of cognitive decline. Fewer than 5% of patients with cognitive impairment will have a potentially treatable or reversible cause (17), but the impact of early detection and treatment may be significant for those patients.

Delirium, a syndrome of acquired impairment of attention, alertness, and perception, is a common cause of cognitive impairment among older adults who are acutely ill or who receive certain types of medications likely to impair cognition. Approximately one-third of patients aged 70 or older admitted to a general medical service experience delirium—half are delirious on admission to the hospital, and the others develop delirium in the hospital. One-third of older patients presenting to the emergency department are delirious. Although delirium, like dementia, involves global cognitive impairment, de-

The Mini-Mental State Examination

Patient _____ Examiner _____ Date _____

Maximum	Score	
		Orientation
5	( )	What is the (year) (season) (date) (day) (month)?
5	( )	Where are we (state) (country) (town) (hospital) (floor)?
		Registration
3	( )	Name 3 objects: 1 second to say each. Then ask the patient all 3 after you have said them. Give 1 point for each correct answer. Then repeat them until he/she learns all 3. Count trials and record. Trials _____
		Attention and Calculation
5	( )	Serial 7's. 1 point for each correct answer. Stop after 5 answers. Alternatively, spell "world" backward.
		Recall
3	( )	Ask for the 3 objects repeated above. Give 1 point for each correct answer.
		Language
2	( )	Name a pencil and watch.
1	( )	Repeat the following "No ifs, ands, or buts"
3	( )	Follow a 3-stage command: "Take a paper in your hand, fold it in half, and put it on the floor."
1	( )	Read and obey the following: CLOSE YOUR EYES
1	( )	Write a sentence.
1	( )	Copy the design shown.

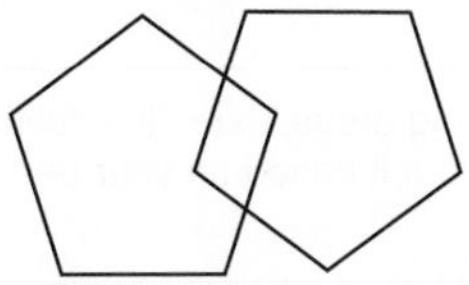

_____ Total Score

ASSESS level of consciousness along a continuum _____

Alert Drowsy Stupor Coma

Figure 42.2 • The Mini-Mental State Examination.

lirium is characterized by an acute onset, fluctuations in mental status over time, impaired consciousness and attention, and altered sleep cycles. Table 42.5 lists and describes common symptoms of delirium.

The Confusion Assessment Method (see Table 42.6) is a validated clinical tool to screen for and diagnose delirium. Major risk factors for delirium include age and the presence of dementia. Causes include infection, pain, sleep or sensory deprivation, and use of multiple concurrent medications or medication/substance withdrawal.

Depression can produce cognitive changes that often make patients fear that they are developing dementia, and symptoms of both may overlap. A common symptom of depression is the inability to concentrate, which can result in memory difficulties. Depressed patients can often display lack of interest in things and decreased energy, symptoms that are also common in dementia. The cognitive complaints in depression are often much greater than actual deficits on testing, however, though patients may often show a tendency to give up early

when completing assessment tools. Use of a formal screening tool such as the Geriatric Depression Scale (see Figure 42.5) is very valuable. When any doubt exists, a trial of treatment with a well-tolerated antidepressant (often an selective serotonin reuptake inhibitor [SSRI]) is essential; an early partial response is encouraging, but full therapeutic effect can take 8–12 weeks.

Hypothyroidism is a common clinical condition that occasionally presents as a dementia-like syndrome. Neurological manifestations include sleepiness or sluggish thought processes. Patients may respond slowly to questions and have difficulty retrieving information from memory. The history and physical should, however, reveal clues of fatigue, cold intolerance, constipation, weight gain, bradycardia, and non-pitting edema (myxedema). Occult hyperthyroidism in older adults can occasionally be associated with cognitive symptoms as well. Therefore, thyroid function studies should be part of the evaluation of all patients with suspected dementia.

Manifestations of severe *vitamin B12 deficiency* can in-

Step 1: Ask the patient to remember three items: "I am going to tell you the names of three items and I would like you to remember them…[Give three unrelated words, e.g. banana – sunrise – chair]. Now try to remember those three things – I will ask you later."

Step 2: Ask the patient to draw a clock face placing all the numbers and the hands in the correct position: "I would like you to draw a picture of the face of a clock on this paper, with all the numbers and with the hands showing a time of 10 minutes past 11."

Step 3: Ask the patient to recall the three items (without cueing): "I asked you to remember the names of three items that I told you earlier – Please tell them to me now."

SCORING:

Three-item recall: One point for each item recalled after the clock drawing test.

Clock drawing test: Two points for a normal clock drawing.

      Normal: All numbers in appropriate quadrants and hands indicate correct time.

      Abnormal: Any variation from above requirements.

INTERPRETING RESULTS:

0-2 Points: Positive screen for dementia

3-5 Points: Negative screen for dementia

Performance in a population-based sample(12): SENSITIVITY = 76%   SPECIFICITY = 89%

Figure 42.3 • Mini-Cog: A brief screen for cognitive impairment.

Please rate the individual's ability in each of the following areas, using the scale at the right to circle the best response. [Note: if he or she never did the activity, score it based on your best guess as to whether he or she could do it if they had to now.]

Activity	Ability to Do the Activity			
	Normal	Has difficulty, but does it him/herself	Requires assistance	Someone else needs to do it
1. Writing checks, paying bills, balancing checkbook.	0	1	2	3
2. Assembling tax records, business affairs, or papers.	0	1	2	3
3. Shopping alone for clothes, household necessities, or groceries.	0	1	2	3
4. Playing a game of skill, working on a hobby.	0	1	2	3
5. Heating water, making a cup of coffee, turning off stove.	0	1	2	3
6. Preparing a balanced meal.	0	1	2	3
7. Keeping track of current events.	0	1	2	3
8. Paying attention to, understanding, discussing TV, books, magazines.	0	1	2	3
9. Remembering appointments, family occasions, holidays, medications.	0	1	2	3
10. Traveling out of neighborhood, driving, arranging to take buses.	0	1	2	3

Scoring
A total score is computed by simply summing the scores across the 10 items. Scores range from 0 to 30. Scores of 9 or above indicated significant cognitive impairment

Figure 42.4 • Functional Activities Questionnaire (FAQ).

TABLE 42.4 Red Flags Suggesting Potentially Treatable and/or Reversible Causes of Cognitive Impairment

Potential Cause	Key Characteristics	Diagnostic Method
Delirium	Acute change in mental status	History and physical
		Mental status exam
	Fluctuating course	
	Inattention	
	Disorganized thinking or altered level of consciousness	
Depression	Concern about treatment out of proportion to clinical deficits.	Depression screening and diagnosis
	Frustration during testing with cognitive assessment tools.	Response to treatment
Hypothyroidism	Fatigue, cold intolerance, constipation	History and physical
		Thyroid function tests
	Weight gain, bradycardia, and nonpitting edema (myxedema)	
Vitamin B12 deficiency	Neuropathy	Vitamin B12 level
	Paresthesias	
	Loss of vibration and position sense	
	Ataxia	
Neurosyphilis	Delusions of grandeur	Serum FTA
	Emotional lability	Spinal fluid FTA
	Argyll Robertson pupils	
Brain tumor	Headache	MRI or CT
	Seizures	
	Nausea/vomiting	
	Muscle weakness	
Normal pressure hydrocephalus	Triad of incontinence, wide-based gait, and dementia.	MRI or CT
		Radioisotope flow studies of CSF
		Therapeutic lumbar puncture
Subdural hematoma	History of trauma (only 50%)	MRI or CT
	Headache	
	Hemiparesis	
	Focal neurologic signs	

CSF, cerebrospinal fluid; FTA, fluorescent treponemal antibody.

clude memory loss, irritability, psychosis, and dementia. Other neurologic findings also may be present; these include symmetrical neuropathy (paresthesias, loss of vibration and position sense) and ataxia. Dementia may also contribute to vitamin B12 deficiency due to changes in food choices (e.g., dropping animal foods because of expense, complex preparation, or forgetfulness) or reduced overall food intake. Therefore, a Vitamin B 12 level should be obtained in all patients evaluated for dementia.

Previously a common cause of dementia syndromes, *neurosyphilis*, is now quite rare. However, with a resurgence of early syphilis in the 1980s and 1990s, late syphilis may become more common again. As a result of inflammation of the meninges and cerebral cortex, a dementia syndrome called general paresis can result. Personality changes include delusions of grandeur, emotional lability, and paranoia. The syndrome can progress to memory loss and dementia. A classic physical finding is the Argyll Robertson pupil, where the pupils do not react to strong light but do constrict with convergence gaze (accommodation). The usual serum and cerebrospinal fluid (CSF) serologies may be negative; therefore, a serum fluorescent treponemal antibody (FTA) and a CSF FTA are recommended as part of the diagnostic assessment for suspected dementia. Many clinicians are not recommending rou-

TABLE 42.5 Risk Factors for Delirium

Predisposing factors
  Advanced age
  Dementia
  Functional impairment in activities of daily living
  High medical comorbidity
  History of alcohol abuse
  Male sex
  Sensory impairment (blindness, deafness)
Precipitating factors
  Acute cardiac events: myocardial infarction, congestive heart failure exacerbation, arrhythmia
  Acute pulmonary events: asthma or chronic obstructive pulmonary disease exacerbation, pulmonary embolism, hypoxemia, hypercarbia
  Bed rest
  Drug withdrawal (sedatives, alcohol)
  Fluid or electrolyte disturbances, including dehydration, hyponatremia, hypernatremia
  Infections (especially respiratory, urinary)
  Intracranial events (stroke, bleeding, infection)*
  Medications
  Severe anemia (hematocrit <30%)
  Uncontrolled pain
  Urinary retention, fecal impaction
  Use of indwelling devices, such as urinary catheters
  Use of restraints

*Intracranial factors are rare and should be considered only when all other factors have been excluded or if there are new focal neurologic signs.
Source: Cobbs EL, Duthie EN, Marcantonio ER, Murphy JB. Delirium: Geriatric Review Syllabus. Blackwell Publishing 2002:134.

TABLE 42.6 The Confusion Assessment Method

The diagnosis of delirium requires the presence of features 1 and 2, and either 3 or 4.
1. Acute change in mental status and fluctuating course
   —Is there evidence of an acute change in cognition from the patient's baseline?
   —Does the abnormal behavior fluctuate during the day, i.e., tend to come and go, or increase and decrease in severity?
2. Inattention
   —Does the patient have difficulty focusing attention, e.g., being easily distractible, or having difficulty keeping track of what was being said?
3. Disorganized thinking
   —Is the patient's thinking disorganized or incoherent, e.g., rambling or irrelevant conversation, unclear or illogical flow of ideas, or unpredictable switching from subject to subject?
4. Altered level of consciousness
   —Is the patient's mental status anything besides alert, i.e., vigilant (hyperalert), lethargic (drowsy, easily aroused), stuporous (difficult to arouse), or comatose (unarousable)?

Adapted from: Inouye SK, van Dyck CH, Alessi CA, et al. Clarifying confusion: the Confusion Assessment Method. Ann Intern Med. 1990; 113(12):941–948.

tine evaluation for neurosyphilis in all patients with symptoms of dementia, but selective screening should be considered if suggested by clinical findings and a high risk history.

Brain tumors can present in many ways, with cognitive impairment among them. For example, memory problems and/or mood or personality changes are the presenting complaint in 30%–35% of persons with brain metastases. Other complaints, such as headaches, nausea and vomiting, muscle weakness, seizures, or loss of consciousness, in the presence of cognitive impairment, should prompt neuroimaging studies. Focal brain tumors (e.g., in the temporal lobe), may cause subtle cognitive changes that a physician who knows the patient well may recognize but that are undetectable with short cognitive screens.

Normal pressure hydrocephalus (NPH) should be considered when the triad of gait disturbance, urinary incontinence, and cognitive dysfunction occur together. Although these same findings can occur in other dementia syndromes, evaluation for NPH should be considered since the findings may be reversible—especially early in the disease. CT or MRI may not be specific but should be obtained first. Radioisotope diffusion studies in the CSF may help with the diagnosis. MRI is much more useful than CT in searching for signs of brain disease, which can cause enlarged ventricles, since lobar patterns of atrophy—which should be absent in NPH—can be identified with this method.

Subdural hematoma is a collection of blood between the dura and the arachnoid and is bilateral in about 15% of cases. The incidence of chronic subdural is 7.4 per 100,000 for persons in their 70s, and in 50% of these persons, there is no history of head injury. Symptoms can include headache, slight to severe impairment in cognition, and (in advanced cases) hemiparesis. Focal neurologic signs, such as weakness and sensory changes, may also be present. Diagnosis is by neuroimaging with CT or MRI.

Laboratory and Other Diagnostic Testing

Because the diagnosis of Alzheimer's dementia is based on clinical criteria, laboratory testing and neuroimaging are used to rule out other causes of dementia, not to make a diagnosis. Recommendations for laboratory evaluation of patients with cognitive impairment vary. The American Academy of Neurology Practice recommends only a vitamin B12 level and thyroid function tests (18). The Second Canadian Consensus Conference on Dementia recommends a complete blood count, serum electrolytes, serum calcium, and serum glucose (19). Other tests, such as serology for syphilis, human immunodeficiency virus testing (HIV), urinalysis, serum toxicology and heavy metal screening, erythrocyte sedimentation rate, liver function, and serum folate, should be performed only when clinical suspicion indicates. Testing for genetic risk fac-

Choose the best answer for how you felt over the past week.

1. Are you basically satisfied with your life? — yes/**no**
2. Have you dropped many of your activities and interests? — **yes**/no
3. Do you feel that your life is empty? — **yes**/no
4. Do you often get bored? — **yes**/no
5. Are you in good spirits most of the time? — yes/**no**
6. Are you afraid that something bad is going to happen to you? — **yes**/no
7. Do you feel happy most of the time? — yes/**no**
8. Do you often feel helpless? — **yes**/no
9. Do you prefer to stay at home, rather than going out and doing new things? — **yes**/no
10. Do you feel you have more problems with memory than most? — **yes**/no
11. Do you think it is wonderful to be alive now? — yes/**no**
12. Do you feel pretty worthless the way you are now? — **yes**/no
13. Do you feel full of energy? — yes/**no**
14. Do you feel that your situation is hopeless? — **yes**/no
15. Do you think that most people are better off than you are? — **yes**/no

NOTE: Score bolded answers. One point for each of these answers. Cut-off: normal = 0–5; above 5 suggests depression. For additional information on administration and scoring, refer to the following references:
1. Sheikh JI, Yesavage JA. Geriatric Depression Scale: recent evidence and development of a shorter version. *Clin Gerontol.* 1986;5:165–172.
2. Yesavage JA, Brink TL, Rose TL, et al. Development and validation of a geriatric depression rating scale: a preliminary report. *J Psych Res.* 1983;17:27.

Figure 42.5 • The Geriatric Depression Scale (short form, GDS).

tors, such as apolipoprotein E alleles, is not recommended due to inadequate sensitivity and specificity.

Lumbar puncture is not recommended for routine evaluation but should be considered if HIV, neurosyphilis, cerebral vasculitis, Lyme disease, or prion disease (e.g., Creutzfeld-Jakob disease) are suspected on clinical grounds.

There is no consensus on whether primary care physicians should routinely order neuroimaging studies in the work-up of typical cases of Alzheimer's disease or other dementias for which a surgical cause is not suspected on other grounds. However, the American Academy of Neurology Practice recommends structural neuroimaging (CT or MRI) for all patients undergoing a dementia workup (18), although the yield of reversible conditions (subdural hematoma, abscess, or tumors) is below 3% (17).

CASE STUDY (PART 2)

Mrs. H. states that she has noted gradually increasing fatigue, decreased energy, and difficulty concentrating over the past 6 months. Her physical exam is normal. She scores 25 on her MMSE; the Mini-Cog reveals a normal clock drawing, 3/3 on registration, and 1/3 on recall; and the Geriatric Depression Scale indicates severe depression. Thyroid stimulating hormone, complete blood count, and B12 are all normal. An imaging study is not done.

Treatment for depression is initiated with citalopram (Celexa), and she is followed closely. At 8 weeks she reports that she feels "back to normal." Her Geriatric Depression

Scale is normal, and her MMSE is 29. The medication is continued for 12 months, after which it is discontinued without recurrence of her symptoms.

Six years later her husband brings her to the office with renewed concern about memory problems and her loss of ability to perform some previously routine tasks, such as balancing the checkbook and paying bills. Her MMSE is 23 and her Mini-Cog score is 1. Neurologic screening examination and laboratory evaluation are normal, and a CT scan of the head suggests mild diffuse atrophy. A diagnosis of mild dementia of the Alzheimer's type is made. She and her husband would like to try any treatments or regimens that might help regain some function or slow further decline, so that she remain at home and avoid institutional care as long as is practical.

CLINICAL QUESTIONS

1. What management strategies are available to slow the course of Alzheimer's disease?
2. What additional strategies are available to help a person with the disease remain at home as long as possible, and to promote quality of life?

MANAGEMENT

Cognitive impairment is a syndrome that requires medical management as well as management of the social impact of the loss of cognitive abilities. The medical management is

and side effects of medications. Numerous types of interventions have been studied (39). Only behavior management therapies, specific types of caregiver education, and possibly cognitive stimulation have demonstrated lasting effectiveness, but not all caregivers are able or willing to participate in behavior management training—and not all locales provide expert training options. Adult day centers offer useful approaches to sharing the burden of care and can help foster behavioral improvements in patients (40) that can translate into greater happiness at home.

In counseling families and caregivers about managing specific behaviors, prioritizing those that are the most distressing or dangerous is the best starting place. A useful strategy is the following:

1. Identify the target symptoms.
2. Determine when the symptoms are most likely to occur.
3. Determine events that precede, and therefore may precipitate or contribute to, the symptoms.
4. Set up a planned intervention.
5. Continue to evaluate and alternate treatment approach as necessary (41).

One difficult aspect of treatment is deciding what option to try. For example hunger may be a trigger for a patient who becomes agitated and wanders in the mid to late morning, so a snack could be scheduled at 10 AM each day. The behavior decreases, and the intervention is continued and monitored for ongoing effectiveness. Alternatively, boredom or loneliness may trigger behavior changes; in these cases, providing company and simple diversions may be quite effective. Pain, a difficult symptom to assess in moderate to severe Alzheimer's, should also be considered as causes of behavior changes. In such cases, a behavior may respond to treatment with an appropriate analgesic, including acetaminophen.

Depression is a common symptom in Alzheimer's dementia. Estimates range from 9%–60% (38). In spite of the high prevalence of depressive symptoms and the frequent use of antidepressants in dementia, there is a paucity of clinical trial data to address drug effectiveness (42, 43). Activity programs for the patient, caregiver training, and treating depression in caregivers, when present, can be quite helpful. The role of medications in treating depression in demented patients remains uncertain except when depression is quite severe and closely resembles major depression in nondemented patients. In such situations, SSRIs are most commonly used because of their lower incidence of anticholinergic and other side effects. Antidepressants with anticholinergic side effects should be avoided.

MEDICATIONS FOR BEHAVIORAL SYMPTOMS

At times, behavioral and environmental strategies are insufficient to control behavioral symptoms, and the use of pharmacologic agents is considered. Table 42.9 summarizes these medications and their use. They should be reserved for situations where there is either clear distress to the patient or risk of physical harm to the patient, caregivers, or others.

The scientific evidence for effectiveness of medication in dementia-related behavioral disturbances is remarkably weak (44). Antidepressants have generally not been shown to be effective other than for depression. Three RCTs of the mood-stabilizer valproate (Depakote) showed no efficacy or intolerable side effects. Two small RCTs of carbamazepine (Tegretol) had conflicting results. Two meta-analyses and six RCTs of cholinesterase inhibitors generally showed small, although statistically significant results, and two RCTs of memantine had conflicting results for neuropsychiatric symptoms of dementia. It is important, however, to recognize that patients enrolled in such clinical trials generally had low-severity behavioral problems, and results may not generalize to the minority of patients with more severe behavioral problems that require specialized treatment. Typical antipsychotics (neuroleptic agents such as haloperidol [Haldol]) were evaluated in two meta-analyses and two RCTs, with small efficacy compared to placebo, significant side effects, and no differences among specific agents. Of the pharmacologic agents reviewed, the atypical antipsychotics risperidone (Risperdal) and olanzapine

TABLE 42.9 Pharmacologic Management of Behavioral Symptoms in Dementia*

Drug Class and Examples	Target Symptoms
Antipsychotics (Usually atypicals: olanzapine, quetiapine risperidone)	Psychosis (hallucinations, delusions), aggression, violent behavior, agitation.
Antidepressants	
Trazodone	Sleep-wake cycle disturbances, agitation aggression, anxiety.
Selective serotonin reuptake inhibitors	Depressive syndromes, depression-associated agitation, emotionality, irritability.
Mirtazapine	Depressive syndromes, sleep-wake cycle disturbances, reduced appetite.
Benzodiazepines	Anxiety, agitation, sleep disturbance.
Anticonvulsants (Valproic acid, carbamazepine)	Agitation, aggression, sleep-wake cycle disturbance, symptoms of mania.

*Note: Behavioral management is always first line and a part of management of all symptoms.

(Zyprexa) showed modest effectiveness in randomized trials in nursing home populations. Unfortunately, concerns have arisen about an increased incidence of stroke in dementia patients taking atypical antipsychotics, and a recent meta-analysis suggests that a small increase in risk of death may be associated with their use, resulting in black-box warnings for all such agents (45). It is important to recognize that the data justifying this warning were acquired in studies of nursing home residents of advanced age, and that the risks identified may vary in other groups. Based on the existing data, it is prudent to use these agents with caution, not rely exclusively on medications to manage behavior, and carefully review the risks and benefits with families and caregivers. Nevertheless, antipsychotic agents do have a place in managing some of the more severe behavioral complications of dementia and can be very effective in treating properly selected patients.

CASE STUDY (PART 3)

Over the next 3 years Mrs. H. continues to decline. At her office visit today, her husband reports that she requires more help with dressing and bathing and is often incontinent of urine but resists application of protective undergarments, saying she's not a baby. She no longer recognizes her daughter's voice on the phone. She tends to wander around in the house during the day mumbling repetitively to herself, and she has fallen several times. Mr. H. is losing sleep at night for fear that his wife will leave the house and get lost. He is not sure how long he can continue. Her repeat MMSE is 15.

LONG-TERM MONITORING

Most dementias, and Alzheimer's disease in particular, are chronic and progressive. Dementia shortens survival, but the magnitude of the effect varies widely among patients, and is strongly influenced by age and comorbid diseases (46, 47).

As the disease progresses, the patient's function decreases, and more assistance with ADLs is required. Often caregivers barely notice, as they take on each new responsibility that the patient formerly managed alone, increasing the proportion of family resources that must be devoted to care of the demented individual. In addition, neuropsychiatric symptoms associated with dementia add further burden to family members and caregivers, as does mourning the progressive loss of the person that they knew. Increasing requirements for care may ultimately result in admission to a long-term care facility.

Care Options

Although many people with Alzheimer's are cared for in the home, sole care by the family member or other caregiver throughout the entire course of the disease is generally not practical. Assistance with home care can come from a variety of sources. Home health agencies tend to be most helpful in addressing acute care issues. Health aides can be very valuable but are often not covered by insurance, and companion care is covered only by some long-term care insurance. Physician home care is a growing area of clinical medicine, with some physicians moving to home-care-only practices.

Some communities have Program of All-Inclusive Care for the Elderly (PACE) available. PACE is a capitated model of care that pools funds from Medicare and Medicaid to provide acute and long-term care to frail older people eligible for both. The goal is to keep the person in the community as long as is medically, socially, and financially feasible. An interdisciplinary team of health care providers provides care across the spectrum of hospital, home, and other institutions. Adult day services, respite care, transportation, medication coverage, and rehabilitation are included. This inclusive system of care provides for the complex social as well as the medical needs of the patient. The effectiveness of PACE has not been tested in an RCT, but research has shown that it provides a high standard of quality, although with significant site-to-site variation. PACE is not available to the majority of older adults, whose incomes are too high to qualify.

Assisted living may be an option for patients in the milder stages of dementia. Patients who are ambulatory and require limited assistance with ADLs may be good candidates. Demented patients fail in these environments when lack of suitable activity programs leaves them alone for too much of the day. Not all facilities have the capacity to handle patients with wandering or other mild behavioral problems, but specialized dementia units are becoming more common. Small care homes are an increasingly important component of the long-term care spectrum as well, as states increasingly offer special licensing for homes with caregivers trained in caring for patients with dementia.

Nursing home care is often the option of choice during the late stages of disease and for some patients with milder dementia and other medical problems or behavioral disturbances. Indeed, dementia is the most common reason for long-term placement in nursing homes; 50% to 80% of nursing home patients have dementia. Thus, in Alzheimer's disease and related dementias, the transition to palliative care and the final months or years of life are often spent in a nursing home or other long-term care setting.

CASE STUDY (PART 4)

As a result of incontinence and continued wandering, Mrs. H. was admitted to a long-term care facility close to her home, where her husband visited almost daily. Over the next 2½ years she continued to decline.

She is now unable to walk or speak, and spends her time in bed and in a chair. Recently she has had trouble coordinating swallowing and has begun to lose weight despite attempts to supplement and fortify her diet. After discussion of options, Mr. H. and his daughter agree not to have a feeding tube placed. A hospice consult is arranged that will augment the care provided by the nursing home, support the family, and help provide comfort in this final stage of Mrs. H's disease.

End-of-Life Care

Many patients with dementia progress steadily to the point where they are no longer able to perform even the most basic

TABLE 42.10 Key Recommendations for Practice

Recommendation	Strength of Recommendation *
Screening for dementia using a formal instrument, such as the Mini-Cog	C
Counseling of family and patient (including support groups)	C
Treatment of comorbid conditions and risk factors	
Rx of depression with medication	B
Treatment of cognitive decline in Alzheimer's disease:	
With acetylcholinesterase inhibitors	B
With neuraminidase (NMDA) inhibitors	C
With antihypertensive treatment	B
Treatment of behavioral symptoms in Alzheimer's disease:	
With nonpharmacological methods	A
With acetylcholinesterase inhibitors	B
With antipsychotics	C
Treatment of vascular dementia:	
With acetylcholinesterase inhibitors	C
With antihypertensive medications	B
By controlling other risk factors (e.g., serum lipids)	C
Treatment of Lewy body disease with acetylcholinesterase inhibitors	B
Hospice care to improve quality of end-of-life care	C

*A = consistent, good-quality patient-oriented evidence; B = inconsistent or limited-quality patient-oriented evidence; C = consensus, disease-oriented evidence, usual practice, expert opinion, or case series. For information about the SORT evidence rating system, see *http://www.aafp.org/afpsort.xml*.

functions of swallowing food or fluids. Studies have shown that artificial ("tube") feeding does not prevent aspiration and does not lead to recovery or improvement for patients with dementia.

Once used primarily for cancer patients, hospice services have begun to be used more widely for end of life care for chronic diseases, including dementia. Services are available for patients at home or in long-term care facilities. One challenge is determining when hospice care is appropriate. The patient with severe dementia, who is consistently losing weight despite attempts to supplement orally, has a limited prognosis and can be considered a good candidate for hospice services.

CASE DISCUSSION

The case of Mrs. H. illustrates many of the characteristics of Alzheimer's disease. Her dementia had an insidious onset and was relentlessly progressive despite attempts to modify its course. It strained the capacity of her family, eventually leading to placement in a nursing home. The main weapons that were available to ease suffering and promote health were nonspecific treatments, avoidance of iatrogenic disease, and support for the patient, family, and caregivers, with a focus on comfort and quality of life. After 6 years of living with Alzheimer's disease, Mrs. H. dies quietly and comfortably in her nursing home bed, with her husband at her side.

CONCLUSION

Cognitive impairment is a major issue in the primary care of older persons. Screening for early cognitive impairment, though still controversial, is important and is likely to be increasingly more so as additional treatments for dementia become available. Skill at diagnosis and management of cognitive symptoms is critical, as dementia and fear of the disease has immense impact on older patients and their families. Much scientific evidence has been accumulated to guide our approach to cognitive impairment; Table 42.10 summarizes many of the key recommendations. The coming decades will bring additional advances, and management of cognitive symptoms will become an increasingly important and sophisticated area of primary care medicine.

Acknowledgment

Thanks to Mollie Scott, PharmD, for preparation of Table 42.8 and to Neil Hall, MD, for reviewing the manuscript.

REFERENCES

1. Hendrie HC. Epidemiology of dementia and Alzheimer's disease. Am J Geriatr Psychiatry. 1998;6(suppl 1); S3–S18.

2. Evans DA, Funkenstein HH, Albert MS, et al. Prevalence of Alzheimer's disease in a community population of older persons; higher than previously reported. JAMA. 1989;262:2551–2556.

3. Sampson EL, Warren JD, Rossor MN. Young onset dementia. Postgrad Med J 2004;80:125–139.

4. American Psychiatric Association. 1994. Diagnostic and Statistical Manual of Mental Disorders, 4th ed. Washington, DC: American Psychiatric Association.

5. Small S. Age-related memory decline. Arch Neurol. 2001;58:360–364.

6. Valcour VG, Masaki KH, Curb JD, Blanchette PL. The detection of dementia in the primary care setting. Arch Intern Med. 200;160:2964–2968.

7. Ballard CG. Definition and diagnosis of dementia with Lewy bodies. Dement Geriatr Cogn Disord. 2004;17(suppl 1):15–24.

8. Snowden JS, Neary D, Mann DA. Frontotemporal dementia. Br J Psychiatry. 2002;180:140–143.

9. Bennett DA. Update on mild cognitive impairment. Curr Neurol Neurosci Rep. 2003;3:379–384.

10. Geslani DM, Tierney MC, Herrmann N, Szalai JP. Mild cognitive impairment: an operational definition and its conversion rate to Alzheimer's disease. Dement Geriatr Cogn Disord. 2005;19:383–389.

11. Boustani M, Peterson B, Hanson L, Harris R, Lohr N; U.S. Preventive Services Task Force. Screening for dementia in primary care: a summary of the evidence for the U.S. Preventive Services Task Force. Ann Intern Med. 2003;927–937.

12. Borson S, Scanlan JM, Chen P, Ganguli M. The Mini-Cog as a screen for dementia: validation in a population-based sample. J Am Geriatr Soc. 2003;51:1451–1454.

13. Borson S, Scanlan JM, Watanabe J, Tu SP, Lessig M. Simplifying detection of cognitive impairment: comparison of the Mini-Cog and Mini-Mental State Examination in a multiethnic sample. J Am Geriatr Soc. 2005;53:871–874.

14. Borson S, Scanlan JM, Watanabe J, et al. Improving identification of cognitive impairment in primary care. Int J Geriatr Psychiatry 2006;21:568–580.

15. Lorentz WJ, Scanlan JM, Borson S. Brief screening tests for dementia. Can J Psychiatry. 2002;47:723–733.

16. Pfeffer RI, Kurosaki TT, Harrah CH, Jr, Chance JM, Filos S. Measurement of functional activities in older adults in the community. J Gerontol. 1982;37:323–329.

17. Freter S, Bergman H, Gold S, Chertkow H, Clarfield AM. Prevalence of potentially reversible dementias and actual reversibility in a memory clinic cohort. CMAJ. 1998;159:657–662.

18. Knopman DS, DeKosky ST, Cummings JL, et al. Practice parameter: diagnosis of dementia (and evidence-based review). Neurology. 2001;56:1143–1153.

19. Chertkow H, Bergman H, Schipper HM, et al. Assessment of suspected dementia. Can J Neurol Sci. 2001;28(suppl 1):S28–41.

20. Alexopoulos GS, Meyers BS, Young RC, Mattis S, Kakuma T. The course of geriatric depression with "reversible dementia": a controlled study. Am J Psychiatry. 1993;150(11):1693–1699.

21. Parks SM, Novielli KD. A practical guide to caring for caregivers. Am Fam Physician. 2000;62:2613–2622.

22. Veld BA, Ruitenberg A, Hofman A, et al. Nonsteroidal antiinflammatory drugs and the risk of Alzheimer's disease. N Engl J Med. 2001;345:1515–1521.

23. Birks JS, Harvey R. Donepezil for dementia due to Alzheimer's disease (Cochrane Review). In: The Cochrane Library. Chichester, UK: John Wiley and Sons, Ltd.; 2005:Issue 1.

24. Birks J, Grimley Evans J, Iakovidou V, Tsolaki M, Rivastigmine for Alzheimer's disease (Cochrane Review). In: The Cochrane Library. Chichester, UK: John Wiley and Sons, Ltd.; 2005:Issue 1.

25. Loy C, Schneider L. Galantamine for Alzheimer's disease (Cochrane Review). In: The Cochrane Library. Chichester, UK: John Wiley and Sons, Ltd.; 2005:Issue 1.

26. Areosa Sastre A, McShane R, Sherriff F. Memantine for dementia (Cochrane Review). In: The Cochrane Library. Chichester, UK: John Wiley and Sons, Ltd.; 2005:Issue 1.

27. Tariot PN, Farlow MR, Grossberg GT, Graham SM, McDonald S, Gergel I. Memantine treatment in patients with moderate to severe Alzheimer disease already receiving donepezil. A randomized controlled trial. JAMA. 2004;291:317–324.

28. Malouf R, Birks J. Donepezil for vascular cognitive impairment (Cochrane Review). In: The Cochrane Library. Chichester, UK: John Wiley and Sons, Ltd.; 2005:Issue 1.

29. McKeith I, Del Ser T, Spano P, et al. Efficacy of rivastigmine in dementia with Lewy bodies: a randomized, double-blind placebo-controlled international study. Lancet. 2000;356:2031–2036.

30. Sano M, Ernesto C, Thomas RG, et al. A controlled trial of selegiline, alpha-tocopherol, or both as treatment for Alzheimer's disease. N Engl J Med. 1997;336:1216–1222.

31. Tabet N, Birks J, Grimley-Evans J, Orrel M, Spector A. Vitamin E for Alzheimer's disease (Cochrane Review) In: The Cochrane Library. Chichester, UK: John Wiley and Sons, Ltd.; 2005:Issue 1.

32. Miller ER III, Pastor-Barriuso R, Dalal D, Riemersma RA, Appel LJ Guallar E. Meta-analysis: high-dosage vitamin E supplementation may increase all cause mortality. Ann Intern Med. 2005;142:37–46.

33. Birks J, Flicker L. Selegiline for Alzheimer's disease. (Cochrane Review). In: The Cochrane Library. Chichester, UK: John Wiley and Sons, Ltd.; 2005:Issue 1.

34. Hogervorst E, Yaffe K, Richards M, Huppert F. Hormone replacement therapy to maintain cognitive function in women with dementia (Cochrane Review). In: The Cochrane Library. Chichester, UK: John Wiley and Sons, Ltd.; 2005:Issue 1.

35. Tabet N, Feldman H. Indomethacin for Alzheimer's disease. (Cochrane Review). In: The Cochrane Library. Chichester, UK: John Wiley and Sons, Ltd.; 2005:Issue 1.

36. Birks J, Grimley Evans J. Ginkgo Biloba for cognitive impairment and dementia (Cochrane Review). In: The Cochrane Library. Chichester, UK: John Wiley and Sons, Ltd.; 2005:Issue 1.

37. Feigin V, Ratnasabapathy Y, Anderson C. Does blood pressure lowering treatment prevent dementia or cognitive decline in patients with cardiovascular and cerebrovascular disease? J Neurol Sci. 2005;229–230:151–155.

38. Finkel SI. Behavioral and psychologic symptoms of dementia. Clin Geriatr Med. 2003;19:799–824.

39. Livingston G, Johnston K, Katona C, Paton J, Lyketsos CG. Systematic review of psychological approaches to the management of neuropsychiatric symptoms of dementia. Am J Psychiatry. 2005;162:1996–2021.

40. Woodhead EL, Zarit SH, Braungart ER, Rovine MR, Femia EE. Behavioral and psychological symptoms of dementia: effects of physical activity at adult day service centers. Am J Alzheimers Dis Other Demen. 2005;20:171–179.

41. Teri L, Logsdon R. Assessment and management of behavioral disturbances in Alzheimer's disease patients. Compr Ther. 1990;16:36–42.

42. Bains J, Birks JS, Dening TR. Antidepressants for treating depression in dementia (Cochrane Review). In: The Cochrane Library. Chichester, UK: John Wiley and Sons, Ltd.; 2005:Issue 1.

43. Snowden M, Sato K, Roy-Byrne P. Assessment and treatment of nursing home residents with depression or behavioral symptoms associated with dementia: a review of the literature. J Am Geriatr Soc. 2003;51:1305–1317.

44. Sink KM. Pharmacological treatment of neuropsychiatric symptoms of dementia: a review of the evidence. JAMA. 2005;293:596–608.

45. Schneider LS. Risk of death with atypical antipsychotic drug treatment for dementia: a meta-analysis of randomized placebo-controlled trials. JAMA. 2005;294:1934–1943.

46. Wolfson C, Wolfson DB, Asgharian M, et al. A reevaluation of the duration of survival after the onset of dementia. N Engl J Med. 2001;344:1111–1116.

47. Larson EB, Shadlen MF, Wang L. Survival after initial diagnosis of Alzheimer disease. Ann Intern Med. 2004;140:501–509.

CHAPTER 43

Dizziness

Kathleen Klink

CASE 1

A 30-year-old woman presents with new onset acute dizziness, with no history of prior or coexisting medical illness. She awoke from sleep with an intense feeling of spinning associated with severe nausea provoked by moving her head, and relieved within seconds by keeping still. She cites no other symptoms. She takes no medications including over-the-counter or herbal preparations, and denies any substance use. She is employed as an administrative assistant and is happy at home without domestic conflict. Review of systems is negative, with particular emphasis on neurological symptoms. Physical exam is essentially normal, except the symptoms were reproduced with the Dix-Hallpike maneuver.

CASE 2

A 45-year-old woman with a history of anxiety complains of recurring dizziness, described as a feeling of lightheadedness, made worse when feeling overwhelmed, anxious or stressed, and not relieved by meclizine. Past medical history includes about one episode of vertigo a year, lasting about a day, without hearing loss or tinnitus, for which she takes meclizine. She has no history of high blood pressure, cardiac disease, or cardiac risk factors. She has a high pressure job, and two active teenagers at home. Review of symptoms reveals chronic insomnia. Physical exam is normal.

CASE 3

A 70-year-old man with long standing diabetes and coronary artery disease complains of recurring dizziness, particularly after moving from a supine position. He was recently discharged from the hospital. His medications include a β-blocker, an angiotensin-converting enzyme inhibitor, and a diuretic. On physical exam he has orthostatic hypotension and lower extremity sensory neuropathy.

CLINICAL QUESTIONS

1. How should your clinical approach to a patient with dizziness vary based on the age of the patient, onset and specific history of dizziness, and comorbidity?

2. In what way should a psychological and emotional evaluation contribute to the differential diagnosis, evaluation, and treatment plan?

Dizziness is a term that includes many symptoms and presentations. It is difficult for patients to describe and for clinicians to define, making the diagnosis challenging. Even with an accurate diagnosis, effective treatment can be elusive.

Patients may describe feelings such as vertigo, (an illusory sensation of movement), lightheadedness, unsteadiness, or faintness. They may have instability with sitting, standing or walking. Symptoms may be acute in onset, chronic, new or recurrent. There may or may not be associated symptoms such as nausea or vomiting, neurologic deficits, headache, anxiety, or other physical and psychological complaints. Life-threatening causes are relatively uncommon, but the astute clinician must be aware of them in order to remediate or intervene appropriately (1).

Dizziness is one of the more common presenting symptoms in primary care, accounting for 8 million outpatient visits annually (2), the majority in the primary care setting. It is estimated that 1 in 3 adults will have had an episode of dizziness, more commonly occurring with increased age (3). The range varies from 23% in all adults to 34% over age 60. In the over-65 age group, 12.5 million are affected, with a reported prevalence of 28% to 34% (4).

In the elderly, dizziness, compounded by falls, contributes significantly to reduced quality of life and morbidity (4, 5). The complaint is one of the top 10 causes for emergency room referrals (6). Persons complaining of dizziness make up 6.7% of emergency department visits and 2.6% of patients seen in primary care practices (7).

Patients complaining of dizziness are seen commonly by cardiologists, neurologists and otolaryngologists as well as primary care clinicians, and it is important for the primary provider to know why and when to refer for specialty care.

DIFFERENTIAL DIAGNOSIS

It is instructive to begin to think about dizziness by thinking about the mechanisms in the body that contribute to a sense of stability. A solid grounding in this knowledge will facilitate understanding of disruption of normally functioning mechanisms. The systems used to provide stability include vision, the peripheral vestibular and auditory systems, proprioceptive receptors in joints of the spine and extremities, the cerebral cortex, the vestibular nuclei, the brainstem (including vestibular ocular and vestibular spinal reflex pathways), and the cerebellum. The other major system is the cardiovascular system, which maintains vascular tone. The subject's medical and psychological history is a key element, including all medications (over-the-counter, herbals, and prescribed), history of anxiety or panic, and an assessment of current psychological and emotional well-being.

The differential diagnosis of dizziness is immense, and the first step in narrowing it involves trying to identify which of the above body systems are most likely to be involved. There are four generally accepted subtypes or categories of dizziness: vertigo, presyncope, disequilibrium and "nonspecific."

- Vertigo is the sensation of moving, often described as spinning, when at rest. It usually reflects problems of the central or peripheral vestibular system (although some patients with dizziness due to migraine or panic disorder can also complain of vertigo).
- Presyncope is a feeling of lightheadedness or faintness, usually due to cerebral hypoperfusion. Diagnoses include any causes that decrease blood delivery to the head: low blood pressure or volume, decreased cardiac output (e.g., resulting from congestive heart failure or aortic stenosis), and severe or acute anemia.
- Disequilibrium is a feeling of imbalance when standing and especially when walking. The cause is often multi-factorial, frequently related to neuromuscular problems, proprioceptive disorders, visual impairment, or central nervous system disease.
- Nonspecific dizziness includes two general types of dizziness: 1) persons (usually elderly with multiple morbidities, on multiple medications) who have more than one dizziness complaint (e.g., presyncope plus imbalance) and whose dizziness is generally multifactorial; and 2) persons whose dizziness is difficult to define and is associated with symptoms suggesting anxiety and/or depression.

Table 43.1 provides an overview of the differential diagnosis of dizziness. Table 43.2 summarizes data on the relative frequency of various dizziness diagnoses depending on setting.

Differential Diagnosis of Vertigo

Causes of vertigo are grouped into peripheral and central disorders. Peripheral causes are far more common, but central causes are more serious.

PERIPHERAL CAUSES

The peripheral vestibular system includes the vestibular end-organs: three semi-circular canals (SCCs) and two otolith organs in each ear, the vestibular portion of the eighth cranial nerve (CN8), and the CN8 root entry zone to the brain stem. Damage to these vestibular elements will cause acute vertigo, spontaneous nystagmus with the fast phase away from affected side, and nausea. The two most common peripheral causes of vertigo in primary care are benign paroxysmal positional vertigo (BPPV) and vestibular neurinititis. These and other peripheral causes are briefly described below:

- Benign paroxysmal positional vertigo (BPPV). Patients with BPPV give a story that is almost pathognomonic: " . . . suddenly, when turning in bed, or looking up, or down" . . . an acute short lived severe vertigo occurs, which resolves with not moving the head. It is so predictable it can almost be diagnosed over the phone (8). The cause is one or more free-floating particulates within the endolymph of one of the semicircular canals (9).
- Vestibular neuronitis (VN). VN is known by several other names, including acute unilateral vestibular paralysis, acute labyrinthitis, vertibular neuritis, neurolabyrinthitis, and acute unilateral peripheral vestibulopathy. VN is a clinical diagnosis. The patients will have acute vertigo that is prolonged and severe. They may have nystagmus, imbalance and nausea. They will not have hearing problems or other neurological symptoms. The cause is unknown and controversial. A viral etiology is supported by detection of herpes simplex type 1 in vestibular ganglia and nuclei, although evidence for this is limited (8, 10).
- Meniere's disease. Meniere's disease is characterized by repeated vertigo attacks lasting for several hours or even days. The attacks occur over many years, with unilateral low frequency tinnitus and low frequency hearing loss, often accompanied by a feeling of blockage in the affected ear. The pathophysiology of the disorder, located in the semicircular canal system or peripheral labyrinth, is presumed to be endolymphatic hypertension or hydrops, caused by impaired resorption of endolymph by the endolymphatic sac (10). The vertigo is often devastating and associated with vomiting and may precede the other symptoms by years. Patients may not be aware of the tinnitus and hearing loss due to the overwhelming symptoms of vertigo. Conversely tinnitus and hearing loss may continue after the vertigo has resolved.
- Perilymph fistula. Perilymph fistula and its' variant, superior canal dehiscence syndrome, are very rare disorders characterized by recurrent attacks of vertigo and oscillopsia as a result of changes in intracranial or middle ear pressure during Valsalva maneuvers (e.g., coughing, sneezing, or shouting) or loud noises. It is due to endolymphatic leakage with resultant pressure changes in the superior semi-circular canal (SCC), and often associated with trauma to the head or ear (10).
- Physiologic vertigo (motion sickness). Physiologic vertigo is fairly common, and occurs when there is discordance between physiological systems, such as between vision and vestibular excitation. For example, after getting off a merry-go-round, the vestibular system has been excited by the movement, but the visual system recognizes there no longer is physical spinning.

CENTRAL CAUSES

The central system is made up of four vestibular nuclei clustered closely together in the medulla and caudal pons and their associated pathways to the ocular, autonomic, spinal, cerebellar, cerebral systems, and the peri-hypoglossal nuclei. Disorders originating in these structures result in what is referred to as a central lesion (10). Central nervous system causes of dizziness generally are accompanied by positive findings on a careful neurological examination. The central causes of vertigo include:

TABLE 43.1   Differential Diagnosis of Dizziness

Predominant Dizziness Symptom	Common Causes

Vertigo (spinning or lateral motion of the person or environment)	<u>Peripheral vestibular disorders:</u>
	Benign paroxysmal positional vertigo (BPPV)
	Vestibular neuritis
	Labyrinthitis
	Meniere's disease
	Physiologic (e.g., sea-sickness)
	Less common:
	   Superior canal dehiscence syndrome
	   Drug related ototoxicity
	   Peripheral vestibulopathy of unknown cause
	<u>Central causes:</u>
	Strokes and transient ischemic attacks
	Migraine
	Trauma: includes post-concussion, labyrinthine concussion, whiplash injuries, any injury from which the central nervous system is impaired in locating the position of the head on the torso
	Less common:
	   Benign tumors (acoustic neuromas or posterior fossae tumors)
	   Multiple sclerosis
	   Vestibular epilepsy
	   Cerebellar degeneration

Presyncope (lightheadedness, as if about to pass out)	Orthostatic hypotension (e.g., hypovolemia, autonomic neuropathy, including diabetic neuropathy) Cardiac arrhythmia Cardiac valvular disorders including aortic stenosis Carotid sinus syndrome Viral syndromes Anemia; acute blood loss Other cardiovascular causes
Dysequilibrium (sense of imbalance; more in the legs than in the head)	Cerebellar disorders (e.g., infarction, degeneration) Peripheral neuropathies (without orthostasis) Physical deconditioning

Nonspecific (giddiness, or vague lightheadedness; difficult to describe)	<u>Psychiatric disorders</u>
	   Panic disorder
	   Generalized anxiety disorder
	   Hyperventilation
	   Depression
	<u>Other disorders</u>
	   Medication-related
	   Metabolic (e.g., hyper- or hypoglycemia, electrolyte disturbance, thyrotoxicosis)
	   Non-vestibular neurological causes, e.g., Parkinsons's disease

Adapted from Kroenke K, Hoffman RM, Einstadter D. How common are various causes of dizziness, a critical review. South Med J. 2000 Feb;93(2): 160–167.

TABLE 43.2 Influence of Practice Setting and Patient Age on the Relative Frequency of Various Diagnoses Among Patients Presenting with Dizziness

Variable	Frequency, by Diagnostic Category, as Percent of Patients				
	Peripheral Vestibular	Central Vestibular	Psychiatric	Non-Vestibular and Non-Psychiatric	Unknown
Clinical setting					
All settings	44	11	16	26	13
Primary care office	43	9	21	34	4
Emergency department	34	6	9	37	19
Dizziness clinic	46	7	20	20	18
Neurology clinic	49	19	10	17	10
Patient age					
Any age	37	7	16	33	14
Older patients only	53	17	10	17	14

Adapted from Sloane PD, Coeytaux RR, Beck RS, Dallara J. Dizziness: state of science. Ann Intern Med. 2001 May 1;134(9, part 2, suppl):823–832.

- Central nervous system ischemia. Both vertebral-basilar insufficiency and brainstem stroke can present as vertigo. Other brainstem signs and symptoms, such as cranial nerve abnormalities, are often present. Presentation may include a combination of peripheral and central symptoms because, an artery, as in the case of the anterior inferior cerebellar artery, may supply both peripheral and central territories (10).
- Vestibular migraine. Dizziness and vertigo in the setting of migraine is complex, not well studied, and is a relatively newly recognized etiology for episodic vertigo (8). Onset appears to be any time in life, but is frequently in the fourth decade. During the acute phase, vestibular imbalance has been documented in all patients, with 10 to 30% showing unilateral hypoexciteability to caloric stimulation. Involvement of the contralateral ear is detectable in 30% to 60% of cases, and over half of the patients have central vestibular dysfunction during the acute migrainous vertigo (11). Vertigo may last a few seconds to hours to (rarely) days, with a small percentage of patients experiencing auditory symptoms. In some cases vertigo is the aura prior to the typical hemicranial headache (8); but one-third have vertigo without headache. In the symptom free period, mild central oculomotor deficits without brainstem or cerebellar findings can be revealed by neuro-ophthalmological evaluation, but neurological examination is generally normal.
- Trauma. Patients may present with dizziness after traumatic brain injury or concussion (post-traumatic vertigo). The most common clinical finding is a positive Romberg test, without nystagmus. Classical tests of vestibular function may be normal and will not necessarily predict ability to return to work (12). Individuals reporting dizziness after head injury, in one study fell into three categories: post-traumatic vestibular migraines (41%), post-traumatic positional vertigo (28%), and post-traumatic spatial disorientation (19%) (13).

- Cerebellar infarction. Uncommon in primary care settings, cerebellar infarction presents with vertigo, nausea, vomiting, and acute disequilibrium so severe that the patient often cannot stand up independently with eyes open. Examination will reveal nystagmus and severe ataxia.
- Familial periodic vertigo. There are families in which multiple members have periodic bouts, typically lasting hours, of either vertigo or ataxia, or both. Although rare, this condition is treatable with acetazolamide.
- Vestibular epilepsy. A rare form of epilepsy may be associated with vertigo. The focality is in the temporal lobe or parietal association cortex (10).
- Neurosyphilis. Presentation may include dizziness along with other central nervous system features, including, at times, dementia.

Differential Diagnosis of Presyncope

Central nervous system hypoperfusion is the cause of most faintness or presyncope. Common diagnoses include hypovolemia, orthostatic hypotension secondary to diabetic or other autonomic neuropathies, cardiac valve disorders (particularly aortic stenosis), arrhythmias and general deconditioning.

Acute orthostatic hypotension can occur after blood volume loss such as an acute gastro-intestinal bleed, or with dehydration, such as with prolonged sun exposure. Chronic orthostasis is frequently due to diuretic or anti-hypertensive medications or to chronic hypovolemia, both of which are most often seen in persons who are elderly or systemically ill. Diagnosis is made by observing a 10–15 mm Hg drop in mean blood pressure associated with assuming an erect posture. Autonomic dysfunction is inferred if, with the drop in blood pressure, the heart rate does not elevate. Test for sympathetic tone by checking pulse and blood pressure after the Valsalva maneuver in the supine position for 30 seconds. A normal response is a decrease in heart rate and a 10–30 mm Hg elevation in mean blood pressure. Treatment is based on the identified cause.

Diabetic patients offer unique challenges, as they may have several factors contributing to either presyncope or disequilibrium. Diabetic autonomic neuropathy, a subset of which is cardiac autonomic neuropathy (CAN), is associated with hear rate irregularity, resting tachycardia, exercise intolerance, orthostatic hypotension, and silent myocardial ischemia. CAN is estimated to be present in 20% of asymptomatic diabetics and is often overlooked. Other peripheral neuropathies, along with hypoglycemia, may contribute to dizziness symptoms as well (14).

Cardiac dysrhythmias can also cause presyncope. Any disorder that compromises cardiac output, including atrial fibrillation or flutter, severe bradycardia, and heart block, can lead the patient to feel lightheaded. The symptom may be relieved by rest or lowering the head to allow improved cerebral perfusion.

Differential Diagnosis of Disequilibrium

A wide variety of problems cause disequilibrium, most of which fall into the neuromuscular category. Common causes include:

- Proprioceptive and somatosensory loss, including the peripheral neuropathies seen in diabetes and spinal stenosis;
- Post-stroke residual deficits. For example, a small infarction in the brainstem or cerebellum, that initially presents with vertigo, will often leave a residual disequilibrium.
- Medication adverse effects. Aminoglycoside toxicity is the classical cause of disequilibrium, because these drugs are toxic to the peripheral vestibular system. However many drugs with central or peripheral nervous system effects can cause disequilibrium.
- Cerebellar degeneration. This leads to a gradual onset of disequilibrium, a tendency to fall, and positive cerebellar neurological signs on examination. Chronic alcoholism is the most common cause; other causes include degenerative disorders, such as Friedreich ataxia, olivopontocerebellar atrophy, and cerebellar-cortical atrophy.

Other causes of disequilibrium include Parkinson's disease, normal pressure hydrocephalus, early progressive supranuclear palsy, primary orthostatic tremor, and posterior fossa tumors. Primary orthostatic tremor typically causes no problems with walking but a feeling of imbalance while standing; neither the patient nor the clinician may notice the fine high frequency tremor.

Frequently the cause of disequilibrium is multifactorial; contributing factors can include visual impairment, physical de-conditioning, medication side effects, unilateral or bilateral vestibular hypofunction, cervical spine disease, and peripheral neuropathy. In addition to the involvement of multiple neurosensory systems, multifactorial dizziness in the elderly is often associated with anxiety, depression, use of five or more medications, impaired balance, previous myocardial infarction, postural hypotension and impaired hearing. The use of a function-oriented approach to patient evaluation, combined with anticipatory management to prevent deconditioning and falls, may improve outcomes (15).

Nonspecific Dizziness

Psychiatric disorders, particularly anxiety and panic attacks, cause symptoms referred to by patients as dizziness. One study identified three equally prevalent patterns: anxiety only, vestibular disorders exacerbating a psychiatric disorder, and neurotologic conditions triggering new anxiety or depression. Depression was not found to be a primary cause of dizziness in any patient (16). Panic attacks, associated with severe anxiety and possibly hyperventilation, commonly cause dizziness that is not true vertigo. Patients with undiagnosed vertigo may develop anxiety in response to the recurrent symptoms. "Phobic postural vertigo" is a variant where patients describe a mild disturbance of balance with brief illusions of motion, usually happening in disturbing or distressful settings. These symptoms may be more common in patients with a peripheral vestibulopathy in the past. Although the term phobic postural vertigo is not universally accepted, these patients do well with support and education (8).

Another frequent cause of nonspecific dizziness symptoms is multiple neurosensory impairment of the elderly (discussed above under disequilibrium). In addition, it should be remembered that virtually any cause of dizziness can present nonspecifically, especially in patients who are chronically ill or whose language or observational skills are limited.

Finally, though posterior fossa tumors (i.e. acoustic neuromas or schwannomas) are often described as causing vertigo, more commonly they lead to vague dizziness and hearing loss (8). In one series 43% presented with total deafness on the affected side, and a large percentage with some hearing loss. Diagnosis requires keeping this cause in the differential diagnosis and, when suspicious, conducting audiometry. Patients with a suspicious history and unilateral hearing loss should be referred for neuroimaging (17).

CLINICAL EVALUATION

The clinician caring for the dizzy patient must be prepared to deal with uncertainty. Empirical guidelines for diagnostic strategies do not exist and are unlikely to be developed in the near future (18). However, the typical patient's symptoms can usually be placed into one of the four categories listed above, and selection of physical examination maneuvers and diagnostic tests should be based on the history. Nearly all patients, however, deserve a simple neurological and otoneurological examination looking for central nervous system and vestibular signs, and an assessment of cardiac risk.

The Clinical History

The history of the presenting symptoms should be obtained in the patient's own words, preferably without using the word "dizzy." It is the history that will point to the system or systems that are most likely to be involved. Included in the history must be the temporal course, whether this episode is the first or recurrent, severity of symptoms, associated symptoms, and precipitating or alleviating activities or movements. A complete medical history, including medications, familial, psychological, and social history, is required to determine predisposing factors.

The initial task is to place the patient's complaint into

one of the four types: vertigo, presyncope, disequilibrium or nonspecific. This differentiation guides the focus of the history:

- If the person has a sensation of movement (commonly, spinning), vertigo is likely. In such cases the history should attempt to differentiate between peripheral and central vertigo (see Table 43.3). In patients with episodic vertigo, the duration of episodes can provide important clues to the most likely diagnoses (see Table 43.4).
- If the patient's symptoms refer more to a sensation of near-faint, or if lightheadedness occurs with movement from supine to standing, presyncope is present. In such cases, the history should inquire about cardiac problems, diabetes, neurological disorders, and medications (including herbals and over the counter preparations). In addition, the psychological and social history should probe for anxiety.
- If the patient's symptoms primarily involve disequilibrium, then the history needs to be broad. It should focus on neurological and vascular complaints, especially in the extremities, plus a general history for central neurological symptoms, cardiovascular symptoms, and medical problems. Rare disorders to keep in mind include aminoglycoside vestibulotoxicity (particularly after a hospitalization), post-stroke syndromes, and a posterior fossa tumor, and orthostatic tremor (8).

The neurological history should include asking about oscillopsia (illusory movement of the environment when walking), diplopia, weakness, sensory deficits, gait and coordination, and mental status changes. These point to a central nervous system disorder. Question if any triggers such as hyperventilation or Valsalva precede symptoms, as this may suggest anxiety or panic disorder. Ask about a history of head trauma; post-trauma patients may have chronic symptoms, including diplopia, unsteadiness, vertigo with head movement, psychological disorders, and cognitive problems (12).

A general rule of thumb, which initially seems paradoxical, is that the more acute and severe the symptoms, the more benign the prognosis. This is because peripheral vestibular problems, which tend to resolve completely, often begin

TABLE 43.4 Relationship Between the Duration of Dizziness Episodes and the Likely Cause of Dizziness in Patients with Vertigo

Duration of Dizziness	Cause
Seconds	Benign paroxysmal positional vertigo
Minutes	Vertebrobasilar insufficiency
Hours	Meniere syndrome
Days	Vestibular neuritis, labyrinth infarction
Minutes	Panic disorder
Longstanding and fluctuating	Generalized anxiety or depression
Days to months (diminishing with time)	Posterior circulation stroke

Adapted from Furman JM, Whitney SL. Central causes of dizziness. Phys Ther. 2000 Feb;80(2):179–187.

TABLE 43.3 Differences Between Peripheral and Central Vertigo*

Symptom	Anatomic Source of Vertigo†	
	Peripheral Vestibular System	**Central Vestibular System**
Vertigo severity	Varies; usually more severe	Varies; usually less severe
Nausea and vomiting	Severe	Moderate
Imbalance	Mild	Severe
Hearing loss	Common	Rare
Oscillopsia‡	Mild	Severe
Neurological symptoms§	Rare	Common
Speed of compensation¶	Rapid	Slow

* Note: These are general principles, and some crossover occurs. For example, severe vertigo, nausea, and vomiting are common as initial symptoms of some cerebellar or brainstem strokes
†Peripheral vestibular structures include the middle ear, inner ear, and the vestibular nerve; central vestibular structures include the vestibular nuclei and related structures and pathways in the brainstem and cerebellum.
‡Oscillopsia refers to a feeling that the environment moves up and down, bounces, or rocks when the person walks.
§Positive neurological findings on physical examination may also be present.
¶Compensation refers to the ability of neurosensory systems to adapt to a disorder, thereby reducing or eliminating symptoms.
Adapted from Furman JM, Whitney SL. Central causes of dizziness. Phys Ther. 2000 Feb;80(2):179–187.

acutely and severely. In contrast, central disorders often develop slowly (e.g. cerebellar ataxia or acoustic neuroma), and are accompanied by reflex compensation mechanisms (19).

In applying this concept, however, one must keep in mind that certain red flags suggest a progressive or life-threatening disorder (see Table 43.5).

Physical Examination

The purpose of the initial evaluative physical examination is to further identify and confirm the system or systems involved in the patient's complaint, and to plan further workup, referral, or treatment. The exam should be tailored based on the history; however, most exams should include a general assessment (e.g. of nutritional and psychological status) and a brief cardiovascular, neurological, and otological evaluation. The sensitivity, specificity, and other properties of much of the physical examination has not undergone scientific evaluation. Table 43.6 summarizes data on physical examination maneuvers for which systematic evaluation is available.

The following outline provides a guide to performing an individualized examination. Maneuvers in *italics* are recommended as part of a screening examination; additional maneuvers should be performed if indicated based on the history. Those marked with an asterisk (*) are explained in greater detail later in the chapter.

General examination:
  Overall assessment of condition, nutrition, level of discomfort
  Vital signs
  Neck range of motion
  Mental status including language, speech, mood
Cardiovascular examination
  Orthostatics (BP and HR supine/standing)

  Cardiac auscultation
  Cervical bruits
Vision/ophthalmological:
  Visual acuity with correction at distance
  *Dynamic visual acuity with 2-Hz passive head movement
  Confrontation with visual fields
  Pupil size and reactivity
  Optic nerve heads and retina
  *Observe for spontaneous nystagmus: may use Frenzel glasses or occlusive funduscopic exam
Eye movements and lids:
  *Ptosis, lid lag, *head tilt*
  Fixation: spontaneous nystagmus, saccadic intrusions
  Extraocular movement range
  Ocular alignment: cover/uncover test
  *Fixation suppression of vestibular nystagmus
Otological exam
  External ear canals
  Gross audiological response
  *Rinne and Weber responses
Vestibular-ocular reflexes (VOR)
  *Slow passive head rotation with fixation of stationary target
  *Rapid 15-degree head rotation (thrusts) with fixation on stationary target
  *Frenzel Examination
  *Dix-Hallpike maneuver-positional testing
Remaining cranial nerves
Motor and sensory examination
  Muscle strength and tone
  Deep tendon reflexes and plantar responses
  Cerebellar: finger to nose to finger, heel-knee-shin, rapid alternating movements

TABLE 43.5 Red Flags for Patients with Dizziness Suggesting That the Patient May Have a Serious, Possibly Urgent Underlying Disease

Red Flag	Suggested Diagnoses	Appropriate Intervention
Cardiovascular symptoms (e.g., chest pain, dyspnea, palpitations)	Any acute cause of heart failure (e.g., AMI, CHF, arrhythmia, or valvulopathy)	EKG, Holter monitor, echocardiogram, appropriate lab evaluation, eg troponin level
Central nervous system symptoms (e.g. numbness, weakness, loss of vision, other nerve palsies)	Brainstem or cerebellar stroke, TIA, tumor, post-traumatic symptoms, demyelination	MRI of brain, vascular ischemia risk evaluation and treatment, neurology consult
Gradual hearing loss and tinnitus	Acoustic neuroma	MRI, audiogram, BAER
Propensity to fall and/or severe lightheadedness on standing	Hypovolemia, orthostatic hypotension, peripheral neuropathy, over-medication, multiple deficits (common in older persons)	Medical assessment for volume depletion, anemia, poly-pharmacy, deconditioning, gait or balance disturbance
Acute or gradual onset of weakness and lightheadedness, possibly with shortness of breath, near-syncope, especially in patients with risk factors for GI bleed (e.g., anticoagulation, prior bleed, or NSAID use)	Upper or lower GI bleed	Complete blood count, stool for occult blood

AMI, acute myorcardial infarction; BAER, brainstem auditory evoked response; CHF, congestive heart failure; EKG, electrocardiogram; GI, gastrointestinal; MRI, magnetic resonance imaging; NSAID, nonsteroidal anti-inflammatory drugs; TIA, transient ischemic attack.

TABLE 43.6 Characteristics of Selected Physical Examination Maneuvers and Laboratory Tests Used to Evaluate Patients with Dizziness

Test or Combination of Findings	Target Diagnosis	Population Studied	Test Characteristics
(+) Nylen-Barany (head-hanging test), plus nausea or vomiting	Lesion involving peripheral vestibular system	Dizzy, lightheaded, or "faint" patients presenting to an emergency department	Sensitivity 43 Specificity 94 LR+ = 7.17 LR− = 0.61
Absence of vertigo or age >69 or neurological deficit	"Serious" cause of vertigo	Dizzy, lightheaded, or "faint" patients presenting to an emergency department	Sensitivity 87 Specificity 43 LR+ = 1.53 LR− = 0.3
Pulse increase >30 or severe dizziness during orthostatic testing	Orthostatic hypotenstion	Various—meta-analysis of variable quality diagnostic studies.	Sensitivity 97 Specificity 98 LR+ = 48 LR− = 0.03
Orthostatic blood pressure	Orthostatic hypotension	Dizziness and syncope patients	Sensitivity 50.7%–57.5% Specificity 72.2%–80.3% LR+ 1.82–2.92
Dix-Hallpike maneuver	Paroxysmal positional vertigo	Referral patients with chronic dizziness	Sensitivity 60.0% Specificity 98.6% LR+ = 42.8 LR− = 0.41
Head-shaking nystagmus	Unilateral vestibular dysfunction	8 studies from multiple settings, mostly in otolaryngology	Mean sensitivity 58.1 Mean specificity 62.1 Mean LR+ 1.97
Routine blood testing	Anemia, renal failure, electrolyte and/or glucose abnormalities, liver function abnormalities, thyroid disorders	Chronic and acute dizziness	Yield is low: none in a study of chronic dizziness; 0.57% positive rate in a review of 4,538 patients.

Hilton M, Pinder D. The Epley (canalith repositioning) manoeuvre for benign paroxysmal positional vertigo (Cochrane Review). In: The Cochrane Library. Oxford, England: Update Software; 2005:Issue 1.

Maarsingh OR, van der Horst HE, Stalman WA, Dros J, van Weert HCPM, Bindels PJE. Developing a diagnostic protocol for dizzy patients in primary care: A Delphi procedure. Amsterdam, Netherlands, 2005. Unpublished working paper.

Sloane PD, Baloh RW. Persistent dizziness in geriatric patients. J Am Geriatr Soc. 1989;37:1031–1038.

Sensory: joint position, pinprick, vibration
Proprioception
Gait and balance:
Walking and turning, heel and toe walking, squatting, rising
Tandem forward and backward
*Fukuda stepping test
*Standing feet together, tandem, either foot eyes open and closed (Romberg)

ORTHOSTATIC HYPOTENSION

Orthostatic hypotension is defined by a fall in blood pressure by 20 mm Hg systolic or 10 mm Hg diastolic in response to standing from the supine position, when accompanied by symptoms. Patients with orthostatic hypotension will complain of lightheadedness, dizziness, weakness, and visual blurring with change of position.

NEURO-OTOLOGICAL EVALUATION

A complete neuro-otological assessment should include inspection of tympanic membranes, the Weber and Rinne tests, cerebellar function testing, examination of the cranial nerves, general balance tests (i.e., Romberg test and gait assessment), extraocular movements, visual fixation, smooth pursuit, and the Hallpike positional test.

Vestibulo-ocular reflexes (VOR) can be tested by passively moving the patient's head slowly (2 rotations per second) or quickly (quick movement by about 15 degrees); a normal response is for the eyes to be able to remained fixed on an object during the manuevers. A sluggish VOR is associated with central nervous system diseases; will cause the patient's gaze to move away from the target and then catch up in a saccadic (rapid) movement (8, 20).

Saccades are rapid refixating movements that are examined by having the patient quickly look from one visual target to another while noting the latency, accuracy, speed, and conjugance. Saccadic dysmetria is seen in cerebellar disease, or pontine lesions. Smooth pursuit is tested by having patient visually pursue a target slowly (20 degrees per second), noting the presence of asymmetry manifesting by reduced gain and corrective catch-up. Severe dysfunction could indicate a cerebellar lesion, while a mild disorder may be due to inattention or a medication side effect.

Note how the patient holds his or her head. Head tilt is a phenomenon that may result from peripheral vestibular dysfunction or a lesion of vestibular nuclei. The tilt is toward the side of the lesion, with hypertropia (relative elevation) of the eye on the upper side the head.

People use three modalities to maintain balance: vision, the vestibular system, and proprioception. Two out of three are necessary to maintain posture. If there is sway with eyes open, consider a cerebellar origin. By closing the eyes (Romberg test), one system is removed; therefore, if a patient sways with eyes closed, the problem is either proprioceptive or vestibular in origin, and the test is considered positive. If the Romberg is positive and the complaint is vertigo, consider a vestibular origin; if positive without vertigo, examine proprioception further. Keep in mind, however, that balance may be impaired with deconditioning or any neuromuscular disease of the lower extremities (21).

Tandem gait and the Romberg test evaluate balance. Vestibular lesions generally cause patients to fall toward the side of the lesion, more severely with eyes closed, and less reliably as central mechanisms compensate over a period of time. In the Fukuda stepping test, the patient marches in place with eyes closed for 30 seconds. Excessive rotation suggests vestibular imbalance (8).

A complete peripheral sensory examination including proprioception, is especially important for patients complaining of disequilibrium symptoms, as neuropathies are prominent in the differential diagnosis and relatively common, especially in older persons and diabetics.

NYSTAGMUS

Vestibulo-ocular reflex (VOR) pathways, located in the brainstem, help to stabilize gaze during times of body movement and help maintain the body's position in space relative to gravity. Nystagmus is the hallmark of VOR instability. The direction of nystagmus is, by convention, named for the quick phase. The slow phase, however, points toward the source of the vestibular imbalance.

In peripheral vestibular disorders (e.g. vestibular neuronitis), nystagmus tends to be horizontal and to fade with time (20). In central vestibular disorders, nystagmus is often (but not always) vertical. Nystagmus due to peripheral causes may be inhibited by patient visual fixation on an object; central nystagmus is not improved with fixation. To remove visual fixation, use Frenzel glasses or funduscopic examination in a dark room.

THE DIX-HALLPIKE MANEUVER

The Dix-Hallpike maneuver, also referred to as the Barany maneuver, is a cornerstone of diagnosis of BPPV. With the patient in a sitting position, turn the patient's head 30 degrees to the side. Move the patient quickly to the supine position,

keeping the head turned, until the patient's head is hanging 30 degrees off the table, a position that places the lower ear's posterior semicircular canal—that most commonly involved in BPPV—in a plane relative to gravity, thereby causing the endolyph to spin and symptoms to be provoked. The hallmarks of a positive response are:

- provocation of the patient's dizziness bout
- torsional nystagmus during the episode
- latency of 2–10 seconds (i.e. symptoms take a few moments to develop)
- symptoms tending to lessen if the maneuver is repeated several times

Figure 43.1 illustrates the Dix-Hallpike maneuver.

OTHER ASPECTS OF THE PHYSICAL EXAMINATION

If anxiety with hyperventilation is suspected, the patient should be instructed to hyperventilate for 60 seconds to attempt reproduction of the symptoms (22).

The most common clinical exam following trauma is finding is a positive Romberg test, without nystagmus. Classical tests of vestibular function may be normal and will not necessarily predict ability to return to work (12).

Diagnostic Testing

Laboratory tests should only be ordered to confirm or rule out suspected diagnoses; no test should be considered "routine" in patients with dizziness. Data on the sensitivity, specificity, and positive likelihood ratios of most laboratory tests performed for dizziness are not available for general patients with dizziness; Table 43.6 summarizes the available data. Among the tests for which systematic data are not available are: formal balance assessment, ambulatory ECG monitoring, and most serologic tests. Since carotid sinus massage is part of the "gold standard" diagnosis of carotid sinus sensitivity, its' sensitivity, specificity and likelihood ratio cannot be computed.

One study found no significant differences between 149 subjects with chronic dizziness and matched community controls in results of laboratory testing, including complete blood count (CBC), erythrocyte sedimentation rate, blood urea nitrogen, electrolytes, glucose, cholesterol, liver function tests, and thyroid function tests (23). In another review of 4,538 patients, only 0.57% of patients had a diagnosis made by laboratory tests; most prominent were glucose disorders and anemia (24).

TESTS TO CONSIDER IN PATIENTS WITH VERTIGO

A variety of tests are available to assess patients with vertigo. The more important ones are discussed briefly below:

- Audiometry. Formal audiogram assessment is important in ruling out an acoustic neuroma (unilateral hearing loss should raise your suspicion) and in helping diagnose Meniere's disease (unilateral or bilateral low frequency hearing loss is common).
- Electronystagmography (ENG). This refers to a combination of tests to evoke eye movements, including vestibular nystagmus. It includes ocular-motor and caloric testing. Each ear is irrigated with water at 30°C and 44°C with eyes open in darkened room or with Frenzel glasses in place. Eye movements are recorded using electro-oculography, through electrodes placed on the eye orbits. If caloric testing

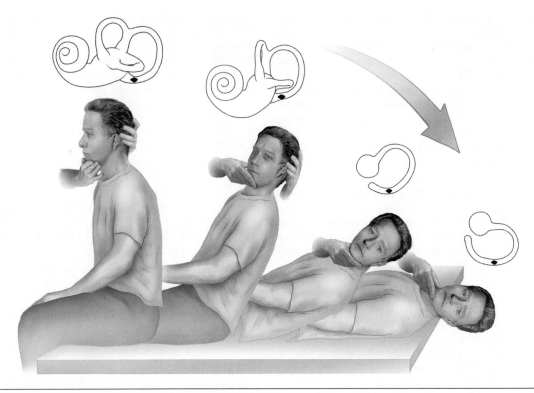

Figure 43.1 • Dix-Hallpike maneuver illustration. (Illustration Copyright © 2006 Nucleus Medical Art, All Rights Reserved. www.nucleusinc.com.)

is positive and if no other brainstem signs have been elicited, the damage is considered to be unilateral peripheral vestibular disease located somewhere between the end organ and the nerve root entry at the lateral medulla.

- Rotational testing. This requires specialized equipment and is generally used primarily as a research tool. However, because it is more sensitive than caloric testing, rotational testing can be a valuable test for bilateral vestibular loss, for example, due to ototoxic drugs (20).
- Neuroimaging. Magnetic resonance imaging (MRI) is the recommended modality to look for central disorders or those related to the internal auditory canal or vestibulocochlear nerve. Gadolinium enhancement may be useful to diagnose vestibular neuromas (i.e., schwannomas or meningiomas). Computed tomography (CT) is useful for middle ear disease, using thin sections for temporal bone assessment. The diagnosis of superior canal dehiscence is made by high resolution temporal bone CT scan, which shows the defective bone overlying the superior SCC (10).
- Brainstem auditory evoked response. This test measures the speed at which impulses move from the external ear to the brainstem. An acoustic neuroma may delay conduction.

TESTS TO CONSIDER IN PATIENTS WITH PRESYNCOPE

- Passive head-up tilting, or tilt table testing. This test provides a more precise evaluation of orthostatic responses than the traditional measurement of blood pressure and pulse in the supine and upright positions. In tilt table testing, the patient is supported by a table tilted at about 60 degrees, thus reducing compensatory muscle contraction in the legs.

The tilt can be maintained for up to 1 hour, or until the patient experiences symptoms. Tilt table testing is controversial because it may be too sensitive and at the same time not specific enough to diagnose neurocardiogenic presyncope.

- Cardiac monitoring. A 24-hour Holter monitor, useful for detecting asymptomatic arrhythmias, will often miss intermittent heart block (14). Therefore, if arrhythmia is suspected, an event monitor (worn for several weeks by the patient) may detect the problem.
- ECG. Atrial fibrillation (AF) is diagnosed using a 12-lead electrocardiogram with a one minute rhythm strip. If paroxysmal atrial fibrillation is being considered, a 24-hour Holter monitor or event monitor should be obtained. All patients with atrial fibrillation should have an echocardiogram to discern any cardiac structural abnormalities causing the dysrhythmia, along with appropriate non-cardiac causes including thyroid function tests, particularly in the elderly where apathetic hyperthyroidism may present with AF (25).
- Laboratory tests. If hypoglycemia is suspected, a glucose monitor can be used to check blood glucose when symptoms occur. A CBC will identify anemia, and a metabolic profile will identify electrolyte disorders if suspected because of underlying renal or cardiovascular disease, or use of certain medications.

TEST TO CONSIDER IN PATIENTS WITH DISEQUILIBRIUM

This category is generally multi-factorial in etiology, manifested by peripheral or autonomic neuropathies, deconditioning and possibly complicated by gait disorders, for example in Parkinson's disease. Electromyographic testing may further elucidate suspected peripheral neuropathies.

Recommended Diagnostic Strategy

In the initial evaluation of a dizzy patient the clinician must discern if there is a serious cause, begin to manage the chronically disabled patient, and determine what, if any, referral is needed (15). Diagnostic strategy is based on the differential diagnosis of dizziness outlined above. Acuity and severity of onset of the patient's complaints, along with risk factor assessment, are central in narrowing the differential. Dizziness may be difficult to diagnose, especially in the elderly, who often have multiple contributing factors; in these cases, a function-oriented approach should be considered, rather than diagnosis-focused strategies (18). Figure 43.2 provides a graphical depiction of a general approach to evaluating the patient with dizziness.

Remember that only a small proportion of patients presenting with dizziness have life threatening illnesses. Therefore, discretion should be used in deciding whether and when to order a laboratory test or prescribe a medication. Quality of life, risk of falling, and associated fears and anxiety are important to address, particularly in the elderly.

MANAGEMENT

Because most patients presenting with the complaint of dizziness have diagnoses that are benign, and self limited, treatment of dizziness for only a small percentage of patients will involve preventing death or severe morbidity. In the elderly, most management strategies have been studied retrospectively or in referral settings, making an evidence-based management approach difficult at best. However, expert opinion and disease-specific research do allow us to approach dizziness management in a systematic manner, following general principles for all and providing specific therapies when they are available.

General Principles

Management of the patient with dizziness should follow these general principles:

1. If the patient has a clear diagnosis, treat the underlying cause.
2. If the problem is self-limited, provide reassurance. Symptomatic relief can be provided, but beware of using medications with significant side effects that may place the patient at risk for complications.
3. All patients, including those with permanent deficits, can be helped by approaches that focus on quality of life and improving function. Strategies include strengthening compensatory mechanisms, treating secondary (usually psychological) symptoms, providing symptom relief, and giving appropriate reassurance.
4. There are patients whose histories and physical examinations do not fall neatly into a well-defined diagnosis. In these cases the clinician should educate the patient about risks and benefits of various approaches to diagnosis and

treatment, and follow the patient closely as a therapeutic guide and partner.

Patients with dizziness are often suffering quite a bit, but do not appear to be in distress. Furthermore, chronic dizziness symptoms, like chronic pain, can be fatiguing and can lead to depression. An empathic approach is important in beginning the course of management. Since most cases of dizziness improve with time, usually days to weeks, the clinician should provide appropriate reassurance that symptoms will be ameliorated. If there appears to be a large psychological component, as there often is, even when there is physiological dysfunction, it is very important to address this as well.

Vestibular disorders cause people to lose independence in self care and activities of daily living. Many patients with chronic dizziness are at increased risk for falls and have serious functional impairment, including anxiety and fear, sometimes leading to depression. In the function-oriented approach to management, improvement of quality of life is the major motivating factor, in that the clinician must manage the multifactorial aspects contributing to the patient's symptoms, including improving vision, anxiety, or muscle strength (18). Many patients, particularly the elderly, are under-referred for specialty consultation and do not receive timely treatment (15). Consult with a neurologist or otolaryngologist for patients with no apparent cause for their dizziness, particularly when it is chronic or recurrent (4).

Medications should be used judiciously, as there is no "dizziness medicine." The following classes of drugs can be helpful if the patient has vertigo: antihistamines, phenothiazines, anticholinergics, and benzodiazepines. However, all of these medications have significant side-effects, and therefore, must be used with discretion, at the lowest effective dose, and for a short period of time (4). Furthermore, because they tend to make presyncope and dysequilibrium worse, they are only indicated for selected vertiginous disorders. Finally, because the symptoms of BPPV are short lived and intermittent, treatment with a high side-effect profile drug is not appropriate for this diagnosis.

A word about meclizine (Antivert) is in order, because it is often used inappropriately. It is an antihistamine that dulls the normal vestibular response. By doing so the two vestibular systems may come into more balance, thus averting some of the symptomatology of acute vestibulitis. There is no place, however, for meclizine in patients who clearly have dizziness secondary to disequilibrium of other etiologies, and it can cause harm to the elderly deconditioned patient who may also be taking other medications. Therefore, meclizine should be prescribed only for peripheral vestibular diseases, and with caution if at all in older persons.

As in other chronic conditions, it is often helpful to track symptoms in a quantitative or semiquantitative manner. The Vestibular Disorders Activities of Daily Living Scale (VADL) may provide a useful objective scale to assess disability and progression in rehabilitation that can be applied along with clinical functional assessment of perceptual and motor function of the patient (26).

Treatment of Selected Diagnoses

Most treatments for vestibular disorders have not been evaluated by randomized controlled trials. The positioning maneu-

Determine which of the four major categories apply:
Vertigo, **Pre-syncope**, **Dysequilibrium**, or **Non-specific**,
then use one of the following algorithms.

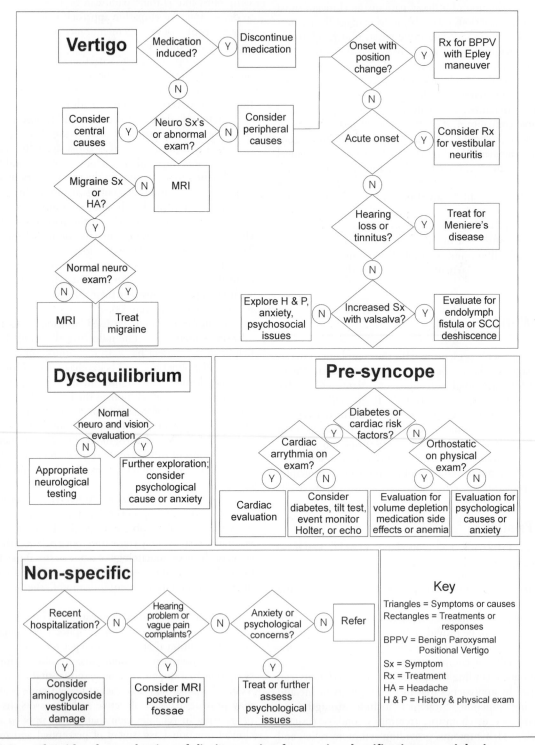

Figure 43.2 • Algorithm for evaluation of dizziness using four major classifications or etiologies.

TABLE 43.7 Key Therapies for Selected Dizziness Diagnoses

Diagnosis and Intervention	Strength of Recommondation*	Comment
BPPV		
Epley maneuver	A	Recommended as first line treatment
Modified Epley maneuver	B	May be taught for patients to do at home
Vestibular neuritis		
Vestibular exercises	B	Exercises for acute symptoms help central compensation mechanisms
Methylprednisone	—	Number needed to treat is two, start with high dose and taper quickly
Meniere's disease		
Low-salt diet/diuretic	C	Lack of evidence that low salt diet or diuretic are effective treatment
Migrainous vertigo		
Vestibular rehabilitation exercises	B	Prophylaxis, migraine abortive medicines and treatment for migraine effective along with vestibular rehabilitation exercises

*A = consistent, good-quality patient-oriented evidence; B = inconsistent or limited-quality patient-oriented evidence; C = consensus, disease-oriented evidence, usual practice, expert opinion, or case series. For information about the SORT evidence rating system, see *http://www.aafp.org/afpsort.xml*.
Sources:
Swartz R, Longwell P. Treatment of Vertigo. Am Fam Physician. 2005 Mar 15;71(6):1115–1122.
Sloane PD, Coeytaux RR, Beck RS, Dallara J. Dizziness: state of science. Ann Intern Med. 2001 May 1;134(9, part 2 suppl):823–832.
Strupp M, Zingler VC, Arbusow V, et al. Methylprednisolone, valacyclovir, or the combination for vestibular neuritis. N Engl J Med. 2004;351:354–361.

ver for BPPV (Epley) and vestibular rehabilitation for chronic vertigo have made some progress in that regard (27). Table 43.7 summarizes existing data on key therapies for selected dizziness diagnoses, and Table 43.8 summarizes medication prescribing information for selected dizziness diagnoses. Treatment of selected diagnoses is discussed briefly below.

BENIGN PAROXYSMAL POSITIONAL VERTIGO

Epley and Semont developed maneuvers to relocate loose particles from the utricular macula to the vestibule of the vestibular labyrinth where they do not cause symptoms. The Epley maneuver (see Figure 43.3), as it has come to be known, has a success rate of 75% at 1 week, with the majority of patients being cured after one office visit. (8). A literature review in 2004 concluded that the scientific evidence is adequate (strength of recommendation [SOR] = B) to support its value in providing symptom relief, but it is unknown if the effectiveness persists over a long period of time. There is no good evidence comparing the Epley maneuver and other modalities of treatment (21).

Recent attention has been placed on treatment of BPPV in the home via self treatment using a modified Epley maneuver. It may be more useful to treat in the office, however, a lack of symptom resolution reduces the chance of there being benign etiology of the vertigo (28).

Additional treatment principles include symptom relief through vestibular habituation exercises (i.e., provoking the dizziness in a controlled setting, such as in bed) (10) or, in severe or persistent cases, by using vestibular suppressant medication.

VESTIBULAR NEURITIS

The vertigo caused by inflammation of the vestibular nerve may last several days to weeks. One series found methylprednisone more effective than placebo, with number needed to treat (NNT) in order to improve symptoms being two. Dosage begins at 100 mg daily for 3 days, then tapers to 10 mg daily by 3 weeks (29).

In the severely acute patient, the following medical therapies have been recommended, though in many cases the level of evidence supporting them is largely anecdotal: 1) metoclopramide 10 mg orally or intramuscularly once or twice daily, to decrease neurovegetative symptoms; 2) diazepam 2 to 10 mg orally, intravenously or intramuscularly 2 to 4 times daily, to decrease oscillopsia, nystagmus, and activation of sensory substitution phenomena; 3) magnesium sulfate solution twice daily, intravenously, to decrease vestibular damage; 4) gabapentin 300 mg orally twice or three times daily, to stabilize visual fields and reduce nystagmus; 5) vestibular electrical stimulation (VES) by means of transcutaneous electrical nerve stimulation (TENS) electrodes placed on the paravertebral muscles opposite the affected side and the trapezius of the affected side for 1 hour daily, to provide symptomatic relief; and 6) lying on the healthy side with head raised to 20 degrees (30).

After the acutely vertiginous stage, specific vestibular habituation exercises improve central nervous system adaptation and hasten rehabilitation. The exercises require about 30 minutes of instruction by either a vestibular physical therapist or someone who has been trained in vestibular rehabilitation (31).

TABLE 43.8 Medication Prescribing Information for Selected Dizziness Diagnoses

Diagnosis	Drug Class/Drugs	Contraindications/ Cautions/Adverse Effects	Dosage	Relative Cost*
BPPV				
	Anticholinergics			
	Meclizine (Antivert)	Sedation, dry mouth, constipation, urinary retention, acute glaucoma	12.5–50 mg every 6–8 hours orally	$
	Dimenhydrinate (Dramamine)	Sedation, blurred vision, nausea	25–100 mg every 6–8 hours, orally or IM or slow IV; no more than 400 mg/day	$
	Benzodiazapines			
	Diazepam (Valium)	Sedation, ataxia, confusion, dizziness, weakness, respiratory depression, hypotension, bradycardia	2–10 mg every 6–8 hours orally or 2–10 mg IV or IM every 3–4 hr; no more than 30 mg/8 hr	$
	Lorazepam (Ativan)	Sedation, dizziness, weakness	0.5–2 mg every 4–8 hrs orally, no more than 10 mg/day; 0.05 mg/kg IM × 1 dose; no more than 4 mg/dose	$
	Nonselective Phenothiazines			
	Metoclopramide (Reglan)	Dystonic reaction, fatigue, sedation, restlessness	5–10 mg every 6 hrs, orally or by slow IV; no more than 80 mg/day	$
	Promethazine (Phenergan)	Sedation, confusion, dry mouth, blurred vision	12.5–25 mg orally, IM, or per rectum every 4–12 hours	$
Vestibular neuritis				
	Prednisone	Insomnia, fluid/electrolyte imbalance, incr. ICP, adrenal suppression, psychosis, pancreatitis	1 mg/kg/day and taper over 2 to 3 weeks until drug is discontinued	$
	Meclizine	As above	As above	
	Diazepam	As above	As above	
Meniere's disease				
	Triamterene 37.5 mg/ hydrochlorothizide 25 mg	Electrolyte imbalance, hypotension, hyperkalemia, hypokalemia, nausea, vertigo, hyperglycemia, lipid increase	1–2 caps daily	$
	Meclizine (Antivert)	As above	As above	
	Dimenhydrinate (Dramamine)	As above	25–50 mg every 8 hrs maintenance; 50 mg IM acute attack	$

ICP, intracranial pressure; IM, intramuscularly; IV, intravenously.
*Relative cost: $ = <$33.00; $$ = $34.00–$66.00; $$$ = >$67.00
Eaton, DA, Roland PS. Dizziness in the older adult, part 2. Geriatrics. 2003 Apr; 58(4):48–52.
Swartz R, Longwell P, Treatment of vertigo. Am Fam Physician. 2005 Mar 15;71(6):1115–1122.

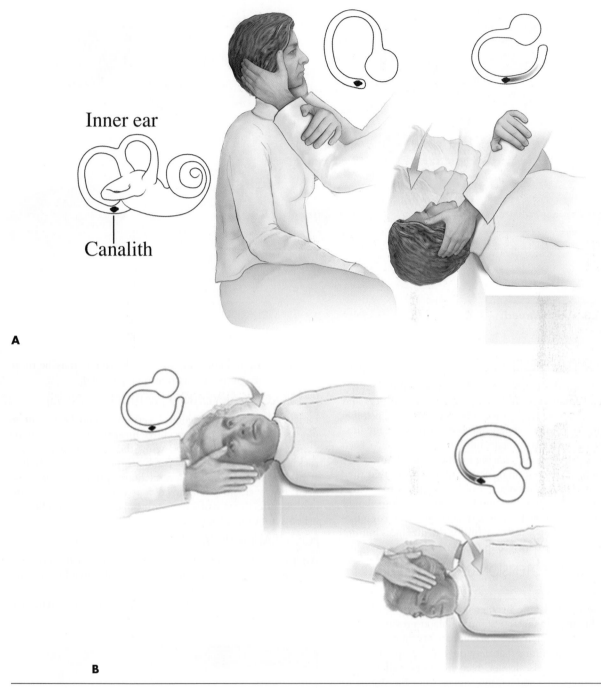

Inner ear

Canalith

A

B

Figure 43.3 • Epley maneuver illustration. (Illustration Copyright © 2006 Nucleus Medical Art, All Rights Reserved. www.nucleusinc.com.) (*continues*)

MENIERE'S DISEASE

The theory behind treatment for Meniere's Disease is to lower the endolymphatic pressure within the inner ear. Traditional management involves a low-salt diet (1 to 2 g daily) and diuretics, commonly a combination of hydrochlorothiazide and triamterene (Dyazide) (32). There are no randomized controlled trials that support either of these treatments, although in one study, diuretics appeared to be more effective in treating the vertigo than the hearing loss or tinnitus (33).

MIGRAINOUS VERTIGO

The first step in management of migrainous vertigo is the recognition of the overlying and complex relationship among migraine headaches, dizziness, and balance disorders. Treatment does not usually include physical therapy, but it has been found to be helpful in some series (7). The natural history is benign with spontaneous remission of four out of five patients within 5 to 10 years (10). Treatment for migraine effectively treats the dizziness, when the diagnosis iz correct.

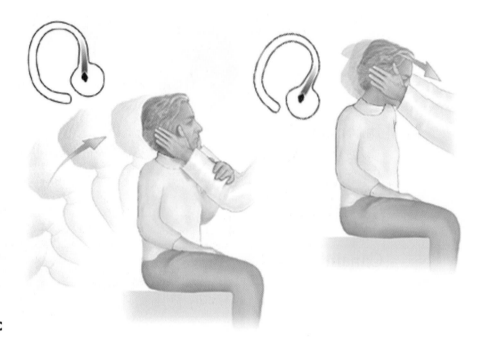

Figure 43.3 • (continued)   **C**

ANXIETY AND DEPRESSION

Many patients with dizziness have anxiety or depression. Because patients may have underlying vestibular disorders and have anxiety as a result, they should be evaluated, and possibly treated with vestibular exercises and/or suppressive medication. Selective serotonin reuptake inhibitors (SSRI's) have been reported to be effective in reducing symptoms over time. Care should be taken in prescribing SSRIs, however, in that they may cause nausea, sedation and dizziness—the same symptoms being treated. Slow titration to an effective dose should be employed. Combined vestibular therapy with cognitive therapy has been shown to be useful for the dizziness but not the anxiety of this patient group (32, 34).

ORTHOSTATIC HYPOTENSION OR AUTONOMIC DYSFUNCTION

If the cause is orthostatic hypotension, treatment goals will consist of therapies to increase standing blood pressure, without causing hypertension. In addition, patients should be educated regarding situations that may provoke symptoms, such as hot baths, large meals, alcohol, over-the-counter allergy and cold medications, and sudden movement from the supine to standing position. Cardiovascular autonomic testing may be indicated if the etiology is still unclear.

VASCULAR ISCHEMIA OR STROKE

Patients whose dizziness is cause by cerebrovascular disease should have therapy aimed at preventing future occurrences. This should include blood pressure management, addressing other cardiovascular risk factors (e.g., smoking and elevated lipids), physical activity, and possibly antiplatelet therapy or stent placement. Patients who have had a stroke and experience dizziness are at high risk for falling. Interventions to reduce balance problems when patients are doing complex tasks (for example, dressing) may play a significant role in reducing fall incidence. Improving postural stability and per-

ceptual skills, and encouraging safer behaviors may be more useful than cognitive behavioral therapies (35).

PHYSIOLOGICAL VERTIGO (MOTION SICKNESS)

Patients prone to physiological vertigo should be taught to use visual and other proprioceptive measures to overcome the vestibular deficit, such as viewing the horizon when on a rocking boat. A scopolamine patch behind the ear may reduce symptoms, when applied several hours prior to anticipated need; however, no randomized controlled trials have examined the effectiveness of scopolamine in the treatment of established symptoms of motion sickness (36).

POST-TRAUMATIC VERTIGO

After trauma, patients often require a primary care physician to oversee and coordinate the required multidisciplinary management including neurotological, neurologic, ophthalmologic, psychiatric specialists who may be involved. Many patients never return to work (12).

CASE 1 DISCUSSION

This patient's history and physical exam suggest the diagnosis of benign paroxysmal positional vertigo. Management should include the Epley maneuver in the office, and if unsuccessful, home exercises with follow-up. The patient should be educated about the cause and benign natural history of the disorder.

CASE 2 DISCUSSION

This patient has a mixed diagnosis of anxiety and a vestibular disorder, each triggered by stressful situations. Management should include further evaluation and treatment of anxiety. An SSRI may improve quality of life and give some symptom relief. Complementary strategies for anxiety and improved quality of sleep should be recommended including relaxation, visualization, sleep hygiene, and dietary and exercise counseling.

CASE 3 DISCUSSION

This patient has multiple causes for his dizziness, including cardiac autonomic neuropathy, sensory neuropathy secondary to diabetes, and the medications being used to treat his heart and blood pressure. Additionally, he likely has deconditioning, which was worsened by his recent hospitalization. Management must include a team approach to functionally oriented assessment and management, focusing on improving performance of activities of daily living, aiding compensation for his deficits, adjustment of medications, and improved fitness. Recommendations include physical therapy, assistive devices, and patient and family education regarding reducing fall risks.

REFERENCES

1. Kroenke K, Hoffman RM, Einstadter D. How common are various causes of dizziness, a critical review. South Med J. 2000 Feb;93(2):160–167.
2. Simon NM, Pollack MH, Tuby BA, Stern TA. Dizziness and panic disorder: A review of the association between vestibular dysfunction and anxiety. Ann Clin Psychiatry. 1998;10(2):
3. Luxon LM. Evaluation and management of the dizzy patient. J Neurol Psychiatry. 2004;75:iv45–iv52
4. Eaton, DA, Roland PS. Dizziness in the older adult, part 1. Geriatrics. 2003 Apr; 58(4):28–36.
5. Sloane PD. Dizziness in primary care: results from the National Ambulatory Medical Care survey J Fam Pract. 1989 Jul;29(1):33–38.
6. Crespi V. Dizziness and vertigo: an epidemiological survey and patient management in the emergency room. Neurol Sci. 2004;24:S24–S25,
7. Furman JM, Whitney SL. Central causes of dizziness. Phys Ther. 2000;80(2):179–187
8. Halmagyi GM, Cremer PD. Assessment and treatment of dizziness. J Neurol Neurosurg Psychiatry. 2000;68:129–136
9. Furman JM, Cass SP. Benign paroxysmal positional vertigo. N Engl J Med. 1999;341: 1590–1596.
10. Arbusow V. Acute vestibulopathy. Curr Opin Neurol. 2001; 14:11–20
11. Neuhauser H, Lempert T. Vertigo and dizziness related to migraine: a diagnostic challenge. Cephalalgia. 2004;24:83–91
12. Marzo SJ, Leonetti JP, Raffin MJ, Letarte P. Diagnosis and management of post-traumatic vertigo. Laryngoscope. 2004 Oct;114(10):1720–1723
13. Hoffer ME, Gottshall KR, Moore R, Balough BJ, Wester D. Characterizing and treating dizziness after mild head trauma. Otol Neurol. 2004 Mar;25(2):135–138
14. Vinik AI, Maser RE, Mitchell BD, Freeman R. Diabetic autonomic neuropathy. Diabetes Care. 2003;26:1553–1579.
15. Kwong EC, Pimlott NJ. Assessment of dizziness among older patients at a family practice clinic: a chart audit study. BMC Fam Pract. 2005 Jan 6;6:2.
16. Staab JP, Ruckenstein MJ. Which comes first? Psychogenic dizziness versus otogenic anxiety. Laryngoscope. 2003;113:1714–1718.
17. Kennedy RJ, Shelton C, Salzman KL, Davidson HC, Harnsberger HR. Intralabyrinthine schwannomas: diagnosis, management, and a new classification system. Otol Neurotol. 2004 Mar;25(2):160–167
18. Sloane PD, Coeytaux RR, Beck RS, Dallara J. Dizziness: state of science. Ann Intern Med. 2003 May 1;134(9 part 2, suppl): 823–832
19. Eaton DA, Roland PS. Dizziness in the older adult, part 2, Geriatrics. 2003 Apr; 58(4):48–52
20. Eggers SDZ, Zee DS. Evaluating the dizzy patient: bedside examination and laboratory assessment of the vestibular system. Semin Neurol. 2003;23(1):47–57.
21. Hilton M, Pinder D. The Epley (canalith repositioning) manoeuvre for benign paroxysmal positional vertigo (Cochrane Review). In: The Cochrane Library. Oxford, England: Update Software; 2005:Issue 3.
22. Bath AP, Walsh RM, Ranalli P. Experience from a multidisciplinary "dizzy" clinic. Am J Otol. 2000 Jan;21(1):92–97.
23. Colledge NR, Barr-Hamilton RM, Lewis SJ, Sellar RJ, Wilson JA. Evaluation of investigations to diagnose dizziness in elderly people: a community based controlled study; BMJ. 1996;313(7060):788–792.
24. Hoffman RM, Einstadter D, Kroenke K. Evaluating dizziness. Am J Med. 1999;107:468–478.
25. Aronow WS. Atrial fibrillation. Heart Dis. 2002;4:91–101.
26. Cohen HS, Kimball KT, Adams AS. Application of the vestibular disorders activities of daily living scale. Laryngoscope. 2000 July 110(7):1204–1209.
27. Lempert T, Brevern M. Episodic vertigo. Curr Opin Neurol. 1995 Feb;18(1):5–9.
28. Furman J, Hain TC. "Do try this at home": self treatment of BPPV. Neurology 2004;63:8–9.
29. Strupp M, Zingler VC, Arbusow V, et al. Methylprednisolone, valacyclovir, or the combination for vestibular neuritis. N Engl J Med. 2004;351:354–361.
30. Cesarani A, Alpini D, Monti B, et al. The treatment of acute vertigo. Neurol Sci. 2004;24:S26–S30
31. Yardley L, Beech S, Zander L, et al. A randomized controlled trial of exercise therapy for dizziness and vertigo in primary care. Br J Gen Pract. 1998;48:1136–1140.
32. Swartz R, Longwell P. Treatment of vertigo. Am Fam Physician. 2005 Mar 15;71(6):1115–1122.
33. James A, Thorp M. BMJ Clinical Evidence E-Journal: Conditions: ENT: Meniere's Disease: Interventions: Diuretics. *http://www.clinicalevidence.com/ceweb/conditions/ent/0505/0505 _I4.jsp* accessed Feb. 27, 2007.
34. Horii A, Mitani K, Kitahara T, Uno A, Takeda N, Kubo T. Paroxetine, a selective serotonin reuptake inhibitor, reduces depressive symptoms and subjective handicaps in patients with dizziness. Otol Neurotol. 2004 Jul;25(4):536–543.
35. Lamb SE, Ferrucci L, Volpato S, et al. Risk factors for falling in home-dwelling older women with stroke: the Women's Health and Aging Study. Stroke. 2003;34:494–501.
36. Spinks AB, Wasiak, J, Villanueva EV, Bernath V. Scopolamine for preventing and treating motion sickness (Cochrane Review). In: The Cochrane Library. Oxford, England: Update Software; 2005:Issue 4.
37. Sloane PD, Baloh RW. Persistent dizziness in geriatric patients. J Am Geriatr Soc. 1989;37:1031–1038.
38. Maarsingh OR, van der Horst HE, Stalman WA, Dros J, van Weert HCPM, Bindels PJE. Developing a diagnostic protocol for dizzy patients in primary care: A Delphi procedure. Amsterdam, Netherlands, 2005. Unpublished working paper.

CHAPTER 44

Fatigue, Tiredness, and Sleep Problems

Philip D. Sloane, Thomas Agresta, David Little, David Henderson, and Saloni Anand

CASE 1

Ms. K. is a 48-year-old woman who presents to your office as a "work-in" patient because of a 3-month history of tiredness. She is a school administrator and typically works 50 to 60 hours per week, including several evening meetings. She reports that her ability to concentrate is diminished, and that she's too tired to use her exercise bicycle when she gets home in the evening, although some days are better than others. She worries that she is losing interest in her professional work and her physical appearance.

She is married without children. Her husband, a bank manager, is supportive but sometimes distant. She recalls a 6-month "nervous breakdown" while she was in college, but has otherwise been in good emotional health. She does not drink alcohol or use illicit drugs.

She had an upper respiratory illness 2 weeks ago and for the past year has had heavy, irregular menstrual periods. She typically gets 7 hours of sleep and occasionally experiences a problem falling asleep at night. She takes acetaminophen for intermittent joint pains that mainly involve the shoulders and knees.

On examination she is moderately overweight, afebrile, and normotensive. There are several 0.5- to 1.0-cm anterior cervical lymph nodes. Her affect is somewhat flat, her thought content is normal, and she is without suicidal ideation. Otherwise her general health appears to be good.

CASE 2

H.B. is a 46-year-old man who presents for evaluation of fatigue and daytime drowsiness. He has had this problem for a number of years. He generally wakes in the morning feeling fatigued, even after sleeping 7 or 8 hours. He has a long history of falling asleep at work, especially in meetings, so much so that it has become a running joke with his coworkers. He fell asleep recently while driving and almost had an accident.

H.B. works in human resources and is sedentary. His medical history is notable for hypertension diagnosed 4 years ago, which is poorly controlled on two medications. On previous office visits he has been encouraged to lose weight, but he has actually gained 5 lbs in the past 6 months. His medical record also shows that he is being followed for borderline fasting blood sugars (he was 115

six months ago), and that he screened positive for snoring on a systems review. He denies abnormal sensations or movement in his legs at bedtime.

On examination, he is alert, cheerful, and cooperative. He weighs 245 pounds (body mass index = 33), with broad shoulders, truncal obesity, and a thick neck. His blood pressure is 150/92. His heart is normal except for a faint S4, and his respiratory examination is normal.

CLINICAL QUESTIONS

1. What is at the top of your differential diagnosis in each of these two cases? How and why do the lists differ?
2. What additional history and what physical examination findings would you seek to obtain in each case?
3. If, at this point in the encounter, the patient asked "So, doctor, why am I so tired?" how would you reply?

Fatigue, tiredness, and sleep problems represent an interrelated group of symptoms and diagnoses that are common, complex, and challenging. Occasionally, though the differential diagnosis is extensive, your initial evaluation will point strongly to a single underlying diagnosis, and you can proceed directly to treatment. More commonly, however, such patients will require a comprehensive approach, during which the diagnosis and management are arrived at over multiple visits.

Fatigue is common both in the community and among primary care patients. Community surveys have documented that 14% to 42% of people report some degree of fatigue, but that only a small percentage bring their symptom to the doctor for evaluation (1). In primary care settings, between 6.7% and 9.9% of adults report fatigue as a chief complaint, making it one of the ten most common symptoms presenting to family practice offices (2–6).

Sleep disorders are also quite common, though they less often surface as a chief complaint. Between 30% and 40% of respondents to community surveys report some level of insomnia within the prior year, with between 10% and 15% rating this as chronic or severe (7, 8). Yet nearly 70% of Americans who have sleep problems do not discuss their concerns with physicians. Therefore, keeping attuned to this fact will allow for more prompt recognition and treatment of these disorders (8).

The prognosis of fatigue depends on whether it is acute or chronic. Acute fatigue is often due to self-limited or reversible conditions, such as viral illnesses, acute stressful situations, or medication side effects. Chronic fatigue (defined as fatigue lasting ≥6 weeks) has a more ominous prognosis—between 50% to 70% of patients fail to improve after a year of follow-up (9–11). As a result, family physicians, with their longitudinal responsibility for patient care, will need to help many individuals cope with a disabling symptom. This includes using strategies such as chronic illness management, in which the doctor and patient share responsibility for symptom control and aim to enhance functional ability.

Excessive sleepiness and the sleep disorders are also often chronic, in part because they are often linked to chronic health problems such as hypertension, heart disease, diabetes, musculoskeletal problems, depression and polypharmacy. In approaching sleep disorders, it is important to remember that a) night-time sleep problems can affect relationships with the patient's spouse or partner—partners of sleep disordered patients average an hour less sleep per night and report reduced sexual and personal intimacy; and b) daytime sleepiness can lead to accidents, decreased productivity, and reduced effectiveness in work or school (8,12). Thus, all sleep complaints should be taken seriously and approached in a systematic manner.

DIFFERENTIAL DIAGNOSIS

There are many causes of fatigue, and many types of sleep disorders. In this section we overview the extensive differential diagnosis that exists for these complaints.

Causes of Fatigue

The underlying causes of fatigue can be placed into several categories: psychological, physical, lifestyle and idiopathic. Table 44.1 illustrates the broad differential diagnosis you should consider when evaluating a patient with fatigue. During your evaluation, keep in mind that some patients will have more than one contributing factor.

PSYCHOLOGICAL CAUSES

Community surveys have shown that patients with psychiatric disorders have a threefold to sixfold increased risk of feeling fatigued and that premorbid psychological symptoms predispose patients to fatigue after infections (1). Depression is the most common psychiatric illness associated with fatigue in the outpatient setting, affecting at least 5% of outpatients in any

TABLE 44.1 Common Causes of Fatigue in Primary Care

Diagnosis	As a Primary Diagnosis*	In Patients with Recent-Onset Fatigue	In Patients with Chronic Fatigue
		Frequency in Primary Care	
Depression	15.0%	Very common	Very common
Diabetes	10.6%	Very common	Very common
Acute infection	10.1%	Very common	Rare
Adjustment reaction	9.6%	Common	Uncommon
Cardiovascular disease	7.9%	Common	Common
Sleep disorders and lifestyle issues	7.8 %	Very common	Common
Chronic pain or dizziness	— †	Common	Very common
Anxiety	6.1%	Common	Very common
Lung disease (COPD, asthma)	4.9%	Common	Common
Connective tissue disease	4.7%	Uncommon	Common
Malignancy	3.2%	Uncommon	Common
Medication side effects	2.8%	Common	Common
Anemia	2.8%	Common	Uncommon
Hypothyroidism	2.6%	Uncommon	Uncommon
Substance abuse	2.2%	Common	Uncommon
Chronic infection (HIV, TB)	1.8%	Rare	Uncommon
GI causes—hepatitis, inflammatory bowel disease	1.6%	Rare	Rare
Neuromuscular disease (MS, etc.)	0.4 %	Rare	Rare
Psychosis	0.1%	Rare	Rare
No diagnosis made	30–40 %	Very common	Common

* Note that patients often will have more than one disease contributing to the symptom of fatigue, and distinguishing the primary reason can be difficult.
†Previous studies of the causes of fatigue did not evaluate the extent to which other symptoms, such as pain and dizziness, may have been contributing factors.
COPD, chronic obstructive pulmonary disease; GI, gastrointestinal; HIV, human immunodeficiency virus; MS, multiple sclerosis; TB, tuberculosis.

6-month period (13). Patients with depressive disorders often complain of fatigue as part of a symptom complex that includes loss of energy, sleep problems, and poor appetite (14). However, although most depressed patients are fatigued, not every fatigued patient has depression (15).

Anxiety disorders are another common psychiatric illness in outpatients presenting with fatigue. Adjustment reactions to life changes (such as marital status change, birth or departure of children, death of a family member, job change) and substance abuse (caffeine, alcohol, illicit drugs) are also common causes of psychologically mediated fatigue.

PHYSICAL CAUSES

Biomedical disorders are the cause of a contributing factor in about half of primary care patients presenting with fatigue (2, 3, 5, 16, 17). The most common physical disorders causing fatigue are diabetes, acute infections, cardiovascular disease, and lung disease. In addition, physicians need to be alert for medication side effects as possible causes of tiredness. Common drug causes of fatigue include analgesics, psychotropics, antihypertensives, and antihistamines.

Connective tissue disorders are another important cause of fatigue. Rheumatoid arthritis and systemic lupus erythematosus, for example, can lead to tiredness and be accompanied by chronic anemia. Another musculoskeletal disorder that contributes to fatigue is fibromyalgia, a chronic condition associated with a history of widespread pain and focal tenderness on digital palpation. Less common disorders presenting as fatigue, which are easy to miss and, therefore, should be kept in mind, are listed and described in Table 44.2.

LIFESTYLE CAUSES

Alterations in lifestyle often cause fatigue, particularly in young and middle-aged adults. Some of the causes to consider include an increase in physical exertion over the patient's established habits, inadequate rest, sleep pattern disruption, and effects of recent surgery or trauma. Studies show that fatigue may also be associated with environmental stresses such as excessive noise, heat, or cold (18).

Ironically, people who have a sedentary lifestyle are more likely to report fatigue than those who are physically active. This is probably because exercise has some inherent anti-depressant and anti-anxiety effects, and can contribute to improved sleep.

UNEXPLAINED FATIGUE AND THE CHRONIC FATIGUE SYNDROME

Over time, with careful follow-up, the number of undiagnosed patients should be quite small, but nonetheless some will remain undiagnosed. Others will meet the criteria for chronic fatigue syndrome (CFS), itself a poorly-understood syndrome that may represent more than one disease process. Table 44.3 lists the official diagnostic criteria for this syndrome. Patients must have unexplained persistent or relapsing fatigue that is not relieved by rest and is severe enough to significantly reduce daily activity levels; in addition, they must have four additional symptoms. Because there is no specific diagnostic test that clearly separates this group of patients from others with chronic fatigue who may not meet these criteria, CFS probably represents more than one specific cause. Research studies to

TABLE 44.2   Causes of Fatigue that May Stump the Clinician

Cause	Comments
Adrenal insufficiency	Clues include increased cutaneous pigmentation, severe postural hypotension, loss of pubic and axillary hair in women, hyponatremia, and hypokalemia. Be suspicious if hx of metastatic cancer (especially lung), or recent discontinuation of steroids.
Hypopituitarism	Be especially suspicious if there is a history of hypotension (e.g., postpartum) or of headaches or breast discharge (in women, suggesting prolactinoma)
Thyroid disease	Have high index of suspicion; remember that in the elderly "apathetic hyperthyroidism" as well as hypothyroidism can cause fatigue.
Hypercalcemia	Be sure to include serum calcium in laboratory evaluation of fatigue.
Anemia	Can be insidious; always check blood count in persons with unexplained fatigue.
Carbon monoxide poisoning	Symptoms are often vague; headache is common. Suspect if using wood stove or gas heater in the winter.
Intimate partner violence	Suspect this in patients with fatigue and multiple somatic complaints or depression.
Malignancy	Suspicious symptoms include weight loss, abdominal pain, and iron deficiency anemia, especially in the elderly.
Obstructive sleep apnea	History or morning tiredness, snoring, and headaches, especially in obese patients
Depression	So common it is often missed. Remember that many chronic illnesses and medications can cause secondary depression, and that postpartum depression is common.

Adapted from Morrison RE, Keating HJ. Fatigue in primary care. Obstet Gynecol Clin North Am. 2001;28(2):225–240.

TABLE 44.3 Centers for Disease Control Criteria for Diagnosis of Chronic Fatigue Syndrome

1. Severe chronic fatigue of 6 months or longer duration, which is not cause by other known medical conditions excluded by clinical diagnosis.

   AND

2. Four or more of the following symptoms, each of which must have persisted or recurred during 6 or more consecutive months of the illness and must not have predated the fatigue:

   - sore throat
   - tender lymph nodes
   - muscle pain (myalgias)
   - multi-joint pain without swelling or redness
   - headaches of a new type, pattern or severity
   - unrefreshing sleep
   - post-exertional malaise lasting more than 24 hours.

Adapted from *http://www.cdc.gov/ncidod/diseases/cfs/about/what.htm.*

date have not identified a viral etiology but have suggested both qualitative and quantitative abnormalities of immunologic function (19). Although no specific treatment yet exists, making a diagnosis of CFS has several benefits: reducing unnecessary investigations, providing an explanation to the patient, providing support for disability (in some cases), and identifying an approach to treatment.

Common Sleep Disorders

The scientific literature on sleep disorders is complex and confusing, with several different categorizations and many rare syndromes and diseases. From a primary care perspective, it may be useful to focus on common sleep symptoms and a few diagnostic categories. The most common symptoms are insomnia and excessive daytime sleepiness. Diagnoses can be divided into those that are secondary to a medical, psychological, or lifestyle cause, and the primary sleep disorders, of which obstructive sleep apnea (OSA), restless leg syndrome (RLS), and narcolepsy are the most important. Table 44.4 provides a list of the common sleep diagnoses.

Insomnia and excessive daytime sleepiness are the most common sleep-related symptoms. Insomnia is a complaint regarding the quantity, quality, or timing of sleep. The most common issues patients report as "insomnia" include: waking up frequently at night, trouble getting to sleep (delayed sleep onset), waking up feeling un-refreshed, and snoring or stopping breathing at night (sleep disordered breathing). Chronic insomnia is defined as occurring several times per week for at least six months (7, 20, 21). Excessive daytime sleepiness (EDS) presents as fatigue, decreased energy, grogginess, and a tendency to fall asleep at inappropriate times. Its frequency increases with age. Persons with EDS are at risk for work-related injuries, motor vehicle accidents, decreased cognitive performance, and adverse health outcomes (22, 23).

In developing a differential diagnosis, it is helpful to think of primary and secondary sleep disorders (Table 44.4). Primary disorders, although less common, should be searched for because patients may benefit from specific therapies and/or evaluation by a specialist in sleep medicine. The three primary sleep disorders that are particularly important are described briefly below:

- Obstructive sleep apnea (OSA)—a condition characterized by episodes of apnea (cessation of breathing for >10 seconds) and of hypopnea (30% reduction in airflow with 4% oxygen desaturation or greater lasting >10 seconds) that occur during sleep. OSA is the most significant of the sleep disorders, because it carries with it a substantial burden in terms of morbidity, mortality, and costs to the health care system. People with OSA tend to complain of frequent awakenings during the night and chronic EDS; their partners often report observing episodes of choking, apneic spells and abrupt arousals from sleep (24–27). The pathophysiology involves periodic airway occlusion as result of decreased pharyngeal muscle tone and/or of airway narrowing. This occlusion results in oxygen desaturation, hypoventilation, and fluctuations in heart rate and blood pressure that, in chronic, severe disease, lead to right-sided congestive heart failure and cor pulmonale. Risk factors for OSA include obesity, smoking, and increased age.

- Restless leg syndrome (RLS)—a sensorimotor neurologic condition characterized by an irresistible urge to move the legs or arms, that interferes with sleep onset. This urge may be associated with pain or sensations such as "creeping, crawling, jittery, worms moving, or an electric current." Because these sensations interfere with sleep onset or maintenance, they impair daytime functioning. The urge to move one's limbs is most prominent at rest and is relieved with activity. Family history is a significant risk factor. Secondary causes of RLS are pregnancy, Parkinson's disease, peripheral neuropathy, anemia (iron deficiency), and end stage renal disease (28).

- Narcolepsy—a rare disorder of REM sleep, characterized by shortened sleep latency and abnormally early entry into REM sleep. Symptoms include episodes of cataplexy (sudden loss of muscle tone), sleep-related hallucinations and sleep paralysis in the transition from sleep to wakefulness. A positive family history greatly increases risk (29).

Secondary sleep disorders, which are far more common than primary disorders, are sleep problems that arise due to medical, psychological, or lifestyle causes. These categories, and their associated diagnoses, are described briefly below:

- Medical—people with chronic illness can be prone to a variety of sleep problems, due to a variety of mechanisms. The natural sleep cycle involves episodes of awakening or near-awakening about every 90 minutes; at these points in the sleep cycle chronic pain or nocturia can bring about a full awakening and difficulty returning to sleep. Medications that are activating, cause nightmares, or lead to nocturia or abdominal discomfort can similarly affect sleep. Medications with sedative properties can lead to EDS and, as a consequence, poor sleep at night. Finally, many chronic illnesses, particularly chronic pulmonary and cardiac disease, are associated with sleep syndromes, such as OSA.

TABLE 44.4   Differential Diagnosis of Patients Complaining of Difficulty with Sleep

Category	Diagnosis	Frequency Among Primary Care Patients with Sleep Complaints*
Adults		
Primary sleep disorders	Obstructive sleep apnea (OSA)	Common ($\leq 10\%$)
	Restless leg syndrome (RLS)	Common ($\leq 15\%$)
	Narcolepsy	Rare
Secondary to medical, psychological, or lifestyle causes	Depression and/or anxiety	Very common ($\leq 50\%$)
	Other drug or alcohol use or abuse (including caffeine)	Common
	Chronic pain (e.g., arthritis)	Common
	Polyuria (e.g., prostatic hyperplasia, diabetes)	Common in elderly
	Dyspnea due to chronic heart or lung disease	Common
	Medications (e.g., diuretics, antidepressants, prescription or OTC sleep aids)	Common
	Sleep restriction (due to lifestyle or schedules)	Common
	Circadian rhythm disturbances (jet lag, shift work)	Somewhat common
Idiopathic	Idiopathic insomnia	Common ($\leq 10\%$)
Children		
Sleep disordered breathing	Primary snoring	Very common—3%–12% of children
	Obstructive sleep apnea	Common 1%–10%
	Adenotonsillar hypertrophy or nasal obstruction	Common
	Macroglossia (Trisomy 21) or micrognathia	Uncommon
Parasomnias†	Night terrors	Common
	Somnambulism	Somewhat common

*Many patients have more than one cause or contributing factor
†Parasomnias in children usually resolve spontaneously

- Psychological—disturbed sleep is one of the cardinal signs of depressive and anxiety disorders, and treatment of one often improves the other.
- Lifestyle—many people today, because of work schedules or lifestyle choices, have variable and/or restricted sleep hours, a situation that disturbs the body's natural circadian rhythms, contributing to disturbed sleep. In addition, many substances—particularly caffeine, alcohol, illicit drugs, and over-the-counter sleep aids—can contribute to chronic sleep-related symptoms.

CLINICAL EVALUATION

An important first step in creating a manageable differential diagnosis is to try to identify whether the patient's predomi-

nant symptom is fatigue or daytime sleepiness. *Fatigue* is present when the patient's main complaints are weariness, weakness, depleted energy, tiredness, and/or exhaustion. Daytime sleepiness is the predominant symptom when the patient's main complaints include drowsiness, a tendency to fall asleep at inappropriate times, and/or decreased alertness at work (30). Daytime sleepiness is a cardinal symptom of many primary and secondary sleep disorders, and its presence should prompt the initial evaluation to focus on those causes. In contrast, a primary complaint of fatigue should lead to a diagnostic approach that focuses on medical and psychological causes of decreased energy.

The evaluation of fatigue will often take more than one visit, and will involve an extensive history and physical examination, rather than the focused examination that is used for some other presenting complaints. When you perform this evaluation, you should keep in mind psychological, physical, and lifestyle causes. The extent of your evaluation, including laboratory investigations, depends on the likely causes suggested by the history and physical examination.

A sleep disorders evaluation will be similarly comprehensive. Input from the patient's partner or family members may be very helpful in this process; so the partner should be included in the first or second visit. Initially, the history should focus on high-risk diagnoses, impact on daily function, and potential secondary causes.

Part of the early patient evaluation should be a search for certain red flags that suggest a problem that might be life-threatening. Because the differential diagnosis of fatigue, tiredness, and sleep complaints is extensive, the list of potential red flags can be quite broad. Table 44.5 lists the most prominent red flags and discusses the implication of each.

The Clinical History

The key elements listed in Table 44.6 should guide your approach to interviewing a patient with fatigue. Because chronic and acute illness is a frequent cause or contributing factor to fatigue and sleep disruption, a careful medical history and symptom review should be taken. Because of the high prevalence of psychological and lifestyle causes, you should take a careful psychosocial history, focusing on symptoms of depression and probing for aspects of the patient's lifestyle, such as environmental stresses, impaired sleep, and inactivity, that can contribute to feeling fatigued. Unless you are already familiar with the patient's family and occupational history, you should cover these areas in your interview. You may want to ask your patient to keep a daily diary to help you determine precipitating factors and associations; such strategies have the added benefit of actively involving your patient in the diagnostic process.

Elements of the history that suggest a psychological diagnosis include:

- A history of a dysfunctional family setting and/or a previous history of functional health problems.

- The onset of the fatigue is associated with stress and accompanied by multiple, nonspecific symptoms.
- The tiredness is worse in the morning and fluctuates rather than progresses in intensity over the course of the day.
- The fatigue is relieved by physical activity.

If your initial history suggests that the patient's fatigue might be psychological, consider screening tests such as the Beck Depression Inventory (31). Explore other expectations or concerns, such as desire for referral, an excuse from work, symptom relief, domestic or substance abuse, and sexual or social problems.

Interviewing a family member, or, more specifically, the patient's bed partner, is particularly critical in conducting a sleep disorders evaluation. As part of this process of interviewing the patient and bed partner, you should:

- Screen for OSA by asking about: frequent snoring, choking or sudden awakening from sleep, spells where breathing stops, and if the partner is afraid that the patient might stop breathing.
- Screen for RLS by asking the patient about unusual sensations and an urge to move the legs while trying to get to sleep, and by asking bed partners about sudden jerking movements that awaken them and not the patient.
- Screen for narcolepsy by asking about dozing or falling asleep while driving, on the job or in school, or in uncomfortable social situations.

In diagnosing children with sleep disorders, it is important to recognize—as in adults—that snoring is not diagnostic of OSA. In addition to snoring, parents should be asked about apnea, mouth breathing, and frequent nocturnal waking. In children over 5 years of age, behavioral problems, enuresis, and attention deficits are important associated findings. Also, it is important to note that hypnagogic hallucinations associated with narcolepsy can easily be confused with night terrors (a benign, self-limited condition that is common in children).

TABLE 44.5 Red Flags Suggesting Progressive or Life-Threatening Disease in Patients with Fatigue, Tiredness, or Sleep Complaints

Red Flag(s)	Diagnosis Suggested
Suicidal ideation, marked social withdrawal	Major depressive episode; high suicide risk
History of alcohol, narcotic, or psychotropic drug abuse with recent discontinuation of use	Withdrawal syndrome
Fever >39.5°C, chills, hypotension, and/or neck stiffness	Life-threatening infection
Recent onset of severe or worsening fatigue, especially if accompanied by pallor, jaundice, or a history of recent blood loss	Severe anemia due to blood loss or hemolysis
Gradual onset of fatigue in a patient with prominent risk factors for HIV exposure	Acquired Immunodeficiency Syndrome (AIDS)
Orthopnea, edema, cardiomegaly, auscultatory crackles	Severe left-sided congestive heart failure
Polydipsia, polyuria	Poorly controlled diabetes
Peripheral edema, especially in the setting of chronic dyspnea and hypoxemia or hypercapnia	Pulmonary hypertension due to severe obstructive sleep apnea with cor pulmonale
Falling asleep during activities, in conversation, or while driving	Significant accident risk; possible narcolepsy

TABLE 44.6   Key Elements of the History and Physical Examination for Fatigue

Question/Maneuver	Purpose
Psychosocial history (sadness or agitation, substance abuse, life and environmental stresses, activity/exercise level, sleep habits, appetite, anhedonia, inability to concentrate, feelings of worthlessness/hopelessness)	Screen for psychological and lifestyle causes
Look for red flags (see Table 44.5)	Screen for suicidal ideation, withdrawal syndromes, life-threatening infections, heart failure or diabetes
Look for features differentiating physical from psychological causes (see text)	Assess likelihood of psychological cause
Medication use	Evaluate for medication side effects
Fever	Screen for acute infections
Weight loss	Screen for cancer, HIV disease
Pallor	Screen for anemia
Cough	Screen for TB, HIV disease, COPD
Joint pains/inflammation	Screen for connective disease disorder
Widespread pain, trigger points (see Chapter 36)	Screen for fibromyalgia
Exertional dyspnea	Screen for heart failure, COPD
Lymphadenopathy/hepatosplenomegaly	Screen for malignancy, infections
Thyromegaly, dry skin, delayed reflexes	Screen for hypothyroidism
Ear-nose-throat examination	Screen for otitis, pharyngitis, sinusitis, allergies
Cardiopulmonary examination	Screen for CHF, COPD, pneumonia

CHF, congestive heart failure; COPD, chronic obstructive pulmonary disease; TB, tuberculosis.

Physical Examination

The physical examination of the patient with fatigue needs to be broad, and should include the cardiovascular, respiratory, endocrine, lymphatic, gastrointestinal, neurological, and musculoskeletal systems. Fever and weight loss may be seen in infections, malignancy, or chronic pulmonary disease. The musculoskeletal examination will screen for signs of connective tissue disorder, such as widespread pain and the presence of trigger points (suggesting fibromyalgia). Search for signs of hypothyroidism by palpating the thyroid gland, and examining for dry, coarse skin and delayed deep-tendon reflexes. Check for lymphadenopathy (suggesting infection or malignancy) and hepatic or splenic enlargement (suggesting an underlying malignancy or a viral infection such as infectious mononucleosis). The ear-nose-throat examination will screen for upper respiratory infections, as well as for chronic allergies that impair sleep. Also, perform a careful cardiopulmonary examination to screen for signs of heart failure, pneumonia, or chronic obstructive lung disease. You may need a second visit to allow sufficient time for performing these examinations.

In patients with sleep problems, the physical examination should concentrate on the cardiac and respiratory systems; however, because many chronic medical conditions are associated with disturbed sleep, a comprehensive exam is often appropriate, as in the evaluation of fatigue. OSA is the only primary sleep condition that has associated physical exam findings; independent risk factors from the physical exam are:

- a body mass index (BMI) ≥ 30
- a neck circumference >16.5 inches in men and >16 inches in women

All suspected OSA patients should be assessed for hypertension and diabetes as well, because one or both conditions often coexist with OSA.

In children the physical exam should include assessment of overall growth and development (in younger children) and obesity, as measured by age-adjusted BMI standards. A careful head and neck exam should be conducted to evaluate craniofacial abnormalities such as micronagthia (Pierre Robin syndrome) and nasal obstruction. Tonsillar size should be assessed for hypertrophy and the soft palate and uvula inspected for movement and tendency to collapse. Adenoidal hypertrophy may be assessed by nasopharyngoscopy or lateral neck radiographs. Neurologic assessment is also appropriate to look for evidence of hypotonia, which can be present in metabolic, primary neurologic or neuromuscular disorders (24, 32).

Diagnostic Testing

Because of the high incidence of psychological causes and the broad differential diagnosis of physical causes, laboratory tests have a low yield in the workup of patients presenting with tiredness (2, 9, 33). The only laboratory test that has been shown to have a greater yield in fatigued patients than in age/gender–matched controls is the mono spot test for infectious mononucleosis. The yield, however, is no greater than 20%, and it is highly dependent on age and associated symptoms (34).

Despite the low predictive utility of laboratory tests, most physicians order a limited initial evaluation that includes a complete blood count (CBC), erythrocyte sedimentation rate, serum glucose (if the patient is obese), and thyroid-stimulating hormone (if the patient is over age 40). This combination of tests will help you to confirm or rule out the most common physical causes of fatigue, which are listed in Table 44.1. You may order other studies based on risk as defined during the initial history and physical examination. Examples of the latter include HIV serology, skin tests for tuberculosis, and Lyme disease serology. Because some women with low ferritin and unexplained fatigue who are not anemic respond to iron supplemtation, iron studies (including ferritin) should also be considered (35).

In evaluating the patient with sleep complaints, the most effective diagnostic tool is the sleep diary. There are a number of readily printable examples available on the Internet. Patients should record about 2 weeks of data that include questions about sleep hygiene (what they do to get ready for sleep, and the environment in which they try to sleep), sleep onset, nighttime awakenings, and symptoms of sleep disorders. In reviewing a sleep diary, take note of the following:

- Total sleep time—most adults require between 7 and 9 hours in order to feel rested (7,8)
- Sleep onset latency (the time it takes to initially fall asleep)—normally, this ranges from 10 to 20 minutes, with times greater than 30 minutes considered abnormal
- Sleep efficiency (the amount of time actually spent asleep, divided by the time in bed)—this affects how patients perceive the symptoms they experience; and
- Arousal earlier than desired

Diagnosis of RLS is mainly dependent on the history and usually does not require further testing. However, serum ferritin and total iron binding capacity should be measured, as iron deficiency can cause RLS, in which case symptoms will often resolve with therapy. Other tests, such as nerve conduction velocity and electromyography, can be done in a patient without a family history or atypical presentation of RLS to differentiate other neurologic disorders (28, 36, 37).

Polysomnography and evaluation by a sleep specialist is usually recommended for patients you suspect might have OSA or narcolepsy. During polysomnography a patient's airflow, abdominothoracic movements, oximetry, and ECG are monitored. The stage of sleep is also assessed using a combination of electroencephalography (EEG), electromyography (EMG), and electro-oculography (EOG). Persons with suspected narcolepsy will often need an additional study, the multiple sleep latency test (27, 38).

For children, polysomnography remains the most accurate diagnostic tool, however logistically it is not always possible to obtain. Nocturnal oximetry and nap polysomnography are alternatives in pediatric populations. Children have higher respiratory rates and shorter periods of apnea, thereby experiencing less oxygen desaturation; so, criteria for OSA are somewhat different.

Recommended Diagnostic Strategy

Figure 44.1 graphically presents a general approach to patients with fatigue and sleep-related complaints. As was noted earlier in this section, the first step is to differentiate between fatigue and daytime sleepiness.

If fatigue is the main complaint, it is useful to think of a two-office-visit evaluation (18). The priorities for the initial visit are to establish a therapeutic relationship, to briefly assess elements of the history and physical examination that may indicate urgent problems, to order laboratory studies, to emphasize need for a comprehensive assessment (in which you introduce the idea that stress may be involved), and to schedule a return visit of adequate length to conduct a comprehensive history and physical examination. Occasionally, this initial evaluation will identify an obvious treatable cause, such as a new medication or a viral illness, in which case you can proceed directly to therapy. If not, the second visit is used to gather additional information regarding the patient's social profile, medical history, family history, review of systems, current medications, and lifestyle issues, as well as to conduct a comprehensive physical examination and to review the laboratory studies. Toward the end of this visit, you should summarize the findings to the patient and make treatment suggestions based on the data. In many cases, a specific diagnosis will be evident and plans can proceed to begin appropriate therapy, but in others either no specific diagnosis will be found or more studies will be needed.

If the patient's problem seems to be a sleep disorder, the approach should be similar, often taking place over two or more visits. Your initial history and examination should screen for red flags (Table 44.5), OSA, RLS, and narcolepsy. If OSA or narcolepsy seems likely, referral to a sleep laboratory for polysomnography should be considered. If not, the initial visit should seek to identify symptoms and signs of chronic illness, psychological conditions (e.g., anxiety, depression, or an acute life stress), or use of medications that adversely affect sleep. You should then order laboratory tests that are suggested by this initial evaluation, and schedule a return visit. In addition, identification of symptoms consistent with depression should usually lead to initiation of antidepressant therapy at the initial visit. Between the first and second visit, ask your patient to keep a daily sleep and symptom log, which you will review as part of that second visit. As is true for fatigue, care should be taken to communicate your thoughts in a sensitive manner, and to develop a therapeutic partnership with the patient.

MANAGEMENT

In the majority of patients with fatigue and sleep problems, you will be able to identify one or more medical, psychological, or lifestyle diagnoses for which specific treatment can be prescribed. A significant minority of patients will, however, have persistent symptoms in spite of the best efforts by the provider(s) and patient to treat the underlying conditions and reduce the risk factors. Management of these individuals should follow the principles of chronic disease management—creation of a therapeutic partnership, involvement of a care team, maximizing medical therapy, monitoring carefully, and provision

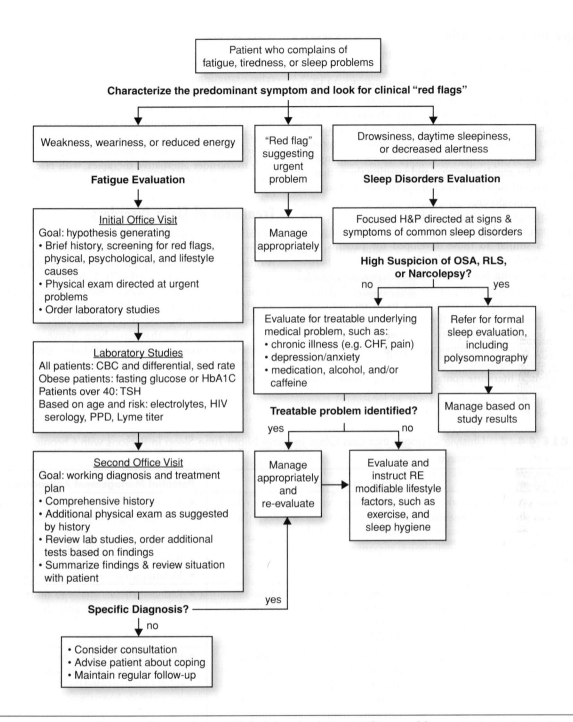

Figure 44.1 • General approach to patients with fatigue, tiredness, or sleep problems. Abbreviations: sed rate, erythrocyte sedimentation rate; TSH, thyroid stimulating hormone; PPD, purified protein derivative; HIV, human immunodeficiency virus; HbA1C, hemoglobin A1C.

of active support. In these circumstances, you should discuss plans with the patient in order to develop understanding, enhance cooperation, and maintain a broad perspective on biomedical and psychosocial issues.

Follow-up plans should be based on mutual agreement. If the cause seems to be physical, further investigation may be indicated. A consultation may be helpful to confirm a suspected diagnosis or to reassure you and your patient that no

medical cause has been overlooked, although continuing to search for a cure may delay effective therapy and create unrealistic expectations. For those patients in whom the pattern of the illness suggests a psychological cause, the specific approaches recommended in Chapters 47 (Anxiety) and 48 (Depression) should be considered. In all cases, you should fully discuss plans and make a commitment to continuing care through follow-up visits.

TABLE 45.1   Differential Diagnosis of the Patient with Headache

Headache Type	Primary or Secondary	Frequency in Primary Care (% of Headaches in Office)
Migraine	Primary	45–50
Tension-type headache	Primary	20–25
Cluster	Primary	2–3
Sinusitis	Secondary	5–7
Withdrawal from caffeine, opiates, alcohol, marijuana	Secondary	5–8
Arthritis/joint disease: osteoarthritis of cervical spine, temporomandibular joint	Secondary	2–4
Posttraumatic headache	Secondary	2–5
Fever	Secondary	2–4
Ophthalmologic (glaucoma, eye strain)	Secondary	1–2
Meningitis/encephalitis	Secondary	<1
Temporal arteritis	Secondary	<1
Subarachnoid/subdural bleeds	Secondary	<1
Brain tumor	Secondary	<1

Data from Becker LA, Iverson DC, Reed FM, Calonge N, Miller RS, Freeman WL. Patients with new headaches in primary care. J Fam Pract. 1988; 27:41–46; and Dubose CD, Cutlip AC, Cutlip WD. Migraines and other headaches: approach to diagnosis and classification. Am Fam Physician. 1995; 51:1498–1504.

aches usually present in late childhood or early adulthood, but the diagnosis may be delayed several years. The incidence is much higher in women than men among adults, but the ratio is equal in children.

Migraine is the most common type of headache to present in the primary care setting. Because patients with migraine often report pain in the face or around (or behind) one eye, they are often misdiagnosed as having sinus headaches. Migraine is primarily a neuronal (not vascular) event; the etiology is not completely known, but there appears to be neurochemical disruption, specifically involving serotonin, dopamine, and norepineprine metabolism. Neurogenic inflammation and regional disruption of cerebral or extracranial blood flow may cause some of the related symptoms. The autonomic nervous system, the trigeminal nerve, and the vagus nerve are also implicated in the etiology of migraine (6).

The frequency, severity, and associated symptoms of migraine can vary between patients and within a given patient's lifetime. Fluctuations in serum estrogen concentration in women (as may occur during menarche, menstrual periods, pregnancy, or menopause) are often associated with onset, remission, or change in severity of migraine-related symptoms. Other known "triggers" include certain foods, caffeine, sleep deprivation, psychosocial stressors, or changes in weather or barometric pressure (see Table 45.2). Daily pain diaries can help identify such triggers.

Tension-Type Headache

Tension-type headache (T-TH) is the most common cause of headache, with a prevalence of between 30%–80% in the general community (7–10). T-THs are usually mild or moderate in severity and are often self-treated. They are usually episodic, but can develop into daily or near-daily headaches. Many patients with TTH describe bilateral symptoms or a "band-like" pain. In some patients, both TTH and migraine are present.

Cluster Headache

Cluster headaches are not common, with a prevalence estimated at about 0.3%–0.4% of the general population (11, 12). This is one of the few headache types more prevalent in males. The name cluster is given to this primary headache disorder due to its classic presentation as a series of headaches occurring close together over 6–12 weeks. Persons with cluster headaches describe a severe, and intense, unilateral pain lasting from several seconds to many minutes. Concurrent symptoms include ipsilateral lacrimation, rhinorrhea, and ptosis. The headache is also always on the same side, no matter how many months are between episodes.

Secondary Headaches

Secondary headaches are caused by an infectious, vascular, traumatic, or other etiology. The headache is typically one among a constellation of symptoms that suggests a specific etiology. To not miss the diagnosis, the provider must be alert to atypical presentations, abrupt new onset, or associated focal physical findings in patients with a possible *organic* cause to the headache. These include:

- Infectious causes. Headache is a significant presenting complaint for a variety of different infectious diseases. Persons

TABLE 45.2 Common Headache Triggers

Categories of Triggers	Specific Triggers	Comments
Alcoholic beverages	Tyramine in red wines, sulfites in white wines. Dehydration, "hangover."	Variable response
Caffeine and/or caffeine withdrawal	May be related to changes in vasomotor tone.	
Food additives	MSG, Aspartame, tyramine (found in aged cheeses, some red wines, smoked fish, *etc.*), sodium nitrite (found in processed meats).	Food diaries may be helpful, as may food challenges
Foods	Chocolate, fruits, dairy, onions, beans, nuts.	As above
Environmental changes	Light, odors (perfume, paint, etc.), travel, abrupt changes in weather or altitude.	May present as "stuffiness" (sinus symptoms)
Lifestyle factors	Insufficient, excessive, disrupted, or irregular sleep. Tobacco or alcohol use. Fasting Physical activity Head injury Schedule changes Stress or release from stress Anger Exhilaration	Very common. Some people increase tobacco or alcohol use to try to alleviate headaches, thereby contributing to the problem.
Hormone changes, or addition of estrogen-containing medication	Timing of headache with menses or change/addition of hormones	Headaches may worsen or improve

with influenza, particularly influenza A, may present with a headache and fever. Other milder viral syndromes may also present with a headache; treatment with analgesics is often helpful in such cases. More concerning infectious etiologies include meningitis or encephalitis. Meningitis generally presents as fever, headache, neck pain and stiffness. Encephalitis may present with headache and global mental status changes, as well as fever. Workup of the infectious cause will be guided by the presenting history and physical, and may include a CT scan, lumbar puncture, and specific blood tests for a bacterial or viral origin.

- Rheumatologic causes. The most concerning of these is giant cell arteritis (temporal arteritis), characterized by pain in the region of the temporal artery, age >50, and a history of polymyalgia rheumatica (PMR). A temporal artery biopsy is diagnostic. Other rheumatologic problems that may present with headache include temporomandibular joint disorders, degenerative disc disorders of the cervical vertebra, and neuritis, or neuralgia of the greater occipital nerve.
- Intracranial mass. A presentation of an abrupt onset of headache along with focal neurologic findings may suggest an intracranial lesion. Although rare, tumors can account for new onset headaches. Subdural hematomas should be suspected in the elderly with a new onset of headache or in a patient with a recent history of trauma.
- Other causes. Vascular events, including stroke, aneurysm leak or rupture, or subarachnoid hemorrhage may present with sudden onset, severe headache, and focal neurologic

changes, often with other systemic findings related to the event. A high clinical suspicion and a head scan (CT or MRI) are indicated. Disorders of the cerebrospinal fluid (CSF) circulation can present with headache and visual changes. The cause of the CSF abnormalities may be iatrogenic, such as a lumbar puncture or spinal or epidural anesthesia or it may be idiopathic, as in pseudotumor cerebri.

Sinusitis and "Sinus Headache"

Many people with headache or facial pain incorrectly diagnose themselves with "sinus headache." Migraines and cluster headaches have symptoms related to the nose and sinuses, with rhinorrhea, pain behind the eye (frontal sinus), and facial tenderness. Rhinosinusitis must also have findings of purulence in the nasal cavity, nasal obstruction, altered smell (hypo or anosmia) and/or fever. Persons treating presumed sinus headaches with decongestants often report incomplete resolution of their pain, and present in the primary care office seeking antibiotics. It is the case that 70%–80% of patients presenting with sinusitis causing a headache may actually have migraine headaches, or could be classified as *probably migraine* based on the presence of most but not all of the IHS criteria for migraine (13).

Chronic Daily Headache

Between 3% and 5% of adults worldwide experience headaches daily or nearly daily (14–17).

Paradoxically, the very medications commonly used to

treat episodic headaches (including over-the-counter (OTC) analgesics and migraine-specific medications such as triptans) are implicated in the transformation of episodic to chronic headaches (18–20), especially if consumed more often than 2 days per week over several months (21). Family physicians should be aware that this is a common condition associated with a significant burden of suffering, and that effective treatment of migraine and TTH without the overuse of medication may help prevent the development of this difficult-to-treat condition.

CLINICAL EVALUATION

An important initial task for the family physician in the evaluation of a patient presenting with headache is to determine whether the patient's symptoms are a manifestation of a secondary headache. Diagnosing a secondary headache usually involves looking for and investigating red flags that may serve as clues to the etiology of the headache (see Table 45.3).

Questions that may be asked as part of the history of present illness to identify red flags include:

- Have you ever experienced a headache like this before (to establish whether the current episode represents a new onset)?
- What other symptoms or problems do you experience along with the headache (to help identify or rule out systemic illness, and to help with the diagnosis of a primary headache)?
- Are you experiencing any changes in your vision or do you have strange or uncomfortable sensations in your arms or legs or other parts of you body? (The purpose of this is to explore the possibility of a cerebral vascular accident.)

Vital signs, including temperature and blood pressure, are important elements of the physical examination of a patient with headache. An exam of the head, eyes, ears, nose, and throat (HEENT) is warranted if the history suggests vision change, ear pain, sore throat, or other symptoms in that region. Neck range of motion and palpation should be performed if the patient reports neck pain or has a fever, to evaluate for possible meningitis. The presence of fever in conjunction with headache may indicate an infectious condition, thereby necessitating a thorough physical exam. Headache is a common symptom of many infectious conditions including influenza, sinusitis, streptococcal pharyngitis, and many viral syndromes, so the source of the fever must be identified. Most importantly, a central nervous system infection must be either identified or ruled out. The neurologic exam should include a cranial nerve survey (including fundoscopic exam) and should be dedicated to looking for any focal or lateralizing signs. Palpation of the temporal artery and assessing the temporomandibular joint may provide useful clues, while evaluation of gait and looking for lateralizing weakness will help in assessing for an intracranial process such as a bleed or stroke.

Laboratory and Radiologic Testing

A systematic review of the literature published in 2000 (22) concluded that there is insufficient evidence to recommend any routine diagnostic testing (beyond a history and physical) for nonacute headache syndromes, with the possible exception of neuroimaging. Presence or absence of neurological findings on exam was the strongest predictor of an abnormal imaging study (see Table 45.4). The likelihood ratio of an abnormal imaging study in patients with a normal neurological exam is estimated at 0.7 (95% confidence interval [CI]: 0.52, 0.93), whereas the likelihood ratio of a finding a significant abnormality on an imaging study in the presence of an abnormal neurological examination is estimated to be 3.0 (95% CI: 2.3, 4.0). The authors' concluded that the decision to use neuroimaging in a patient with nonacute headache (present for at least 4 weeks) should be made on a case-by-case basis, and medical-legal considerations or alleviation of patients' anxiety may need to be factored into the decision-making process.

Other Diagnostic Tools

Inexpensive and noninvasive diagnostic tools such as headache diaries or headache questionnaires often prove more useful than laboratory or radiological tests.

A sample headache diary can be downloaded free of charge from the American Headache Society (AHS) at *http://achenet.org/resources/diary.php*. Patients may be instructed to use either a 4-point scale (0 = headache free, 3 = severe head-

---

TABLE 45.3 Red Flags Suggestive of a Secondary Cause of Headaches

Red Flag	Suggested Diagnosis
1. Sudden onset severe headache ("thunderclap" headache) 2. "Worst headache of my life" 3. Headache first occurring with exercise	Ruptured aneurysm
New onset HA after age 50	Arteritis, intracranial mass
Headache with fever, stiff neck or other systemic signs	Meningitis, encephalitis
Headache after history of trauma	Subdural hematoma
Headache with focal neurologic signs or symptoms, or papilledema	Tumor, subdural hematoma, epidural bleed
Similar, new-onset of headaches in an acquaintance or family member	Environmental exposure such as carbon monoxide

Adapted from Clinch R. Evaluation of acute headache in adults. Am Fam Physician. 2001;63:685–692.

TABLE 45.4 Signs and Symptoms that Suggest Neuroimaging May Be Indicated in Patients with Headache

Clinical Feature	Sensitivity	Specificity	LR+	LR−
Focal findings on neurologic examination	1.0	0.76	4.21	0
Abrupt onset of headache	0.55	0.79	2.5	0.57
Change or alteration in the characteristics of headache	0.67	0.67	2.0	0.49
Increased intensity and frequency of headaches	0.39	0.73	1.44	0.83
Persistence despite analgesics	0.60	0.56	1.36	0.71

Modified from Aygun D, Bildik F. Clinical warning criteria in evaluation by computed tomography the secondary neurological headaches in adults. Eur J Neurol. 2003; 10(4):437–442.

ache, normal activity is not possible) or an 11-point scale (0 = headache free, 10 = extremely severe headache) to indicate the presence and severity of headaches. Other pertinent data, such as duration of headaches, onset and duration of menstrual period and medications taken, can also be recorded on the diaries. This information may help both the patient and provider identify trends or triggers, which in turn may help prevent or treat the headaches. The two most commonly used headache questionnaires are the Migraine in Disability Scale (MIDAS) (see Figure 45.1) and the Headache Impact Test (HIT-6) (see Figure 45.2). These instruments may be used both to assess the level of disability associated with headaches at the time of initial evaluation and to monitor clinical change over time (23–25).

MANAGEMENT

The management of headache depends on the diagnosis, frequency, and surrounding circumstances. The discussion here will be geared toward primary headaches, as secondary headaches require a management plan tailored to the particular cause. Management will also be reviewed on the basis of acute (abortive) therapy, and preventive (prophylactic) therapy.

Once a primary headache diagnosis has been made, a discussion of treatment strategies can begin. Discussion points to cover may include what interventions were attempted in the past, and the patient's concerns about a given treatment. Concerns such as work impact, medication side effects, expense of treatments, etc. should be reviewed. Patients need to

Question	Number of Days
1. On how many days in the past 3 months did you miss work or school because of your headaches?	_____
2. How many days in the past 3 months was your productivity at work or school reduced by half or more because of your headaches?	_____
3. On how many days in the past 3 months did you not do household work because of your headaches?	_____
4. How many days in the past 3 months was your productivity in household work reduced by half or more because of your headaches?	_____
5. On how many days in the past 3 months did you miss family, social or non-work activities because of your headaches?	_____

Add up the numbers: there are four grades of severity for the MIDAS-
Grade I- minimal disability = 0-5
Grade II- mild or infrequent disability = 6-10
Grade III- moderate disability = 11-20
Grade IV- severe disability = 21+

Figure 45.1 • Migraine Disability Scale (MIDAS). This survey was developed by Richard B. Lipton, MD, Professor of Neurology, Albert Einstein College of Medicine, New York, NY, and Walter F. Stewart, MPH, PhD, Associate Professor of Epidemiology, Johns Hopkins University, Baltimore, MD.

1. When you have headaches, how often is the pain severe?

          Never   Rarely   Sometimes   Very Often   Always

2. How often do headaches limit your ability to do usual daily activities including household work, work, school, or social activities?

          Never   Rarely   Sometimes   Very Often   Always

3. When you have a headache, how often do you wish you could lie down?

          Never   Rarely   Sometimes   Very Often   Always

4. In the past 4 weeks, how often have you felt too tired to do work or daily activities because of your headaches?

          Never   Rarely   Sometimes   Very Often   Always

5. In the past 4 weeks, how often have you felt fed up or irritated because of your headaches?

          Never   Rarely   Sometimes   Very Often   Always

6. In the past 4 weeks, how often did headaches limit your ability to concentrate on work or daily activities?

          Never   Rarely   Sometimes   Very Often   Always

I = 6 pts each	II = 8 pts each	III = 10 pts each	IV = 11 pts each	V = 13 pts each

Scores are calculated by summing the points from each column.

KEY

60 or >	High impact on quality of life
56–59	Substantial impact on life, missing work, school or family time
50–55	Some impact, but not losing time at work or with family
49 or <	Little impact, at present

Figure 45.2 • Headache Impact Test (HIT-6).

know that others suffer similar headaches and that they are not alone in their suffering. They need to be informed that many effective treatments are available, and that there are a number of different treatment strategies from which to choose.

Migraine

Education about identifying and avoiding triggers should be the first treatment explored with the patient (see Table 45.2). Medication treatment may be "stepwise," going from basic or simplest to more complex, or "stratified," with the aim of identifying the most effective treatment, and using it as the first-line intervention (see Table 45.2) (26). Triptans are generally considered the first-line medications for moderate to severe migraine. OTC medications such as acetaminophen, aspirin, nonsteroidal anti-inflammatory drugs (NSAIDs), or combination anti-migraine drugs (which usually include caffeine) may be helpful, especially for milder episodes and when taken early. Behavioral strategies include resting in a dark, quiet place, meditation, massage, or heat or ice applied to the head or neck. Treatment in some cases may be chosen to treat symptoms, e.g., antiemetics.

Specific pain medications may be chosen to provide quick relief, (NSAIDs, barbiturate and caffeine compounds, or nar-

cotics, which are not recommended in most cases), or migraine-specific medications (ergotamines, triptans, or Isometheptene compounds) (see Tables 45.5 and 45.6). Persons suffering from two or more headaches a week may benefit from prophylactic or preventative therapies (1,38) (see Table 45.7). Migraines in children often respond well to NSAIDs such as Naproxen, ibuprofen, or aspirin, in the highest appropriate doses. Women with menstrual-related migraines also often respond well to the prostaglandin inhibition of NSAIDs.

Because of the debility of migraines for many patients, the goals of therapy for the acute episode should be clear to both the provider and the patient. They are:

- Treat the headache rapidly
- Prevent recurrence
- Provide symptom relief or at least increased level of function in two hours.
- Minimize the use of second-line drugs
- Optimize in-home care
- Minimize the utilization of healthcare resources, including hospitalization
- Minimize the adverse effects from the therapies

Stepwise care has been used in migraine treatment. Recent recommendations suggest, however, that this may not be

TABLE 45.5 Medications for Acute Migraine Therapy (35, 36, 37)

Medications	Action	Efficacy	Sample Medications and Adult Dosages	Cost*
Nonsteroidal anti-inflammatory agents (NSAIDs)	Analgesia, prostaglandin blockade	Effective in many patients; children, and women with menstrual migraines.	Ibuprofen 800 mg Naproxen OTC 375–500 mg every 8–12 hrs Toradal IM 60 mg IX	$$$
Acetaminophen	Analgesia	Effective for mild episodes, early treatment of migraines.	Tylenol 500–650 mg	$
Combinations-analgesics with caffeine or isometheptene	Analgesics, regulation of vasomotor tone.	Weak evidence for efficacy.	Midrin 1 every hr. up to 5 caps in 24 hrs. Duradrin 1 g hr. up to 5 in 24 hrs.	$$
Opiod	Analgesia	Use for acute episodes if no other therapy effective, P.O., IM, IV	Oxycodone, metochlopramide hydrocodone	$–$$$
Antiemetics	Controls nausea, may potentiate opiates or other analgesics	Adjunctive P.O., P.R., IM, IV	Promethazine Metoclopramide Zofran	$–$$
Triptans: Almotriptan Eletriptan Frovatriptan Naratriptan Rizatriptan Sumatriptan Zolmatriptan	Serotonin (5HT) receptor agonists. Actions include vasoconstriction, peripheral neuronal inhibition and inhibition of transmission through the trigeminocervical complex.	Abortive. Several routes of delivery (e.g., oral, intranasal, subcutaneous, etc.) are available. The various triptans differ in their onset and duration of action (see Table 45.6).	See Table 45.6	$$$
Ergot derivatives	Vasoconstriction, (has a long half-life, and cannot be combined with triptans or SSRIs).	Effective, but often not well tolerated because of nausea and other side effects. DHE 45	Cafergot (ergotamine/caffeine)	$$–$$$
Metoclopramide -IV		Works well IV in ER/Office		$$–$$$

*$ = <$1.00/dose; $$$ = >$10.00 per dose.

cost-effective in many cases, and may result in patients suffering for longer than is necessary. Stratified care involves a more individualized, patient-centered approach to treatment, and it takes into account the severity of the headache. The objective is to select treatment options based upon attack-related disability and patient goals. For persons whose headache pain is relieved by the early or first treatments, the stepwise approach is fine; these would be persons with mild disability from the headache. For persons reporting moderate disability, with the headache interrupting the ability to work or care for daily needs, migraine-specific therapy should be employed at headache onset. If there is not rapid improvement (within 2 hours), the person may require "rescue" treatment, including repeating a dose of a triptan, employing antiemetics (intramuscularly or per rectum), or using intramuscular ketorolac, or even opiods. Persons with a known history of severe disability with the headache attack should always start with the most effective non-addictive medications that abort the headache (26, 38, 39).

If migraine attacks are frequent, prophylaxis should be employed (1). Clinical criteria for migraine prophylaxis include:

• Headaches >2 days a week, on average
• Recurring migraines that, in the patient's opinion, significantly interfere with his or her daily routine
• Failure of, or contraindication to, acute therapies
• Patient preference
• Significant cost of acute therapies
• Presence of uncommon headache conditions including hemiplegic migraine, basilar migraine, migraine with prolonged aura or migrainous infarction

Cognitive-behavioral therapy, acupuncture, biofeedback, relaxation and stress management training also have known benefit (1, 27–29). Table 45.7 reviews prophylactic medications and the usual dosage ranges.

TABLE 45.6 Available Triptan Medications for Migraine

Drug (product name)	Halflife	Onset of Action	Dose/Route Oral, SC, etc.	Max Dose/Spacing
Sumatriptan (Imitrex)	2.5 hrs	30min–1 hr	PO, SC, or nasal	100 mg PO or 6 mg SQ/dose 200 mg PO/24 12 mg/24 SC
Naratriptan (Amerge)	6 hrs	>/=2 hrs	PO	2.5 mg/dose 5 mg/24 hrs
Zolmatriptan (Zomig)	3 hrs	< 1hr	PO, or nasal hard tablet or dissolving (ODT)	2.5–5 mg/dose; max 10 mg/24 hrs
Rizatriptan (Maxalt)	2–3 hrs	30 min–1 hr	PO hard tablet or ODT	5 mg–10 mg/dose max 30 mg/24 hrs
Eletriptan (Relpax)	4 hr, metabolite 13 hrs	30 min–1 hr	PO	20–40 mg/dose max 80 mg/24 hrs
Frovatriptan (Frova)	26 hrs	<2 hrs	PO	2.5 mg/dose max 7.5 mg /24 hrs
Almotriptan (Axert)	3–4 hrs	30 min–1 hr	PO	6.25–12.5 mg/dose max 25 mg/24 hrs

1. Most recommendations say no more than two separate 24 hour treatments per week due to risk of precipitating coronary disease.
2. Potential life-threatening, but rare side effects include: chest pain, arrhythmias, severe hypertension, stroke.
Source:
Taylor F, Hutchinson S, Graff-Radford S, Cady R, Harris L. Diagnosis and management of migraine. In Family Practice.Supplement to JFP Jan 2004
Lenaerts ME. Pharmacoprophylaxis of tension-type headache. Curr Pain Headache Rep. 2005;9(6);442–447.

Tension-Type Headache (T-TH)

T-THs tend to not be debilitating, but patients often bring them to the attention of their health care providers. Medication treatment with acetaminophen or NSAIDs has been successful (29). Complementary or alternative approaches such as nutritional supplements or acupuncture have been shown to be effective in the treatment of T-TH (30, 31), but the data about the efficacy of manipulative treatments or botox injections is ambiguous (32, 33). Prophylaxis should be considered for persons who experience 15 or more T-THs per month (34).

Cluster Headaches

Cluster headaches are infrequently seen, but are invariably debilitating. Treatment options for acute episodes include oxygen therapy (first-line treatment), triptans, ergot derivatives, and intranasal lidocaine (35). Verapamil may be used for prophylaxis (35).

CASE DISCUSSION

CASE 1

The history of patient L.S. is reassuring for a benign primary headache, but it is remotely possible that she has temporal arteritis. The differential diagnosis, given the available information about L.S., is probably limited to migraine and tension-type headache. The patient's history, combined with the observation that she is sitting in the shadows and speaks softly, indicates that L.S.'s symptoms are aggravated by light (photophobia) or loud noises (phonophobia), thereby suggesting migraine. Additional information is needed however, including the patient's description of the quality, severity, onset, length, and recurrence rate of the headache, along with associated symptoms and apparent triggers. You may also want to ask if there are external factors that make the headache worse, such as light, loud noises, or physical activity, and what alleviates the headaches, such as rest or sleep or medication. As with any initial evaluation of a new patient with headache, you would look for the presence of any red flags (see Table 45.3). If further information confirms your initial diagnosis of migraine, first-line treatment options include identifying and avoiding triggers, judicious use of OTC medications, prescription of a triptan medication, and consideration of one or more nonpharmacological interventions, such as acupuncture.

CASE 2

You don't yet know what R.B.'s cluster headaches are like, but you note that he is neurologically impaired, that he has recently fallen, and that this represents a "new and different" headache. All of these are red flags. Your differential diagnosis includes such secondary etiologies as a subdural hematoma or an intracranial lesion. You perform a focused neurological examination, including pupil size and reactivity, motor and sensory exams and gait, paying particular attention to the symmetry of the findings. Unless further history or examination effectively rules out the pos-

TABLE 45.7 Drugs Used in the Prophylaxis for Migraine Headaches

Medication	Dose	Onset of Action	Side Effects
Antidepressants: Tricyclic- Amitriptyline Nortriptyline	10–150 mg/day 10–150 mg/day	3–4 weeks (at appropriate dose)	Sedation, dry mouth, constipation
SSRI's-most	variable	" "	caution with triptans or ergotamines
Anti-convulsants:		All require titration to effect	Nausea, tremor, hair loss, VA
Valproic acid (VA) Gabapentin (GBP)	500–1500 mg/day 900–1800 mg/day	2–3 weeks 2–3 weeks-titrate to dose	Sedation-dizziness GBP Weight loss, memory (Tolpiromate)
Topiramate (T) Pregabalin (PG)	50–200 mg/day 150–300 mg/day	" "	Similar to GBP-PG
Beta-blockers: Propranolol-P Timolol-T Nadolol-N Metoprolol-M	80–240 mg/day (LA if possible) P 10 mg BID–20 mg 1x a day (T) 20–260 mg/day(N) 200 mg/day(M)	3–4 weeks (titrating up to affective dose)	Fatigue, drowsiness, may worsen asthma, impotence, may worsen depression (P)
Calcium channel blockers: Verapamil Nimodipine	120–240mg/day 40 mg BID	3–4 weeks	A-V block(verapamil), constipation, edema, hypotension
Muscle relaxants Tizanidine(zanaflex)	8 mg BID	?	Drowsiness
Botulinum toxin	25 to 75 mcg/injection	After injections	Very expensive, requires injections of trigger areas.
Opoids-long acting: Methadone Morphine controlled release Oxycodone (OxyContin)	*last resort* 5–20 mg/day 20–50 mg/day 10–20 mg (or more)/day	Titrate to effect over weeks.	Drowsiness, impairment, withdrawal symptoms after chronic use. Constipation

Source:
Taylor Frederick, Hutchinson S, Graff-Radford S, Cady R, Harris L. Diagnosis and Management of Migraine; In Family Practice.Supplement to JFP Jan 2004
Woolhouse M. Migraine and tension headache—a complementary and alternative medicine approach. Aust Fam Phys. 2005;34(8):647–651.

sibility of subdural hematoma, brain imaging (preferably CT) is indicated emergently. Laboratory testing, including a protime, is also indicated. If this patient has a subdural hematoma, he should be referred for urgent neurosurgical evaluation.

REFERENCES

1. Taylor F, Hutchinson S, Graff-Radford S, Cady R, Harris L. Diagnosis and management of migraine. J Fam Pract. 2004;(suppl):S3–S24.
2. Clinch R. Evaluation of acute headaches in adults. Am Fam Physician. 2001;63:685–692.
3. Headache Classification Committee of the International Headache Society. Classification and diagnostic criteria for headache disorders, cranial neuralgias and facial pain. Cephalalgia. 1988;8(suppl 7):1–96.
4. Martin V, Elkind A. Diagnosis and Classification of headache disorders. In Standards of Care for Headache Diagnosis and Treatment. Chicago, IL: National Headache Foundation; 2004:4–18. Available at *www.guideline.gov/summary/*.
5. Headache Classification Subcommittee of the International Headache Society. The international classification of headache disorders. Cephalalgia. 2004;24(suppl 1):1–160.
6. Jay, GW. The Headache Handbook: Diagnosis and Treatment. Boca Raton, FL: CRC Press; 1999.
7. Lipton RB, Stewart WF, Diamond S, Diamond ML, Reed M. Prevalence and burden of migraine in the United States: data from the American Migraine Study II. Headache. 2001; 41(7):646–657.
8. Pryse-Phillips W, Findlay H, Tugwell P, Edmeads J, Murray TJ, Nelson RF. A Canadian population survey on the clinical, epidemiologic and societal impact of migraine and tension-type headache. Can J Neurol Sci. 1992;19(3):333–339.
9. Lavados PM, Tenhamm E. Epidemiology of tension-type headache in Santiago, Chile: a prevalence study. Cephalalgia. 1998;18(8):552–558.
10. Lyngberg AC, Rasmussen BK, Jorgensen T, Jensen R. Has the prevalence of migraine and tension-type headache changed over a 12-year period? A Danish population survey. Eur J Epidemiol. 2005;20(3):243–249.
11. Sjaastad O, Bakketeig LS. Cluster headache prevalence. Vaga

Left margin (partially visible)

CHAPTER

Addictio

Adam O. Golds

CASE

A 51-year-old tru
physical. He has
hypertension, is 3
is borderline hig
and a full pack o
he drinks beer w
does not use any
for 25 years, has
nor children hav
died of lung ca
severe emphysen
azide. In the off
addition to perf
weight loss, disc
ance with medic
tests, you decide

CLINICAL QUESTIC

1. How should
   of this clinic
   minutes at m
2. How can yo
   dency?
3. What behavi
   natives are a
   bacco, alcoho
   tiveness and

The American S
tion as "a disease
of a specific psyc
logical, or social
tive consequence
the association, a
cians and other
While addiction
practices, eating
strategies for tre
will deal specific
tions because of
defines terms ass
stances.
More than
tobacco, alcohol.

study of h[...]
528–533.

12. Torelli P, [...]
lence in the [...]
469–74.

13. Grayson S, [...]
headache?–[...]

14. Mehle ME, [...]
otolaryngol[...]
489–496.

15. Lanteri-Mi[...]
and descrip[...]
ulation in [...]

16. Scher AI, S[...]
of frequent [...]
38:497–506.

17. Castillo J, [...]
chronic dai[...]
1999;39(3):1[...]

18. Zwart JA, [...]
use: a predi[...]
ache: the [...]
160–164.

19. Bahra A, W[...]
headache a[...]
analgesics?[...]

20. Tepper SJ. [...]
quence, of [...]
cause of c[...]
543–547.

21. Dodick D[...]
Engl J Me[...]

22. Frishberg [...]
based guid[...]
in patients [...]
www.aan.c[...]

23. Stewart W[...]
and testing [...]
Questionna[...]
ogy. 2001;5[...]

24. Headache [...]
healthy.com[...]

25. Coeytaux [...]
Four meth[...]

TABLE 47.3 Diagnostic Criteria for Post-traumatic Stress Disorder

I. The person has been exposed to a traumatic event in which both of the following were present:
   a. The person experienced, witnessed, or was confronted with an event or events that involved actual or threatened death or serious injury, or a threat to the physical integrity of self or others
   b. The person's response involved intense fear, helplessness, or horror. **Note:** In children, this may be expressed instead by disorganized or agitated behavior

II. The traumatic event is persistently re-experienced in one (or more) of the following ways:
   a. Recurrent and intrusive distressing recollections of the event, including images, thoughts, or perceptions. **Note:** In young children, repetitive play may occur in which themes or aspects of the trauma are expressed.
   b. Recurrent distressing dreams of the event. **Note:** In children, there may be frightening dreams without recognizable content.
   c. Acting or feeling as if the traumatic event were recurring (includes a sense of reliving the experience, illusions, hallucinations, and dissociative flashback episodes, including those that occur on awakening or when intoxicated). **Note:** In young children, trauma-specific reenactment may occur.
   d. Intense psychological distress at exposure to internal or external cues that symbolize or resemble an aspect of the traumatic event
   e. Physiological reactivity on exposure to internal or external cues that symbolize or resemble an aspect of the traumatic event

III. Persistent avoidance of stimuli associated with the trauma and numbing of general responsiveness (not present before the trauma), as indicated by three (or more) of the following:
   a. Efforts to avoid thoughts, feelings, or conversations associated with the trauma
   b. Efforts to avoid activities, places, or people that arouse recollections of the trauma
   c. Inability to recall an important aspect of the trauma
   d. Markedly diminished interest or participation in significant activities
   e. Feeling of detachment or estrangement from others
   f. Restricted range of affect (e.g., unable to have loving feelings)
   g. Sense of a foreshortened future (e.g., does not expect to have a career, marriage, children, or a normal life span)

IV. Persistent symptoms of increased arousal (not present before the trauma), as indicated by two (or more) of the following:
   a. Difficulty falling or staying asleep
   b. Irritability or outbursts of anger
   c. Difficulty concentrating
   d. Hypervigilance
   e. Exaggerated startle response

V. Duration of the disturbance (symptoms in Criteria B, C, and D) is more than 1 month.

VI. The disturbance causes clinically significant distress or impairment in social, occupational, or other important areas of functioning.

Reprinted with permission from the American Psychiatric Association. Diagnostic and Statistical Manual of Mental Disorders, 4th ed. Washington, DC: American Psychiatric Association; 2000.

depression. With hypertension, for example, patients who report side effects not related to the antihypertensive medications they are taking, or patients who have switched among many antihypertensives, are more likely to have anxiety, panic, or depression (16).

Discussing mental health often is difficult, and the language is unfamiliar to most patients. Physicians also should be aware that patients who tend to normalize or "explain away" their anxiety symptoms are harder to diagnose (17). Yet,

breaking through patient barriers to disclosure, and getting a thorough history is vital. Anxiety disorders seldom improve without interventions to reduce isolation. Finding a non-threatening way to broach the subject, e.g., using the terms such as "worry," "stress," or "tension" instead of anxiety, is important.

Should physicians screen all patients for mental health disorders? Although the prevalence data presented above suggest physicians underdiagnose anxiety disorders, it is unclear

TABLE 47.4 Typical Symptoms of Panic Attacks

Shortness of breath or a smothering sensation
Dizziness, unsteady feelings, or faintness
Palpitations or accelerated heart rate
Trembling or shaking
Sweating
Choking
Nausea or abdominal upset
Feeling that your body is not real
Numbness or tingling in a body part
Hot flashes or chills
Chest pain or discomfort
Fear of dying
Fear of going crazy or losing self control

Reprinted with permission from the American Psychiatric Association. Diagnostic and Statistical Manual of Mental Disorders, 4th ed. Washington, DC: American Psychiatric Association; 2000.

whether screening each patient actually improves patient outcomes. A well-done evidence-based review (Cochrane Review) of depression screening suggests general screening, with questionnaires, of all patients is not worthwhile (18); therefore, formal screening for anxiety currently lacks a consensus statement. If you choose to screen, use a few brief questions (see Table 47.5) or a brief questionnaire that screens for both anxiety and depression (19). However, until studies demonstrate the benefits of general screening in primary care, recommendations to do so are speculative.

TABLE 47.5 Effective Screening Questions for Anxiety Disorders

1. Do you ever feel anxious, stressed or fearful? (screen for generalized anxiety disorder)

2. In the past 4 weeks, have you had an anxiety attack-suddenly feeling fear or panic? (single question screen for panic disorder) (40)

3. In the past 6 months, did you ever have a spell or an attack when all of a sudden you felt frightened, anxious, or very uneasy?

   In the past 6 months, did you ever have a spell or an attack when for no reason your heart suddenly began to race, you felt faint, or you couldn't catch your breath?

   Did any of these spells or attacks ever happen in a situation when you were not in danger or not the center of attention?

   (3 question screen for panic disorder) (41).

4. Do you ever find that certain thoughts or images keep coming into your head even though you try to keep them out? (screen for obsessive compulsive disorder)

A better approach may be to screen only patients who are at high risk for developing anxiety disorders i.e., persons who have experienced a traumatic event, chronic illness, or dementia. Women who experience a stillbirth, neonatal loss, or a sudden infant death syndrome (SIDS) loss may have incidences of PTSD as high as 21% during a subsequent pregnancy (20). Refugees relocated to western countries also have higher rates of PTSD (9%) (21). Alzheimer's patients exhibit clinically significant anxiety in 25% to 75% of cases (22); in contrast, the elderly have lower overall rates of anxiety disorders than younger age groups (23). Thus, knowing your patients' background confers a great advantage in screening. Laboratory studies or imaging studies are not generally useful in screening or diagnosing anxiety disorders other than to exclude other conditions, such as hyperthyroidism.

As stated previously, many medical conditions mimic anxiety, which makes anxiety difficult to isolate during a single office visit. Accordingly, there are no easy-to-follow diagnostic algorithms. Some common conditions are listed in Table 47.6. Other conditions may cause anxiety, but treatment should be directed at the underlying condition. For example, a patient with Parkinson's disease may appear agoraphobic by avoiding public places because of embarrassment about a tremor. Many symptoms, such as dyspnea, chest pain, and palpitations directly overlap with panic symptoms. Physicians must examine these and other symptoms appropriately while simultaneously considering anxiety. Red flags for patients needing separate or concurrent evaluation and treatment for other conditions are shown in Table 47.7. The importance of follow up in the evaluation of anxiety cannot be overstated.

MANAGEMENT

Figure 47.1 shows one approach to managing anxiety disorders. It is important to recognize comorbidities that warrant treatment prior to or concurrently with treatment of anxiety. Alcoholism is one common example, as alcohol abuse often accompanies anxiety disorders. Even if patients are self-medicating their anxiety symptoms with alcohol, they should be referred for standard alcohol treatment before or during

TABLE 47.6 Medical Conditions that Mimic Anxiety

Hyperthyroidism
Menopause
Cardiac arrythmias
Asthma
Angina
Transient ischemic attacks
Alcohol withdrawal
Medication side effects
Substance abuse
Neurologic disorders
Stuttering
Bipolar Disorder
Attention Deficit Hyperactivity Disorder
Bulimia

TABLE 47.7 Clinical Red Flags Suggesting a Serious Additional Problem in Patients Presenting with a Suspected Anxiety Disorder

Suicidality
Alcohol abuse
Substance abuse
Sexual/ physical abuse
Bulimia/ anorexia
Weight loss
Syncope
Focal, persistent weakness
Neurologic physical exam findings
Hallucinations—although reliving experiences in post-traumatic stress disorder can be very vivid
Delusions
Developmental delay

is important. Common features of anxiety management are described below, and therapies unique to individual disorders are provided under specific subject headings.

One key element of treatment for any anxiety disorder is effective patient education. This includes:

- Suggesting the possibility as part of a differential diagnosis
- Explaining the illness using terms and mechanisms that make sense to the patient
- Describing the course, prognosis, effectiveness, and side effects of therapy
- Providing written resources, such as those available at *http://www.nimh.nih.gov/health*

Antidepressants alone are highly effective in reducing symptoms and improving quality of life, with selective serotonin reuptake inhibitors (SSRIs) and tricyclic antidepressants (TCAs) generally showing equal efficacy. Each class of antidepressant has side effects, and patients' tolerance of any therapy may vary. Therefore, a follow-up appointment to assess for side effects is important. Patients should generally stay on an antidepressant for 6 months after the reduction of symptoms and be followed closely for recurrence after stopping antidepressants. Regarding children, both sertraline and fluvoxamine have been shown to improve anxiety scores in children ages 6–17 with severe anxiety or OCD; however, decisions to start children on psychoactive medications typically warrant consultation with a specialist.

Benzodiazepines are effective in all anxiety disorders and should be used to stabilize patients over the short-term. Symptoms such as extreme agitation or insomnia are reasonable indications for benzodiazepines. Although long-term studies have shown that they are effective at reducing anxiety symptoms, benzodiazepines have long-term side effects (e.g., addic-

anxiety treatment (24). Sexual or physical abuse is another situation that requires a separate intervention to ensure safety while initiating anti-anxiety therapy. All patients with suspected anxiety should be asked about suicidal thoughts or plans.

Table 47.8 describes treatment options for each disorder and provides an evidence rating for each option. The therapeutic options for all anxiety disorders are remarkably similar, suggesting common pathophysiologic mechanisms. Therefore, the initial management choices in anxiety disorders are fairly straightforward for family physicians, unless one wants to develop skills in providing cognitive-behavioral therapy (CBT). Patient choice in determining which therapy to use

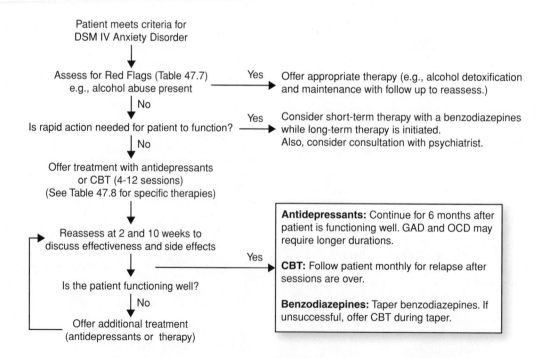

Figure 47.1 • General algorithm for the management of anxiety disorders.

TABLE 47.8 Key Therapies for Treating Anxiety Disorders

Condition and Intervention	Efficacy	Strength of Recommendation*
Generalized Anxiety Disorder		
Antidepressants	Reduce anxiety symptoms (NNT 5) compared to placebo.	A
Anxiolytics	Benzodiazepines and buspirone effective in reducing anxiety measures compared to placebo.	B
Cognitive Behavioral Therapy (CBT)	Effective in reducing anxiety measures compared to control groups. More effective than benzodiazepines in improving depression measures.	B
Herbal	Kava extract effective but safety concerns limit use. Other herbals studied but not proven effective.	B
Alternative	Acupuncture, massage, dance therapy, exercise, meditation are mildly effective.	B
Panic Disorder		
CBT	Improves global functioning.	B
Antidepressants	SSRIs and TCAs appear equally efficacious.	A
Benzodiazepines	Reduce panic severity.	A
Self-Help Videos & Books	These reduce panic severity when used with at least minimal (1–2 session) therapist contact.	B
Exercise	Exercise reduces panic severity, but not as well as antidepressants.	B
Social Anxiety Disorder		
Beta Blockers for Performance Anxiety	Effective for subclinical "performance anxiety" but less evidence for use in true social anxiety disorder.	B
CBT	CBT with exposure or cognitive restructuring reduces distress and avoidant behavior.	B
Antidepressants	SSRIs superior to placebo.	B
Specific Phobias		
Benzodiazepines	Recommended for stabilization of symptoms if necessary.	C
Antidepressants	Pilot studies of sertraline and paroxetine suggest effectiveness.	C
CBT	Reduces phobic response.	C
Post-Traumatic Stress Disorder and Acute Stress Disorder		
Psychotherapy after event	No proven benefit.	B
CBT	Reduces disability for 6 months.	B
Antidepressants	Effective at reducing symptoms compared to placebo.	A
Benzodiazepines	Effective compared to placebo. Use for stabilization (insomnia, agitation) and progress to other therapies.	B
Obsessive Compulsive Disorder (OCD)		
Antidepressants	Both SSRIs and TCAs (clomipramine) are effective compared to placebo.	B
CBT	CBT especially using exposure techniques is effective at reducing symptoms in >80% of patients.	B
Sertraline in children	Improves OCD rating scales (NNT 6 vs. placebo).	B

NNT, number needed to treat; SSRIs, selective serotonin reuptake inhibitors; TCAs, tricyclic antidepressants.

*A = consistent, good-quality patient-oriented evidence; B = inconsistent or limited-quality patient-oriented evidence; C = consensus, disease-oriented evidence, usual practice, expert opinion, or case series. For information about the SORT evidence rating system, see *http://www.aafp.org/afpsort.xml*.

tion, increased risk of falls, domestic violence) that make them inferior to CBT and antidepressants in improving overall patient quality of life, decreasing disability, and in measures of comorbid depression. Family physicians often prescribe benzodiazepines frequently for insomnia, agitation, and other anxieties; however, the goal should be to transition to a better long-term therapy. For patients on benzodiazepines, imipramine and buspirone are effective (number needed to treat (NNT) = 2) as adjuvant therapy during a successful benzodiazepine taper (25).

Family physicians may wish to refer patients with anxiety disorders to a therapist. Most children merit referral. In adults, there is evidence to support the benefits of 9–12 sessions with a therapist skilled in CBT for panic disorder, GAD, specific phobias, social anxiety disorder, OCD, and PTSD. It is important to distinguish CBT from generally supportive psychotherapy, which is less effective in anxiety disorders. Although long-term data are lacking as to whether CBT is more effective with or without simultaneous treatment with antidepressants, it is reasonable to combine CBT with antidepressant treatment. For patients who are having a difficult time weaning off antidepressants or benzodiazepines, CBT is an effective way to continue anxiety remission while tapering medications. CBT is especially useful in patients intolerant of medications; it should, therefore, be considered for elderly patients (23).

GAD

It is difficult to know which antidepressant should be first-line treatment for GAD without information from direct comparison trials; however, the antidepressants shown in Table 47.9 have been well studied (26). Benzodiazepines (alprazolam and clonazepam) are useful for stabilization and may be used long-term, however, transition to other therapies such as CBT has been shown to be more effective. The anxiolytic buspirone is of equal or superior efficacy compared to benzodiazepines for GAD (27, 28). Small studies have found that several alternative therapies, such as exercise, acupuncture, massage, dance therapy, and meditation, are moderately effective (29). Because GAD often is chronic, lifestyle changes, including diet and exercise, should be recommended. The herbal supplement "kava root extract" has been shown effective compared to

TABLE 47.9 Effective Medications and Doses in Anxiety Disorders

Drug	Contraindications/Cautions/Adverse Effects	Dosage	Cost per Course $*
Selective Serotonin Reuptake Inhibitors			
Citalopram	Avoid with monoamine oxidase inhibitors (MAOIs), decreased libido	20–60 mg daily	$$
Escitalopram	Same as citalopram	10–20 mg daily	$$
Fluoxetine**	Same as for citalopram	10–60 mg daily	$
Fluvoxamine**	Same as for citalopram	50–300 mg daily	$$
Paroxetine**	Same as for citalopram	10–60 mg daily	$
Sertraline**	Same as for citalopram	25–200 mg daily	$$
Selective Norepinephrine Reuptake Inhibitors			
Venlafaxine	Same as above, plus nausea and risk of increased blood pressure	37.5–150 mg daily	$$
Benzodiazepines			
Alprazolam	Alcohol intoxication, sleep apnea, substance abuse, withdrawal seizures	0.25–0.5 two to three times daily	$
Clonazepam	Same as for alprazolam	0.25–0.5 two times daily	$
Tricyclic Antidepressants			
Clomipramine**	Same as for imipramine	Start 25 mg and increase to 150–250 mg daily	$$
Imipramine	Avoid in heart block, cardiovascular disease, glaucoma, prostatic hypertrophy, and urinary retention	Start 25 mg and increase to 75–150 daily	$
Miscellaneous Anti-anxiety Agent			
Buspirone	Decreased clearance in renal and liver disease, avoid with MAOIs	7.5–30 mg twice daily	$$

*$ = <$33, $$ = $34–$66, $$$ = >$67.
**Doses may be higher in obsessive-compulsive disorder.

placebo (30); however, safety concerns limit any conclusions about this therapy.

Panic Disorder

As shown in Table 47.9, SSRIs and TCAs are effective antidepressants and have been well studied. There are no clear indications as to which antidepressant works most effectively, and the side effect profile should be considered when selecting which antidepressant to use. TCAs and benzodiazepines may be less well tolerated in the elderly. CBT remains an effective therapy alone or in combination with antidepressants or benzodiazepines; CBT may, in fact, offer the best chance at long-term remission from panic attacks. In patients with non-cardiac chest pain, for example, CBT reduces severity and occurrences of pain (31). In addition to the therapies mentioned for anxiety disorders, self-help books and videos should be considered as options for panic disorder. Where referral options to therapists skilled in CBT are limited, it appears that self-help treatment is effective, but only when combined with at least 1 or 2 face-to-face or telephone sessions with a therapist. Self-help treatment, however, is a good option for patients needing to travel long distances for therapy. (32).

PTSD and Acute Stress Disorder

The goal of treatment in PTSD and acute stress disorder (ASD), as with other anxiety disorders, is stabilization and decreased dysfunction. What to do after a traumatic event is unclear. American Psychiatric Association guidelines recommend psychological debriefing; however, a Cochrane Review of the literature did not show any benefit in psychological morbidity, depression, or anxiety (33). In the immediate crisis setting, after addressing medical stabilization, safety, food, shelter, clothing and family support concerns, physicians may treat anxiety symptoms with pharmacotherapy, psychotherapy, or both. CBT beginning 2–3 weeks after the trauma exposure may speed recovery and prevent PTSD (34).

The most important initial intervention after trauma and stabilization may be to arrange follow up to evaluate for a stress disorder. Once a diagnosis of ASD or PTSD is made, benzodiazepines and antidepressants, such as SSRIs and TCAs, have been shown to be effective first-line agents in doses equivalent to those used in other anxiety disorders (35). Antipsychotic or mood stabilizing medications may be helpful as second-line agents or for patients with comorbid psychotic disorders. CBT is also effective at reducing anxiety symptoms in PTSD and ASD.

OCD

Antidepressants such as SSRIs and TCAs are effective compared to placebo in treating OCD. Of the SSRIs, fluvoxamine, sertraline, and fluoxetine have been extensively studied, and among TCAs, clomipramine has been studied the most in randomized-controlled trials. The doses of antidepressants needed to treat OCD appear higher than those used with depression or other anxiety disorders (36). Antidepressants appear more effective than benzodiazepines, although alprazolam has been shown highly effective compared to placebo. Referral of patients for 10–12 weeks of CBT, particularly with a therapist skilled in exposure and response prevention techniques, also is effective. It is reasonable to combine antidepressants with CBT, although, long-term data on which ther-

apy best maintains remission are lacking. Because this disorder can present during adolescence, physicians may initiate sertraline, which has been shown effective in patients aged 6–16 (37). Consultation with a psychiatrist is highly recommended before starting any psychotropic medications in children.

Social Anxiety Disorder

Therapies for social anxiety disorder (see Table 47.8) improve measures of anxiety and social functioning. CBT using exposure techniques in particular improves patients' distress and avoidant behavior. Combining CBT with antidepressants does not appear to add benefit when compared to psychotherapy or antidepressants alone. SSRIs appear effective both short- and long-term (treatment for at least one year is recommended) (38). Benzodiazepines are effective anxiolytics for social anxiety disorder. Buspirone has not been shown to be any more effective than placebo (39). It should be noted that, although not necessarily meeting the criteria for social anxiety disorder, "performance anxiety" may respond to beta-blockers (38).

Specific Phobias

It is unclear whether specific phobias are the exception to the rule suggested above that all anxiety disorders usually respond to the same therapies. CBT (with exposure technique) is effective in both adults and children and is the mainstay of therapy for debilitating specific phobias. Data on antidepressants are largely limited to pilot studies. However, pilot data from small trials show promise that antidepressants may also be broadly effective (2).

LONG-TERM MONITORING

There is no long-term evidence to suggest whether one particular therapy is better than another at maintaining remission in GAD. There are some data showing CBT is effective in preventing panic disorder relapse for up to 2 years. Until long-term data are available, follow up at 3–6 month intervals, especially during periods of stress, to evaluate for relapse is warranted. Patients should be familiar with the signs and symptoms that indicate that anxiety is returning. CBT may be more effective than other treatments at sustaining remission because symptom education is part of the therapy. When patients discontinue anti-anxiety medication, they should be followed up by a physician within 2 months of stopping treatment to assess for symptoms. All follow-up visits provide opportunities to educate patients about relapse symptoms and therapeutic options.

CASE DISCUSSIONS

1. It is difficult to tell that this patient is having panic attacks, but the patient meets the criteria. Cardiac ischemia should be considered and fully explored. However, as many as 17%–25% of patients presenting with chest pain in the ED have panic disorder and initiating early consultation or starting anti-anxiety therapy benefits these patients. Advising the patient that "There is also a possibility that

stress is a factor in your chest pain" is a nonthreatening way of broaching the subject of anxiety. Briefly asking about life stressors or past experiences may engage the patient in this idea. Suggesting antidepressants or benzodiazepines by asking the patient "Are you willing to try . . ." in addition to the cardiac workup and ongoing follow up may dramatically improve this patient's quality of life.

2. Knowing when bereavement progresses to a mood disorder is difficult. Stabilization and assessment for suicidality are the mainstays of treatment, until a full assessment can be made. For patients exhibiting anxious symptoms such as insomnia, restlessness, or irritability, short- acting anxiolytics, such as alprazolam, are reasonable options; follow up by phone or in the office should occur within a few days.

3. This case initially appears to involve a patient whose anxiety is related to mammography, which, while treatable, is not a disorder. Yet anxious patients often initially present with plausible reasons for worry (what will the mammogram find?), but further questioning elicits the diagnosis. In this case, missing a week of work once a year is out of proportion to the event, and should trigger other questions. Many patients who worry about mammograms will not fall neatly into a DSM-IV box. However, in this case, the patient's broad pattern of worry is the hallmark of generalized anxiety disorder.

REFERENCES

1. Weissman MM, Klerman GL, Markowitz JS, Ouellette R. Suicidal ideation and suicide attempts in panic disorder and attacks. N Engl J Med. 1989;32:1209–1214.
2. Barlow DH, Esler JL, Vitali AE. Psychosocial treatments for panic disorders, phobias, and generalized anxiety disorder. In: Nathan PE, Gorman JM, eds. A Guide to Treatments that Work. New York, NY: Oxford University Press; 1998: 288.
3. Abramowitz JS. Effectiveness of psychological and pharmacological treatments for obsessive-compulsive disorder: a quantitative review. J Consult Clin Psychol. 1997;65(1):44–52.
4. Karno M, Golding JM, Sorenson SB, Burnam, MA. The epidemiology of obsessive-compulsive disorder in five US communities. Arch Gen Psychiatry. 1988;45:1094–1099.
5. Lepine JP. The epidemiology of anxiety disorders: prevalence and societal costs. J Clin Psychiatry. 2002;63(Suppl 14):4–8.
6. Roy-Byrne PP, Wagner A. Primary care perspectives on generalized anxiety disorder. J Clin Psychiatry. 2004;65(Suppl 13):20–26.
7. Allgulander C, Nilsson B. A nationwide study in primary health care: One out of four patients suffers from anxiety and depression. Lakartidningen. 2003;100(10):832–838.
8. Strine TW, Chapman DP, Kobau R, Balluz L. Associations of self-reported anxiety symptoms with health-related quality of life and health behaviors. Soc Psychiatry Psychiatr Epidemiol. 2005;40(6): 432–438.
9. Strine TW, Chapman DP, Kobau R, Balluz L, Mokdad AH. Depression, anxiety, and physical impairments and quality of life in the U.S. noninstitutionalized population. Psychiatr Serv. 2004;55(12):1408–1413.
10. Yingling KW, Wulsin LR, Arnold LM, Rouan GW. Estimated prevalences of panic disorder and depression among consecutive patients seen in an emergency department with chest pain. J Gen Intern Med. 1993;8(5):231–235.
11. Fleet RP, Dupuis G, Marchand A, Burelle D, Arsenault A, Beitman BD. Panic disorder in emergency department chest

pain patients: prevalence, comorbidity, suicidal ideation, and physician recognition. Am J Med. 1996;101:371–380.
12. Mikkelsen RL, Middelboe T, Pisinger C, Stage KB. Anxiety and depression in patients with chronic obstructive pulmonary disease (COPD). Nord J Psychiatry. 2004;58(1):65–70.
13. Kunik ME, Roundy K, Veazey C. Souchek J, Richardson P, Wray NP, Stanley MA. Surprisingly high prevalence of anxiety and depression in chronic breathing disorders. Chest. 2005;127(4): 1205–1211.
14. McNaughton-Collins M, Fowler FJ, Caubet JF, et al. Psychological effects of a suspicious prostate cancer screening test followed by a benign biopsy result. Am J Med. 2004;117: 719–725.
15. Rimer BK, Bluman LG. The psychosocial consequences of mammography. J Natl Cancer Inst Monogr. 1997;22:131–138.
16. Davies SJC. Drug intolerance due to non specific adverse affects related to psychiatric morbidity in hypertensive patients. Arch Intern Med. 2003;163:592–600.
17. Kessler D, Lloyd K, Lewis G, Gray DP. Cross sectional study of symptom attribution recognition of depression and anxiety in primary care. BMJ. 1999; 318:436–440.
18. Gilbody S, House AO, Sheldon TA. Screening and case finding instruments for depression. Cochrane Database Syst Rev. 2005;4:CD002792.
19. Spitzer RL, Kroenke K, Williams JBW. Validation and utility of a self-report version of PRIME-MD. The PHQ primary care study. JAMA. 1999;282:1737–1744.
20. Boyle FM, Vance JC, Najman JM, et al. The mental health impact of stillbirth, neonatal death or SIDS: prevalence and patterns of distress among mothers. Soc Sci Med. 1996;43: 1273–1282.
21. Fazel M, Wheeler J, Danesh J. Prevalence of serious mental disorder in 7000 refugees resettled in western countries: a systematic review. Lancet. 2005;365(9467):1309–1314.
22. Porter VR, Buxton WJ, Fairbanks LA, Strickland T, O'Connor SM, Rosenberg-Thompson S, et al. Frequency and characteristics of anxiety among patients with Alzheimer's disease and related dementias. J Neuropsychiatry Clin Neurosci. 2003;15:180–186.
23. Nordhus IH, Pallesen S. Psychological treatment of late-life anxiety: an empirical review. J Consult Clin Psychol. 2003; 71(4):643–651.
24. Bowen R, D'Arcy C, Keegan D and Senthilselvan A. A controlled trial of cognitive behavioral treatment of panic in alcoholic patients with comorbid panic disorder. Addict Behav. 2000;25(4):593–597.
25. Rickels K, DeMartinia N, Garcia-Espana F, Greenblatt DJ, Mandos LA, Rynn M. Imipramine and buspirone in treatment of patients with generalized anxiety disorder who are discontinuing long-term benzodiazepine therapy. Am J Psychiatry. 2000;157:1973–1979.
26. Kapczinski F, Lima MS, Souza JS, Schmitt R. Antidepressants for generalized anxiety disorder. Cochrane Database of Syst Rev. 2003;2:CD003592.
27. Mahe V, Balogh A. Long-term pharmacological treatment of generalized anxiety disorder. Int Clin Psychopharmacol. 2000;15(2):99–105.
28. Gould RA, Otto MW, Pollack MH, Yap L. Cognitive behavioral and pharmacologic treatment of generalized anxiety disorder: a preliminary meta-analysis. Behav Ther. 1997;28: 285–305.
29. Jorm AF, Christensen H, Griffiths KM, Parslow RA, Rodgers B, Blewitt KA. Effectiveness of complementary and self-help treatments for anxiety disorders. Med J Aust. 2004;181: s29–s46.
30. Pittler MH, Ernst E. Kava extract for treating anxiety (Coch-

rane Review). In: The Cochrane Library. Chichester, UK: John Wiley and Sons, Ltd; 2004:Issue 2.

31. Kisely S, Campbell LA, Skerritt P. Psychological interventions of non-specific chest pain in patients with normal coronary anatomy (Cochrane Review). In: The Cochrane Library. Chichester, UK: John Wiley and Sons, Ltd; 2004:Issue 2.

32. Bower P, Richards D, Lovell K. The clinical and cost-effectiveness of self-help treatments for anxiety and depressive disorders in primary care: a systematic review. Br J Gen Pract. 2001;51(471):838–845.

33. Rose S, Bisson J, Wessely S. Psychological debriefing for preventing post traumatic stress disorder (PTSD) (Cochrane Review). In: The Cochrane Library, Chichester, UK: John Wiley and Sons, Ltd; 2004: Issue 2.

34. American Psychiatric Association—Practice Guideline for the Treatment of Patients with Acute Stress Disorder and Posttraumatic Stress Disorder. Arlington, VA: American Psychiatric Association; 2004. Available at *www.psych.org/ psych_pract/treatg/pg/prac_guide.cfm.*

35. Stein DJ. Pharmacotherapy for posttraumatic stress disorder (PTSD) (Cochrane Review). In: The Cochrane Library. Chichester, UK: John Wiley and Sons, Ltd; 2004:Issue 2.

36. Eddy MF, Walbroehl GS. Recognition and treatment of obsessive-compulsive disorder. Am Fam Physician. 57(7): 1623–1628.

37. March JA. Sertraline in children and adolescents with obsessive-compulsive disorder. A multicenter randomized controlled trial. JAMA. 1998;280:1752–1756.

38. Stein DJ, Ipser JC, Balkom AJ. Pharmacotherapy for social phobia. Cochrane Database Syst Rev. 2004;4: CD001206.

39. Stravynski A, Greenberg D. The treatment of social phobia: a critical assessment. Acta Psychiatr Scand. 1998;98(3): 171–181.

40. Lowe B, Grafe K, Zipfel S, et al. Detecting panic disorder in medical and psychosomatic outpatients: comparative validation of the Hospital Anxiety and Depression Scale, the Patient Health Questionnaire, a screening question, and the physician's diagnosis. J Psychosom Res. 2003;55:515–519.

41. Stein MB, Roy-Byrne PP, McQuaid JR, et al. Development of a brief diagnostic screen for panic disorder in primary care. Psychosom Med. 1999;61:359–364.

CHAPTER 48

Depression

Donald E. Nease, Jr.

CASE

J.F. is a 51-year-old woman who presents with an acute complaint of depression and a request for treatment. She relates that her live-in boyfriend of 15 years moved out 5 days ago, severing the relationship because of another woman. This separation resulted in not only emotional but also financial distress, as her former boyfriend had assisted with mortgage payments on J.F.'s home. J.F.'s daughter accompanies her to the physician's visit and expresses a great deal of concern about her mother's emotional state. She is under the impression that her mother is suffering from depression.

On questioning, J.F. has experienced a marked decrease in her appetite, is sleeping poorly, and has missed several days of work because of emotional distress. She denies suicidal thoughts. Her medical history is negative for any mental health disorders, and she has never taken psychotropic medication, received mental health counseling, or tried any herbal products for emotional distress. She has no history of alcohol use or any other substance abuse. She has no chronic medical problems other than occasional seasonal allergies that she manages with loratadine on an as-needed basis. Family history is also negative for mental health disorders.

You defer the physical examination, noting in her record that she has a cheerful affect, somewhat pressured speech, and thought patterns that are clear and not disordered. She shows no evidence of tearfulness.

The working diagnosis is acute grief reaction or adjustment reaction with depressed mood. Lorazepam 1 mg three times daily is prescribed, with a 2-week supply, and she is scheduled for follow-up in 3 days.

At her follow-up visit, J.F. reports that she is doing much better. She has been taking 1/2 to 1 tablet three times daily, and reports greatly increased ability to cope with her emotions as a result. Sleep has improved; she has been attending work without difficulty; and she has applied for a home equity loan to assist with short-term finances. You assess her to be improving steadily and ask to see her for follow-up in 1 week. J.F. follows up 11 days later, because of scheduling difficulties, and reports continued improvement. She admits to one crying episode per day but denies any other depressive symptoms. You broach the possibility of counseling, which J.F. agrees to consider. Follow-up plans are made for 2 weeks.

J.F. follows up 3 weeks later, a month and a half after her separation from her boyfriend. At this visit, there is evidence of marked tearfulness, depressed affect, and inability to think positively about the future. J.F. expresses a great deal of concern that she is no longer getting better and in fact seems to be getting worse. She is again having difficulty maintaining her composure at work and has problems with sleep. There are no thoughts of suicide, but feelings of worthlessness are beginning to manifest.

A change in diagnosis is made to major depressive disorder (MDD). She is prescribed sertraline at 50 mg/d, and a counseling referral is initiated. She follows up in 1 week, and the sertraline is increased to 100 mg/d.

Three weeks later, J.F. reports improvement in her depressive symptoms, and her therapist reports improvement in her coping skills. She continues on sertraline and sees her therapist every other week for another 2 months.

CLINICAL QUESTIONS

1. Why not agree with the patient and make the diagnosis of depression at the first visit?
2. What enabled the family physician to revise the diagnosis at follow-up?
3. Should the patient have been maintained longer on the starting dose of the antidepressant to give her more of an chance to respond?

The various depressive or mood disorders that present in individuals are defined by diagnostic criteria set forth in the *Diagnostic and Statistical Manual of Mental Disorders* (DSM) of the American Psychiatric Association (1). The most common are listed in Tables 48-1 through 48-5.

Major Depressive Disorder

Major depressive disorder (MDD) is a chronic, relapsing illness and causes significant impairment in patients who experience the illness. Initial episodes often occur in adolescence, although MDD sometimes first occurs late in life. Periods of MDD exacerbation are marked by anhedonia, feelings of failure, inability to think positively about current life events or the future, and suicidal thoughts. Both genetic and environmental influences increase an individual's risk of MDD (2). Periods of remission can last years, during which patients lead normal lives; stressful life events have been associated with relapse (3, 4).

Mood Disorder Secondary to a General Medical Condition

Many chronic medical conditions have a significant impact on patients' affect and sense of well-being. Patients who have

TABLE 48.1 Diagnostic Criteria for Major Depression

<u>Criteria for an Episode of Major Depression</u>

A. Five (or more) of the following symptoms have been present during the same 2-week period and represent a change from previous functioning; at least one of the symptoms is either (1) depressed mood or (2) loss of interest or pleasure.
   Note: Do not include symptoms that are clearly due to a general medical condition, or mood-incongruent delusions or hallucinations.

   (1) depressed mood most of the day, nearly every day, as indicated by either subjective report (e.g., feels sad or empty) or observation made by others (e.g., appears tearful).
      Note: In children and adolescents, can be irritable mood.
   (2) markedly diminished interest or pleasure in all, or almost all, activities most of the day, nearly every day (as indicated by either subjective account or observation made by others)
   (3) significant weight loss when not dieting or weight gain (e.g., a change of more than 5% of body weight in a month), or decrease or increase in appetite nearly every day. **Note:** In children, consider failure to make expected weight gains.
   (4) insomnia or hypersomnia nearly every day
   (5) psychomotor agitation or retardation nearly every day (observable by others, not merely subjective feelings of restlessness or being slowed down)
   (6) fatigue or loss of energy nearly every day
   (7) feelings of worthlessness or excessive or inappropriate guilt (which may be delusional) nearly every day (not merely self-reproach or guilt about being sick)
   (8) diminished ability to think or concentrate, or indecisiveness, nearly every day (either by subjective account or as observed by others)
   (9) recurrent thoughts of death (not just fear of dying), recurrent suicidal ideation without a specific plan, or a suicide attempt or a specific plan for committing suicide

B. The symptoms do not meet criteria for a mixed Episode.

C. The symptoms cause clinically significant distress or impairment in social, occupational, or other important areas of functioning.

D. The symptoms are not due to the direct physiological effects of a substance (e.g., a drug of abuse, a medication) or a general medical condition (e.g., hypothyroidism).

E. The symptoms are not better accounted for by Bereavement, i.e., after the loss of a loved one, the symptoms persist for longer than 2 months or are characterized by marked functional impairment, morbid preoccupation with worthlessness, suicidal ideation, psychotic symptoms, or psychomotor retardation.

<u>Criteria for 296.2x: Major Depressive Disorder, Single Episode</u>

A. Presence of a single Major Depressive Episode

B. The Major Depressive Episode is not better accounted for by Schizoaffective Disorder and is not superimposed on Schizophrenia, Schizophreniform Disorder, Delusional Disorder, or Psychotic Disorder Not Otherwise Specified.

C. There has never been a Manic Episode, a Mixed Episode, or a Hypomanic Episode.
   Note: This exclusion does not apply if all of the manic-like, mixed-like, or hypomanic-like episodes are substance or treatment-induced or are due to the direct physiological effects of a general medical condition.

<u>Criteria for 296.3x: Major Depressive Disorder, Recurrent</u>

A. Presence of two or more Major Depressive Episodes.
   Note: To be considered separate episodes, there must be an interval of at least 2 consecutive months in which criteria are not met for a Major Depressive Episode.

B. The Major Depressive Episodes are not better accounted for by Schizoaffective Disorder and are not superimposed on Schizophrenia, Schizophreniform Disorder, Delusional Disorder, or Psychotic Disorder Not Otherwise Specified.

C. There has never been a Manic Episode, a Mixed Episode, or a Hypomanic Episode.
   Note: This exclusion does not apply if all of the manic-like, mixed-like, or hypomanic-like episodes are substance- or treatment-induced or are caused by the direct physiological effects of a general medical condition.

TABLE 48.2   Diagnostic Criteria for Dysthymic Disorder

A. Depressed mood for most of the day, for more days than not, as indicated either by subjective account or observation by others, for at least 2 years.
   Note: In children and adolescents, mood can be irritable, and duration must be at least 1 year.

B. Presence, while depressed, of two (or more) of the following:
   (1) poor appetite or overeating
   (2) insomnia or hypersomnia
   (3) low energy or fatigue
   (4) low self-esteem
   (5) poor concentration or difficulty making decisions
   (6) feelings of hopelessness

C. During the 2-year period (1 year for children or adolescents) of the disturbance, the person has never been without the symptoms in Criteria A and B for more than 2 months at a time.

D. No Major Depressive Episode has been present during the first 2 years of the disturbance (1 year for children and adolescents); i.e., the disturbance is not better accounted for by chronic Major Depressive Disorder, or Major Depressive Disorder, In Partial Remission.
   Note: There may have been a previous Major Depressive Episode provided there was a full remission (no significant signs or symptoms for 2 months) before development of the Dysthymic Disorder. In addition, after the initial 2 years (1 year in children or adolescents) of Dysthymic Disorder, there may be superimposed episodes of Major Depressive Disorder, in which case both diagnoses may be given when the criteria are met for a Major Depressive Episode.

E. There has never been a Manic Episode, a Mixed Episode, or a Hypomanic Episode, and criteria have never been met for Cyclothymic Disorder.

F. The disturbance does not occur exclusively during the course of a chronic Psychotic Disorder, such as Schizophrenia or Delusional Disorder.

G. The symptoms are not due to the direct physiological effects of a substance (e.g., a drug of abuse, a medication) or a general medical condition (e.g., hypothyroidism).

H. The symptoms cause clinically significant distress or impairment in social, occupational, or other important areas of functioning.

recently suffered a myocardial infarction, stroke, trauma, hospitalization, or a diagnosis of cancer are at risk for developing depression. This depression can present in the same way as MDD, and is often difficult to distinguish from a primary depressive disorder. Although improvement of the underlying medical condition may be enough to resolve the depressive symptoms, specific treatment of the depressive symptoms is often needed.

Dysthymia

This disorder is generally less severe than MDD, yet is more resistant to treatment. Patients with dysthymia experience a persistent, chronic depressed mood that is less likely to be relieved by periods of remission or by antidepressant treatment.

Bipolar Disorder, Type II

Bipolar disorder appears to be more common in primary care than previously had been reported; a higher prevalence of the disorder has been seen in recent reports from primary care samples (5, 6). Bipolar type II disorder is easy to overlook, as it only requires the presence of one hypomanic episode along with features of an MDD diagnosis.

Seasonal Patterns

The most recent revision of the DSM, DSM IV-TR (the primary care version), has subsumed the diagnosis of seasonal affective disorder (SAD) under the "Seasonal Pattern Specifier" designation within MDD and bipolar disorder. A seasonal pattern should be suspected when patients present with depressive symptoms during winter months in regions that experience a marked decrease in ambient light during the winter. Symptoms of hypersomnia, hyperphagia, and psychomotor slowing are part of the symptom complex. A history of remission during the summer months is helpful in making the diagnosis. These patients often respond to high-intensity light therapy; therefore, pharmacologic treatment is reserved for cases that are severe or are resistant to phototherapy.

PUBLIC HEALTH SIGNIFICANCE

Depression is highly prevalent within the general population. Annually, 9.5 percent of adults will experience mood disorders, 6.7 percent will experience MDD, and 2.6 percent will experience bipolar disorders (7). Depression has a high impact

TABLE 48.3 Diagnostic Criteria for Mood Disorder Due to . . . [Indicate the General Medical Condition]

A. A prominent and persistent disturbance in mood predominates in the clinical picture and is characterized by either (or both) of the following:

  (1) depressed mood or markedly diminished interest or pleasure in all, or almost all, activities

  (2) elevated, expansive, or irritable mood

B. There is evidence from the history, physical examination, or laboratory findings that the disturbance is the direct physiological consequence of a general medical condition, such as myocardial infarction, stroke, or cancer.

C. The disturbance is not better accounted for by another mental disorder (e.g., Adjustment Disorder With Depressed Mood in response to the stress of having a general medical condition).

D. The disturbance does not occur exclusively during the course of a delirium.

E. The symptoms cause clinically significant distress or impairment in social, occupational, or other important areas of functioning.

on patient well-being and function, including an estimated $26.1 billion in direct medical costs and $51.5 billion in workplace costs in the year 2000 (8). There also is increasing evidence of depression's impact as a comorbid condition on other chronic medical conditions such as coronary artery disease and diabetes (9–11).

Depressive disorders continue to rank among the top ten diagnoses given by family physicians in patients aged 18–65 according to the 2002 National Ambulatory Medical Care Survey (12). Prevalence estimates of depression within primary care patients range from 6 to 9 percent, with up to 50 percent of these being unrecognized (13), indicating that in a busy practice of 20 to 30 patient visits a day, as many as 2 to 3 may be depressed; of these patients, one or more may be undiagnosed. The importance of clinical suspicion cannot be overemphasized.

Depression is important in primary care not only because of its high prevalence, but also because primary care is often the only source of care chosen by patients suffering from this condition (14). Unfortunately, recognizing depression in primary care is complicated because patients often present with somatic complaints (e.g., palpitations, abdominal pain, or fatigue) (15). Other factors that may contribute to underrecognition of depression in primary care include patients' concerns about being labeled with a mental health diagnosis (16); the burden of many competing demands in primary care also makes diagnosing depression difficult. (17–19).

Family physicians should maintain a high level of watchfulness for symptoms or functional impairment that may suggest anxiety or depression. Tiredness or fatigue as a presenting complaint should trigger the clinician to suspect depression,

whereas agitation or difficulty maintaining concentration may indicate the presence of an anxiety disorder. Prolonged somatic symptoms that do not appear to have a recognizable, physiologic etiology and do not resolve with several weeks of watchful waiting may indicate the presence of depression. Pursue any suspicion of depression with careful, yet tactful, questioning to confirm or rule out a diagnosis.

Screening for depression remains a topic of controversy. The US Preventive Services Task Force (USPFTF)recommended screening in 2002, but only where systems are in place to ensure appropriate treatment and follow-up (20), whereas the 2004 United Kingdom National Institute for Clinical Excellence recommended screening only those patients with significant risk factors (21). A 2005 Cochrane Review also questioned the usefulness of general screening for depression (22). Therefore, watchfulness in individuals at risk and a high index of suspicion appear to be the most appropriate approach. Significant risk factors include a past history of depression, significant physical illness causing disability, substance abuse, and other mental health problems.

Experienced clinicians use a variety of clinical clues to help them determine the presence of depression (23). The following clues suggest depression:

- Complaints that involve multiple organ systems or are physiologically unrelated
- Emotional flatness, or worry that is not consistent with the severity of the presenting problem
- Sleep disturbance that is persistent or unrelated to obvious stressors
- Frequent office visits for unclear or seemingly trivial reasons
- Frequent emergency department visits for unexplained physical symptoms
- Patients who are "difficult" for unclear reasons
- Patients who express thoughts or emotions that are inappropriate to the context
- Patients with a previous history of emotional disturbances or breakdowns

INITIAL EVALUATION

If initial clinical clues cause you to suspect depression, discuss it with the patient as part of the differential diagnosis. When the clinician fails to discuss concerns about depression initially, proceeding instead with an intensive biomedical evaluation, the patient may assume there is a physical cause for his/her symptoms; the patient later may have difficulty accepting a diagnosis of depression. If, instead, primary care physicians open the door early to considering depression or anxiety in a nonjudgmental fashion, patients will often admit to having a concern themselves. It is helpful, therefore, to develop a way of introducing the possibility early in the discussion of a patient's illness. For example: "Just as physical symptoms sometimes have what people think of as a 'medical' cause, physical symptoms are often caused by stress or other fears. It is important that we keep an open mind about the role these may play in your symptoms. Have you wondered about whether stress or similar issues might be causing your symptoms?"

TABLE 48.4 Diagnostic Criteria for Bipolar II Disorder

Criteria for Hypomanic Episode

A. A distinct period of persistently elevated, expansive, or irritable mood, lasting throughout at least 4 days, that is clearly different from the usual nondepressed mood.

B. During the period of mood disturbance, three (or more) of the following symptoms have persisted (four if the mood is only irritable) and have been present to a significant degree:

    (1) inflated self-esteem or grandiosity

    (2) decreased need for sleep (e.g., feels rested after only 3 hours of sleep)

    (3) more talkative than usual or pressure to keep talking

    (4) flight of ideas or subjective experience that thoughts are racing

    (5) distractibility (i.e., attention too easily drawn to unimportant or irrelevant external stimuli)

    (6) increase in goal-directed activity (either socially, at work or school, or sexually) or psychomotor agitation

    (7) excessive involvement in pleasurable activities that have a high potential for painful consequences (e.g., the person engages in unrestrained buying sprees, sexual indiscretions, or foolish business investments)

C. The episode is associated with an unequivocal change in functioning that is uncharacteristic of the person when not symptomatic.

D. The disturbance in mood and the change in functioning are observable by others.

E. The episode is not severe enough to cause marked impairment in social or occupational functioning, or to necessitate hospitalization, and there are no psychotic features.

F. The symptoms are not due to the direct physiological effects of a substance (e.g., a drug of abuse, a medication, or other treatment) or a general medical condition (e.g., hyperthyroidism).

    Note: Hypomanic-like episodes that are clearly caused by somatic antidepressant treatment (e.g., medication, electroconvulsive therapy, light therapy) should not count toward a diagnosis of Bipolar II Disorder.

Criteria for 296.89: Bipolar II Disorder

A. Presence (or history) of one or more Major Depressive Episodes.

B. Presence (or history) of at least one Hypomanic Episode.

C. There has never been a Manic Episode or a Mixed Episode.

D. The mood symptoms in Criteria A and B are not better accounted for by Schizoaffective Disorder and are not superimposed on Schizophrenia, Schizophreniform Disorder, Delusional Disorder, or Psychotic Disorder Not Otherwise Specified.

E. The symptoms cause clinically significant distress or impairment in social, occupational, or other important areas of functioning.

Clinical History

Once a depressive disorder is suspected, evaluation should proceed in a logical fashion. Unfortunately, laboratory evaluation is not usually helpful except to rule out suspected contributing or underlying medical conditions. However, a formal evaluation of the patient using the DSM criteria for depression should be performed. The DSM criteria may be rapidly assessed using the Nine-Item Patient Health Questionnaire (PHQ-9) (24). A downloadable version of the PHQ-9, with scoring instructions, is available at the MacArthur Initiative on Depression in Primary Care Web site (*http://www.depression-primarycare.org/clinicians/toolkits/materials/forms/phq9/*). The PHQ-9 is particularly useful because it permits a simultaneous assessment of both DSM criteria and severity (25), and therefore can be used as a guide to treatment and management.

In situations in which a specific DSM diagnosis is impor-tant for treatment or billing decisions, use the diagnostic criteria from the DSM as listed in Tables 48-1 to 48-5.

Because depression often presents as a manifestation of an underlying medical condition, the patient with depressive symptoms should undergo a careful medical evaluation. If the patient has recently suffered a major illness, consider whether the depressive symptoms are secondary. Medications should also be considered as a potential cause of depressive symptoms. Table 48.6 provides a list of medications frequently associated with depression. Beta-blocker medications are no longer included in this list because of a recent study that showed no association with their use and depression, after controlling for confounders (26). If medications are suspected, minimize their use; be on the alert for substance abuse, mania, hypomania, or anxiety (see Table 48.7).

After reviewing underlying medical conditions and med-

TABLE 48.5 Criteria for Seasonal Pattern Specifier

With Seasonal Pattern (can be applied to the pattern of Major Depressive Episodes in Bipolar I Disorder, Bipolar II Disorder, or Major Depressive Disorder, Recurrent)

A. There has been a regular temporal relationship between the onset of Major Depressive Episodes in Bipolar I or Bipolar II Disorder or Major Depressive Disorder, Recurrent, and a particular time of the year (e.g., regular appearance of the Major Depressive Episode in the fall or winter). **Note:** Do not include cases in which there is an obvious effect of seasonal-related psychosocial stressors (e.g., regularly being unemployed every winter).

A. Full remissions (or a change from depression to mania or hypomania) also occur at a characteristic time of the year (e.g., depression disappears in the spring).

B. In the last 2 years, two Major Depressive Episodes have occurred that demonstrate the temporal seasonal relationships defined in Criteria A and B, and no nonseasonal Major Depressive Episodes have occurred during that same period.

C. Seasonal Major Depressive Episodes (as described above) substantially outnumber the nonseasonal Major Depressive Episodes that may have occurred over the individual's lifetime.

TABLE 48.6 Medications that Often Cause or Worsen Depression

Category	Examples
Drugs of abuse	Alcohol Amphetamines Cocaine Marijuana
Steroid hormones	Prednisone (or any glucocorticoids) Oral contraceptives
Psychoactive drugs	Opiate analgesics (e.g., codeine) Sedative-hypnotics (e.g., triazolam) Barbiturates Anxiolytics (e.g., diazepam)
Antihistamines	Chlorpheniramine Diphenhydramine
Cancer chemotherapy	

TABLE 48.7 Red Flags Suggesting More Serious or Complex Disease in Patients Presenting with Depression

Red Flag	Significance
Personal or family history of mania, hypomania, or formal diagnosis of bipolar disorder	Consider a diagnosis of bipolar disorder
Personal or family history of substance abuse	Screen for co-occurring substance abuse disorder
Prominent anxiety symptoms	Consider co-occurring diagnosis of an anxiety disorder and/or management of anxiety symptoms as antidepressant is taking effect.

ications as potential causes, next consider whether the symptoms may be secondary to another psychiatric condition. Frequently, substance abuse manifests in this way. Traditional wisdom suggests that treating a comorbid depression is extremely difficult in the face of a substance abuse condition, and the Agency for Health Care Policy and Research (AHCPR) Depression Guideline (13) recommends treating the underlying substance abuse disorder before treating the depression. However, the results of several studies have begun to question this practice (27–29).

In considering a specific diagnosis for your patient, remember that anxiety and depressive disorders overlap, with many patients meeting criteria for both. In fact, patients meeting criteria for a depressive disorder may have a symptom profile that favors anxiety (30). Finally, when considering a diagnosis of depression, assess for a personal or family history of mania. This is important because patients with hypomania or a bipolar disorder are at high risk for developing acute mania if treated with a selective serotonin reuptake inhibitor (SSRI) (30).

MANAGEMENT

Effective management of patients with depression should proceed through stages of shared agreement on the diagnosis, preferred treatment modalities, plans for follow-up, monitoring, and duration of treatment.

A strong, trusting relationship and a therapeutic alliance between the physician and patient is the foundation for managing depression or anxiety. This has been shown in a referral population (31, 32), and is reasonable to infer in family medicine. A strong therapeutic alliance facilitates discussion and development of a diagnosis, choice and monitoring of treatment modalities, discussion of referral if needed, and agreement on long-term treatment when necessary. It is important at the beginning to emphasize your commitment to see a patient through the treatment, even if you decide at some point that referral is necessary.

This discussion lays the groundwork for the supportive counseling and education that is a cornerstone of treatment. Much of this activity is undocumented and, therefore, difficult to study in terms of its effectiveness (33). However, it is in this context that much of the primary care treatment of depression occurs.

If the depression is secondary to an underlying medical condition, supportive counseling as part of treatment for the underlying condition is always appropriate. Beyond this, encouraging the patient to seek out a local support group for people suffering from the condition may also be helpful. If the depression is severe enough to interfere with the patient's daily life or ability to participate in treatment of the medical condition, specific pharmacologic treatment should be initiated. The PHQ-9 can guide decisions about pharmacologic versus psychotherapeutic treatment modalities. Generally, patients with PHQ-9 scores of 15 or above should have pharmacologic treatment.

Answer any questions patients may have about their diagnosis because a mental health diagnosis often carries with it fears of "losing one's mind" or "being crazy." Reassure the patient and emphasize the effectiveness of treatment. A variety of books are available to help patients understand their condition. Two excellent ones are: *Feeling Good: The New Mood Therapy,* by David Burns (34) and *How to Heal Depression* by Harold Bloomfield and Peter McWilliams (35). For patients with Internet access, the National Institute of Mental Health (NIMH) Web site (*http://www.nimh.nih.gov*) has excellent information for patients about depression and its treatment. NIMH also has excellent patient education brochures that are available for download or purchase.

Assessment of Suicide Risk

Risk factors for suicide are listed in Table 48.8. An open discussion of suicidal thoughts does not increase the likelihood that patients will act on their thoughts, but does give you a chance to intervene if needed. Because the PHQ-9 includes a question on suicidal thoughts, this may facilitate identification and discussion of the topic. Patients may feel shame about having suicidal thoughts. When these thoughts are disclosed, you should remind them that most, if not all, patients with depression experience them. When several risk factors for suicide are present, consider referral to a mental health specialist.

Choice of Treatment Modality

The primary, proven modalities for treating depression are prescription medication and formal psychotherapy. The choice of either single or combination therapy is one that should be made with your patient after considering the severity of their depression. Table 48.9 summarizes the evidence for the common treatments.

Selecting an Antidepressant Medication

Medication should be initiated when:

- A patients' symptoms have been present for more than 1 month
- Symptoms result in significant interference with a patient's ability to function at work or home
- A patient's score on the PHQ-9 is 15 or greater

Fortunately, your decisions about which medication to use do not need to be based on considerations of efficacy. Instead, you should base your choice primarily on adverse effects, potential for drug interactions, and considerations of cost and insurer formularies. All available medications in the SSRI classes have good rates of response to treatment for depression. Tricyclics are not commonly used because of their side-effect profile and related risk for discontinuation. Hypericum (St. John's wort) continues to show evidence for efficacy in mild to moderate depression when compared to placebo and may be an option for those who have a preference for a complementary substance. A list of commonly prescribed antidepressants with their contraindications and/or adverse effects is provided in Table 48.10.

Points to consider when selecting a medication include:

- History of good response to previous use
- Successful use of an agent in a close relative (use by a parent or sibling may enhance compliance)
- Presence of chronic pain or severe sleep disturbance (if so, consider using a tricyclic antidepressant [TCA])
- Coexisting medical conditions (e.g., avoid TCAs in patients with known cardiac conduction disturbances)
- Hypersomnia (if so, consider an SSRI)
- Cost

Once a specific medication has been chosen, enough time is needed to adequately assess its effectiveness. Included in this is a willingness to increase the dose to a level at which the drug is effective. Allow at least 4 to 6 weeks of treatment at a known effective dose before abandoning the drug. If there is no response by 6 weeks, switch medication and/or consider referral. It is important to emphasize to the patient that the failure of one medication does not mean that the condition is untreatable. The monitoring strategies discussed below are helpful in guiding decisions about advancing, augmenting, or switching treatments.

For initial episodes of depression, continue treatment for 9 to 12 months. At that point, consider discontinuance of the

---

TABLE 48.8	Factors Increasing the Risk of Suicide in Depressed Patients*

1. Increased age (over 70 years in men, 60 years in women)
2. Gender (women make more attempts; men are successful more often)
3. Poor social support
4. Lack of marital support and absence of children
5. Chronic physical illness or chronic pain
6. Alcoholism or substance abuse
7. History of prior attempts
8. Specific plan or explicit communication about intent
9. Family history of successful suicide

*Several risk factors together are particularly significant; for example, a recently widowed, 70-year-old man who drinks excessively is an extremely high suicide risk and requires specific assessment.

TABLE 48.9 Recommended Treatments for Depression

Intervention	Efficacy	Strength of Recommendation*	Comment
Moderate to severe MDD			
Prescription antidepressants vs. placebo	69% of placebo users had worse outcomes than average antidepressant users over 6 weeks	A	
SSRIs vs. other antidepressants	No difference in efficacy	A	Some evidence exists that the lower side-effect profile reduces non-adherence in SSRIs
Formal psychotherapy in combination with medication	OR for improvement 1.86 (95% CI 1.38 to 2.52) vs. medication alone	A	
Mild to moderate MDD			
Cognitive therapy (CBT) and Interpersonal Therapy (IPT)	OR for recovery vs. usual care 3.4 (95% CI 2 to 6); IPT vs. usual care OR 3.45, (95% CI 1.91 to 6.51)	A	
Nondirective counseling	OR for worse symptoms vs. usual care at 1–6 months: SMD −0.28, 95% CI −0.43 to −0.13	A	No proven benefit beyond 6 months

MDD, major depressive disorder; SSRIs, selective serotonin reuptake inhibitors
*A = consistent, good-quality patient-oriented evidence; B = inconsistent or limited-quality patient-oriented evidence; C = consensus, disease-oriented evidence, usual practice, expert opinion, or case series. For information about the SORT evidence rating system, see *http://www.aafp.org/afpsort.xml.*

medication (via taper), but be aware that one-third of MDD patients will relapse within a year. For those who do, consider chronic therapy in an effort to prevent or decrease the severity of relapses (36).

Role of Psychotherapy

Studies continue to show the effectiveness of psychotherapy in the treatment of depression (37, 38). There is also evidence for enhanced relapse prevention when cognitive behavioral therapy (CBT) has been used in conjunction with medication (38, 39). Occasionally, family physicians have obtained enough experience and training in brief psychotherapy to provide this to their patients, but time and poor insurance reimbursement often result in patients being referred for these treatments. It is helpful to have familiarity with therapy modalities, however. Two of the most studied therapies are briefly described below.

INTERPERSONAL THERAPY

Interpersonal therapy (IPT) focuses on practical resolution of problematic interpersonal relationships or other stressful events. The therapist seeks to:

- Identify events or relationships that stimulate abnormal amounts of stress or grief

- Encourage discussions about the nature and origin of the stress reaction
- Move through strategies to resolve the stressful situation or relationship

For example, a common source of interpersonal stress is social isolation. Practical suggestions for such a situation might include: calling a friend with whom the patient has lost contact, joining a social club specific to an interest the patient may have, volunteering for a community or religious group, or enrolling in adult education classes.

IPT is often directed toward marital stress, which may be somewhat more complicated, but still benefits from engaging with an outside person (e.g., the primary care physician) in mutual problem solving. IPT may seem simplistic at times, but patients can be very appreciative of this problem-solving approach when they have lost the motivation or cognitive function to identify and resolve the source of their distress.

CBT

CBT is based on the observation that depressed patients suffer from an unrelenting and unjustifiably negative view of the world around them. CBT has been tested in both MDD and panic disorder patients and found to be as effective as antidepressant medication in mild to moderate disease (40). The main function of the therapist is to provide "homework" as-

TABLE 48.10 Common Antidepressants

Drug	Contraindications/Cautions/Adverse Effects	Dosage	Relative Cost*
Selective Serotonin Reuptake Inhibitors (SSRIs)			
Citalopram	Avoid with monoamine oxidase inhibitors (MAOIs)	20–60 mg once daily	$$
Escitalopram	Avoid with MAOIs	10–20 mg	$$
Fluoxetine	Initial nervousness/arousal/insomnia; avoid with MAOIs	20–80 mg once daily	$
Paroxetine	Drowsiness; avoid with MAOIs	10–50 mg once daily	$
Sertraline	Insomnia; avoid with MAOIs	25–200 mg once daily	$$
Other agents			
Buproprion	Contraindicated with history of seizures, eating disorders or substance abuse; avoid with MAOIs	100–150 mg BID-TID	$$
Duloxetine	Contraindicated with history of uncontrolled narrow angle glaucoma	20–60 mg once daily or 20–30 mg twice daily	$$$
Mirtazapine	Drowsiness, marked weight gain; avoid with MAOIs	15–45 mg at bedtime	$$
Nefazodone	Black-box warning for liver disease; avoid with MAOIs	100–300mg bid	$$
Venlafaxine	Risk of hypertension (dose-dependant); avoid with MAOIs	37.5–150 mg/day divided BID-TID with max. of 225 mg/day or extended-release daily	$$
Tricyclics			
Amitriptyline	Contraindicated in patients with cardiac conduction abnormalities, benign prostatic hypertrophy, glaucoma, orthostatic hypotension and seizures/Marked sedation & anticholenergic effects	25–300 mg at bedtime	$
Nortriptyline	Contraindicated in patients with cardiac conduction abnormalities, benign prostatic hypertrophy, glaucoma, and seizures/Marked sedation & anticholenergic effects	25–150 mg at bedtime	$
Trazodone	Marked drowsiness	50–600 mg at bedtime	$
Complementary therapy			
Hypercium	Contraindicated in conjunction with SSRIs; many drug interactions	300 mg tid (0.3% standardized extract)	$

*$ = <$33, $$ = $34-$66, $$$ = >$67.

signments to the patient. These assignments require the patient to gather and process information about his or her situation and relationships in a way that leads to new cognitive views of their surroundings, new relationships, or new social skills. This may require the therapist to provide basic information in a didactic way, such as knowledge about the origin of panic symptoms.

Therapists also teach patients new ways of self-talk—positive self-statements made before, during, and after stressful events that would normally provoke significant symptoms. Sometimes the therapist actually encourages the patient to seek stressful events, after much practice and prepa-

ration, as a way of testing new skills and achieving new levels of comfort in daily responsibilities. CBT is most successful if it is framed as exercises or assignments; the therapist is very specific about the assignments, the patient is seen frequently to provide appropriate feedback, and the patient is deeply engaged in the problem-solving process.

PROBLEM-SOLVING THERAPY

Problem-solving therapy (PST) is a recently developed therapy that is designed for the primary care setting (41). Patients are led through stages of identifying their primary problems, generating solutions, and trying out these solutions. Early trials show promising results in treatment of mild to moderate depression using this technique in the primary care outpatient setting (42–44).

Indications for Referral

Patients with a history of severe, chronic symptoms often benefit from referral. Also consider referral of patients who have a history of unresponsiveness to treatment or bipolar disorder or of patients who are at high risk for suicide. Again, early establishment of a strong therapeutic alliance with the patient will greatly facilitate the referral process and enhance the likelihood that the patient will experience a successful result from the referral. When not restricted by a patient's health insurance plan, direct referral and close communication with the mental health specialist is desirable. Comanagement with a mental health specialist is frequently promoted as a model for primary care; a recent survey of family physicians in Michigan found that collaborative treatment actually occurred in about 30% of their cases. Managed care carve-outs and lack of geographic proximity were seen as barriers to collaborative care by respondents (45).

LONG-TERM MONITORING

Once you begin treating a patient with depression, monitoring their course is essential. Depression is often a long-term illness, with periods of waxing and waning, of relapse and remission. The critical nature of systematic follow-up is evident from its inclusion in the USPFTF depression screening recommendations (20). There is evidence that systematic follow-up is best accomplished through a combination of telephone contact and regular scheduled office visits.

Consider monitoring the patient with a structured instrument such as the PHQ-9. This allows you and the patient to review current and previous scores. Whether or not you use a monitoring instrument, assess current stressors, response to treatment, and the presence of suicidal thoughts at each office visit. Patients under treatment often respond initially to questions about treatment response with a general statement such as, "I'm doing better." It is useful to elicit a description of exactly what "doing better" means. Find out how the patient is responding to stressful situations because these rarely go away simply because treatment was started. This questioning will guide the patient into a discussion about how response to previously stressful situations has or has not changed after initiation of treatment or changes in treatment. Also ask patients whether spouses or significant others have noted changes. Any specific areas of improvement should be noted in the record and can provide useful markers of relapse for both the physician and patient.

It is also important to inquire about medication side effects. Patients may withhold mentioning these unless prompted, especially if they include sexual side effects such as erectile dysfunction or loss of libido. You can reassure patients that information from them on side effects they may be experiencing is important to you, and that if the side effects do not improve, a change in medication can be made. Monitoring should be monthly during treatment; once a patient has returned to baseline functioning and symptoms, monitoring and visits may be performed at decreased intervals. Regularly monitoring patients helps to ensure that treatment remains matched to their symptoms and helps reinforce the importance of relapse prevention once recovery has occurred.

SPECIAL DIAGNOSIS AND TREATMENT CONSIDERATIONS FOR ADOLESCENTS

Adolescent depression has received considerable attention recently because of the high prevalence of adolescent depressive symptoms (46), and concerns about risks of SSRI treatment. Certainly, monitoring adolescent patients for depression is prudent. Adolescents tend to present somewhat differently, however, especially regarding the cardinal DSM symptom of depressed mood. Adolescents often exhibit this as heightened irritability. Suicide risk is also important to consider. The 2003 National Youth Risk Behavior survey reported that 17% of youth in grades 9–12 had considered suicide (47). Treatment of adolescent depression was recently assessed in a large NIMH-sponsored trial. The trial demonstrated that fluoxetine combined with CBT provided the most favorable benefit versus risk profile (48). Although there have been concerns that SSRIs increase the risk of suicide in adolescents, this was not demonstrated in the NIMH trial (48). Clinicians that treat depressed adolescents should stay abreast of this topic, however. NIMH maintains regularly updated information for both clinicians and concerned parents on their Web site [*http://www.nimh.nih.gov/publicat/medicate.cfm#ptdep16*].

CASE DISCUSSION

Despite initial concerns voiced by J.F. and her daughter, an initial diagnosis of depression would have been premature. *Diagnostic and Statistical Manual of Mental Disorders* criteria require at least 2 weeks of depressive symptoms before making a diagnosis of MDD, and this is confirmed by clinical experience. Also a lack of prior history in either J.F. or her family made an early diagnosis of MDD problematic. Indeed, J.F. responded well to a benzodiazepine early in her course, and it seemed that her grief reaction would resolve without further intervention.

The clinician treating a mood disorder must, however, remain open to changes or additions in the diagnosis, as occurred 1.5 months after J.F.'s first episode. When a change occurs in the patient's condition, the family physician's therapeutic alliance with the patient can permit an adjustment in the diagnosis, and treatment to occur smoothly. In J.F.'s case, the appropriate changes were instituted with effective results.

Finally, note the rapid increase in the antidepressant dose. Often clinicians shy away from such rapid increases, initiating follow-up only after a patient has been on an antidepressant for 2 to 3 weeks. However, follow-up after 1 week of treatment affords the advantage of quick monitoring for adverse effects, and rapid adjustment of the dose to a therapeutic level.

REFERENCES

1. American Psychiatric Association. American Psychiatric Association—Task Force on DSM-IV. Diagnostic and Statistical Manual of Mental Disorders: DSM-IV, 4th ed. Washington, DC: American Psychiatric Association; 2000.

2. Sullivan PF, Neale MC, Kendler KS. Genetic epidemiology of major depression: review and meta-analysis. Am J Psychiatry. 2000;157(10):1552–1562.

3. Brown GW, Harris TO. Social origins of depression: a study of psychiatric disorder in women. (1st US ed.) New York, NY: Free Press; 1978.

4. Kendler KS, Kessler RC, Neale MC, Heath AC, Eaves LJ. The prediction of major depression in women: toward an integrated etiologic model. Am J Psychiatry. 1993;150(8):1139–1148.

5. Manning JS, Haykal RF, Connor PD, Akiskal HS. On the nature of depressive and anxious states in a family practice setting: the high prevalence of bipolar II and related disorders in a cohort followed longitudinally. Compr Psychiatry. 1997;38(2):102–108.

6. Hirschfeld RM, Cass AR, Holt DC, Carlson CA. Screening for bipolar disorder in patients treated for depression in a family medicine clinic. J Am Board Fam Pract. 2005;18(4):233–239.

7. Kessler RC, Chiu WT, Demler O, Merikangas KR, Walters EE. Prevalence, severity, and comorbidity of 12-month DSM-IV disorders in the National Comorbidity Survey Replication. Arch Gen Psychiatry. 2005;62(6):617–627.

8. Greenberg PE, Kessler RC, Birnbaum HG, et al. The economic burden of depression in the United States: how did it change between 1990 and 2000? J Clin Psychiatry. 2003;64(12):1465–1475.

9. Ferketich AK, Schwartzbaum JA, Frid DJ, Moeschberger ML. Depression as an antecedent to heart disease among women and men in the NHANES I study. National Health and Nutrition Examination Survey. Arch Intern Med. 2000;160(9):1261–1268.

10. Ford DE, Mead LA, Chang PP, Cooper-Patrick L, Wang NY, Klag MJ. Depression is a risk factor for coronary artery disease in men: the precursors study. Arch Intern Med. 1998;158(13):1422–1426.

11. Lustman PJ, Anderson RJ, Freedland KE, de Groot M, Carney RM, Clouse RE. Depression and poor glycemic control: a meta-analytic review of the literature. Diabetes Care. 2000;23(7):934–942.

12. American Academy of Family Physicians. Facts about family practice. Kansas City, MO: American Academy of Family Physicians.

13. Depression Guideline Panel. Depression in primary care. Rockville, MD: Agency for Health Care Policy and Research. US Department of Health and Human Services; 1993.

14. Regier DA, Goldberg ID, Taube CA. The de facto US Mental Health Services system: a public health perspective. Arch Gen Psychiatry. 1978;35:685–693.

15. Suh T, Gallo JJ. Symptom profiles of depression among general medical service users compared with specialty mental health service users. Psychol Med. 1997;27(5):1051–1063.

16. Rost K, Smith R, Taylor JL. Rural-urban differences in stigma and the use of care for depressive disorders. J Rural Health. 1993;9(1):57–62.

17. Klinkman MS. Competing demands in psychosocial care. A model for the identification and treatment of depressive disorders in primary care. Gen Hosp Psychiatry. 1997;19(2):98–111.

18. Nutting PA, Rost K, Smith J, Werner JJ, Elliot C. Competing demands from physical problems: effect on initiating and completing depression care over 6 months. Arch Fam Med. 2000;9(10):1059–1064.

19. Rost K, Nutting P, Smith J, Coyne JC, Cooper-Patrick L, Rubenstein L. The role of competing demands in the treatment provided primary care patients with major depression. Arch Fam Med. 2000;9(2):150–154.

20. The US Preventive Services Task Force. Screening for depression: recommendations and rationale. Ann Intern Med. 2002;136(10):760–764.

21. National Institute for Clinical Excellence. Depression: management of depression in primary and secondary care. 2004. Accessed December 1, 2005. Available at: *http://www.nice.org.uk/pdf/CG023quickrefguide.pdf*.

22. Gilbody S, House A, Sheldon T, Gilbody S. Screening and case finding instruments for depression. Cochrane Database Syst Rev. 2005(4):CD002792.

23. Klinkman MS, Coyne JC, Gallo S, Schwenk TL. False positives, false negatives, and the validity of the diagnosis of major depression in primary care. Arch Fam Med. 1998;7(5):451–461.

24. Kroenke K, Spitzer RL, Williams JB. The PHQ-9: validity of a brief depression severity measure. J Gen Intern Med. 2001;16(9):606–613.

25. Nease DE, Jr, Maloin JM. Depression screening: a practical strategy. J Fam Pract. 2003 Feb;52(2):118–124.

26. Bright RA, Everitt DE. Beta-blockers and depression. Evidence against an association. JAMA. 1992;267(13):1783–1787.

27. Mason BJ, Kocsis JH, Ritvo EC, Cutler RB. A double-blind, placebo-controlled trial of desipramine for primary alcohol dependence stratified on the presence or absence of major depression. JAMA. 1996;275(10):761–767.

28. Roy-Byrne PP, Pages KP, Russo JE, et al. Nefazodone treatment of major depression in alcohol-dependent patients: a double-blind, placebo-controlled trial. J Clin Psychopharmacol. 2000;20(2):129–136.

29. Moak DH, Anton RF, Latham PK, Voronin KE, Waid RL, Durazo-Arvizu R. Sertraline and cognitive behavioral therapy for depressed alcoholics: results of a placebo-controlled trial. J Clin Psychopharmacol. 2003;23(6):553–562.

30. Nease DE Jr, Aikens JE. DSM depression and anxiety criteria and severity of symptoms in primary care: cross sectional study. BMJ. 2003;327(7422):1030–1031.

31. Weiss M, Gaston L, Propst A, Wisebord S, Zicherman V. The role of the alliance in the pharmacologic treatment of depression. J Clin Psychiatry. 1997;58(5):196–204.

32. Klein DN, Schwartz JE, Santiago NJ, et al. Therapeutic alliance in depression treatment: controlling for prior change and patient characteristics. J Consult Clin Psychol. 2003;71(6):997–1006.

33. Rost K, Smith R, Matthews DB, Guise B. The deliberate misdiagnosis of major depression in primary care. Arch Fam Med. 1994;3(4):333–337.

34. Burns DD. Feeling Good: The New Mood Therapy. Revised and updated. New York, NY: Avon; 1999.

35. Bloomfield HH, McWilliams P. How to Heal Depression. Los Angeles, CA: Prelude Press; 1994.

36. Geddes JR, Carney SM, Davies C, et al. Relapse prevention with antidepressant drug treatment in depressive disorders: a systematic review. Lancet. 2003;361(9358):653–661.

37. Chambless DL, Sanderson WC, Shoham V, et al. An update on empirically validated therapies. Clinical Psychologist. 1996;29(2):5–18.

38. Gloaguen V, Cottraux J, Cucherat M, Blackburn IM. A meta-analysis of the effects of cognitive therapy in depressed patients. J Affect Disord. 1998;49(1):59–72.

39. Fava GA, Ruini C, Rafanelli C, Finos L, Conti S, Grandi S. Six-year outcome of cognitive behavior therapy for prevention of recurrent depression. Am J Psychiatry. 2004;161(10):1872–1876.

40. Robinson LA, Berman JS, Neimeyer RA. Psychotherapy for the treatment of depression: a comprehensive review of controlled outcome research. Psychol Bull. 1990;108(1):30–49.

41. Mynors-Wallis L. Problem-solving treatment: evidence for

effectiveness and feasibility in primary care. Int J Psychiatry Med. 1996;26(3):249–262.

42. Mynors-Wallis L, Davies I, Gray A, Barbour F, Gath D. A randomised controlled trial and cost analysis of problem-solving treatment for emotional disorders given by community nurses in primary care. Br J Psychiatry. 1997;170:113–119.

43. Mynors-Wallis L, Gath D. Predictors of treatment outcome for major depression in primary care. Psychol Med. 1997;27(3):731–736.

44. Mynors-Wallis LM, Gath DH, Day A, Baker F. Randomised controlled trial of problem solving treatment, antidepressant medication, and combined treatment for major depression in primary care. BMJ. 2000;320(7226):26–30.

45. Valenstein M, Klinkman M, Becker S, et al. Concurrent treatment of patients with depression in the community: provider practices, attitudes, and barriers to collaboration. J Fam Pract. 1999;48(3):180–187.

46. Rushton JL, Forcier M, Schectman RM. Epidemiology of depressive symptoms in the National Longitudinal Study of Adolescent Health. J Am Acad Child Adolesc Psychiatry. 2002;41(2):199–205.

47. Grunbaum JA, Kann L, Kinchen S, et al. Youth risk behavior surveillance—United States, 2003. MMWR Surveill Summ. 2004;53(2):1–96.

48. March J, Silva S, Petrycki S, et al. Fluoxetine, cognitive-behavioral therapy, and their combination for adolescents with depression: Treatment for Adolescents With Depression Study (TADS) randomized controlled trial. JAMA. 2004;292(7):807–820.

CHAPTER 49

Allergies and Asthma

Dorothy E. Vura-Weis

CASE

S. is an 11-year-old girl who is being seen for severe nasal congestion and clear discharge, itchy watery eyes, and a cough that wakes her several times each night. Her mother had been giving her over-the-counter (OTC) antihistamine/decongestant medication in the spring for several years for similar but milder nasal symptoms, but it's not helping now. When questioned about respiratory difficulty with physical activity, she reports that she doesn't like running so she doesn't know. Her little sister interrupts to say that sometimes S. won't walk fast to school because it makes her short of breath. The mother comments that right before the new symptoms started they bought a pet rabbit that stays in the kitchen. Physical exam is notable for inflamed watery conjunctiva, swollen pale nasal mucosa, and mild diffuse expiratory wheezing.

CLINICAL QUESTIONS

1. What are the common causes and manifestations of allergies in children and adults?
2. How is asthma identified, classified, and treated?
3. How can the patient or family monitor asthma in order to initiate early intervention for exacerbations?

Asthma and respiratory allergies are closely linked; they share many of the same precipitants, mechanisms, and treatments, and often occur in the same patients, so they are considered together in this chapter. Chronic obstructive pulmonary disease (COPD), which includes chronic bronchitis and emphysema, is also linked with asthma by sharing a number of symptoms, physical findings, and treatments. Asthma is usually completely reversible (although with longer duration and greater severity it may develop a chronic component) while COPD by definition is not completely reversible, and the two diagnoses can coexist in the same patient. COPD is covered in Chapter 51, Chronic Obstructive Pulmonary Disease. Atopic dermatitis is often present in patients with allergic rhinitis and asthma; its treatment is addressed in Chapter 40, Dermatology.

ALLERGIES

Respiratory allergies and hay fever affect approximately 28 million Americans and were responsible for 14.1 million physician office visits in 2003 (1). They result in sneezing, runny nose, nasal itching and congestion, and a sense of fullness in the head. Eye symptoms such as itching, watering, and blurred vision, with pink edematous conjunctiva, may also be present, indicating allergic conjunctivitis. The triggers of allergic rhinitis are primarily inhaled allergens that interact with cells in the nasal passages.

Allergic symptoms are caused by a cascade of events after pollens or other allergens come in contact with the nasal mucosa. Allergenic molecules are processed by macrophages and dendritic cells, which present them to Helper T (T_H) cells and then to B cells. People with an allergic diathesis have a large population of T_H2 cells which stimulates B cells to secrete allergen-specific IgE. The IgE attaches to basophils and mast cells which, when exposed again to the same antigen, release histamine, leukotrienes, and cytokines. Eosinophils and additional T_H2 cells are recruited to the area; the allergic response is amplified for the original antigen and facilitated for new antigens, creating a positive feedback loop (2).

In people without an allergic tendency, a high proportion of T_H cells are T_H1 cells, which participate in cell-mediated immune responses. T_H1 cells produce substances that limit the allergic response. Conversely, T_H2 cells limit production of T_H1 cells. This suggests that exposure to infections that stimulate T_H1 responses might prevent allergic reactions. In fact, there is some evidence that early exposure to infections, by having older siblings or by attending day care in the first 6 months of life, results in lower rates of allergies and/or asthma in school-age children (3).

Allergen exposure may cause an immediate response of sneezing, watery eyes, and nasal discharge that resolves within an hour after removal of the stimulus. Symptoms may return 4 to 12 hours later. The early phase symptoms are associated with the initial histamine release, while the late phase symptoms are related to the recruitment of additional inflammatory cells and mediators. Ongoing or recurrent exposure to allergens can cause continuous symptoms. Irritants such as ozone, tobacco and wood smoke, perfumes, and cleaning chemicals can cause similar symptoms.

Initial Evaluation

Ask patients about the symptoms listed above and in Table 49.1, about any particular exposure or time of year when symptoms are usually worse, any medications that have been tried, and their effects. Specific exposures to pets such as cats and dogs, molds, and dust are important, as is a family history of asthma or allergies. Patients whose symptoms recur at a particular time of year have seasonal rhinitis, usually related to specific pollens. Symptoms lasting more than 9 months

TABLE 49.7 Management of Asthma

Treatment Strategy	Efficacy	Strength of Recommendation*	Comments
Prevention			
Exclusive breastfeeding for at least 3 or 4 months decreases risk of developing asthma	OR of asthma up to age 6: 1.25 if not exclusively breastfed for 4 months (14) ; OR of developing asthma 0.70 if exclusively breastfed at least 3 months (58)	A	Note: This does not imply a shortening of the standard recommendations for exclusive breastfeeding for six months.
Avoid exposure to tobacco smoke, including prenatally	Fourfold increase in wheezing illness in infants whose mothers smoke (16)	A	Although wheezing illnesses increased, no increase in atopic sensitization. Tobacco smoke is also a trigger for those who already have asthma.
Education and Monitoring			
Self-management education programs including written asthma management plan and regular physician review	Compared to "usual care", RR 0.64 for hospitalization, RR 0.82 for emergency room visits, RR 0.79 for missed work or school (27, 28)	A	
Action plans based on symptoms or peak flow equally effective in adults (59)		B	
Routine peak expiratory flow monitoring useful for patients with moderate and severe asthma (10)		C	Although difficult to separate from other program components, peak flow monitoring beneficial in several studies and recommended
Controlling chronic home environmental triggers may reduce asthma symptoms	In comprehensive individually tailored programs, days with symptoms were 3.2 per 2 weeks in control group and 2.6 per 2 weeks in treatment group (30).	B	Comprehensive interventions appear effective but expensive: $750–$1,000 for 34 fewer days of symptoms per year. Single interventions not as effective. (It's still important to avoid obvious intermittent triggers, like tobacco smoke or a pet that causes symptoms.)
Long-Term Control			
Inhaled corticosteroids most effective as long-term controller	RR of exacerbation 0.46 compared to placebo (60)	A	Effective in children and adults. Appears to prevent structural changes in airways that would cause chronic obstruction.
Inhaled LABA effective as add-on medicine when ICS don't provide adequate control	When added to ICS, RR of exacerbation 0.76 compared to addition of placebo (60)	A	Most effective therapy to add to ICS. (Note: Initial treatment with ICS/LABA no better than ICS alone (61)
Leukotriene antagonists are second-line as single agent.	Less effective than ICS (RR for exacerbations$^{1.65}$) (62) but more effective than placebo (RR for exacerbations 0.59) (60)	A	LTRAs decrease β_2 agonist use.

Recommendation	Rating	Evidence	Comments
LABA better than leukotriene antagonists as add-on to ICS	A	LABA more effective (RR for exacerbations 0.83 compared to LTRA) (37)	
Specific immunotherapy (allergy shots) effective for high IgE asthma patients with positive skin tests	A	NNT = 5 to prevent need for increased meds in meta-analysis	Useful in patients whose symptom pattern and allergen tests match. Risk of anaphylaxis needs to be balanced.
Anti-IgE effective for mild-severe asthma in patients with high IgE	A	Decreased risk of exacerbation - OR 0.49; More likely to be able to reduce steroids by 50% compared to placebo—OR 2.50 (38)	Requires subcutaneous injection every 2–4 weeks, very expensive.
Treatment of acute symptoms and exacerbations			
MDI with spacer at least as effective as nebulizer for albuterol delivery	A	RR hospitalization 0.42 compared to nebulizer in children under 5 (33, 66)	At least as effective with fewer side effects for most patients.
Ipratropium bromide added to albuterol for moderate to severe exacerbations	A (63, 64)	RR 0.68–0.75 for hospitalization if multiple doses ipratropium given with albuterol in ED	Effectiveness seen for both children and adults.
Systemic corticosteroids for exacerbations	A	7–10 day courses of systemic steroids reduce admissions and decrease relapse rates (65)	
ICS for acute exacerbations	B	OR for hospitalization 0.30 compared to placebo (43).	Metanalysis on studies done in emergency departments.

Abbreviations: ED, emergency department; FH, family history; ICS, inhaled corticosteroids; LABA, long-acting β₂ agonist; LTRA, leukotriene antagonist; MDI, metered dose inhaler; NNT, number needed to treat; OR, odds ratio; RR, relative risk

*A = consistent, good-quality patient-oriented evidence; B = inconsistent or limited-quality patient-oriented evidence; C = consensus, disease-oriented evidence, usual practice, expert opinion, or case series. For information about the SORT evidence rating system, see *http://www.aafp.org/afpsort.xml*

TABLE 49.8 Medications Used for Asthma

Generic Name (Trade Name)	Usual Adult Dosing Range–For Steroids: Low Dose [Medium Dose] {High Dose}	Main Adverse Drug Events	Cost Per Month or Course or per Inhaler, Usual Dose*	Comments
Inhaled Corticosteroids (usually split BID) **Children's doses are usually ~ 2/3 of adult dose in each dosage range*				
Beclomethasone-HFA (QVAR®, 40 or 80 mcg/puff)	For 40 mcg/puff form: 2–6 puffs/day [6–12 puffs/day] {> 12 puffs/day}	Sore throat, dry mouth; oropharyngeal candidiasis. (gargle afterwards)	$$	5 yrs and up
Budesonide (Pulmicort Turbuhaler®) (DPI-dry powder inhaler—200 mcg/dose)	1–2 puffs/day [2–3 puffs/day] {>3 puffs/day}	Same	$$$	6 yrs and up for inhaler
Budesonide (Pulmicort Respules®) solution for inhalation	0.25 mg BID [0.5 mg BID] {1 mg BID} For children	Same	$$$	12 months to 8 years
Flunisolide (Aerobid®) 250 mcg/puff	2–4 puffs [4–8 puffs] {> 8 puffs}	Same	$$	6 yrs and up
Fluticasone (Flovent ® –44, 110, or 220 mcg/puff MDI)	88–264 mcg/day [264–660 mcg/day] {>660 mcg/day}	Same	$$	12 yrs and up
Fluticasone-Salmeterol combination (Advair®)	100/50 BID [250/50 BID] {500/50 BID}	Same	$$$	4 yrs and up
Triamcinolone (Azmacort®, 100 mcg/puff)	4–10 puffs/day [10–20 puffs/day] {> 20 puffs/day}	Same	$$	Same.
Mometasone(Asmanex®) 220 mcg/puff DPI	1–2 puffs/day [2–4 puffs/day] {>4 puffs/day} Split BID or once daily in evening	Same	$$$	12 yrs and up

	Dose	Side Effects	Cost	Notes
Leukotriene Antagonists				
Montelukast (Singulair®)	10 mg QHS (adults) 5 mg QHS (5–12 yo) 4 mg QHS (6 mo–5 yo) (4 & 5 mg chewable, 4 mg granules)	None common. Rare itching or tingling, sinus inflammation	$$	6 mo and up
Zafirlukast (Accolate®)	20 mg BID	Rare headaches, nausea	$$	5 yrs and up
Long-Acting β₂ Agonists				
Salmeterol Xinafoate (Serevent®)	1 inhalation Q 12 hrs. (DPI)	Occasional tachycardia, tremor, nervousness	$$	NOT to be used as quick-relief medicine. 4 yrs and up
Formoterol fumarate (Foradil®)	1 inhalation Q 12 hrs (DPI)	Same	$$	5 yrs and up
Albuterol-SR tablets	4–8 mg Q 12 hrs.	Tachycardia, tremor, nervousness	$$	More systemic effects than inhaled β₂ agonists
Methylxanthines				
Theophylline	300–400 mg Q 12 hrs.	Nausea, tremor, tachycardia, nervousness, seizures at high doses	$	Adjust dosage by blood levels. Other medications may raise level.
Anti IgE				
Omalizumab (Xolair ®)	Dose determined by serum IgE and weight	Injection site reactions.	$$$	12 years and up
Short-Acting β₂ Agonist				
Albuterol ***	2–4 puffs as directed in asthma management plan (also available as nebulizer solution)	Tachycardia, tremor, nervousness.	$	Use with a spacer to decrease side effects.
Anticholinergic				
Ipratropium Bromide *** (Atrovent®)	2 puffs with albuterol prn exacerbations	Cough, sore throat, rare palpitations; if sprayed in eye can precipitate glaucoma	$$	Used for severe asthma exacerbations

* Relative cost: $ = <$33.00; $$ = $34.00–$66.00; $$$ = >$67.00

**Inhaled corticosteroid dosages in "high dose" range are over FDA approved levels, but are recommended in major guidelines such as NAEPP and GINA.

***Also available as solution for nebulizer.

How to position the inhaler:

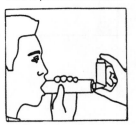

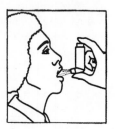

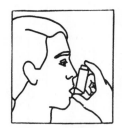

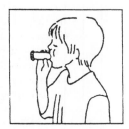

A. Use spacer. This is especially recommended for young children, for others who have difficulty coordinating inhaler use, and for all corticosteroid inhalers.

B. Open mouth with inhaler 1–2 inches away.

C. In the mouth. Do not use with inhaled corticosteroids. Use this position for breath-activated inhalers.

D. Dry powder inhalers (DPIs) require a different inhalation technique. To use a dry powder inhaler, it is important to close the mouth tightly around the mouthpiece of the inhaler and to inhale rapidly

How to Use Your Inhaler

A. With a spacer (this is the preferred method for most inhalers):
1. Remove the cap, hold the inhaler upright, and shake it.
2. Insert the inhaler into one end of the spacer.
3. Breathe out slowly.
4. Put the other end of the spacer in your mouth.
5. You can press the inhaler to release the medication either just before or right as you begin to *breathe in slowly* all the way. Hold your breath for 10 seconds.
6. Wait a minute, and then repeat if using more than one puff.

B and C. If you use your inhaler without a spacer:
1. Remove the cap, hold the inhaler upright, and shake it.
2. Tilt your head back slightly and *breathe out slowly*.
3. Position the inhaler as in sketches A or C.
4. As you start to breathe in (or within a second after starting the breath) press down on the inhaler to release the medication.
5. Continue to *breathe in slowly* (over 3 to 5 seconds), then hold your breath for 10 seconds to allow the medicine to reach deeply into your lungs.
6. Wait a minute, and then repeat if using more than one puff.

D. Using a breath-activated inhaler (or DPI):
1. Follow the instructions for your inhaler to prepare it for use.
2. *Breathe out slowly.*
3. Put the inhaler in your mouth with your lips making a tight seal.
4. *Breathe in rapidly to activate the inhaler.*
5. Hold your breath for 10 seconds to allow the medicine to reach deeply into your lungs.
6. Wait a minute, and then repeat if using more than one puff.

Figure 49.3 • How to use the inhaler. Adapted from National Asthma Education and Prevention Program. Expert Panel Report II: guidelines for the diagnosis and management of asthma. Washington, DC: US Department of Health and Human Services, 1997.

pituitary-adrenal axis and also increase the risk of cataracts. Studies on the impact of ICS on growth in children have shown a short-term decrease in growth velocity but no difference in height at age 20 years compared to controls (16, 36). Many effective inhaled corticosteroids are available, and the choice for a particular patient is based on a combination of convenience of dosing schedule, ease of use of delivery device, insurance coverage and cost (see Table 49.8).

In severe chronic asthma, oral steroids may be needed to deliver a higher total dose and to reach small airways inaccessi-ble to inhaled medications in the presence of obstruction. In view of the serious adverse effects of long-term systemic ste-roids, they should be replaced by inhaled forms as soon as possible or reduced to the lowest effective dose (e.g. 5 to 10 mg of prednisone) given in the morning to decrease adrenal suppression.

OTHER ANTI-INFLAMMATORY MEDICATIONS

Leukotriene modifiers block part of the inflammatory cascade in both the early and late asthmatic response. They are not as effective as ICS so they are not first-line therapy, and they are less effective as add-on therapy than inhaled long-acting beta agonists (37). When used as add-on therapy, the dosage of inhaled corticosteroid needed for effective control can sometimes be reduced. Leukotriene modifiers come in oral formulations, which some patients prefer, and they are helpful for some patients with coexisting allergic rhinitis. Montelukast (Singulair ®) is given once a day in the evening, and is available for children over 2 years as well as adults. Zafirlukast (Accolate ®) is given twice a day. It has minor adverse effects (headache, nausea, diarrhea) but does have several drug interactions (e.g. it increases the effect of warfarin and may cause bleeding, and increases erythromycin and theophylline levels). Leukotriene modifiers are often useful for asthma triggered by aspirin and nonsteroidal anti-inflammatory drugs (NSAIDs).

The mast cell stabilizers cromolyn (Intal ®) and nedocromil (Tilade®) are considered alternative anti-inflammatory medications. They are less effective than inhaled corticosteroids. They may be useful as pretreatment before exposure to allergens and before exercise.

Omalizumab (Xolair®) is an anti-IgE antibody that binds free IgE, thus preventing the IgE from binding to basophils and mast cells and causing their degranulation. It is used for patients 12 years of age and older with moderate to severe persistent allergic asthma that is not controlled with inhaled corticosteroids and other medications. Dosage is based on serum IgE levels and patient weight. It is given subcutaneously and is very expensive, so it is reserved for patients with severe asthma (38).

LONG-ACTING BRONCHODILATORS

Long-acting bronchodilators are used as controller medications if low to medium doses of inhaled corticosteroids (ICS) do not provide adequate relief. Inhaled forms are preferred because they have fewer side effects than systemic versions. Salmeterol (Serevent®) or formoterol (Foradil®), long-acting inhaled β_2 agonists, can be added to an inhaled corticosteroid to improve control. Neither is recommended for use without an ICS because such use was associated with small but significant increased risk of severe asthma attacks and death in a single randomized double-blind controlled study of salmeterol (39). Sustained-release albuterol in tablet form can improve control, especially for nighttime symptoms, but it is more likely to cause systemic adverse effects such as tremor and palpitations than inhaled long-acting bronchodilators. Sustained-release theophylline can also be used to improve control; it is much less expensive than salmeterol or formoterol, but is more likely to cause adverse effects such as tremors, palpitations, nausea, and, rarely, seizures at high serum concentrations. Serum theophylline levels should be monitored periodically with a target range of 5–15 mcg/mL.

Managing Acute Exacerbations

Three types of quick-relief medications are commonly used to control acute symptoms. The short-acting β_2 agonist albuterol acts directly on the smooth muscle of the bronchioles to oppose the bronchoconstriction caused by inflammatory mediators. Onset of action is rapid, and it can be repeated as often as every 20 minutes during an exacerbation if needed, or used continuously in a monitored setting. Ipratropium bromide (Atrovent®) is an inhaled anticholinergic medication that blocks the bronchoconstriction caused by cholinergic stimulation of the more proximal bronchioles. It is effective in decreasing the need for hospitalization when used with albuterol in urgent care/emergency settings for severe acute asthma exacerbations in both children and adults (40, 41). Levalbuterol, the R-isomer of albuterol, can be used for patients with unacceptable side effects from albuterol. It is available as a solution for a nebulizer (Xopenex ®) or as an MDI (Xopenex HFA ™), and is more expensive than albuterol.

Corticosteroids are used to treat exacerbations that do not respond adequately to the short-acting bronchodilators. Either an oral steroid (most commonly prednisone or prednisolone) or intravenous corticosteroid (usually methylprednisolone) is commonly used. A typical adult dose is 40 to 60 mg of prednisone per day for 3–10 days, or until the peak flow has returned to over 80% of the patient's personal best. It can be stopped abruptly without danger of adrenal suppression if it has been used for less than 2 weeks. For children, 1–2 mg/kg/day of prednisolone liquid is used. Alternatively, a patient's dose of ICS can be doubled to quadrupled for 1–2 weeks to regain control—this has been effective in both emergency department settings and as part of instructions on Asthma Action Plans (42, 43).

Patients can manage most asthma exacerbations themselves if they have medication (albuterol MDI and spacer), a peak flow meter, instructions in the form of an asthma action plan, and know how to interpret either their symptoms or their peak-flow reading. See Figures 49.1 and 49.2 for standard regimens. A well-educated patient can use albuterol, adjust doses of ICS, and if needed begin an oral corticosteroid at home (if the latter is used, the patient should also call the physician immediately.)

When patients come to the office or emergency room with a more severe acute exacerbation, higher or more frequent doses of β_2 agonists, often with ipratropium bromide, are given either by MDI and spacer or by using a nebulizer with a mouthpiece or a mask. Corticosteroids are prescribed to break the cycle of inflammation and airway hyper-responsiveness. If the patient's symptoms don't respond adequately hospitalization may be necessary.

Frequent asthma exacerbations are a sign that the long-term management plan is not adequate. The physician should review the environmental measures to decrease asthma triggers, and add or increase the dosages of long-term control medications.

Patient Education

Asthma differs from most other chronic diseases in that the exacerbations may be dramatic and even terrifying, thus posing a true challenge to the patient to respond calmly and appropriately. Several points deserve special mention.

- The difference between dosage schedules for chronic versus acute management is confusing to patients. An asthma action plan needs clear instructions identifying the controller medicines that should be taken daily, both when asthma is controlled and during exacerbations, and listing the steps to follow during exacerbations with addition of quick relief medication and adjustment of controller medications. Make photocopies for the patient to keep in several locations.
- Few asthma patients use their MDIs or peak flow meters correctly on a regular basis. Have patients demonstrate them at every visit and review their technique.

- Similarly, reinforce use of the peak-flow meter and the importance of keeping a diary if they have moderate or severe asthma. If they realize that a decrease in peak-flow value or an increase in symptoms can predict an asthma attack, they may be motivated to check their peak flow and use medication more appropriately.
- Remind patients to bring the peak-flow meter and diary to each visit for review of technique and results. They should measure and record peak flow twice a day for 1–2 weeks when medications are changed. In addition, patients with moderate-to-severe asthma should maintain a record of their peak flow readings for early detection of deterioration.
- Parents become understandably frantic if their child does not respond to quick-relief medications in his or her usual manner. It is important to let them know ahead of time that each attack is likely to be a little different, that the written instructions will indicate the proper response, and that a phone consultation with the physician is encouraged whenever they are unsure how to proceed.
- Asthma has a major impact on family relationships, especially when the patient is a child. Parents often need to be encouraged to be consistent in their expectations and their response to any unacceptable behavior and to provide frequent positive feedback to the child separate from dealing with the asthma. Providing education and clear-cut guidelines for the asthma management can help to reduce their

anxiety level. They should be reassured that most children with asthma can maintain normal activity levels and keep up with their peers.
- Environmental measures to decrease exposure to allergens and irritants should be reviewed every 6 to 12 months to reinforce their importance. If asthma is difficult to control, the possibility of environmental tobacco should be reassessed (44, 45).
- Health educators, nurses, respiratory care practitioners, and community workers can reinforce and expand on the education done in physicians' offices, both in classes and in individual sessions, in an office setting or in the patient's home.

Special Considerations

Pregnant women with asthma can be treated according to the same protocols as other patients. All of the inhaled asthma medications can be used in pregnancy. Montelukast and zafirlukast are Category B for pregnancy. Very little prednisone crosses the placenta, so it is also considered safe in pregnancy. Conversely, poorly controlled asthma is a known risk factor for intrauterine growth retardation.

Psychosocial stress and negative family dynamics may affect asthma control. In a study of patients with asthma, those who wrote about stressful experiences for 20 minutes 3 days in a row had improved FEV_1 up to 4 months later compared to those who wrote about neutral experiences, suggesting that

---

TABLE 49.9 Red Flags for Increased Risk of Death from Asthma

1. History of previous life-threatening exacerbation with
   - sudden onset
   - intensive care unit admission
   - intubation
2. Frequent unscheduled care manifest as
   - two or more hospitalizations in past year
   - three or more emergency visits in past year
   - emergency visit or hospitalization within past month
3. High medication need, as evidenced by
   - use of two or more MDIs of β_2 agonists per month
   - current use or recent withdrawal from systemic corticosteroids
4. Behavioral issues
   - serious psychiatric disease (including depression and psychosis)
   - illicit drug use
5. Social factors
   - low socioeconomic status
   - urban residence
   - limited access to ongoing medical care
6. Cognitive problems
   - difficulty perceiving changes in airflow obstruction
   - inability of patient or caretaker to understand instructions

Adapted from National Asthma Education and Prevention Program. Expert Panel Report II: Guidelines for the Diagnosis and Management of Asthma. Washington DC: US Department of Health and Human Services, 1997.

writing about the stresses was therapeutic (46). In another study of children aged 5 to 12 years old, analysis of family reports showed that severity of asthma was worse when fathers made more critical comments of their children and when fathers spent less time with their children (47). Maternal depression increases a child's likelihood of emergency department visits for asthma (48). These studies reinforce the importance of helping families and individuals address psychosocial issues.

Many of the environmental triggers for asthma are beyond the control of the individual patient and can only be controlled by changes in public policy. Family physicians can have a significant impact in these areas by advocating for laws to limit environmental tobacco smoke exposure and outdoor air pollution and for programs that provide assistance to schools, landlords, and families to improve indoor air quality.

Family physicians can manage asthma in the majority of their patients. Consultation with a pulmonary or allergy specialist is indicated if a patient's diagnosis is in doubt, the history suggests that immunotherapy may be beneficial, the asthma does not come under control within 3 to 6 months of appropriate treatment, or the patient has severe asthma. If the patient has any of the red flags that indicate increased risk of death (see Table 49.9), management should be coordinated with appropriate specialists, health educators, and home health or school nursing clinicians.

CASE DISCUSSION

S. has allergic rhinitis and conjunctivitis as well as asthma. The history of previous milder symptoms indicates an existing atopic tendency. Her allergic rhinitis can best be controlled with a daily nasal steroid spray and use of an oral antihistamine as needed. If these medications don't control the conjunctivitis, topical treatment would be indicated.

S. also has asthma. The history of symptoms with normal childhood activity (walking fast) suggests that there's a persistent component; the lack of baseline night-time cough and the presence of daytime symptoms some days but not daily indicate the severity is probably mildly persistent. S. should be taught to do peak flow measurements twice a day and record them in a diary, and spirometry should be scheduled. Appropriate treatment is to gain control of her symptoms quickly with a 5–7 day course of prednisone, use albuterol via MDI and spacer, 2–4 puffs every 4 hours as needed, and initiate low-dose inhaled corticosteroids. S. and her family should receive additional education about asthma and an asthma action plan describing her monitoring and medication regimen (a copy for her school should be provided as well). Initial follow-up should be in 1–2 weeks to determine her response to medications. Further follow-up visits will be needed to confirm the level of asthma severity and to review monitoring, trigger control, medication use, and response to treatment. It is likely that S. will be able to enjoy more physical activity after her asthma is controlled.

REFERENCES

1. National Center for Health Statistics. Fast stats A to Z—allergies/hayfever. Available at *http://www.cdc.gov/hcsh/ fastats/allergies.htm.* Accessed January 22, 2006.

2. Busse WW, Lemanske RF. Advances in immunology: asthma. N Engl J Med. 2001;344:350–362.

3. Karmaus W, Botezan C. Does a higher number of siblings protect against the development of allergy and asthma? A review. J Epidemiol Community Health. 2002;56:209–217.

4. Institute for Clinical Systems Improvement. Rhinitis, 5th ed. 2003. Available at *www.icsi.org,* enter search term "rhinitis." Accessed February 25, 2007.

5. Weiner JM, Abramson MJ, Puy RM. Intranasal corticosteroids versus oral H_1 receptor antagonists in allergic rhinitis: systematic review of randomized controlled trials. BMJ. 1998; 317:1624–1629.

6. Weber RW. Immunotherapy with allergens. JAMA 1997; 278:1881–1887.

7. Huggins JL, Looney RJ. Allergen Immunotherapy. Am Fam Physician. 2004;70:689–696,703–704.

8. National Center for Health Statistics. Asthma prevalence, health care use and mortality, 2002. Available at *www.cdc.gov/ nchs/products/pubs/pubd/hestats/asthma/asthma.htm.* Accessed February 25, 2007.

9. National Asthma Education and Prevention Program. Expert Panel Report II: guidelines for the diagnosis and management of asthma. Washington, DC: US Department of Health and Human Services, 1997.

10. NAEPP Expert Panel Report: guidelines for the diagnosis and management of asthma—ipdate on selected topics 2002. NIH Publication No. 02-5074. Available at www.nhlbi.nih. gov/guidelines/asthma Accessed February 25, 2007.

11. Young S, O'Keeffe PT, Arnott J, Landau LI. Lung function, airway responsiveness, and respiratory symptoms before and after bronchiolitis. Arch Dis Child. 1995;72:16–24.

12. Ball TM, Castro-Rodriguez JA, Griffith KA, et al. Siblings, day-care attendance, and the risk of asthma and wheezing during childhood. N Eng J Med 2000;343:538–543.

13. Salam MT, Li YF, Langholz B, Gilliland FD. Early-life environmental risk factors for asthma: findings from the Children's Health Study. Environ Health Perspect. 2005;112: 760–765.

14. Oddy WH, Holt PG, Sly PD, et al. Association between breast feeding and asthma in 6 year old children: findings of a prospective birth cohort study. BMJ 1999;319:815–819.

15. Ram FSF, Ducharme FM, Scarlett J. Cow's milk protein avoidance and development of childhood wheeze in children with a family history of atopy (Cochrane Review). In: The Cochrane Library. Oxford, England: Update Software; 2005: Issue 1.

16. Global Initiative for Asthma. Global Strategy for Asthma Management and Prevention. Availble at *http://www. ginasthma.org/Guidelineitem.asp??11 = 2&12 = 1&intId = 60.*

17. Martinez FD, Wright AL, Taussig LM, et al. Asthma and wheezing in the first six years of life. N Engl J Med. 1995; 332:133–138.

18. Soyseth V, Kongerud J, Boe J. Postnatal maternal smoking increases the prevalence of asthma but not of bronchial hyperresponsiveness or atopy in their children. Chest. 1995;107: 389–394.

19. Brooke AM, Lambert PC, Burton PR, Clarke C, Luyt DK, Simpson H. The natural history of respiratory symptoms in preschool children. Am J Respir Crit Care Med. 1995;152: 1872–1878.

20. Simon PM, Schwartzstien RM, Weiss JW, Fencl V, Teghtsoonian M, Weinberger S. Distinguishable types of dyspnea in patients with shortness of breath. Am Rev Respir Dis. 1990;142:1009–1014.

21. Sinha T, David AK. Recognition and management of exer-

cise-induced bronchospasm. Am Fam Physician. 2003:
769–774, 776.

22. Li JT, O'Connell E. Clinical evaluation of asthma. Ann Allergy Asthma Immunol. 1996;76:1–14.

23. Turcotte H, Boulet L. Perception of breathlessness during early and late asthmatic responses. Am Rev Respir Dis. 1993; 148:514–518.

24. van Schayck CP, van Weel C, Harbers HJM, van Herwaarden CLA. Do physical signs reflect the degree of airflow obstruction in patients with asthma or chronic obstructive pulmonary disease? Scand J Prim Health Care. 1991;9: 232–238.

25. King DK, Thompson BT, Johnson DC. Wheezing on maximal forced exhalation in the diagnosis of atypcal asthma. Ann Intern Med. 1989;110:451–455.

26. Nowak RM, Pensler MI, Sarkar DD, et al. Comparison of peak expiratory flow and FEV_1 admission criteria for acute bronchial asthma. Ann Emerg Med 1982;11:64–69.

27. Gibson PG, Powell H. Written action plans for asthma: an evidence-based review of the key components. Thorax. 2004 Feb;59(2):94–99.

28. Gibson PG, Powell H, Coughlan J, et al. Self-management education and regular practitioner review for adults with asthma (Cochrane Review). In: The Cochrane Library. Oxford, England: Update Software; 2005:Issue 1.

29. Evans R, Gergen PJ, Mitchell H, et al. A randomized clinical trial to reduce asthma morbidity among inner-city children: results of the National Cooperative Inner-City Asthma Study. J Pediatr. 1999;135:332–338.

30. Morgan WJ, Crain EF, Gruchalla RS, et al. Results of a home-based environmental intervention among urban children with asthma. N Engl J Med. 2004;351:1068–1080.

31. Abramson MJ, Pay RM, Weiner JM. Is allergen immunotherapy effective in asthma? A meta-analysis of randomized clinical trials. Am J Respir Crit Care Med. 1995;151:969–974.

32. Abramson MJ, Puy RM, Weiner JM. Allergen immunotherapy for asthma. (Cochrane Review). In: The Cochrane Library. Oxford, England: Update Software; 2003:Issue 4.

33. Castro-Rodriguez JA, Rodrigo GJ. Beta-agonists through metered-dose inhaler with valved holding chamber versus nebulizer for acute exacerbation of wheezing or asthma in children under 5 years of age: a systematic review with meta-analysis. J Pediatr. 2004 Aug;145(2)172–177.

34. Newman KB Milne S, Hamilton C, Hall K. A comparison of albuterol administered by metered-dose inhaler and spacer with albuterol by nebulizer in adults presenting to an urban emergency department with acute asthma. Chest. 2002;121: 1036–1041.

35. Dompeling E, van Schayck CP, van Grunsven M, et al. Slowing the deterioration of asthma and chronic obstructive pulmonary disease observed during bronchodilator therapy by adding inhaled corticosteroids. Ann Intern Med. 1993;118: 770–778.

36. Price J, Hindmarsh P, Hughes S, Efthimiou J. Evaluating the effects of asthma therapy on childhood growth: what can be learnt from the published literature? Eur Respir J. 2002 Jun;19(6):1179–1193.

37. Ram FS, Cates CJ, Ducharme FM. Long-acting beta2-agonists versus anti-leukotrienes as add-on therapy to inhaled corticosteroids for chronic asthma (Cochrane Review). In: The Cochrane Library. Oxford, England: Update Software; 2005:Issue 1.

38. Walker S, Monteil M, Phelan K, Lasserson TJ, Walters EH. Anti-IgE for chronic asthma in adults and children (Cochrane Review). In: The Cochrane Library. Oxford, England: Update Software; 2003:Issue 3.

39. FDA Medical Officer Review of Salmeterol, September 2004.

Available at *http://www.fda.gov/ohrms/dockets/ac/05/briefing/2005-4148B1_03_02-FDA-Smart-Study.pdf*. Accessed February 25, 2007.

40. Rodrigo G, Rodrigo C, Burschtin O. A meta-analysis of the effects of ipratropium bromide in adults with acute asthma. Am J Med. 1999;107:363–370.

41. Plotnick LH, Ducharme FM. Should inhaled anticholinergics be added to beta2 agonists for treating acute childhood and adolescent asthma? A systematic review. BMJ. 1998;317: 971–977.

42. Foresi A, Morelli MC, Catena E. Low-dose budesonide with the addition of an increased dose during exacerbations is effective in long-term asthma control. Chest. 2000;117:440–446.

43. Edmonds ML, Camargo CA Jr, Pollack CV Jr, Rowe BH. Early use of inhaled corticosteroids in the emergency department treatment of acute asthma (Cochrane Review). In: The Cochrane Library. Oxford, England: Update Software; 2005: Issue 1.

44. Thomson NC, Spears M. The influence of smoking on the treatment response in patients with asthma. Curr Opin Allergy Clin Immunol. 2005 Feb;5(1):57–63.

45. Chaudhuri R, Livingston E, McMahon AD, Thomson L, Borland W, Thomson NC. Cigarette smoking impairs the therapeutic response to oral corticosteroids in chronic asthma. Am J Respir Crit Care Med. 2003 Dec 1;168(11):1308–1311.

46. Smyth JM, Stone AA, Hurewitz A, Kaell A. Effects of writing about stressful experiences on symptom reduction in patients with asthma or rheumatoid arthritis: a randomized trial. JAMA 1999;281:1304–1309.

47. Gartland HJ, Day HD. Symptoms: expressed emotion, medication, parent contact, and life events. J Clin Psychol. 1999; 55(5):573–584.

48. Bartlett SJ, Kolodner K, Butz AM, Eggleston P, Malveaux FJ, Rand CS. Maternal depressive symptoms and emergency department use among inner-city children with asthma. Arch Pediatr Adolesc Med. 2001 Mar;155(3):347–353.

49. Sheikh A, Hurwitz B. House dust mite avoidance measures for perennial allergic rhinitis (Cochrane Review). In: The Cochrane Library. Oxford, England: Update Software; 2005: Issue 1.

50. Yanez A, Rodrigo GJ. Intranasal corticosteroids versus topical H1 receptor antagonists for the treatment of allergic rhinitis: a systematic review with meta-analysis. Ann Allergy Asthma Immunol. 2002 Nov;89(5):479–484.

51. Hore I, Georgalas C, Scadding G. Oral antihistamines for the symptom of nasal obstruction in persistent allergic rhinitis—a systematic review of randomized controlled trials. Clin Exp Allergy. 2005 Feb;35(2):207–212.

52. Allergic Rhinitis, Guidelines for clinical care. University of Michigan Health System. July 2002. Available at *http://cme.med.umich.edu/pdf/guideline/allergic.pdf*. Accessed February 25, 2007.

53. Wilson AM, O'Byrne PM, Parameswaran K. Leukotriene receptor antagonists for allergic rhinitis: a systematic review and meta-analysis. Am J Med. 2004 Mar 1;116(5):338–344.

54. Meltzer EO, Malmstrom K, Lu S, et al. Concomitant montelukast and loratadine as treatment for seasonal allergic rhinitis: A randomized, placebo-controlled clinical trial. J Allergy Clin Immunol 2000;105:917–922.

55. Greiner JV, Udell IJ. A comparison of the clinical efficacy of pheniramine maleate/naphazoline hydrochloride ophthalmic solution and olopatadine hydrochloride ophthalmic solution in the conjunctival allergen challenge model. Clin Ther. 2005 May;27(5):568–577.

56. Ross RN, Nelson HS, Finegold I. Effectiveness of specific immunotherapy in the treatment of allergic rhinitis: an analy-

sis of randomized, prospective, single- or double-blind, placebo-controlled studies. Clin Ther. 2000 Mar;22(3): 342–50.

57. Wilson DR, Torres Lima M, Durham SR. Sublingual immunotherapy for allergic rhinitis (Cochrane Review). In: The Cochrane Library. Oxford, England: Update Software; 2005: Issue 1.

58. Gdalevich M, Mimouni D, Mimouni M. Breast-feeding and the risk of bronchial asthma in childhood: a systematic review with meta-analysis of prospective studies. J Pediatr. 2001 Aug; 139(2):261–266.

59. Powell H, Gibson PG. Options for self-management education for adults with asthma (Cochrane Review). In: The Cochrane Library. Oxford, England: Update Software; 2004: Issue 1.

60. Sin DD, ManJ, Sharpe H, et al. Pharmacological management to reduce exacerbations in adults with asthma: a systematic review and meta-analysis. JAMA. 2004 Jul 21;292(3): 367–376.

61. Ni CM, Greenstone IR, Ducharme FM. Addition of inhaled long-acting beta2-agonists to inhaled steroids as first line therapy for persistent asthma in steroid-naïve adults (Cochrane Review). In: The Cochrane Library. Oxford, England: Update Software; 2005:Issue 2.

62. Duchamme FM, Hicks GC. Anti-leukotriene agents compared to inhaled corticosteroids in the management of recurrent and/or chronic asthma in adults and children. (Cochrane Review). The Cochrane Library, Issue 1, 2004. Chichester UK: John Wiley & Sons, Ltd.

63. Plotnick LH, Ducharme FM. Combined inhaled anticholinergics and beta2-agonists for initial treatment of acute asthma in children (Cochrane Review). In: The Cochrane Library. Oxford, England: Update Software; 2000:Issue 3.

64. Rodrigo GJ, Castro-Rodriguez JA. Anticholinergics in the treatment of children and adults with acute asthma: a systematic review with meta-analysis. Thorax. 2005 Sep;60(9): 740–746.

65. Fitzgerald JM, Dennis RJ, Solarte I. Asthma. Clin Evid Concise. 2005;13:432–435.

66. Cates CJ, Bara A, Crilly JA, Rowe BH. Holding chambers versus nebulisers for beta-agonist treatment of acute asthma. (Cochrane Review). In: The Cochrane Library. Oxford, England: Update Software; 2003:Issue 2.

CHAPTER 50

Acute Respiratory Infections

Arch G. Mainous III and William J. Hueston

CASE STUDY

Mr. S. is a 48-year-old man who has been seeing you for several years for routine health maintenance. He works as an accountant and is in good health, is taking no medications, and has no allergies. He comes in to see you one afternoon feeling ill with a productive cough that started yesterday. He has felt hot at home and occasionally had sweats, but has not taken his temperature. He says he had some nasal congestion 3 weeks ago, but that seemed to have cleared before these problems started. He is not having any nausea or vomiting, but feels run down and tired. On physical examination, he looks moderately ill with a fever of 101.5°F. His heart rate is 90, and respiratory rate is 16. His tympanic membranes are normal, his nose is clear, and his sinuses transilluminate well bilaterally. His throat shows no erythema or tonsillar exudates. His neck is supple, and he has no cervical nodes. On lung examination, he has decreased breath sounds at the left base, with rales heard. Your nurse conducts a pulse oximetry reading, which shows his oxygen saturation at 97%. You explain to Mr. S. that he probably has a community-acquired pneumonia. Mr. S. is concerned because both his mother and father were hospitalized for pneumonia later in their lives; he wonders if this means he will have to go into the hospital as well. He says he doesn't have time to be sick, since tax season is coming up. You arrange for a chest radiograph to confirm your clinical suspicion and suggest some simple blood work before you can make a firm recommendation about hospitalization. Mr. S. leaves to have his chest radiography and lab work done, while you contemplate whether he should be hospitalized.

Mr. S. returns and you find that he has a well-defined lobar infiltrate in his left lower lobe. His laboratory work, which included a chemistry profile and complete blood count, reveals that his white blood count is elevated at 15,300 with 73% neutrophils, but his hemoglobin, electrolytes, and creatinine are all normal.

You confirm that Mr. S. is still married, and that his wife is available to help during his illness. Mr. S. has been a reliable patient, so you have no concerns about his ability to follow up with you within the week so you can monitor his illness. Because you are suspicious that he has pneumococcal pneumonia, you prescribe a respiratory quinolone for him and arrange a recheck in 4 days. Mr. S. returns feeling significantly better and notes that he was able to return to work the day before. You are relieved to see that he is better, especially because he has done your taxes for the last 8 years!

CLINICAL QUESTIONS

1. How are upper respiratory tract infections distinguished from each other?
2. When are antibiotics indicated as treatment?
3. How are serious lower respiratory tract infections distinguished from self-limited respiratory infections?

Acute respiratory infections range from self-limited conditions such as uncomplicated upper respiratory infections (URI, common cold) to serious life-threatening conditions like pneumonia. URIs and acute bronchitis are among the most common reasons for visits in ambulatory care; they account for significant morbidity and absenteeism from work and school. Management of these infections has been complicated by recent evidence indicating a rise in the prevalence of antibiotic-resistant pathogens (1). The vast majority of antibiotics prescribed in ambulatory settings are for respiratory tract infections (2). The injudicious use of antimicrobial agents creates an environment for developing resistance, placing the population and individual patient at risk. Consequently, appropriate treatment of acute respiratory tract infections has become a challenge to the clinician. This chapter reviews the common infections of the upper and lower respiratory tract.

Bacterial or viral pathogens invade the respiratory tract and grow rapidly and aggressively. The physiological responses to viral or bacterial pathogens in respiratory tract infections tend to be similar. It is important to be aware that the majority of colonized bacteria found in the respiratory tract do not cause any problems for individuals with normal immune systems, until there is a breakdown in the immune system. For example, a significant proportion of children are colonized by *Streptococcus pneumoniae*, the leading cause of pneumonia, otitis media, and bacteremia. Yet *S. pneumoniae* bacteria tend not to cause illness in people with normally functioning immune systems; treating children with antibiotics, therefore, to eradicate *S. pneumoniae* has been incapable of preventing illness.

Infection can exist throughout the respiratory tract, with inflammation and involvement of the mucosal surfaces of the nose, the paranasal sinuses, pharynx, Eustachian tube, middle ear, epiglottis, larynx, trachea, bronchi, bronchioles, and alveoli. The inflammatory response to the infectious agent produces mucosal swelling, discharge, and local pain. Many diagnoses used for respiratory tract infections have significant symptom overlap with others (e.g., acute sinusitis and common

769

cold; common cold and acute bronchitis). It may be useful to conceptualize these entities in more general terms (3). For example, infections localized in respiratory structures above the larynx can be conceptualized as URIs, and correspondingly those below the larynx as lower respiratory tract infections. An advantage to focusing on different primary sites of infection is that different pathogens are more common at certain sites than others thereby providing a guide for treatment.

SINUS AND NASAL PROBLEMS

Generally, viruses are the most common causes of respiratory complaints, and the history and physical examination are meant to detecting other reasons for these symptoms. The most common causes of noninfectious nasal discharge include allergic rhinitis and foreign bodies. Key historical findings that suggest causes other than infection for a runny nose include unilateral nasal discharge (as seen with a foreign body or necrotic tumor) or a clear nasal discharge that has persisted for several weeks (suggesting allergy).

Differentiating bacterial from viral URIs is very difficult. Evidence suggests that many of the symptoms that are typically ascribed to bacterial sinusitis occur just as often with sinus inflammation associated with common colds. Two studies have been helpful in identifying clinical cues that can be used to differentiate these two conditions. Combined, these studies suggest that patients with sinusitis are more likely to have a constellation of maxillary toothache, purulent nasal discharge by history or examination, poor sinus transillumination, and a lack of response to decongestants, along with a phenomenon termed "double sickening" (4, 5). Double sickening refers to patients who say they started with the symptoms of a common cold, but a few days later they "got sicker" (5). One or two of these symptoms alone are not predictive of a sinusitis, but the presence of the entire spectrum increases the likelihood of a secondary sinusitis (4).

SORE THROATS

Sore throats or hoarseness may be caused by a limited number of other conditions. These are primarily laryngeal inflammation from acute insults such as smoke inhalation, chronic abuse from smoking, or singing. Vocal cord neoplasms may also be suspected in patients with chronic hoarseness, especially if risk factors such as cigarette smoking or alcohol use are present.

Pharyngeal infections are even more difficult to differentiate into bacterial- or viral-based on clinical criteria. Decision rules using fever, tonsillar exudate, cervical adenopathy, and the lack of either a runny nose or cough have been evaluated to identify patients with streptococcal pharyngitis, but have had mixed success (6). Another difficulty in evaluating decision rules is that a large segment of the population (up to 20%) can be colonized with group A *Streptococcus*; so a positive culture may not indicate infection with this agent in a fairly large group of patients. However, at this time either rapid or conventional throat cultures remain the best way to differentiate a strep throat from pharyngitis associated with a cold. See Chapter 21 for a detailed discussion of sore throat.

COUGH AND LOWER RESPIRATORY SYMPTOMS

For lower respiratory symptoms such as cough, additional noninfectious causes should be considered. Congestive heart failure, aspiration of gastric contents or foreign bodies, lung neoplasms, asthma, and other inflammatory pulmonary conditions can produce a cough and shortness of breath. Congestive heart failure and pulmonary embolism also can cause pulmonary infiltrates and effusions that can be confused with pneumonia. Medications, most notably angiotensin-converting enzyme inhibitors, may cause a cough as well.

If a lower respiratory infection is suspected, several possible conditions should be considered. First, it is important to differentiate acute bronchitis, a self-limited condition, from pneumonia. The presence of rales and/or a localized decrease in breath sounds suggest pneumonia, but may not be sensitive. Patients who appear to be ill yet have no abnormal physical findings on lung examination that suggest pneumonia should have a chest radiograph.

In addition to pneumonia, other infectious conditions can cause rales and productive cough. Pulmonary abscesses may produce undulating fevers, shortness of breath, and cough. Abscesses are associated with certain types of pneumonia-causing organisms such as *Staphylococcus sp*. Bronchiectasis is a bronchial wall disease that allows accumulation of large amounts of secretions in the diseased bronchus. The copious secretions result in a chronic productive cough. Furthermore, these pooled secretions often become infected and can produce a fever, shortness of breath, and purulent sputum production consistent with pneumonia.

DIFFERENTIAL DIAGNOSIS

Uncomplicated URI/Common Cold

URIs, or the "common cold," are common infectious conditions often seen in the ambulatory care setting (7, 8). Adults typically have two to four URIs annually, and children in day care have as many as six or seven (9, 10). Although URIs are mild, self-limited, and of short duration, they are a leading cause of acute morbidity, and industrial and school absenteeism (11). Each year, URIs account for 170 million days of restricted activity, 23 million days of school absence, and 18 million days of work absence. And while colds may be viewed as benign, the impact of URIs on quality of life is similar in magnitude to such chronic illnesses as chronic lung disease, depression, or osteoarthritis (12).

The mechanisms of transmission suggest that URIs can be spread through contact with inanimate surfaces (13) as well as direct hand-to-hand contact (14). URIs have a seasonal variation, with an increased prevalence in the United States between September and March. It is unclear why this variation exists although it may be related to increased crowding of indoor populations in the colder months. Temperature is not the key to seasonal variation without the presence of a pathogen. Evidence from Antarctica showed that spacious well-ventilated rooms reduced transmission of URIs compared to crowded poorly-ventilated rooms regardless of temperature (15).

One study was able to identify the specific virus believed

to cause a URI in 69% of all URI cases (16). Rhinoviruses were the most prevalent virus and were seen in 52% of the patients. Coronaviruses were the second most common group of causative agents, followed by influenza A or B virus. Identified bacterial pathogens were *Chlamydia pneumoniae, Haemophilus influenza, Streptococcus pneumoniae,* and *Mycoplasma pneumoniae.* None of the patients had beta-hemolytic group A *Streptococcus.* In terms of bacterial pathogens, infections without evidence of a viral infection occurred in only 0.05% of the cases.

Uncomplicated URIs are characterized by rhinorrhea, nasal congestion, sneezing, sore or "scratchy" throat, and cough (17). The incubation period varies between 48 and 72 hours. In some cases a low-grade fever is present, but temperature elevation is rare in adults. The early symptoms may be minimal and limited to malaise and nasal symptoms. The nasal discharge is initially clear and watery. There is a subsequent transition period where the nasal discharge becomes viscous, opaque, and discolored (white, yellow, green) (17). The color of the secretions alone is not predictive of a bacterial infection. The clinical presentation is similar in both adults and children. The episode tends to be self-limited. The median duration of a cold is 1 week, with most patients improving by day 10, but lingering symptoms may last up to two weeks.

Acute Sinusitis

Because sinusitis usually is a complication of upper respiratory viral infections, the incidence peaks in the winter. Among children, sinusitis is frequently found as a comorbidity with otitis media (18). Children are also more likely to have posterior ethmoidal and sphenoid inflammation, while adults have mainly maxillary and anterior ethmoidal sinusitis (19).

Some medical conditions may increase the risk for sinusitis. These include cystic fibrosis, asthma, immunosuppression, and allergic rhinitis (19). Cigarette smoking may also increase the risk of bacterial sinusitis during a cold because of reduced mucociliary clearance.

Sinus inflammation can be caused by viral, fungal, and bacterial infections as well as allergies. Most acute sinusitis is caused by viral infection. The inflammation associated with viral infections clears without additional therapy.

Cultures from patients with sinusitis show that the most prevalent organisms are *S. pneumoniae* and, especially in smokers, *H. influenza.* These two organisms are present in 70% of bacterial acute sinusitis cases (20). When antibiotics are used to treat bacterial sinusitis, selection criteria should include sufficient coverage of these two organisms.

Fungal sinusitis is very rare and usually occurs in immunosuppressed individuals or those with diabetes mellitus.

Acute sinusitis has considerable overlap in its constellation of signs and symptoms with URIs. One half to two thirds of patients with sinus symptoms seen in primary care are unlikely to have sinusitis (21). URIs are often precursors of sinusitis, and at some point symptoms from each condition may overlap. Sinus inflammation from a URI without bacterial infection is also common. In a series of 60 children undergoing computerized tomography (CT) for nonsinus-related diagnoses, 47% had evidence of sinus inflammation with no clinical signs of sinusitis, and with complete resolution following their viral illness (22).

Acute sinusitis tends to start with a URI that leads to sinus ostial obstruction. The signs and symptoms that increase the likelihood that the patient has acute sinusitis are a "double sickening" phenomenon, maxillary toothache, purulent nasal discharge, poor response to decongestants, and a history of discolored nasal discharge (4, 23). Other authors have stressed that the symptoms need to persist longer than 1 week to distinguish sinusitis from a URI (24). It should be pointed out that the commonly used sign of facial pain or swelling has low sensitivity for acute sinusitis (4).

Acute Bronchitis

Acute bronchitis in the otherwise healthy adult is one of the most common medical problems encountered in primary care. The prevalence of acute bronchitis peaks in the winter and is much less common in the summer.

Viral infection is the primary cause of most episodes of acute bronchitis. A wide variety of viruses have been shown as causes of acute bronchitis including influenza, rhinovirus, adenovirus, coronavirus, parainfluenza, and respiratory syncytial virus (25). Nonviral pathogens including *Mycoplasma pneumoniae* and *Chlamydia pneumoniae* have also been identified as causes (26, 27).

The etiologic role of bacteria like *H. influenza* and *S. pneumoniae* in acute bronchitis is unclear because these bacteria are common upper respiratory tract flora. Sputum cultures for acute bronchitis are therefore difficult to evaluate since it is unclear whether the sputum has been contaminated by pathogens colonizing the nasopharynx.

Acute bronchitis is an inflammatory condition of the tracheobronchial tree usually associated with a generalized respiratory infection. Cough begins early in the course of the illness and is the most prominent feature of the condition. An initially dry cough may later result in sputum production, which characteristically changes from clear to discolored in the later stages of the illness. The cough may last for a significant time. Although the duration of the condition is variable, one study showed that 50% of patients had a cough for more than 3 weeks, and 25% had a cough for more than 4 weeks (28).

Patients with acute bronchitis usually have a viral respiratory infection with transient inflammatory changes that produce sputum and symptoms of airway obstruction. Acute bronchitis is essentially a diagnosis of exclusion. The history should include information on cigarette use, exposure to environmental toxins (e.g., dust, beryllium, volatile organic compounds, asbestos), as well as medication history (e.g., use of angiotensin converting enzyme inhibitors). The chronicity of the cough should be established to distinguish acute bronchitis from chronic bronchitis since they have different treatments.

Both acute bronchitis and pneumonia can present with fever, constitutional symptoms, and a productive cough. While patients with pneumonia often have rales, this finding is neither sensitive nor specific for the illness. When pneumonia is suspected because of a high fever, constitutional symptoms, severe dyspnea, and certain physical findings or risk factors, a chest radiograph should be obtained to confirm the diagnosis.

Asthma and allergic bronchospastic disorders can mimic the productive cough of acute bronchitis. When obstructive symptoms are not obvious, mild asthma may be misdiagnosed as acute bronchitis. Further, since respiratory infections can trigger bronchospasm in asthma, patients with asthma that occurs only in the presence of respiratory infections may present as patients with acute bronchitis.

Asthma should be considered in patients with repetitive episodes of acute bronchitis. Patients who repeatedly present with cough and wheezing can be given pulmonary function testing with and without a bronchodilator. For patients for whom routine pulmonary function testing is equivocal but asthma is highly suspected, further or provocative testing with a methacholine challenge test may help differentiate asthma from recurrent bronchitis.

Finally, nonpulmonary causes of cough should enter the differential diagnosis. In older patients, congestive heart failure may cause cough, shortness of breath, and wheezing. Reflux esophagitis with chronic aspiration can cause bronchial inflammation with cough and wheezing. Bronchogenic tumors may produce a cough and obstructive symptoms.

Bronchiolitis

Acute bronchiolitis is a distinct syndrome occurring in young children with a peak incidence at 6 months of age. It is an acute respiratory illness resulting from inflammation of small airways and characterized by wheezing. Children generally acquire the infection from family members or other children in day care who are infected with an upper respiratory tract infection. Bronchiolitis is not uncommon, with approximately 15% of children experiencing this illness during the first 2 years of life.

Respiratory syncytial virus (RSV) is the most common cause of bronchiolitis accounting for between 50% and 90% of cases. The majority of the cases occur during the winter and early spring mirroring the prevalence of the viral pathogens in the community.

The diagnosis of bronchiolitis is based on clinical findings and on the knowledge of the prevalence of viral pathogens prevalent in the community. The classic signs of bronchiolitis are wheezing and hyperexpansion of the lungs. Bronchiolitis begins as a URI, but soon the patient develops a cough, audible wheezing, irritability, listlessness, dyspnea, and cyanosis. Chest radiographs may reveal atelectasis, hyperinflation, or both. Untreated, infants with bronchiolitis can die from hypoxemia, dehydration, or apnea; less than 1% of affected infants die, however. Most recover but suffer recurrent wheezing episodes, usually precipitated by viral infections.

Influenza

Approximately 10% to 20% of the population in the United States develops influenza annually, with influenza season usually peaking between late December and early March. In recent influenza seasons, especially when influenza A type H3N2 predominated, 80% to 90% of influenza-related deaths occurred in individuals older than 65 years of age. It is the fifth leading cause of death in individuals over 65, and the most common infectious cause of death in this country. Rates of disease are increased in individuals 65 years of age or older and in those with underlying health problems, such as diabetes mellitus and coronary artery disease (29, 30).

Influenza is caused by highly infectious RNA viruses of the orthomyxovirus family. Influenza A viruses are classified into subtypes based on two surface antigens—hemagglutinin (H) and neuraminidase (N). Changes in the H or N antigen account for the epidemiologic success of these viruses. Infec-

tion with one subtype however, provides little protection against infection with other subtypes, and infection or vaccination with one strain does not result in immunity to distantly related strains of the same subtype because of antigenic drift. Consequently, major epidemics of respiratory disease are caused by influenza virus strains not represented in that year's vaccine.

Occasionally, there are major shifts in the antigenic composition of the influenza virus. Such shifts are believed to be associated with the deadly pandemic of influenza in 1917–1918 as well as pandemics in 1957 and 1968 (31, 32). What made the 1918 influenza pandemic so remarkable was the high fatality rate in young to middle-age adults. Concerns about emerging antigen shifts associated with avian flu viruses compare possible consequences to the 1918 pandemic, although there is no evidence that an avian strain was associated with this prior epidemic.

During the initial evaluation of an influenza-like illness, the following entities must be considered in the differential: respiratory syncytial virus, parainfluenza, adenovirus, enterovirus, *mycoplasma*, *chlamydia*, and streptococcal disease. Influenza is extremely contagious and is transmitted from person to person through small particles of virus-laden respiratory secretions that are propelled into the air by infected persons during coughing, sneezing, and talking. The abrupt onset of fever, myalgia, sore throat, and a nonproductive cough characterize the typical influenza infection. Symptoms usually last 1 to 5 days. Unlike other common respiratory illnesses, influenza viruses cause severe malaise lasting several days. The symptoms vary by age, with children commonly presenting with cough, rhinorrhea, and croup, while adults present with cough, myalgia, sore throat, and headache. The elderly usually complain of cough alone or in combination with headache. A key to diagnosis is being aware of influenza outbreaks in the community at the time of presentation.

The availability of rapid tests to identify influenza has made it possible to evaluate patients quickly for this disorder. However, the cost-benefit of this approach is questionable (33). Most studies show that during flu season when influenza is highly likely, it is most economical to simply treat the patient. The value of office-based testing is probably during the "shoulders" of flu season when the probability of influenza is lower.

Community-Acquired Pneumonia

Pneumonia is one of the most common reasons for hospitalization and is the sixth leading cause of death in the United States. Pneumonia causes over 10 million visits to physicians annually and accounts for 3% of all hospitalizations in the United States (34). Pneumonia occurs in about 12 people/1,000 per year, but is much higher in the elderly population (35). In the United States, hospitalizations for pneumonia in adults over age 65 rose by 20% between 1990 and 2000 (36). Pneumonia is even more common in the very-elderly. One of every 20 individuals over the age of 85 will be hospitalized for pneumonia in a given year (36). In addition to age, institutionalization and debilitation increase the risk for acquiring pneumonia (37). Smokers and patients with chronic respiratory diseases are more likely to require hospitalization for pneumonia (38).

Comorbidities in a patient are strongly linked to survival from pneumonia. Patients with underlying comorbidities such as congestive heart failure, cerebrovascular diseases, cancer, diabetes mellitus, and poor nutritional status are more likely to die from pneumonia if they are infected. Thus, age and comorbidities are important factors to consider when deciding whether to hospitalize a patient with pneumonia.

In the past, over 80% of confirmed pneumonia cases were caused by *Streptococcus pneumoniae* with mortality rates between 20% and 40% (34). While pneumococcal disease still represents the largest single cause of pneumonia in large recent studies, other bacterial causes and nonbacterial pathogens now represent the majority of cases. Prevalence data from a number of North American studies estimate that pneumococcal pneumonia now represents about 20%–60% of documented cases. Atypical agents such as Legionella and *Mycoplasma* are identified in 10%–20% of infections while less common causes include viruses (2%–15%), *Haemophilus influenza* (3–10%), *Staphylococcus aureus* (3–5%), and gram negative organisms (3%–10%) (34).

Primary care physicians must be cautious when interpreting the data on the prevalence of causative agents for pneumonia. These data are generally derived from a few academic medical centers and may only include cases in which a causative agent was identified. The increase in the number of patients who are immunosuppressed from drug therapy or HIV disease and the trend towards treating less severely ill individuals as outpatients has skewed the spectrum of illness cared for in the hospital setting. An example of this are data from Johns Hopkins Hospital in 1991 in which *S. pneumoniae* was the most common cause of pneumonia, but was followed in frequency by *Pneumocystis carinii,* which accounted for 13% of all cases (34).

The most common presenting complaints for patients with pneumonia are fever and a cough, which may be either productive or nonproductive. In one study, 80% of patients with pneumonia had a fever. Other symptoms that suggest pneumonia include dyspnea and pleuritic chest pain. However, none of these symptoms is specific for pneumonia.

Symptoms of pneumonia may be very nonspecific in older patients. Elderly individuals who suffer a general decline in their function, become confused or have worsening dementia, or experience frequent falls should receive a chest radiograph even if no pulmonary symptoms or physical findings are present (39). Elderly patients who have preexisting cognitive impairment or depend on someone else for support of their daily activities are at highest risk for not exhibiting typical symptoms of pneumonia (39).

The most consistent sign of pneumonia is tachypnea. In one study of elderly patients, tachypnea was observed to be present 3 to 4 days before the appearance of other physical findings of pneumonia (40). Rales or crackles are often considered the hallmark for pneumonia, but these may be heard in only 75%–80% of patients (35, 37). Other signs of pneumonia, such as dullness to percussion or egophony, which are usually believed to indicate consolidation, occur in less than a third of patients with pneumonia (34).

Chest radiography is the diagnostic standard for pneumonia. In rare cases, the chest radiograph may be falsely negative. This generally occurs in profound dehydration, early pneumonia (first 24 hours), infection with *Pneumocystis,* and severe neutropenia (34). Not every infiltrate is an infectious pneumonia, however. Other conditions such as postobstructive pneu-

monitis, pulmonary infarct from an embolism, radiation pneumonitis, and interstitial edema from congestive heart failure may produce infiltrates that are indistinguishable from an infectious process.

Adequate specimens for sputum evaluation may be difficult to obtain, especially on an outpatient basis. Even for those who can produce sputum that is sufficient for culture, 30% to 65% of specimens do not grow out a predominant organism. For patients admitted to the hospital, sputum cultures may be useful because when the results are positive, they can help guide initial therapy (41).

Blood cultures are controversial for patients with pneumonia. In ambulatory patients who will be treated on an outpatient basis, blood cultures rarely produce clinically useful data. Even in hospitalized patients, the clinical usefulness and cost-effectiveness of blood cultures in otherwise healthy nonimmunosuppressed patients is controversial (42). For patients in whom hospitalization is considered, serum electrolytes, blood urea nitrogen/creatinine, and arterial oxygen saturation should be determined. For patients who appear well and for whom hospitalization is not expected, assessment of oxygen saturation with a pulse oximeter may be sufficient.

CLINICAL EVALUATION

Patients with acute respiratory infections need a focused history that includes current and recent symptoms, duration of episode, prior episodes and treatment, other family members affected, risk factors, and smoking history. In addition, several red flags in the history and physical examination may alert the clinician to noninfectious or life-threatening emergencies (see Table 50.1).

History and Physical Examination

Fever is a nonspecific sign, but can be used to discriminate mild, self-limited problems, such as acute bronchitis, from more significant infections such as pneumonia. Both the height of the temperature and the pattern of its development can give clues to the diagnosis. For example, URI ("colds") generally cause little or no fever in older children and adults. However, a child with symptoms of a common cold but who also has a high fever might be suspected of having otitis media, sinusitis, or another bacterial infection. Fever also can be used to discriminate between different types of virally-mediated illnesses such as the common cold and influenza, since influenza generally produces a high fever.

Rhinorrhea, either watery or purulent, indicates inflammation in the nasal cavities from either an infectious or noninfectious source. Although viral illnesses commonly cause runny noses, noninfectious conditions such as allergic rhinitis (hay fever) and a foreign body in the nose can also present with rhinorrhea. In viral illnesses, the nose is usually red and swollen with patchy areas of exudates. In contrast, in allergic rhinitis, the mucosa usually is swollen (boggy) and often pale with a clear, glistening surface and little exudate. With foreign bodies, generally only one nostril is affected and the drainage is usually purulent and foul-smelling.

Headache is another symptom that can arise from respiratory and nonrespiratory structures. Frontal headache, particularly if it gets worse by bending over, suggests sinus inflamma-

TABLE 50.1 Red Flags in the History and Physical Examination

Red Flag	Other Conditions to Consider
Unilateral purulent nasal drainage	Occult nasal foreign body
Severe sore throat with deviation of the uvula laterally	Peritonsillar abscess
Difficulty swallowing with stridor	Epiglottitis
Hoarseness persisting greater than 30 days	Laryngeal cancer or nodule
Cough persisting greater than 30 days	Lung cancer
Hemoptysis	Bronchial lung cancer
Cough with unilateral wheezing	Bronchial foreign body
Early morning cough with hoarseness	Reflux esophagitis
Shortness of breath with unilateral decreased breath sounds	Spontaneous pneumothorax

tion from either a cold or sinusitis. Facial pain is another symptom of sinus disease, since portions of the sinuses, the ear, and the skin of the face are all supplied by the trigeminal nerve. However, as noted below, facial pain alone is not a good discriminator of sinusitis since many patients with common colds also have sinus inflammation. Sinus inflammation also can cause maxillary toothache because the superior alveolar nerve passes through that sinus.

Sore throats can result from direct inflammation of the throat caused by a variety of different pathogens. The type of pain associated with streptococcal pharyngitis is not helpful in differentiating strep throat from virally mediated infections. However, very severe pain with difficulty swallowing may be indicative of a peritonsillar abscess. Severe pain and swallowing difficulty also is common with herpangina, a Coxsackie viral infection of the throat, palate, and posterior tongue. Pharyngeal inflammation also can cause referred pain to the ear because the middle ear shares innervation from the glossopharyngeal nerve.

Hoarseness generally indicates narrowing of the airway in the region of the larynx. Typically, the cause is inflammation of the vocal cords from laryngitis. In small children, narrowing of the same air passage leads to stridor.

Cough is the most common symptom observed in lower respiratory tract infections, but is common in URIs as well; Table 50.2 lists causes of cough that should be considered. Inflammation of the trachea, bronchi, bronchioles, or alveoli causes cough regardless of the etiology of the inflammation. Infections also cause hypersecretion of and production of infectious exudates that are cleared with coughing. Some infections, such as mycoplasma influenza and other viral infections, produce inflammation without a great deal of exudate and are typified by a nonproductive or dry cough. The degree of cough provides little indication of disease severity; many viral respiratory infections cause severe, persistent cough, even when they are largely resolved.

Chest pain can occur with some respiratory infection, but it is a rare symptom in isolation. Usually chest pain is present with coughing, shortness of breath, fever, or some other sign of infection. Chest pain with infection is usually pleuritic in nature and represents pleural inflammation from the infectious process. The pleuritis can be mild as seen in some cases of acute bronchitis, severe as with some Coxsackie B virus infections, or associated with significant pleural effusions and respiratory compromise in pneumonias. Because other conditions, such as a pulmonary embolism, can cause chest pain and low grade fever, clinicians should consider non-infectious causes as well as respiratory infections when patients complain of chest discomfort. Finally, cough can lead to chest pain by straining or otherwise injuring the muscles and bones of the chest wall or by irritating an inflamed trachea or bronchi. Red flags in the history that suggest other disorders are shown in Table 50.1.

For patients with respiratory tract disease, a thorough physical examination often confirms the diagnosis that was suspected after a careful history. When evaluating a patient with a potential respiratory infection, a first step is to assess the overall appearance of the patient, and his or her vital signs. Patients who are comfortable, breathing easily, and afebrile are unlikely to have a life-threatening disease. However, tachycardia, tachypnea, and alterations in mental status are ominous signs that are associated with much higher death rates from respiratory infections such as pneumonia.

After initial assessment, careful attention should be paid to the ears, nose, throat, neck, and chest. As noted earlier, the appearance of the nasal mucosa may be helpful in determining if rhinorrhea is caused by infection as opposed to allergy. Palpation of the sinuses is sometimes performed, but since this maneuver offers little value in differentiating sinusitis from a common cold and is likely to be highly operator-dependent, it is of little value. Transillumination of the sinuses has a much higher value in differentiating a sinusitis from a cold (4).

Pharyngeal findings of erythema, tonsillar enlargement, and exudate are useful in identifying a likely infection. Exudative tonsillitis is common with streptococcal pharyngitis, but is seen just as frequently in adenoviral throat infections; exudative tonsillitis also is a feature of mononucleosis. Uvular deviation is another important sign to look for during the pharyngeal examination. Deviation of the uvula is an early sign of a peritonsillar abscess; in these cases, the uvula points away from the side with the abscess.

Cervical adenopathy, which is common with streptococcal pharyngitis and mononucleosis, should be searched for during the neck examination. Palpation of the neck also may be useful in detecting an enlarged thyroid or other mass that may be compressing the trachea and producing stridor.

TABLE 50.2 Causes of Cough

Upper respiratory tract
  Acute rhinitis/pharyngitis (common cold)
  Allergic rhinitis
  Sinusitis
  Tracheolaryngitis (croup)
  Epiglottitis
Lower respiratory tract
Infectious causes
  Acute bronchitis
  Pneumonia
  Tuberculosis
  Pneumocystis carinii
  Bronchiectasis
  Lung abscess
Noninfectious causes
  Asthma
  Chronic bronchitis
  Allergic aspergillosis
  Bronchogenic neoplasms
  Sarcoidosis
  Pulmonary fibrosis
  Chemical or smoke inhalation
Cardiovascular causes
  Congestive heart failure/pulmonary edema
  Enlargement of left atrium
Gastrointestinal tract
  Reflux esophagitis
  Esophageal-tracheal fistula
Other causes
  Medications, especially angiotensin converting
  enzyme (ACE) inhibitors
  Psychogenic cough
  Foreign body aspiration

Reprinted with permission from Hueston WJ. Cough. In: Weiss BD, 20 Common Problems in Primary Care. New York, NY: McGraw Hill; 1999:181–206.

A complete lung examination is crucial in patients with suspected lower respiratory infections. Auscultation over all areas of the lungs is important to detect rales or a rub from pleuritis. Percussion of the lower lung fields may be useful in detecting pleural effusions.

Diagnostic Testing

Routine laboratory testing is not indicated for the vast majority of respiratory infections (43). The most helpful tests for URIs are a throat culture and serum testing for mononucleosis. Because of delays in the appearance of antimononucleosis anti-bodies, the commonly used mononucleosis tests may be falsely negative in the first week of symptoms, so testing should be delayed until symptoms have been present for a week or longer. Sinus radiographs or CT scans offer little benefit over clinical criteria for sinusitis and should be reserved only for patients with very confusing clinical pictures or fever without a clear origin.

For lower respiratory infections, the most valuable test is a chest radiograph. This is useful in differentiating pneumonia from acute bronchitis or other causes of shortness of breath and cough. The appearance of the infiltrate on the chest radiograph is sometimes helpful in predicting the etiologic agent as well (see Table 50.3). However, clinicians should be wary of false negative chest radiographs, which can occur in patients who are dehydrated or neutropenic.

Sputum cultures are less helpful. Cultures are often unreliable or contaminated. Many studies have found that only about one third of hospitalized patients with pneumonia are able to produce adequate specimens for culturing. Empiric treatment based on the age of the patient, severity of illness, and other risk factors is the most cost-effective strategy.

MANAGEMENT

Patient management and treatment is based on the condition. Table 50.4 summarizes the evidence for treatment options for most acute respiratory infections.

Uncomplicated URI/Common Cold

The most effective symptomatic treatments are over the counter decongestants (44). Preparations containing pseudoephedrine are effective in treating the nasal congestion associated with the common cold. However, several states have begun regulating the purchase of pseudoephedrine because of its integral role in the illicit manufacture of methamphetamine.

Despite the viral etiology of common colds, several studies have shown that the majority of common cold cases seen by physicians are treated with antibiotics (45, 46). It should be noted that many individuals do not seek care from physicians for colds and therefore are limited in their ability to use antibiotics. Controlled trials of antibiotic treatment of URIs have consistently demonstrated no benefit (47–53). In seven trials of antimicrobial treatment of URIs, six found no difference in improvement or further complications between the groups. Complications tend to be minimal and occur at a rate of 1%–15%. One trial found a slight benefit in decreasing purulent rhinitis (53). Similarly, an additional trial attempted to isolate "bacterial colds," for which antibiotics might be effective treatments (54). Although there was some indication of patient improvement at day 5, the differences were gone by day 10. It should be noted that the normal presentation of a URI is 1 to 2 weeks. In addition, it is important to emphasize that the use of antibiotics for URIs does not prevent bacterial complications such as otitis media (55).

Many alternatives to antibiotics for URIs have been investigated and have their advocates, if not strong evidence of effectiveness. Zinc gluconate lozenges are available without a prescription and have been suggested as effective in decreasing the duration of the common cold (56). However, one meta-analysis of eight randomized trials and another of seven trials

TABLE 50.3 Appearance of Infiltrates on Chest Radiograph

Immunocompetent Host	Immunosuppressed Host
Focal opacity	*Focal opacity*
Streptococcus pneumoniae	Same as immunocompetent plus:
Haemophilus influenzae	*Cryptococcus neoformans*
Mycoplasma pneumoniae	*Nocardia*
Chlamydia pneumoniae	Kaposi sarcoma
Staphylococcus aureus	
M. tuberculosis	
Gram-negative bacteria	
Anaerobic bacteria	
Interstitial/Miliary pattern	*Interstitial/Miliary pattern*
Viruses	Same as immunocompetent plus:
Mycoplasma pneumoniae	*Pneumocystis carinii*
M. tuberculosis	*Leishmania donovani*
Fungi	Cytomegalovirus
Hilar adenopathy +/− infiltrate	*Hilar adenopathy +/− infiltrate*
Epstein-Barr virus	Same as immunocompetent plus:
Chlamydia psittaci	*Cryptococcus neoformans*
Mycoplasma pneumoniae	Fungi
M. tuberculosis	Lymphoma
Fungi	Kaposi's sarcoma
Atypical rubella	

Reprinted with permission from Bartlett JC. Approach to the patient with pneumonia. In: Gorbach SL, Bartlett JG, Blacklow NR. Infectious Disease, 2nd ed. Philadelphia, PA: WB Saunders. 1998:554–557.

concluded that zinc lozenges were not effective in reducing the duration of cold symptoms (57, 58).

Echinacea has shown mixed results as a treatment for URIs in both children and adults. Although several smaller studies have observed some benefit, larger studies have tended to find no significant benefit for using echinacea (59). Several recent studies have found echinacea beneficial when compounds are used that mix echinacea with other treatments such as vitamin C or tea (60, 61).

Vitamin C also has been advocated for URIs; systematic reviews of the literature, however, provide only weak support for its effectiveness (62). Antihistamines, with a few exceptions, have not been shown to be effective treatments (63–65).

Other treatments also are being evaluated for use in URIs. Ipratropium bromide has demonstrated use in controlling congestion and rhinorrhea (66, 67), but its cost has limited its usefulness to date. Other treatments that are being investigated for URIs include acupuncture (68), nitric oxide (69), vitamin E (70), and North American ginseng (71). Some appear promising, but it is premature to recommend them as treatments because of limited evidence of their benefits.

Acute Sinusitis

Antibiotics are commonly prescribed for adult patients who present with complaints consistent with acute sinusitis. The effectiveness of antibiotics is unclear, although some evidence supports their use. Four recent placebo-controlled, double-blind, randomized trials of antibiotics for acute sinusitis encountered in general practice settings have yielded mixed results (5, 72–74). Two of these trials showed no beneficial effect of antibiotics, but two demonstrated significant effects of penicillin and amoxicillin. The trials demonstrating effects suggested that patients with more severe signs and symptoms, as well as radiographic or CT confirmation, may benefit from an antibiotic. A meta-analysis of 32 randomized trials of antibiotics versus placebo and antibiotics of different classes captured in computerized databases such as MEDLINE and studies from pharmaceutical companies indicated that acute maxillary sinusitis may benefit from treatment with penicillin or amoxicillin for 7 to 14 days (75).

If an antibiotic is used, evidence using trimethoprim/sulfamethoxazole suggests that short duration treatment (e.g., 3 days) is as effective as longer treatment (76). Further, a meta-analysis indicates that narrow spectrum agents are as effective as broad spectrum agents (77).

Acute Bronchitis

Antibiotic treatment for acute bronchitis is quite common, with evidence indicating that 60%–75% of adults visiting a doctor for acute bronchitis receive an antibiotic (78). Clinical trials of the effectiveness of antibiotics in treating acute bronchitis have had mixed results. One reason for the lack of con-

TABLE 50.4 Evidence Supporting Management of Common Respiratory Tract Infections

Treatment Strategy	Strength of Recommendation*	Recommendations/Conclusions
Upper respiratory tract infections		
Antibiotic therapy	A	No benefits seen and complications higher in treated group
Use of decongestants	A	Assist in symptom control, no effect on duration of illness
Echinacea products	B	Early trials demonstrated modest benefit, better controlled trials show no benefit
Zinc lozenges	A	Effectiveness in adults not shown; one randomized trial showed no benefit in children
Antihistamine therapy	A	No benefit at relieving symptoms or altering duration of disease
Acute bronchitis		
Use of routine antibiotics	A	Meta-analyses show weak/modest benefit; no evidence of effectiveness in single trials of individual drugs
Use of short-acting bronchodilators	A	Two randomized trials showed benefit in cough duration
Influenza		
Use of amantadine/rimantadine	A	Useful in influenza A only if started in first 48 hours
Use of neuraminidase inhibitors	A	Useful in influenza A and B but only if started in first 30–36 hours
		Beneficial in preventing complications in high-risk patients
Acute sinusitis		
Antibiotic therapy	A	Useful, but benefit limited to small number of patients; highly dependent on accurate diagnosis
Community-acquired Pneumonia		
Routine use of antibiotics	C	Antibiotic selection depends on situation and patient risks
ATS/ISDA guidelines for antibiotic selection	B	ATS guideline adherence decreased morbidity and hospitalizations

ATS/IDSA, American Thoracic Society and Infectious Disease society of America.

*A = consistent, good-quality patient-oriented evidence; B = inconsistent or limited-quality patient-oriented evidence; C = consensus, disease-oriented evidence, usual practice, expert opinion, or case series. For information about the SORT evidence rating system, see *http://www.aafp.org/afpsort.xml*.

sensus is that in each of the nine trials, different antibiotics were used as well as different outcomes. In an effort to quantitatively review the data, three different meta-analyses were recently conducted (79–81). In one meta-analysis, neither resolution of cough nor clinical improvement at reexamination was affected by antibiotic treatment. Importantly, the side effects were more common in the antibiotic groups compared to placebo. The other two meta-analyses concluded that antibiotics may be modestly effective for acute bronchitis. All of the meta-analyses agreed that the benefits of antibiotics in a general population are marginal and should be weighed against the impact of excessive use of antibiotics on the development of antibiotic resistance.

Data from clinical trials suggests that bronchodilators may provide effective symptomatic relief to patients with acute bronchitis (82, 83). Treatment with bronchodilators demonstrated significant relief of symptoms including faster resolution of cough, as well as return to work. However, one study evaluated the effect of albuterol in a population of patients with undifferentiated cough and found no beneficial effect (84). Since a variety of conditions present with cough, there may have been some misclassification in generalizing this to acute bronchitis.

Bronchiolitis

The mainstay of therapy consists of respiratory support, nutrition, and hydration. Bronchodilators have been suggested as treatments for bronchiolitis, but a meta-analysis of eight trials of bronchodilators versus placebo indicated that bronchodilators produce only limited short-term improvement in clinical scores (85). This small benefit must be weighed against the costs of these agents.

The use of antivirals in the treatment of RSV infections remains controversial. Ribavirin is the only antiviral agent licensed for the treatment of RSV infections and should be considered in severely affected children. Patients undergoing therapy should be placed in negative pressure rooms with frequent air exchanges and scavenging systems to decrease ribavirin exposure of health care providers and to minimize release into the surrounding environment. Uncontrolled trials show that early therapy with ribavirin aerosol may be beneficial (86). In a systematic review of 10 trials of ribavirin for RSV, it was concluded that the trials lack sufficient power to provide reliable estimates of the effects (87). The cumulative results of three small trials show that ribavirin reduces length of mechanical ventilator support, and may reduce days of hospitalization.

Vaccines against RSV are under development but not currently available. Hand washing is currently the most effective preventive measure.

Influenza

Treatment of influenza infection is targeted toward symptoms, with spontaneous recovery within 5 to 7 days. The typical therapy includes bed rest, oral hydration, acetaminophen or NSAIDs to reduce fever, headache, and myalgias, over the counter throat lozenges, intranasal anticholinergics, and systemic antihistamines and anticholinergics. Preventative measures along with antiviral drugs are used to shorten the disease course and decrease secondary complications (88).

In addition to symptomatic medications, influenza may be treated with antiviral agents. First generation antiviral agents effective against influenza A are amantadine hydrochloride and rimantadine hydrochloride (see Table 50.5). These drugs have no effect on influenza B viruses, however. A meta-analysis of the randomized and quasi-randomized trials indicate that both amantadine or rimantadine are effective in reducing the severity and duration of symptoms, particularly if given within 48 hours of illness onset (89). Unfortunately these drugs have shown substantial rates of adverse events (90).

Two neuraminidase inhibitors, zanamivir and oseltamivir, have been successful against both influenza A and B. An analysis of six randomized placebo-controlled trials of zanamivir indicated a decrease in illness duration ranging from 1 to 3 days in different populations (91). The greatest benefit was found in patients >50 years of age. Randomized trials of oseltamivir have also demonstrated reduced duration of illness (92, 93). The treatments must be given within 36 hours, and preferably within 24 hours, of onset for maximum effectiveness.

PREVENTION

Vaccination for influenza is the most common and effective way to prevent influenza. Each year's vaccine contains three virus strains representing the viruses that are predicted to circulate in the United States during the upcoming influenza season. Unfortunately, sometimes the supply of influenza vaccine is delayed or insufficient to cover all patients recom-

TABLE 50.5 Pharmacotherary Treatment for Influenza

Drug	Dosage	Adverse effects	Cost per course ($)*	Comments
Amantadine	• 100 mg BID for 3 to 5 days • Reduced dose in elderly (100 mg/D) • Dose in children 5 mg/kg/D in 2 divided doses	Confusion, insomnia, depression, nervousness, nausea, anorexia, dry mouth	$	Start within 48 hours; Type A only shortens symptoms by 1 day
Rimantidine	• 100 mg BID for 3 to 5 days • Reduced dose in elderly (100 mg/D) • Dose in children under 10 is 5 mg/kg once a day	Nausea, dizziness	$	Start within 48 hours; Type A only shortens symptoms by 1 day
Zanamivir	• 2 inhalations Q12 hours for 5 days • Approved in children ≥7 years of age	Cough	NA	Start within 30 hours; Types A & B shortens symptoms by 1.5 days
Oseltamivir	• 75 mg BID for 5 days • Approved in children ≥1 years of age, ≤ 15 kg, 30 mg BID; >15–23 kg, 45 mg BID; >24–40 kg, 60 mg BID; >40 kg, 75 mg BID	Nausea and vomiting; insomnia; vertigo; bronchitis	$$$	Initiate treatment within 2 days of symptoms; Types A&B shortens symptoms by 1.5 days

*$ = <$33, $$ = $34-$66, $$$ = >$67

mended for immunization (94). It is recommended that the following individuals receive the influenza vaccine:

- persons aged 65 years and older
- residents at least 6 months of age in nursing homes or chronic care facilities
- individuals 6 months or older who have underlying medical conditions
- individuals 6 months to 18 years of age who receive long-term aspirin therapy and have an increased risk for developing Reye's syndrome after being infected with influenza virus
- women who will be at or beyond 14 weeks gestation during the influenza season or at any stage, if underlying medical conditions may result in secondary complications
- employees of hospitals, outpatient settings, nursing homes, and other chronic care facilities that care for high-risk patients.

Because of the decline of immunity during the year and antigen variation from year to year within the influenza virus, individuals should receive the vaccine every year. The optimal time for vaccination is October to mid-November.

Community-Acquired Pneumonia

In prior decades, penicillin was the foundation for pneumonia therapy. *Streptococcus pneumoniae* was the most common bacterial pathogen, and the drug was very sensitive to penicillin. However, with the emergence of other pneumonia-causing agents and the development of drug resistance to penicillin and other antibiotics used in *S. pneumoniae,* treatment decisions have become more complex.

A Centers for Disease Control and Prevention working group on drug-resistant *S pneumoniae* (DRSP) released recommendations on management of community-acquired pneumonia (CAP) (95) (see Table 50.6). These recommendations are similar to more recent recommendations from the American College of Chest Physicians (96). For outpatient treatment of CAP, suitable empiric oral antimicrobial agents include a macrolide (e.g., erythromycin, clarithromycin, or azithromycin), doxycycline (or tetracycline) for children aged 8 years or older, or an oral β-lactam with good activity against pneumococci (e.g., cefuroxime axetil, amoxicillin, or a combination of amoxicillin and clavulanate potassium).

In addition to appropriate antibiotic management, several other factors influence whether the patient with pneumonia

TABLE 50.6 Oral Pharmacotherapy for Ambulatory Management of Community-Acquired Pneumonia

Drug	Adult Dosage	Adverse Effects	Cost per Course ($)*	Comments
Macrolides				
Azithromycin	500 mg day 1, then 250 mg for 4 d	Diarrhea, nausea	$$	
Tetracylcines				
Doxycycline	100 mg twice daily for 10–14 d	Diarrhea, nausea, skin photosensitivity	$	Contraindicated in children and pregnancy; avoid calcium or dairy products within 2 hrs of dose
Oral β-lactams				
Cefuroxime axetil	250–500 mg twice daily for 10 d	Diarrhea, nausea, elevated liver enzymes	$$$	
Amoxicillin-clavulanate potassium	500 mg three times daily or 875 mg twice daily for 10–14 d	Diarrhea, nausea	$$$	Diarrhea may be reduced by taking with food; reduce dose needed with renal impairment
Fluoro-quinolones				
Levofloxacin	250–500 mg once a day for 10–14 d	Diarrhea, nausea	$$$	Contraindicated in children and pregnancy Reduced dose needed with renal impairment. Avoid use of calcium, magnesium or iron products within 2 hr or more of dose.

*$ = <$33, $$ = $34-$66, $$$ = >$67
Reprinted with permission from Heffelfinger JD, Dowell SF, Jorgensen JH, et al. Management of community-acquired pneumonia in the era of pneumococcal resistance: a report from the Drug-Resistant *Streptococcal pneumoniae* Therapeutic Working Group. Arch Intern Med. 2000;160:1399–1408.

should be cared for at home or in the hospital (96). Generally, home care should be considered for younger, previously healthy individuals with no signs of cardiopulmonary compromise, such as hypoxia, hypotension, or tachycardia. The patient's primary caregiver(s) should be instructed in the management plan and be capable of carrying out the plan. Additionally, the patient should be able to carry on with their usual activities of living and have adequate oxygenation either on room air or with supplemental oxygen. Suitable follow up should be arranged, and the patient should be reliable about returning for subsequent care or if problems arise.

If patients are at high risk for mortality based on their age, clinical condition, or pre-existing comorbidities, the patient should be hospitalized for treatment. Suitable empiric antimicrobial regimens for inpatient pneumonia have been recommended depending on the patient's severity of illness and the risk for pseudomonas (97). For lower risk patients who are not severely ill, therapy can include an intravenous β-lactam, such as cefuroxime, ceftriaxone sodium, cefotaxime sodium, or a combination of ampicillin sodium and sulbactam sodium, plus a macrolide. New fluoroquinolones with improved activity against *S pneumoniae* can also be used to treat adults with CAP. To limit the emergence of fluoroquinolone-resistant strains, the new fluoroquinolones should be limited to adults 1. for whom one of the above regimens has already failed; 2. who are allergic to alternative agents; or 3. who have a documented infection with highly drug-resistant pneumococci (e.g., penicillin mean inhibitory concentration (MIC) 4 µg/mL). Vancomycin hydrochloride is not routinely indicated for the treatment of CAP or pneumonia caused by DRSP.

PREVENTION

Pneumococcal pneumonia may be prevented through immunization with multivalent pneumococcal vaccine. Pneumococcal vaccination is indicated for individuals over age 65, and those 2 years of age or older with diabetes mellitus, chronic pulmonary or cardiac disease, and those without a spleen. Additionally, people in certain high-risk populations, such as Native American, Alaska Native populations, and those people over age 50 living in chronic care facilities should be vaccinated. Immunosuppressed patients including those with HIV, alcoholism, cirrhosis, chronic renal failure, sickle cell disease, or multiple myeloma may benefit from immunization, but the evidence is less convincing.

In addition to initial vaccination, clinicians should advise patients that the duration of protection is uncertain. For those at particularly high risk of mortality from pneumococcal pneumonia, such as patients over age 75 and those with chronic pulmonary disease or lacking a spleen, revaccination every 5 years is a worthwhile precaution.

Currently, pneumococcal vaccination is ineffective for children under the age of 2 because infants will not mount an adequate immune response to the antigens in the polyvalent vaccine. Efforts at producing a conjugated pneumococcal vaccine similar to the *Haemophilus influenza* vaccine are currently under development. In the next few years, a conjugated pneumococcal vaccine may be marketed that will offer protection not only from pneumonia, bacteremia, and meningitis caused by pneumococcus, but also from the most common cause of otitis media.

CASE DISCUSSION

This case involves three decisions made by clinicians when faced with patients with acute respiratory infections. First, clinicians must decide which respiratory infection is present. Cough can be a symptom of a common cold or allergy, influenza, tracheitis, or a lower respiratory tract infection such as acute bronchitis or pneumonia. The absence of any upper respiratory tract symptoms and the presence of rales on the physical examination point in the direction of pneumonia. This was confirmed with a chest radiograph.

The second decision with this individual was whether his clinical condition warranted hospitalization or if he could be treated as an outpatient. Since he is under the age of 50, has no comorbidities, and has stable vital signs with good oxygenation, he meets the clinical criteria for a low-risk patient. Additionally, in assessing his social situation, the clinician learned that he has support at home, is likely to be reliable about taking his medications and following up, and understands the instructions for home care. Based on the clinical and social situations in this case, this gentleman should be able to have his pneumonia managed as an outpatient.

The third clinical decision in this case is the selection of an appropriate antibiotic for outpatient management of pneumonia. Options according to the Infectious Disease Society of America include an advanced-spectrum macrolide, doxycycline, or a respiratory quinolone. Because of the rapid onset of his symptoms, his high fever, and the lobar pattern of his pneumonia, the clinician was highly suspicious of pneumococcus as the etiology of the pneumonia. A respiratory quinolone was selected in this case, which will help cover the patient if he has an intermediate-resistant strain of pneumococcus, but either of the other two medications also would have been adequate.

REFERENCES

1. Tenover FC, Hughes JM. The challenge of emerging infectious diseases: development and spread of multiply resistant bacterial pathogens. JAMA. 1996;275:300–304.
2. McCaig LF, Hughes JM. Trends in antimicrobial drug prescribing among office-based physicians in the United States. JAMA. 1995;273:214–219.
3. Hueston WJ, Mainous AG III, Dacus EN, Hopper JE. Does acute bronchitis really exist? A reconceptualization of acute viral respiratory infections. J Fam Pract. 2000;49:401–406.
4. Williams JW Jr, Simel DL. Does this patient have sinusitis? Diagnosing acute sinusitis by history and physical examination. JAMA. 1993;270:1242–1246.
5. Lindbaek M, Hjortdahl P, Johnsen U. Randomised, double blind, placebo controlled trial of penicillin V and amoxycillin in treatment of acute sinus infection in adults. BMJ. 1996; 313:325–329.
6. Poses RM, Cebul RD, Collins M, Fager SS. The accuracy of experienced physicians' probability estimates for patients with sore throats. Implications for decision making. JAMA. 1985; 254:925–929.
7. Woodwell DA. National Ambulatory Medical Care Survey: 1995 Summary. Advance data from Health and Vital Statistics (286). Hyattsville, MD: National Center for Health Statistics; 1997.
8. Woodwell DA. National Ambulatory Medical Care Survey: 1996 Summary. Advance data from Health and Vital Statis-

tics. Hyattsville, MD: National Center for Health Statistics; 1997.

9. Croughan-Minihane MS, Petitti DB, Rodnick JE, Eliaser G. Clinical trial examining effectiveness of three cough syrups. J Am Board Fam Pract. 1993;6:109–115.

10. Sperber SJ, Levine PA, Sorrentino JV, Riker DK, Hayden FG. Ineffectiveness of recombinant interferon-beta serine nasal drops for prophylaxis of natural colds. J Infect Dis. 1989;160:700–705.

11. Adams PF, Hendershot GE, Marano MA. Current estimates from the National Health Interview Survey, 1996. National Center for Health Statistics. Vital Health Stat 10. 1999; 10(200):1–40.

12. Linder JA, Singer DE. Health-related quality of life of adults with upper respiratory tract infections. J Gen Intern Med. 2003;18:802–807.

13. Sattar SA, Jacobsen H, Springthorpe VS, Cusack TM, Rubino JR. Chemical disinfection to interrupt transfer of rhinovirus type 14 from environmental surfaces to hands. Appl Environ Microbiol. 1993;59:1579–1585.

14. Ansari SA, Springthorpe VS, Sattar SA, Rivard S, Rahman M. Potential role of hands in the spread of respiratory viral infections: studies with human parainfluenza virus 3 and rhinovirus 14. J Clin Microbiol. 1991;29:2115–2119.

15. Warshauer DM, Dick EC, Mandel AD, Flynn TC, Jerde RS. Rhinovirus infections in an isolated Antarctic station. Transmission of the viruses and susceptibility of the population. Am J Epidemiol. 1989;129:319–340.

16. Makela MJ, Puhakka T, Ruuskanen O, et al. Viruses and bacteria in the etiology of the common cold. J Clin Microbiol. 1998;36:539–542.

17. Gohd RS. The common cold. N Engl J Med. 1954;250: 687–691.

18. Gordts F, Clement PA, Destryker A, Desprechins B, Kaufman L. Prevalence of sinusitis signs on MRI in a non-ENT paediatric population. Rhinology. 1997;35:154–157.

19. Henriksson G, Westrin KM, Kumlien J, Stierna P. A 13-year report on childhood sinusitis: clinical presentations, predisposing factors and possible means of prevention. Rhinology. 1996;34:171–175.

20. Evans KL. Diagnosis and management of sinusitis. Lancet. 1994;309:1415–1422.

21. Holleman DR Jr, Williams JW Jr, Simel DL. Usual care and outcomes in patients with sinus complaints and normal results of sinus roentgenography. Arch Fam Med. 1995;4: 246–251.

22. Manning SC, Biavati MJ, Phillips DL. Correlation of clinical sinusitis signs and symptoms to imaging findings in pediatric patients. Int J Pediatr Otorhinolaryngol. 1996;37:65–74.

23. Lindbaek M, Hjortdahl P, Johnsen ULH. Use of symptoms, signs and blood tests to diagnose acute sinus infections in primary care: comparison with computed tomography. Fam Med. 1996;28:183–186.

24. Shapiro GG, Rahelefsky GS. Introduction and definition of sinusitis. J Allergy Clin Immunol. 1992;90:417–418.

25. Tyrrell DAJ. Common Colds and Related Diseases. Baltimore, MD: Williams & Wilkins; 1965.

26. Mogabgab WJ. *Mycoplasma pneumoniae* and adenovirus respiratory illnesses in military and university personnel. Am Rev Resp Dis. 1968;97:345–358.

27. Falck G, Heyman L, Gnarpe J, Gnarpe H. *Chlamydia pneumoniae* (TWAR): a common agent in acute bronchitis. Scand J Infect Dis. 1994;26:179–187.

28. Williamson HA. A randomized, controlled trial of doxycycline in the treatment of acute bronchitis. J Fam Pract. 1984; 19(4):481–486.

29. Centers for Disease Control and Prevention. Prevention and control of influenza: recommendations of the Advisory Committee on Immunization Practices (ACIP). MMWR Morb Mortal Wky Rep. 1998;47(RR-6):1–26.

30. Cox NJ, Fukuda K. Influenza. Infect Dis Clin North Am. 1998;12(1):27–38.

31. Kilbourne ED. Influenza pandemics of the 20th century. Emerg Infect Dis. 2007;12:9–14.

32. Taubenberger JK, Morens DM. 1918 influenza: the mother of all pandemics. Emerg Infect Dis. 2006;12:15–22.

33. Hueston WJ, Benich JJ. A cost-benefit analysis of testing for Influenza A in high-risk adults. Ann Fam Med. 2004;2: 33–40.

34. Bartlett JG, Mundy LM. Community-acquired pneumonia. N Engl J Med. 1995;333:1618–1624.

35. Brown PD, Lerner SA. Community-acquired pneumonia. Lancet. 1998;352:1295–1302.

36. Fry AM, Shay DK, Holman RC, et al. Trends in hospitalizations for pneumonia among persons aged 65 or older in the United States, 1988–2002. JAMA. 2005:294:2712–2719.

37. Sims RV. Bacterial pneumonia in the elderly. Emerg Med Clin North Am. 1990;8:207–219.

38. LaCroix AZ, Lipson S, Miles TP, White L. Prospective study of pneumonia hospitalizations and mortality of U.S. older people: the role of chronic conditions, health benefits and nutritional status. Public Health Rep. 1989;104:350–360.

39. Harper C, Newton P. Clinical aspects of pneumonia in the elderly veteran. J Am Geriatr Soc. 1989;37:867–872.

40. McFadden JP, Price RD, Eastweek HD, et al. Raised respiratory rate in elderly patients: a valuable physical sign. BMJ. 1982;1:626–628.

41. Gleckman R, DeVita J, Hilert D, et al. Sputum gram-stain assessment in community-acquired bacteremic pneumonia. J Clin Microbiol. 1988;26:846–849.

42. Chalasani NP, Valdecanas AL, Gopal AK, McGowen JE, Jurado RL. Clinical utility of blood cultures in adult patients with community-acquired pneumonia without defined underlying risks. Chest. 1995;108:932–936.

43. Carroll K, Reimer L. Microbiology and laboratory diagnosis of upper respiratory tract infections. Clin Infect Dis. 1996; 23:442–448.

44. Smith MBH, Feldman W. Over-the-counter cold medications: a critical review of clinical trials between 1950 and 1991. JAMA. 1993;269:2258–2263.

45. Mainous AG III, Hueston WJ, Clark JR. Antibiotics and upper respiratory infection: do some folks think there is a cure for the common cold? J Fam Pract. 1996;42:357–361.

46. Gonzales R, Steiner JF, Sande MA. Antibiotic prescribing for adults with colds, upper respiratory tract infections, and bronchitis by ambulatory care physicians. JAMA. 1997;278: 901–904.

47. Cronk GA, Naumann, DE, McDermott K, Menter P, Swift MB. A controlled study of the effect of oral penicillin G in the treatment of non-specific upper respiratory infections. Am J Med. 1954; 16:804–809.

48. Hardy LM, Traisman HS. Antibiotics and chemotherapeutic agents in the treatment of uncomplicated respiratory infections in children. J Pediatr. 1956;48:146–156.

49. Townsend EH. Chemoprophylaxis during respiratory infections in a private pediatric practice. J Dis Child. 1960; 99: 566–573.

50. Townsend EH, Radebaugh JF. Prevention of complications of respiratory illnesses in pediatric practice. N Engl J Med. 1962; 266: 683–689.

51. Gordon M, Lovell S, Dugdale AE. The value of antibiotics in minor respiratory illness in children. Med J Aust. 1974;1: 304–306.

52. Lexomboon U, Duangmani C, Kusalasai V, Sunakorn P,

Olson LC, Noyes HE. Evaluation of orally administered antibiotics for treatment of upper respiratory infections in Thai children. J Pediatr. 1971; 78: 772–778.

53. Taylor B, Abbott GD, Kerr MM, Fergusson DM. Amoxycillin and co-trimoxazole in presumed viral respiratory infections of childhood: placebo-controlled trial. BMJ. 1977;2: 552–554.

54. Kaiser L, Lew D, Hirschel B, et al. Effects of antibiotic treatment in the subset of common-cold patients who have bacteria in nasopharyngeal secretions. Lancet. 1996;347:1507–1510.

55. Autret-Leca E, Giraudeau B, Ployet MJ, Jonvillle-Bera AP. Amoxicillin/clavulanic acid is ineffective at preventing otitis media in children with presumed viral upper respiratory infection: a randomized, double-blind equivalence, placebo-controlled trial. Br J Clinical Pharmacol. 2002;54:652–656.

56. Mossad SB, Macknin ML, Medendorp SV, Mason P. Zinc gluconate lozenges for treating the common cold: a randomized, double-blind, placebo-controlled study. Ann Intern Med. 1996;125:81–88.

57. Jackson JL, Lesho E, Peterson C. Zinc and the common cold: a meta-analysis revisited. J Nutr. 2000;130(5S Suppl): 1512S–1515S.

58. Marshall I. Zinc for the common cold. Cochrane Database Syst Rev. 2000;2:CD001364.

59. Melchart D, Linde K, Fischer P, Kaesmayr J. Echinacea for preventing and treating the common cold. Cochrane Database Syst Rev. 2000;2:CD00530.

60. Cohen HA, Varsano I, Kahan E, Sarrell EM, Uziel Y. Effectiveness of an herbal preparation containing echinacea, propolis, and vitamin C in preventing respiratory tract infections in children: a randomized, double blind, placebo-controlled, multicenter study. Arch Pediatr Adolesc Med. 2004;158: 217–221.

61. Lindenmuth GF, Lindenmuth EB. The efficacy of echinacea compound herbal tea preparation on the severity and duration of upper respiratory and flu symptoms: a randomized, double-blind placebo-controlled study. J Altern Complement Med. 2000;6:327–334.

62. Hemila H. Does vitamin C alleviate the symptoms of the common cold? A review of current evidence. Scand J Infect Dis. 1994;26:1–6.

63. Luks D, Anderson MR. Antihistamines and the common cold: a review and critique of the literature. J Gen Intern Med. 1996;11:240–244.

64. Gwaltney JM Jr, Park J, Paul RA, Edelman DA, O'Connor RR, Turner RB. Randomized controlled trial of clemastine fumarate for treatment of experimental rhinovirus colds. Clin Infect Dis. 1996;22:656–662.

65. Aitkin M, Taylor JA. Prevalence of clinical sinusitis in young children followed up by primary care pediatricians. Arch Ped Adolesc Med. 1998;152:244–248.

66. Ecles R, Jawad MS, Jawad SS, Angello JT, Druce HM. Efficacy and safety of single and multiple doses of pseudoephedrine in the treatment of nasal congestion associated with common cold. Am J Rhinol. 2005;19:25–31.

67. Kim KT, Kerwin E, Landwehr L, et al. Pediatric Atrovent Nasal Spray Study Group. Use of 0.06% ipatroprium bromide nasal spray in children aged 2 to 5 years with rhinorrhea due to a common cold or allergies. Ann Allergy Asthma Immunol. 2005;94:73–79.

68. Kawakita K, Shichidou T, Inoue E, et al. Preventive and curative effects of acupuncture on the common cold: a multicentre randomized controlled trial in Japan. Complement Ther Med. 2004;12:181–188.

69. Proud D. Nitric oxide and the common cold. Curr Opin Allergy Clin Immunol. 2005;5:37–42.

70. Meydani SN, Leka LS, Fine BC, et al. Vitamin E and respiratory tract infections in elderly nursing home residents: a randomized controlled trial. JAMA. 2004;292:828–836.

71. Predy GN, Goel V, Lovlin R, Donner A, Stitt L, Basu TK. Efficacy of an extract of North American ginseng containing poly-furanosyl-pyranosyl-saccharides for preventing upper respiratory tract infections: a randomized controlled trial. CMAJ Can Med Assoc J. 2005;173:1043–1048.

72. Van Bucham FL, Knottnerus JA, Schrijnemaekers VJJ, Peeters MF. Primary-case-based randomised placebo-controlled trial of antibiotic treatment in acute maxillary sinusitis. Lancet. 1997;349:683–687.

73. Stalman W, van Essen GA, van der Graaf Y, de Melker RA. The end of antibiotic treatment in adults with acute sinusitis-like complaints in general practice? A placebo-controlled double-blind randomized doxycycline trial. Br J Gen Pract. 1997;47:794–799.

74. Hansen JG, Schmidt H, Grinsted P. Randomized, double blind, placebo controlled trial of penicillin V in the treatment of acute maxillary sinusitis in adults in general practice. Scand J Prim Health Care. 2000;18:44–47.

75. Williams JW Jr, Aguilar C, Makela M, et al. Antibiotics for acute maxillary sinusitis. Cochrane Database Syst Rev. 2000; 2:CD000243.

76. Williams JW Jr, Holleman DR Jr, Samsa GP, Simel DL. Randomized controlled trial of 3 vs 10 days of trimethoprim/sulfamethoxazole for acute maxillary sinusitis. JAMA. 1995; 273:1015–1021.

77. De Bock GH, Dekker FW, Stolt J, et al. Antimicrobial treatment in acute maxillary sinusitis: a meta-analysis. J Clin Epidemiol. 1997;50:881–890.

78. Mainous AG III, Zoorob RJ, Hueston WJ. Current management of acute bronchitis in ambulatory care: the use of antibiotics and bronchodilators. Arch Fam Med. 1996;5:79–83.

79. Fahey T, Stocks N, Thomas T. Quantitative systematic review of randomised controlled trials comparing antibiotic with placebo for acute cough in adults. BMJ. 1998;316: 906–910.

80. Bent S, Saint S, Vittinghoff E, Grady D. Antibiotics in acute bronchitis: a meta-analysis. Am J Med. 1999;107:62–67.

81. Smucny JJ, Becker LA, Glazier RH, McIsaac W. Are antibiotics effective treatment for acute bronchitis? A meta-analysis. J Fam Pract. 1998;47:453–460.

82. Hueston WJ. Albuterol delivered by metered-dose inhaler to treat acute bronchitis. J Fam Pract. 1994;39:437–440.

83. Melbye H, Aasebo U, Straume B. Symptomatic effect of inhaled fenoterol in acute bronchitis: a placebo-controlled double-blind study. Fam Pract. 1991;8:216–222.

84. Littenberg B, Wheeler M, Smith DS. A randomized controlled trial of oral albuterol in acute cough. J Fam Pract. 1996;42:49–53.

85. Kellner JD, Ohlsson A, Gadomski AM, Wang EE. Bronchodilators for bronchiolitis. Cochrane Database Syst Rev. 2000; 2:CD001266.

86. Englund JA, Piedra PA, Whimbey E. Prevention and treatment of respiratory syncytial virus and parainfluenza viruses in immunocompromised patients. Am J Med. 1997;102: 61–70.

87. Randolph AG, Wang EE. Ribavirin for respiratory syncytial virus infection of the lower respiratory tract. Cochrane Database Syst Rev. 2000;2:CD000181.

88. Mossad SB. Underused options for treating and preventing influenza. Cleve Clin J Med. 1999;66:19–23.

89. Jefferson TO, Demicheli V, Deeks JJ, Rivetti D. Amantadine and rimantadine for preventing and treating influenza A in adults. Cochrane Database Syst Rev. 2000;2:CD001169.

90. Kucers A, Crowe SM, Grayson ML, Hoy JF, eds. The Use of Antibiotics: A Clinical Review of Antibacterial, Antifun-

gal, and Antiviral drugs. Oxford, England: Butterworth-Heinmann;1997:1834–1854.

91. Monto AS, Webster A, Keene O. Randomized, placebo-controlled studies of inhaled zanamivir in the treatment of influenza A and B: pooled efficacy analysis. J Antimicrob Chemother. 1999;44(Suppl B):23–29.

92. Nicholson KG, Aoki FY, Osterhaus AD, et al. Efficacy and safety of oseltamivir in treatment of acute influenza: a randomised controlled trial. Neuraminidase Inhibitor Flu Treatment Investigator Group. Lancet. 2000;355(9218):1845–1850

93. Treanor JJ, Hayden FG, Vrooman, et al. Efficacy and safety of the oral neuraminidase inhibitor oseltamivir in treating acute influenza: a randomized controlled trial. US Oral Neuraminidase Study Group. JAMA. 2000;283(8):1016–1024.

94. Advisory Committee on Immunization Practices. Delayed supply of influenza vaccine and adjunct ACIP influenza vaccine recommendations for the 2000–01 influenza season. MMWR Morb Mortal Wky Rep. 2000;49:619–622.

95. Heffelfinger JD, Dowell SF, Jorgensen JH, et al. Management of community-acquired pneumonia in the era of pneumococcal resistance: a report from the Drug-Resistant *Streptococcus pneumoniae* Therapeutic Working Group. Arch Intern Med. 2000;160:1399–1408.

96. Ramsdell J, Narsavage GL, Fink JB. American College of Chest Physicians' Home Care Network Working Group. Management of community-acquired pneumonia in the home: an American College of Chest Physicians clinical position statement. Chest. 2005:127:1752–1763.

97. Bartlett JG, Dowell SF, Mandell LA, File Jr, TM, Musher DM, Fine MJ. Practice guidelines for the management of community-acquired pneumonia in adults. Infectious Diseases Society of America. Clin Infect Dis. 2000;31:347–382.

CHAPTER 51

Chronic Obstructive Pulmonary Disease

David L. Gaspar and Dorothy E. Vura-Weis

CASE

Mr. R.L. was first seen at our office in 2001 at age 55 for leg pain and known chronic obstructive pulmonary disease (COPD). He was smoking 1/2 to 2 packs of cigarettes per day, as he had for 40 years. He had worked as a carpenter and at one time in a shipyard, with possible asbestos exposure. Medications were albuterol and ipratropium inhalers, 2 to 4 puffs of each, 4 times per day. Pulmonary function tests (PFTs) showed forced vital capacity (FVC) at 67% of the predicted value; forced expiratory volume in one second (FEV$_1$) at 36% of the predicted value; and an FEV$_1$/FVC ratio of 39%. Arterial blood gas results were pH, 7.38; Pco$_2$, 41; Po$_2$, 62. He was referred for smoking cessation classes.

CLINICAL QUESTIONS

1. What are his predisposing factors for COPD?
2. What category of COPD do his findings suggest?
3. What other tests, if any, should be done?
4. What would be done differently if his Po$_2$ were 52 instead of 62?

Chronic obstructive pulmonary disease (COPD) is a chronic respiratory disorder primarily caused by smoking. It is characterized by progressive airflow obstruction that is not fully reversible and is associated with systemic manifestations.

COPD is both a common and costly medical condition. The monetary and social costs include consumption of health care resources, lost workplace productivity due to disability, caregiver burden, and a negative impact on the quality of life of COPD patients. Since so many of the interventions in COPD are aimed at improving quality of life and decreasing symptoms rather than simply improving objective tests of lung function, a patient-centered orientation is crucial. In addition, since the disease is linked closely with smoking and air pollution, public health strategies to improve air quality and to encourage smoking cessation and avoidance of tobacco can do much to reduce the burden of disease. Family physicians can play a key role not only in the management of this condition but in providing family support, advocating for public policy changes to reduce air pollutants and to encourage smoking cessation.

Patients with COPD have a poorer quality of life as their breathing difficulties progress and disease progression has significant effects on their ability to satisfactorily perform activities of daily living. Even patients with minimal or no apparent symptoms may appear so because they have modified their activities and life in ways to compensate for their respiratory symptoms. Along with their pulmonary difficulties, patients with COPD are more likely to have other significant medical co-morbidities since smoking is also a risk factor for cardiovascular, neoplastic, and other systemic diseases (1). These can add to the overall burden of disease that the patient and his family experience and to the cost and complexity of treatments. As with many chronic diseases, there is an increased risk of concurrent depression, which can cause further deterioration in quality of life. As COPD progresses other non-respiratory effects are seen that contribute to a reduction in exercise tolerance and a worsening quality of life. Extrapulmonary systemic inflammation with activation of circulating inflammatory cells and increased levels of pro-inflammatory cytokines is associated with skeletal muscle dysfunction, nutritional abnormalities, and weight loss (2). Gradual worsening of airway obstruction occurs in patients who continue to smoke and COPD is the one top five killer whose mortality is increasing. COPD patients experience acute exacerbations of their disease that can vary in severity from mild worsening that requires only a change in medication regimen to severe exacerbations that require hospitalization, intubation, or can result in death.

Physicians need to ask smokers about symptoms and be prepared to conduct spirometry to confirm the diagnosis of COPD and assess severity. The Global Initiative for Chronic Obstructive Lung Disease (GOLD) Criteria (see Table 51.1) classifies patients according to severity and helps guide management. The only intervention that changes the course of the illness is smoking cessation, and targeting smokers to encourage them to quit is the most important element of COPD management. While rehabilitation programs and pharmacologic treatments can improve symptoms and quality of life, none of our existing treatments have been shown to arrest disease progression of or reduce mortality. Exacerbations need to be managed promptly with the goal to avoid hospitalization and serious respiratory compromise. Chronic disease management principles apply to COPD, and a partnership with our patients needs to be established so they may take an active part in the decisions involved in the management of their disease (3). In addition to negotiating goals of therapy, advanced directives should be discussed and documented.

There is a high prevalence of known COPD, and it would be difficult for family physicians to not encounter these patients weekly. The most recent data from the United States National Center for Health Statistics (NCHS) notes that 5.5% of persons 18 years and older reported that they had been told

TABLE 51.1 Stages of Chronic Obstructive Pulmonary Disease

Stage	Symptoms	Spirometry
I—Mild	With or without chronic symptoms: cough, sputum production	$FEV_1/FVC < 70\%$ $FEV_1 \geq 80\%$ predicted
II—Moderate	With or without chronic symptoms: cough, sputum production	$FEV_1/FVC < 70\%$ $FEV_1 < 80\%$ predicted $FEV_1 \geq 50\%$ predicted
III—Severe	With or without chronic symptoms: cough, sputum production	$FEV_1/FVC < 70\%$ $FEV_1 < 50\%$ predicted $FEV_1 \geq 30\%$ predicted
IV—Very Severe		$FEV_1/FVC < 70\%$ $FEV_1 < 30\%$ predicted OR $FEV1 < 50\%$ predicted plus respiratory failure

ABG, arterial blood gases; ATS, American Thoracic Society; FEV_1, forced expiratory volume in one second; FVC, forced vital capacity.
Source: GOLD Report Classification update November.

they had COPD. Adding to these numbers, it is also estimated that about 50% of patients with COPD have not been identified (4). Of those adults who report that they have COPD, 15 % state that their activities are limited because of their breathing problems. Chronic lower respiratory diseases including COPD, asthma, and bronchiectasis, were the fourth leading cause of death with nearly 120,000 adults dying of COPD. Death rates increase with age with a mortality rate of 0.5 per 100,000 in the 18 to 44 age group, while in the 75 and over group the death rate is 440 per 100,000. Prevalence is associated with socioeconomic status. Adults who live below the poverty line were 75% more likely to report that they had COPD than those in higher socioeconomic brackets (5).

A significant portion of health resources are used in caring for patients with COPD. The most recent NCHS data indicate over 6 million inpatient hospital stays and nearly 21 million visits to physicians and hospital outpatient departments were made by patients with a diagnosis of COPD. Total direct treatment cost is highly correlated with disease severity (6). Indirect costs of COPD are similarly high. One study of work force participation found that COPD patients in GOLD Stages I, II and III were associated with a 3.4%, 3.9%, and 14.4% reduction in the labor force participation rate relative to those without COPD. This adverse impact on work force participation was responsible for work loss estimated at $9.9 billion in the United States in 1994 (7).

Understanding the pathophysiology of COPD helps explain its manifestations and the rationale for treatment. The airways in COPD patients have a number of characteristics that are similar to those in asthma: hypertrophy and overactivity of the mucus glands, increased numbers of goblet cells, smooth muscle hypertrophy, small airways clogged with mucus, and sloughing of the ciliated epithelium. During COPD exacerbations, the mucus contains primarily neutrophils rather than the eosinophils seen in asthma. Tobacco smoke and other irritants increase the number and activity of macrophages in the lungs, which initiate the inflammatory and destructive processes. Chemical substances elaborated in the inflammatory cells (such as neutrophil elastase) destroy the supporting attachments of the alveoli and small bronchioles, resulting in decreased elastic recoil; they may also destroy the alveolar cells themselves, resulting in less surface area for gas exchange.

Airflow obstruction is caused by several factors. Acutely, there are increased secretions and bronchoconstriction. In addition, with lack of external support, the small bronchioles collapse even with the normal increase in intrathoracic pressure that occurs during expiration. As obstruction increases and intrathoracic pressure during expiration increases, this effect is even more pronounced.

Most COPD occurs in smokers. The incidence and severity increase with longer duration of smoking and higher number of packs smoked per day. A normal nonsmoker loses 15 to 30 ml/year of forced expiratory volume in the first second of expiration (FEV_1); the rate of loss is doubled to quintupled in people with COPD who continue to smoke. If they stop smoking, the rate of decline will return to normal, but they do not regain lost function.

Approximately 1% of people with COPD have a severe deficiency of alpha$_1$-antitrypsin (AAT), an inhibitor of neutrophil elastase; without adequate amounts of AAT, the elastase destroys alveolar tissue. COPD tends to occur earlier in these patients, often without smoking exposure, and it progresses more rapidly. Screening by testing AAT serum levels is indicated only if a patient has unusually severe disease compared with age and smoking history (before age 50 in smokers and in any nonsmoker) or has a positive family history of AAT deficiency. Only patients with severe deficiency, consistent with homozygous disease, benefit from AAT replacement therapy.

COPD is also more common in people exposed to certain occupational dusts and chemicals or to high concentration of indoor particulate pollutants such as wood-burning stove smoke. Passive smoking and outdoor environmental pollutants (such as sulfur dioxide in smog) are possible but not definite causes of COPD, but they are known to contribute to exacerbations in people with the disease.

INITIAL EVALUATION

The initial evaluation should establish the diagnosis and severity of COPD based on symptoms and spirometry. While the treatment of COPD shares common elements with other respiratory diseases such as asthma, it is important to make a correct diagnosis in order to select appropriate therapy. Treatment guidelines follow disease severity and patients should be categorized by GOLD severity. This guides treatment that is proven to improve symptoms and quality of life and avoids using therapy that has not been shown to provide benefit. The evaluation should also focus on identifying possible comorbidities that like COPD are also caused by smoking such as coronary artery disease (CAD), peripheral vascular disease (PVD), and lung neoplasms as well as associated conditions such sleep apnea and depression. In addition to these disease-related indices and conditions, a functional assessment is necessary to determine how the disease is affecting our patients' daily lives. Since almost all recommended treatments for COPD are aimed at improving patient-oriented outcomes such as exercise tolerance, perception of dyspnea, and quality of life rather that spectrometric improvements, having a metric to determine patient-oriented responses is important.

Testing using spirometry to establish an early diagnosis in individuals at risk for COPD should be carried out based on symptoms and predisposing factors. Patients with possible COPD who require spirometry for confirmation include (8):

1. A smoker or ex-smoker, patients with exposure to occupational dusts and chemicals and those exposed to home cooking and heating fuels.
2. Patients with chronic intermittent or daily cough
3. Patients with a pattern of chronic sputum production,
4. Patients who report progressive activity-related shortness of breath.

A family history of severe early-onset emphysema increases the possibility of α_1 antitrypsin deficiency. Smokers over age 50 are also at risk for CAD and lung cancer, which can cause similar symptoms; therefore, it is important to question the patient about chest pain, palpitations, hemoptysis, or weight loss, which would point to these conditions. Occupational exposure to a variety of dusts and chemicals can cause both obstructive and restrictive lung disease, so an occupational history is essential. Other elements of the history include family and social support systems, past medical history of asthma, sinusitis, allergy, or nasal polyps.

While spirometry is important in diagnosis, even patients with mild to no abnormalities on spirometry can still have significant symptoms and disability (9). Therefore an important element of the initial evaluation of a COPD patient is to determine how the disease is affecting the patients' life and activities. This also includes determining the impact of the disease on the patient's family routines as well as missed work and the social impact of their symptoms. Many patients modify their lifestyle and activities to minimize their symptoms. Some may relate their difficulties to poor conditioning or advancing age instead if their COPD. Physicians should ask about breathing difficulties and if they cause curtailment of exercise or activities. One measure of breathing difficulty is the Medi-

TABLE 51.2 Medical Research Council Grading of Functional Limitation Due to Dyspnea

1. "I only get breathless with strenuous exercise."
2. "I get short of breath when hurrying on the level or walking up a slight hill."
3. "I walk slower than most people of the same age on the level because of breathlessness or have to stop for breath when walking at my own pace on the level."
4. "I stop for breath after walking about 100 yards or after a few minutes on the level."
5. "I am too breathless to leave the house" or "I am breathless when dressing."

cal Research Council dyspnea scale (see Table 51.2). Studies have shown that this scale can help identify patients with a poor quality of life and provides prognostic information on survival with COPD (10). In addition, using this one possible metric can help determine response to treatment.

Additional history should include previous hospitalizations for respiratory disorders and an assessment of the frequency and severity of exacerbations. Most definitions of acute exacerbation include increased dyspnea and an increase in sputum purulence or volume, or both. One classification rates exacerbation severity on the basis of presenting symptoms, ranging from mild (type I) to severe (type III) (see Table 51.3).

The evaluation of a COPD patient presenting for the first time or presenting with worsening symptoms of breathlessness may pose challenges since it may initially be difficult to determine if the symptoms are due to COPD or whether they are caused by other common conditions or comorbid diseases. Asthma, coronary vascular disease (CVD), pulmonary vascular diseases such as thromboembolic disease, and other lung

TABLE 51.3 Classification of acute exacerbations of COPD (33)

Type I	One of three cardinal symptoms: 1. Worsening dyspnea 2. Increase in sputum purulence 3. Increase in sputum volume *and* One of the following: Upper respiratory tract infection in the past 5 days Fever without other apparent cause Increased wheezing Increased cough Increase in respiratory or heart rate by 20% above baseline
Type II	Two of three cardinal symptoms
Type III	All three cardinal symptoms

TABLE 51.4 Differential Diagnosis of Chronic Respiratory Conditions

COPD	Mid-life onset Slowly progressive symptoms Smoking history Dyspnea with exertion Largely irreversible airway obstruction
Asthma	Early onset Symptoms vary day to day Atopic conditions often present Family Hx of asthma Airflow obstruction is largely reversible
Congestive heart failure (CHF)	Fine basilar crackles on exam Dilated heart, pulmonary edema on chest X-ray Volume restriction on PFT
Bronchiectasis	Large volume of purulent sputum Commonly associated with bacterial infection Coarse crackles and clubbing on exam Bronchial dilatation and bronchial wall thickening on imaging
Tuberculosis	Onset at all ages Lung infiltrate or granulomata (nodular lesions) on chest X-ray AFB positive
Sarcoidosis	Dry cough Fever present Symptoms and signs of systemic inflammation present
Obliterative bronchiolitis	Onset at younger age and in non-smokers Hx of RA or fume exposure CT on expiration shows hypo-dense areas

AFB, acid fast bacilli; CT, computed tomography; PFT, pulmonary function test; RA, rheumatoid arthritis.

diseases all can be in the differential diagnosis. Cues pointing to alternative cardiac or pulmonary diagnoses are presented in Table 51.4.

Screening for depression is important in all chronic diseases. A large number of COPD patients have depression and this is a significant complication that diminishes quality of life, can affect morbidity and mortality, and has an important impact on treatment compliance (11). Depressed COPD patients have a poorer quality of life and more frequent hospital admissions, with longer in-patient stays compared with non-depressed patients (12).

Sleep apnea is common in COPD patients. The combination of COPD and sleep apnea (labeled Overlap syndrome in pulmonology literature) has an understandably big effect on patients' oxygenation, gas exchange, and breathing patterns. The 5 year survival of patients with Overlap syndrome is lower than that of patients with sleep apnea alone (13) and COPD patients should be should be assessed for signs and symptoms of sleep apnea.

Take a medication history that includes a patient's use of inhalers, their use of spacers for the delivery of metered dose inhaler (MDI) aerosols and other prescribed drugs. Inhaler technique should be assessed. One clinical question that can arise in caring for COPD patients who are on beta-blockers or who are considered for beta-blocker therapy for associated cardiovascular diseases is the safety of this treatment. It appears that patients with COPD who use cardio selective beta-blockers do not experience a significant worsening of their short-term pulmonary status as measured by FEV_1, or by changes in patients' self-reported symptoms (14).

The physical exam in COPD is not diagnostic. Even a careful examination can underestimate airflow limitation, especially in the early stages of the illness. Examination helps identify comorbid conditions and can aid in the diagnosis of other respiratory diseases. As the disease advances more signs of hyperinflation, right heart failure and general muscle wasting may be present. Table 51.5 lists key elements of the history and physical examination for COPD.

While there are no commonly used decision rules for COPD, forced expiratory time can be used as a clinical screening test for COPD. The test is performed by having the patient take a deep breath and then exhale as hard and long as possible while listening with a stethoscope placed over the trachea in the suprasternal notch until the last moment that sounds are audible. A result of more than 6 seconds has been shown to have a sensitivity of 74% and a specificity of 75% in detecting obstructive disease in patients over 60 years of age (15).

Diagnostic Testing

Pulmonary function tests (PFTs) are the best objective measurement of lung impairment. They are used to identify airway obstruction as the cause of chronic dyspnea, to classify

TABLE 51.5 Key Elements in the History and Physical Examination for Chronic Obstructive Pulmonary Disease (COPD)

Question or Maneuver	Purpose
Detailed history of shortness of breath, wheezing, cough, and character of sputum	To identify symptoms and their time patterns, including aggravating factors such as tobacco smoke, pollution, or infection, and to identify frequent mucus production
Smoking history—by either the patient or household members	To identify contributing factors and to begin the process for helping the patient stop smoking
Family history of chronic obstructive pulmonary disease, including age at onset and whether any family member smoked	To determine probability of α_1-antitrypsin deficiency
History of atopy (allergic rhinitis, eczema or asthma) in the patient or family members	To assess likelihood of a significant reversible (asthmatic) component
History of exposure to asbestos, silica, and other dusts or chemicals that damage lungs	To determine the risk for restrictive disease as coexisting or alternative diagnosis
History of hypertension, palpitations, chest pain, or hyperlipidemia	To determine the likelihood of cardiac disease as a cause of symptoms
Assessment of heart rate, respiratory rate, cyanosis, and use of accessory muscles	To identify patients needing prompt intervention
Lung examination for decreased breath sounds, wheezing, prolonged expiration, increased resonance to percussion, or low diaphragm	These findings support a diagnosis of obstructive airway disease
Lung examination for fine basilar or other localized rales, or decreased resonance	These findings would suggest congestive heart failure, infection, tumor, or pleural effusion

the severity of the disease, and to establish a baseline. The basic test is spirometry, which can be performed either in the office or in a pulmonary function laboratory. The patient breathes in fully and then out as fast as possible through tubing connected to sensors that measure and record air flow. The test is repeated after administering two puffs of a short-acting bronchodilator such as albuterol. Results are compared with normal predicted values for people of the same age, height, and gender.

The key values in the PFTs are the FVC, FEV_1, and the ratio of FEV_1/ FVC. In obstructive diseases, the problem is getting the air out of the lungs at a normal speed, and the FEV_1/FVC is <70%. If this ratio returns to >70% with the inhaled bronchodilator, the patient has asthma; if it stays <70%, the patient has COPD. If it increases by more than 15% but is still below 70%, the patient has a combination of reversible and irreversible components. While indices of airway obstruction can fluctuate over time, testing must show persistent obstruction that is not fully reversible in order to make the diagnosis of COPD. Volume/time graphs comparing asthma and COPD are presented in Figure 51.1. Other tests of lung function are not used routinely, but if spirometry suggests restrictive or mixed disease, full pulmonary function tests with total lung capacity and inspiratory and expiratory reserve are measured.

Chest X-rays and CT imaging are not routinely used to diagnose COPD and are more important for ruling out other lung and chest conditions. They are also recommended in patients who have acute exacerbations in the emergency department or hospital setting (16). In early COPD the chest X-ray is normal, but later it shows hyperinflation with flattened diaphragms. Bullae or blebs that predispose the patient to pneumothorax would indicate more severe disease. In AAT deficiency, there may be increased radiolucency in the bases.

A complete blood count (CBC) is not always needed, but may show evidence of infection (elevated white blood cell count), or chronic hypoxia (elevated hematocrit) that also raises the possibility of pulmonary hypertension.

Arterial blood gases (ABGs) are obtained in patients with an FEV_1 of less than 40 % of the predicted value, based on age, sex, and height, or in patients where respiratory failure is suspected. In severe COPD it has value in determining baseline status and identifies "CO_2 retainers." These are people with longstanding, severe COPD whose respiratory drive is stimulated only by low blood oxygen levels and not by increased carbon dioxide levels. If they are given enough supplemental oxygen to achieve normal blood oxygen levels, they have no stimulus to breathe and progressively retain more carbon dioxide. They become acidotic and stuporous. A low PO_2 on ABG may indicate a need for continuous oxygen therapy. Sputum Gram stain is sometimes used to guide antibiotic therapy during exacerbations, although most often antibiotics are chosen empirically. Sputum culture and sensitivity are indicated only in patients who are severely ill and require hospitalization, especially if pneumonia is suspected.

MANAGEMENT

Manage COPD to achieve patient oriented outcomes. The goals of management of COPD are the following:

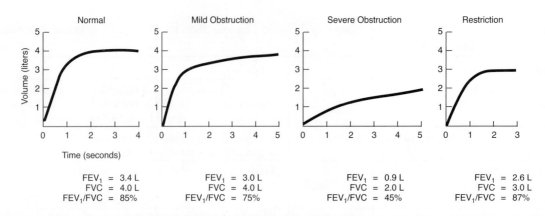

Figure 51.1 • Interpreting basic pulmonary function tests (spirometry). FEV_1, forced expiratory volume in the first second of expiration; FVC, forced vital capacity. (Adapted from National Institutes of Health. Guidelines for the Diagnosis and Management of Asthma. EPR Report No. 1. Bethesda, MD: National Institutes of Health; August 1991:91–3042, Figure 2.1, Interpretation of Results of Spirometry.)

1. To prevent disease progression
2. To alleviate breathlessness and other respiratory symptoms
3. To improve exercise tolerance
4. To prevent and treat acute exacerbations
5. To improve health status
6. To reduce mortality

Therapy follows the stage of disease. An approach to the COPD patient is presented in Figure 51.2. All patients including at risk patients who have normal spirometry, should receive annual influenza immunization, (17) exercise training, patient education (18) and avoidance of risk factors especially smoking. Cigarette smoking is the single most important cause of COPD, accounting for approximately 85%–90 % of cases. As exposure increases, the risk of developing airway obstruction increases. Smoking cessation programs are the most effective intervention to reduce the risk of COPD. This is also the only intervention that has been shown to slow its progression. COPD patients who continue smoking will see accelerated deterioration of airway obstruction. Smoking cessation produces only a small improvement in the FEV_1, however the rate of decline after stopping smoking returns to that of a non-smoker (19). Smoking cessation results in diminishing cough, less sputum production, shortness of breath and wheezing. Brief intervention and advice on quitting smoking from physicians, non-physician health professionals, nicotine replacement treatment, bupropion, and individual group counseling will all increase cessation rates (20).

Improvement in FEV1 in response to drug therapy correlates poorly with improvements in dyspnea, exercise tolerance, and quality of life. Since seemingly minor improvements in pulmonary function can result in significant improvements of these patient-oriented outcomes, assessing symptom improvement is more meaningful than measuring changes in pulmonary function (21). Bronchodilators are the mainstay of treatment and they improve patient symptoms. Short-acting bronchodilators such as the beta-agonist albuterol, the anticholinergic ipratropium, or a combination of the two (Combivent)

are used first (22). For mild (Stage I) disease intermittent use is appropriate. Regular treatment with the short acting agents combined with a long acting beta agonist, salmeterol, or the long acting anticholinergic agent, tiotropium, is recommended for patients with Stage II disease and greater (23, 24). The methylxanthine bronchodilator theophylline can be used in a long acting form in more severe disease (25). Besides its bronchodilatory action it has an effect of diaphragmatic strength. However it has a narrow therapeutic index and toxicity limits its use. A summary of commonly prescribed drugs is presented in Table 51.6.

In spite of the role that inflammation plays in COPD, inhaled corticosteroids generally have no consistent effect on patient oriented outcomes and are not recommended. However, a smaller subset of patients, those in Stage III with frequent exacerbations of COPD, may benefit from inhaled corticosteroids (26). Frequent exacerbations are defined as at least one acute exacerbation a year for 3 years. Oral corticosteroids also have been shown to improve COPD symptoms but the significant side-effects associated with oral steroids preclude long term use. It is also seen that response to oral steroids does not predict response to inhaled corticosteroids.

Therapies that may be considered in Very Severe (Stage IV) disease include, long term home oxygen therapy and surgical therapy (lung volume reduction surgery) on emphysematous lung tissue. A summary of the strength of recommendation for COPD therapies is presented in Table 51.7.

All patients with Stage II and greater should be recommended for formal pulmonary rehabilitation. Patients show improved exercise tolerance, less dyspnea and improved quality of life compared to standard care (27). This benefit is lost after 6 months however, unless patients continue their exercise program.

End of life care and discussion of advance directives are important in the later stages of this illness. Patients with moderate to severe COPD deserve a discussion (when they still feel well, if at all possible) of their preferences regarding their care. Specifically, would they want to be intubated if they develop respiratory failure? It is often very difficult to wean

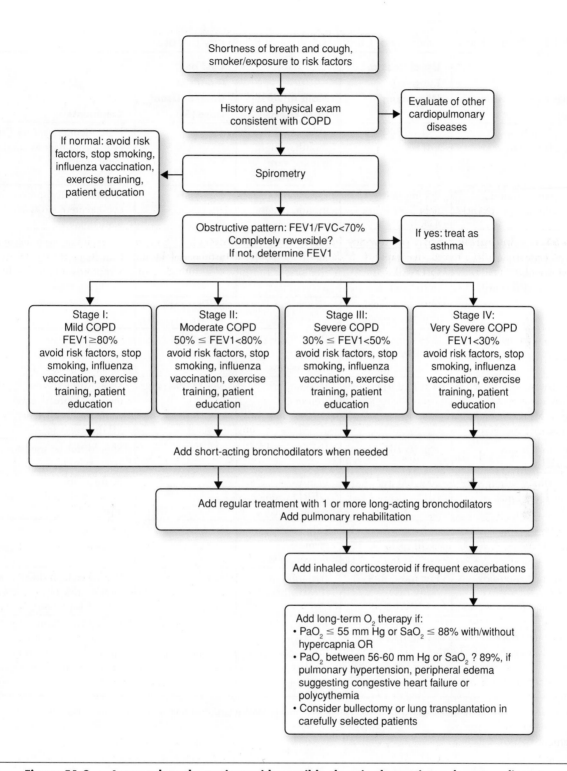

Figure 51.2 • Approach to the patient with possible chronic obstructive pulmonary disease.

TABLE 51.6 Pharmacotherapy of Chronic Obstructive Pulmonary Disease

Generic Name (Trade Name)	Usual Dosing Range (Maximum Dose)	Main Adverse Drug Effects	Cost per Month or Course, Usual Dose ($)*	Comments
Ipratropium bromide 0.03% MDI (Atrovent)	2–4 puffs TID-QID	Occasional dry mouth, cough, nausea; rare palpitations	$$	If accidentally sprayed in eyes, acute narrow-angle glaucoma
Ipratropium bromide 0.02% solution (Atrovent)	0.5 mg in nebulizer every 4–8 h	Occasional dry mouth, cough, nausea; rare palpitations	$/25 vials	If accidentally sprayed in eyes, acute narrow-angle glaucoma
Albuterol MDI [outside United States: salbutamol] (Proventil, Ventolin)	2–4 puffs TID-QID (max 12 puffs/day)	Palpitations, tremors, nervousness	$ (generic) $$	Can be used either for acute symptoms or as scheduled medication
	(6–8 puffs every 1/2–2 h acutely)		$$(Proventil HFA)	
Albuterol nebulizer solution	2.5–5 mg in nebulizer every 1/2–2 h acutely	Palpitations, tremors, nervousness	$/25 vials	
Combination ipratropium and albuterol MDI (Atrovent or Duoneb)	2 puffs QID	Palpitations, tremors, nervousness	$$$ $$/30 vials	Some studies show increased effectiveness compared with separate MDIs
Salmeterol Diskus (Serevent)	1 puffs BID	Palpitations	$$$	Should not be used for acute symptoms
Theophylline, sustained release (Theo-Dur)	200–400 mg BID	Nausea, GERD, tremor, palpitations	$	In toxic doses, causes seizures; desirable serum level 5–12 μg/L
Albuterol, sustained-release tablets	4–8 mg every night or BID	Palpitations, tremors, nervousness	$	
Inhaled corticosteroids inhaler (e.g., beclomethasone)	For most, 2–4 puffs BID	Irritation of throat, thrush	$$$	If used in high doses, can increase risk of cataracts and adrenal suppression
Prednisone, short-term	40–60 mg daily for 5–10 d	Increased BP, hyperglycemia, hypokalemia, irritability or euphoria	$$ 5mg tabs	If used for less than 14 d, can be stopped without taper

BP, blood pressure; GERD, gastroesophageal reflux disease; MDI, metered-dose inhaler; QID, four times daily; TID, three times daily. Based on prices at *www.drugstore.com*
*Relative cost: $ = <$33.00; $$ = $34.00–$66.00; $$$ = >$67.00

COPD patients off of a ventilator, so determining the patient's preference in advance is very helpful to the patient and family.

Education

A number of studies are underway to evaluate the impact of various educational interventions. While education alone is not associated with improved pulmonary function or exercise tolerance, combining it with a self- management program and smoking cessation has been shown to improve patient oriented outcomes (17). In addition, while self management plans improve outcomes in asthma, no studies consistently support this intervention in COPD (28).

Patients with moderate COPD may have mortality and health related quality of life gains from a nursing outreach program, but there are no data about reductions in hospital utilization due to this intervention. Patients with severe

TABLE 51.7 Strength of Recommendation for Management of Chronic Obstructive Pulmonary Disease

Indications	Treatment Strategy	Strength of Recommendation*	Comments
For all patients	Influenza Immunization	A	Reduces rate of hospitalization
For all patients	Patient Education and Self-Management Information	A	Reduces health costs, Improves quality of life
For all patients	Stop smoking	A	Improves long-term outcome Use of nicotine substitutes and bupropion doubles cessation rate
Chronic management			
Stage I COPD	Inhaled beta-agonist (albuterol) or anticholinergic (Ipratropium) as needed for symptoms up to 2–4 puffs four times daily	A	Improves dyspnea, exercise tolerance. No consistent effect on quality of life
	Consider combined ipratropium and albuterol metered-dose inhaler (Combivent)	C	Easier to use, improves adherence but not superior for dyspnea, exercise tolerance or quality of life compared to individual components
Stage II COPD	Add long-acting bronchodilator Salmeterol (long-acting inhaled beta-agonist)	A	Improves dyspnea and quality of life but not shown to improve exercise tolerance
	or Tiotropium bromide (Spiriva) a long acting anticholinergic.	A	Improves dyspnea and quality of life Decreases the number of acute exacerbations
Stage II–IV COPD	Pulmonary Rehabilitation	A	Improves dyspnea, exercise tolerance and quality of life
Stage III–IV COPD	Consider trial of inhaled corticosteroid if frequent exacerbations	A	No improvement in dyspnea, exercise tolerance or quality of life Reduces severity but not the frequency of exacerbations
	Combination inhaled corticosteroid and long-acting bronchodilator. e.g. Fluticasone and Salmeterol (Advair)	C	Use for convenience if on both a long-acting beta-agonist and inhaled corticosteroid.
	Consider long-acting theophylline	B	Improves dyspnea and exercise tolerance
Stage IV COPD	Long-term oxygen therapy (>15 hours per day) if $PO_2 \leq 55$ mm Hg with or without hypercapnia If PO_2 56–60 mm Hg if pulmonary hypertension, CHF or polycythemia	A	Improved survival Improved sense on well-being
Management of exacerbations			
For all exacerbations	Add inhaled beta-agonist or Ipratropium	A	Improves symptoms more than the small improvements in FEV1 seen
Moderate-severe type II	Systemic glucocorticoids	A	Reduce severity of exacerbation and shorten recovery
If purulent exacerbation	Antibiotics	A	Symptomatic improvement

CHF, congestive heart failure; COPD, chronic obstructive pulmonary disease; FEV_1, forced expiratory volume in one second.
*A = consistent, good-quality patient-oriented evidence; B = inconsistent or limited-quality patient-oriented evidence; C = consensus, disease-oriented evidence, usual practice, expert opinion, or case series. For information about the SORT evidence rating system, see *http://www.aafp.org/afpsort.xml*.

TABLE 51.8 Red Flags Suggesting Progressive or Life-Threatening Disease in Patients with COPD

Red Flag	Condition of Concern	Comments
Hemoptysis	Pulmonary neoplasm, Pulmonary embolus, CHF	Further pulmonary imaging warranted
Hypoxia	Impending respiratory failure	Usually a determinant of need for hospitalization in the setting of acute exacerbations
Peripheral Edema	Heart failure, Thromboembolic disease	Consider PE if exacerbation occurs associated with unilateral edema and CHF with bilateral edema
Hypercapnia	Impending respiratory failure	Rising hypercapnia may occur with O_2 treatment, cautious titration is advised
Hypotension, confusion	Sepsis	Usually a determinant of need for hospitalization in the setting of acute exacerbations

CHF, congestive heart failure; PE, pulmonary embolism.

COPD do not appear to have benefit from such programs and one large study found no reduction in hospital admissions in such patients (29).

Depression is commonly associated with COPD as well as other chronic diseases (30). Treatment with antidepressants may improve quality of life and exercise tolerance but the effects of treatment on these parameters do not appear until treatment has been in effect for at least 3 months. These effects occur in the absence of any change in spirometry (31).

Very little research has been published on alternative/complementary therapies in COPD. One study concluded that neither beta-carotene nor Vitamin E given as supplements affected COPD symptoms. The study did indicate that a diet rich in these nutrients appeared to lower the risk of developing COPD.

Most patients with COPD can be cared for by family physicians. Some reasons to consider specialist consultation include uncertainty over the diagnosis, severe symptoms, symptoms disproportionate to airway obstruction, accelerated decline in function, and the development of COPD at a young age (<40 years of age).

Acute Exacerbations

No standardized guidelines have been developed to define acute exacerbations of COPD. Most definitions include increased dyspnea and an increase in sputum purulence or volume, or both (see Table 51.3). Mild exacerbations may be treated on an outpatient basis, whereas moderate to severe flares may require hospitalization and possibly admission to the intensive care unit. Moderate exacerbations of COPD are treated by increasing the frequency of inhaled ipratropium (6 to 8 puffs up to every 3 to 4 hours) and albuterol (up to 6 to 8 puffs every 2 to 4 hours if tolerated) to decrease bronchospasm, while initiating a course of oral corticosteroids at 40 to 60 mg of prednisone per day. The inhaled medications should be decreased to 4 times per day as soon as possible. Prednisone can be stopped abruptly, without tapering, if given for fewer than 2 weeks. Many clinicians provide 5 days of prednisone and then stop it; others prefer to taper it after the patient's disease has stabilized in order to decrease the likelihood of recurrence.

Infections can cause COPD exacerbations by causing mucus production and bronchoconstriction. Although many of the infections are viral, it is a possible practice to prescribe antibiotics for patients to keep at home so they can initiate treatment when mucus production increases and changes to a yellow or green color (32). Be aware of red flags (see Table 51.8) that the patient's symptom exacerbation may not be due solely to COPD.

If the above measures are not effective or the patient's condition deteriorates rapidly, hospitalization may be necessary to give more intensive bronchodilator therapy, intravenous antibiotics, steroids, and oxygen therapy. Intubation and mechanical ventilation may be necessary, but should be avoided if possible because of the difficulty in weaning a COPD patient off of the ventilator. It should be noted that guidelines related to management of acute exacerbations refer to patients who present to hospital emergency departments or those who require hospitalization. A management algorithm is described in Figure 51.3.

CASE DISCUSSION

Mr. R.L.'s most serious predisposing factor was the heavy smoking history. Particulate exposures in the shipyard and as a carpenter may also have been significant. The low FVC suggests a possible restrictive component to his disease. The FEV_1 was almost low enough to be classified as severe disease. The other indicated tests were repeat PFTs with bronchodilators (which showed 18% to 20% improvement); a chest radiograph, which did not have any evidence of lung cancer; and an electrocardiogram, which was normal. A $Po_2 < 55$ would be an indication for continuous home oxygen, which Mr. L. needed 3 years later. Follow-up over the next 8 years included an annual influenza vaccine, a pneumonia vaccine, and addition of theophylline to his regimen. He had several episodes of increased productive cough and dyspnea, which were treated with broad-spectrum antibiotics. He did not require hospitalization until an episode of pneumonia in 2004. After discharge, he was more conscientious in continuous use of his

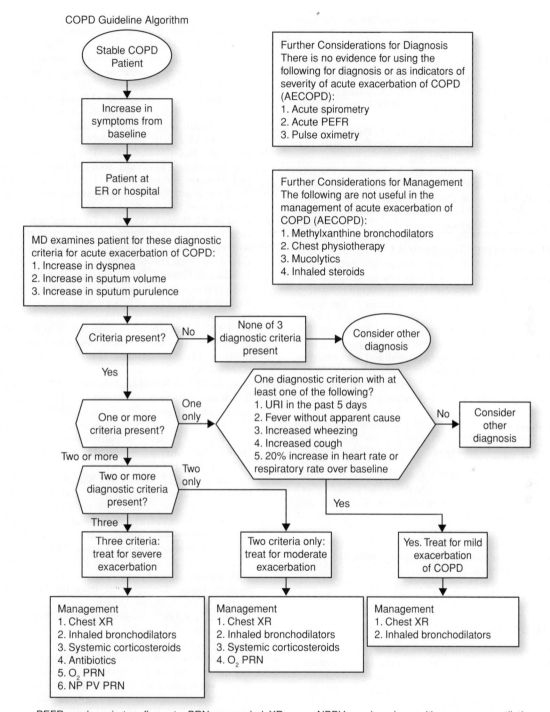

PEFR, peak expiratory flow rate; PRN, as needed; XR, x-ray; NPPV, non-invasive positive pressure ventilation.

Figure 51.3 • Acute exacerbation of COPD Guideline Algorithm. (From Bach PB, et al. Position Paper: Management of Acute Exacerbations of Chronic obstructive pulmonary disease: A Summary and Appraisal of Published Evidence. Ann Intern Med. 2001;134:600–620, with permission.)

oxygen, and about 3 months later he was symptomatically back to his baseline.

REFERENCES

1. Mapel DW, Dedrick D, Davis K. Trends in cardiovascular co-morbidities of COPD patients in the Veterans Administration Medical System 1991–1999. COPD: J Obstruct Pulm Dis. 2005;2:35–41.
2. Agusti AGN, Noguera A, Sauleda J, Sala E, Pons J, Busquets X. Systemic Effects of Chronic Obstructive Pulmonary Disease. Eur Respir J. 2003;21:347–360.
3. Oliver SM, Living with failing lungs: the doctor–patient relationship. Fam Pract. 2001;18:430–439.
4. Calverley P, Bellamy D. The challenge of providing better care for patients with chronic obstructive pulmonary disease: The poor relation of airway obstruction. Thorax. 2000;55:78–82.
5. NCHS Data on COPD. Available at *http://www.cdc.gov/nchs/data/factsheets/copd.pdf*. Accessed February 15, 2006.
6. Hilleman DE, Dewan N, Malesker M, Friedman M. Pharmacoeconomic evaluation of COPD. Chest. 200;118:1278–1285.
7. Sin DD, Stafinshi T, Ng YC, Bell NR, Jacobs P. The impact of chronic obstructive pulmonary disease on work loss in the United States. Am J Respir Crit Care Med. 2002;165:704–707.
8. Global initiative for chronic obstructive lung disease. Global strategy for the diagnosis, management and prevention of chronic obstructive pulmonary disease. NHLBI/WHO workshop report. Bethesda,MD: National Heart, Lung and Blood Institute; 2001. Available at *www.goldcopd.com*. Accessed January10, 2006.
9. Stewart AL, Greenfield S, Hays RD, et al. Functional status and well-being of patients with chronic conditions. Results from the Medical Outcomes Study. JAMA. 1989;262:907–913.
10. Bestall JC, Paul EA, Garrod R, Garnham R, Jones PW, Wedizcha JA. Usefulness of the Medical Research Council (MRC) dyspnoea scale as a measure of disability in patients with chronic obstructive pulmonary disease. Thorax. 1999; 54:581–586.
11. Isoaho R, Keistinen T, Laippala P, Kivela SL. Chronic obstructive pulmonary disease and symptoms related to depression in elderly persons. Psychol Rep. 1995;76:287–297.
12. Yohannes AM, Roomi J, Baldwin RC, Connolly MJ. Depression in elderly outpatients with chronic obstructive pulmonary disease. Age Aging. 1998;27:155–160.
13. Bhullar S, Phillips B. Sleep in COPD Patients. COPD. 2005; 3:355–361.
14. Salpeter SS, Ormiston T, Salpeter E, Poole P, Cates C. Cardioselective beta-blockers for chronic obstructive pulmonary disease (Cochrane Review). In: The Cochrane Library. Oxford, England: Update Software; 2005:Oct 19;(4):CD003566.
15. Schapira FM, Schapira MM, Funahashi A, McAuliffe T, Barkdy B. The value of the forced expiratory time in the physical diagnosis of obstructive airways disease. JAMA. 1993;270:731–736.
16. Tsai TW, Gallagher EJ, Lombardi G, et al. Guidelines for the selective ordering of admission chest radiography in adult obstructive airway disease. Ann Emerg Med. 1993;22:1854–1858.
17. Poole PJ, Chacko E, Wood-Baker RWB, Cates CJ. Influenza vaccine for patients with chronic obstructive pulmonary disease (Cochrane Review). In: The Cochrane Library. Oxford, England: Update Software; 2004:Issue2.
18. Bourbeau J, Julien M, Maltais F, et al. Reduction of hospital utilization in patients with chronic obstructive pulmonary disease: a disease-specific self-management intervention. Arch Intern Med. 2003;163:585–591.
19. Anthonisen NR, Connett JE, Murray RP, for the Lung Health Study Research Group. Smoking and lung function of lung health study participants after 11 years. Am J Respir Crit Care Med. 2002;166:675–679.
20. Fiore MC, Bailey WC, Cohen SJ, et al. Treating tobacco use and dependence. Rockville, MD: US Department of Health and Human Services, Public Health Service, June 2000. Available at *http://www.surgeongeneral.gov/tobacco/smokesum.htm*. Accessed
21. Belman MJ, Botnick WC, Shin JW. Inhaled bronchodilators reduce dynamic hyperinflation during exercise in patients with chronic obstructive pulmonary disease. Am J Resp Crit Care Med. 1996;153:967–975.
22. Jaeschke R, Guyatt GH, Willan A, et al. Effect of increasing doses of β agonists on spirometric parameters, exercise capacity, and quality of life in patients with chronic airflow limitation. Thorax. 1994;49:479–484.
23. Ulrik CS. Efficacy of inhaled salmeterol in the management of smokers with chronic obstructive pulmonary disease, double-blind, placebo controlled, crossover study. Thorax. 1995;50:750–754.
24. Vincken W, van Noord JA, Greefhorst APM, et al. Improved health outcomes in patients with COPD during 1 yr's treatment with tiotropium. Eur Respir J. 2002;19:209–216.
25. Murciano D, Auclair M-H, Pariente R, Aubier M. A randomized, controlled trial of theophylline in patients with severe chronic obstructive pulmonary disease. N Engl J Med. 1989;320:1521–1525.
26. Lacasse Y, Wong E, Guyatt GH, King D, Cook DJ, Goldstein RS. Meta-analysis of respiratory rehabilitation in chronic obstructive pulmonary disease. Lancet 1996;348:1115–1119.
27. Lacasse Y, Wong E, Guyatt GH, King D, Cook DJ, Goldstein RS. Meta-analysis of respiratory rehabilitation in chronic obstructive pulmonary disease. Lancet. 996;348:1115–1119.
28. Monninkhof EM, van der Valk PDLPM, van der Palen J, et al. Self-management education for chronic obstructive pulmonary disease (Cochrane Review). In: The Cochrane Library. Oxford, England: Update Software; 2004:Issue 2.
29. Smith B, Appleton S, Adams R, Southcott A, Ruffin R. Home care by outreach nursing for chronic obstructive pulmonary disease (Cochrane Review).). In: The Cochrane Library. Oxford, England: Update Software; 2004:Issue 2.
30. Lacasse Y, Rousseau L, Maltais F. Prevalence and impact of depression in patients with severe chronic obstructive pulmonary disease. J Cardiopulm Rehabil. 2001;21:80–86.
31. Eiser N, Harte R, Karvounis S, Phillips C, Isaac MT. Effect of treating depression on quality-of-life and exercise tolerance in severe COPD. COPD. 2005;2:233–241.
32. Snow V, Lascher S, Mottur-Pilson C. Evidence base for management of acute exacerbations of chronic obstructive pulmonary disease. Ann Intern Med. 2001 Apr 3;134(7):595–599.
33. Anthonisen NR, Manfreda J, Warren CP, et al. Antibiotic therapy in exacerbations of chronic obstructive pulmonary disease. Ann Intern Med. 1987;106:196–204.

INDEX

Note: Page numbers followed by *f* denote figures; those followed by a *t* denote tables; those followed by *b* indicate a box.

AAP/AAFP guideline, OM and, 297
AAT. *See* Alpha₁-antitrypsin
Abdominal pain, 325–340, 511
  case, 325
  case discussion, 337
  causes, 326*t*
  clinical evaluation, 326–327
  constipation, 375
  diagnosing, 327, 328*f*
    algorithm for, 328*f*
  diagnostic tests, characteristics of, 330*t*–331*t*
  differential diagnosis, 326, 326*t*
  history for, key elements, 329*t*
  life-threatening, red flags in, 327*t*
  management, 334–336
  pathophysiology, 325–326
  physical examination for, key elements, 327, 329*t*
  structures causing, by type and site, 326*f*
ABG. *See* Arterial blood gas
Abnormal uterine bleeding (AUB), 447–452
  adolescent patients and, 448
  case, 447, 452
  clinical evaluation, 448–450
  diagnostic tests, 440*t*
  elements in, 440*t*
  general approach, 450*f*
  management, 443*t*–444*t*, 450–452
  pathophysiology, 448
  progressive/life-threatening disease, red flags, 441*t*
Abortion, 57. *See also* Medical abortion
  unintended pregnancy, 396
Abortion ratio, 396
Abrasions, evaluation and management, 635
Abscess, 623
Abscess-causing organisms, pneumonia and, 770
Absorbable sutures, 637
Abuse, during pregnancy, 63
Abuse Assessment Screen, 502
AC compression test, AC joint and, 607–608
AC distraction test, AC joint and, 607
AC joint
  injury, 613–614
  testing, 607–608
Academic medicine, 23–24
Acamprosate, alcohol dependence and, 716
ACC/AHA guidelines, chronic stable angina and, 154, 154*t*
ACE inhibitors (Angiotensin-converting enzyme inhibitors)
  adverse effects, 173
  CAD and, 154
    mortality, 153, 153*t*
  diastolic heart failure and, 157*f*, 158–159
  DM and, 231, 232
  HTN and, 173, 174*t*, 175*t*
  systolic heart failure, 156, 157*f*, 158
Acetaminophen
  arthritis and, 564
  febrile children and, 223
  fever reduction and, 222
  musculoskeletal chest pain, 144
  myofascial trigger points, 573
Acetaminophen with codeine, medical abortion and, 417
Achilles tendinitis, 544
  imaging, 547
  long-term management, 548
ACMG. *See* American College of Medical Genetics
Acne, 627–628
  benzoyl peroxide, 628
  therapy, by severity, 628*t*

ACOG. *See* American College of Obstetricians and Gynecologists
Acoustic reflectometry, 296
ACR. *See* American College of Radiology
ACS. *See* American Cancer Society
Actinic keratoses (AKs), 629
Activated partial thromboplastin time (APTT), VTE and, 189
Active compression test. *See* O'Brien test
Active range-of-motion (ROM), Apley scratch test and, 604, 605*f*
Activities of daily living (ADLs)
  cognitive impairment, case study, 659
  COPD and, 785
Activity
  chronic health conditions, 92*t*
  DVT and, 191
Actuate salpingitis, gonorrhea and, 514
Acupuncture, migraine, 701
Acute urinary retention (AUR), *See* Urinary retention
Acyclovir, 624
  recurrent HSV infection, 521
ADA. *See* American Diabetes Association
Addictions, 705–719. *See also* Substance abuse; Withdrawal syndromes
  algorithm for, 715*f*
  case, 705
  case discussion, 718, 729–730
  diagnosis, 707
  family intervention, 717–718
  initial evaluation, 706–707
  long-term monitoring, 716–718, 729
  pathophysiology of, 705–706
  red flag diagnosis, 706–707
  treatment
    current effectiveness, 718
    modalities, 714–715
    therapeutic options, 710*t*–711*t*
  withdrawal symptoms, 714*t*
Adenoma, breast skin changes, 386
Adenoviruses, pharyngitis and, 313
Adequate Intakes, 279
ADHD. *See* Attention deficit-hyperactivity disorder
Adhesive capsulitis, 614
ADLs. *See* Activities of daily living
Adolescent patients. *See also* Teenagers
  anovulatory menorrhagia and, 451
  AUB, 448
  counseling, 82–85, 82*t*
  depression and, diagnosis/ treatment considerations, 742
  pregnancy and, 396
  screening, 74*t*, 77
  weight management in, 290
Adoption, 396
ADT. *See* Androgen deprivation therapy
Advance care planning, cognitive impairment, 654
Advance directives, 106
Adverse reaction pharmacotherapy, addiction and, 715
Aerobic activity, HF and, 156
AF. *See* Atrial fibrillation
Aging population, 26
AHS. *See* American Headache Society
AIDS syndrome, HIV disease and, 518
Airflow obstruction, causes, COPD and, 786
Airway obstruction, asthma and, 747
Airway resistance, 747
AKP in children, Osgood-Schlatter's disease, 551
AKP of knee, 550–551
AKs. *See* Actinic keratoses

Alanine transaminase (ALT) abnormalities
  abnormal, 341
  management, 342*f*
Albuterol, COPD and, 752, 794
Alcohol, 705, 706, 718. *See also* Substance abuse
  abuse
    algorithm for, 715*f*
    Cyr-Wartman questions, 706, 708*t*
  acute pancreatitis, 332
  addiction, managing, 709, 711–716
  chronic gout, 573
  dependence, acamprosate and, 716
  detoxification regimens, 716*t*
  HTN and, 172–173, 172*t*
  use
    counseling and, children and, 83
    NASH *v.*, 343
    preconception care and, 53, 55
    USPSTF and, 101
  withdrawal syndromes, 711–712, 716*t*
Alcoholic hepatitis, 341
  biopsy, 342
  NASH *v.*, 343
Alendronate (Fosamax), osteopenic women and, 460
Alfuzosin, 471
Algorithmic reasoning, diagnosis and, 122
Allergen
  asthma, 753
  identification, 747, 748*t*
Allergic conjunctivitis, 302
  drugs for, 310, 310*t*
Allergic rhinitis, 747, 749*t*
  history/physical examination for, key elements, 746*t*
  medications for, 750*t*–751*t*
Allergic vaginosis, 538
Allergies, 745–747
  case, 745
  initial evaluation, 745–746, 746*t*
  management, 746–747
  "triggers," 747
Allopurinol, chronic gout, 573
Alpha 2 blockers
  ADHD and, 204
  CD and, 206
Alpha₁-antitrypsin (AAT), COPD and, 786
Alpha-adrenergic blockers, BPH and, 471
Alprazolam
  dyspnea and, 111
  GAD and, 728, 728*t*
ALT. *See* Alanine transaminase
Alternative therapy. *See* Complimentary and alternative medicine
Alzheimer's Association, 655
Alzheimer's disease, 643, 647
  behavioral/psychological symptoms, 656–659
    nonpharmacological treatment, 656–658
    pharmacological treatment, 658–659
  pharmacological treatment, 656, 657*t*
  stages of dementia, 644, 645*t*
  testing, 652
  treatment, 655–656
Amantadine hydrochloride, influenza, 778
AMBRI mnemonic, shoulder instability and, 612
Amenorrhea
  breast pain and, 387
  pregnancy and, 55–56
American Cancer Society (ACS), prostate cancer, 479
American College of Medical Genetics (ACMG), 53
American College of Obstetricians and Gynecologists (ACOG)
  genetic screening, 52–53
  PMS and, 445

American College of Radiology (ACR), mammogram abnormality, 393
American Diabetes Association (ADA), monitoring, 241
American Headache Society (AHS), patient education and, 698
American Society of Addiction Medicine, 705
American Urologic Association Symptom Score, 471
    BPH and, 470, 471*t*
Amine test (Whiff test), BV and, 531
Amino acid supplements, 490
Aminoglycosides, conjunctivitis and, 310
Amiodarone
    AF and, 160
    hormone release and, 263
Amniocentesis, 61
    threshold age, 62
Amoxicillin
    acute pyelonephritis, 431
    ear pain, 299
    OM and, 298
    UTI and, 430
Amoxicillin/clavulanate, UTI and, 430
    infants and children, 433
Amphetamine-dextroamphetamine, ADHD and, 203
Ampicillin
    acute pyelonephritis, 431
    infants and children, UTIs and, 433
Amputations, DM and, 227
AN. *See* Anorexia nervosa
ANA. *See* Antinuclear antibody
Anabolic Steroids Control Act of 1990, 488
Analgesic ladder, WHO and, 110, 111*f*
Analgesics, corneal abrasions, 310
Anaphylaxis, polio vaccine, 81
Androgen deprivation therapy (ADT), prostate cancer and, 479
Androgens
    adverse effects, 488*t*
    performance enhancing supplements and, 487–489
    postmenopausal women, 463
Androstenedione, 487, 489
Anemia
    medical abortion and, 417
    occult bleeding, 368
Anemia screening, pregnancy and, 66
Anesthesia, facet joints and, 590
Angina pectoris, 149
Angina symptoms, medication for, 154
Angiotensin receptor blockers, HTN and, 173, 174*t*, 175*t*
Angiotensin-converting enzyme inhibitors. *See* ACE inhibitors
Animal bites, 636
Ankle
    anatomy, 543–544, 544*f*
    injury, 543
    joint, 543
    OAR and, case discussion, 550
    stress testing, 546*f*
Ankle fracture
    diagnostic testing, 545
    long-term management, 548
Ankle pain, 543–550
    case, 543
    clinical evaluation, 544–547
    differential diagnosis, 545*t*
    drugs for, 549*t*
    history and physical examination, key elements of, 547*t*
    management, 547–548
    progressive/life-threatening disease, red flags for, 545*t*
Ankle sprain
    fracture *v.*, 544
    initial management, 547–548
    management, 548*t*
Anorexia nervosa (AN), 207
Anovulatory bleeding, approach to, 451*f*
Anovulatory menorrhagia, adolescents and, 451
Antabuse. *See* Disulfiram
Anterior dislocation, 612–613
Anterior tibiofibular ligaments (ATFL), 543, 544, 545
Anthralin, psoriasis, 627
Antibiotic(s)
    acute bronchitis, 776–777
    acute sinusitis, 776

asymptomatic bacteriuria, 434
catheter-associated infections, 434
diarrhea disorders, 371, 372*t*
disseminated gonococcal infection, 516
ear pain, 299, 300
GABHS pharyngitis, 319–320, 320*t*
ointments
    blepharitis and, 311
    hordeolum, 311
OM and, 297, 298*t*
ophthalmic, 309*f*
SBI and, children, 223–224, 223*t*
sore throat, 313
Sputum Gram stain, 789
URI and, 775
UTI and, 429, 430
wounds, 640
Antibody screen, pregnancy and, 65
Anticoagulation
    AF and, 160, 161*t*
    DVT and, 182
    long-term
        DVT and, 193*t*
        PE and, 193*t*
Antidepressants
    CD and, 206
    dementia, behavioral symptoms, 658, 658*t*
    ED and, 483
    selection of, depression, 739–740, 741*t*
Antifungals
    CVV and, 537
    tinea cruris, 625
Antihistamines, URI and, 776
Antihypertensive medication, 165
    adverse effects, 173, 175
    coexistent medical problems and, 173
    cost, 175
    DM and, 231
    dosing, 175
    ED and, 483
    HTN and, 173, 174*t*, 175*t*
Anti-inflammatory medications
    asthma and, 756, 762–763
    shoulder pain and, 610*t*
Antimicrobial agents
    acute prostatitis, 474
    CAP and, 779
    URI and, 775
Antinuclear antibody (ANA), SLE and, 575
Antiplatelet agents
    ACS and, 139
    CAD mortality and, 153, 153*t*
Antipsychotics
    ADHD and, 204
    CD and, 206
Antipyretic therapy, fever reduction and, 222
Antiretroviral therapy, HIV disease, 519
Antithyroid drugs (ATDs), 268
    side effects, 269
Antithyrotropin antibodies, 268
Antivert, dizziness and, 673
Antivirals, recurrent HSV infection, 521
Anxiety, 678, 689, 721–730
    cases, 721
    end-of-life care, 113–114
    medical conditions mimicking, 725*t*
Anxiety disorder(s)
    algorithm, 726*f*
    diagnostic criteria, 723*t*
    fatigue, 682*t*, 683
    initial evaluation, 723–725
    medications and doses, 728*t*
    public health significance, 722–723
    red flags, 725, 726*t*
    screening questions, 725*t*
    sleep disorder and, 685
    spectrum of, 721–722
    therapies for, 727*t*
Anxiolytics, dyspnea and, 111
Aortic regurgitation (AR), 162–163
Aortic stenosis (AS), 162
Apley scratch test, active ROM and, 604, 605*f*
Appendectomy, spiral CT and, 333
Appendicitis, 331*t*333
    management, 336

Appendix rupture, 333
Apprehension test, 605*f*, 608
    laxity/instability testing and, 608
APTT. *See* Activated partial thromboplastin time
AR. *See* Aortic regurgitation
ARBs (Angiotensin receptor blockers)
    DM and, 231, 232
    systolic heart failure, 156, 157*f*, 158
Area Agency on Aging, 655
Aredia. *See* Pamidronate
Arm abduction test, cervical disc herniation, 591
Arnold's nerve, 293
Arrhythmias, common, 160–162
Arterial blood flow, ED and, 483
Arterial blood gas (ABG)
    asthma and, 753
    COPD and, 789
Arthralgia, PMR and, 575
Arthritis, 557–558, 562, 562*t*
    acetaminophen, 564
    case discussion, 576
    radiographic findings in, 563, 563*t*
Arthritis Foundation, patient education, 576
Arthrocentesis, septic joint and, 574
Arthroscopic debridement, OA and, 566
AS. *See* Aortic stenosis
ASB. *See* Asymptomatic bacteriuria
Ascites, cirrhosis and, 347
ASD. *See* Acute stress disorder; Autistic spectrum disorder
Aspartame, phenylketonuria and, 63
Aspartate transaminase (AST) abnormalities
    abnormal, 341
    management, 342
Aspirin
    AF, 160
    arthritis and, 564
    CAD and, 153, 153*t*
    DM and, 232
    febrile children and, 223
    nonvalvular atrial fibrillation and, 161*t*
    RA and, 568
Aspirin chemoprophylaxis, USPSTF, 94
Assisted living, cognitive impairment, 659
AST. *See* Aspartate transaminase
Asthma, 747–749, 751–756, 762–765
    acute bronchitis, 772
    acute exacerbations, managing, 763
    case discussion, 765
    COPD *v.*, 789, 790*f*
    death from, 755*t*
        red flags, 764*t*
    diagnostic tests, 752–753
    home management, 755*f*
    initial evaluation, 751–752, 752*t*
    lung function and, measurements, 756, 757*t*–761*t*
    management, 753, 754*t*
    medications, classification/long-term control, 756, 757*t*–761*t*
    persistent, long-term control, 756
    severity of, factors affecting, 753, 755–756
    "triggers," 747
Asthma Action Plan, 753, 754*t*
Asthma-related death, 755*f*
Asymptomatic bacteriuria (ASB), 434
    prenatal care and, 60
Asymptomatic disease, screening for, 97
ATDs. *See* Antithyroid drugs
ATFL. *See* Anterior tibiofibular ligaments
Atopic dermatitis, 626–627
    popliteal fossa and, 625*f*
    treatment, 626
Atrial fibrillation (AF), 159–160, 159*f*
    rhythm *vs.* rate control, 160
Atrophic vaginitis, 538
    low-dose estrogen and, 458, 459*t*
Attention deficit-hyperactivity disorder (ADHD), 201, 202*t*, 203–204
    long-term monitoring, 204
    medications for, 204*t*
    recommendations, 205*t*
AUB. *See* Abnormal uterine bleeding
Audiometry
    nonspecific dizziness, 667
    vertigo, 671
AUDIT questionnaire, 101

AUR. *See* Acute urinary retention
Auscultation, asthma, 750
Autistic spectrum disorder (ASD), 200
Autoimmune disease, PMS and, 445
Autonomic dysfunction, dizziness and, 678
Axial traction test, cervical disc herniation, 591
Azathioprine, RA and, 569
Azithromycin, viral pharyngitis, 317

B12 deficiency. *See* Vitamin B12 deficiency
Babinski reflex, low back pain, 583
Bacitracin
    abrasions, 635
    corneal abrasions, 310
Bacitracin-polymyxin B, conjunctivitis and, 309
Backache. *See also* Low back pain
    pregnancy and, 66
Bacteremia, children, 217, 221
Bacterial infections, 621–622. *See also* Serious
            bacterial infection
    treatment of, 622t
Bacterial pathogens, 769
Bacterial vaginosis (BV), 527–528
    clinical evaluation, 529
    diagnostic criteria, 530
    office testing, 530–531
    in pregnancy, 533, 537
    treatment, 533, 534t
Balance, cognitive impairment, 647f
Balneotherapy, RA and, 570
Bankart lesion, 613
Bariatric surgery, 290t
Barium swallow, goiter and, 271
Barrett's esophagus, 356, 360
Barrier contraceptive methods, 410–412
BAS. *See* Bile acid sequestrants
Basal body temperature (BBT), natural family
            planning, 414
Basal cell carcinoma (BCC), 619, 628, 629f
Basal insulin therapy, HbA1c goals and, 238
BBT. *See* Basal body temperature
BCAA. *See* Branched chain amino acids
BCC. *See* Basal cell carcinoma
Behavior
    disorders, 197–213
    management
        DM and, 233
        hypoglycemic medications, 236–238, 240f
    modification, Alzheimer's disease and, 658
    monitoring, DM and, 238, 241t
    therapy
        ADHD and, 204
        weight-loss diet, 286
Behavioral and developmental screening
    case discussion, 210–211
    initial evaluation, 197–198, 198t
Behavioral medicine, primary care and, 507–508
Benign paroxysmal positional vertigo (BPPV), 664,
            675, 677f
Benign prostatic hyperplasia (BPH), 469–474
    case, 469, 473–474
    diagnosis and treatment, algorithm, 472f
    diagnostic testing, 470
    initial evaluation, 469–470
    management, 470–474
    medications, 473t
    pharmacotherapy, 471–472, 473t
    referral indications, 473t
    treatments, strength of recommendation for, 474t
    urologic referral, indications, 472–473
Benzathine penicillin G, syphilis and, 522
Benzodiazepines
    delirium and, 654
    GAD and, 728, 728t
Benzoyl peroxide, acne, 628
Beta human chorionic gonadotropin (β-HCG), 56
β-HCG. *See* Beta human chorionic gonadotropin
Beta-blockers
    ADHD and, 204
    adverse effects, 173
    AF and, 159f, 160
    CAD and, 143, 153–154, 153t
        mortality and, 153, 153t
    chest pain, 143

diastolic heart failure and, 159
    DM and, 232
    HTN and, 173, 174t, 175t
    MI and, 153–154, 153t
    SVT and, 162
    systolic heart failure, 156, 157f, 158
Beta-lactam, CAP and, 779
Bias, clinical studies and, 41
Biceps tendinitis, 614
Biceps testing, 608–609
Bile acid sequestrants (BAS), 254–255, 256t
    cholesterol and, 253
Biliary pain, gallbladder disease, 331–332
Bimanual examination, 511
Binge eating disorder, 207
Biofeedback, migraine, 701
Biologic response modifiers, RA and, 569
Biomechanical neck pain, 589
Biomedical disorders, fatigue, 683
Biopsy
    alcoholic hepatitis, 342
    NAFLD, 342
    skin cancers and, 630
BiPAP (Bilevel positive airway pressure), 691
Bipolar disorder, type II, 735
    diagnostic criteria, 737t
Birth control method
    algorithm for, 418f, 419
    decision-making, 417–419
Birth plan, pregnancy and, 67
Births, 396
Bladder outlet obstruction (BOO), 469
Blended family, 504
Blepharitis, 303, 305, 306f, 310–311
Blocking agents, addiction and, 715
Blood, UTI and, 428
Blood cultures, pneumonia and, 773
Blood glucose
    DM and, 233
    sulfonylureas, 235
Blood lead concentration. *See* Lead toxicity
Blood pressure (BP), 279
    age and gender, percentile cutoffs for, 76t
    birth control method, 417–418
    contraceptive use and, 421
    DM and, 229, 229t
        monitoring and, 241
    Ephedra plus caffeine, 492
    measurement, HTN cut-offs, 166, 168t
    prenatal visits and, 65
BMD. *See* Bone mineral density
BMI. *See* Body mass index
BN. *See* Bulimia nervosa
B-natriuretic peptide levels (BNP levels), HF and,
            155–156
BNP levels. *See* B-natriuretic peptide levels
Body mass index (BMI), 286, 291
    AUB and, 449
    children and, 76
    classification of, 282t
    DM monitoring, 241
    HTN and, 168, 170
    nutrition and, 281
    surgery, 288
    weight and, 284
    weight gain, IOM recommendations, 57, 57t, 58
Bone mineral density (BMD), medroxyprogesterone
            acetate, 406
Bone remodeling, eating disorders, 208
Bone spurs, OA and, 564
Boniva. *See* Ibandronate
BOO. *See* Bladder outlet obstruction
Botulism toxin, neck pain, 595
Bowel habits, children and, counseling, 84–85
Bowel obstruction, 332–333
    management, 336
BPH. *See* Benign prostatic hyperplasia
BPPV. *See* Benign paroxysmal positional vertigo
Braces, ankle sprain management, 548t
Braided sutures, 637
Brain tumors, 652, 654
Brainstem auditory evoked response, vertigo, 671,
            672
Branch retinal vein occlusion, 304
Branched chain amino acids (BCAA),
            supplementation of, 490

"Breaking bad news," SPIKES protocol for, 108,
            109t
Breast. *See also* Breast cancer; Clinical breast
            examination; Postsurgical breast pain
    pain, 381–384
        clinical evaluation of, 382–383
        differential diagnosis, 381–382, 382t
        management, 383–384, 385t
    problems, 381–394
        case discussions, 393
        cases, 381
    skin changes, adenoma and, 386
Breast cancer, 386, 388. *See also* Malignant breast
            masses
    breast pain and, 382
    contraceptive use and, 421
    HT and, 462
    OC and, 401–402
    red flags, 390t
    tamoxifen and, 464
Breast examination, prenatal care, first trimester, 58
Breast mass. *See also* Malignant breast masses
    birth control method, 417–418
    palpable
        clinical evaluation, 389–391
        differential diagnosis, 388–389, 389t
        history and physical examination, 390t
        management, 391
        algorithm for, 392f
Breast milk
    counseling, 84
    WHO and, 67
Breastfeeding. *See also* Lactating breast
    mastitis and, 392
    progestin-only contraceptives, 407
Breath sounds
    asthma, 752
    asthma and, 752
Bromocriptine
    cyclic mastalgia, 383, 383t, 384
    nipple discharge, 387–388
Bronchiolitis, 772, 777–778
    children and, 217
Bronchitis, acute, 771–772, 776–777
Bronchodilators
    acute bronchitis, 777
    bronchiolitis, 777–778
    COPD and, 790
    long-acting, asthma and, 763
Brown, V., multispecialty health systems, 22–23
Bruits, chest pain and, 137
BSCS. *See* Short Blessed Cognitive Status Screen
B-sitosterol, BPH and, 472
Bulging disk, 579, 580
Bulimia nervosa (BN), 207
Bupropion, ADHD and, 203
Buried suture technique, 639f
Bursitis, 575
Business, health care as, 24–25
Butoconazole, CVV and, 537
BV. *See* Bacterial vaginosis

Cabergoline, nipple discharge, 387–388
CABG (Coronary artery bypass graft)
    CAD and, 143–144
    chronic stable angina and, 155
CAD. *See* Chronic cardiac disease
Caffeine. *See also* Ephedra plus caffeine
    during pregnancy, 63
CAGE questionnaire, 101
    alcohol abuse, 706, 708t
    preconception screening, 55, 55t
Calcific tendinitis, 614
Calcium antagonists. *See* Calcium channel blockers
Calcium channel blockers (CCBs)
    AF and, 159f, 160
    angina and, 154
    CAD and, 143
    chest pain, 143
    DM and, 231
    HF and, 156
Calcium supplements
    PMS, 446
    during pregnancy, 62

Calorie restriction, weight loss and, 284
CAM. *See* Complimentary and alternative medicine
Campylobacter jejuni infection, 370
CA-MRSA. *See* Community acquired methicillin-resistant S. aureus
CAN. *See* Cardiac autonomic neuropathy
Canadian C-Spine Rule, neck pain, 593, 595*f*
Cancer. *See also specific i.e. breast cancer*
    breast discharge and, 387
    HRT and, 458
    hyperthyroidism and, 272
    OCs and, 397
Candida culture
    central laboratory testing, 532–532
    molecular testing, 533
Candida vulvovaginitis (CVV), 528
    clinical evaluation, 529
    self-diagnosis of, 533
    treatment, 534*t*–535*t*, 537
CAP. *See* Community-acquired pneumonia
Carbamazepine
    ADHD and, 204
    dementia, behavioral symptoms, 658, 658*t*
Cardiac auscultation, chest pain and, 137
Cardiac autonomic neuropathy (CAN), presyncope v., 667
Cardiac diagnoses, COPD v., 788
Cardiac dysrhythmias, presyncope v., 667
Cardiac medications, hypothyroidism, 265
Cardiac monitoring, presyncope, 672
Cardiac murmurs, valvular heart disease and, 162
Cardiac stress imaging, chronic stable angina and, 154
Cardiac troponins, cardiac injury and, 138–139
Cardiologists, dizziness and, 663
Cardiovascular disease
    obesity284, 283*t*
    OC and, 398
Cardiovascular mortality, OSA and, 692
Caregiving, family, chronic illness and, 506
Cash-only medical practice, 28
Catheter-associated UTI, 433–434
Cauda equina syndrome, 580
CBC. *See* Complete blood count
CBE. *See* Clinical breast examination
CBT
    depression and, 740–741
    OCD, 729
CCBs. *See* Calcium channel blockers
CD. *See* Conduct disorder
CD4 count, HIV disease, 519
CDC. *See* Centers for Disease Control
Cefotaxime, CAP and, 779
Cefotetan, PID and, 517
Cefoxitin, PID and, 517
Ceftriaxone
    CAP and, 779
    chlamydia and, 516
    disseminated gonococcal infection, 516
    parenteral, acute pyelonephritis, 431
    pharyngeal gonococcal infections, 516
Cefuroxime, CAP and, 779
Celiac disease, 281
Cellulitis, 622
Centers for Disease Control (CDC)
    chlamydia and, 512
    chronic fatigue syndrome, 683–684, 684*t*
    drug-resistant *S. pneumoniae* and, 779
    gonococcal infections, treatment for, 516, 516*t*
    hepatitis and, 346
    STIs, screening and prevention, 523
    travel immunization, 92, 93
Central laboratory testing, BV and, 531–533
Central nervous system (CNS), vertigo and, 664, 666
Central nervous system hypoperfusion, dizziness and, 666
Central nervous system ischemia, 666
Central retinal artery occlusion (CRAO), 304, 307, 308–309
Central retinal vein occlusion, 304
Central system, vertigo and, 664, 666
Central vertigo, peripheral vertigo v., 668*t*
Cephalexin, bacterial infections, 621
Cephalosporin
    asymptomatic bacteriuria, 434
    infants and children, UTIs and, 433
    parenteral, acute pyelonephritis, 431

Cerebellar degeneration, disequilibrium, 667
Cerebellar infarction, central system and, 666
Cerebral palsy (CP), 200–201
    subtypes, 200–201
Cerumen impaction, 293, 296–297
Cervical adenopathy, URIs and, 774
Cervical cancer, OC and, 402
Cervical cap, 410–412
Cervical disc herniation, tests for, 591
Cervical dysplasia, adolescents screening, 77
Cervical neuropathy, breast pain and, 382
Cervical polyps, 440
Cervical radiculopathy, 591
Cervical spine, pain and, 589, 591*f*
Cervical spondylosis, 590
Cervical spondylotic myelopathy, 591, 596–597
Cervical stenosis, dysmenorrhea, 439
Cervical vertebra, secondary headaches and, 697
Cervicitis, 537
    central laboratory testing, 531–532
Cervix, evaluation of, 512
Cesarean deliveries, 51
CF. *See* Cystic fibrosis
Chalazion, 304, 305, 307, 307*f*
    management, 311
Challenging patient encounter, 31–38
    approach guidelines for, 32*t*
    management goals, 37*t*
    management strategies, 36–38, 36*t*
    outcomes improvement, strategies for, 32
    reassurance therapy and, 37*t*
    research literature and, 31–32
CHD. *See* Coronary heart disease
Chemoprophylaxis, 94, 97
Chest infections, acute, 217
Chest pain, 131–147
    case discussions, 144–145
    categories of, 151, 151*t*
    by cause, pharmacotherapy for, 142*t*
    chronic stable angina and, 151
    clinical evaluation for, 133–139, 134*t*, 135*t*
    complete evaluation phase, 137
    diagnostic testing, 137–139, 138*t*
    differential diagnosis, 131–133, 133*t*, 185*t*
    management, 139, 140*t*, 141, 142*t*, 143–145
        by cause, 140*t*
    medical therapy, 143
    pathophysiology, 131–132
    patient approach, 141*f*
    rare causes, 133
    red flags for, 136*t*
    URIs and, 774
Chest percussion, asthma, 752
Chest radiographs
    bronchiolitis and, 772
    chest pain, 138
    goiter and, 271
    pneumonia and, 773
    URIs and, 775, 776*t*
Chickenpox, VZV and, 624
Child
    maltreatment, 208–211
    preventive services to, 73
Childhood obesity, 76
Children. *See also* Failure to Thrive
    asthma and, 751
    bronchiolitis and, 772
    CAP vaccination, 779
    chlamydia and, 512–514
    chronic constipation, 375
    counseling, 82–85, 82*t*
    divorce and, 504
    ear pain, 298–299, 300
    with fever, therapeutic options, 223*t*
    gonorrhea and
        diagnostic testing for, 515
        treatment, 516
    OAR and, 547
    PFTs, 753
    physical examination
        dysuria and, 426–427
        fatigue, 687, 687*t*
    polysomnography and, 688
    RSV and, 778
    screening tests, 73–78, 74*t*
    sleep disorder and, 686

URIs, 773
UTIs in, 432
    clinical evaluation of, 432–433
    weight management in, 290
    wounds and, 636
Children with special healthcare needs (CSHCN), 500–501
Chlamydia, 511, 512
    birth control method, 418
    contraceptive use and, 421
    diagnosis and treatment, 512–514, 513*t*
    screening and prevention, 523
    systemic antibiotics, 309, 309*t*
Chlamydia trachomatis eye infection, 304
Chloasma, pregnancy and, 56
Chlorpromazine, drug related lupus, 575
Cholecystitis, cholescintigrams for, 329*t*, 331
Cholesterol, ezetimibe and, 257
Cholinesterase inhibitors, Alzheimer's disease, 656, 657*t*
Chondroitin, OA and, 564
Chondroitin sulfate, OA and, 565
Chondromalacia patellae, 551
Chorionic villus sampling (CVS), pregnancy and, 61
Chromium, 490
Chronic abdominal pain, causes, outpatient pharmacologic management, 337*t*
Chronic cardiac disease (CAD), 149–164
    case study, 149
    management, 152*f*
Chronic constipation, 375
    case discussion, 379
    management, 37*t*, 377–379
    treatment options, 378*t*
Chronic daily headache, 697–698
Chronic diarrhea, 372–374
    diagnostic strategy, 373, 374*t*
    differential diagnosis, 372, 373*t*
Chronic diseases
    epidemiology, 506
    management, 124–126
Chronic dyspnea, 788–789
Chronic fatigue, 681–682
    therapy, 690
Chronic fatigue syndrome, 683–684
    CDC and, 683–684, 684*t*
Chronic gout, 572, 573
Chronic health conditions, limitation of activity and, 92*t*
Chronic illness
    family and, 506
        case, 507
    sleep disorder and, 684
Chronic infection, hepatitis as, 344
Chronic insomnia, lifestyle changes and, 690*t*
Chronic liver disease (CLD), 341–349
    case discussions, 348
    cases, 341
    recommendations, 348*t*
Chronic low back pain, management, 584–385
Chronic obstructive pulmonary disease. *See* COPD
Chronic pelvic pain, 334
    management, 336
Chronic prostatitis/Chronic pelvic pain syndrome (CP/CPPS), 474
Chronic respiratory conditions, differential diagnosis of, 788*t*
Chronic stable angina, 149–155
    with chest pain, evaluation, 150*f*
    diagnosis, 151–152
    long-term monitoring, 154–155, 154*t*
    management, 152*f*
Chronic viral hepatitis, 343–346
CHT therapy, 462
Cigarette smoking. *See also* Substance abuse; Tobacco cessation
    CAD and, 143
        stable angina and, 152
    clinical intervention for, "5-As," 712*f*
    community-acquired pneumonia, 772–773
    COPD and, 786
    counseling for, 101
    menopause, 455, 458
    preconception care and, 53, 55
Ciprofloxacin, UTI and, 430

Cirrhosis
  complications, 346–347
  prognosis, Modified Child-Pugh Score, 346, 347t
CIWA-Ar scores, withdrawal syndromes, 712
CK. See Creatine kinase
CK-MB. See MB isoenzyme
CLD. See Chronic liver disease
Clindamycin, BV treatment, 533
  pregnancy, 533, 537
Clinical breast examination (CBE), 382, 386–387
  breast mass, 389–391
Clinical decision making. See Decision making
Clinical decision rule
  DVT and, 181
  PE and, 185, 186t
Clinical experience, EBM and, 46–47
Clinical pelvimetry, prenatal care, first trimester, 58
Clinical prediction rule
  ECG and, 135, 135t
  streptococcal pharyngitis, 315, 316t
Clinical studies, bias and, 41
Clinical uncertainty, 126
Clinician's Handbook of Preventive Services Task Force,
    preventive program, office setting, 88
Clomiphene, ovulatory dysfunction and, 500
Clonazepam, GAD and, 728, 728t
Clonidine
  ADHD and, 204
  adverse effects, 173
  CD and, 206
  hot flashes and, 456
Clopidogrel, CAD and, 153, 153t
Cluster headache, 696
  treatment, 702
CNS. See Central nervous system
Coagulopathy, medical abortion and, 417
Cochrane database, 46
Cochrane Systematic Review
  Alzheimer's disease, 656
  lacerations and, 636
  medical abortion, 415
  overweight children and, 76
Cognitive history, 647–648
Cognitive impairment, 643–662
  case study, 643, 653, 659, 660
  comorbid illness and, treating, 654–655
  diagnostic and screening tools, 648
  diagnostic approach, 647f
  diagnostic testing and, laboratory and, 652–653
  differential diagnosis of, 643–646, 646t
  initial evaluation, 646–649, 651–653
  long-term monitoring, 659–660
    case study, 659
  management, 653–656, 658–659
  recommendations for practice, 660t
  treatable/reversible causes, 651t
Cognitive therapy, panic disorder, 144
Cognitive-behavioral therapy
  addiction, 715
  migraine, 701
Colchicine
  acute gout, 572, 573
  chronic gout, 573
Cold. See Common cold
Collagen vascular disease, 558
Collateral ligament injuries, 551
Cholecystitis, cholescintigrams for, 329t, 331
Colon cancer
  colonoscopy, 376–377
  flexible sigmoidoscopy, 376–377
Colonic angiodysplasia, management, 368–369
Colonoscopy
  bleeding and, 368
  constipation, 376
  guidelines for, 376
Colony count infections, UTI and, 428
Combination therapy
  acne, 628
  DM and, 232
  psoriasis, 627
Combined contraceptives, 397
Combined hormone therapy (CHT), risks/benefits,
    463t
Combined oral contraceptives (OC), 397–398,
    401–404
Combined vestibular therapy, depression, dizziness
    and, 678

Common cold, 770–771, 775–776
Communication
  challenging patient encounter and, 37t
  couples and, 504, 504t
  end-of-life care and, 114
Community
  EBM and, 39
  physician and, 8, 9b
Community acquired methicillin-resistant S. aureus
    (CA-MRSA), 621–622
Community health centers (CHCs), 16–18
Community intervention, addictions, 718
Community-acquired pneumonia (CAP), 772–773,
    779–780
  pharmacotherapy for, 779t
  prevention, 779
Comorbid illness, cognitive impairment and, treating,
    654–655
Complementary and alternative medicine (CAM). See
    also Nutritional supplements
  arthritis and, 564
  hyperlipidemia, 258–259
  low back pain, 385
  during pregnancy, 63
  RA, 570
  URI and, 776
Complete blood count (CBC), LGI bleeding, 366,
    366t
Complete evaluation phase, chest pain, 137
Comprehensiveness of care, 7
Compresses, warm, hordeolum, 311
Compression, venous stasis ulcers, 641
Compression stockings, VTE and, 192
Computed tomography. See CT
Conception. See also Preconception
  infertility and, 499
Condoms, 396
  male and female, 412–413
  side effects, follow-up and managing, 420
Conduct disorder (CD), 201, 204–205, 206t
Condylomata acuminata, therapy for, 623
Conflict Tactics Scale (CTS), IPV and, 502
Confrontation, patient encounters and, 35
Confusion Assessment Method, delirium, 649, 652t
Congenital adrenal hyperplasia, infertile couple and,
    499
Congenital heart disease, newborns, 74
Congenital malformations, diabetes mellitus and, 53
Congestive heart failure. See heart failure
Conjunctivitis, 302, 309–310, 747, 749t
  causes, 303t
  history/physical examination for, key elements,
    746t
  medications for, 750t–751t
  topical ophthalmic antibiotics, 309, 309t
Connective tissue disorders
  fatigue, 683
  immunologic tests, 562
Constipation, 374–379
  alarm symptoms, 375, 377t
  diagnostic testing, 375–377, 377t
  differential diagnosis, 375, 376t
  end-of-life care and, 112, 113t
  management, 377–379
  recommendations, 369t
Contact dermatitis, 626
Contact lens wearers, corneal abrasion and,
    antibiotics for, 310
Contact sports, infectious mononucleosis, 321
Continuity of Care, 6–7, 8t
  patient outcomes v., 8t
Continuous positive airway pressure. See CPAP
Contraception
  barriers to use, 397
  methods, 397–398, 399t, 400t–401t, 401–415
  transdermal patch (OrthoEvra patch), 404–405
    missed or late, management of, 405t
    side effects, follow-up and managing, 420
  unintended pregnancy and, 395–397
Contraceptive sponge (Today sponge), 412
Contraceptives. See also Emergency contraceptive;
    specific types i.e. condom
  methods, 400t–401t
    algorithm for, 418f, 419
    future choices, 420
  side effects, follow-up and managing, 419–20

Contusions, evaluation and management, 635
Coordination of care, 5, 7–8
COPD (Chronic obstructive pulmonary disease),
    785–796
  acute exacerbations, 794t
    guideline algorithm, 795t
  albuterol, 752
  approach to patient, algorithm, 791f
  asthma v., 789, 790f
  case, 785
  case discussion, 794
  classification of, 787t
  GOLD criteria and, 785, 786t
  initial evaluation, 787–789
  insomnia and, 691
  management, 789–790, 792
    strength of recommendation, 793t
  metformin and, 235
  pharmacotherapy, 792f
  progressive/life-threatening disease, red flags, 794t
Corneal abrasions, 303, 310
Coronary angiography, CAD and, 152
Coronary artery bypass graft. See CABG
Coronary artery disease (CAD), See Coronary heart
    disease (CHD)
Coronary heart disease (CHD), 143–144, 149, 247
  ACSs and, 135–136, 136f
  case discussion, 163
  DM and, 232
  exercise ECG and, 139
  "gold standard" evaluation, 152
  fibric acid derivatives, 257
  history and physical examination, 151
  lipid lowering medication therapy, prevention
    trials and, 254t
  mortality, medications and, 153–154, 153t
  nicotinic acid and, 255
Coronary risk factor assessment, 137
Coronary syndromes (ACSs), 131
  CAD history and, 135–136, 136f
  chest pain and, 132
  management, 139–144
Corticosteroids
  acute gout, 573
  asthma and, 756, 762, 763
  COPD and, 790
  Meibomian gland dysfunction, 311
  shoulder pain and, 610, 610t
Coryza pharyngitis, 315
Costochondritis, 381
Cotton test, sprains and, 544
Coughing
  persistent, 313, 770
  URIs and, 774, 775
Counseling. See also Patient education; Subsequent
    counseling
  Alzheimer's disease and, 658
  physical activity, 101
  pregnancy and, 52–53
  well child care and, 82–85, 82t
Cover-uncover test, infancy and, early childhood and,
    75, 75f
COX-2 inhibitors
  ankle sprain, 547
  CAD and, 144
CP. See Cerebral palsy
CPAP (Continuous positive airway pressure), OSA
    and, 691
CP/CPPS. See Chronic prostatitis/Chronic pelvic pain
    syndrome
Craniofacial abnormalities, ear and, 294
Crank test. See O'Brien test
CRAO. See Central retinal artery occlusion
C-reactive protein (CRP), inflammation and, 562
Creatine, 489
  performance enhancing supplements and, 487
Creatine kinase (CK), MI and, 138
Crepitus
  OA and, 564
  rheumatic disorders, 559, 561f
Cromolyn nasal spray, allergies, 747
Cross-over impingement test, AC joint and, 607
Crying babies, counseling, 84
CT (Computed tomography)
  low back pain, 583–584
  neck pain, 593
  OA and, 565
  PE and, 186

CT venography, DVT and, 182
CTS. See Conflict Tactics Scale
Cutaneous flushing, nicotinic acid and, 257
CVS. See Chorionic villus sampling
CVV. See Candida vulvovaginitis
CXR, febrile child and, 221
Cyanocobalamin
    Alzheimer's disease, 656
    vitamin B-12 deficiency, 654
Cyclic breast pain
    nonpharmacotherapy, 383
    pharmacotherapy, 383, 383t
Cyclic mastalgia, 381, 382
    pharmacotherapy, 383, 383t
Cyclophosphamide, RA and, 569
Cyclosporine, RA and, 569
Cyr-Wartman questions, alcohol abuse, 706, 708t
Cyst aspiration, breast mass and, 390
Cystic fibrosis (CF), 53
Cytology smear, 533
    nipple discharge, 388
Cytomegalovirus infection, 313

D (Rh) factor, prenatal care, 58
Danazol
    cyclic mastalgia, 383, 383t
    endometriosis, 336
    noncyclic breast pain and, 384, 384f
Darkfield examination, syphilis, 521–522
DASH diet, 88, 279–280
    DM and, 231, 233
    HTN and, 170, 172t, 173
DASH study, 290–291
DBP. See Diastolic BP
DCCBs. See Non-dihydropyridine calcium channel
        blockers
D-dimer assays
    DVT and, 184
    PE and, 186
D-dimer testing, DVT and, 182
Death. See also End-of-Life care; SIDS
    actual causes of, 91t
    from asthma, 755t
        red flags, 764t
    CAD and, 149
    chronic illness and, 506–507
    COPD and, 786
    grief and bereavement, 115
    immediately after, 115
    leading causes, 90t
    management, 114–115
    stroke and, 165
Death, Dying, and Bereavement, 506–507
Decision making, steps in, 120–122
Deep suture technique, 639f
Deep vein thrombosis (DVT), 179, 180
    case study, 193
    diagnostic testing, 123, 124
    evaluation of, algorithm for, 184f
    history and physical examination, 181
    laboratory testing, 181–182, 183t, 184
    pathophysiology and differential diagnosis of, 180,
        180t
    patient approach, 184, 184f
    red flags for, 181t
    tamoxifen and, 463
Degenerative disc disorders, secondary headaches
        and, 697
Degenerative joint disease, 603
Dehydroepiandrosterone. See DHEA
Delirium, 648–649
    Confusion Assessment Method, 649, 652t
    end-of-life care and, 114
    management, 654
    risk factors, 649, 652t
Dementia, 643, 646
    behavioral symptoms, pharmacologic management,
        658–659, 658t
    functional lapses, 647
    normal cognitive lapses v., differentiating, 644t
    stages of, Alzheimer's disease, 644, 645t
Dental health, 101
    counseling and, 83, 83t

Depo-subQ Provera 104, 406
Depot medroxyprogesterone acetate (DMPA), 397
Depression, 689, 733–744
    adolescent patients, diagnosis/ treatment
            considerations, 742
    Alzheimer's disease and, 658
    case, 733
    case discussion, 742
    clinical clues, 736
    COPD, 794
    divorce and, 505
    dizziness and, 678
    ED and, 483, 483t
    end-of-life care, 114
    fatigue, 682, 682t
    initial evaluation, 736–738
    IPV and, 501
    long-term monitoring, 742
    management, 654, 738–739
    medications causing, or worsening, 738t
    nonspecific dizziness, 667
    screening, 91, 93t
    serious/complex disease, red flags for, 738t
    treatment modality, 739, 740t
    treatments, 740t
Depressive disorder, sleep disorder and, 685
Dermatitis, 625–629
Dermatologic preparations, vehicles for, 621f
Dermatology, 617–631
    cases, 617, 630
    diagnostic testing, 620
    family in, 618–619
    initial evaluation, 617–620
    management principles, 620–621
Dermatophytes, tinea infections and, 624
Desipramine, ADHD and, 203
Desquamative inflammatory vaginitis (DIV), 538
Detoxification, addiction and, 711–712, 716t
Development disorders, 197–213
Development screening, children and adolescents, 76
Developmental delay, 197
    management, 198, 198t
    screening, 198t
Dexamethasone, GABHS pharyngitis, 320, 320t
Dextroamphetamine, ADHD and, 203
DHEA (Dehydroepiandrosterone), 487, 489
    postmenopausal women, 463
    sexual interest and, 458
Diabetes mellitus (DM), 227–245, 655
    case, 238
    CLD and, 347
    clinical presentation, 227–231
    complications, screening for, 241, 244
    congenital malformations and, 53
    conveying diagnosis, 230–231
    diagnostic criteria, 228, 229t
    management, 231–233, 231t
        over time, 238–244
        practice recommendations, 243t, 244
    monitoring, 238, 240–241, 241t
    pharmacologic management, 233, 234t
    presyncope v., 667
    screening, pregnancy and, 65
    self-care activities, 240
    self-care questionnaire, 242f
    type 1, 227
        insulin therapy and, 236
    type 2, 227
        basal insulin therapy and, nighttime, 236, 237t
        hypoglycemic medications, use strategy,
            236–238, 240f
        insulin therapy and, 235–236
Diabetic foot ulcers, 641
Diabetic kidney disease, microalbuminuria and, 241
Diagnosis
    making, 119, 121t
    studies and, 43–44
Diagnostic and Statistical Manual of Mental
        Disorders (DSM-IV) criteria, 201
    ADHD and, 201, 202t
    anxiety and, 721
    depression, 737
    panic disorder, 722t
    SAD, 735
Diagnostic process, pitfalls, 122–123

Diagnostic testing, 123–124, 124f, 125, 125f
    allergies, 746
    asthma, 752–753
    chronic stable angina and, 151–152
    DVT and, 183t
    ear pain, 295–296
    fatigue, 687–688, 687t
    febrile children and infants, 220–221
    HF and, 155–156
    HTN and, 169
    LGI bleeding, 366, 366t
    URIs and, 775, 776t
Diaphragm, 410–412
    fitting and insertion, 411
    patient education, 411–412
    side effects and contraindications, 411
Diarrhea, acute, 369–372, 369t
    diagnostic strategy, 371, 371t
    differential diagnosis, 370
    exposures and symptoms, 370, 370t
    infectious
        antibiotic treatment, 371, 372t
        exposures and symptoms, 370t
    recommendations, 369t
    stool specimen testing, diarrhea category and, 374t
Diary
    asthma and, 764
    headache, 698, 698t
    sleep, 688
Diastolic BP (DBP), HTN and, 166, 167, 168
Diastolic heart failure, 157f, 158–159
Diclofenac, cyclic mastalgia, 383, 383t
Dicloxacillin, bacterial infections, 621
Diet, 279, 284–285
    counseling and, children and, 83
    prostate cancer, 481
    stable angina and, 152, 153
Dietary fiber, chronic constipation, 378t
Dietary history, 280–281
Dietary supplements. See also Protein supplements;
        Sports supplements; Supplementation
    brand names, 490, 491t
    calcium, PMS, 446
    cost, 492t
    PMS, 446
    side effects, 491t
Diethylpropion, weight loss and, 287
Digit examination, rheumatic disorders, 559
Digital rectal examination, enlarged prostate and,
        469, 470
Digitalis glycosides, systolic heart failure, 158
Digoxin, AF and, 159f, 160
Diphtheria immunization, 78–79
Dipstick urinalysis, infants and children, UTIs and,
        433
Dipyridamole, CAD and, 153, 153t
Dipyridamole stress test, HF and, 156
Disease modifying antirheumatic drugs. See
        DMARDs
Disease-oriented evidence. See DOEs
Diseases, preconception screening for, 54t
Disequilibrium, 664
    clinical history, 668
    differential diagnosis, 667
    tests, 672–673
Disopyramide, AF and, 160
Disordered eating. See Eating disorders
Disruptive behavior, 204–206
Disseminated gonococcal infection
    ceftriaxone and, 516
    diagnostic testing, 515
    treatment, 516, 516t
Disulfiram (Antabuse)
    addiction and, 715
    alcohol cessation and, 55
    pregnancy and, 55
Diuretics
    DM and, 231, 232
    HF and, 156
    HTN and, 173, 174t, 175t
    MS and, 163
    systolic heart failure, 156, 157f, 158
DIV. See Desquamative inflammatory vaginitis
Diverticular bleeding, management, 368–369
Diverticulitis, 333
    management, 336

Divorce, 503–505
Dix-Hallpike maneuver, 671, 672f
Dizziness, 663–679
　case discussions, 678–679
　cases, 663
　cause of v., episode duration and, 668t
　clinical evaluation, 667–673
　clinical history, 667–669
　diagnostic strategy, algorithm for, 673, 674f
　differential diagnosis, 663–664, 665t
　frequency of diagnoses, practice setting/patient age
　　and, 666t
　management of, 673, 675, 677–679
　medication for, 676t
　neuro-otological evaluation, 670–671
　nonspecific, 667
　therapies, 675t
　urgent disease and, red flags, 669t
DM. See Diabetes mellitus
DMARDs (Disease modifying antirheumatic drugs),
　RA and, 568, 569, 570
DMPA. See Depot medroxyprogesterone acetate
DMPA-IM (Intramuscular medroxyprogesterone
　acetate), 406, 407–408, 419
　contraceptive use and, 421
DOEs (Disease-oriented evidence), 41
　POEMs v., 42t
"Dog ear" lacerations, repair, 639, 640f
Domestic violence, 101. See also Intimate partner
　violence
　reporting of, 502
Donepezil, Alzheimer's disease, 656, 657t
Doppler flow studies, HF and, 155
Doubling sickening, 770
Down syndrome
　risks, 62
　screening, pregnancy and, 61
Doxazosin, 471
Doxazosin with finasteride, prostate and, 471
Doxycycline
　Meibomian gland dysfunction, 311
　PID and, 517
　viral pharyngitis, 317
"Drop arm" test, 604
Drospirenone, 397
DRSP. See Drug-resistant S. pneumoniae
Drug(s). See also Drug abuse; Medication history;
　Substance abuse; specific i.e.
　Erythromycin(s)
　acute migraine, 701t
　for addiction, 710t–711t, 715–716
　adverse effects, disequilibrium, 667
　allergic conjunctivitis, 310, 310t
　Alzheimer's disease, 656, 657t
　ankle pain, 549t
　antidepressants, selection of, 739–740, 741t
　arthritis and, 564
　asthma, classification/long-term control, 756,
　　757t–761t
　AUB and, 448
　BPH, 471–472, 473t
　CAD mortality and, 153–154, 153t
　causing depression, or worsening, 738t
　chest pain, by cause, 142t
　chronic insomnia, 690t
　for community-acquired pneumonia, 779t
　comparison of, HPV, 624t
　COPD, 792f
　dizziness, 676t
　DM and, 231
　and doses, anxiety disorders, 728t
　dyspepsia, 358, 358t
　ED and, 483, 483t
　GABHS pharyngitis, 321t
　HF and, 156
　hyperthyroidism and, 268–269
　for influenza, 778t
　knee pain, 549t
　oral, ED and, 484, 486
　for osteoporosis, 460, 461t
　panic disorder and, 144
　during pregnancy, 63
　risk factors, 483, 483t
　UTIs, 431t
　weight loss and, 286–288, 289t

Drug abuse. See also Recreational drugs
　algorithm for, 715f
　common terms in, definitions of, 705, 706t
　counseling and, children and, 83
　USPSTF and, 101
Drug addiction
　managing, 709, 711–716
　pharmacological interventions, 717t
Drug related lupus, 575
Drug-resistant S. pneumoniae (DRSP), CDC and, 779
DTP. See Pertussis vaccine
DUB. See Dysfunctional uterine bleeding
Duct papilloma, 385–386
Ductal diseases, 385
Duodenal ulcer, 361
Duplex venous ultrasound, DVT and, 182
DVT. See Deep vein thrombosis
Dying process, 114–115
Dynamic restraints, 602
Dysfunctional uterine bleeding (DUB), 448
Dyslipidemia, 247. See also NCEP ATP III lipid
　　classification system
　DM and, 232–233
　secondary causes, 249t
Dysmenorrhea, 437–442
　approach to, 442f
　cases, 437
　clinical evaluation, 438–439
　diagnostic tests, 440t
　management, 443t–444t
　NSAIDs for, 444t
　pathophysiology, 437–438
Dyspepsia, 351–363
　case discussion, 361
　cases, 351
　diagnosis and management, algorithm of, 357f
　diagnostic strategy, 356–357
　differential diagnosis, 351–352, 352t
　history and physical examination, 353
　life-threatening diseases, red flags, 353t
　pathophysiology, 351
　pharmacotherapy options, 358, 358t
Dyspnea, end-of-life and, 110–111
Dysthymic disorder, diagnostic criteria, 735, 735t
Dysuria, 425–436
　case, 425
　case discussion, 434
　management, algorithm, 429f
　urine tests, characteristics of, 428t

E. coli
　diaphragm and, 411
　UTIs and, 425, 428
Ear infection, 293–294
Ear pain, 293–300
　case, 293, 299–300
　causes, management of, 298t
　diagnostic strategy, 296, 296f
　differential diagnosis, 293–294, 294t
　elements in, 295t
　life-threatening disease, red flags for, 296t
　long term monitoring, prevention and, 298
　management, 296–298
Earlobe creases, chest pain and, 137
Eating disorder not otherwise specified (EDNOS),
　207
Eating disorders, 207–208
　gastrointestinal symptoms, 208
　initial evaluation, 207–208
　laboratory abnormalities, 208t
　long-term monitoring, 208
EC. See Emergency contraceptive
ECG (Electrocardiogram)
　ACIs, predictors of, 137–138
　AF and, 160
　cardiac murmurs, 162
　chronic stable angina and, 154
　clinical prediction rule, 135, 135t
　premature beats and, 161
　presyncope, 672
　PVCs and, 162
　simultaneous nuclear imaging, 139
　trauma and, 671
Echinacea, URI and, 776

Ectopic pregnancy, 56, 334
　management, 336
　medical abortion and, 417
　transvaginal ultrasound, 334
Eczema, 625, 625f, 626f
　treatment, 626
ED. See Erectile dysfunction
EDD. See Estimated date of delivery
Edema, end-of-life care and, 112
EDNOS. See Eating disorder not otherwise specified
EDS. See Excessive daytime sleepiness
Education. See Patient education
Educational interventions, postmenopausal women,
　464, 465t
EE. See Ethinyl estradiol
EF. See Ejection fraction
EGD (Esophagogastroduodenoscopy)
　LGI bleeding and, 365, 367
　occult bleeding, 367
Ejection fraction (EF), HF and, 155
Elderly patients
　cognitive impairment, 643
　disequilibrium, 667
　dizziness and, 663
　hypothyroidism, 267
　obesity and weight management, 290–291
Elective abortion, 57
Elective repeat cesarean delivery (ERCD), 67
Electrocardiogram. See ECG
Electrodiagnostic tests, neck pain, 593
Electromyography. See EMG
Electronic communication, with patients, family
　　medicine and, 27–28
Electronic medical records (EMR), 25
　family medicine and, 27
　photographs and, 633
Electronic prescribing software, prescription writing
　　and, 126
Electronystagmography. See ENG
ELISAs (Enzyme-linked immunosorbent assays)
　DVT and, 184
　HIV disease, 519
　PUD and, 356
Ellipse, closure of, 638f
E-mail services, 45
Emergency contraceptive (EC), 396, 397, 408–409,
　　421
　DMPA and, 408
　drug interactions, 408
　patient education, 408–409
EMG (Electromyography)
　neck pain, long-term management, 597
　rotator cuff, 604
EMR. See Electronic medical records
EMS. See Extramarital sex
Endocarditis prophylaxis
　MR and, 163
　MVP and, 163
Endocervix, gonorrhea and, 514
Endocrine system, eating disorders, 208
End-of-Life care, 105–116
　COPD and, 790
　dementia and, 659–660
　ethical and legal issues, 112–113
　psychosocial issues and, 113–114
　symptom management, 108–112
Endometrial biopsy
　AUB and, 449
　PID and, 517
Endometriosis, 334, 440
　dysmenorrhea, 439
　management, 336
Endoscopic retrograde cholangiopancreatography
　　(ERCP), gallbladder disease, 331–332
Endoscopy, dyspepsia, 354t
Endothelial dysfunction, DM and, 232
Enema, chronic constipation, 379
ENG (Electronystagmography), vertigo, 671
Environment, asthma and, 764, 765
Enzyme-linked immunosorbent assays. See ELISAs
Ephedra, 492
　weight loss and, 287
Ephedra plus caffeine, BP and, 492
Ephedrine, weight loss and, 287
Epicondylitis, 575

Epididymitis
  chlamydia and, 512
  in men, gonorrhea and, 514
Episodic therapy, recurrent HSV infection, 521
Epley maneuver, BPPV and, 675, 677f–678f
EPO. *See* Evening primrose oil
Epstein-Barr virus, infectious mononucleosis, 315, 317
ERCD. *See* Elective repeat cesarean delivery
ERCP. *See* Endoscopic retrograde cholangiopancreatography
Erectile dysfunction (ED), 481–487
  BPH and, 470
  case, 486–487
  causes, 482–483
  initial evaluation, 483–484
  management, 484, 486
  management/treatment, algorithm for, 485f
  medications associated with, 483, 483t
Eruptive xanthomas, triglycerides and, 248
Erysipelas, 622
Erythrocyte sedimentation rate (ESR), inflammation and, 562
Erythromycin(s)
  BV treatment, 537
  conjunctivitis and, 309
  corneal abrasions, 310
  hordeolum, 311
Esomeprazole, 361
Esophageal pH monitoring, dyspepsia, 354t
Esophageal spasm, chest pain and, 132
Esophagogastroduodenoscopy. *See* EGD
ESR. *See* Erythrocyte sedimentation rate
Estimated date of delivery (EDD), pregnancy and, 56
Estradiol, 455
Estriol, 455
Estrogen(s), 397
  bone maintenance, 458
  hot flashes and, 456
  for perimenopausal women, 459t–460t
Estrogen and testosterone, HRT and, 458
Estrone, 455
Estrostep, 421
ESWT. *See* Extracorporeal shock wave therapy
Etanercept, RA and, 569
Ethinyl estradiol (EE), 397
Ethnic diversity, 26
Eustachian tube, 294
Euthyroid, 263
Evening primrose oil (EPO)
  cyclic mastalgia, 383, 383t
  noncyclic breast pain and, 384, 384f
  during pregnancy, 63
Evidence-based clinical information, web-based sources, 40, 41t
Evidence-based medicine (EBM), 25, 39–40
  preventive health services and, 88, 90
  primary care office, 10, 11b
Evidence-based practice, 8, 10
Excessive daytime sleepiness (EDS), 684
Excisional biopsy, breast mass and, 391
Exercise, 279. *See also* Activity
  counseling and, children and, 83
  HTN and, 170, 172t
  low back pain, 385
  OA and, 566–567
  during pregnancy, 63
Exercise ECG. *See* Exercise stress test
Exercise stress test
  CAD and, 139, 151–152
  HF and, 156
Exercise therapy, low back pain, 386
Exhaustive methods, diagnosis and, 122
Exogenous insulin, DM and, 235
Experts, 46
Exposures, asthma and, 749
External beam radiation therapy, prostate cancer and, 479–480
Extracorporeal shock wave therapy (ESWT), 614
Extramarital sex (EMS), 503
Eye problems. *See also* Antibiotic(s)
  case discussion, 311–312
  cases, 301
  clinical evaluation, 304–305, 307–308
  common, 301–312
  management, 308–312

Eyelid disorders, differential diagnosis of, 303–304
Eyelids, 302
Ezetimibe, cholesterol and, 257

Facial lacerations, 639
Factitious hyperthyroidism, 267
Fagerstrom Test for Nicotine Dependence, 708
Failure to Thrive, 199–200
  long-term monitoring, 200
Famciclovir, 624
  recurrent HSV infection, 521
Familial periodic vertigo, central system and, 666
Family, 497
  asthma and, 764
  care, 5
  grief and bereavement, death and, 115
  history
    asthma and, 749
    prenatal care, first trimester, 57
    rheumatic disorders, 559–560, 560t
  intervention, addiction, 717
  issues, end-of-life care and, 114
  primary care and, 10–12
Family caregivers, resources for, Alzheimer's disease, 655t
Family medicine practice
  future, 27–28
  principles, 6–12, 7t
    case study, 11–12, 12f
  today, 12–24
Family physician
  approach to maternity care, 68
  obstetric consultants, 68, 70
Family practice
  common problems seen, 119–129
  DM management, 243t, 244
Family relationships, disabling chronic illness, impact of, 505–507
Family violence, prevention and, 102
FAQ (Functional Activities Questionnaire), cognitive impairment, 648, 650f
Farmington study, 250, 252f
Fast lipid monitoring, DM and, 241
Fatigue, 681
  case discussions, 691–692
  causes of, 682t, 683t
  clinical evaluation, 685–688
  diagnostic strategy, 688, 689f
  differential diagnosis, 682–684
  end-of-life care and, 112
  management, 688, 689f
  physical examination and, 687, 687t
  progressive/life-threatening disease, red flags for, 686t
  summary of, 691
  unexplained, 683–683, 683t
FDA (Food and Drug Administration), fetal risk categories, 64t
Febrile child. *See also* Fever in infants
  appearance, 216t
  follow-up, 224
Febrile infant
  age 3–36 months, 222
  age 28–90 days, 222
  fever reduction, 222–223
  managing, 222t
Feeding, counseling, 84
Feet, OA and, 565
Female condoms, 412–413
Female sterilization, 397
Fertility awareness methods, natural family planning, 414–415
Fetal heart rate (FHR), 65
Fetal risk categories, FDA, 64t
FEV1, drug therapy and, 790
Fever
  assessment, 215–216
  infants and preschool children, 215–226
    cases, 215
  reducing, febrile child and, 222
  rheumatic disorders, 559, 560

Fever in infants and children, 215–226. *See also* Febrile child; Febrile infant
  case discussions, 224
  management, 221–224
    algorithm, 218f
    preschool children, clinical evaluation and protocols, 217–221
FHR. *See* Fetal heart rate
Fibric acid derivatives, 257
  cholesterol and, 253
Fibrocystic masses, 390
Fibromyalgia, 574
  fatigue, 683
Finasteride, BPH and, 472
Fine needle biopsy (FNB)
  breast and, 393
  solitary thyroid nodule, 273
Fine-needle aspiration (FNA), breast mass and, 390–391
Finger deformities, RA and, 567f
Fish oil supplements, 257
5-alpha-reductase inhibitors, BPH and, 471–472
Flat warts, therapy for, 623
Flecamide, AF and, 160
Flexible sigmoidoscopy
  constipation, 376
  guidelines for, 377
Flucytosine, CVV and, 537
Fluid retention
  HF and, 156
  thiazolidinediones and, 235
Fluorescein staining, 305
Fluorescent treponemal antibody absorb (FTA-ABS), syphilis, 522
Fluoroquinolone(s)
  acute pyelonephritis, 431–432
  CAP and, 779
  catheter-associated infections, 434
  chlamydia and, 516
  UTIs and, 430
    infants and children, 433
Fluoxetine, PMS, 446
FNA. *See* Fine-needle aspiration
FNB. *See* Fine needle biopsy
Folic acid
  epilepsy and, 53
  pregnancy and, 52
Follicle stimulating hormone (FSH)
  eating disorders, 208
  menopause and, 455
    diagnosis, 456
  PMS and, 445
Folliculitis, 623
Follow-up, febrile children and, 224
Fondaparinux, VTE and, 190–191
Food and Drug Administration. *See* FDA
Foods, during pregnancy, 62
Foot ulcers. *See also* Diabetic foot ulcers
  screening, 241–242
Forced expiration time, COPD and, 788
Forced vital capacity. *See* FVC
Forced vital capacity in 1 second. *See* FVC₁
Forceps deliveries, 51
Formoterol, asthma and, 763
Fosamax. *See* Alendronate
Fractured clavicle, 613
Fractures. *See also specific i.e. vertebral compression fractures*
  ankle sprain *v.*, 544
  HRT, 458
  management, 553–554, 554t
Free fatty acids, nicotinic acid and, 256
Frontotemporal dementia, 644–645
FSH. *See* Follicle stimulating hormone
FT4. *See* Serum free thyroxine
FTA-ABS. *See* Fluorescent treponemal antibody absorb
Functional Activities Questionnaire. *See* FAQ
Functional dyspepsia, 352, 354t, 356
  H. pylori, 360–361
  history and physical examination, 353
Fundal height, 65
Fundus examination, 3–7
Fungal infections, 624–625

Furunculosis, 294, 297
FVC (Forced vital capacity), 752, 789
FVC$_1$ (Forced vital capacity in 1 second), 752, 753, 789

Gabapentin, hot flashes and, 456
GABHS bacteria (Group Aβ-hemolytic streptococcal bacteria), sore throat, 313, 314
GABHS pharyngitis, 314–315, 319–320
   antibiotics, 319–320, 320t
   diagnostic testing, 317, 318t
   pharmacotherapy, 321t
GAD. See Generalized anxiety disorder
Galactorrhea, 386, 387
Gallbladder
   disease, 331–332
      management, 334–335
   HT and, 462
Gallstones, ultrasonography, 329t, 331
Gamma-linolenic acid (GLA), RA and, 570
Gardnerella evaluation, central laboratory testing, 532
Gardnerella vaginalis, 527
Gas exchange, COPD and, 786
Gastroenteritis, fever in children and, 217
Gastro-esophageal reflux disease. See GERD
Gastroesophageal varices, cirrhosis and, 347
Gastrointestinal bleeding, 353
   differential diagnosis, 366, 366t
   DM and, 232
   lower gastrointestinal bleeding (LGI bleeding), 365–369
      diagnostic studies, 366, 367t
      differential diagnosis, 366, 366t
      recommendations, 369, 369t
Gatekeeping systems, 7
GBS. See Group B streptococcus
Generalized anxiety disorder (GAD), 721, 728–729, 728t
   diagnosis of, 722
   diagnostic criteria, 723t
Genetic testing
   pregnancy and, 52–53, 61–62
   second-trimester, 61
Genetics, rheumatic disorders, 559–560
Genital examination, men, 511
Genital herpes, 623–624
Gentamicin
   acute pyelonephritis, 431
   contact lens wearers and, 310
   infants and children, UTIs and, 433
   ocular allergic reaction and, 310
GERD (Gastro-esophageal reflux disease), 131, 351–352
   chest pain and, 132, 136
   diagnostic testing, 353–354, 356
   dyspepsia and, 351
   history and physical examination, 353
   management, 358–360
   pharyngeal tissue and, 313
Geriatric Depression Scale, 649, 653f
Gestational age
   mean serumβ-HCG levels and, 56
   mifepristone and, 415
Gestational diabetes mellitus (GMD), 65, 229
Giant cell arteritis, secondary headaches and, 697
Gibbons, E., 14–16
Gibbons, G., 14–16
Gilmer-Scott, M., CHCs and, 16–18
Ginger, during pregnancy, 63
Ginkgo biloba, Alzheimer's disease, 656
Glargine insulin, 236
Glaucoma, acute narrow angle, 302
Gleason histologic grading system, prostate cancer and, 479, 480t
Glenohumeral joint, 601, 612
Glenohumeral joint capsule, 602
Global cardiovascular risk, assessing, 168
Global Initiative for Chronic Obstructive Lung Disease criteria (GOLD criteria), COPD and, 785, 786t
Globalization, 25–26
Glucocorticoids, RA and, 569
Glucosamine, OA and, 555, 564
Glucose, fetus and, 62

Glucose challenge test (GTT), GMD and, 65
Glucose monitoring, DM and, 241
Glycemic control, preconception care, 53
Glycosylated hemoglobin (HgA1c), preconception care and, 53
GMD. See Gestational diabetes mellitus
Goiter (Thyroid enlargement), 270–272
   case discussion, 272
   laboratory testing, 271
   long-term monitoring, 271–272
Goitrogens, foods and drugs as, 270
GOLD criteria. See Global Initiative for Chronic Obstructive Lung Disease criteria
Gonadotropin-releasing hormones antagonists, endometriosis, 336
Gonococcal infections. See also Disseminated gonococcal infection
   systemic antibiotics, 309, 309t
   treatment for, 516, 516t
Gonorrhea, 512, 514–517
   clinical evaluation, 514–515
   prenatal care, 60
Goserelin, cyclic mastalgia, 383, 383t, 384
Gout, 572–573
   diagnostic criteria, 568t
   differential diagnosis, 572t
Gram stain, BV and, 530
Grapefruit juice, estrogen degradation and, 462
Graves' disease, 267
   thyroiditis v., 268
Gravidity, 57
Grief and bereavement, death and, 115
Group Aβ-hemolytic streptococcal bacteria. See GABHS bacteria
Group B streptococcus (GBS), fetus and, 66
Group visits, family medicine and, 27
Growth hormone, performance enhancing supplements and, 487
Growth screening, children and adolescents, 75–76
GTT. See Glucose challenge test
Guanfacine, ADHD and, 204
Guillain-Barré syndrome, 370

H. influenza type B immunization, children, 224
H. pylori, 361
   eradication, 360
   gastritis, dyspepsia and, 352
   infection, PUD and, 356–357
H$_2$RAs. See Histamine$_2$ receptor antagonists
Haemophilus influenzae, vaccine, 780
Haemophilus influenzae type B (HiB), 81
Haloperidol, dementia, behavioral symptoms, 658, 658t
Hand washing, RSV and, 778
Hands, OA and, 565
Hashimoto's thyroiditis, 270, 271
Hawkins-Kennedy test, 605, 606f
HbA1c
   DM and, 233
   goals, basal insulin therapy and, 238
HCC. See Hepatocellular cancer
HDL. See High-density lipoproteins
Head tilt, peripheral vestibular dysfunction and, 671
Head trauma, dizziness and, 668
Headache(s)
   case discussion, 702–703
   cases, 695
   classification, 695–698
   clinical evaluation, 698–699
   differential diagnosis, 695, 696t
   laboratory testing, 698
   management, 699–700
   nicotinic acid and, 257
   questionnaire, 698, 699f
   red flags for, 698, 698t
   triggers, 696, 697
   URIs and, 773–774
Headache diary, 698, 698t
Headache Impact Test (HIT-6), 700f
Health, priorities, national perspective, 3–6
Health care system
   benefits, contraception and, 397
   changing, 24–27
   expenditures, 25

family medicine in, 3–48
   response of, 26–27, 26b
U.S.
   changing, 24–27
   trends affecting, 24t
Health educators, asthma and, 764
Healthy People 2010
   unintended pregnancy and, 396, 420
   U.S. health priorities and, 3
Hearing loss, 294
Heart attack, low-dose OCs, 398
Heart disease
   children and, 78
   children and adolescents, 76, 76t
Heart failure (HF), 155–156, 158–159
   initial evaluation, 155–156
   symptoms, 157f
   systolic heart failure, 156, 157f, 158
   systolic v. diastolic dysfunction, 156, 157f, 158t
   treatment, 156–159
HEENT examination, prenatal care, first trimester, 58
Hegar's sign, pregnancy and, 56
Helical computed tomography, PE and, 186, 187f
Hemarthrosis, knee pain and, 551
Hematochezia (Nonmassive gross bleeding), 368, 368t
Hemochromatosis, 341
Heparin
   chest pain, 143
   PE and, 187
Hepatica encephalopathy, cirrhosis and, 347
Hepatitis, 341
   hepatotoxic medications, 346t
   screening and prevention, 345–346
Hepatitis A virus, vaccine, 81
Hepatitis B virus
   infection
      epidemiology, 343–344
      hepatitis C v., 343t
      laboratory markers for, 344, 344t
      prenatal care, 60
      prenatal screening, 345
      treatment, 344, 345t
   vaccine, 81, 92, 346
Hepatitis C virus, infection, 348
   epidemiology, 343–344
   hepatitis B v., 343t
   prenatal care, 60
   treatment, 344–345, 345t
Hepatocellular cancer (HCC), 341
   screening for, 347
Hepatotoxic medications, 346t
Hepatotoxicity, nicotinic acid and, 257
Herbal medicine
   GAD and, 728, 728t
   PMS, 446
Herbal supplements, weight loss and, 287
Herniated disc syndrome, 580
Herniated nucleus pulposus (HNP), 580
Herniation of intervertebral discs, 581f
Herpes simplex virus (HSV), 519–521, 623
   cell culture, 521
   febrile infants and, 217
   pregnancy and, 66
Herpes zoster, VZV and, 624
Herpesviruses, 623–624
HFA. See Hydrofluoralkane
HgA1c. See Glycosylated hemoglobin
HiB. See Haemophilus influenzae type B
Hidden agendas, diagnostic process and, 123
High-density lipoproteins (HDL), 248. See also Nicotinic acid
   CAD and, 154
   DM and, 232
   performance enhancing supplements and, 487–489
High-dose opioids, ethical issues, 113
Hips, OA and, 565
Histamine$_2$ receptor antagonists (H$_2$RAs)
   arthritis, 564
   GERD, 358, 359
History
   abdominal pain, key elements, 326–327, 329t
   accuracy of, functional dyspepsia, 354t
   acute diarrhea, 370
   ankle pain, 544, 545t
   AUB and, 449

History (*contd.*)
  breast pain, 382–383, 382*t*
  chronic diarrhea, 372, 373*t*
  chronic stable angina and, 151
  depression, 737–738
  domestic violence, 502
  dysmenorrhea, 439, 440*t*
  dysuria and, 426, 427*t*
  eating disorders, 207
  eye problems, 305*t*
  Failure to Thrive, 199
  fatigue, examination for, 686, 687*t*
  fever in infants/children, 218, 220*t*
  functional dyspepsia, 353
  GERD, 353
  HF and, 155
  HTN and, 168, 168*t*
  knee pain, 551–552
  LGI bleeding, 366, 366*t*
  menopause, 456
  neck pain, 591, 593
  patient nutrition and, 280
  PUD, 353
  rheumatic diseases, 558–559, 560*t*
  shoulder pain, 602–603
  skin wounds and, 633
  sore throat, 314–315, 316*t*
  URIs, 773–774
  vulvovaginal complaints, 528, 530*t*
HIT-6. *See* Headache Impact Test
HITS. *See* Hurt, Insulted, Threatened and Screamed
    scale
HIV disease, 10, 512, 652, 653
  addiction and, 718
  AIDS syndrome and, 518
  birth control method, 419
  case, 498
  clinical evaluation, 518–519
  community-acquired pneumonia, 773
  counseling, 101–102
  diagnostic testing, 519
  diaphragm, 411
  nevirapine, 60
  pregnant women and, 60
  primary dysmenorrhea, 439
  screening and prevention, 523
  spermicides, 413
HMG-CoA reductase inhibitors. *See* Statins
HNP. *See* Herniated nucleus pulposus
Hoarseness, URIs and, 774
Home oxygen, COPD exacerbations and, 794
Home-Care
  CAP and, 779
  practices, 28
Homosexuality, 497–498
Hordeolum, 303, 305, 307*f*
  management, 311
Hormonal contraceptives, 397–409
Hormonal emergency contraceptives, 408–409
Hormone(s)
  nipple discharge, 385
  supplementation, hypothyroidism, 264
Hormone replacement therapy (HRT)
  chemoprophylaxis and, 94
  fractures and, 458
  menopause, 462–464
Hormone therapy (HT)
  breast cancer, 462
  cardiovascular effects, 462
  PMS, 446
  WHI and, 462
Hospice care, 105, 507
  dementia and, 659–660
Hospitalization
  criteria for, PID and, 518, 518*t*
  Failure to Thrive, 199
Hot flashes, 456
  tamoxifen and, 463
HPV. *See* Human papilloma virus
HRT. *See* Hormone replacement therapy
HSG. *See* Hysterosalpingogram
HSV. *See* Herpes simplex virus
HT. *See* Hormone therapy
HTN. *See* Hypertension
Human bites, 636, 640

Human chorionic gonadotropin testing, medical
    abortion, 416
Human herpes virus 6, infants and, 217
Human papilloma virus (HPV), 402, 519, 623
  therapies, comparison of, 624*t*
  treatment, 519, 520*t*
  vaccine, 92
    children and, 81
β-HCG. *See* Beta human chorionic gonadotropin
Hurt, Insulted, Threatened and Screamed (HITS)
    scale, 502
Hydrofluoralkane (HFA), asthma and, 756
Hydroxy-methylbutyrate, weight loss and, 288
Hyperglycemia
  DM and, 233
  nicotinic acid and, 257
Hyperglycemic crises, DM and, 228, 228*t*
Hyperlipidemia, 247–261
  case discussion, 259
  initial evaluation, 247–248
  long-term monitoring, 260
  management, 248, 250–259
  pharmacotherapy, 250, 253, 254*t*
  recommendation summary, 258*t*, 259
Hyperprolactinemia, nipple discharge, 385
Hypersomnia, SSRI and, 739
Hypertension (HTN), 165–178, 168, 170*t*
  CAD and, 151
  case studies, 176–177
  children and adolescents, 76, 76*t*
  clinical assessment, 166–169
  cut-offs, BP and, 168*t*
  diagnosis algorithm, 166, 167*f*
  DM and, 231–232
  evaluation, key features, 169*t*
  initial evaluation, 168, 168*t*
  laboratory tests and, 169, 170*t*
  long-term management, 175–176, 176*t*
  recommendations, 176*t*
  screening, 166
  secondary causes, ABCDE mnemonic and, 168,
    170*t*
Hyperthyroidism (Thyrotoxicosis), 265–270
  case, 265, 270
  initial evaluation, 267–268
  long-term monitoring, 270
  management, 268–270
  management algorithm, 268*f*
  signs and symptoms, 267*t*
  subclinical, management algorithm, 276*f*
  surgery and, 269–270
Hyperuricemia, nicotinic acid and, 257
Hypoglycemia, sulfonylureas, 235
Hypoglycemic medications, DM type 2, use strategy,
    236–238, 240*f*
Hypokalemia, ACE inhibitors and, 173
Hypothesis generation and testing, 121
Hypothyroidism, 649
  case, 263
  causes, 264*t*
  initial evaluation, 263–264
  laboratory testing, 264
  levothyroxine and, 654
  long-term monitoring, 265
  management, 264–265
  signs and symptoms, 265*t*
  subclinical, management algorithm, 275*f*
Hysterectomy, menopause and, 455–456
Hysterosalpingogram (HSG), infertile couple and,
    500
Hysteroscopy, infertile couple and, 500

I & D. *See* Incision and drainage
"I got burned once." *See* IGBO
Ibandronate (Boniva), osteopenic women and, 460,
    462
IBS. *See* Irritable bowel syndrome
Ibuprofen
  febrile children and, 223
  fever reduction and, 222
ICS. *See* Inhaled corticosteroids
IDEA. *See* Individuals with Disabilities Education
    Act
IDM. *See* Informed decision making

IGBO ("I got burned once"), diagnostic process and,
    123
IGF-1. *See* Insulin-like growth factor-1
IgG "blocking" antibodies, allergies and, 747
IHS. *See* International Headache Society
Imaging studies. *See also specific imaging modality i.e.
    CT*
  acute pancreatitis, 332
  bowel obstruction, 332–333
  CAD, 139
  comparison of, DVT diagnosis and, 184
  COPD and, 789
  infants and children, UTIs and, 433
  joint pain and, 563
  solitary thyroid nodule, 272–273
Imipramine, ADHD and, 203
Immunizations
  adults and, 91–93
    recommendations for, 91–93, 95*t*–100*t*
  childhood, 78–82, 224
    contraindications and precautions, 78, 78*t*
    schedule for, 78, 79*t*–80*t*
  preconception screening, 55
  well adult care, 95*t*–96*t*
Immunologic tests, connective tissue disorders, 562
Immunotherapy, allergies and, 747
Impetigo, 622
Impingement testing, 604–605, 614
Implanon, 420
Implantable defibrillators, premature beats and, 162
Inactivated poliovirus vaccine (IPV), 81
Incision and drainage (I & D), abscess, 623
Incontinence, pregnancy and, 66
Individuals with Disabilities Education Act (IDEA),
    198
Indomethacin, Alzheimer's disease, 656
Infant stimulation, counseling, 84
Infants
  chlamydia and, 512
  with fever
    frequent diagnosis, 216*t*
    therapeutic options, 223*t*
  human herpes virus 6 and, 217
  mortality, 3, 51
  screening tests, 74–75
  testicular examination, 77
Infections. *See also specific i.e. vaginal infections;
    specific i.e. viral infections*
  asthma and, 752
  COPD exacerbations and, 794
  of eyelids, 302
  middle ear, 294
  middle ear inflammation and, 293
  respiratory, 769
  secondary headaches and, 696–697
  skin shaving and, 637
  wounds, 640
Infectious disease screening, pregnancy and, 66
Infectious disorders, affecting joints, 573–574
Infectious mononucleosis, 314, 315, 317
  diagnostic testing, 317, 318*t*
  Epstein-Barr virus, 315
  management, 320–321
Infertile couple, 498–500
  discussion case, 500
  history-taking for, 499*t*
Infertility, 498
Infidelity, case, 503
Inflammation. *See also* Dermatitis
  ESR, 562
  eyelid, 302
Inflammatory response, 769–770
Infliximab, RA and, 569
Influenza, 772
  medications for, 778*t*
  prevention, 778–779
  SBI and, 217
  treatment, 778
Influenza A virus, 772
Influenza vaccine (TIV), 81, 92
  recommendations for, 779
Information
  relevance and validity evaluation, 40–47
  responsible, 47–48
  using, changing practice with, 47, 47*t*

Information sources, 44–47
Informed decision making (IDM), prostate cancer, 479
Ingledue, V., rural practice and, 13–14
Inhaled β₂ agonists, asthma and, 763
Inhaled corticosteroids (ICS), asthma and, 763
Inhaled medications, asthma and, 756
Inhaler, asthma and, 762f
Inhibin, menopause and, 455
Injury
  care instructions, for patients, 641t
  prevention, counseling and, 83
  unintentional, 101
Inpatient detoxification, 713–714
Inpatient interventions, outpatient interventions v., for addiction, 712–714
INR. See Normalized ratio
Institutes of Medicine (IOM), prenatal care and, 51
Insulin
  preparations, pharmacology and use, 239t–240t
  therapy
    DM and, 235–236
    DM type 1, 236
    DM type 2, twice-daily-bolus, 236
    guidelines, 237t–239t
Insulin-like growth factor-1 (IGF-1), testosterone levels and, 489
Insurance. See Medicaid; Medicare; Private insurers
Interactive dermatology atlas, 630b
Internal hordeolum, 307f
International Headache Society (IHS), headache classification and, 695
International travel, vaccines for, 92
Interpersonal therapy (IPT), depression and, 740
Interventions
  alcohol addiction, 709
  drug addiction, 709
Interview, rambling patient and, 33–34, 33t
Intestinal brush boarder inhibitors, cholesterol and, 253
Intestine, lower, symptoms, 365–380
  cases, 365
Intimate partner violence (IPV), 501–502
  case, 501, 502
  screening tools, 501–502
Intra-articular steroid injections, joints and, 566
Intracorporeal injection therapy (ICI), 486
Intracranial mass, secondary headaches and, 697
Intracystic carcinoma, 390
Intramuscular medroxyprogesterone acetate. See DMPA-IM
Intranasal calcitonin (Miacalcin), osteoporosis, 462
Intraurethral alprostadil (MUSE), 486
Intrauterine device (IUD), 397
  side effects, follow-up and managing, 420
  side effects and contraindications, 410
Intubation, COPD exacerbations and, 794
Iodine ingestion, excess, 267
IOM. See Institutes of Medicine
IPG, DVT and, 182
Ipratropium bromide, URI and, 776
IPT. See Interpersonal therapy
IPV. See Inactivated poliovirus vaccine; Intimate partner violence
Iron deficiency anemia, infancy and, early childhood and, 74–75
Irritable bowel syndrome (IBS), 333–334
  diagnosis, 372, 373t
  management, 336, 337t
  physical examination and history, 372, 373t
  tegaserod, 374
ISDN. See Isosorbide dinitrate
ISMN. See Isosorbide mononitrate
Isoflavones, cyclic mastalgia, 383, 383t
"Isolated systolic hypertension," 167
Isoniazid, drug related lupus, 575
Isosorbide dinitrate (ISDN), angina and, 154
Isosorbide mononitrate (ISMN), angina and, 154
Isotretinoin, acne, 627
Itraconazole
  CVV and, 537
  tinea capitis and, 625
IUD. See Intrauterine device
IUD and Copper T-380A, 409, 410

Joint(s)
  intra-articular steroid injections, 566
  pain
    history/physical examination for, 560–562, 560t
    imaging studies, 563
    management, 563–564
    problems, initial approach, 561f
    replacement, RA and, 571
    ROM, 561
Joint custody, 504
Joint fluid analysis, 562, 563t

Keratitis, 303
Ketoconazole cream, seborrhea, 627
Knee(s)
  disorders, long-term management, 554–555
  ligaments and cartilage injuries, 550
  OA and, 565
Knee joint, anterior view, 550, 550f
Knee pain, 550–555
  clinical evaluation, 551–553
  diagnostic testing, 552–553
    characteristics of, 553t
  differential diagnosis, 545t, 550–551
  drugs, 549t
  history and physical examination, key elements of, 547t
  management, 553–555
  progressive/life-threatening disease, red flags for, 545t
KOH. See Potassium hydroxide

Laboratory tests
  AUB and, 449–450
  birth control method, 419
  breast mass and, 390–391
  characteristics of, dizziness and, 670t
  children, dysuria and, 427–429
  DM and, 230
  goiter and, 271
  HTN and, 169, 170t
  hyperthyroidism, 267–268, 268f
  hypothyroidism, 264
  infants and children, UTIs and, 433
  insufficient evidence in, children and, 77–78
  MI and, 138
  patient nutrition and, 281
  PE and, 185–186
  prenatal care, first trimester, 58, 59t, 60–61
  presyncope, 672
Labral pathology, 613
Labral tests, 609
Labrum, 601
Laceration repair, supplies for, 637t
Lacerations. See also specific i.e. facial lacerations
  aftercare, 640–641
  evaluation and management, 635–636
  repair, goals of, 635
Lachman test, 551
Lactate acidosis, metformin and, 235
Lactating breast, 392–393
  trichomonas vaginalis, 537
Lamivudine, HIV disease, pregnant women and, 60
Language and learning disorders (LLD), 206–207
Laparoscopic examination of pelvis, PID and, 517
Latin abbreviations, prescription writing and, 126
Laxative agents, chronic constipation, 378–379
Laxity/instability testing, 608
LDLs. See Low-density lipoprotein levels
Lead toxicity (Blood lead concentration), infancy and, early childhood and, 75
Lectures, new information and, 45–46
Leflunomide, RA and, 569
Left ventricular ejection fraction (LVEF), HF and, 155
Left ventricular failure, HF and, 155
Leg pain, differential diagnosis of, 180, 180t
Leukorrhea, 66
Leukotriene, asthma and, 762–763
Leuprolide, endometriosis, 336
Leuteinizing hormone, eating disorders, 208
Levonorgestrel, EC and, 408–409, 410

Levothyroxine, hypothyroidism and, 654
Lewy body dementia, 644
LGI bleeding. See Lower gastrointestinal bleeding
LHRH agonists. See Luteinizing hormone releasing hormone agonists
Libido, 483
Lichen sclerosus, 538
Lid hygiene, 310–311, 311
Lidocaine
  lacerations and, 636
  nasal, cluster headache, 702
Lidocaine/epinephrine combinations, wounds, 636
Life expectancy, national targets for, 3, 4t
Lifestyle
  chronic insomnia, 690t
  fatigue, 683
  GERD, 358–360
  HTN and, 169, 170–171, 172t
  modification, PMS, 446
  sexual dysfunction and, 482t
  skin and, 630
  sleep disorder and, 685
  stable angina and, 152–153
"Lift-off" test, subscapularis and, 604
Likelihood ratios, interpreting, 44, 44b, 44t
Lipemia retinalis, 248
Lipid profiles, subclinical thyroid disease, 276
Lipid-lowering agents
  algorithm for, 253f
  CAD and, 153t, 154
    mortality and, 153, 153t
  CHD and, prevention trials and, 254t
Lipids, medications and, 247, 249t
Lipoprotein levels, CAD and, 143
Lithium, hormone release and, 263
Liver disease, metformin and, 235
Liver function tests, 342, 342f
Liver transaminases, abnormal, causes of, 341–343
Living wills, 106
LMWH. See Low-molecular-weight heparin
LNG-IUS, 409, 452
  AUB and, 450
Load and shift, laxity/instability testing and, 608
Long-term monitoring, addiction, 716–718
Long-term suppressive therapy, recurrent HSV infection, 521
Low back pain
  accuracy of findings, history/physical exam and, 583t
  acute, 585f
  case, 579
  case discussion, 586–587
  clinical evaluation, 581–582
  diagnostic testing, 583–584
  differential diagnosis, 579–581, 580t
  neurologic examination findings, 583t
  physical examination, 582–583
  prevention, 386
  red flags for, 582, 582t
Low birth weight, 64–65
Low-density lipoprotein levels (LDLs), 250, 251f
  CAD and, 154
  DM and, 232
  NIH and, 247
Low-dose estrogen, atrophic vaginitis and, 458, 459t
Low-dose oral contraceptives, 398, 399t
Low-dose steroids, PMR and, 575
Low-level laser therapy, RA and, 570
Low-molecular-weight heparin (LMWH)
  DVT and, 190–191, 192
  VTE and, 190–191
Low-overhead practices, 28
Lumbar puncture, cognitive impairment, 653
Lumbar strain, 580
  management, 584
Lung
  examination, URIs and, 775
  function, measures of, 756, 757t–761t
Luteinizing hormone releasing hormone agonists (LHRH agonists), prostate cancer and, 479–480
LUTS. See Lower urinary tract symptoms
LVEF. See Left ventricular ejection fraction
Lybrel, 420
Lyme disease, 574

Magnetic resonance imaging. *See* MRI
Major depressive disorder (MDD), 733
    diagnostic criteria, 734*t*
Male condoms, 412–413
Malignancy
    CBE and, 382
    goiter and, 271
    PUD and, 356
    solitary thyroid nodule, 272
    VTE and, 192–193
Malignant breast masses, 390
Malignant otitis externa, seventh nerve palsy *v.,* 295
Malnutrition, Failure to Thrive, 199
Mammary duct ectasia, 384, 386
Mammogram. *See* Mammography
Mammography
    abnormal screening, 393
    breast mass and, 390
    nipple discharge, 387
Management plan
    deciding on, 125–126
    symptoms, diagnosis and, 119
Manipulation, neck pain, 593, 595
Manning criteria, IBS and, 333–334
Marital separation, 503–505
    case, 503
Maslow, Abraham, patient needs and, 10, 11*f*
Massachusetts Male Aging Study (MMAS), ED and, 481
Massive lower intestinal bleeding, 368
Mastalgia, 381
    algorithm for, 384*f*
Mastitis, 386, 392
Maternal blood glucose levels, 53
Maternal mortality, 51
Maternity care, family physician approach, 68
Mattress sutures, 638, 639*f*
Maximum bone density, 458
MB isoenzyme (CK-MB), MI and, 138, 139
MCI. *See* Mild cognitive impairment
McMurray test, knee pain, 551–552, 552*f*
MCV. *See* Mean corpuscular volume
MCV4. *See* Meningococcal vaccine
MDI (Metered dose inhaler)
    asthma and, 756
    COPD and, 788
Mean corpuscular volume (MCV), thalassemia and, 53
Mean serumβ-HCG levels, gestational age and, 56
Measles, mumps, and rubella (MMR), 81, 92
    preconception screening, 55
Mechanical conjunctivitis, 302
Mechanical ventilation, COPD exacerbations and, 794
Medicaid, hospice and, 108
Medical abortion, 415–417, 420
    patient education, 417
    procedure, 416
    regimen comparison, 416*t*
    side effects and contraindications, 416–417
Medical care
    etiology of, 5*f*
    high-tech *v.* high touch, 25
Medical history
    birth control method, 417
    chest pain and, 137
    prenatal care, first trimester, 57
Medical information, usefulness, 40–42
Medical Research Council dyspnea scale, breathing
        difficulty and, 787, 787*t*
Medical stability, for addiction, 711
Medicare, hospice and, 108
Medication history, preconception screening, 55
Medications. *See* Drug(s)
Mediterranean diet, stable angina and, 153
Megestrol acetate, hot flashes and, 456
Meibomian gland dysfunction, 311
Melanoma, 628, 629, 629*f*
    diagnosis, ABCDE guidelines for, 629*t*
MELD score. *See* Model for End-Stage Liver Disease
        score
Memory, HT and, 462
Meniere's disease, 664, 677
Meningitis, children and, 217
Meningococcal vaccine (MCV4), 81
Meniscus tears, 554

Menopause. *See also* Perimenopause; Postmenopausal
        women
    case, 455
    case discussion, 464–465
    diagnosis, 456–458
    hormone therapies, 462–464
    mood disturbances, 457
    natural history, 455–456
    patient medical history and, 456
    vasomotor symptoms, 456
    women at, health for, 455–467
Menorrhagia, 448
Men's health, 469–495
Menstrual bleeding, IUD, 410
Menstrual cycle
    history, pregnancy dating and, 56
    modulation, PMS, 446
    period, progestin-only contraceptives, 406
    problems, differential diagnosis of, 438*t*
    related pain, 440*t*
    symptothermal variations, 414*f*
Menstrual syndromes, 437–453
Mental health status, 5, 724
    screening, 91, 93*t*
Mental retardation (MR), 201
Message therapy, low back pain, 385
Meta-analyses, 45
Metabolic syndrome, 151
Metered dose inhaler. *See* MDI
Metformin, 65, 235, 237
    DM and, 233, 235
    insulin therapy and, 236
    ovulatory dysfunction and, 500
Methadone
    addiction and, 715
    long-term monitoring, 716
Methotrexate
    oral ulcers and, 417
    psoriasis, 627
    RA and, 568
Methyldopa
    adverse effects, 173
    drug related lupus, 575
Methylphenidate, ADHD and, 203
Metronidazole
    BV treatment, 533
        pregnancy and, 537
    trichomonas vaginalis, 537
Metrorrhagia, 448
MI. *See* Myocardial infarction
Miacalcin. *See* Intranasal calcitonin
Microalbuminuria, diabetic kidney disease and, 241
Micronized progesterone, 462
MIDAS. *See* Migraine Disability Scale
Middle ear
    infections, 294
    throat pain and, 293
Midfoot fractures, 547
Mifepristone (RU-486), medical abortion, 415
Migraine Disability Scale (MIDAS), 699*f*
Migraine headache, 695–696, 699*f,* 700.
    medications for, 701*t*
    OCs and, 398
    prophylaxis, clinical criteria for, 701
    prophylaxis for, drugs used as, 703*t*
    triptan medications for, 702*t*
Migraine-specific medications, 700
Migrainous vertigo, 677
Mild cognitive impairment (MCI), 645–645
    management, 654
Military medicine, 18–19
MINI-COG, cognitive impairment, 648, 650*f*
Mini-Mental State Examination. *See* MMSE
Minipres. *See* Prazosin
Minnesota model, addiction, 714–715
Minocycline, drug related lupus, 575
Miscommunication, management, 35–36, 35*t*
Misoprostol, NSAID-induced gastric ulcers and, 564
Mitral regurgitation (MR), 163
Mitral stenosis (MS), 163
Mitral valve prolapse (MVP), 163
    chest pain and, 132
Mixed dementia, 644
MMAS. *See* Massachusetts Male Aging Study
MMR. *See* Measles, mumps, and rubella

MMSE (Mini-Mental State Examination), cognitive
        impairment, 648, 649*f*
Mobiluncus evaluation, central laboratory testing, 532
Model for End-Stage Liver Disease score (MELD
        score), 346
Modified Child-Pugh Score, cirrhosis prognosis, 346,
        347*t*
Mohs, J., public health service and, 19–20
Monofilament nylon sutures, 637
Monofilament testing, DM and, 244
Monosodiumurate crystals, synovial fluid and, gout
        and, 572
Montelukast, asthma and, 763, 764
Mood
    disorders
        diagnostic criteria, 736*t*
        general medical condition, secondary to, 733,
            734
    disturbances, menopause, 457
    stabilizers, CD and, 206
Motion sickness. *See* Physiologic vertigo
MR. *See* Mental retardation; Mitral regurgitation
MRI (Magnetic resonance imaging)
    Achilles tendinitis and, 547
    breast pain and, 387
    bulging disk, 579, 580
    DVT and, 182
    goiter and, 271
    knee pain, 552–553
    low back pain, 583–584
    neck pain, 593
    primary dysmenorrhea, 439
    shoulder pain, 609
MS. *See* Mitral stenosis
Mucous membranes, pregnancy and, 56
Multinodular goiters, 270, 271
Multisensory impairment, nonspecific dizziness, 667
Multispecialty health systems, 22–23
Musculoskeletal chest pain, management, 144
Musculoskeletal disorder, fatigue, 683
Musculoskeletal pain, chest pain and, 132
MUSE. *See* Intraurethral alprostadil
MVP. *See* Mitral valve prolapse
Myocardial infarction (MI)
    beta-blockers, 153, 153*t,* 154
    tests for, 138
Myofascial junction, pain at, 590
Myofascial trigger points, 573

N. gonorrhoeae eye infection, 304
Naegele's rule, 56
NAFLD. *See* Nonalcoholic fatty liver disease
Nail changes, psoriasis, 627
Naltrexone
    addiction and, 716
    alcohol cessation and, 55
Narcolepsy, 684, 686
Nasal examination, asthma, 752
Nasal polyps, 747
Nasal problems, 770
NASH. *See* Nonalcoholic steatohepatitis
National Cholesterol Education Project (NCEP), DM
        and, 232
National Consensus Project, palliative care, practice
        guidelines, 106, 107*t*
National Institutes of Health (NIH)
    CF and, 53
    HIV disease, 519
    LDL and, 247
    obesity and, 281
Natural family planning, fertility awareness methods,
        414–415
Nausea and vomiting
    end-of-life care and, 111–112
    pharmacologic management of, 112*t*
Nausea gravidarum, pregnancy and, 55–56
NCEP. *See* National Cholesterol Education Project
NCEP ATP III lipid classification system, 247, 248*t*
Nebulizer, asthma and, 756
Neck, URIs and, 774
Neck pain, 589–599
    acute thyroiditis, 313
    case, 589
    case discussion, 597

clinical evaluation, 591, 593
diagnostic testing, 593
differential diagnosis, 589–591, 590t
long-term management, 597–598
management, 593, 595
flow sheet for, 593, 596f
therapeutic options for, 597t
prevention, 597–598
with radiculopathy, 595–596
clinical findings, 592t
red flags for, 593, 594t
treatments for, 593, 595f
Necrotizing fasciitis, 623
Neer's test (Neer's sign), 604–606
Negative predictive values (NPV), studies and, 44
Neglect, children and, 209–210
Neonatal herpes, 521
Neonatal morbidity. See Herpes simplex virus
Neonates
chlamydia in, 512
gonorrhea and, 515
UTIs in, clinical evaluation of, 432–433
Nerve block, wounds, 636
Neural tube defects (NTDs), folic acid and, 52
Neuroaminidase inhibitors, influenza, 778
Neuroblastoma, children and, 77
Neurogenic pain, 590
Neuroimaging
dementia workup and, 653
headache and, 698, 699t
nonspecific dizziness, 667
vertigo, 672
Neurologic examination
DM and, 230
low back pain, 583t
Neuropathic pain, 110
Neurosyphilis, 522, 651, 652
central system and, 666
penicillin G and, 655
Nevirapine, HIV disease, pregnant women and, 60
New York Heart Association classification scale, 163
chest pain, 151, 151t
HF and, 156
systolic heart failure, 156, 157f, 158
Newborns. See also Neonates
screening tests for, 73–74
Newsletters, 45
Niacin. See Nicotinic acid
Nicotine, Fagerstrom Test for Nicotine Dependence
and, 708t
Nicotinic acid (Niacin), 255–257
cholesterol and, 253
Night sweats, 457
Nighttime insulin therapy, 236, 239t
NIH. See National Institutes of Health
Nipple discharge
algorithm, 388f
bloody, 385
clinical evaluation, 386–387
differential diagnosis, 385–386, 386t
fibrocystic changes, 386
history and physical examination, elements of,
387t
management, 387–388
Nitrates
angina, 154
CAD and, 143
Nitrofurantoin
asymptomatic bacteriuria, 434
infants and children, 433
UTIs and, 430
Nitroglycerin, chest pain, 143
NMDA receptor antagonist, Alzheimer's disease,
656, 657t
NNT. See Numbers needed to treat
"No test/test threshold," 124, 124f, 125f
Nociceptive pain, 110
Nocturnal penile tumescence (NPT), 484
Nonalcoholic fatty liver disease (NAFLD), 341
biopsy, 342
red flags for, 342t
risk factors, 343, 343t
Nonalcoholic steatohepatitis (NASH), 341, 343
risk factors, 343, 343t
Noncyclic breast pain, 384, 384f
Noncyclic mastalgia, 381, 382

Nondegenerative disorders, 645
Non-dihydropyridine calcium channel blockers
(DCCBs)
diastolic heart failure and, 159
DM and, 232
SVT and, 162
Nonmassive gross bleeding. See Hematochezia
Non-oral combined hormone contraceptives, 404–406
Nonrhegmatogenous retinal detachment, 304
Nonspecific dizziness, 664
Non-ST elevation myocardial infarction (NSTEMI),
131, 143
Nonsteroidal anti-inflammatory drugs. See NSAIDs
Nontraumatic ankle pain, 543
Nontreponemal tests, syphilis, 522
Nonvalvular atrial fibrillation, warfarin v. aspirin,
161t
Normal pressure hydrocephalus (NPH), 652
disequilibrium, 667
Normal saline microscopic evaluation, BV and, 531
Normalized ratio (INR), VTE and, 189
Northern Navajo Medical Center, 20
NPH. See Normal pressure hydrocephalus
NPT. See Nocturnal penile tumescence
NSAID-induced gastric ulcers, misoprostol, 564
NSAIDs (Nonsteroidal anti-inflammatory drugs)
Achilles tendinitis, 548
acute gout, 572, 573
acute prostatitis, 474
ankle sprain, 547
arthritis and, 564
AUB and, 450
CAD and, 144
contusions, 635
corneal abrasions, 310
dysmenorrhea, 440t, 444t
endometriosis, 336, 440
H. pylori, 360–361
HF and, 156
infectious mononucleosis, 321
influenza, 778
IUDs and, 420
medical abortion and, 417
migraine, 700
musculoskeletal chest pain, 144
myofascial trigger points, 573
neck pain, 593
OA and, 555, 565
patient education, 322
PMS, 446
RA and, 568, 569
shoulder pain and, 610, 610t
skin wounds, 633–634
T-TH, 702
viral pharyngitis, 317, 319
whiplash, 597
NSTEMI. See Non-ST elevation myocardial
infarction
NTDs. See Neural tube defects
Numbers needed to treat (NNT)
examples, 43t
hyperlipidemia and, 250, 253f
Nummular eczema, 625
Nurse practitioners, family medicine and, 27
Nursing home care
catheter-associated infections, 434
cognitive impairment, 659
Nutrients, during pregnancy, 62
Nutrition
education, 279–280, 280f
initial evaluation, 280–281
management, 279–292
poor
evaluation of, 280t
red flags for, 281t
USPSTF and, 101
Nutrition and Your Health: Dietary Guidelines for
Americans, evidence-based advise,
279–280
Nutritional supplements
athletes and, 489–490
protein content of, 490t
NuvaRing. See Vaginal ring
Nystagmus, 671

OA. See Osteoarthritis
OAR. See Ottawa Ankle Rules
Obese patients, 279
counseling, 101
treatment, evidence-based guidelines, 285t
Obesity, 281–282, 284
childhood, 76
classification of, 282t
diagnostic evaluation of, 282, 283t
risks of, 283t
treatment methods, comparison, 286t
O'Brien test (Active compression test), 609
Obscure bleeding, 368
Obsessive-compulsive disorder (OCD), 721
diagnosis, 722
initial evaluation, 723
treatment, 729
Obstetric consultants, family physician and, 68, 70
Obstetric history, documentation of, first trimester,
57
Obstructive sleep apnea (OSA), 684, 686
Occult bleeding, LGI bleeding, 367
Occupational exposures
COPD and, 786
pregnancy and, 52
Occupational health specialists, RA and, 571
OCD. See Obsessive-compulsive disorder
OCs. See Oral contraceptives
ODD. See Oppositional defiant disorder
Office medical assistants, family medicine and, 27
Office testing, BV and, 530–531
Ofloxacin, pharyngeal gonococcal infections, 516
OGTT. See Oral glucose tolerance test
Olanzapine, dementia, behavioral symptoms,
658–659
Older adults, prevention and, 102
Oligomenorrhea, 448
OM. See Otitis media
Omacor, 257
Omalizumab, asthma and, 763
Omega 3 fatty acids, 257–258
cholesterol and, 253
Omeprazole, GERD, 359
Onychomycosis, 625
tinea pedis, 625f
Opacification, ear and, 296
Open access scheduling, 27
Open prostatectomy, 472
Ophthalmia neonatorum, gonorrhea and, 515
Ophthalmic allergy drugs, 310t
Ophthalmic ointment, hordeolum, 311
Ophthalmologist
eye problems and, 308
referral to, 304, 305t
Opiates, 110, 111t
adverse effects, 110
detoxification regimens, 716t
skin wounds, 633–634
Opioids, dyspnea and, 111
Oppositional defiant disorder (ODD), 204–206, 206t
OPV. See Oral polio vaccine
Oral anticoagulation, extended, VTE, 191–192, 192t
Oral contraceptives (OCs), 397
benefits, 398
contraindications, 402, 402t
drug interactions, 402–403, 403t
efficacy, 398
endometriosis, 336
mechanism of action, 398
missed, management of, 404t
pregnancy and, 56
side effects, follow-up and managing, 419–420
side effects and contraindications, 398, 401–402
Oral glucose tolerance test (OGTT), DM and, 228
Oral health, 101
Oral polio vaccine (OPV), 81
Oral rehydration, acute diarrhea, 371, 371t
Oral ulcers, methotrexate, 417
OrthoEvra patch. See Contraception
Orthostatic hypotension, 670
dizziness and, 678
presyncope versus, 666–667
Ortho-Tricyclen, 421
Ortolani-Barlow maneuver, 77
OSA. See Obstructive sleep apnea
Oscillopsia, 668

Oseltamivir, influenza, 778
Osgood-Schlatter's disease, AKP in children and, 551
Osteoarthritis (OA), 555, 557, 564–567
　clinical evaluation, 564–565
　joint involvement in, distribution of, 565f
　laboratory tests, 565
　management, 565–566
　therapies, level of evidence for, 566t
Osteoporosis
　drugs for, 460, 461t
　preventing, 461t
　prevention and treatment, 458, 460, 462
　risk factors, 460t
OTC drugs (Over-the-counter drugs)
　allergies, 746–747
　chronic daily headache, 697–698
　CVV, 533
　decongestants, common cold, 775
　endometriosis, 440
　GERD, 358
　migraine, 700
　patient education, 322
　tinea corporis, 625
　viral pharyngitis, 317
Otitis externa, 294, 295, 297
Otitis media (OM), 295, 297–298
　children and, 217
Ottawa Ankle Rules (OAR), 544, 547
　knee pain, 552–553, 553t
　radiographic series, acute injuries, 546f
Outcome-based management, of chronic diseases, 27
Outpatient
　detoxification, 713
　management, 119
Outpatient interventions, inpatient interventions v.,
　　for addiction, 712–714
Outsourcing, 25–26
Ovarian cysts, 440
Over-the-counter drugs. See OTC drugs
Overweight
　children and, Cochrane review, 76
　classification of, 282t
　diagnostic evaluation of, 282, 283t
　risks of, 283t
　treatment, evidence-based guidelines, 285t
Ovulation, natural family planning and, 415
Ovulatory menorrhagia, treatment, 452
Ovum, fertilization of, 395
Oxygen
　chest pain, 143
　supplemental, dyspnea and, 111
　therapy, cluster headache, 702

PACE. See Program of All-Inclusive Care for the
　　Elderly
PACs. See Premature atrial contractions
Pain. See also Referred pain; specific i.e. Knee
　assessment, 110t
　control, medical abortion and, 417
　end-of-life and, 110
　endometriosis, 440
　receptors, zygapophyseal joints and, 590
　relief, patient management and, 34–35, 34t
　skin injuries and, 633
　skin wounds, 633–634
Painful arc test, 605
Palliative care, 105–116, 506–507
　continuum of curative to, 109f
　explanation of, 108t
Palpable breast mass, 388–393
Pamidronate (Aredia), osteoporosis, 461t
Pancreatic cancer, 332
Pancreatic disease, 332
　management, 335–336, 336
Pancreatitis, acute
　alcohol and, 332
　prognosis in, Ranson criteria for, 335, 335t
Panic attack, symptoms of, 725t
Panic disorder, 721, 722, 722t
　chest pain and, 132
　treatments, 144, 728t, 729
PAP. See Prostatic acid phosphatase
Pap screening. See Papanicolaou screening
Pap smear. See Papanicolaou screening

Papanicolaou screening (Pap smear), 421, 533
　birth control method, 418
　BV and, 530
　cervical HPV and, 519
　prenatal care and, 60
Papaverine, penile injections and, 486
Papulosquamous skin rash, reactive arthritis and, 574
Parenteral gold, RA and, 569
Parity
　cervical cap, 410
　mnemonics for, 57
Parkinsonian signs, 647
Parkinson's disease, disequilibrium, 667
Paroxetine
　hot flashes and, 456
　PMS, 446
Partner Violence Screen (PVS), 502
Parvovirus serology, 562
PAS. See Physician-assisted suicide
Passive head-up tilting, presyncope, 672
Passive range-of-motion (ROM), 604
　exercises, ankle sprain, 547
Patellar dislocations, 554
Patient
　EBM and, 39, 40
　management, case studies, 127–129
　outcomes, Continuity of Care v., 8t
Patient education, 5
　AHS and, 698
　Alzheimer's disease, 655
　Arthritis Foundation and, 576
　asthma and, 763–764
　condom use, 412–413
　contraceptive patch, 404–405
　contraceptive sponge, 412
　COPD, 792
　diaphragm and, 411–412
　ear pain, 298–299
　EC, 408–409
　hormonal emergency contraceptives, 408–409
　hyperlipidemia, 260
　insulin therapy and, 235–236
　IUD, 410
　medical abortion and, 417
　natural family planning, 415
　OC and, 403–404
　POP, 407
　pregnancy and, 62–63
　preventive medicine and, 97
　RA and, 569
　sore throat, 321–322
　spermicides, 413–414
　thiazolidinediones and, 235
　vaginal contraceptive ring, 405–406
　vaginal symptoms and, 538
　VTE and, 193
Patient history
　chest pain and, 134–137, 134t
　diagnostic test and, 125, 125f
　EBM and, 39
　prenatal care, first trimester, 57
Patient-oriented evidence that matters. See POEMs
Pattern recognition, diagnosis and, 121–122
PCI. See Percutaneous coronary intervention
PCOS. See Polycystic ovary syndrome
PCR studies. See Polymerase chain reaction studies
PDD. See Pervasive developmental disorder
PDD-NOS, 200
PDE5 inhibitors
　comparison of, 485t
　ED and, 484
PE. See Pulmonary embolism
Peak flow measurements, asthma and, 753
Peak flow meter, asthma and, 764
Pelvic examination
　birth control method, 417–418
　prenatal care, first trimester, 58
　STI and, 511
Pelvic infections, IUD, 410
Pelvic inflammatory disease (PID), 440–441, 517,
　　517t
　dysmenorrhea, 439
　gonorrhea and, 514
　hospitalization criteria, 518t
　treatment regimens, 518t

Pelvic pain, 511
　diagnostic tests, characteristics of, 330t–331t
　life-threatening, red flags in, 327t
　progressive/life-threatening disease, red flags, 441t
Penicillamine, RA and, 569
Penicillin
　GABHS pharyngitis, 320, 320t
　sore throat, 313
Penicillin G, neurosyphilis, 655
Penile erection, normal physiology, 482
Penile injections, 486
Penile prosthesis, ED and, 486
Peptic ulcer disease (PUD), 352
　clinical evaluation, 352–353
　dyspepsia and, 351
　H. pylori, 360
　history and physical examination, 353
　malignancy and, 356
Percutaneous coronary intervention (PCI), 139
　ACS and, 141–143
Percutaneous transcutaneous coronary angioplasty
　　(PTCA), chronic stable angina and, 155
Percutaneous transluminal coronary angioplasty
　　(PTCA), ACS and, 141
Performance-enhancing supplements, 487–489
　case, 487–489
Pericarditis pain, 135
Perichondritis, 294, 297
Perilymph fistula, 664
Perimenopause, WHO and, 455
Periodic health evaluation (PHE), well adult care
　　and, 88, 89t
Peripheral neuropathy
　B12 deficiency and, 648
　DM and, 229, 229t
Peripheral sensory examination, dizziness and, 671
Peripheral vertigo, central vertigo v., 668t
Peripheral vestibular dysfunction, head tilt and, 671
Peripheral vestibular system, vertigo and, 664, 666
Pertussis, prevention and, 8, 10f
Pertussis vaccine (DTP), 78–79
Pervasive developmental disorder (PDD), 200
PFTs. See Pulmonary function tests
pH assessment test, BV and, 530
Pharmaceutical representatives, 46, 46t
　sales techniques and, 46, 46t
Pharmaceuticals. See Drug(s)
Pharmacotherapy. See Drug(s)
Pharyngeal infections, 770
　gonococcal treatment, 516
　gonorrhea and, 514
Pharyngeal tissue, GERD and, 313
Pharyngitis, viruses and, 313
PHE. See Periodic health evaluation
Phenylketonuria, Aspartame and, 63
Phobias, 721
　specific, 722
　　treatment for, 729
Photodocumentation, sexual abuse, 209
Photographs, electronic medical records, 633
Photopsia, 304
Physical abuse, children and, 209
Physical activity
　counseling, 101
　weight control and, 285–286
Physical examination, 123, 687
　abdominal pain, key elements, 329t
　accuracy of, functional dyspepsia, 354t
　acute diarrhea, 370
　allergies, 746, 746t
　ankle pain, 544, 545t
　AUB and, 449
　birth control method, 417–418
　breast pain, 382–383, 382t
　chest pain and, 134–137, 134t, 137
　child and, 73
　chronic diarrhea, 372, 373t
　chronic stable angina and, 151
　cognitive impairment, 647f
　constipation, 375
　diagnostic test and, 125, 125f
　dizziness and, 669–671, 670t
　DM and, 229, 229t
　dysmenorrhea, 439, 440t
　dysuria and, 426–427
　eating disorders, 207

EBM and, 39
ED and, 484
eye problems, 305, 305*t*
fever in infants/children, 218–219, 220*t*
findings, STI and, 419*t*
functional dyspepsia, 353
GERD, 353
HF and, 155
HTN and, 168
knee pain, 551–552, 552*f*
LGI bleeding, 366, 366*t*
lower extremity examination, DM and, 230
male, infertile couple, 499
menopause, 456
neck pain, 591, 593
obesity, 283*t*
patient nutrition and, 281
prenatal care, first trimester, 57–58
PUD, 353
sexual abuse, 209
shoulder pain, 602–603
skin wounds and, 633
sore throat, 314–315, 316*t*
URIs, 773–774
vulvovaginal complaints, 528, 530*t*
Physical therapy
    low back pain, 385
    RA and, 571
Physician assistants, family medicine and, 27
Physician-assisted suicide (PAS), 106, 112
Physiologic vertigo (Motion sickness), 664
    dizziness and, 678
Phytoestrogens, postmenopausal women, 463
Phytotherapies. *See* Plant extracts
PID. *See* Pelvic inflammatory disease
Pimecrolimus, atopic dermatitis, 626
Pioglitazone, DM and, 235
PIOPED study. *See* Prospective Investigation of
    Pulmonary Embolism Diagnosis
Plain abdominal radiographs, constipation, 375–377
Plain radiograph, low back pain, 583–584
Plan B, EC and, 408, 409
Plant extracts (Phytotherapies), BPH and, 472
Plantar warts, therapy for, 623
Platelet inhibition, ACS and, 143
Pleural pain, chest pain and, 132
PMDD. *See* Premenstrual dysphoric disorder
PMR. *See* Polymyalgia rheumatica
PMS. *See* Premenstrual syndrome
Pneumococcal immunization, children, 224
Pneumococcal polysaccharide vaccine (PPV), 92
Pneumonia
    abscess-causing organisms, 770
    acute bronchitis, 771–772
    children and, 217
POEMs (Patient-oriented evidence that matters), 41
    DOEs *v.,* 42*t*
Polio vaccine, 81
Polyarthritis, viral causes, 574
Polyarticular gout, 572
Polycystic ovary syndrome (PCOS), 448
    infertile couple and, 499–500
Polymenorrhea, 448
Polymerase chain reaction studies (PCR studies),
    febrile infants and, 217
Polymyalgia rheumatica (PMR), 574–575
    secondary headaches and, 697
Polysomnography, children and, 688
Polysporin, abrasions, 635
POP. *See* Progestin-only pill
Popliteal fossa, atopic dermatitis, 625*f*
Positive predictive values (PPV), studies and, 44
Postdates pregnancy, 67–68
Postdates Pregnancy Surveillance, testing methods
    for, 68*t*
Posterior dislocation, 613
Posterior fossa tumors, nonspecific dizziness, 667
Postmenopausal women, educational interventions,
    464, 465*t*
Post-stroke, disequilibrium, 667
Postsurgical breast pain, 381
Post-traumatic stress disorder (PTSD), 721, 722, 729
    diagnostic criteria, 724*t*
Post-traumatic vertigo, dizziness and, 678
Potassium hydroxide (KOH)
    microscopic preparation, BV and, 531
    skin scraping with, 625

Poverty
    Failure to Thrive, 199
    patient nutrition and, 280
Power of attorney, health care, 506
PPIs. *See* Proton pump inhibitors
PPTCA. *See* Percutaneous transluminal coronary
    angioplasty
PPV. *See* Pneumococcal polysaccharide vaccine
Prazosin (Minipres), BPH, 471
Precancers, 628–629
Preconception
    care, medical conditions and, 53–55
    genetic counseling, 52–53
    screening, for diseases, 54*t*
Preconception visit. *See* Randomized control trials
Predictive values, studies and, 44
Prednisone
    asthma and, 764
    COPD, 794
Pregnancy. *See also* Ectopic pregnancy; Maternity
        care; Pregnancy dating; Unintended
        pregnancy
    abuse, 63
    Abuse Assessment Screen, 502
    adolescent patients, 396
    asthma and, 764
    backache, 66
    BMI and, 62
    BV treatment, 533, 537
    CAM, 63
    chlamydia and, 512–514
    chloasma and, 56
    counseling and, 52–53
    dating, diagnosing and, 55–56
    diabetes screening, 65
    disulfiram and, 55
    DVT and, 184
    EDD, 56
    EPO, 63
    exercise, 63
    family practice settings and, 51
    genetic testing, 52–53, 61–62
    gonorrhea and, treatment, 516–517
    HSV, 66
    isotretinoin, 627
    loss, 56
    metformin and, 235
    metronidazole, 537
    nausea gravidarum, 55–56
    nutrients, 62
    OCs, 56
    patient education, 62–63
    planning, risk assessment, 52–53, 55
    prostaglandins, 67
    psychosocial support, 62–63
    quadruple screening, 61, 62
    reversible contraception method, 396
    round ligament pain, 66
    skin and, 56
    SLE and, 575
    sulfonylureas, 65
    testing
        progesterone, 56
        rubella, 60
        transvaginal ultrasound, 56
    travel during, 63
    trichomonas vaginalis, 537
    ultrasound, 61*t*
    unintended pregnancy
        abortion, 396
        case discussion, 420–421
        contraception, 395–397
        counseling for, 101–102
        health risks, 396
    urine dipstick tests, 65
    weight-gain, 57*t*
        IOM recommendations, 57*t*
Premature atrial contractions (PACs), 161–162
Premature closure, diagnostic process and, 122–123
Premature ventricular contractions (PVCs), 161
Premenstrual dysphoric disorder (PMDD), 437, 445
Premenstrual syndrome (PMS), 437
    cases, 442, 445–447, 446–447
    clinical evaluation, 445
    diagnostic strategy, 445
    differential diagnosis, 438*t,* 445

management, 443*t*–444*t,* 446
    psychotropic drugs, 447*t*
Prenatal care, 51–72
    evidence-based recommendations, 68, 69*t*–70*t*
    first trimester, 57–58, 60–63
    in office, 56–63
Prentif Cavity -Cervical Cap, 410
Prescription writing, 126
    standard form, 127*f*
Pressure ulcers, end-of-life care and, 112
Presyncope, 664
    clinical history, 668
    differential diagnosis, 666–667
    tests, 672
Preterm delivery, 57
Prevention
    Alzheimer's disease, family members and,
        655–656
    CAP and, 779
    chronic gout, 573
    ear pain, 298
    examination, skin and, 619–620
    family physician and, 4–5*b*
    focus, 8, 10*f*
    influenza, 778–779
    low back pain, 386
    neck pain, 597–598
    OA and, 566–567
    prostate cancer, 481
    special considerations, 102
Preventive care, 49–116, 124
    case study, 103
    electronic resources for, 103
    implementing, 87–88
    rationale for, 87
Preventive health services
    child and, 73
    risk assessment, 90*t,* 91, 91*t,* 92*t*
Priapism, ICI and, 486
Primary amenorrhea, infertile couple and, 499
Primary care
    delivery, innovations in, 27–28
    principles, 6–12, 7*t*
    subspecialty-based care *v.,* 5–6, 7*f*
Primary care health professions shortage areas
    (PCHPSAs), 13*f*
Primary care office, evidence-based medicine and, 10,
    11*b*
Primary care physicians
    activities, study of, 4–5
    working with couples, 504, 504*t*
Primary care practice, information flow, 121, 122*f*
Primary dysmenorrhea
    case, 441–442
    diagnostic testing, 439
    pathophysiology, 437–438
Primary hyperthyroidism, 263
Primary orthostatic tremor, disequilibrium, 667
Primary skin lesions, 619*t*
Private insurers, hospice and, 108
Problem-solving therapy (PST), depression and,
    740–741
Procainamide, AF and, 160
Progesterone
    endometriosis, 336
    pregnancy testing and, 56
Progestin-only contraceptives, 397, 399*t,* 406–408
    anovulatory menorrhagia, 451
    drug interactions, 403*t,* 407
    efficacy, 406
    mechanism of action, 406
    side effects and contraindications, 406–407
Progestin-only pill (POP), 406, 419
    patient education, 407
Progestins, 397
Program of All-Inclusive Care for the Elderly
    (PACE), cognitive impairment, 659
Progress note, problem-oriented, writing, 126
Prokinetic drugs, GERD, 358–359
Prolonged QT interval, eating disorders, 208
Propafenone, AF and, 160
Propothiouracil (PTU), hyperthyroidism and, 269
Propranolol, CAD and, 154
Proprioceptive loss, disequilibrium, 667
Prospective Investigation of Pulmonary Embolism
    Diagnosis (PIOPED), PE and, 186

Prostaglandin
    dysmenorrhea and, 437
    medical abortion, 415
Prostaglandin E1, ED and, 486
Prostaglandins, pregnancy and, 67
Prostate biopsy
    complications of, 479
    positive, predicting nomograms for, 477f
Prostate cancer, 475–481
    advanced, 479–480
    case, 475, 481
    early, 480–481
    lead time bias, 477–478, 478f
    length- time bias, 478, 478f
    management, 479–481
    prevention, 481
    risk factors, 475, 476t
    screening, 477–479
    screening recommendations, current, 479
    staging, 479
        TNM and, 479, 480t
Prostatic acid phosphatase (PAP), prostate cancer
    and, 476
Prostatitis syndromes, 475t
    antimicrobials and, 474
    case, 475
Prosthetic joint infections, 574
Protectaid, 420
Protein content, nutritional supplements, 490t
Protein supplements, 490, 490t
Proteus, otitis externa, 297
Proton pump inhibitors (PPIs)
    GERD and, 354, 359, 360
    H. pylori, 360–361
PSA (Serum prostate specific antigen) testing, 102,
    476, 478
    BPH and, 470
    prostate cancer and, 475, 476, 476t
    screening recommendations, current, 479
Pseudoclaudication, 580
Pseudomonas, otitis externa, 297
Psoriasis, 627
PST. *See* Problem-solving therapy
Psychiatric disorders
    fatigue, 682–683, 682t
    nonspecific dizziness, 667
Psychiatric illness, challenging patient encounter and,
    32, 37t
Psychologic stress, asthma and, 764
Psychological abuse, children, 210
Psychological disorders, diagnosis for, fatigue and,
    685
Psychological factors, Failure to Thrive, 199
Psychological stability, for addiction, 711
Psychological therapy, ADHD and, 204
Psychosocial distress, rambling patient and, 33, 33t
Psychosocial support, pregnancy and, 62–63
Psychotherapeutic agents, PMS, 446
Psychotherapy, role of, depression and, 740–742
Psychotropic drugs, PMS, 447t
Psyllium, chronic constipation, 378
PTCA. *See* Percutaneous transcutaneous coronary
    angioplasty; Percutaneous transluminal
    coronary angioplasty
PTSD. *See* Post-traumatic stress disorder
PTU. *See* Propothiouracil
Puberty, girls, mean age of onset, 76t
Public health
    anxiety disorder and, 722–723
    depression, 735–736
Public health service, 19–20
Public schools, LLDs and, 207
PUD. *See* Peptic ulcer disease
Pulmonary diagnoses, COPD *v.,* 788
Pulmonary embolism (PE), 179
    chest pain and, 132
    evaluation algorithm, 188f
    initial evaluation, 185–186
    laboratory testing, 185–186
    management, 187, 189–191
    symptoms and signs, 185t
Pulmonary function tests (PFTs). *See also* Spirometry
    asthma, 752–753
    COPD and, 788
    goiter and, 271
    interpreting, 790f

Pulmonary pain, chest pain and, 132
Pulmonary rehabilitation, COPD and, 790
Pulse oximetry
    asthma and, 753
    fever in infants, 219
Pulse palpation, chest pain and, 137
PVCs. *See* Premature ventricular contractions
PVS. *See* Partner Violence Screen
Pyelonephritis, younger women and, 431–432
Pygeum africanum, BPH and, 472
Pyramid regimen, RA and, 569
Pyridoxine, PMS, 446
Pyruvate, weight loss and, 288
Pyuria, UTI and, 428

QALY. *See* Quality adjusted life years
Quadruple screening, pregnancy and, 61, 62
Quality adjusted life years (QALY), prostate cancer
    and, 479–480
Quality of care, 25
Quality of Life, national targets for, 3, 4t
Quinidine, drug related lupus, 575
Quinolones
    conjunctivitis and, 309
    contact lens wearers and, 310

RA. *See* Rheumatoid arthritis
RAAS (Renin-angiotensin-aldosterone system), HF
    and, 155
Racial diversity, 26
Radiation therapy (RT), early prostate cancer, 480
Radical prostatectomy, mortality and, 481
Radioactive iodine therapy (RAI), 269, 270
Radiographs, acute pancreatitis, 332
Radiography, shoulder pain, 609
Radiologic testing, headache, 698, 698t
Radionuclide scanning, solitary thyroid nodule, 273
RAI. *See* Radioactive iodine therapy
Rales, fever in infants, 218–219
Raloxifene, 463
    osteoporosis, 462
    postmenopausal women, 463
Rambling patient, management, 33–34, 33t
Randomized control trials (RCTs), prenatal care and,
    52
Range-of-motion (ROM). *See also* Active range-of-
        motion; Passive range-of-motion
    joint, 561
    rotator cuff tendons, 602
Rapid evaluation phase, chest pain and, 134–137
Rare disease rule, diagnostic process and, 123
RAST, asthma and, 753
Raynaud's syndrome, SLE and, 575
RCTs. *See* Randomized control trials
Reactive arthritis (Reiter's syndrome), 574
    Chlamydia infection and, 514
Reason for visit, 119, 120t
Reassurance therapy, challenging patient encounter
    and, 37t
Recommended Dietary Allowances, 279
Recreational drugs, adverse effects of, 705, 707t
Rectal bleeding, 368
Recurrent HSV infection, 521
Red eye, 301–302
    differential diagnosis, 302–303, 302t
    evaluation, algorithm, 305, 306f
Referral, indications for, depression and, 742
Referred pain
    ear and, 294
    shoulder, 603t
Refractory pain, 555
Rehabilitation
    Achilles tendinitis, 548
    ankle joint and, 548
    exercises, shoulder pain, 610, 612
Reiter's syndrome. *See* Reactive arthritis
Relationships
    difficult, types of, 32–36
    evidence-based recommendations, 507t
    personal, 497–509
Relative rest, 610, 610t
Relative risk reduction (RRR), 43

Relaxation therapy, migraine, 701
Relevance, 40–47
Relocation sign, laxity/instability testing and, 608
Remission, hyperthyroidism and, 269
Renal insufficiency, metformin and, 235
Renin-angiotensin-aldosterone system. *See* RAAS
Reperfusion therapy, ACS and, 139, 141, 143
Replens, menopause, 458
Reproductive health education, young adults and,
    396
Research journals, 44
Research literature
    challenging patient and, 31–32
    EBM and, 40
Research reports, deciphering, 42–44, 43b
Resort setting medicine, 20–22
Respiratory infections, case, 780
Respiratory syncytial virus (RSV), 772, 778
    asthma and, 749
    children and, 217
    ribavirin and, 778
Respiratory tract infections, 769–783
    case, 780
    case study, 769
    clinical evaluation, 773–775
    emergencies, 773, 774t
    evidence supporting, 777t
    lower, symptoms, 770
    management of, 775–780
    upper, uncomplicated, 770–771, 775–776
Respite care, Alzheimer's disease, 655
Resting tremor, Parkinsonian signs, 647
Restless leg syndrome (RLS), 684, 688
Reticent patient, management, 35–36, 35t
Retinal artery occlusion, 308f
Retinal detachment, 304, 307–308
Retinal hemorrhage, 304, 308f
    examination findings, 307
Retinal tears, trauma, 308f
Retinal vein occlusion, 307
Retinoid therapy
    isotretinoin, 627–628
    psoriasis, 627
Retinopathy, DM and, 241
Revascularization
    CAD and, 143–144
    chronic stable angina and, 155
Reversible contraception method, pregnancy and, 396
Review articles, 45
Rhegmatogenous retinal detachment, 304
Rhegmatogenous tears, 304
Rheumatic diseases
    case, 557
    initial evaluation, 558–563
Rheumatic disorders
    laboratory tests, 562, 562t
    nonarticular features, 559t
    prevalence of, 558t
Rheumatoid arthritis (RA), 558, 567–571
    diagnostic criteria, 568t
    differential diagnosis, 561f, 567
    fatigue, 683
    finger deformities, 567f
    joint involvement in, distribution of, 565f
    laboratory tests, 567–568
    long-term care, 570–571
    management, 568–571
    prognosis, 571
    supportive management, 571
Rhinitis, 745
Rhinorrhea
    uncomplicated URI and, 771
    URIs and, 773
RhoGAM. *See* Rho(D) immune globulin
Rho(D) immune globulin (RhoGAM), 65
    prenatal care and, 58
Ribavirin, RSV and, 778
Rimantadine hydrochloride, influenza, 778
RISE mnemonic, 90
Risedronate, 460
Risk assessment
    pregnancy planning and, 52–53, 55
    prenatal care, first trimester, 57
    preventive health services and, 90t, 91, 91t, 92t
Risk stratification, genetic conditions and, 52

Risperidone
    ADHD and, 204
    dementia, behavioral symptoms, 658
RLS. *See* Restless leg syndrome
Rofecoxib, ankle sprain, 547
ROM. *See* Range-of-motion
Romberg test, trauma and, 671
Rome II Criteria, IBS, 372, 373*t*
Rosiglitazone, DM and, 235
Rotational testing, vertigo, 671, 672
Rotator cuff
    pain and weakness, assessment for, 604
    problems, 614–615
    tear, 604
    tendonitis, 603, 614
    tendons, ROM and, 602, 602*t*
Rotavirus vaccine, 81–82
Round ligament pain, pregnancy and, 66
Roux-en-Y gastric bypass, weight loss and, 289*t*
RRR. *See* Relative risk reduction
RSV. *See* Respiratory syncytial virus
RU-486. *See* Mifepristone
Rubella, pregnancy testing and, 60
Rural practice, 13–14

Saccadic dysmetria, 671
SAFE screen, 102
Salmeterol, asthma and, 763
Salt water gargles, patient education, 322
SAM-e, OA and, 565
Satcher, D., 26*b*
Saw palmetto, BPH and, 472
Sawin, S., resort setting medicine, 20–22
Saw-tooth regimen, RA and, 569
SBI. *See* Serious bacterial infection
SBP. *See* Systolic BP
Scalp lacerations, 639
Scarlatina rash, GABHS pharyngitis, 315
SCC. *See* Squamous cell carcinoma
Scleritis, 303
Screening. *See also* Universal screening
    anxiety disorder, 725*t*
    intervention
        anxiety, 725
        criteria, 97, 98*t*–100*t*
    tests
        addictions, 706
        asymptomatic disease, 97, 98*t*
        children, 73–78
        HTN and, 166
        infants, 74–75
        insufficient evidence in, children and, 77–78
        LLDs and, 207
        vertigo, 671–672
SDM. *See* Shared decision making
Seasonal affective disorder (SAD), DSMIV and, 735, 738*t*
Seborrhea, 626–627, 626*f*
Seborrheic keratosis, 629
Secondary amenorrhea, infertile couple and, 499
Secondary dysmenorrhea, 440–447
    pathophysiology, 438, 438*t*
Secondary headaches, 696–697
Secondary hyperthyroidism, 263
Secondary skin lesions, 619*t*
Selective serotonin reuptake inhibitors. *See* SSRI's
Selegiline, Alzheimer's disease, 656
Self blood glucose monitoring, insulin therapy and, 236
Self-help groups, addiction, 714
Self-management program, COPD and, 792
Semen analysis, infertile couple, 499*t*
Sensitivity (Sn), studies and, 43–44
Serious bacterial infection (SBI)
    age less than 28 days, 221–222
        medications, 223*t*
    children/infants, 218–220
        management, 221
    differential diagnosis, 216–217
    fever in infants and, 218
    prevention, children and, 224
    risks by age, 216*t*
SERMs, postmenopausal women, 463
Sertraline, PMS, 446

Serum albumin, nutrition and, 281
Serum CA-125 level, primary dysmenorrhea, 439
Serum free thyroxine (FT4), hypothyroidism, 263, 264
Serum lipase, acute pancreatitis, 332
Serum prostate specific antigen. *See* PSA testing
Serum proteins, nutrition and, 281
Serum transferrin, nutrition and, 281
17-alpha-alkylated androgens, 487, 488
Seventh nerve palsy, malignant otitis externa *v.,* 295
Severe acute lower gastrointestinal bleeding, clinical risk factors, 368*t*
Severe bladder dysfunction, 469
Sexual abuse
    children and, 209
    gonorrhea and, 515
Sexual activity, menopause, 458
Sexual behavior, counseling and, children and, 83–84
Sexual dysfunction
    antihypertensive medication, 173
    MMAS and, 481
Sexual function, menopause and, 458
Sexual Health Inventory for Men, ED and, 483
Sexual identity, relationships and, 497
Sexual orientation, 497–498
Sexual partners, *trichomonas* vaginalis, 537
Sexuality, 497–498
Sexually transmitted disease (STDs). *See* Sexually transmitted infections (STIs)
Sexually transmitted infections (STIs), 396, 511–, 511–525
    adolescents screening, 77
    birth control method, 418
    BV and, 528
    case discussion, 523
    condom use, 412–413
    counseling, 101–102
    EMS and, 503
    HIV disease, 519
    initial evaluation, 511–512
    IUD, 410
    physical examination findings, 419*t*
    primary dysmenorrhea, 439
    screening and prevention, 523
    treatment for, 515–517
    urethritis, 425
    USPSTF and, 60
Shared decision making (SDM), prostate cancer, 479
Short Blessed Cognitive Status Screen (BSCS), 94*f*, 102
Short-acting dextroamphetamine, ADHD and, 203
Short-acting methylphenidate, ADHD and, 203
Shortness of breath, differential diagnosis, 185*t*
Shoulder
    anatomy, 601, 602*f*
    referred pain, 603*t*
    ROM and, 602, 602*t*
Shoulder pain, 601–616
    algorithm, 611*f*
    anti-inflammatory medications, 610*t*
    case discussion, 615
    cases, 601
    clinical evaluation, 602–609
    clinical tests, characteristics of, 608*t*
    diagnostic testing, 609
        accuracy of, 609*t*
    differential diagnosis, 602, 603*t*
    incidence, 601
    management, 610, 612–615
    physical examination, elements of, 608*t*
    special tests for, 604, 605*f*–607*f*, 608
    treatments, strength of recommendations, 612*t*
Sibutramine, weight loss and, 287
Sick sinus syndrome (SSS), 162
SIDS (Sudden infant death syndrome), counseling and, 83
Silastic prostheses, RA and, 571
Sildenafil (Viagra), ED and, 484
Simultaneous nuclear imaging, ECG abnormalities and, 139
Sinus bradycardia, 162
"Sinus headache," 697
Sinus problems, 770
Sinus rhythms, 162
    AF and, 159, 160
Sinus tachycardia, 162

Sinusitis, 771, 776
    headache and, 697
Sjögren's syndrome, 575
Skeletal injury, physical abuse, 209
Skin
    infections, 621–625
    lesions, 617–618
        primary and secondary, 619*t*
    physical abuse, 209
    pregnancy and, 56
    surgery, skin cancers and, 630
    testing, asthma, 753
    ulcers, 641
    wounds, 633–642
Skin cancers
    counseling, 102
    risk for, 619
    skin surgery, 630
Skin suture technique, 638*f*
Skincare, children and, counseling, 84
Skochelak, S., academic medicine and, 23–24
SLAP lesion, 613
SLE. *See* Systemic lupus erythematosus
Sleep
    counseling, 84
    difficulty, differential diagnosis, 685*t*
    disorders, 681, 682, 684–685
        differential diagnosis, 684–685
        treatment, 690–691, 690*t*
    disturbance, menopause, 457
    progressive/life-threatening disease, red flags for, 686*t*
Sleep apnea, COPD *v.,* 788
Sleep-related complaints
    diagnostic strategy, 688, 689*f*
    management, 688, 689*f*
Slit-lamp examination, 305
Smokers. *See* Cigarette smoking
Smoking. *See* Cigarette smoking; Tobacco
Social anxiety disorder, 722
    therapies, 727*t*, 729
Sodium restriction, HTN and, 172, 172*t*
Soft tissue syndromes, 573–576
Somatic dysfunction, 573
Somatosensory loss, disequilibrium, 667
Sore throat, 770
    case, 313
    case discussion, 322
    clinical evaluation, 314–315, 317
    diagnostic strategy, 314*t*, 317
    differential diagnosis, 313–314, 314*t*
    general approach, 319*f*
    life-threatening/progressive disease, red flags, 314, 315*t*
    treatment, 320*t*
    URIs and, 774
Sotalol, AF and, 160
Spacer
    asthma and, 762*f*, 763
    COPD and, 788
Specificity (Sp), studies and, 43–44
Specimen collection, UTI and, 427
Speed's test, biceps testing, 608–609
Spermicides, 413–414
    diaphragm and, 411
    drug interactions, 413
    side effects, follow-up and managing, 420
Spinal fluid analysis, children, 220–221
Spinal manipulation, low back pain, 385
Spinal stenosis, 580
Spine, OA and, 565
Spiral CT (Computed tomography), appendectomy, 333
Spiritual issues, end-of-life care and, 114
Spirometry, COPD and, 787
Spironolactone, PMS, 446
Spontaneous abortion, documentation, 57
Spontaneous bacterial peritonitis, cirrhosis and, 347
Sports supplements, 487. *See also* Performance-enhancing supplements
    case, 492
Spurling test, cervical disc herniation, 591
Sputum
    COPD and, 789
    pneumonia and, 773
    URIs and, 775

Sputum Gram stain, antibiotic therapy and, 789
Squamous cell carcinoma (SCC), 628, 629f
Squeeze test, ankle pain, 544–545
SSRI's (Selective serotonin reuptake inhibitors)
    depression, 654, 739, 741t
        dizziness and, 678
    ED and, 483
    OCD, 729
    panic disorder and, 144, 728t, 729
    PMS, 446
SSS. See Sick sinus syndrome
St. John's Wort, OC and, 403
Stable angina
    chest pain and, 132
    treatment, 152–155, 152f
Staphylococcus, otitis externa, 297
Statin with niacin, 256
    DM and, 232
Statins (HMG-CoA reductase inhibitors), 253–254
    cholesterol and, 250, 253
STDs. See Sexually transmitted disease
ST-elevation myocardial infarction (STEMI), 131
STEMI. See ST-elevation myocardial infarction
Step-down Bridge regimen, RA and, 569
STEPS approach, antibiotics, children and, 223–224,
        223t
Steroid use. See Insulin-like growth factor-1
Steroids. See also Insulin-like growth factor-1
    chalazion, 311
    COPD and, 790
    psoriasis, 627
    seborrhea, 627
    vehicles for, 621f
STI. See Sexually transmitted infections
Stool specimen testing, diarrhea category and, 374t
Streptococcal pharyngitis
    clinical prediction rule, 315, 316t
    signs and symptoms, 315, 316t
Streptococcal vaginitis, 538
Streptococcus pneumoniae, OM and, 297, 298t
Stress disorder, acute, 722, 729
Stress testing, ankle, 546f
Stroke
    dizziness and, 678
    OC and, 398
Subconjunctival hemorrhage, 302, 310
Subdural hematoma, 652, 655
Subsequent counseling, pregnancy and, 66–67
Subsequent prenatal care, 63–68
Subspecialty-based care, primary care v., 5–6, 7f
Substance abuse
    adolescents screening, 77
    diagnosis, 707
    red flag diagnosis, 706–707
    withdrawal symptoms, 714t
Subtotal thyroidectomy, ATDs v., 269
Suffering, end-of-life and, 108–109
Suicide. See also Physician-assisted suicide
    adolescents screening, 77
    depression and, 739, 739t
Sulcus sign, laxity/instability testing and, 608
Sulfacetamide, conjunctivitis and, 310
Sulfonylureas, 237, 238
    DM and, 235
    pregnancy and, 65
Sun damage, 628–629
Sunscreen, SLE and, 575
Supplementation, infancy and, early childhood and,
        74–75
Supplements. See Dietary supplements
Support systems
    Alzheimer's disease, 655
    challenging patient encounter and, 37t
Suppressive therapy, recurrent HSV infection, 521
Supraventricular tachycardias (SVTs), 162
Surgery, for weight loss, 288, 289f
Surgical endometrial destruction techniques, 452
Surgical history, prenatal care, first trimester, 57
Sustained-release albuterol, asthma and, 763
Suture(s)
    placement, 638
    removal, guidelines, 637t
    selection and timing, guidelines, 637t
    techniques, 638–639, 638f
Suture needle, grasping, position for, 638f
SVTs. See Supraventricular tachycardias

Swelling, differential diagnosis of, 180, 180t
Symptoms, diagnosis and, 119
Syndesmosis sprains, management, 547
Synovectomy, RA and, 571
Synovial fluid
    analysis, 562, 563t
        OA and, 565
    monosodiumurate crystals, gout and, 572
Syphilis
    clinical evaluation, 521–522
    diagnostic testing, 522
    personality changes and, 651
    prenatal care, 58, 59
    treatment, 522, 522t
Systematic reviews, 45
Systemic lupus erythematosus (SLE), 558, 575–576
    fatigue, 683
Systolic BP (SBP), HTN and, 166, 167

T. pallidum particle agglutination (TP-PA), syphilis
        and, 522
Tacrolimus, atopic dermatitis, 626
Tadalafil, ED and, 486
Talar tilt test, 544
Tamoxifen, 463
    cyclic mastalgia, 383, 383t, 384
Tamsulosin, 471
Tandem gait, dizziness and, 671
Tazarotene gel, acne, 628
TCA. See Tricyclic antidepressants
TdaP vaccines. See Tetanus-diphtheria-acellular
        pertussis vaccines
Teenagers, abortion and, 396
Tegaserod
    chronic constipation, 379
    chronic diarrhea, 374
Temperature, children and infants, 220
"Ten Commandments of Divorcing Parents," 505t
Tendonitis/tendinopathy, 575
TENS. See Transcutaneous electrical nerve
        stimulation
Tension-type headache (T-TH), 696
    treatment, 702
Terazosin, 471
Terbinafine, tinea capitis and, 625
Terconazole, CVV and, 537
Testicular examination, infants and, 77
Testosterone
    postmenopausal women, 463
    supplements and, 489
"Test/treat threshold," 124, 124f, 125f
Tetanus
    immunizations, skin wounds, 634
    vaccine, 78–79
Tetanus-diphtheria-acellular pertussis (TdaP)
        vaccines, 92
Tetracycline, Meibomian gland dysfunction, 311
Textbooks, 45
TH1 cells, 745
Thalassemia, MCV and, 53
Theophylline, COPD and, 790
Therapeutic lifestyle changes (TLC), hyperlipidemia
        and, algorithm, 250, 253f
Thiazide diuretics, HTN and, 173, 174t, 175t
Thiazolidinediones, 237–238
    DM and, 235
Thiomersal
    childhood immunizations and, 78
    conjunctivitis and, 302
3-D imaging, pregnancy and, 61t
Thrombolysis
    ACS and, 139, 141, 143
    DVT and, 191
Thrombophilia, VTE and, 192–193
Thyroid cancer, thyroid nodules and, red flags for,
        273t
Thyroid disease, 263–2778
    treatment, 266t
Thyroid disease, subclinical, 275–277
    case, 274–275, 277
    initial evaluation, 275–276
    long-term monitoring, 277
    management, 276–277
Thyroid enlargement. See Goiter

Thyroid nodules
    management algorithm, 274f
    thyroid cancer and, red flags for, 273t
Thyroid nodule, solitary, 272–274
    case discussion, 273–274
    laboratory testing, 272–273
    management and long-term monitoring, 273
Thyroid ultrasound, 271
    hypothyroidism, 264
Thyroidectomy, 269–270
    solitary thyroid nodule, 273
Thyroiditis, 267
    Grave's disease v., 268
    neck pain and, 313
Thyroid-stimulating hormone (TSH), 265
    AUB and, 449
    dyslipidemia and, 247
    hyperthyroidism, 267
    hypothyroidism, 265t
    subclinical thyroid disease, 275–276
Thyrotoxicosis. See Hyperthyroidism
L-thyroxine, 272
    hypothyroidism, 264, 265
    solitary thyroid nodule, 273
    subclinical thyroid disease, 276–277
Tilt-table testing, presyncope, 672
Time-out, behavior disorder and, 205
Tinea capitis, 624
Tinea corporis, 625
Tinea cruris, 625
Tinea pedis, 625
    onychomycosis and, 625f
Tinidazole, trichomonas vaginalis, 537
TIPS procedure. See Transjugular intrahepatic
        portosystemic shunt
Tiredness, progressive/life-threatening disease, red
        flags for, 686t
TIV. See Influenza vaccine
TLC. See Therapeutic lifestyle changes
TMP/SMX. See Trimethoprim/sulfamethoxazole
TNF receptor blockers, RA and, 568
TNM. See Tumor-node-metastasis
Tobacco, 705, 706, 718
    addiction
        Fagerstrom Test for Nicotine Dependence and,
                708t, 709
        managing, 709, 712f, 713t
    preconception care and, 53, 55
    use
        CHD and, 248
        counseling and, children and, 83
        DM and, 232
        OC and, 403–404
Today sponge. See Contraceptive sponge
TOLAC (Trial of Labor after Cesarean), 51, 67, 70
Tongue lacerations, 639
Tophus, gout and, 572
Topical corticosteroids
    choosing and dispensing, 620, 621t
    dermatology, 620
Topical ophthalmic antibiotics, conjunctivitis and,
        309, 309t
Topical tar, psoriasis, 627
Toremifene, 463
Total cholesterol, 248
Total estrogen, menopause and, 455
Toxic child, management of, algorithm, 219f
Toxic nodular goiter, 267
Toxic shock syndrome (TSS)
    diaphragm, 411
    medical abortion and, 417
Toxicity, peripheral neuropathy, 648
TP-PA. See T. pallidum particle agglutination
Tramadol, OA and, 566
Transcutaneous electrical nerve stimulation (TENS),
    vestibular neuritis, 675
Transdermal progesterone cream, hot flashes and,
        456
Transillumination of sinuses, URIs and, 774
Transjugular intrahepatic portosystemic shunt (TIPS
        procedure), 347
Translation journals, 44–45
Transrectal ultrasound-guided biopsy (TRUS),
        prostate cancer and, 479
Transthoracic two-dimensional echocardiogram, HF
        and, 155–156

Transurethral drugs, ED and, 486
Transurethral incision of prostate (TUIP), 472
Transurethral needle ablation (TUNA), 472
Transurethral resection of prostate (TURP), 472–473
Transvaginal ultrasound
   ectopic pregnancy and, 334
   PID and, 517
   pregnancy testing and, 56
   primary dysmenorrhea, 439
Trauma
   ear and, 293, 294
   retinal tears, 308*f*
   Romberg test and, 671
   vertigo and, 666
Traumatic ankle pain, 543
Travel
   immunization, CDC and, 92, 93
   during pregnancy, 63
Tretinoin, acne, 628
Trial of Labor after Cesarean. *See* TOLAC
Trichomonas culture, central laboratory testing, 533
Trichomonas vaginalis
   molecular testing, 533
   treatment, 535*t*–536*t*, 537
Trichomonas vaginitis (TV), 528
   clinical evaluation, 529–530
Tricyclic antidepressants (TCA)
   ADHD and, 203
   depression, 739, 741*t*
   OCD, 729
   panic disorder, 144, 728*t*, 729
Trigger points, 590
Triglycerides, 248
Trimethoprim/sulfamethoxazole (TMP/SMX)
   acute pyelonephritis, 431
   acute sinusitis, 776
   asymptomatic bacteriuria, 434
   OM and, 298
   UTIs and, 430
      infants and children, 433
      older adults and, 432
Triptan medications, migraine and, 702*t*
TRUS. *See* Transrectal ultrasound-guided biopsy
TSH. *See* Thyroid-stimulating hormone
TSS. *See* Toxic shock syndrome
T-TH. *See* Tension-type headache
Tuberculosis
   children and adolescents, 76–77
   screening, biologic response modifiers and, 569
Tubo-ovarian abscess, 441
TUBS mnemonic, shoulder instability and, 612
TUIP. *See* Transurethral incision of prostate
Tumor-node-metastasis (TNM), prostate cancer
   staging, 479, 480*t*
TUNA. *See* Transurethral needle ablation
TURP. *See* Transurethral resection of prostate
TV. *See* Trichomonas vaginitis
Tympanic membrane examination, 294–295

UKPDS. *See* United Kingdom Preventive Diabetes
   Study Group
Ulceration, 641
Ultrasonography
   Achilles tendinitis and, 547
   gallstones, 329*t*, 331, 332
Ultrasound
   breast mass and, 390
   indications for, pregnancy and, 61*t*
   prenatal care and, 61
Underweight patient, 284
   management of, 290
Unfractionated heparin (UFH), VTE and, 189–190
United Kingdom Preventive Diabetes Study Group
   (UKPDS), medications and, 233
United States Preventive Services Task Force
   (USPSTF)
   cholesterol and, 247
   hepatitis and, 345
   preventive services and, 73
Universal screening, conditions for, early childhood
   and, 75*t*
University of Rochester criteria, SBI, 221
Unna wrappings, venous stasis ulcers, 641
Unplanned pregnancy. *See* Pregnancy

Unstable angina (UA), 131, 143
Upper respiratory infections (URIs), 217, 769,
   775–776
   differential diagnosis, 770–773
Urate renal stones, gout and, 572
Urban private practice, 14–16
"Urethral syndrome," 425
Urethritis
   chlamydia and, 512, 513
   STIs and, 425
Uric acid levels, gout and, 572
Uricosuric drugs, chronic gout, 573
Urinalysis
   BPH and, 470
   children, sensitivity and specificity, 220, 221*t*
   UTI and, 427–428
Urinary incontinence, HT and, 462
Urinary retention, 469
Urinary tract infections (UTIs), 469
   acute prostatitis, 474
   adult men with, 432
   case discussion, 434
   children and, 217, 220, 432
   complicated infection, red flags, 427*t*
   differential diagnosis, 425–426, 426*t*
   effectiveness evidence, 430*t*
   evaluation of, 426–429
   management, 429–432, 430*t*
   older adults with, 432
   oral drugs for, 431*t*
   pathophysiology, 425
   prostatitis, 474
   risk factors, clinical epidemiology and, 426
   symptoms, lower urinary tract, 469, 470*t*
   therapy for, effectiveness evidence, 430*t*
   uncomplicated lower tract, healthy women and,
      430, 430*t*
Urinary uric acid study, chronic gout, 573
Urine culture, UTI and, 428–429
Urine dipstick tests
   children and, 77
   pregnancy and, 65
Urine tests, characteristics of, dysuria and, 428*t*
URIs. *See* Upper respiratory infections
Urogenital symptoms, menopause, 457–458
US Preventive Services Task Force (USPSTF)
   alcohol misuse and, 97
   chemoprophylaxis and, 94, 97
   depression, 736
   health habit messages, 5, 6*b*
   Nutrition, 101
   patient education, 97
   preventive health services and, 88, 90
   PSA screening, 479
   STIs, screening and prevention, 523
USPSTF. *See* US Preventive Services Task Force
Uterine bleeding. *See* Abnormal uterine bleeding
UTIs. *See* Urinary tract infections
Uveitis, 303

Vaccination
   CAP and, 779
   influenza, 778
VACTERL syndrome, disulfiram and, 55
Vacuum extraction, 51
Vacuum-assist devices, ED and, 486
VADL. *See* Vestibular Disorders Activities of Daily
   Living Scale
Vaginal atrophy, 458
Vaginal birth after cesarean (VBAC), 67
Vaginal bleeding, 511
Vaginal infections, historical and physical
   examination, 530*t*
Vaginal lubricants, menopause, 458
Vaginal ring (NuvaRing), 404–406
Vaginal symptoms
   case discussion, 538
   differential diagnosis, 528, 528*t*
   patient education, 538
Vaginitis, 527–541
   case, 527
   diagnostic tests for, 532*t*
   differential diagnosis, 527–528, 528*t*

Valacyclovir, 624
   recurrent HSV infection, 521
Valproate, dementia, behavioral symptoms, 658, 658*t*
Valproic acid, ADHD and, 204
Valsalva precede symptoms, 668
Valvular heart disease, 162–163
Vancomycin hydrochloride, CAP and, 779
Vardenafil, ED and, 484, 486
Varicella, preconception screening, 55
Varicella vaccine. *See* Measles, mumps, and rubella
Varicella-zoster virus (VZV), 623
Vascular dementia, 644
   treatments, 656
Vascular events, secondary headaches and, 697
Vascular ischemia, dizziness and, 678
Vascular system, DM and, 232
Vasculogenic impotence, 483
Vasoconstriction, primary dysmenorrhea, 438
Vasodilation, primary dysmenorrhea, 438
Vasomotor symptoms
   menopause diagnosis, 456
   nonestrogen treatment, 456, 457*t*
   treatment, 456–457
VBAC. *See* Vaginal birth after cesarean
Vena cava filter replacement, DVT, 191
Venlafaxine
   ADHD and, 203
   hot flashes, 456
Venous stasis dermatitis, 641
Venous stasis ulcers, treatment, 641, 641*t*
Venous thromboembolism (VTE), 179–196
   case studies, 179
   initial management, 189–191
   long-term management, 191–194
   OCs and, 401
   treatment algorithm, 189*f*
Ventricular rate, AF and, 159*f*, 160
Ventricular-perfusion scanning. *See* V/Q scanning
Verapamil, cluster headache, 702
Vertebral compression fractures, 581
Vertical banded gastroplasty, weight loss and, 289*t*
Vertical mattress sutures, 638, 639*f*
Vertigo, 663, 664
   central causes, 664, 666
   clinical history, 668, 668*t*
   differential diagnosis, 664, 666
   peripheral causes, 664
   tests, 671–672
Very-low density lipoproteins (VLDL), fibric acid
   derivatives and, 257
VES. *See* Vestibular electrical stimulation
Vestibular disorders, treatments, 673
Vestibular Disorders Activities of Daily Living Scale
   (VADL), 673
Vestibular electrical stimulation (VES), vestibular
   neuritis, 675
Vestibular epilepsy, central system and, 666
Vestibular migraine, 666
Vestibular neuronitis (VN), 664
Vestibulo-ocular reflexes (VOR)
   dizziness, 670–671
   nystagmus and, 671
Viagra. *See* Sildenafil
Viral infections, 623–624
   acute bronchitis, 771–772
   fever in children and, 217
Viral pathogens, 769
Viral pharyngitis, management, 317, 319
Viral shedding
   HSV and, 520–521
   recurrent HSV infection, 521
Viruses, pharyngitis and, 313
Viscosupplementation, OA and, 566
Vision screening, infancy and, early childhood and,
   75, 75*f*
Visual acuity examination, 305
Visual loss, differential diagnosis, 304
Vital signs, fever in infants, 218
Vitamin B12 deficiency
   cyanocobalamin and, 654
   peripheral neuropathy and, 648, 649, 651
Vitamin C, URI and, 776
Vitamin D
   OA and, 566–567
   psoriasis, 627

Vitamin E
  Alzheimer's disease, 656, 657*t*
  PMS, 446
Vitreous hemorrhage, 304
  examination findings, 307
VLDL. *See* Very-low density lipoproteins
VN. *See* Vestibular neuronitis
VOR. *See* Vestibulo-ocular reflexes
V/Q scanning (Ventricular-perfusion scanning), PE
    and, 185–186
V-shaped lacerations, repair, 639, 640*f*
VTE. *See* Venous thromboembolism
Vulvar intraepithelial neoplasia, 538
Vulvodynia, 538
Vulvovaginal complaints
  clinical evaluation, 528–533
  evaluation algorithm, 529*f*
VZV. *See* Varicella-zoster virus

Warfarin
  AF and, 160
  nonvalvular atrial fibrillation and, 161*t*
  PE and, 187
  VTE and, 191–192, 192*t*
Warts, 623
"Watchful waiting," BPH and, 470
WBC. *See* White cell blood count
WBC/hpf. *See* White blood cells per high-power
    field
Weight. *See also* Overweight; Underweight patient
  management, 279–292
  physical activity, 285–286
  problems, management of, 284
Weight-based IV heparin nomogram, 190, 190*t*
Weight-gain
  BMI and
    IOM recommendations, 57, 57*t,* 58
    pregnancy and, 62

fetus and, 64–65
  in pregnancy, IOM recommendations, 57*t*
  progestin-only contraceptives, 406
Weight-loss, 207
  case, 291
  diet
    behavior therapy and, 286
    guidelines, 286*t*
    HTN and, 170–171, 172*t*
    medications and, 286–288
    tips, 287*f*
    vertical banded gastroplasty, 289*t*
Well adolescent care, 73–85
  case study, 85
Well adult care, 87–104
  immunization recommendations, 95*t*–96*t*
  preventive services, 98*t*–100*t*
Well child care, 73–85
Wells Clinical Decision Rule
  case studies, 193–194
  DVT and, 182*t*
  PE and, 186*t,* 187*f,* 188*f*
    and ventilation-perfusion lung scan, 188*f*
Western blot, HIV disease, 519
Wheezing, non-asthma causes, 753
WHI. *See* Women's Health Initiative study
Whiff test. *See* Amine test
Whiplash, 591
  management, 597
White blood cells per high-power field (WBC/hpf),
    UTI and, 428
White cell blood count (WBC)
  bacteremia in children and, 220
  diverticulitis, 333
WHO (World Health Organization)
  analgesic ladder, 110, 111*f*
  breast milk and, 67
Withdrawal syndromes, treatment, 711–712, 716*t*
Women's Health Initiative study (WHI), HT and,
    462

Work-site exposures, asthma, 755*f*
World Health Organization. *See* WHO
Wound(s)
  assessment, essentials of, 636*t*
  cleaning, 636
  closure
    contraindications, 636
    timing, 637
  contaminated, 640
  healing phases, 635–636
  repair, preparing for, 637–638
  skin, 633–642
    case discussion, 641–642
    diagnostic testing, 633
    management, 633–634
      red flags in, inspection of, 635*t*
    treatment algorithm, 633, 634*f*
Wright, J., military medicine and, 18–19

X-rays, asthma and, 753

Yale Observation Scale, fever in infants, 219
Yasmin, 421
Yergason's test, biceps testing, 609
Yogurt, culture-positive, CVV and, 537
Yohimbine, ED and, 486
Youth violence, 77
Yuzpe regimen, EC and, 408

Zafirlukast, asthma and, 763
Zanamivir, influenza, 778
Zebras, diagnostic process and, 123
Zidovudine, HIV disease, pregnant women and, 60
Zinc gluconate lozenges, URI and, 775
Zoledronic acid, osteoporosis, 462
Zung self-rating depression scale, 91, 93*t*